Knee Surgery

Springer
New York
Berlin
Heidelberg
Barcelona
Hong Kong
London
Milan
Paris
Singapore
Tokyo

M. Mike Malek, M.D.
Washington Orthopaedic and Knee Clinic, Inc.
Vienna, Virginia
Editor-in-Chief

Section Editors
Gregory Fanelli, M.D.
Darren Johnson, M.D.
Don Johnson, M.D.

KNEE SURGERY
COMPLICATIONS, PITFALLS, AND SALVAGE

Foreword by Frank R. Noyes, M.D.

With 537 Illustrations, 108 in Full Color

Springer

M. Mike Malek, M.D.
Washington Orthopaedic and Knee Clinic, Inc.
Tyson's Professional Building
8206 Lessburg Pike, #201
Vienna, VA 22182
USA
info@wokc2.com

Library of Congress Cataloging-in-Publication Data

Knee surgery : complications, pitfalls, and salvage / M. Mike Malek, [editor].
p. cm.
Includes bibliographical references and index.
ISBN 0-387-98294-9 (hardcover : alk. paper)
1. Knee—Surgery—Complications. I. Malek, M. Mike.
[DNLM: 1. Knee—surgery. 2. Arthroplasty, Replacement, Knee—adverse effects. 3. Intraoperative Complications—prevention & control. 4. Postoperative Complications—therapy. WE 870 K6819 2000]
RD561.K5847 2000
617.5′82059—dc21
DNLM/DLC 99-40673

Printed on acid-free paper.

Production coordinated by WordCrafters Editorial Services, Inc., and managed by Lesley Poliner; manufacturing supervised by Jeffrey Taub.
Typeset by Matrix Publishing Services, Inc., York, PA.
Printed and bound in China by Everbest Printing Company, through Four Colour Imports, Louisville, KY.

9 8 7 6 5 4 3 2 1

ISBN 0-387-98294-9 SPIN 10634217

Springer-Verlag New York Berlin Heidelberg
A member of BertelsmannSpringer Science+Business Media GmbH

To my wife, Feri,
and my children Ali and Bobby,
for their love, support, and understanding.

Foreword

Frank R. Noyes, M.D.
Director, Cincinnati Sportsmedicine and Orthopaedic Center
Director, Cincinnati Sportsmedicine Research and Education Foundation
Professor, Orthopaedic Surgery, University of Cincinnati
Adjunct Professor, Noyes Giannestras Biomechanics Laboratory, University of Cincinnati

A view of the advances in knee surgery with the sheer amount of new information, procedures, techniques, and treatment algorithms is somewhat staggering. Consider the past ten years: the number and development of newer arthroscopic procedures, knee ligament reconstructions, meniscus repairs and transplants, revision knee surgery, ligament allografts, total knee arthroplasties, and treatment of articular cartilage abnormalities. All of these advances have resulted in corresponding needs for education, training, and knowledge. The knee joint is one of the most frequently operated joints in the human body, and functional abnormalities to the knee joint are one of the most frequent causes for referral to an orthopaedic specialist. Given the frequency of knee joint problems and newer sophisticated procedures, it is not surprising that complications may arise requiring the skill and judgment of the orthopaedic specialist.

The expansion in knee treatment options and approaches introduces challenging problems to the practicing orthopaedic surgeon and orthopaedic resident in training. What are the objective and functional results, as well as the patient-perceived outcomes of newer knee operative procedures? Most importantly, and the subject of this textbook, what are the associated complications and their treatment? Is the incidence of an associated complication acceptable with regard to the benefits to be derived? Are there scientifically based treatment algorithms that allow a complication to be treated with minimum chance of interfering with the anticipated results? The answers to these questions provide a basis for patient selection and indications for newer treatment modalities. Most importantly, this knowledge provides the basis upon which an orthopedist counsels a patient regarding the risks and benefits of operative treatment, to provide informed patient consent.

This textbook provides needed and important knowledge to address these issues. The 35 chapters are divided into major knee disease or treatment categories, discussing the prevention, recognition, and treatment of knee complications. Complications are discussed related to a variety of arthroscopic procedures: meniscus surgery, reconstruction of knee ligaments, patellofemoral surgery, articular cartilage transfer and regeneration procedures, knee fractures, and prosthetic knee arthroplasty. An additional section describes the treatment of unusual complications by surgeons around the world—interesting and provocative material.

A textbook of complications and surgical treatment deals, for the most part, with two major groups. One group of complications represents events that are often unpredictable and difficult to prevent. For example, a complication of a postoperative infection may be extremely serious and alter the intended result, and it may develop despite all of the expertise of the surgeon and the surgical team. The surgeon is responsible for the immediate recognition of the complication and the assembly of other specialists to assess the gravity of the complication, combining clinical experiences and data, to implement a logical, scientifically based treatment protocol. Hopefully the treatment plan will lead to a satisfactory patient result. This textbook represents an excellent opportunity to obtain the knowledge and combined clinical expertise of many highly skilled and experienced surgeons.

A second group of complications after knee surgery is based on the experience and expertise of the surgeon. Perhaps the major importance of a textbook devoted to complications of the knee joint is to provide the insight and knowledge of newer treatment advances and surgical procedures, to present the collective wisdom of experienced surgeons. Every surgeon should question the necessary clinical and surgical experience required for total management of a patient treatment protocol, including all of the potential complications that may result. Is the patient best treated by another colleague who has more experience in a newer treatment arena? Not all orthopedists should necessarily feel competent to undertake the many varied and sometimes complex treatment programs and surgical procedures covered in this textbook.

Complications diminish with clinical experience, and the clinical experience in treating complications provides the expertise and skill of the highly seasoned and knowledgeable surgeon. It is unfortunate that this truism cannot be avoided. Certainly the knowledge contained in this textbook—imparted by experts who have been through this circle of clinical experience and desire to share their knowledge—is beneficial to all of us in achieving superior treatment results for our patients with the lowest possible complication rate.

Decreases in knee complications have been experienced at many centers publishing knee surgery results, due to the team approach of surgeons, physical therapists, athletic trainers, and allied personnel. The physical therapy component of the equation needed to restore muscle strength, endurance, coordination, and functionality is as important to the end result as the successful completion of the actual surgical procedures. I have treated many patients whose treatment results were less than adequate, and complications occurred in which the skilled surgeon functioned without the support of the physical therapy and rehabilitation team.

Hopefully, as knee surgery advances, future textbooks on complications of knee surgery will have fewer topics to cover. However, it is probable that the sophistication of newer surgical procedures will result in new and different types of complications than those treated today.

Dr. Malek was the first sports medicine and arthroscopic fellow to enter and graduate from our fellowship program, and it is a privilege to write the foreword for *Knee Surgery*. I am especially pleased that Dr. Malek provided the leadership, energy, and expertise to bring together so many experienced clinicians.

PREFACE

Any surgical procedure is associated with a certain degree of risk and complication. Unfortunately, in this medicolegal environment, any unexpected complication can be labeled the surgeon's negligence or deviation from the standard of care.

Over the last 20 years we have witnessed an explosion in arthroscopic and related techniques as well as many other nonarthroscopic procedures for the knee.

Arthroscopic surgery developed very rapidly and with it brought numerous new surgical procedures that required an above-average degree of skill and manual dexterity as well as the need to deal with many new and, at times, complicated instrumentation systems. These new techniques also entailed a higher learning curve. It was easier for the younger generation of orthopedic surgeons to learn those techniques during training as a resident or fellow, and harder for those who had no opportunity to learn those techniques while they were training.

I have always been interested in investigating the cause of complications, particularly those that I have had in my own practice, as well as collecting examples of complications from colleagues who shared them with me. I have learned a great deal from these complications. I have come to realize that complications occur despite the best of care and do not necessarily indicate deviation from standard of care or the surgeon's poor judgment.

We also have to be realistic and recognize that a poor surgical result does not always indicate the presence of a complication. Many other factors are involved. Individuals are different and with this comes different biologic responses to injury and to nonoperative and operative treatment. There are those who are fast healers and those who are slow healers. To prevent any postoperative complications not directly related to the surgical procedure performed, our postoperative care should be supervised by knowledgeable and skilled clinicians.

With the help of my contributors and the dedicated effort of section editors, we have compiled this volume to help our readers identify the potential complications of the most frequently performed knee surgeries and the steps to avoid them, as well as procedures to deal with them once they have occurred.

I hope our readers find this volume beneficial in their day-to-day practice and learn from the complications reported here by surgeons from around the world and the ways and means to reduce their own rate of complications by meticulous attention to detail and, above all, patient selection.

ACKNOWLEDGMENTS

A volume like this is the reflection of hard work of many people. I am grateful to the chapter authors for their efforts and expertise. I am indebted to my section editors, Doctors Gregory Fanelli, Darren Johnson, and Don Johnson, for their dedication, energy, and willingness to participate in this project. Many thanks to the editorial staff at Springer-Verlag for bringing this volume to a timely completion. Finally, I would like to thank my office staff; special thanks to Karen Knable for her technical assistance and extra time that she spent on this project.

M. MIKE MALEK, M.D., F.A.C.S.
Potomac, Maryland
2000

CONTENTS

Contributors

HORMOZAN APRIN, M.D., F.A.C.S., F.A.A.P.
Associate Clinical Professor of Orthopaedics
State University of New York at Stony Brook
Great Neck, NY 11021, USA

DAE KYUNG BAE, M.D.
Department of Orthopaedic Surgery
Kyung Hee University School of Medicine
Seoul, South Korea

HARALD BOSZOTTA, M.D.
Department of Trauma Surgery
Krankenhaus der Barmherzigen Brüder Eisenstadt
Esterhazystr .26
Austria

ROBERT B. BOURNE, M.D., F.R.C.S.C.
London Health Sciences Centre
London, Ontario, Canada N6A 5A5

JEFFERSON C. BRAND, JR., M.D.
Sports Medicine Fellow
University of Kentucky School of Medicine
Department of Orthopaedic Surgery
Kentucky Clinic K439
Lexington, KY 40536, USA

PHILIPPE CARTIER, M.D.
Clinique des Lilas
Les Lilas, France

MARK CLATWORTHY, M.D.
Fellow, Sports Medicine & Shoulder Surgery
Department of Orthopaedics
University of Pittsburgh
Pittsburgh, PA 15232, USA

SUSAN CRAIG SCOTT, M.D.
New York, NY 10128, USA

RAMON CUGAT, M.D.
Barcelona, Spain

FRED D. CUSHNER, M.D.
Director, ISK Institute
Beth Israel Hospital
New York, NY 10128, USA

THOMAS M. DEBERARDINO, M.D.
Staff Orthopaedic Surgeon
Research Director, US Army Joint & Soft Tissue Trauma Fellowship
Brooke Army Medical Center
Orthopaedic Surgery Service, Sports Medicine Section
Ft. Sam Houston, TX 78234, USA

GÉRARD P. DESCHAMPS, M.D.
Centre Orthopédique Médico-Chirurgical
Dracy-le-Fort, France

GERARD A. ENGH, M.D.
President, Anderson Orthopaedic Research Institute
Associate Clinical Professor
Department of Orthopaedics
University of Maryland School of Medicine
Alexandria, VA 22306, USA

GREGORY C. FANELLI, M.D.
Chief, Sports Injury & Arthroscopic Surgery Services
Geisinger Clinic Medical Center
Department of Orthopaedic Surgery
Danville, PA 17822, USA

DANIEL D. FELDMANN, M.D.
Department of Orthopaedic Surgery
Geisinger Clinic
Penn State Health System
Danville, PA 17822, USA

PONKY FIRER, M.D.
Highlands North
Republic of South Africa

FRED FLANDRY, M.D., F.A.C.S.
Attendant Surgeon
The Hughston Clinic, PC
Clinical Associate Professor of Orthopedic Surgery
Tulane University School of Medicine
Department of Orthopedic Surgery
Columbus, GA 31904, USA

VITTORIO FRANCO, M.D.
Rome, Italy

MARC J. FRIEDMAN, M.D.
Southern California Orthopaedic Institute
Van Nuys, CA 91405, USA

FREDDIE H. FU, M.D.
Blue Cross Professor of Orthopaedic Surgery
Executive Vice Chairman & Professor
Department of Orthopaedic Surgery
Medical Director, Center for Sports Medicine
University of Pittsburgh
Pittsburgh, PA 15213, USA

MARK GALLAND, M.D.
Senior Resident
Department of Orthopaedic Surgery
Tulane University School of Medicine
Department of Orthopaedic Surgery
New Orleans, LA 70112, USA

MONTSERRAT GARCIA, M.D.
Barcelona, Spain

MARK GETELMAN, M.D.
Southern California Orthopaedic Institute
Van Nuys, CA 91405, USA

GREGORY A. HANKS, M.D.
Orthopaedic Institute of Pennsylvania
Harrisburg Hospital
Camp Hill, PA 17011, USA

CHRISTOPHER D. HARNER, M.D.
Chief, Division of Sports Medicine
Department of Orthopaedic Surgery
University of Pittsburgh
Pittsburgh, PA 15213, USA

MICHAEL T. HAVIG, M.D.
Orthopaedic Surgeon
The Orthopaedic Specialty Hospital
Salt Lake City, UT 84107, USA

JOHN S. HENRY, M.D.
Geisinger Medical Center
Department of Orthopaedic Surgery
Danville, PA 17821, USA

LAURENCE D. HIGGINS, M.D.
Assistant Professor
Department of Surgery, Division of Orthopaedics
Duke University Medical Center
Durham, NC 27710, USA

RAYMOND C. HUI, M.D.
Fellow in Sports Medicine, Knee Surgery & Traumatology
The Hughston Clinic, PC
Columbus, GA 31904, USA

MASAAKI ITO, M.D.
Department of Orthopaedic Surgery
Sapporo Medical University
Sapporo 060, Japan

DARREN L. JOHNSON, M.D.
Chairman, Department of Orthopaedics
University of Kentucky School of Medicine
Department of Orthopaedic Surgery
Kentucky Clinic—K431
Lexington, KY 40536, USA

DERYK G. JONES, M.D.
Sports Medicine/Shoulder Fellow
University of Pittsburgh
Department of Orthopaedic Surgery
Center for Sports Medicine
Pittsburgh, PA 15213, USA

GRANT L. JONES, M.D.
Fellow in Sports Medicine
The Hughston Clinic, PC
Columbus, GA 31908, USA

ALEXANDER KALENAK, M.D.
Attending Orthopaedic Surgery
Pinnacle Health System
Department of Orthopaedics
Camp Hill, PA 17011, USA

KIRK A. KINDSFATER, M.D.
Staff Physician
Orthopaedic Center of the Rockies, Ft. Collins, CO
Assistant Clinical Professor of Orthopaedics
University of Colorado, Denver, CO
Ft. Collins, CO 80525, USA

L. ANDREW KOMAN, M.D.
Professor and Vice-Chair
Department of Orthopaedic Surgery
Wake Forest University School of Medicine
Medical Center Blvd.
Winston-Salem, NC 27157, USA

MARTIN W. KORN, M.D.
Clinical Assistant Professor
University of Rochester
Strong Memorial Hospital
Rochester General Hospital
Department of Orthopaedic Surgery
Rochester, NY 14642, USA

KEVIN L. KUNKLE, M.D.
Private Practice
Trenton Orthopaedic Group
Mercerville, NJ 08648, USA

M. KUROSAKA, M.D.
Department of Orthopaedic Surgery
Kobe Universoty School of Medicine
Kobe, Japan

ROGER V. LARSON, M.D.
Associate Professor
University of Washington
Department of Orthopaedic Surgery
Seattle, WA 98195, USA

WAYNE B. LEADBETTER, M.D.
Clinical Assistant Professor of Orthopaedic Surgery
Georgetown University
Clinical Assistant Professor of Surgery
Uniformed Services University of Health Sciences
Washington, DC, USA

ROBERT E. LEGGON, M.D.
Director, Orthopaedic Traumatology
Department of Orthopaedic Surgery
Geisinger Clinic
Penn State Geisinger Health System
Danville, PA 17822, USA

PHILLIP J. LEWANDOWSKI, M.D.
Crystal Clinic
Akron, OH 44308, USA

RONALD W. LINDSEY, M.D.
Professor of Orthopaedic Surgery
Chief, Section of Orthopaedic Trauma
Department of Orthopaedic Surgery
Baylor College of Medicine
Houston, TX 77002, USA

M. MIKE MALEK, M.D., F.A.C.S.
Director, Washington Orthopaedic and Knee Clinic
Vienna, VA 22182, USA

R.K. MARTI, M.D.
Amsterdam, The Netherlands

ANTONIO MIGUEL, M.D.
Mexico City, Mexico

K. MIZUNO, M.D.
Department of Orthopaedic Surgery
Kobe University School of Medicine
Kobe, Japan

TIMOTHY J. MONAHAN, M.D.
Resident in Orthopaedic Surgery
Geisinger Clinic Medical Center
Department of Orthopaedic Surgery
Danville, PA 17822, USA

MICHAEL A. MONT, M.D.
The John Hopkins University Medical Institution
Department of Orthopaedic Surgery
Division of Arthritis Surgery
The Good Samaritan Hospital
Baltimore, MD 21239, USA

JAMES S. MULHOLLAN, M.D.
Private Practice
Little Rock, AR 72205, USA

HIROSHI NARITA, M.D., PH.D.
Assistant Professor
Department of Orthopaedic Surgery
Sapporo Medical University
Sapporo 060, Japan

CHARLES L. NELSON, M.D.
Assistant Professor of Orthopaedic Surgery
University of Pennsylvania Medical Center
Department of Orthopaedic Surgery
Philadelphia, PA 19104, USA

M. NODA, M.D.
Department of Orthopaedic Surgery
Kobe University School of Medicine
Kobe, Japan

FELICIA OLLIVIERRE, M.D.
Private Practice—Kaiser Permanente
Cumberland, MD 21502, USA

DAVID A. PADDEN, M.D.
The John Hopkins University Medical Institution
Department of Orthopaedic Surgery
Division of Arthritis Surgery
The Good Samaritan Hospital
Baltimore, MD 21239, USA

LONNIE E. PAULOS, M.D.
Medical Director, The Orthopaedic Specialty Hospital & Orthopaedic Biomechanics Institute
The Orthopaedic Special Hospital
Salt Lake City, UT 84107, USA

VINCENT D. PELLEGRINI, JR., M.D.
Professor & Chair, Department of Orthopaedics & Rehabilitation, Pennsylvania State University
Professor & Chief, Department of Orthopaedics & Rehabilitation, Penn State Geisinger Health System
Hershey, PA 18033, USA

LARS PETERSON, M.D., PH.D.
Gothenburg Medical Center
Gothenburg, Sweden

DENNIS J. PHILLIPS, M.D.
Tuckahoe Orthopaedic Associates
Richmond, VA 23226, USA

GARY G. POEHLING, M.D.
Professor & Chair
Department of Orthopaedic Surgery
Wake Forest University School of Medicine
Winston-Salem, NC 27157, USA

DAVID C. POLLOCK, M.D.
Orthopaedic Surgery Resident
Wake Forrest University Baptist Medical Center
Department of Orthopaedic Surgery
Winston-Salem, NC 27157, USA

GIANCARLO PUDDU, M.D.
Rome, Italy

JOHN C. RICHMOND, M.D.
Associate Professor of Orthopaedic Surgery
Tufts University School of Medicine
New England Medical Center
Boston, MA 02111, USA

JOHN B. RYAN, M.D.
Private Practice
Warren, MI 48093, USA

SUSAN CRAIG SCOTT, M.D.
Private Practice
New York, NY 10128, USA

W. NORMAN SCOTT, M.D.
Chairman, Department of Orthopaedic Surgery
Beth Israel Hospital
Associate Professor
Mt. Sinai School of Medicine
New York, NY 10128, USA

THOMAS L. SMITH, PH.D.
Research Assistant Professor
Department of Orthopaedic Surgery
Wake Forest University School of Medicine
Winston-Salem, NC 27157, USA

GLENN C. TERRY, M.D.
Staff Physician
The Hughston Clinic, PC
Columbus, GA 31908, USA

JÜRGEN TOFT, M.D.
Chief Knee Surgery
Alpha-Klinik for Knee & Spine Surgery
Department of Knee Surgery
Munich, 81925 Germany

C.N. VAN DIJK, M.D.
Amsterdam, The Netherlands

TERRY L. WHIPPLE, M.D., F.A.C.S.
Tuckahoe Orthopaedic Associates
Richmond, VA 23226, USA

RUSSELL E. WINDSOR, M.D.
Associate Professor of Orthopaedic Surgery
Hospital for Special Surgery
Cornell University Medical Center
Department of Orthopaedic Surgery
New York, NY 10021, USA

MICHAEL R. WOOLFREY, M.D., F.R.C.S.C.
London Health Sciences Centre
University Campus
London, Ontario, Canada N6A 5A5

CHANG MOO YIM, M.D.
Department of Orthopaedic Surgery
School of Medicine
Kyung Hee University
Seoul, South Korea

S. YOSHIYA, M.D.
Department of Orthopaedic Surgery
Kobe University School of Medicine
Kobe, Japan

Section I

Overview of Complications and Pitfalls in Arthroscopy and Arthroscopic Procedures of the Knee

Chapter 1

Avoiding Complications

Guidelines for Safe Arthroscopic Knee Surgery

Terry L. Whipple and Dennis J. Phillips

Knee arthroscopy is one of the most frequently performed surgical procedures in the field of orthopedics. This procedure has relatively low morbidity, but with the large volume of procedures performed and the evolution of more complex techniques using minimally invasive approaches, complications are bound to occur.

With continued advances in orthopedic surgery of the knee, hospitalization time, medical cost, and time lost from work and recreation have been dramatically reduced and restoration of neuromuscular function has improved.[1–7] Although the benefits of minimally invasive surgery should reasonably include a reduction in the rate of complications, a review of the literature suggests there is room for improvement. DeLee[8] reported in 1985 the results of a national survey conducted by the Arthroscopy Association of North America on 118,600 arthroscopic knee procedures with a complication rate of 0.8%. Sherman et al[9] reported a much higher complication rate of 8.2% on a review of 2,640 cases in 1986. Identifying factors that commonly lead to complications can heighten a surgeon's awareness of risk and invite precautionary measures. This chapter reviews the safety measures and routines that can help avert complications through preparedness, alertness, and routine precautions.

Most complications associated with arthroscopic knee procedures can be attributed to errors that could be avoided during the perioperative period. A complete history and physical exam should establish a working diagnosis preoperatively, so the surgeon has a reasonable expectation of pathology to be encountered, and has immediately at hand the instruments and facilities to address them. Ancillary diagnostic services and studies should be ordered to complement the patient's clinical examination. Too often, residents, fellows, and staff surgeons embark on surgical procedures lacking complete familiarity with the patient's history and physical findings. This leaves them unprepared to perform the procedures in the proper context, and to exercise intraoperative judgment that is most appropriate for a patient's prioritized goals, lifestyle, and physical demands. Rarely is it appropriate for a surgeon to embark on an arthroscopic procedure without having personally examined and interviewed the patient, expecting to deal with whatever abnormal anatomy is encountered intraoperatively.

A preoperative plan should establish the objectives of the arthroscopic procedure. Contingency plans should also be reviewed to ensure the availability of equipment that might be needed, and to properly inform and prepare the patient for possible alternative results and altered plans for recuperation and outcome. Before commencing the procedure, the surgeon should review the availability of required instrumentation personally.

Complications increase with the unnecessary prolongation of surgical procedures. Cases may be prolonged waiting for instruments to be retrieved, sterilized, or even brought into the hospital setting after induction of anesthesia. Lesser delays may result from the surgical team's lack of familiarity with the equipment and its proper operation. The surgical team should make a habit of reviewing the assembly and operation of unfamiliar equipment preoperatively with the surgeon or other staff members to expedite the procedure and minimize operating time. New techniques and equipment are best rehearsed or reviewed in a simulated surgical setting or laboratory, not in the course of a patient's surgery. Operating room personnel should be cognizant of their individual responsibilities and should be accountable for the delivery, maintenance, and sterilization of surgical equipment.

General preparedness for appropriate medical management of patients takes priority over elective surgical repair or reconstruction of the knee. Past medical illnesses, prior difficulties with anesthesia or surgical recuperation, routine medications, and medical allergies should be reviewed preoperatively in detail. A final review of clinical records of the patient's knee history and physical examination are helpful. Preoperative radiographs and films of special procedures should be available for reference intraoperatively if necessary. Before a patient is premedicated, the surgeon should briefly review the planned treatment objectives and invite the patient's questions to allow the patient to feel comfortable, confident, and well informed about his treatment and the expectation of outcomes. The patient should be asked to mark the operative site before premedication to avoid the possibility of wrong-site or wrong-side surgery.

As a final preoperative physical check, the surgeon should inspect the operative site for skin breaks or inflammation, and assess the patient's airway, heart rate and rhythm, peripheral circulation, and mental status before induction of anesthesia. Even if the procedure is to be performed under local or regional anesthesia, intravenous access is advisable. Once the patient is anesthetized, a thorough examination of the knee should be repeated and compared with the opposite extremity for an understanding of the patient's normal range of motion, stability, and laxity. During induction, the surgeon would do well to review the instrumentation he anticipates needing to ensure availability, and should discuss with the staff preparedness for possible contingency plans if unexpected pathology or intraoperative complications are encountered.

It is the surgeon's responsibility to see that no harm befalls the patient intraoperatively. Accordingly, one should double check the patient's proper positioning and stability on the operating table, and be certain that all bony prominences or potential pressure points are well padded (Fig. 1.1). The patient should have no direct contact with metal objects, and particular attention should be paid to nerve pressure points such as the neck of the fibula, the posteromedial aspect of the elbow, and the axilla. The nonoperative leg should be well padded, the table should be slightly flexed to avoid strain on the lumbar spine, and a safety belt should always be applied.

If a tourniquet is used, it should be sufficiently wide and smoothly applied against the skin to avoid pressure points or skin necrosis. One should be sure the tourniquet is placed proximal enough on the thigh to allow

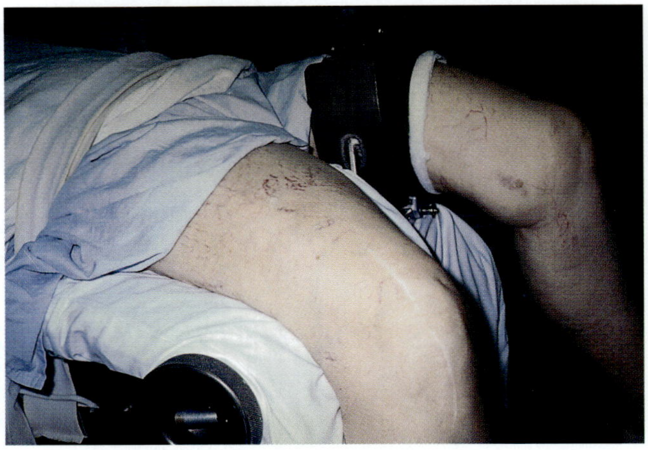

Figure 1.1. In positioning the patient, all possible pressure points are padded, not only on the operated extremity, but the opposite side as well. This is especially important for patients with capillary fragility or any connective tissue disease.

sterile access to exit points for guide pins or sutures without compromising the sterile field.

If a leg holder is used as a fulcrum for stressing the medial or lateral compartments of the knee open for better arthroscopic visualization, the surgeon should be sure that it is placed so as not to interfere with the sterile field, the tourniquet, or electrical grounding, and that it will not place undue pressure on the skin or interfere with the tourniquet. Many thigh-stabilizing devices placed proximally on the extremity pose a risk to the patient's genitalia. A last-minute safety check in the perineum and adequate padding or coverage is imperative. Tourniquet pressure set 100 mm Hg above systolic pressure is usually adequate, but it is almost never necessary to exceed 150 mm Hg above systolic pressure.

Varus or valgus stress in a thigh stabilizer should never be excessive. The patient's advanced age, frailty, or possible history of steroid consumption would indicate greater vulnerability of the collateral ligaments, and surgeons should be cognizant of those conditions (Fig. 1.2). The Arthroscopy Association of North America report of complications in knee arthroscopy in 1985 noted that intraoperative ligament injuries constituted 4.4% of all complications, and occurred in 0.04% of all arthroscopic knee cases.[8]

Prepping and draping must maintain a sterile waterproof barrier for the surgical field, and should allow ample exposure of the knee with the leg, foot, and ankle draped into the field.

Sterile prepping of the skin should not be compromised, even though knee arthroscopy involves no wide surgical exposure, and entails copious irrigation of the

A B
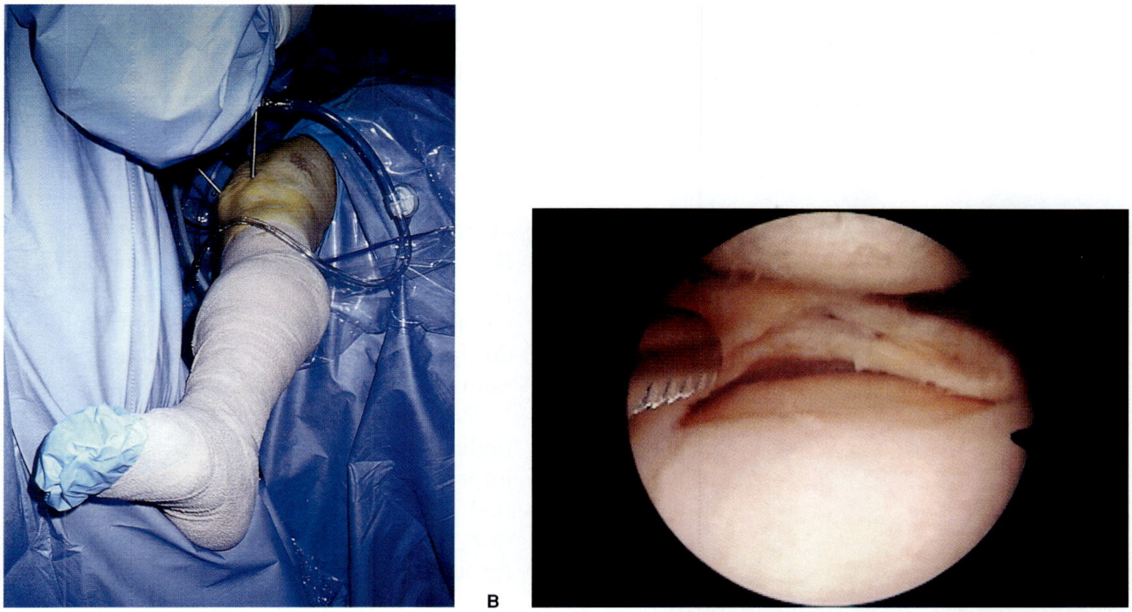

Figure 1.2. **A:** Using one's body weight to apply valgus or varus stress against a fulcrum beneath the drapes requires special precautions, especially in the elderly. **B:** Iatrogenic rupture of the medial collateral ligament creates obvious increase in the intraarticular work space, but complicates recovery from otherwise straightforward arthroscopic procedures.

joint space. Still, skin contaminants pose a risk of infection in arthroscopic procedures, and can usually be avoided with careful compliance with routine sterile technique.

Portal placement in the knee should become routine. Care is taken always to avoid the infrapatellar branch of the saphenous nerve. Initial anteromedial or anterolateral portals should be established directing the scalpel toward the intercondylar notch to avoid accidental contact with the femoral articular cartilage. Avoid the practice of spinning the scalpel in the portal, which can lacerate the joint capsule, patella tendon, or meniscus. If the initial portals are made with the knee passively flexed 90 degrees, it should be easy to follow the path of the capsular incision with the arthroscope sheath and trochar. Extending or flexing the knee after the scalpel insertion allows subcutaneous tissues to obscure the capsular puncture. Inserting the arthroscope sheath and trochar toward the intercondylar notch minimizes risk of scuffing the articular cartilage on entry.

An initial comprehensive arthroscopic survey of the entire knee is imperative, but we recommend the initial inspection be directed to the compartment and anatomic structures where pathology is most expected to be found. This permits the scrub nurse or circulating nurse to prepare instrumentation needed for the definitive procedure while the surgeon completes his survey inspection of the rest of the joint. Time is saved in this way should the preoperative diagnosis be mistaken and different instrumentation be required.

Establishing a coordinated accessory portal can be accomplished most accurately by sounding the portal placement initially with a hypodermic or spinal needle while monitoring the intended portal placement arthroscopically. If a spinal needle can be inserted to directly reach the target structures in the knee, less struggle and easier execution of the procedure will occur with the appropriate instrumentation. It usually helps also to place the anteromedial and anterolateral portals at slightly different levels above the anterior menisci so as to avoid crowding instruments with the arthroscope, especially in the intercondylar notch. Although many surgeons orient their portals transversely in keeping with Langer's skin lines, the authors prefer longitudinally oriented portals that parallel the fibers of the joint capsule (Fig. 1.3). These portals heal readily and cosmetically without suture closure or skin tapes, and seem to minimize the risk of synovial herniation compared with transverse portals that cut fibers of the anterior capsule. Lidge[10] found that problems with the execution of arthroscopic procedures are inversely proportional to the skill of the arthroscopist. Though this is an apparent truism, everyone encounters difficult cases and unexpected obstacles irrespective of experience. Arthroscopy is a visual procedure, and it is folly to proceed with a case unless or until adequate internal visualization is obtained. Visual-

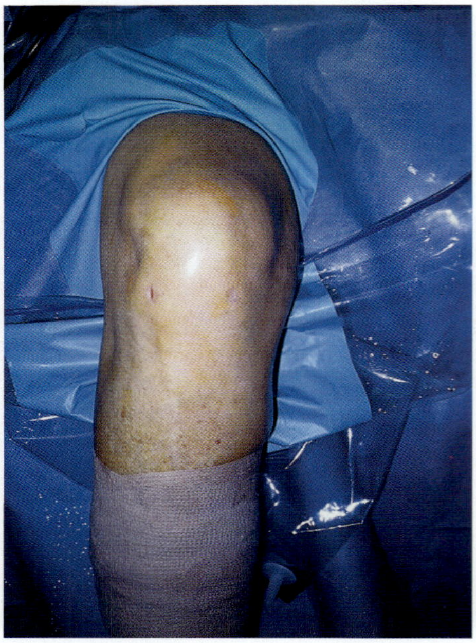

Figure 1.3. Vertically oriented portals for knee arthroscopy parallel the fibers of the joint capsule and are less likely to cause synovial herniation. The portals may pout a bit immediately postoperatively, but require no closing sutures or tapes to produce a very cosmetic scar.

ization may be obscured by internal bleeding, arthritic debris, fatty tissue, or synovial hypertrophy. Establishing optimal visualization must always be the first and important objective in every case. Bleeding problems can be minimized by adding epinephrine to each bag of irrigating solution and by controlling intraoperative hypertension. Arthritic debris and excessive fatty or synovial tissue should be resected patiently until visibility is optimal. One should never compromise on good visualization.

Arthroscopic surgery requires finesse and gentleness. All instruments should be inserted gently with a twisting motion and with an index finger extended along the shaft of the instrument to meet the skin and avoid an inadvertent traumatic plunge into the joint. Articular cartilage must be respected in every circumstance to prevent inadvertent iatrogenic injury.

Some arthroscopic procedures pose particular risk to certain potential complications. Lateral retinacular release, for example, may risk transection of the anterior branch of the lateral geniculate artery and risk excessive bleeding, bruising, or hemarthrosis. This artery can usually be identified during the course of the release, if diligently sought. Cauterizing it minimizes complications associated with excessive postoperative bleeding.

Infusion pumps are now in widespread use to facilitate distention of the joint during arthroscopy and to maintain a clear visual field. Mechanical positive pressure flow has a number of advantages compared with gravity-assisted systems, but complications are more likely to occur with the mechanical systems. Reports in the literature include ruptured suprapatellar pouch, deep posterior compartment syndrome, and skin slough.[11,12] Uncontrolled pressure in the irrigation system should be avoided. Most modern pumps contain both pressure and flow rate sensors that can automatically retard flow when pressure exceeds a safe threshold. The surgeon and the circulating nurse should both be familiar with the pump's design and operation. Pump malfunctions should be recognized and corrected thriftily to avoid overdistention.

Perhaps the three most common intraoperative impediments to a successful arthroscopic knee exam are impaired visibility due to bleeding or to an exuberant fat pad anteriorly, and compromised access to the posterior regions due to ligament contracture. Struggling through a case with poor visibility or difficult access compounds the risk of an incomplete examination or an inadequate procedure, and may result in further injury to articular surfaces or ligaments. Most such risks can be overcome with patience, understanding of the cause of the problem, coaching, experience, finesse, and knowing when to stop.

Bleeding is best controlled with a tourniquet. All knee arthroscopy cases should be performed with a tourniquet in place, whether the surgeon chooses to inflate it electively or not. With the tourniquet deflated, excessive bleeding could be caused by a relative venous tourniquet effect from a tight circumferential thigh stabilizer. Intraoperative hypertension should be controlled to a systolic pressure level of 110 to 120 mm Hg unless the patient has a history of a stroke or myocardial ischemia. Unbalanced inflow and outflow can increase bleeding even from minor synovial punctures from well-placed portals (Fig. 1.4). Any abrasion treatment or intraarticular fractures will cause even worse bleeding with insufficient inflow pressure.

When intraoperative bleeding is encountered, reduce the level of any outflow suction, increase the inflow pressure in 10-mm increments up to the diastolic blood pressure if necessary, or by elevating the irrigation bags if using gravity infusion. These adjustments should tamponade venous bleeding within a few seconds. If not, reduce pressure on the thigh stabilizer and inflate a pneumatic tourniquet to a level of 100 to 150 mm Hg above systolic blood pressure.

If bleeding persists with tourniquet elevation, check the tourniquet connections.

The obstructive fat pad or ligamentum mucosum simply requires a couple of extra minutes for resection. The ligamentum mucosum is most easily removed by detaching it from the roof of the intercondylar notch,

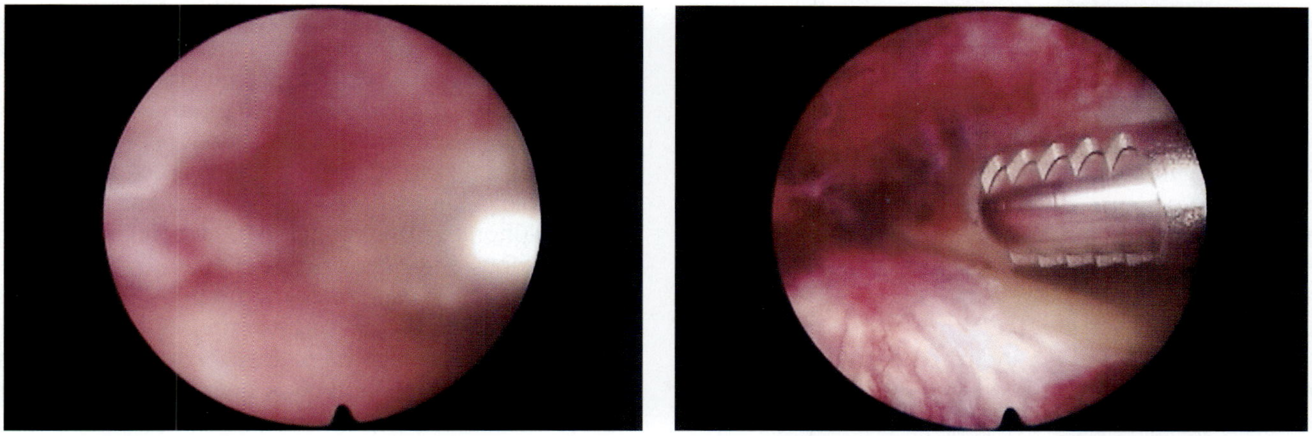

A B

Figure 1.4. Balancing inflow and outflow rates, even in bloody or inflamed joints, is critical to good visualization and efficient operating time. **A:** Before balancing irrigation rates. **B:** After balancing irrigation to maintain a constant slightly positive intra-articular pressure.

which allows the fat pad to float anteriorly and usually out of the way. When resecting the fat pad, remember once its synovial covering has been breached, the fatty tissues will gradually absorb fluid and become enlarged. If one anticipates a more lengthy procedure, therefore, such as anterior cruciate ligament (ACL) reconstruction or stabilization of a tibial plateau fracture, more extensive fat pad resection might be appropriate (Fig. 1.5).

When resecting the fat pad, be careful not to divide the intermeniscal ligament anteriorly. This is especially problematic in the presence of radial meniscus tears where the hoop stresses are further reduced.

Tight compartments that limit access to the posterior regions of the knee require gentleness and cautious applications of varus or valgus stress. Fracture of the femur or a medial collateral ligament tear can almost always be avoided. Elderly patients, paraplegics, patients with metabolic bone disease, or those who have been immobilized for a period of time pose heightened risk of bone or ligament injury, as do rheumatoid patients or others with a prolonged history of steroid treatment. With gentle but sustained varus or valgus stress, collateral ligaments usually elongate gradually. This plastic change may require 5 or 6 minutes of continuous pressure. Remember, the posterior condyles of the femur are longer than the distal condyles, so the posterior compartments are easier to visualize with the knee relatively extended instead of flexed in a figure-four position.

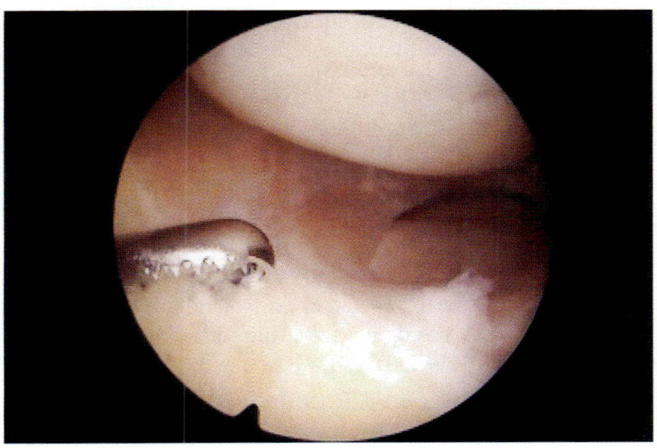

Figure 1.5. Ample resection of the fat pad improves visualization and saves time in all arthroscopic procedures in the anterior compartment or the intercondylar notch.

This is a good opportunity to address the risks of a skin burn from electrocautery utilized under arthroscopic control. In slender patients, the normal fatty buffer between retinaculum and skin is not present, and one should be constantly aware of the depth of the electrocautery tip to avoid skin burns. Although it is tempting to use higher power for faster cutting speed, patience and gentleness will prove effective when cutting tissues or coagulating vessels under arthroscopic control.

At the conclusion of a procedure, attention to exact details can also help prevent complications. Aspirating excess irrigating fluid from the joint before withdrawing instruments enhances postoperative comfort and mobility. Intraarticular Marcaine can provide 4 to 6 hours of pain relief, and Marcaine with epinephrine will help to reduce intraarticular bleeding postoperatively. It is prudent for the surgeon to check with the anesthetist for any contraindication to injecting epinephrine, especially in patients with hypotension or bradycardia.

Injecting 4 to 5 mg of intraarticular Duramorph can provide even longer pain relief, lasting up to 24 hours.

Whereas Marcaine is usually sufficient for a patient to clear the recovery room and make it home, Duramorph may easily last through the first night postoperatively.

Routine portals in the knee rarely require closure even though they may pout at the end of a procedure. Laceration of a superficial vein when establishing a portal may require a suture to reduce bleeding, but most portals will heal more cosmetically without closure. Sutures leave additional puncture and pressure marks, and Steri-Strips often blister the skin if the knee swells postoperatively.

Compressive bandages should be applied with attention to uniform pressure and avoidance of any circumferential fabric with an inelastic edge. Flexion and extension of the knee cause nonelastic bandages to creep and roll, creating strictures around the skin that can compress the peroneal nerve or impede venous return.

Complications from anesthesia have been alluded to earlier with respect to hypotension and cardiac arrhythmias, but somnolence, nausea, and pain control warrant some additional comment.

If the proper medications are given in the correct dosages, admission to the hospital can be minimized. Our surgery center has a 1.8% admission rate for all open and arthroscopic procedures.[13] Somnolence, pain, and nausea are the most frequent issues encountered in the postanesthesia care unit or recovery room following arthroscopic procedures. Most of these can be traced to inappropriate use of narcotics. Anesthesia induction with intravenous propofol has drastically reduced the incidence of nausea, but intraoperative fentanyl often causes nausea anyway. As noted above, immediate postoperative pain can usually be controlled by deflating the tourniquet a few minutes before waking the patient, and by injecting Marcaine or Duramorph intraarticularly. Toradol given in intravenous doses of up to 30 mg can provide additional postoperative analgesia nearly equivalent to narcotics, but without the nausea side effects. Avoidance of narcotics also reduces the postoperative somnolence, which is frequently the cause of prolonged recovery room stays.

Most perioperative complications can be intercepted early if the patient is properly monitored. In an outpatient setting, the patient may become responsible for his own postoperative monitoring. Adequate coaching of a family member before discharge is imperative for patients undergoing ambulatory surgery, and if the patient will be spending all or part of the first 24 hours alone, this coaching should take place preoperatively before administering any medication. Patients and their families must know what to expect, and how to recognize signs of complications that warrant urgent medical attention.

It is helpful to provide patients with written instructions that document signs of infection, bleeding, and nerve or vascular compression. We also like to include specific instructions with respect to diet, ambulation, mobilization of the operated extremity, weight-bearing status, muscle isometrics, management of bandages, and activity level. These specific written instructions not only help avoid complications, but also minimize unnecessary telephone calls postoperatively when the patient is most anxious and most uncomfortable.

Finally, surgical speed is important to reduce costs, infection risk, and sequelae from prolonged anesthesia. Important as speed is, haste that leads to carelessness or increased surgical trauma is never justified. Surgical speed is a function of precision, efficiency of movement, and preparedness. The surgeon should assume some of the responsibility for the readiness of surgical assistants, scrub nurse, circulating nurse, and even the anesthetist by briefing everyone in advance of what he intends to do and what special instrumentation, implants, or ancillary support, such as radiology services, he will need for the case. For unusual or complex cases, rotation of team members in and out of the case is ill advised, as the replacements have not been briefed on the surgical plan, and are unaware of intraoperative contingencies that may be under way. Only a coordinated team of staff members who are prepared for and attentive to the operation can contribute to a well-executed procedure and the avoidance of complications.

References

1. Chana GS, Tubbs N. Early results of arthroscopic surgery of the knee. *Injury* 1981;13:227–229.
2. Dandy OJ. Early results of closed partial meniscectomy. *Br Med J* 1978;1:1099–1101.
3. Hamberg P, Gillquist J, Lysholm J, Oberg P. The effect of diagnostic and operative arthroscopy and open meniscectomy on muscle strength in the thigh. *Am J Sports Med* 1983;11:289–292.
4. Hershman EB, Nisonson B. Arthroscopic meniscectomy: a follow-up report. *Am J Sports Med* 1983;11:253–257.
5. Northmore-Ball MO, Dandy DJ, Jackson RW. Arthroscopic, open partial and total meniscectomy. A comparative study. *J Bone Joint Surg* 1983;65B(4):400–404.
6. Patel O, Fahmy N, Sakayan A. Isokinetic and functional evaluation of the knee following arthroscopic surgery. *Clin Orthop* 1982;167:84–91.
7. Prietto CA, Caiozzo VJ, Prietto PP, McMaster NC. Closed versus open partial meniscectomy: postoperative changes in the force velocity relationship of muscle. *Am J Sports Med* 1983;11:189–194.
8. Delee JC. Complications of arthroscopy and arthroscopic

surgery: results of a national survery. *Arthroscopy* 1985; 1:204–220.

9. Sherman OH, Fox JM, Snyder SJ, et al. Arthrscopy—"no problem surgery." An analysis of complications in 2640 cases. *J Bone Joint Surg* 1986;68A:256–265.
10. Lidge RT. Problems and complications in arthroscopy. In: Cascells SW, ed. *Arthroscopy: Diagnostic and Surgical Practice*. Philadelphia: Lea and Febiger, 1984:81–85.
11. Metcalf RW. An arthroscopic method for lateral release of the subluxing or dislocating patella. *Clin Orthop* 1982; 167:9–18.
12. Noyes FR, Spievack ES. Extraarticular fluid dissection in tissues during arthroscopy. *Am J Sports Med* 1982;10: 346–351.
13. Padgett LR. Personal communication on effective outpatient anesthesia and pain management for orthopaedic procedures in ambulatory surgery center, Residents and Fellows Arthroscopy Conference, Scottsdale, AZ, April 1998.

Chapter 2

Postarthroscopy Septic Arthritis

Gregory C. Fanelli and Timothy J. Monahan

Infection is second only to hemarthrosis in frequency of complications following arthroscopy.[1] The extent may range from superficial wound infection of the portals to septic arthritis of the knee joint, which may result in destruction of articular cartilage, and impairment of joint mobility if not promptly and effectively treated. The reported incidence of septic arthritis following knee arthroscopy is between 0.03% and 0.3%.[2–6] Causes of postarthroscopy septic arthritis include intraarticular steroid injections, prolonged operating time, inadequate equipment sterilization, airborne bacteria, skin lesions, and supracutaneous sutures. This chapter discusses the causes, clinical presentation, prevention, and treatment of postarthroscopy septic arthritis.

CONTRIBUTING FACTORS

Intraarticular Steroids

The use of intraarticular steroids may help to reduce the inflammation and pain of the chronically painful knee; however, intraarticular steroid use during arthroscopy is strongly associated with increased rates of infection.[7] It has also been reported that intraarticular steroid usage is contraindicated within several days preceding joint surgery,[8] and is not recommended for several weeks after arthroscopy.[9] Proposed mechanisms include delaying healing, inhibiting inflammatory effects and immune response, as well as masking signs of infection.

Sterilization Procedures

Gluteraldehyde disinfection is less damaging to arthroscopic equipment than steam sterilization, and has been shown to be bactericidal with 10 minutes of immersion. Strict adherence to a soak time of 15 minutes, and regular changes of the solution are required if this method is used.[4] Improper sterilization techniques, including incomplete arthroscope immersion and failure to change the gluteraldehyde solution on schedule, have been implicated in increased infection rates.[7,10]

Operating Room Environmental Factors

Increased aerosolization of pathogenic bacteria during procedures has been demonstrated by culture plate growth. Attention should be given to minimization of traffic in the operating room, and placement of sterilized arthroscopes, cables, and supplies away from doorways and air vents.[11]

Skin Lesions

Skin lesions such as abrasions, lacerations, and abscesses around the operative site are an absolute contraindication to arthroscopic surgery.[12] We recommend postponing surgery with any potentially infectious remote site such as an ingrown toenail or other source of infection. The skin should be inspected immediately prior to the procedure to rule out the presence of such lesions.

Foreign Material

Introduction of hair into the joint may occur from inserting the arthroscopic equipment into unshaven areas of the skin.[3] This serves as a potential source of infection, and may be prevented by thorough skin preparation and shaving of the operative site.

Supracutaneous Sutures

Sutures tied over the skin were prevalent in previously used meniscus repair techniques, and were associated with frequent infections. Current techniques advocate sutures tied intraarticularly, or sutures tied directly over the capsule deep to the subcutaneous tissue. A substantial decrease in infection rate has been observed since externally tied sutures have been abandoned.[2,13]

CLINICAL PRESENTATION

Armstrong et al[7] reported that septic arthritis tends to present as one of two syndromes: classic or insidious. Classic symptoms of septic arthritis occur in about 25% of infections, and include onset within about 2 days of surgery with rapidly progressive knee pain, swelling, warmth, erythema, fever, and accompanying leukocytosis. The classic presentation is almost always caused by *Staphylococcus aureus;* however, *S. aureus* presents with classic symptoms only approximately 50% of the time.

An insidious presentation occurs in approximately 75% of infected patients with subacute pain, swelling, mild fever, and minimal or no leukocytosis within 1 to 11 days of surgery. Coagulase-negative staphylococci almost always exhibited the insidious presentation.[7] A high degree of suspicion is necessary due to the insidious nature of some infections, and the difficulty in distinguishing them from the normal postoperative synovitis. This high index of suspicion helps to decrease the devastating consequences of untreated infection.

When infection is suspected, synovial fluid aspiration, analysis for leukocytes in the joint fluid, and culture should be performed, and treatment promptly started. Cultures should be repeated if any contamination or doubt exists regarding the pathogen. *Staphylococcus epidermidis* and other coagulase-negative staphylococci are important pathogens, and should not be dismissed as a contaminant.[7,14] Jerosch et al[15] recommend measurement of joint fluid for leukocytes and C-reactive protein (CRP) levels, as CRP is useful for diagnosis within hours of joint infection, and decreases by 50% per day with successful treatment. Peripheral white blood cell counts, synovial fluid Gram stain, and gross appearance were normal in 50% of infected patients,[7] and were especially poor indicators in the group that presented insidiously.

PREVENTION

Antibiotic Prophylaxis

Antibiotic prophylaxis is expected to give a fourfold reduction in infection rate and to decrease morbidity, and was calculated to be cost-effective for infection rates greater than 0.08%.[4] The use of prophylactic antibiotics, however, is controversial. Strict adherence to aseptic technique is cited by Keiser[2] as more important in infection control, and Guhl and Schonholtz[9] recommend against routine use of prophylactic antibiotics in short diagnostic and surgical cases. D'Angelo and Ogilvie-Harris[4] state that reliable prediction of septic complications is not possible using risk factors, but several authors have found that multiple concurrent procedures and long operative times correlate with increased infection rates.[6,7] An extremely large study group would be necessary to determine the efficacy of prophylactic antibiotics because of the small underlying rate of infection, and may be impractical. In the absence of this information, proper attention should be given to sterile technique and other controllable factors. Prophylactic antibiotics may be appropriate during multiple, concurrent, and lengthy surgical procedures.

TREATMENT

Immediate drainage and administration of intravenous antibiotics is necessary to avoid decreased joint mobility and further articular cartilage destruction. DeLee[3] reported that 18 of 95 infections resulted in a permanent loss of flexion to less than 90 degrees in the involved knee. Several options exist for removing purulent material from the knee joint, including arthroscopic lavage and debridement, repeated aspirations, arthrotomy, and suction/irrigation. Smith[16] reported that arthroscopic lavage and debridement within 24 hours of diagnosis resulted in no recurrent infections and decreased morbidity and hospital stay. Armstrong et al[7] reported no secondary infections or immediate relapse following arthroscopic treatment.

The following disadvantages exist with other methods of draining the knee joint: Repeated aspiration of the knee is painful, and concern exists that aspiration does not completely evacuate and decompress the knee.[16] Open arthrotomy is effective at eliminating infection, but has significant morbidity with associated scarring, joint stiffness, and prolonged hospitalization.[16] Suction/irrigation technique has a higher rate of secondary infections and relapse than arthroscopic lavage and debridement,[7] and Jackson[17] reports that it is effective only if the joint is fully distended with fluid, and drained dry in a cyclic fashion.[17] If irrigation and suction are applied at the same time, the fluid flows along a "highway" in the joint, and does not flush remote or localized areas. Armstrong et al[7] report that distention/irrigation is no longer necessary with the advent of arthroscopic lavage.

There is general agreement in the literature that septic arthritis of the knee is best treated initially with arthroscopic lavage and appropriate antibiotic therapy. The effectiveness of this procedure is attributed to decompressing the joint, removing tissue debris that may cause further enzymatic destruction of articular cartilage,[18] and removing any foreign material that may have caused the pyogenic condition. Articular lavage must be prompt once diagnosis of pyarthrosis is made. No recurrence of infection or treatment failures were observed in a series of 30 patients lavaged within 24 hours of diagnosis, and all patients were ambulatory on postoperative day 1 with normal knee range of motion.[16] Failure and recurrence rates have been shown to be higher when treatment is delayed.[18] Williams et al[6] recommend arthroscopic debridement and lavage, combined with open debridement of extraarticular wounds and intravenous antibiotics, as first-line treatment for infections following arthroscopically assisted anterior cruciate ligament surgery. Open arthrotomy and debridement should be considered only if clinical signs of infection persist despite the above treatment.

The recommended duration of antibiotic treatment is variable. Smith[16] started intravenous antibiotics at admission, and continued them postoperatively for 48 to 72 hours in uncomplicated cases. In diabetics or patients with other medical problems such as renal failure, intravenous antibiotics were continued for up to 2 weeks. In all cases, treatment was followed by 1 month of oral antibiotics.[16] Armstrong et al[7] administered intravenous antibiotics for 2 weeks, with an additional 2 weeks of oral therapy. Regardless of the specific regimen of treatment, progress should be closely monitored for recurrence of symptoms, and prompt corrective action taken.

In a national survey of arthroscopy complications Small[1] found that the most commonly isolated infecting organisms were staphylococci, with *S. aureus* and *S. epidermidis* the most common types, followed by *Streptococcus, Pseudomonas,* and other unspecified organisms. In a review of arthroscopic surgery complications, Keiser[2] notes that *Staphylococcus* is the most common pathogen, and *Streptococcus,* meningococcus, and gram-negative organisms including *Pseudomonas* are rarely seen.

Clostridium perfringens has been reported in three cases following disinfection of the arthroscope and cables in gluteraldehyde solution.[2] *Pasteurella multocida* has been documented with animal exposure following arthroscopic surgery.[19] In most cases of *P. multocida* septic arthritis, a history of an animal bite distal to the affected joint is present, but in the above case, and in one-third of reported cases, there is only a history of animal exposure, not a bite. Blastomycosis of the knee and skull was reported in a previously healthy patient following arthroscopy, and did not respond to conventional treatment.[20] When resistant septic arthritis is encountered, unusual organisms should be considered. Finally, Michalska[21] reports that synovial fluid cultures are negative in 10% to 15% of patients with bacterial arthritis, and that synovial biopsy cultures may improve yield in identifying an infecting organism.

OTHER CONSIDERATIONS

Synovial Fistula

Collins[22] reported that synovial fistulas occurred at a portal site in four of 1,500 diagnostic and operative arthroscopies. These synovial fistulas resulted in persistent discharge of synovial fluid with other symptoms, and all fistulas closed spontaneously within 14 days. The most significant issue regarding a fistula is possible misdiagnosis as an infection. If persistent discharge is accompanied by pain, swelling, or fever, then synovial fluid aspirate should be performed. The synovial fluid aspirate should be evaluated for leukocytes, and culture should be performed. In the absence of these symptoms of infection, the fistula may be left to close spontaneously.

Superficial Portal Infection

Collins[22] reported that superficial portal infections occurred in five of 4,200 portal sites used in diagnostic and operative arthroscopies. In all five cases, no infection of the knee joint was found, and the superficial infections responded rapidly to oral antibiotic therapy. Fairclough and Moran[23] state that an increased wound infection rate is observed if subcutaneous tissue is included in the suture, and note that Gristina et al[24] have shown bacterial colonization of suture tracks. Forrester et al[25] reported that the strength and toughness of wounds were comparable when closed with either surgical tape or suture material after about 20 days of healing. Fairclough and Moran observed that it would be preferable to use tape closure of arthroscopy portals in lieu of percutaneous sutures, and reported no complications with tape closure in 168 patients. One superficial portal infection developed in wounds closed with nylon suture.

Williamson and Copeland[26] reported no complications in 140 patients whose portal incisions were treated without sutures, and found that leaving the portal wounds open precludes hematoma by allowing drainage, provides a better cosmetic result, and has the added advantage of suture material cost savings. Maffuli et al[27] corroborated the above findings in a study of 100 patients randomly assigned to suture and sutureless groups. No major complications were encountered in either group, but the incidence of hematoma and superficial abscess formation was lower in the sutureless technique. Based on the current literature, sutureless treatment of portal incisions appears effective, with lower rates of superficial infection, hematoma, and scarring.

CONCLUSION

Postarthroscopy septic arthritis is an uncommon complication. Contributing factors include intraarticular steroids, inadequate sterilization procedures, operating room environmental factors, skin lesions, and supracutaneous suture placement. Strict adherence to sterile technique in the operating room decreases the chances of this complication. Preoperative antibiotics may decrease the incidence further. Arthroscopic surgical lavage, debridement, and drainage, combined with the appropriate intravenous antibiotics, is the treatment of choice for postarthroscopy septic arthritis.

References

1. Small NC. Complications in arthroscopic surgery performed by experienced arthroscopists. *Arthroscopy* 1988; 4(3):215–221.
2. Keiser CH. A review of the complications of arthroscopic knee surgery. *Arthroscopy* 1992;8(1):79–83.
3. DeLee JC. Complications of arthroscopy and arthroscopic surgery: results of a national survey. *Arthroscopy* 1985; 1(4):214–220.
4. D'Angelo GL, Ogilvie-Harris DJ. Septic arthritis following arthroscopy with cost/benefit analysis of antibiotic prophylaxis. *Arthroscopy* 1988;4(1):10–14.
5. Johnson LL, Shneider DA, Austin MD, Goodman FG, Bullock JM, DeBruin JA. Two percent gluteraldehyde: a disinfectant in arthroscopy and arthroscopic surgery. *J Bone Joint Surg* 1982;64A:237–239.
6. Williams RJ, Laurencin CT, Warren RF, Speciale AC, Brause BD, O'Brien S. Septic arthritis after arthroscopic anterior cruciate ligament reconstruction. *Am J Sports Med* 1997;25(2):261–267.
7. Armstrong RW, Bolding F, Joseph R. Septic arthritis following arthroscopy: clinical syndromes and analysis of risk factors. *Arthroscopy* 1992;8(2):213–223.
8. Gray R, Gottlieb NL. Intraarticular corticosteroids: an updated assessment. *Clin Orthop Rel Res* 1983;177:235–263.
9. Guhl J, Schonholtz G. *Foot and Ankle Arthroscopy*, 2nd ed. Thorofare, NJ: Slack, 1993:215.
10. Armstrong RW, Bolding F. Septic arthritis after arthroscopy: the contributing roles of intraarticular steroids and environmental factors. *Am J Infect Control* 1994;22: 16–18.
11. Ajemian E, Andrews L, Hryb K, Klimek JJ. Hospital acquired infection after arthroscopic knee surgery: a probable environmental source. *Am J Infect Control* 1987; 15(4):159–162.
12. Bamford DJ, Paul AS,Noble J, Davies DRA. Avoidable complications of arthroscopic surgery. *J R Coll Surg Edinb* 1993;38:92–95.
13. Small NC. Complications in arthroscopic surgery of the knee and shoulder. *Orthopaedics* 1993;16(9):985–988.
14. Toye A, Thomson J, Karsh J. *Staphylococcus epidermidis* septic arthritis post arthroscopy. *Clin Exp Rheumatol* 1987;5(2):165–166.
15. Jerosch J, Hoffstetter I, Schroder M, Castro WHM. Septic arthritis: arthroscopic management with local antibiotic treatment. *Acta Orthop Belg* 1995;61(2):126–134.
16. Smith MJ. Arthroscopic treatment of the septic knee. *Arthroscopy* 1986;2(1):30–34.
17. Jackson RW. The septic knee—arthroscopic treatment. *Arthroscopy* 1985;1(3):194–197.
18. Thiery JA. Arthroscopic drainage in septic arthritis of the knee: a multicenter study. *Arthroscopy* 1989;5(1):65–69.
19. Bhagat B, Ahmed M, Lovelanet M, Berger B. Knee pain, swelling, and effusion after arthroscopy. *Hosp Pract* 1996;48.
20. Yocum J, Seligson D. Blastomycosis of the knee and skull after arthroscopy. *Am J Sports Med* 1991;19(6):670–673.
21. Michalska M. Knee arthroscopy in the office. *Hosp Pract* 1997;32(3):179–190.
22. Collins JJ. Knee joint arthroscopy—early complications. *Med J Aust* 1989;150:702–706.
23. Fairclough JA, Moran CG. The use of sterile adhesive tape in the closure of arthroscopic puncture wounds: a comparison with single layer nylon closure. *Ann R Coll Surg Engl* 1987;69(3):140–141.
24. Gristina AG, Price JL, Hobgood CD, Webb LX, Costerton JW. Bacterial colonization of percutaneous sutures. *Surg* 1985;98(1):12–19.
25. Forrester JC, Zederfeldt BH, Hayes TL, Hunt TK. Tape-closed and sutured wounds: a comparison by tensiometry and scanning electron microscopy. *Br J Surg* 1970; 57(10):729–737.
26. Williamson DM, Copeland SA. Suturing arthroscopy wounds: brief report. *J Bone Joint Surg* 1988;70B:146.
27. Maffuli N, Pintore E, Petricciuolo F. Arthroscopy wounds: to suture or not to suture. *Acta Orthop Belg* 1991; 57(2):154–156.

Chapter 3

Soft Tissue Complications

Ecchymosis, Hemarthrosis, Chronic Effusion, and Wound Dehiscence

Wayne B. Leadbetter

No matter how well conceived, knee surgery is a deliberate controlled wounding of highly vascularized living tissues. The benefits of any proposed surgical procedure must be constantly weighed against the induced costs of functional recovery from creating an acute injury, namely, hemorrhage, inflammation, pain, muscle inhibition, and possible arthrofibrosis. While the advent of arthroscopic techniques has reduced obvious cutaneous and myotendinous trauma, intraarticular hemorrhage from such procedures as synovectomy, ligament tunneling, burring, retinacular release, or various chondral restoration procedures can lead to significant postoperative disability. Given these circumstances, it is not surprising that most reviews have shown hemarthrosis to be the most frequent complication of knee arthroscopy and, by experience, of knee surgery in general.[1] Postoperative hemarthrosis of the knee along with prominent cutaneous ecchymosis, recurrent effusions, and potential wound dehiscence with synovial fistula pose clinical problems ranging from patient apprehension due to tenderness at wound sites to serious delays in the recovery of joint motion or limb strength.

This chapter discusses these issues primarily in the context of prevalent arthroscopic technique, although the principles are applicable to all knee surgery.

CUTANEOUS ECCHYMOSIS

Nothing alarms a patient more in the immediate postoperative period than the appearance of bleeding, whether on the dressings or in the form of cutaneous ecchymosis (Fig. 3.1). The fear of a "blood clot" as an imminent thromboembolic threat or the perceived onset of "gangrene" stirs patient anxiety. If such cutaneous staining is accompanied by prominent calf swelling and pain, differentiating an actual thrombophlebitis can be difficult and warrants immediate venous plethysmography evaluation.[2] An improperly applied or disheveled Ace bandage may actually contribute to the risk of venous stasis and distal leg edema (Fig. 3.2). The resulting dependent swelling and pain may slow recovery and the ability of the patient to ambulate. A tourniquet or leg holder may also cause prominent skin contusion as well as underlying muscle pain, presumably from either local ischemic effect or direct muscle trauma (Fig. 3.3). Such reactions can be reduced in severity or occurrence, although not completely eliminated, by setting tourniquet pressures to realign to the patient's actual systolic blood pressure and in most cases 250 mm Hg or less for the shortest reasonable time required by the surgical technique. While the decreased use of the tourniquet has been popularized in recent years due to concerns about both muscular and peripheral nerve injury, recent studies have not demonstrated significant functional recovery benefits in such procedures as anterior cruciate ligament reconstruction. It has been the author's experience that the procedural time saved from improved visibility combined with the diminished actual blood loss during the procedure has created fewer problems with postoperative hemorrhage residuals when a tourniquet is used.

A simple bruise reaction at a portal site may occur (Fig. 3.4). This may result from inadvertent damage to a cutaneous vein or to underlying bleeding from penetration of the vastus musculature during portal incisions. Such wounds may remain sensitive and heal with excessive subcutaneous scarring, creating a thickened palpable lump. Patients can be reassured that these will re-

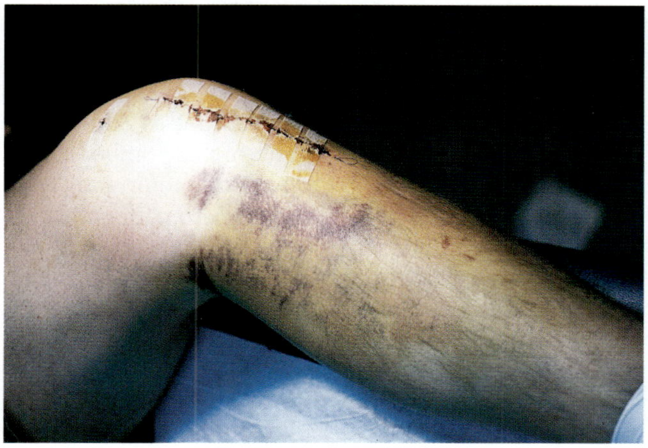

Figure 3.1. Typical degree of ecchymosis that may be seen after an arthroscopic anterior cruciate ligament (ACL) reconstruction, bone–patella–bone, single-incision endoscopic technique. A tourniquet was used for 74 minutes at 250 mm Hg; Cryocuff (Aircast Corp.) and postoperative dressing were applied before tourniquet release.

solve and become less symptomatic, but the process may take several months. Such problems can be reduced by transluminating with the arthroscope cutaneous vessels before actually incising portal sites and by avoiding the superior genicular vessels at outflow portal sites.

Another manifestation of postoperative cutaneous ecchymosis in the author's experience is pruritus. Local itching and irritation as well as pain may result from the biodegradation of hemoglobin to its elemental pigments, biliverdin and bilirubin. These bile salts are in turn stimulating to histamine-bearing cutaneous mast cells. These symptoms resolve gradually with appropriate medication.

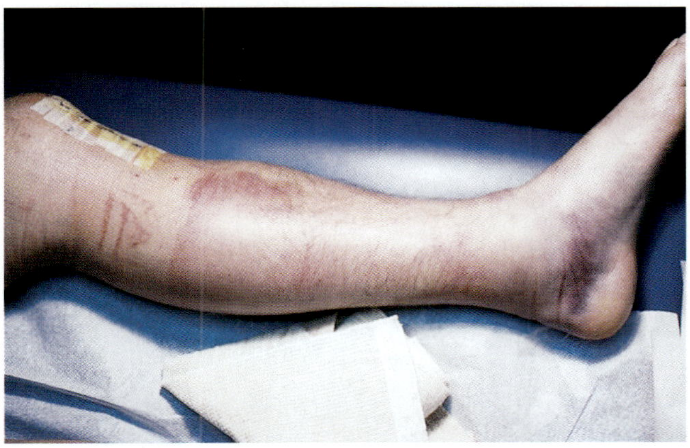

Figure 3.2. Leg appearance 3 days postarthroscopy and ACL reconstruction. Note tourniquet effect caused by Ace wrap bandage below knee with extravasation of bleeding to foot and ankle. Patient complained of tightness and aching pain in lower leg and ankle.

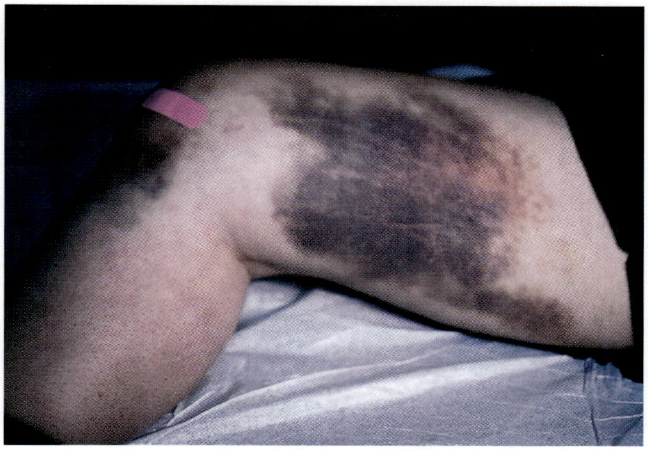

Figure 3.3. Typical bruise effect from tourniquet and leg holder. Such reactions may retard knee rehabilitation.

HEMARTHROSIS AND HEMATOMA

The retrospective incidence of postoperative hemarthrosis in arthroscopic knee surgery varies from 5% to 42%.[2,3] In an often-quoted prospective study of 23 experienced arthroscopists, Small[4] recorded an incidence of hemarthrosis of 1%, which still represented 23.5% of all complications. If one considers that this was a series of reputedly skilled surgeons, then the true incidence of operative hemarthrosis is probably higher in practice. Lateral retinacular release has the highest reported incidence (7.15%) of hemarthrosis.[4]

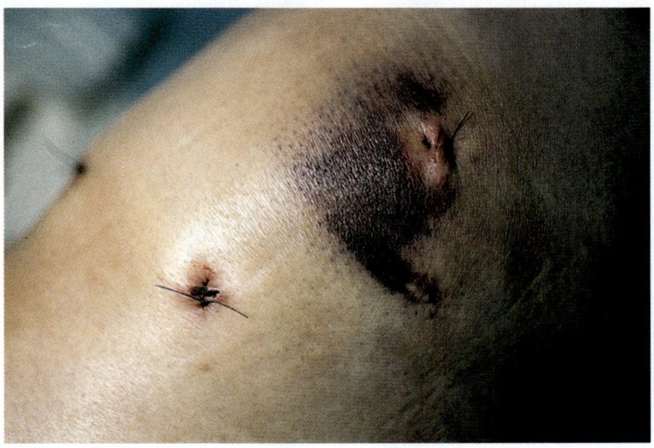

Figure 3.4. Local portal contusion of superomedial cannula site. Such reactions usually resolve uneventfully but may remain tender.

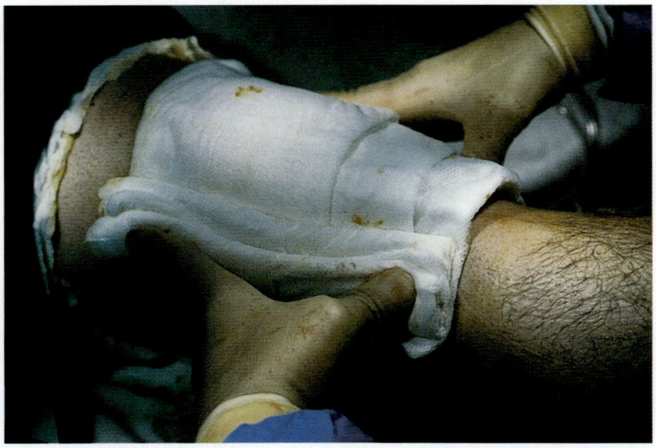

Figure 3.5. Preferred dressing technique. A thick, padded dressing of fluffs, bulk cotton, or similar material is applied to the knee.

Increased risk for this complication is associated with bleeding diathesis, platelet aggregation problems, and chronic renal disease, and with patients who are on warfarin (Coumadin) or have known coagulation defects.[5]

While various medical strategies can alleviate some risk, surgeries involving increased bleeding such as tibial tubercle osteotomy (e.g., Fulkerson procedure) or extensive synovectomy may require preventive measures at the time of surgery in addition to careful surgical hemostasis. These measures include the use of intraarticular Marcaine with epinephrine and careful attention to the postoperative dressing application (Figs. 3.5 and 3.6).

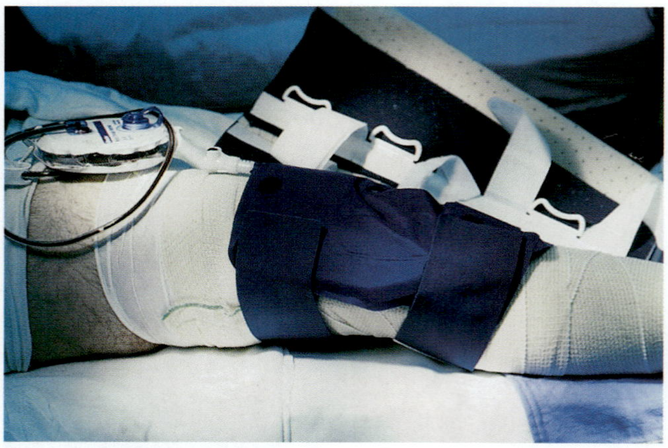

Figure 3.6. Preferred dressing technique. A thigh-high thromboembolic disease (TED) stocking is applied over the dressing. An Ace bandage may be temporarily added for additional compression. A cooling device (Cryocuff, Aircast Corp.) and knee immobilizer complete the treatment. A hemovac suction drain is used and removed 2 to 3 hours postoperatively.

Author's Preferred Technique for Postoperative Dressing in Cases at Risk for Hemarthrosis

The wound is carefully padded; in the case of a lateral retinacular release, a lateral buttress pad is added. The overall dressing consists of a thigh-high thromboembolic disease (TED) stocking with optional temporary Ace bandage overwrap, later removed before discharge; a cooling unit such as a Cryocuff (Aircast Corp., Summit, NJ) and a knee immobilizer. A hemovac drain is inserted through the drainage portal and removed 2 to 3 hours postoperatively, before discharge from recovery.

Paradoxically, Small[4] has reported a higher incidence of hemarthrosis with the use of knee drainage, presumably due to a relative lack of tamponade of capillary bleeding. The author has not observed such a trend. On the contrary, it has been the author's experience that the undrained knee may sequester large amounts of blood before tamponade, leading to severe joint distention, synovial herniation, or subcutaneous hematoma formation (Fig. 3.7). Such a development in the first few days postoperatively may require surgical evacuation but more often can be managed expectantly until aspiration of the clot can be effectively accomplished. Magnetic resonance imaging (MRI) may help assess the extent of the postoperative hematoma.[5]

A concern is the risk of wound dehiscence resulting from extreme intraarticular fluid pressure, with the coincident risk of bacterial contamination of the resulting synovial fistula. Both the patient and support staff should be cautioned that such a development warrants immediate evaluation and oral antibiotic prescription.

Burch and DeHaven[6] reported five cases of hemarthrosis and one subcutaneous hematoma after patello-

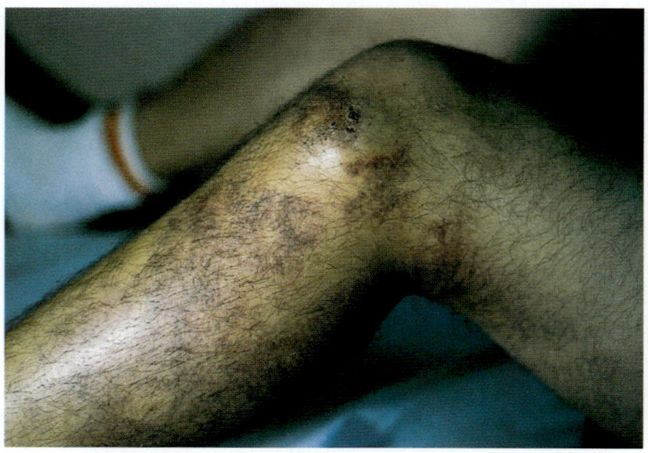

Figure 3.7. Tense hemarthrosis with subcutaneous synovial herniation and hematoma at anterolateral arthroscope portal site. There is prominent secondary distal cutaneous ecchymosis.

femoral lateral release by percutaneous scissors technique. Treated by aspiration for relief of pain or persistent distention, none resulted in long-term poor results.

CHRONIC RECURRENT NONHEMORRHAGIC EFFUSION IN THE POSTOPERATIVE KNEE

Nonhemorrhagic joint effusion postoperatively is the manifestation of a persistent inflammatory response.[7,8] The stimulus of such a synovial response may be recurrent trauma, metabolic disease (e.g., chondrocalcinosis, gout), infection, or arthropathy.[5]

The potential for infection should always be assessed by analyzing a synovial fluid aspirate for cell count, anaerobic and aerobic cultures, and Gram stain. In the author's experience, systemic symptoms may only develop late in the course of joint sepsis, and local inflammatory signs upon knee examination are not always specific for sepsis. A foul odor or turbid fluid (i.e., fluid density through which newsprint cannot be read) should raise immediate clinical suspicion of infection.

Occult or progressive arthritis is the most frequent etiology of recurrent postoperative effusion. Such degenerative articular wear may develop rapidly and unpredictably after meniscectomy or debridement procedures, especially in the mid-life and older patient. Risk factors for progressive osteoarthritis include female gender, overweight body habitus, genu varum malalignment, coincident ligamentous instability, and a high occupational or recreational biomechanical stress profile.

Aspiration in such a setting may reveal particulate articular debris in the synovial fluid. This is a poor prognostic sign indicating degeneration of the articular cartilage matrix and often precedes detectable changes on MRI or plain x-ray (Fig. 3.8).

Chronic synovitis has also been associated with Cidex sterilization of instruments.[9] Thorough instrument rinsing and using alternative sterilizing techniques have lessened this problem.

The use of allograft tissue sterilized by ethylene oxide is now recognized to cause prominent synovitic reactions and is no longer recommended.[10]

WOUND DEHISCENCE AND SYNOVIAL FISTULA

Joint distention from hemarthrosis or chronic effusion can cause disruption of arthroscopic portals or incisions (Fig. 3.9). This development poses an immediate risk of secondary infection. The predominant organisms in arthroscopic wound infection have been reported as *Staphylococcus aureus* and, to a lesser extent, *Staphylococcus epidermidis*.[4]

The incidence of synovial fistula varies from 0.64% to 3.2%.[2,11] Immobilization, sterile dressings and a cephalosporin-derived oral antibiotic usually result in successful outcome. Because of the infection risk posed by such occurrences, I have continued to use suture clo-

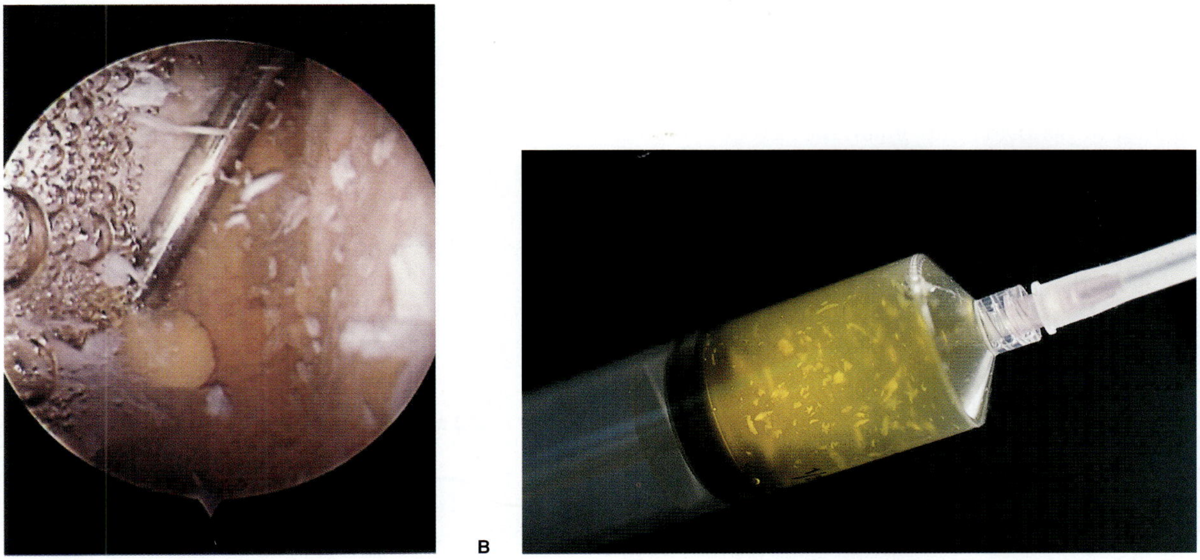

A B

Figure 3.8. **A:** Arthroscopic appearance of articular degenerative fragmentations. Such material may provide autoantigenic chronic inflammatory response. **B:** Synovial fluid aspirate in chronic effusion. Note suspended articular wear fragments, which are best seen by transillumination.

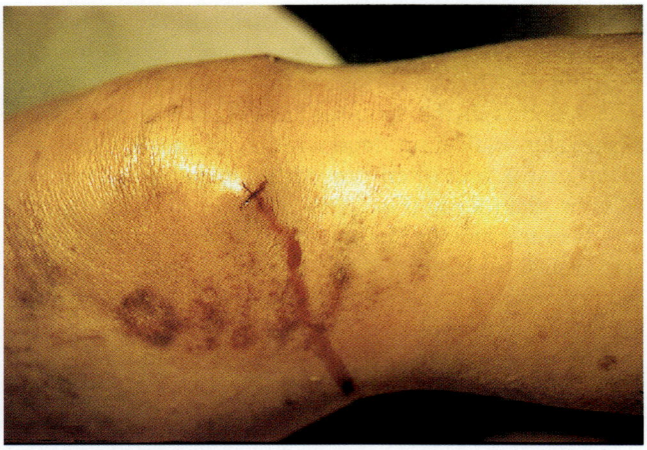

Figure 3.9. Clinical appearance of arthroscopic portal dehiscence of the knee with fistulous drainage.

sure of all portals and wounds when heavy bleeding or effusion is anticipated. Sutures remain for 7 days to obtain secure healing. This may be particularly important in the steroid-dependent patient. While Steri-Strip closures have become popular in some clinics, it has been my experience that sutures provide a more reliable apposition of subcutaneous and capsular layers, affording less opportunity for fluid leakage or synovial herniation with joint distention.

OBSERVATIONS ON THE PATHOPHYSIOLOGY OF HEMARTHROSIS AND CHRONIC EFFUSION—THE RATIONALE FOR CLINICAL TREATMENT

Hemarthrosis of the knee has long been a concern regarding the risk of destruction of articular cartilage due to proliferative synovitis and inflammatory cell infiltration, especially in the setting of hemophiliac disease.[12] Furthermore, most experimental models have shown increased protease activity in particular cartilage, a drop in glycosaminoglycan content of articular surfaces, and associated early cartilage destruction with chronic hemarthrosis.[13] The intraarticular pathologic effects of a single episode of bleeding is unclear but would appear to be associated with lower risk. Safran et. al[14] injected a single dose of blood into the ankle joints of rabbits and found only transient changes in joint stiffness and synovial histology at 28 days after injection. Ishizue et al[15] studied recurrent hemarthrosis in a rabbit knee, by inoculating the joint on 7 consecutive days with assessment on the ninth day and found inflammatory proliferation of the synovium but no effect on the histologic architecture, total collagen content, collagenase activity, or biomechanical properties of the anterior cruciate ligament. This was in contradistinction to a previous study in their laboratories with focus on the medial and lateral menisci demonstrating an increase in degradative activity assessed by collagenase activity.[16] Other series have demonstrated proteoglycan degradation in the presence of a single episode of experimental hemarthrosis.[17] None of these studies attempted to correlate the pathologic effects of hemarthrosis with the actual pressure of hemorrhagic distention of the joint nor did they evaluate the quality of any limb dysfunction that the animal may have suffered. Such observations in the human model are a prominent concern.

In a study of the effects of chronic effusion on knee joint proprioception, Guido et al[18] noted that reflex inhibition of joint proprioception as well as the subtended muscular function is caused by capsular distention. The ability of a knee joint effusion to cause reflex inhibition of the quadriceps musculature has been demonstrated by several authors.[19–21] Guido et al further observed that "aspiration of the effusion may have reset the afferent feedback system of the capsular mechanoreceptors, causing an improvement in the subject's passive repositioning sense." In the presence of effusion, the resting intraarticular pressure of the knee usually becomes positive.[21] Simkin[23] has noted that effusions of significant volume may deprive the joint of the stabilizing effects of subatmospheric pressure and substitute instead a distending force that increases the stress on ligaments and capsule (Fig. 3.10). In contrast to normal

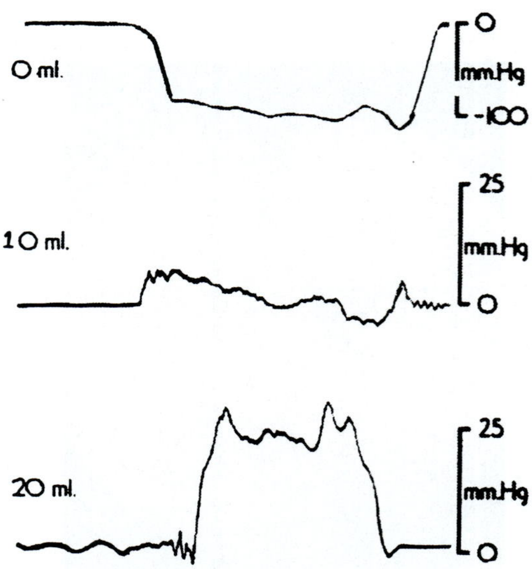

Figure 3.10. Isometric quadriceps contraction in normal knee containing 0, 10, and 20 mL added saline. With no injection, the intraarticular pressure is subatmospheric. This is no longer seen with 10 mL saline, and the pressure becomes positive with a simulated 20-mL effusion.[22]

joints, the pressure of knee effusion is greatest in full flexion and full extension, with lowest intraarticular pressures occurring at 30 degrees of flexion.[24] Hence, it is understandable why the swollen postoperative knee is vulnerable to loss of motion in extension and may have subsequent permanent restriction by fibroarthrosis. Passive range of motion as is often exerted in early rehabilitation of the operated knee may result in extremely high intraarticular pressures. Jayson and Dixon[24] observed a mean pressure of 802 mm Hg in three rheumatoid patients injected with 100 mm of intraarticular fluid. Such high pressures can often cause severe discomfort in effused joints, limit rehabilitation and function, and cause herniation through the capsule and/or fistulous disruption of surgical wounds.

In chronic recurrent nonhemorrhagic effusion, a growing body of literature reflects renewed appreciation for underlying immunologic-mediated responses. Autoreactivity is the generation of immunologic responses specifically against normal endogenous molecules.[25] Autoimmunity is defined as a pathophysiologic process characterized by a loss of self recognition and resulting reaction against autologous molecular structure. Type 2 collagen of articular cartilage, proteoglycan molecules, and their fragments or epitopes have been documented to generate autoimmune synovitis in animals.[8,26] Nonspecific posttraumatic inflammation and progressive joint trauma can result in altered antigenic states of matrix molecules due to enzymatic degradation.[25]

Hypothetical models have been suggested to explain how an initial nonspecific microtraumatic inflammatory process could create the exposure of previously clustered protein antigens and alter native protein structure.[25] Cell membrane, matrix, and collagen provide possible sources of such antigenic stimulation. Autoantibodies to collagen in human synovial fluid have been documented.[27] Specific antigen recognizing T-cell lymphocytes (CD4 helper cells) cooperate with antibody-producing B-cell lymphocytes to initiate a specific cellular immunologic response. In addition, a third subset of dendritic synoviocytes are capable of presenting antigen to subsynovial T cells.[26]

T cells and B cells are not seen in great numbers in normal synovium.[28] T cells have inherent migratory proficiency that explains their ability to accumulate in inflamed synovium.[28] T cells produce cytokines that activate tissue macrophages and macrophage-like cells such as the synovial A cell.[8] Further tissue injury results when activated tissue macrophages give rise to hydrolases and toxic oxygen radicals.[29] Activated synoviocytes are capable of releasing neutral proteinases such as collagenase, gelatinase, and stromolycen.[26] Intimal synoviocytes are also capable of releasing potent cytokines such as interleukin-1 with autocrine and paracrine feedback to synovium and articular cartilage cells,[26] which may lead to further matrix degradation, weakening, and eventual tissue fragmentation. Leadbetter et al[30] have documented the presence of significant T-cell and B-cell lymphocyte populations in the subsynovial layers as well as increased macrophage activity in sports-induced synovial knee inflammation. Such studies provide further support for the observed increased clinical efficacy of corticosteroid injection in synovial inflammation versus oral nonsteroidal medication, namely, greater suppression of lymphocyte and/or macrophage activity. These findings place new emphasis on the role of intrinsic host factors in explaining the refractoriness to conventional medical treatment in chronic synovitis of the knee. Viscosupplementation with high molecular weight sodium hyaluronate injection (Hyalgan, Synvisc) can also be a useful adjunct in reducing postoperative synovitis based on evidence of similar downregulation of inflammatory T-cell and macrophage response.[31]

THERAPEUTIC MEASURES TO EMPLOY WHEN ENCOUNTERING POSTOPERATIVE HEMARTHROSIS OR CHRONIC RECURRENT NONHEMORRHAGIC EFFUSION OF THE KNEE

The principles of rehabilitation of the knee after injury or surgery have been well defined.[32] Current knee rehabilitation programs are designed to decrease symptoms of inflammation, restore motion, improve muscle function, regain agility, improve conditioning, and hasten return to work or sports.[32] The principle of inflammation reduction in the postsurgical knee has been well defined and typically includes both medical modifiers of inflammation as well as the use of physical modalities.[7,8] In the presence of active or recent intraarticular bleeding, the option now exists to use a Cox2-specific inhibitor drug (Celecoxib), thereby avoiding the platelet inhibition effects of nonsteroidal medications.[33] Also, I have found steroid use in the form of an oral Medrol Dosepak to be useful in select cases. While cryotherapy has not always been shown to produce measurable differences in outcome,[34] most authors still promote regional cooling as an important modality in knee surgery recovery and reduction of further bleeding.[7,35]

The value of early motion in the recovery of limb function and conservation of joint motion has also been well established.[36] In addition, the increased clearance of a hemarthrosis from a synovial joint as an effect of continual passive motion treatment has been experimentally validated.[37]

THE IMPORTANCE OF THERAPEUTIC JOINT ASPIRATION IN THE TREATMENT OF SYMPTOMATIC EFFUSION

Therapeutic aspiration and intrasynovial therapy can often be an important adjunct in expediting a more complete recovery after knee surgery. Aspiration should be considered whenever the pain of joint distention creates significant lack of compliance with rehabilitation goals or threatens to contribute to potentially preventable secondary complications such as muscle atrophy or joint contracture (Figs. 3.11 and 3.12). In the case of chronic, nonhemorrhagic recurrent effusion, aspiration provides not only relief of the mechanical disabilities of joint distention but also improves the efficacy of medical management, by diminishing the resident volume of autogenously produced proinflammatory degenerative macromolecules within the joint.

The Author's Preferred Technique for Joint Arthrocentesis

Since the risk of any aspiration is potential infection, it is critical that a fastidious sterile technique and compulsive methodology be used to ensure success. Gloves are worn and the cutaneous sterilization is done as a first step with Betadine or similar antiseptic, allowing it to dry on the skin during further preparation for aspiration. Alcohol swabbing at the moment of arthrocentesis is also done. A 60-cc syringe is initially used with a 16-gauge needle. Smaller-bore needles provide poorer results because of intraluminal clotting. The aspiration site should be clear of all inflammatory signs; generally, the superolateral aspect of the superior patella pouch provides easy access. If resistance to aspiration is encountered, turning of the bevel of the needle while attached to the syringe may be helpful. At no time should the same needle be removed and reinserted.

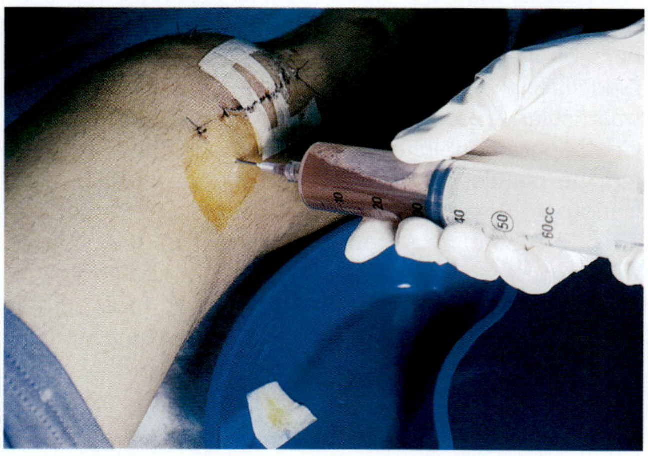

Figure 3.11. Technique of knee joint aspiration, which demands fastidious sterile technique and attention to proper preparation. As such, responsibility should not be delegated to the inexperienced.

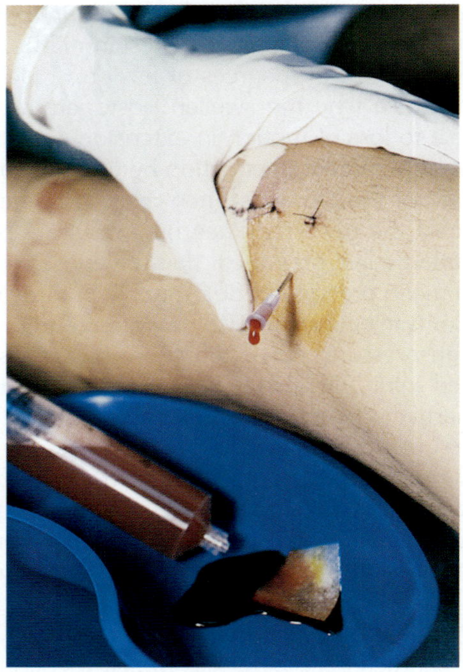

Figure 3.12. Technique of knee joint aspiration. Further decompression of excess blood or synovial fluid can be often improved by gentle manual pressure. With the syringe detached from the needle, careful rotation of the needle bevel will improve fluid flow. Once the needle has been inserted, it should not be removed and reintroduced, to avoid possible contamination of the joint.

Once the maximum amount of aspiration has been achieved by use of the syringe, further removal of blood or synovial fluid can be achieved by manual joint compression with the needle left in place. This milking technique has proved useful many times when conventional aspiration technique has failed. After aspiration is completed, a sterile dressing with adequate padding and compression must be applied, as there is a tendency for the wound to drain spontaneously for a short period of time.

Therapeutic aspiration is generally regarded as having an important role in the management of the acutely or chronically swollen knee.[8,38] As such, it should not be thought of as applicable only to the treatment of rheumatoid-related disease or as a measure of last resort. The selective use of parenteral corticosteroids has proven effective in further reducing the morbidity of these conditions.[8] Two criticisms of aspiration and intrasynovial therapy have been the risk of introducing infection and the potential catabolic harm of corticosteroids to articular cartilage or healing structures. However, a review of the literature reveals only anecdotal evidence for corticosteroid arthropathy when reasonable use is employed.[8] In a series of 400,000 injections over a period of 32 years, Hollander[39] recorded an incidence of rapid joint damage of less than 1%, and an incidence of infection with intrasynovial therapy of 0.0005%. These concerns can be avoided by limiting the use of intrasynovial corticosteroid therapy to acute traumatic inflammation or arthropathy. I specifically avoid injection of knees in which healing processes are intrinsic to the outcome of the procedure, such as anterior cruciate ligament reconstruction, meniscal repair, or chondral regeneration. Injections are used sparingly with 4- to 6-week intervals; often only one injection is required. Triamcinolone hexacetonide in a dosage of 20 mg is the preferable parenteral agent.[8,40] If three injections have not controlled the recurrent effusion, the surgeon should reassess the underlying pathology and seek different solutions.

References

1. Small NC. Complications in arthroscopy: the knee and other joints. *Arthroscopy* 1986;2:253–258.
2. DeLee JC. Complications of arthroscopy and arthroscopic surgery: results of a national survey. *Arthroscopy* 1985; 1:204–220.
3. Sherman O, Fox JM, Snyder SJ, et al. Arthroscopy—no problem surgery. *J Bone Joint Surg* 1986;68A(2):256–265.
4. Small NC. Complications in arthroscopic surgery performed by experienced arthroscopists. *Arthroscopy* 1988;4(3): 215–221.
5. Roberts TS, Terry R. Complications of knee surgery. In: DeLee JD, Drez D, eds. *Orthopedic Sports Medicine: Principles and Practice*. Philadelphia: WB Saunders, 1994:1528–1548.
6. Burch MT, DeHaven KE. Pitfalls of the lateral retinacular release. *Clin Sports Med* 1989;8(2):279–290.
7. Maywood RM, Boland AC. Control of inflammation. *Sports Med Arthrosc Rev* 1996;4:8–15.
8. Leadbetter WB. Anti-inflammatory therapy in sports injury—the role of nonsteroidal drugs and corticosteroid injection. *Clin Sports Med* 1995;4(2):353–408.
9. Harner CD, Mason GC, Fu FH. Cidex induced synovitis. *Am J Sports Med* 1987;15(6):623.
10. Roberts TS, Drez DS Jr, McCarthy W, Paine R. Anterior cruciate ligament reconstruction using freeze-dried ethylene-oxide bone–patellar tendon–bone allografts. Two year results in thirty-six patients. *Am J Sports Med* 1991;19(1):34–51.
11. Proffer DS, Drez DJ, Daus GP. Synovial fistula of the knee: a complication of arthroscopy. *Arthroscopy* 1991; 7(1):98–100.
12. Madhok R, Bennett D, Sturrock RD, Forbes CD. Mechanisms of joint damage in an experimental model of hemophilia or history of arthritis. *Rheumatology* 1988; 31(9):1148–1155.
13. Fabry G. Early biochemical and histological findings in experimental hemarthrosis in dogs. *Am Orthop Trauma Surg* 1982;100:167.
14. Safran MR, Johnston-Jones K, Kabo JM, Meals RA. The effect of experimental hemarthrosis on joint stiffness and synovial histology in a rabbit model. *Clin Orthop Rel Res* 1994;303:280–288.
15. Ishizue KK, Lyon RM, Amiel D, Woo SL-Y. Acute hemarthrosis: a histological biochemical and biomechanical correlation of early effects on the anterior cruciate ligament in a rabbit model. *J Orthop Res* 1990;8: 548–554.
16. Ishizue KK, Lyon R, Amiel D, et al. Hemarthrosis: a biochemical and mechanical evaluation of effects on the anterior cruciate ligament and menisci. *Trans Orthop Res Soc* 1988;13:55.
17. Hibayash H, Shimizue K, Suzuko K, Yamamoto S, Yasuda T, Yamamuro T. Proteoglycan degradation in hemarthrosis—intra-articular blood injection in rat knees. *Acta Orthop Scand* 1995;66(1):73–79.
18. Guido J, Voight ML, Blackburn TA, Kidder JD, Nord S. The effects of chronic effusion on knee joint proprioception: a case study. *J Orthop Sports Physician Ther* 1997;25(3):208–212.
19. deAndrade JR, Grant C, Dixon A. Joint distension and reflex muscle inhibition. *J Bone Joint Surg* 1965;49: 313–322.
20. Kennedy JC, Alexander IJ, Hayes KC. Nerve supply of the human knee and its functional importance. *Am J Sports Med* 1982;6:329–335.
21. Spencer JD, Hayes KC, Alexander IJ. Knee joint effusion and quadriceps reflex inhibition in man. *Arch Phys Med Rehabil* 1984;65:171–177.
22. Jayson MIV, Dixon AStJ. Intra-articular pressure and rheumatoid geodes ("bone cysts"). *Ann Rheum Dis* 1970;29:496–502.
23. Simkin PA. Synovial physiology. In: McCarty DJ, ed. *Arthritis and Allied Conditions—A Textbook of Rheumatology*. Philadelphia: Lea and Febiger, 1989: 207–221.
24. Jayson MIV, Dixon AStJ. Intraarticular pressure in rheumatoid arthritis of the knee. *Ann Rheum Dis* 1970; 29:401–408.
25. Friedlaender GE, Jokl P, Horowitz MC. The autoimmune nature of sports injury: a hypothesis. In: Leadbetter WB, Buckwalter JA, Fordon SL, eds. *Sports-Induced Inflammation*. Park Ridge, IL: American Academy of Orthopaedic Surgeons, 1990:619–628.

26. Rodosky MW, Fu FH. Induction of synovial inflammation by matrix molecules, implant particles, and chemical agents. In: Leadbetter WB, Buckwalter JA, Fordon SL, eds. *Sports-Induced Inflammation*. Park Ridge, IL: American Academy of Orthopaedic Surgeons, 1990: 357–381.

27. Gracelino A, Michaeli D, Goldberg LS, Fudenberg HH. The occurrence of antibodies to collagen in synovial fluids. *Clin Immunol Immunopathol* 1975;3:567–574.

28. Cush JJ, Pietschmann P, Oppenheimer-Marks N, et al. The intrinsic migratory capacity of memory T cells contributes to their accumulation in rheumatoid synovium. *Arthritis Rheum* 1992;35(12):1434–1444.

29. Smith DL, Bakke AC, Campbell SM, Beckstead JH. Immunocytologic characteristics of mononuclear cell populations found in nonspecific olecranon bursitis. *J Rheumatol* 1994;21(2):209–214.

30. Leadbetter WB, Wahl S, Tiah H, Cook K. T-cell infiltration and activation: a possible autoimmune mechanism in chronic sports injury. *Proceedings of the 2nd meeting of the Combined Orthopaedic Research Societies*, San Diego, CA, November 1995:309.

31. Corrado EM, Peluso GF, Gigliotti S, et al. The effect of intra-articular administration of hyaluronic acid on osteoarthritis of the knee: a clinical study of immunological and biochemical evaluations. *Eur J Rheumatol Inflamm* 1995;15:1.

32. Wolff G, Grana WA. Principles of rehabilitation of the knee. *Sports Med Arthrosc Rev* 1996;42:2–7.

33. Trippel SB. The unmet anti-inflammatory needs in orthopedics. *Am J Orthop* 1999;28:3–7.

34. Konrath GA, Lodc T, Goitz HT, Scheidler J. The use of cold therapy after anterior cruciate ligament reconstruction. A prospective randomized study and literature review. *Am J Sports Med* 1996;24(5):629–633.

35. Knight KL. Cold as a modifier of sports-induced inflammation. In: Leadbetter WB, Buckwalter JA, Fordon SL, eds. *Sports-Induced Inflammation*. Park Ridge, IL: American Academy of Orthopaedic Surgeons. 1990: 463–478.

36. Guse TR, Steiner ME. The importance of motion. *Sports Med Arthrosc Rev* 1996;4:16–25.

37. O'Driscoll SW, Kumar A, Salter RB. The effect of continuous passive motion on the clearance of a hematoma from a synovial joint. *Clin Orthop Rel Res* 1983; 176:305–311.

38. Gatter RA. Arthrocentesis technique and intrasynovial therapy. In: McCarty DJ, ed. *Arthritis and Allied Conditions—A Textbook of Rheumatology*, 10th ed. Philadelphia: Lea and Febiger, 1989:207–221.

39. Hollander TL. Intrasynovial therapy. In: McCarthy DJ, ed. *Arthritis and Allied Conditions—A Textbook of Rheumatology*, 10th ed. Philadelphia: Lea and Febiger, 1989:543.

40. Goss JA, Adams RF. Local injection of corticosteroids in rheumatic diseases. *J Musculoskel Med* 1993;10:83–92.

Chapter 4

REFLEX SYMPATHETIC DYSTROPHY FOLLOWING KNEE SURGERY

David C. Pollock, Gary G. Poehling,
L. Andrew Koman, and Thomas L. Smith

Reflex sympathetic dystrophy (RSD) is a complex pathologic entity that may occur following surgery or trauma, resulting in abnormally intense and inappropriately prolonged pain that is not a reflection of actual or impending tissue damage in an affected area. Until recently, the syndrome was not well described in the knee. Persistent knee pain was traditionally thought to be due to various posttraumatic or postoperative conditions.[1] The classification of posttraumatic pain is complicated. RSD is well established in the lay, medical, and legal literature despite the absence of defined pathophysiology or consistent clinical symptoms or signs. The term reflex sympathetic dystrophy, however, may inappropriately imply that the sympathetic nervous system is actively involved without proof of increased sympathetic activity. Disorders considered to be RSD and causalgia are now classified under the term *complex regional pain syndrome* (CRPS) and are based entirely on clinical criteria. The new terminology of CRPS will be used throughout the text except where RSD was originally used by cited authors.

HISTORICAL REVIEW

Silas Weir Mitchell et al[2] first published descriptions of dystrophic pain in a patient following a gunshot wound with partial nerve disruption and unrepaired vascular supply. They used the term *causalgia*, from the Greek word for burning pain to describe this injury. Posttraumatic persistent burning pain, diminished function, and abnormal vasoconstriction/vasodilation were first attributed to abnormal sympathetic nervous system responses by Leriche[3] in 1916.

Regional bone demineralization accompanying posttraumatic pain was described by Sudek[4] in 1900. The term *reflex sympathetic dystrophy* was introduced by Evans[5] in 1947 and expanded by Bonica[6] in 1973. Koman et al[7] in 1984 documented microvascular changes associated with RSD. The term *reflex sympathetic dystrophy* has been used synonymously with a large variety of descriptors and is felt to be inappropriately broad.[8] Dobyns[9] proposed that abnormal function related to pain be grouped broadly under the term *pain dysfunction syndrome*. Others have stressed the importance of differentiating sympathetically maintained pain (SMP) from sympathetically independent pain (SIP) and have defined the former as a better descriptor of RSD.[10,11] In 1991 Janig et al[12] proposed a system that would avoid undocumented emphasis on the sympathetic nervous system. The term *complex regional pain syndrome* (CRPS) was proposed as an inclusive category of subgroups based on clinical and/or pathophysiologic manifestations of dystrophic pain. The subgroups are further differentiated into CRPS type I (no peripheral nerve injury), corresponding to RSD, and CRPS type II (with peripheral nerve injury), corresponding to causalgia.[11] Further differentiation into SMP and SIP has been emphasized,[13] and can be made dependent on sympathetic interventions.[12–14]

The historical reluctance to describe CRPS in the knee may be due to several factors. First, the pathogenesis and natural history of dystrophy is not well defined in any area of the body, even though initial descriptions of the symptoms date from 1864.[15,16] Second, recognition of the syndrome is often delayed by repeated diagnostic and therapeutic interventions that inadequately address the underlying disease process. Third, no treatment for CRPS has proven consistently effective, perhaps because of the dynamic evolution of the disease over time.[17] Finally, the prolongation of symptoms often results in increasing frustration for both patient and physician, culminating in delayed diagnosis, randomly selected therapeutic interventions, and frequent permanent partial disability judgments.

DEFINITION

Schutzer and Gossling[18] have defined RSD as an exaggerated response of an extremity to an injury. This response is manifested by four characteristics: (1) intense or unduly prolonged pain, (2) vasomotor disturbances, (3) delayed functional recovery, and (4) trophic changes in the soft tissues. Another response to CRPS may include psychological problems secondary to pain. We have observed that dystrophy must be suspected when recovery from a traumatic or surgical insult is delayed from what is expected given the magnitude of injury.[19] This may be an abnormal expression of the normal physiologic response to injury.[19]

PAIN

Physiology

Numerous investigators have suggested various theories regarding the pathophysiology of CRPS. Three main areas have been suggested as possible sources of chronic pain and disability of CRPS: (1) central nervous system (CNS) abnormalities, (2) peripheral nerve dysfunction, and (3) abnormal nutritional blood flow in the affected area.

Pain is an unpleasant sensory and emotional event associated with actual or impending cellular damage. In the absence of continued trauma, persistent pain is pathologic. The perception of pain involves the initiating event, afferent information, efferent modulation, and CNS interpretation. Painful peripheral nociceptive experiences associated with cellular damage produce secondary inflammation by the activation of pain receptors (Fig. 4.1). This information is relayed through afferent fibers to the dorsal horn of the spinal cord to higher cognitive centers. Nociceptive input is modulated via descending pathways. Conscious perception of the intensity of pain is related to the physiologic adaptations that modulate and balance afferent and efferent information (Fig. 4.2). Vasomotor disturbances may result from a variety of mechanisms.[20] The presence of nociceptive-induced inappropriate transmitter-receptor activity can affect peripheral microcirculatory control, resulting in impaired nutritive flow.[21–25]

Most individuals who sustain an injury to the knee experience transient symptoms of hyperpathia (increased pain), allodynia (sensation of pain following a nonpainful stimulus), burning discomfort, vasomotor abnormalities, and some degree of functional deficit. These symptoms generally subside as recovery progresses. The CRPS patient's symptoms do not subside and often escalate, leading to unremitting pain, vasospasm, edema, and immobility. Abnormal persistence of these responses is pathologic and may result in permanent structural, functional, anatomic, and physiologic changes in the extremity and CNS (Fig. 4.3).

Perception

CRPS, by definition, does not exist in the absence of pain. Pain requires cognitive recognition. Peripheral injury stimulates endogenous inflammatory mediators via

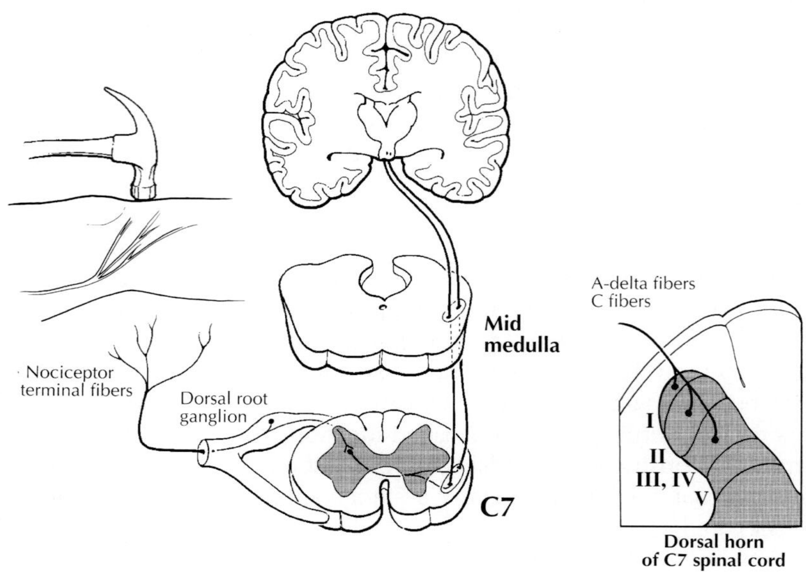

Figure 4.1. Abnormal central nervous system modulation of afferent sensory stimuli may contribute to the development of a dystrophic response after an injury that produces a peripheral nociceptive focus or "trigger." (From ref. 128, with permission.)

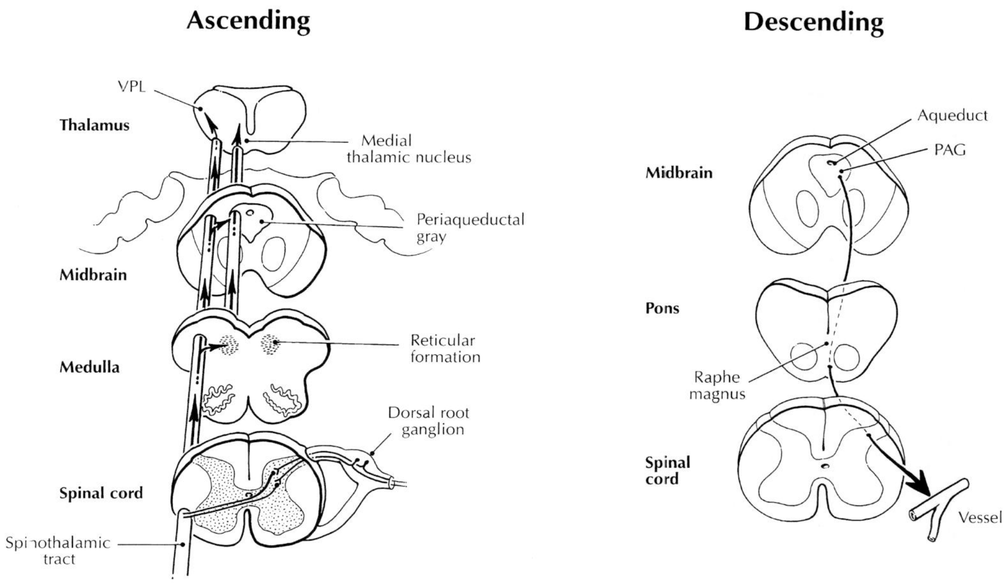

Figure 4.2. Ascending and descending pathways in the spinal cord and brain. (From ref. 128, with permission.)

nociceptive pathways. Repetitive trauma/injury may alter protective responses by producing earlier activation through sensitization. In addition to providing central input, local nociceptors initiate the direct release of peptides and neurotransmitters, control the inflammatory process, and promote tissue repair.

Mediators/Receptor Control

A variety of nonneurogenic and neurogenic mediators participate in the transmission of information interpreted as pain.[26] The role of α-adrenergic receptors and local blood flow in SMP complex regional pain states is well documented,[27–35] and relief of pain after intravenous phentolamine, a nonspecific α-adrenergic receptor antagonist, is considered pathognomonic for SMP.[36–38] Abnormal adrenoreceptor function and/or modulation in neural and vascular structures is the major common control pathway supporting the concept that CRPS is a "receptor disease."[33,34] Pre- and postsynaptic receptors are involved and affect nociceptive foci, blood flow, nutritional perfusion, and peripheral nerve excitability.[21,23,24,33,34,39–41] The potential pathologic mechanisms involved in the compromise of extremity blood flow and neural control include (1) abnormal neurotransmitter release secondary to nociceptive foci, (2) abnormal receptor distribution, and (3) alterations in receptor sensitivity.

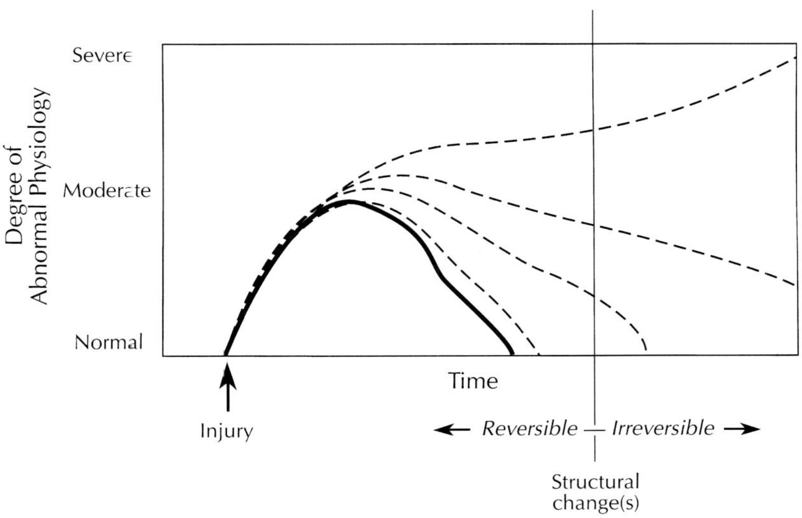

Figure 4.3. Abnormal physiologic events following trauma are normal; the majority of patients (solid line) recover spontaneously from the trauma. An abnormal prolongation of intensity of these events and dystrophic pain of varying magnitude and duration (broken lines) is pathologic. Irreversible changes may occur converting sympathetically maintained pain to sympathetically independent pain. (From ref. 128, with permission.)

Gate Theory

Melzak and Wall[42] were among the first to suggest that awareness of pain is subject to modulation within the substantia gelatinosa of the CNS. Their "gate control system" proposed that stimulation of large, myelinated afferent fibers "close the gate to pain," while stimulation of small, unmyelinated peripheral fibers "open the gate," and allow the subsequent sensation of pain. Wall[43] has refined this theory, and emphasized the difference between acute and chronic pain. The gate theory is an appropriate aid in the conceptualization of pain. It assumes that a finite amount of information can be received at the spinal cord or cortical level. The "gate" is the dorsal horn of the spinal cord. Thus, painful information displaced or modified by less noxious input cannot be processed through the gate. Although as yet unproven, certain general principles relating to pain processing can be conceptualized using this theorem.[42]

Acute Versus Chronic Pain

Acute pain is initiated during tissue injury or destruction. The presence of acute pain may be beneficial or harmful. The beneficial effects of acute pain include maintenance of blood pressure, cardiac output, intravascular volume, and appropriate homeostasis. Acute pain warns the organism of danger, prevents inappropriate motion of an injured extremity, and may diminish additional harm from repetitive injury. Persistence of pain beyond the need for protective action is unpleasant and may induce hypertension, tachycardia, coagulopathy, hyperglycemia, anxiety, fear, and chronic pain. Chronic pain that occurs in the absence of ongoing tissue destruction or that provides an inappropriate reflection of intensity, magnitude, and/or duration of tissue damage/compromise is pathologic. Although the pathophysiology of chronic pain is incompletely understood, the following processes can contribute to its establishment: persistent mechanical irritation of peripheral neural structures, incomplete regeneration of peripheral nerves, abnormal neurotransmitter activity, nutritional deprivation secondary to abnormal arteriovenous shunting, and central imprinting.

Following trauma or surgery, a transient period of extremity dystrophy is normal. However, it is abnormal for hyperpathia, allodynia, vasomotor disturbances, and functional deficiencies to persist. Untreated, these conditions may progress to permanent compromise of the extremity. Posttraumatic alterations in extremity physiology follow a variable time course. Therefore, the abnormal prolongation of these otherwise normal responses is pathologic and, over time, irreversible changes in anatomic structures of physiologic processes may occur. CRPS may therefore be considered an abnormally severe and/or prolonged manifestation of a normal postinjury response. Abnormally prolonged dystrophic events may produce arthrofibrosis,[21,23] cause excessive osteopenia,[44] alter neuroreceptor function,[33,34] and/or result in central pain imprinting.[22]

The true pathogenesis of CRPS probably involves both peripheral and central mechanisms interacting to produce pain with unusual topography and chronicity. Unfortunately, little is known about the etiology of CRPS in the knee. Several investigators have observed that the syndrome is often associated with symptoms about the patellofemoral joint,[17,45–47] and Lagier[48,49] and Lequesne and colleagues[50] have described roentgenographic and bone scan evidence of patellofemoral involvement in patients with RSD of the knee. Despite these observations, the pathogenesis of dystrophy of the knee remains obscure.

DIAGNOSIS

The diagnosis of CRPS must be considered in any patient with unexplained pain about the knee, especially if the patellofemoral joint appears to be involved. Because no sensitive and specific test for CRPS is currently available, the diagnosis must depend on careful scrutiny of presenting symptoms, interpretation of objective tests against the background of the clinical presentation, and a high index of suspicion for the syndrome.

Most patients have a history of either traumatic or surgical injury to the knee.[1,19] The pain associated with RSD is characteristic; burning sensations predominate, but complaints of aching or shooting pains are also common.[51] Limited range of motion and stiffness is invariably noted upon physical examination,[15,47] along with difficulty bearing weight on the extremity. Palpation of the knee often reveals pain localized to the patella, the femoral condyles, or the patellofemoral articulation; the tibia is less often involved.[48–50]

Ficat and Hungerford[46] described three different modes of onset: (1) The pain begins after trauma or surgery and is out of proportion to the inciting trauma. (2) The postinjury/postoperative course is normal but the predicted recovery does not occur. The pain continues and may even increase, resulting in loss of range of motion. (3) The postinjury/postoperative course is as expected, and the patient makes a good recovery and may be symptom free. The pain then reappears with increasing morbidity. Tietjen[15] described three stages of RSD: (1) early, in which pain was the presenting complaint; (2) dystrophic, in which the classic discoloration and skin temperature changes are present; and (3) atrophic, in which muscle atrophy and joint changes occur. He also noted that arthroscopic findings were normal.

Laboratory studies are helpful only in distinguishing CRPS from infection, arthritis, and malignancies. Complete blood count, chemistry profile, erythrocyte sedimentation rate, C-reactive protein, and rheumatoid tests are all normal in the dystrophic patient.

Demographics

Eighty percent of patients with CRPS diagnosed and treated within 1 year of injury improve significantly.[52,53] However, 50% of patients with untreated symptoms lasting more than 1 year have profound residual impairment.[54] Although children and adolescents can develop CRPS, the majority of patients are between 30 and 55 years of age, the median age being 45.[55–61] CRPS specifically in the knee is not well documented. Cooper and DeLee[62] found in 1994 that of 224 cases of RSD of the knee noted in the literature review, 70% occurred in female patients with an average age of 38. In the general literature, women have been affected three times more frequently than men.[58] The incidence of cigarette smoking is higher in RSD patients, and cigarette smoking is statistically linked to RSD.[63] Common nerve injuries associated with operative procedures that may precipitate RSD in the knee include injury to the infrapatellar branch of the saphenous nerve.[64]

Psychological Issues

CRPS is not a psychogenic condition. Extensive reviews of the literature have not supported a psychological causation[65–73] or verifiable personality disorder.[66,74] However, chronic pain is known to play a role in psychologic well-being, with 58% of pain center admissions, regardless of etiology, fulfilling the criteria for personality disorders.[75,76] Dependent, passive-aggressive, and histrionic personality disorders are common in patients with chronic pain and are seen in patients with RSD.[67] Behavioral responses that reduce extremity use exacerbate edema and atrophy.[66]

DIAGNOSTIC TESTING

A variety of objective tests are available to further define the disease process: (1) pain threshold evaluation, (2) plain radiographs of the knee (anteroposterior [AP] and lateral of the knee, and Merchant view of the patella), (3) three-phase technetium bone scan (TcBS), (4) pharmacologic neural blockade, and (5) endurance testing.

Pain Threshold Evaluation

Utilization of specific standardized evaluations and/or tests provides reproducible and objective information with regard to pain-pressure thresholds.[77,78] Rubber-tipped algometers,[79] dolorimetry,[80] monofilaments,[22,81] computer-controlled stimuli,[82] or evaluations of thermal pain threshold[78,83] may be used to provide a quantitative measure of hyperpathia and/or allodynia. For example, pain perception from a 2.83 monofilament (normally not painful) in a specified area or dermatomal distribution defines the extent of allodynia. Success or failure of treatment can be assessed by repeated evaluations during treatment. Decreased pain from the same size or larger-diameter monofilament documents improvement; persistent pain from the same size or smaller-diameter monofilament suggests ineffective management.

Radiographic Evaluation

Radiographs of the knee made early in the course of RSD are uniformly normal.[15] Lequesne and colleagues[50] have described a diffuse and generalized osteoporosis occurring about the knee a few weeks after the onset of symptoms. Genant and associates[84] described five roentgenographic patterns of resorption: irregular resorption of trabecular bone in the metaphysis, creating a patchy appearance; subperiosteal bone resorption; intracortical bone resorption; endosteal bone resorption; and surface erosions in subchondral and juxtachondral bone. The articular margins are not affected, and once symptoms have improved the osteoporosis resolves.[51] This finding has been associated histiologically with active bone remodeling,[49,50,85,86] and has been noted in other conditions besides RSD.[87] Tietjen[15] has stressed the importance of obtaining a skyline view of the patella because of its frequent involvement in the disease precess (Fig. 4.4).

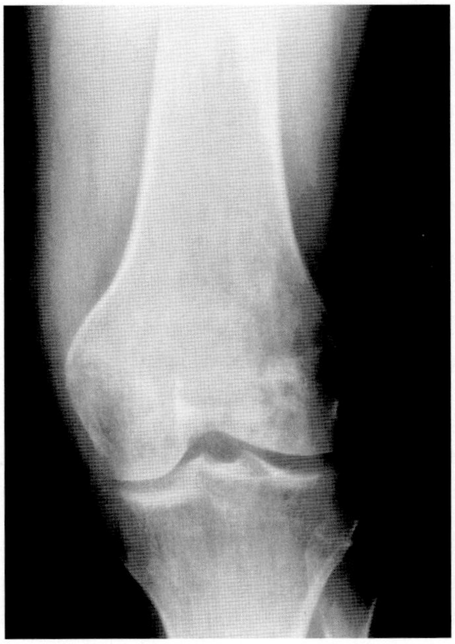

Figure 4.4. Plain roentgenogram of a patient with complex regional pain syndrome (CRPS) type I following arthroscopic knee surgery. There is diffuse osteopenia. (From ref. 128, with permission.)

Three-Phase Bone Scanning (Scintigraphy)

Three-phase technetium 99m bone scanning (TcBS) is performed commonly[88] and has assumed a significant role in the diagnosis of CRPS. Increased periarticular uptake often is present in multiple joints of the affected extremity in patients with RSD of the knee.[1,51,89] The first or "dynamic phase" of the bone scan lasts 2 to 3 minutes and provides an assessment of perfusion. The second phase or "blood pool image/tissue phase" represents total perfusion over a specified time (3 to 5 minutes). The third phase, a standard bone scan, evaluates radiotracer uptake in bony structures. Scans have been considered positive if there is asymmetric flow in phase I, II, or III.[90] However, more recent reports suggest that the diagnostic yield of phase II alone equals the diagnostic yield of the three-phase scan.[91,92] Mackinnon and Holder[91] have observed that a phase III scan showing diffuse increased tracer uptake is diagnostic for CRPS.

The increased technetium uptake is thought to reflect increased blood flow to the bone reflecting hyperemia and increased bone metabolism. The test has been repeatedly shown to have excellent specificity for the presence of RSD.[89,90] However, recent studies of TcBS in both upper and lower extremities have suggested that the sensitivity of the test ranges from 44% to 60%[89,92]; the test is more likely to be positive in the later stages of RSD of the lower extremity.[89] Tietjen[15] noted that two-thirds of the patients in his study had positive TcBS. Although TcBS is employed frequently, there is no evidence to support (1) its diagnostic accuracy, (2) the ability of the scan to predict outcome,[21] or (3) its value in determining management decisions.[53,81,93–95] The presence of a positive phase III bone scan provides objective corroboration for the clinical diagnosis of CRPS (Fig. 4.5).

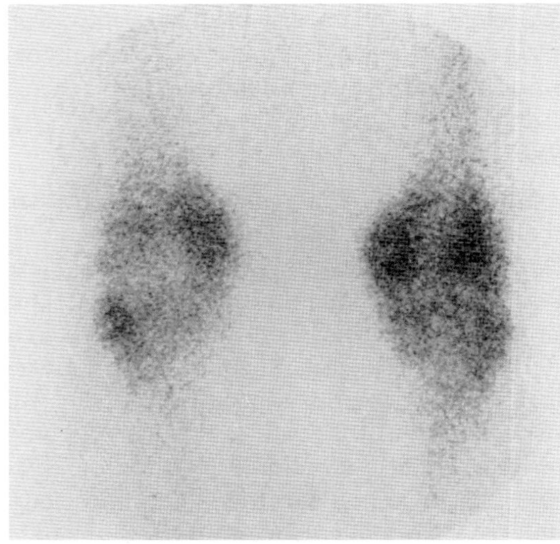

Figure 4.5. Abnormal bone scan of a patient with CRPS type I demonstrating increased uptake throughout the knee. (From ref. 128, with permission.)

Isolated Cold Stress Testing/Laser Doppler Fluxmetry

Autonomic regulation of blood flow is abnormal in patients with CRPS, and peripheral pain is related, in part, to nutritional deprivation associated with arteriovenous shunting.[21,24,96] The evaluations of cutaneous perfusion, thermoregulation, and nutritional flow before, during, and after stress provide both qualitative and quantitative physiologic data. The tests employed are noninvasive, reproducible, and sensitive.[21,97,98] The importance of nutritional flow in the pathogenesis of CRPS is supported by the rapid diminution or elimination of pain associated with the use of sympatholytic drugs or sympathetic blockade. Therefore, an assessment of total flow and of its components (thermoregulatory and nutritional flow) provide important diagnostic information.

Vasomotor and thermoregulatory flow may be evaluated by monitoring temperature and laser Doppler flux during stress. Isolated cold stress testing with laser Doppler fluxmetry (ICST/LDF) assesses the dynamic sympathetic response of an extremity to changes in environmental temperature.[99] Nutritional flow may be assessed directly by vital capillaroscopy in the digits.[21] Quantitative analysis of thermoregulatory and nutritional flow characteristics allows physiologic staging of autonomic-sympathetic control and provides a mechanism for monitoring the effects of specific interventions (Fig. 4.6).

Patents with CRPS of the knee demonstrate asymmetric responses in both temperature curves and LDF of the feet. The test appears to be sensitive to vasomotor disturbances, which occur in 80% to 90% of CRPS patients[19,64]; however, the specificity of the test for CRPS is poor, and its diagnostic value has not been examined in a prospective arena. ICST/LDF may provide a mechanism for monitoring the effects and verifying the physiologic efficacy of specific interventions (Fig. 4.7).

Diagnostic Sympathetic Blockade

Several investigators have suggested that lumbar sympathetic blockade should be used to establish the diagnosis of CRPS. Patman and colleagues[100] have stated that relief of pain following sympathetic blockade was the most important diagnostic criterion in the evaluation of RSD. Others have emphasized that failure to relieve pain with a sympathetic block suggests that the patient does not have RSD.[45,46,48] The test also has

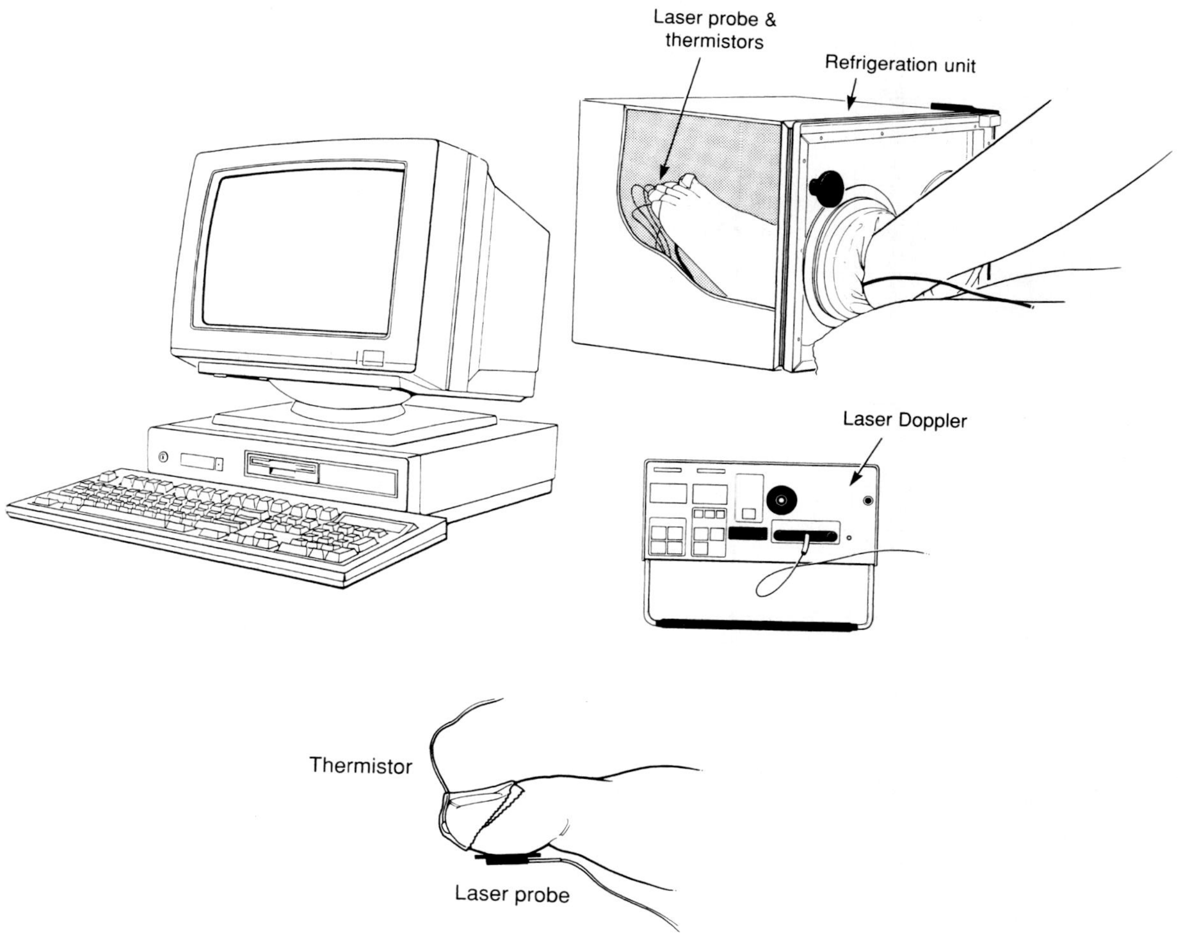

Figure 4.6. Digital microvascular physiology can be evaluated using an isolated cold stress test combining digital temperature and laser Doppler fluxmetry measurements. Digital temperatures are monitored with thermistors attached to each digit of both extremities. Microvascular cutaneous perfusion is assessed with a laser Doppler probe attached to one digit of each extremity. Digital temperature and laser Doppler fluxmetry measurements are sampled using custom computer software, and the results of the test are plotted for analysis. (From ref. 128, with permission.)

prognostic value because the amount of pain relief produced by the block has been reported to correlate with improvement following sympathectomy.[48,101]

Endurance Testing

Endurance testing is an extremely effective means of documenting functional deficits.[19,45,46] Patients are tested with the Cybex II isokinetic dynamometer and are evaluated for strength, power, and endurance in both the affected and normal extremities; comparisons between the two sides then are made. Ogilvie-Harris and Roscoe[45] have reported that deficits are most apparent in endurance testing. The test is difficult to falsify and provides quantitative information about functional impairment in the knee.

AUTHORS' APPROACH (DIAGNOSIS)

Successful treatment of CRPS is influenced by the rapidity of diagnosis and treatment. Early recognition of this syndrome is crucial to the overall prognosis for recovery. A dystrophic process should be considered in any patient experiencing pain that is out of proportion to the traumatic or surgical insult. In the postoperative period, painful and excessive swelling combined with vasoconstriction or vasodilation suggest CRPS. The diagnosis is clinical, and symptoms must include pain, trophic change, autonomic dysfunction, and functional deficit. If the diagnosis is suspected, instruments to quantitate pain (e.g., the McGill Pain Questionnaire and Visual Analog Scale), overall symptoms, and function are administered.[42] Objective measures of hyperpathia/allodynia can be under-

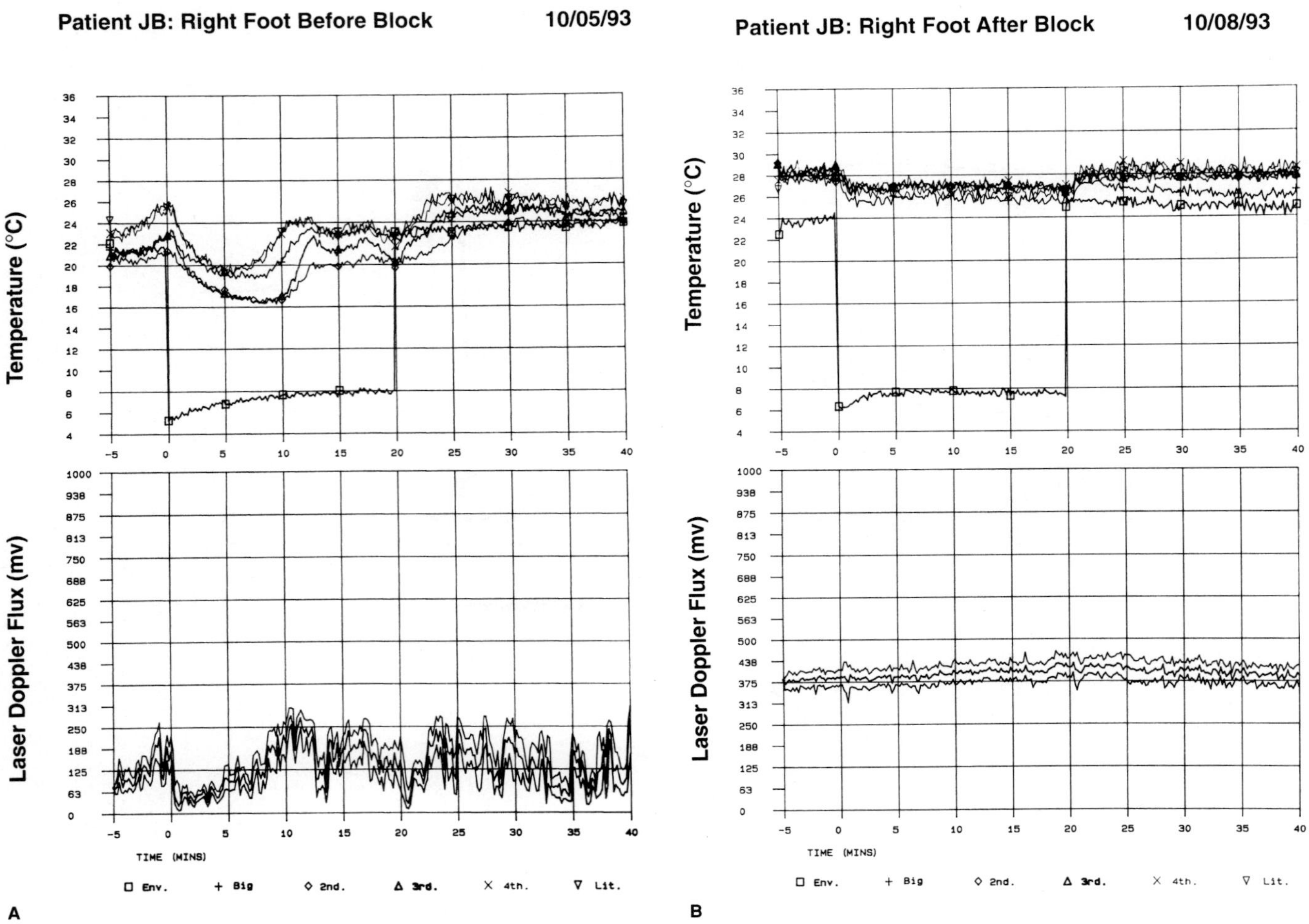

Figure 4.7. Laser Doppler fluxmetry in a patient with clinical CRPS type I, before and after sympathetic blockade. Baseline temperatures and laser Doppler measurements were taken for 5 minutes. For the cooling phase, the feet were inserted into the refrigeration unit for 5 minutes. Following cooling, the feet were removed from the unit and were allowed to rewarm at room temperature. Following the sympathetic block, digital temperatures were increased markedly during all phases of the testing procedure. The amplitude of laser Doppler flux was increased after the block confirming modulation of sympathetic input. (From ref. 128, with permission.)

taken using monofilaments. Edema is estimated or measured by volumetric analysis. The use of standard instruments, appropriate questionnaires, and reproducible objective tests assists in confirming the diagnosis and aids in monitoring the efficacy of interventions.

Three-phase bone scan (TPBS) can provide confirmative information when combined with clinical signs and symptoms. Intravenous phentolamine, stellate ganglion blocks, epidural injections, or somatic nerve blocks can be used to verify the presence of SMP and to predict overall efficacy of oral sympatholytic drugs.

TREATMENT

Effective treatment for CRPS of the knee requires both diligence and patience from both the patient and physician. No treatment has proven to be consistently effective in alleviating pain and restoring function, and multiple therapeutic modalities often are required to promote improvement.

Early treatment has been shown to be the most important factor influencing clinical improvement. Numerous studies have shown that patients treated within 6 to 12 months after the onset of dystrophic symptoms have much better pain relief and functional improvement than those with symptoms of longer duration.[17,45,46,48,64] This observation has also been made in the treatment of dystrophy affecting other areas of the body.[62]

Most treatments are directed toward decreasing the sympathetic hyperactivity characteristic of CRPS. The therapeutic modalities that have proven effective include

(1) physical therapy, (2) various oral medications, (3) pharmacologic sympathetic blockade, (4) surgical or chemical sympathectomy, and (5) various adjuvant therapies.

Therapy and Adaptive Modalities

Active and active-assisted range-of-motion exercises are begun immediately after the diagnosis of CRPS has been made in order to prevent atrophy and stiffness in the knee. Tietjen[15] has emphasized that extreme gentleness and patient cooperation are necessary to effect improvement.

Patients unable to tolerate physical therapy are asked to perform standing stress therapy.[19] The patient bears small amounts of weight on the affected extremity for short periods of time during the day while keeping a log of the amount of time tolerated and the amount of pain experienced. Progress is often slow, but this regimen allows the achievement of limited goals while applying some physiologic loading to the knee.

Pharmacologic Interventions (Oral)

A variety of oral, topical, and parenteral pharmacologic interventions are used to treat CRPS. Theoretical mechanisms of drugs that control pain associated with dystrophic or causalgic responses include membrane stabilization, competitive inhibition of neurotransmitters, receptor blockade, blockade of end-organ effects, desensitization of central pain-signaling neurons, and blockade of sympathetic-somatic coupling. Few of the drugs used in the management of CRPS are listed for pain management in the package insert approved by the Food and Drug Administration. Their usage is based on largely empiric data and an assessment of risk/benefit. Prior to utilizing the drugs discussed in this chapter, each practitioner should be familiar with the pharmacology, side effects, potential complications, indications, and contraindications for each compound.

Antidepressants

Antidepressants are used frequently in the management of chronic pain. They were originally used to relieve posttraumatic depression; however, they also provide analgesia and modulate sympathetic hyperactivity in the peripheral and central nervous systems.[102–107] Medications frequently used in CRPS include tricyclic antidepressants, atypical antidepressants, and selective serotonin reuptake inhibitors.

Tricyclic antidepressants, the most common agents employed in the treatment of CRPS, are useful in treating the "burning " pain. The drug decreases sympathetic outflow by blocking postganglionic reuptake of norepinephrine, by reducing the synthesis and release of norepinephrine, and by downregulating presynaptic alpha and serotonergic receptors.[106,108,109] Each of these drugs produces a different receptor affinity and accounts for the differences noted clinically. Therefore, one antidepressant may prove efficacious in one patient and not in another. The most commonly used tricyclic antidepressants include amitriptyline (Elavil), nortriptyline (Pamelar), and doxepin (Sinequan).

A dosage of amitriptylene 25 to 50 mg taken at bedtime is often effective, and may be adjusted as necessary. Amitriptyline may be used in conjunction with other agents except guanethidine.[19]

Drug selection should be individualized to reduce the potential for side effects. The most common side effects are anticholinergic, cardiovascular, and CNS, and may cause racing heart, insomnia, weight gain, sedation, and hypotension. Long-term treatment is tolerated, and abrupt discontinuation should be avoided because of the potential for side effects. Chronic treatment requires physician monitoring.

Trazodone (Desyrel), an atypical antidepressant, can be used to treat CRPS. It preferentially blocks the reuptake of serotonin and binding to adrenergic receptors.[108] Once per day dosing is possible; however, the side effects (tremor, hypertension, bradycardia, dizziness, and sedation) are often difficult to tolerate.

The use of serotonin reuptake inhibitors, second-generation antidepressants, to treat CRPS has increased significantly over the past decade. The drugs include fluvoxamine (Luvox), paroxetine (Paxil), fluoxetine (Prozac), and sertraline (Zoloft). These drugs bind preferentially to the presynaptic serotonin carrier in the CNS and inhibit serotonin reuptake. Side effects (tremors, weight loss, sexual dysfunction, insomnia, anxiety, anorexia, and nausea) may require several weeks to diminish. Selective serotonin reuptake inhibitors are commonly used synergistically with low-dose tricyclic antidepressants.[108,110,111]

Anticonvulsants

Anticonvulsants were first used to treat hyperpathic pain.[112,113] They are thought to suppress ectopic discharge in the peripheral and CNS neurons[114] and have proven very effective in reducing "shooting" or "stabbing" pain in patients with posttraumatic neuralgia.[115] The drugs most commonly used to treat CRPS include phenytoin (Dilantin), carbemazepine (Tegretol), valproic acid (Depekene), gabapentine (Neurontin), clonazepam, and sodium valproate.

Adrenergic Compounds

Alpha receptor blockade produces arterial vasodilation and may facilitate more normal modulation of afferent signals to the CNS.[114,116] These drugs have been reported to be effective in the treatment of patients with causalgia; their efficacy in patients with CRPS of the knee is unknown.

Corticosteroids

Corticosteroids have been used by a number of investigators to treat CRPS with good success.[117,118] Typical dosages range from 60 to 80 mg daily for 2 weeks, followed by a tapering dosage over another 2-week period. The regimen may be repeated if symptoms recur; reported side effects are rare.[118]

Calcium Channel Blockers

Calcium channel blockers have been shown to improve symptoms in patients with CRPS. Nifedipine has been shown to improve nutritional blood flow[96] and has been used to treat lower extremity dystrophy with good success.[119,120] Although the mechanism of action of calcium channel blockers is unclear in the treatment of CRPS, they decrease sympathetic tone by preventing calcium release following stimulation of adrenergic receptors. This effectively blocks adrenergic agents and leads to vasodilation. Nifedipine (Adalat, Procardia) and amlodipine (Norvasc) are the most commonly employed drugs. Use of these drugs results in decreased pain and may correlate with increased nutritional perfusion.[21,38,121] Nifedipine may be taken in 10- to 20-mg increments three times daily, or once daily in a 30-mg sustained-release preparation.

PHARMACOLIGIC INTERVENTIONS (PARENTERAL)

Pharmacologic Sympathetic Blockade

Three types of pharmacologic sympathetic blockade are available to reduce the elevated sympathetic tone associated with CRPS: (1) intravenous regional blockade, (2) lumbar sympathetic ganglia blockade, and (3) continuous blockade using epidural anesthesia.

Hannington-Kiff[122] has described excellent results using intravenous guanethidine administered under conditions similar to Bier block anesthesia. Because the drug displaces norepinephrine in presynaptic vesicles, it should not be used with amitriptyline, which would inhibit uptake of the drug into the terminal neuron.[18] Pain relief typically lasts 12 to 36 hours, but may last as long as 6 months.[123] This technique may serve both diagnostic and therapeutic functions in the evaluation of CRPS.[114] A randomized, double-blind comparison of intravenous guanethidine, reserpine, and normal saline demonstrated significant and equal improvement with all three at 30 minutes and no differences in outcome at 24 hours. Tourniquet-induced analgesia may be involved in the short-term pain relief observed using the Hannington-Kiff protocol.[124]

Bretylium tosylate (Bretylol) is the only drug approved by the Food and Drug Administration as an intravenous competitive blocking agent. It produces a transient release of norepinephrine from postganglionic sympathetic nerve endings, followed by prevention of the release of norepinephrine.[32,125,126] In rare cases, lasting relief may be obtained following a single intravenous infusion of a sympatholytic drug.

Blockade of lumbar sympathetic ganglia is the most widely recognized treatment for patients with refractory CRPS. Blocks are generally performed with small volumes of long-acting anesthetic agents and are usually well tolerated.[114] Katz and Hungerford[47] reported good relief of pain in 58% of patients who underwent lumbar sympathetic blockade; the remaining 42% had fair relief. However, 89% of patients had recurrence of symptoms. The duration of reduced pain has been reported to outlast the duration of action of the anesthetic agent, especially if the block is performed shortly after symptoms occur.[14,114]

A series of 14 patients with CRPS of the knee were treated with epidural block anesthesia followed by epidural narcotics.[17] All patients underwent physical therapy and continuous passive motion of the knee during hospitalization, and all patents were treated shortly after the onset of symptoms. With over 2 years of follow-up, 11 patients were cured with no functional deficit. Two patients had intermittent aching, and one had no relief of symptoms. This therapeutic technique holds promise for total alleviation of symptoms in patients with CRPS which is recognized and treated promptly.

SURGICAL OR CHEMICAL SYMPATHECTOMY

Surgical or chemical ablation of the lumbar sympathetic ganglion is generally reserved for patients who have experienced only transient relief from intravenous or sympathetic ganglion blockade. Many patients experience good pain relief initially, but recurrence of pain may occur in as many as one-third of patients.[114] Katz and Hungerford[47] noted that in their patents who had sympathectomies, the amount of pain relief provided by the surgery could be predicted by the amount obtained transiently with a sympathetic block.

ADJUVANT THERAPIES

Numerous other modalities have been suggested in the treatment of CRPS. Contrast baths and nonsteroidal antiinflammatory agents have been used with good success during courses of physical therapy.[15] Others have described the benefits of electrical nerve stimulation in patients with causalgia.[42,127] Biofeedback, occupational therapy, and psychiatric testing may aid in pain relief while providing emotional and psychological support.[19] Many of these modalities may be used in conjunction with other treatments.

Tietjen[15] has stressed that the most important therapy that can be offered the patient with dystrophy of the knee is the establishment of a good doctor–patient relationship. Patients will be frustrated by the chronic pain and functional loss associated with CRPS, and will require patience, understanding, and encouragement from physicians, nurses, and therapists to become motivated to work toward improvement.

AUTHORS' APPROACH TO TREATMENT

It is important to reassure the patient that CRPS is a real problem, and not psychosomatic. Explain the natural history of CRPS: 18 to 24 months may pass before some improvement occurs, and patients may always experience some problems. It is important for patients to know that they should expect 30% to 50% improvement in symptoms, not 100%. Only rarely does CRPS completely resolve. Combinations of medication work better than individual drugs alone (tricyclic antidepressant with a serotonin reuptake inhibitor). Finally, patients need to keep as active as possible. The good news is that patients are usually better 5 years after the onset of CRPS than they were at 2 years.

The use of drugs can often break the CRPS cycle so that it may not reestablish itself. Start with Elavil 10 mg once at night (qhs), and Zoloft 25 mg each morning (qam). Recheck in 2 weeks. If the patient is not sleeping well or continues to have burning pain, then increase Elavil to 25 mg. The dosage of Elavil may be increased up to 100 mg/day until the patient experiences relief or side effects become intolerable. Zoloft's major side effect is a hyperactive nervous system. If the patient is tolerating the medication without relief of chronic ache during the day, then gradually increase the medication to 100 mg/day. Remember that every patient reponds differently to each of the recommended medications. You may need to change medications dependent on efficacy and side effects encountered.

CONCLUSION

The pathophysiologic entity known as complex regional pain syndrome (CRPS) includes classic reflex sympathetic dystrophy (RSD) and causalgia. RSD of the knee is a complication that often follows surgical or traumatic insult to the knee. The diagnosis is based on clinical findings and is defined as an exaggerated physiologic response to an injury, and may be characterized by (1) intense or unduly prolonged pain; (2) vasomotor disturbances; (3) delayed functional recovery; and (4) trophic changes in the soft tissues, which may be supported by a variety of objective instruments and tests.. The pain often involves the patellofemoral articulation and produces limited range of motion and stiffness in the knee. No objective testing technique is currently available that provides sensitivity and specificity in the identification of dystrophic patients. However, plain x-rays, bone scans, and ICST/LDF may aid in the diagnostic evaluation of the patient with chronic knee pain. Effective treatment of CRPS is multifaceted, and requires prompt recognition of the syndrome. The use of a combination of modalities designed to maintain lower-extremity strength and range of motion while decreasing symptoms of sympathetic hyperactivity in the extremity is recommended.

References

1. Kim HJ, Kozin F, Johnson RP, et al. Reflex sympathetic dystrophy syndrome of the knee following meniscectomy. *Arthritis Rheum* 1979;22:177–181.
2. Mitchell SW, Morehouse GR, Keen WW. *Gunshot Wounds and Other Injuries of Nerves*. Philadelphia: JB Lippincott, 1864.
3. Leriche R. *The Surgery of Pain*. Young A, trans-editor. London: Bailiere, Tindall & Cox, 1939.
4. Sudek PHM. Uber die acute entzundliche Knochenatrophie. *Arch Klin Chir* 1900;62:147–156.
5. Evans JA. Reflex sympathetic dystrophy: report on 57 cases. *Ann Intern Med* 1947;26:417–426.
6. Bonica JJ. Causalgia and other reflex sympathetic dystrophies. *Postgrad Med* 1973;53:143–148.
7. Koman LA, Nunley JA, Goldner JL, et al. Isolated cold stress testing in the assessment of symptoms in the upper extremity: preliminary communication. *J Hand Surg* 1984;9A:305–313.
8. Amadio PC. Pain dysfunction syndromes. *J Bone Joint Surg* 1988;70A:944–949.
9. Dobyns JH. Pain dysfunction syndrome. In: Gelberman RH, ed. *Operative Nerve Repair and Reconstruction*. Phildelphia: JB Lippincott, 1991:1489–1496.
10. Amadio PC, Mackinnon SE, Merritt WH, et al. Reflex sympathetic dystrophy syndrome: consensus report of an ad hoc committee of the American Association for Hand Surgery on the definition of reflex sympathetic dystrophy syndrome. *Plast Reconstr Surg* 1991;87:371–375.

11. Merskey H, Bogduk N. *Classification of Chronic Pain. Descriptions of Chronic Pain Syndromes and Definitions of Pain Terms.* Seattle: IASP Press, 1994:39–43.
12. Janig W, Blumberg H, Boas RA, et al. The reflex sympathetic dystrophy syndrome. Consensus statement and general recommendations for diagnosis and clinical research. In: Bond MR, Charlton JE, Woalf CJ, eds. *Pain Research and Clinical Management: Proceedings of the VIth World Congress on Pain, Pain Research and Clinical Management*, vol 4. Amsterdam: Elsevier Science, 1991:372–375.
13. Janig W. The puzzle of "reflex sympathetic dystrophy": mechanisms, hypotheses, open questions. In: Janig W, Stanton-Hicks M, eds. *Reflex Sympathetic Dystrophy: A Reappraisal. Progress in Pain Research and Management*, vol 6. Seattle: IASP Press, 1996:1–24.
14. Boas RA. Complex regional pain syndromes: symptoms, signs, and differential diagnosis. In: Janig W, Stanton-Hicks, eds. *Reflex Sympathetic Dystrophy: A Reappraisal. Progress in Pain Research and Management*, vol 6. Seattle: IASP Press, 1996:79–92.
15. Tietjen R. Reflex sympathetic dystrophy of the knee. *Clin Orthop* 1986;209:234–243.
16. Shelton RM, Lewis CW. Reflex sympathetic dystrophy: a review. *J Am Acad Dermatol* 1990;22:513–520.
17. Cooper DE, DeLee JC, Ramamurthy S. Reflex sympathetic dystrophy of the knee: treatment using continuous epidural anesthesia. *J Bone Joint Surg* 1989;71A: 365–369.
18. Schutzer SF, Gossling HR. Current concepts review. The treatment of reflex sympathetic dystrophy syndrome. *J Bone Joint Surg* 1984;66A:625–629.
19. Poehling GG, Koman LA, Pollock FE. Reflex synpathetic dystrophy of the knee. In: Sprague NF, ed. *Complications in Arthroscopy*. New York: Raven Press, 1989: 53–72.
20. Dotson RM. Causalgia—reflex sympathetic dystrophy—sympathetically maintained pain: myth and reality. *Muscle Nerve* 1993;16:1049–1055.
21. Koman LA, Smih BP, Smith TL. Stress testing in the evaluation of upper-extremity perfusion. *Hand Clin* 1993;9:59–83.
22. Koman LA, Smith TL, Smith BP, et al. The painful hand. *Hand Clin* 1996;12:757–764.
23. Kurvers HAJM, Jacobs MJHM, Beuk RJ, et al. Reflex sympathetic dystrophy: evoluton of microcirculatory disturbances in time. *Pain* 1995;60:333–340.
24. Ostergren J, Rosen L, Fagrell B, et al. Skin microvascular circulation in the sympathetic dystrophies evaluated by videophotometric capillaroscopy and laser Doppler fluxmetry. *Int J Microcirc* 1988;7:289.
25. Rosen L, Ostergren J, Fagrell B, et al. Skin microvascular circulation in the sympathetic dystrophies evaluated by videophotometric capillaroscopy and laser Doppler fluxmetry. *Eur J Clin Invest* 1988;18:305–308.
26. Koman LA. Painful upper extremity. In: Manske PR, ed. *Hand Surgery Update*, vol 1. Englewood, CO: American Society for Surgery of the Hand, 1994:24.1–24.8.
27. Campbell JN, Raja SN, Selig DK, et al. Diagnosis and management of sympathetically maintained pain. In: Fields HL, Liebeskind JC, eds. *Progress in Pain Research and Management*, vol 1. Seattle: IASP Press, 1994:85–100.
28. Campbell JN, Meyer RA, Raja SN. Is nociceptor activation by alpha-1 adrenoreceptors the culprit in sympathetically maintained pain? *Am Pain Soc J* 1992;1:3–11.
29. Devor M. Nerve pathophysiology and mechanisms of pain in causalgia. *J Auton Nerv Syst* 1983;7:371–384.
30. Eisenach JC, Rauck RL, Buzzanell C, et al. Epidural clonidine analgesia for intractable cancer pain—phase I. *Anaesthesiology* 1989;71:647–652.
31. Fouch RA, Abram SE, Hogan QH. Neural blockade for upper-extremity pain. *Hand Clin* 1996;12:791–800.
32. Hord AH, Rooks MD, Stephens BO, et al. Intravenous regional bretylium and lidocaine for treatment of reflex sympathetic dystrophy: a randomized, double-blind study. *Anesth Analg* 1992;74:818–821.
33. Raja SN, Davis KD, Campbell JN. The adrenergic pharmacology of sympathetically-maintained pain. *J Reconstr Microsurg* 1992;8:63–69.
34. Raja SN, Meyer RA, Campbell JN. Peripheral mechanisms of somatic pain. *Anesthesiology* 1988;68:571–590.
35. Rauck RL, Eisenach JC, Jackson K, et al. Epidural clonidine treatment for refractory reflex sympathetic dystrophy. *Anesthesiology* 1993;79:1163–1169.
36. Arnold JMO, Teasell RW, MacLeod AP, Brown JE, et al. Increased venous alpha-adrenoceptor responsiveness in patients with reflex sympathetic dystrophy. *Ann Intern Med* 1993;118:619–621.
37. Raja SN, Treede RD, Davis KD, et al. Systemic alpha-adrenergic blockade with phentolamine: a diagnostic test for sympathetically maintained pain. *Anesthesiology* 1991;74:691–698.
38. Raja SN, Turnquist JL, Meleka S, et al. Monitoring adequacy of α-adrenoceptor blockade following systemic phentolamine administration. *Pain* 1996;64:197–204.
39. Bej MD, Schwartzman RJ. Abnormalities of cutaneous blood flow regulation in patients with reflex sympathetic dystrophy as measured by laser Doppler fluxmetry. *Arch Neurol* 1991;48:912–915.
40. Daemen M, Kurvers H, Slaff D, et al. Reflex sympathetc dystrophy: microcirculatory observations in humans. *Int J Microcirc* 1995;15:105.
41. Ecker A. Norepinephrine in reflex sympathetic dystrophy: a hypothesis. *Clin J Pain* 1989;5:313–315.
42. Melzak R, Wall PD. Pain mechanisms: a new theory. *Science* 1965;150:971–979.
43. Wall PD. Mechanisms of acute and chronic pain. In:

Kruger L, Liebeskind JC, eds. *Advances in Pain Research and Therapy*, vol 6. New York: Raven Press, 1984:95–104.

44. Bickerstaff DR, Charlesworth D, Kanis JA. Changes in cortical and trabecular bone in algodystrophy. *Br J Rheumatol* 1993;32:46–51.
45. Ogilvie-Harris DJ, Roscoe M. Reflex sympathetic dystrophy of the knee. *J Bone Joint Surg* 1987;69B:804–806.
46. Ficat RP, Hungerford DS. *Disorders of the Patello-Femoral Joint*. Baltimore: Williams & Wilkins, 1977: 146–169.
47. Katz MM, Hungerford DS. Reflex sympathetic dystrophy affecting the knee. *J Bone Joint Surg* 1987; 69B:797–803.
48. Lagier R. Partial algodystrophy of the knee. *J Rheumatol* 1983;10:255–260.
49. Lagier R, Boussina I, Mathies B. Algodystrophy of the knee. *Clin Rheumatol* 1983;2:71–77.
50. Lequesne M, Kerboull M, Benasasson M, et al. Partial transient osteopososis. *Skeletal Radiol* 1977;2:1–9.
51. Nathan PW. Pain and the sympathetic system. In: Bannister R, ed. *Autonomic Failure: A Textbook of Clinical Disorders of the Autonomic Nervous System*, 2nd ed. Oxford: Oxford University Press, 1988:733–747.
52. Koman LA, Smith TL, Smith BP, et al. Reflex sympathetic and other dystrophies. In: Peimer C, ed. *Surgery of the Hand and Upper Extremity*. New York: McGraw-Hill, 1995:2295–2312.
53. Subbarao J, Stillwell GK. Reflex sympathetic dystrophy syndrome of the upper extremity: analysis of total outcome of management of 125 cases. *Arch Phys Med Rehabil* 1998;62:549–554.
54. Veldman PHJM, Reynen HM, Arntz IE, et al. Signs and symptoms of reflex sympathetic dystrophy: prospective study of 829 patients. *Lancet* 1993;342:1012–1016.
55. Baron R, Blumberg H, Janig W. Clinical characteristics of patients with complex regional pain syndrome in Germany with special emphasis on vasomotor function. In: Janig W, Stanton-Hicks M, eds. *Reflex Sympathetc Dystrophy: A Reappraisal. Progress in Pain Research and Management*, vol 6. Seattle: IASP Press, 1996: 25–48.
56. Carron H, Weller RM. Treatment of post-traumatic sympathetic dystrophy. *Adv Neurol* 1974;4:485–490.
57. Holden WD. Sympathetic dystrophy. *Arch Surg* 1948; 57:373–384.
58. Low PA, Wilson PR, Sandroni P, et al. Clinical characteristics of patients with reflex sympathetic dystrophy (sympathetically maintained pain) in the USA. In: Janig W, Stanton-Hicks M, eds. *Reflex Sympathetic Dystrophy: A Reappraisal. Progress in Pain Research and Management*, vol 6. Seattle: IASP Press, 1996:49–66.
59. Moberg E. The shoulder-hand-finger syndrome. *Surg Clin North Am* 1960;40:367–373.
60. Pak TJ, Martin GM, Magness JL, et al. Reflex sympathetic dystrophy: a review of 140 cases. *Minn Med* 1970;53:507–512.
61. Schwartzman RJ, McLellan TL. Reflex sympathetic dystrophy: a review. *Arch Neurol* 1987;44:555–561.
62. Cooper DE, DeLee JC. Reflex sympathetic dystrophy of the knee. *J Am Acad Orthop Surg* 1994;2:79–86.
63. An HS, Hawthorne KB, Jackson WT. Reflex sympathetic dystrophy and cigarette smoking. *J Hand Surg* 1988;13A:458–460.
64. Poehling GG, Pollock FE Jr, Koman LA. Reflex sympathetic dystrophy of the knee after sensory nerve injury. *J Arthrosc Rel Res* 1988;4:31–35.
65. Bruehl S, Carlson CR. Predisposing psychological factors in the development of reflex sympathetic dystrophy. *Clin J Pain* 1992;8:287–299.
66. Covington EC. Psychological issues in reflex sympathetic dystrophy. In: Janig W, Stanton-Hicks M, eds. *Reflex Sympathetic Dystrophy: A Reappraisal. Progress in Pain Research and Management*, vol 6. Seattle: IASP Press, 1996:191–215.
67. Haddox JD. Psychological aspects of reflex sympathetic dystrophy. In: Stanton-Hicks M, ed. *Pain and the Sympathetic Nervous System*. Boston: Kluwer Academic, 1990.
68. Lynch ME. Psychological aspects of reflex sympathetic dystrophy: a review of adult and pediatric literature. *Pain* 1992;49:337–347.
69. Ochoa JL, Verdugo RJ. The mythology of reflex sympathetic dystrophy and sympathetically maintained pains. *Phys Med Rehabil Clin North Am* 1993;4:151–162.
70. Ochoa JL, Verdugo RJ. Reflex sympathetic dystrophy. A common clinical avenue for somatoform expression. *Neurol Clin* 1995;13:351–363.
71. Ochoa JL, Yarnitsky D, Marchettini P, et al. Interactions between sympathetic vasoconstrictor outflow and C nociceptor induced antidromic vasodilatation. *Pain* 1993;54:191–196.
72. Van Houdenhove B, Vasquez G, Onghena P, et al. Etiopathogenesis of reflex sympathetic dystrophy: a review and biopsychosocial hypothesis. *Clin J Pain* 1992; 8:300–306.
73. Weiss WU. Psychophysiologic aspects of reflex sympathetic dystrophy syndrome. *Am J Pain Manage* 1994; 4:67–72.
74. Hemler DE, McAuley RA, Belandres PV. Common clinical presentations among active duty personnel with traumatically induced reflex sympathetic dystrophy. *Mil Med* 1988;153:493–495.
75. DeGood DE, Cundiff GW, Adams LE, et al. A psychosocial and behavioral comparison of reflex sympathetic dystrophy, low back pain, and headache patients. *Pain* 1993;54:317–322.
76. Fishbain DA, Goldberg M, Meagher BR, et al. Male and female chronic pain patients categorized by DSM-III psychiatric diagnostic criteria. *Pain* 1986;26:181–197.

77. Davidoff G, Morey K, Amann M, et al. Pain measurement in reflex sympathetic dystrophy syndrome. *Pain* 1988;32:27–34.

78. Gracely RH, Price DD, Roberts WJ, et al. Quantitative sensory testing in patients with complex regional pain syndrome (CRPS) I and II. In: Janig W, Stanton-Hicks M, eds. *Reflex Sympathetic Dystrophy: A Reappraisal. Progress in Pain Research and Management*, vol 6. Seattle: IASP Press, 1996:151–172.

79. Bryan AS, Klenerman L, Bowsher D. The diagnosis of reflex sympathetic dystrophy using an algometer. *J Bone Joint Surg* 1991;73B:644–646.

80. Atkins RM, Kanis JA. The use of dolorimetry in the assessment of post-traumatic algodystrophy of the hand. *Br J Rheumatol* 1989;28:404–409.

81. Koman LA, Poehling GG. Reflex sympathetic dystrophy. In: Gelberman R, ed. *Operative Nerve Repair and Reconstruction*. Philadelphia: JB Lippincott, 1990: 1497–1523.

82. Liu S. Kopacz DJ, Carpenter RL. Quantitative assessment of differential sensory nerve block after lidocaine spinal anesthesia. *Anesthesiology* 1995;82:60–63.

83. Price DD, Harkins SW, Rafii A, et al. A simultaneous comparison of fentanyl's analgesic effects on experimental and clinical pain. *Pain* 1986;24:197–203.

84. Genant HK, Kozin F, Bekerman C, et al. The reflex sympathetic dystrophy syndrome. *Radiology* 1975;117: 21–32.

85. Fulkerson JP, Hungerford DS. Reflex sympathetic dystrophy and chronic pain. In: *Disorders of the Patellofemoral Joint*, 2nd ed. Baltimore: Williams & Wilkins, 1990:247–264.

86. Arlet J, Ficat P, Durroux R, et. al. Histopathologie des lesions osseuses et cartilagineuses dans l'algodystrophie sympathique reflexe du genou: a propos de 16 observations. *Rev Rhum Mal Osteoartic* 1981;48:325–331.

87. Kozin F, Genant HK, Beckerman C, et al. The reflex sympathetic dystrophy syndrome. II. Roentgenographic and scintigraphic evidence of bilaterality and of periarticular accentuation. *Am J Med* 1976;60:332–337.

88. Bekerman C, Genant HK, Hoffer PB, et al. Radionuclide imaging of the bones and joints of the hand. *Radiology* 1975;118:653–659.

89. Intenzo C, Kim S, Millin J, et al. Scintigraphic patterns of the reflex sympathetic syndrome of the lower extremites. *Clin Nucl Med* 1989;14:657–661.

90. Kozin F, Soin JS, Ryan LM, et al. Bone scintigraphy in the reflex sympathetic dystrophy syndrome. *Radiology* 1981;138:437–443.

91. Mackinnon SE, Holder LE. The use of three-phase radionuclide bone scanning in the diagnosis of reflex sympathetic dystrophy. *J Hand Surg* 1984;9A:556–563.

92. Werner R, Davidoff G, Jackson MD, et al. Factors affecting the sensitivity and specificity of the three-phase technetium bone scan in the diagnosis of reflex sympathetic dystrophy syndrome in the upper extremity. *J Hand Surg* 1989;14A:520–523.

93. Hoffman J, Phillips W, Blum M, et al. Effect of sympathetic block demonstrated by triple-phase bone scan. *J Hand Surg* 1993;18A:860–864.

94. Koman LA, Barden A, Smith BP, et al. Reflex sympathetic dystrophy in an adolescent. *Foot Ankle* 1993;14: 273–277.

95. Pollock FE, Koman LA, Smith BP, et al. Patterns of microvascular response associated with reflex sympathetic dystrophy of the hand and wrist. *J Hand Surg* 1993; 18A:847–852.

96. Fagrell B. The relationship between macro- and microcirculation: clinical aspects. *Acta Pharmacol Toxicol* 1986;58:67–72.

97. Koman LA, Ruch DS, Smith BP, et al. Reflex sympathetic dystrophy after wrist surgery. In: Levin L, ed. *Problems in Plastic and Reconstructive Surgery*. Philadelphia: JB Lippincott, 1992:300–322.

98. Irazuata JE, Berde CB, Sethna NF. Laser Doppler measurements of skin blood flow before, during, and after lumbar sympathetic blockade in children and young adults with reflex sympathetic dystrophy syndrome. *J Clin Monit* 1992;8:16–19.

99. Pollock FE, Koman LA, Smith BP, et al. Thermoregulatory abnormalities of the foot. *Orthop Clin North Am* 1989;20(4):737–749.

100. Patman RD, Thompson JE, Persson AV. Management of post-traumatic pain syndromes: report of 113 cases. *Ann Surg* 1973;177:780–787.

101. Toumey JW. Occurrence and management of reflex sympathetic dystrophy (causalgia of the extremities). *J Bone Joint Surg* 1948;30A:883–894.

102. Czop C, Smith TL, Rauck R, et al. The pharmacologic approach to the painful hand. *Hand Clin* 1996;12: 633–642.

103. Feinmann C. Pain relief by antidepressants: possible modes of action. *Pain* 1985;23:1–8.

104. Magni G. The use of antidepressants in the treatment of chronic pain: a review of current evidence. *Drugs* 1991;42:730–748.

105. Monks R. Psychotropic drugs. In: Wall P, Melzack R, eds. *Textbook of Pain*. Edinburgh: Churchill Livingstone, 1994:963–989.

106. Tyler DC. Pharmacology of pain management. *Pediatr Clin North Am* 1994;41:59–71.

107. Watson CPN. Antidepressant drugs as adjuvant analgesics. *J Pain Symp Manage* 1994;9:392–405.

108. Hardman JG, Limbird LE, Molinoff PB, et al. *Goodman and Gilman's The Pharmacological Basis of Therapeutics*, 9th ed. New York; McGraw-Hill, 1996.

109. Stoelting RK. Drugs used in treatment of psychiatric disease. In: Stoelting RK (ed.), *Pharmacology and Physi-*

ology in Anesthetic Practice. Philadelphia: JB Lippincott, 1987:347–364.

110. Mitchell PB. Selective serotonin reuptake inhibitors: adverse effects, toxicity and interactions. *Adverse Drug React Toxicol Rev* 1994;13:121–144.

111. Van Harten J. Clinical pharmacokinetics of selective serotonin reuptake inhibitors. *Clin Pharmacokinet* 1993;24:203–220.

112. Chaturvedi SK. Phenytoin in reflex sympathetic dystrophy. *Pain* 1989;36:379–380.

113. Mellick G, Mellicy L. Gabapentine in the management of reflex sympathetic dystrophy. *J Pain Symp Manage* 1995;10:265–266.

114. Payne R. Neurophathic pain syndromes, with special reference to causalgia and reflex sympathetic dystrophy. *Clin J Pain* 1986;2:59–73.

115. Swerdlow M. Anticonvulsant drugs and chronic pain. *Clin Neuropharmacol* 1984;7:51–82.

116. Ghostine SY, Comair YG, Turner DM, et al. Phenoxybenzamine in the treatment of causalgia. *J Neurosurg* 1984;60:1263–1268.

117. Kozin F, McCarty DJ, Sims J, et al. The reflex sympathetic dystrophy syndrome. I. Clinical and histologic studies: evidence for bilaterality, response to corticosteroids and articular involvement. *Am J Med* 1976; 60:321–331.

118. Kozin F, Ryan LM, Carerra GF, et al. The reflex sympathetic dystrophy syndrome (RSDS): III. Scintigraphic studies, further evidence for the therapeutic efficacy of systemic corticosteroids, and proposed diagnostic criteria. *Am J Med* 1981;70:23–30.

119. Prough DS, McLeskey CH, Poehling GG, et al. Efficacy of oral nifedipine in the treatment of reflex sympathetic dystrophy. *Anesthesiology* 1985;62:796–799.

120. Paulson RR. Reflex sympathetic dystrophy in a teenaged girl. *Postgrad Med* 1987;81:66–67.

121. Warfield CA. *Principles and Practice of Pain Management*. New York: McGraw-Hill, 1993.

122. Hannington-Kiff JG. Hyperadrenergic-effected limb causalgia: relief by IV pharmacologic norepinephrine blockade. *Am Heart J* 1982;103:152–153.

123. Loh L, Nathan PW, Schott GD, et al. Effects of guanethidine infusion in certain painful states. *J Neurol Neurosurg Psychiatry* 1980;43:446–451.

124. Blanchard J, Rammamurthy S, Walsh N, et al. Intravenous regional sympatholysis: a double-blind comparison of guanethidine, reserpine and normal saline. *J Pain Symptom Manage* 1990;5:357–361.

125. Ford SR, Forrest WH Jr, Eltherington L. The treatment of reflex sympathetic dystrophy with intravenous regional bretylium. *Anesthesiology* 1988;68:137–140.

126. Hanowell LH, Kanefield JK, Soriano SG III. A recommendation for reduced lidocaine dosage during intravenous regional bretylium treatment of reflex sympathetic dystrophy. *Anesthesiology* 1989;71:811–812.

127. Meyer GA, Fields HL. Causalgia treated by selective large fiber stimulation of peripheral nerve. *Brain* 1972; 95:163–165.

128. Koman LA, ed. Department of Orthopaedic Surgery, Wake Forest University School of Medicine Manual. Winston-Salem, NC: Orthopaedic Press, 1998.

Section II

Complications and Pitfalls in Meniscal Surgery

Chapter 5

COMPLICATIONS OF ARTHROSCOPIC MENISCECTOMY

John B. Ryan and Thomas M. DeBerardino

MENISCAL STRUCTURE AND FUNCTION

The menisci of the knee are semi-circular wedge-shaped fibrocartilagenous disks firmly attached to the tibia and the joint capsule (Fig. 5.1). The medial meniscus is wider posteriorly than anteriorly and forms a half circle. The lateral meniscus is uniform in width and forms almost three-quarters of a circle. The medial meniscus is attached to the capsule, medial collateral ligament, and tibial plateau. The lateral meniscus is attached to the capsule and tibial plateau but not to the fibular collateral ligament. The lateral meniscus also has posterior attachments to the medial femoral condyle (meniscal femoral ligaments), which attaches to the femur near the origin of the posterior cruciate ligament.[1,2] The popliteal tendon courses through the popliteal hiatus at the posterolateral corner of the knee. The anteroinferior popliteomeniscal fascicle, and the posterosuperior popliteomeniscal fascicle attachments to help provide stability to the posterior corner.[3] With knee motion both menisci translate on the tibial plateau, but the lateral meniscus is more mobile than the medial.[4,5] The organic composition of the meniscus is 65% type I collagen. The majority of the collagen fibers are oriented along the long axis of the meniscus (i.e., following the natural curve) with a small number of fibers oriented obliquely, radially, and vertically (Fig. 5.2).[6] The peripheral 10% to 30% of the meniscal tissue is vascularized by synovial branches of the genicular arteries (Fig. 5.3).[7] The central 70% to 90% is nourished by diffusion from synovial fluid.

In 1985 Soren[8] described the etiology of congenitally malformed menisci. Dissections of various vertebrates revealed menisci shaped like a plate, disk, or ring. Lateral menisci have been described in two cases with one meniscus overlying another (double-layered).[9] Another lateral meniscal variant is the ring meniscus (making a complete circle). This ring meniscus has an intercondylar bridge between the two horns attached to the tibial plateau differentiating it from an old bucket-handle tear.[10,11] Hypoplastic menisci have been described both medially and laterally; discoid menisci are more frequent laterally ($n = 29$) than medially ($n = 1$) in symptomatic patients.[12] Three types of lateral discoid menisci are described by Ikeuchi: complete, incomplete, and Wrisberg type.[13]

Functionally, the menisci increase the surface area of the knee by filling the void between the curved femoral surface and the flat tibial surface, thereby decreasing the force per unit area on the femur and the tibia with axial load.[14] Renström and Johnson[15] demonstrated that the knee meniscus tissue acts as a stabilizing shock absorber force as axial loading causes the elongation of the circumferential meniscal collagen fibers and allows some extruding of the edges of the menisci out from underneath the joint surfaces peripherally (tensile strain). This hoop or tensile stress reduces the impulse loading of weight bearing, sparing the articular cartilage and the subchondral bone. The menisci also aid in the lubrication of the knee by extruding free fluid and by distributing synovial fluid over the distal femur with knee motion.[6] Meniscal tissue has been shown to stabilize the knee in the anterior, posterior, and medial/lateral planes by acting as a mechanical stop to translation. However, this finding appears to become significant only when the major stabilizing ligaments of the knee have been injured.[16,17] Biomechanical studies have demonstrated that 50% (knee in extension) to 90% (knee in flexion) of the compression forces across the knee are transmitted through the normal menisci. When the knee is

Figure 5.1. The menisci of the knee are semicircular wedge-shaped fibrocartilaginous disks firmly attached to the tibia and the joint capsule.

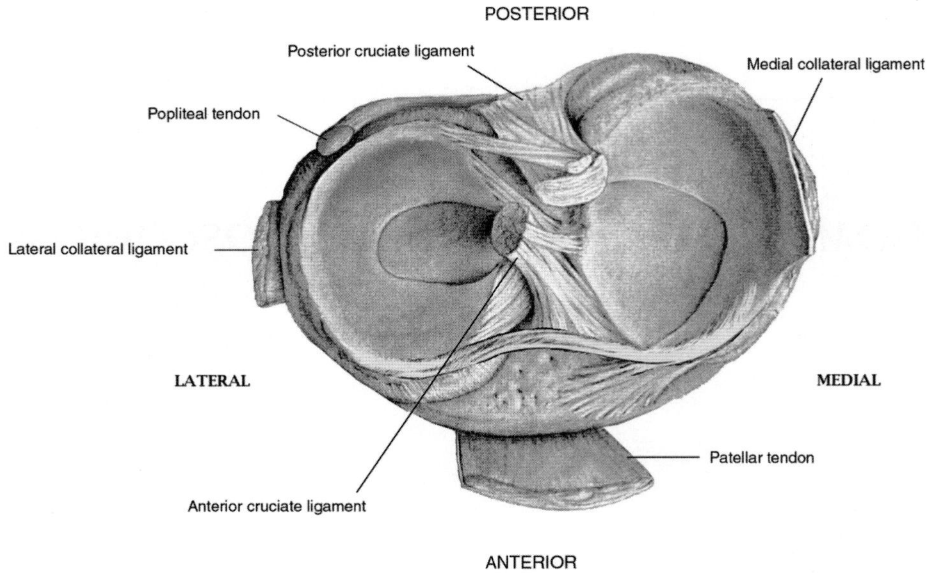

in 70 degrees of flexion, 100% of the load is transmitted through the posterior horn of the menisci.[15,18–21]

MENISCAL TEARS

When compression or shear forces exceed the structural design of the meniscus, clefts are created along naturally occurring planes between bundles of collagen fibers. Some clefts are along the circumferential fibers of the menisci, causing vertical longitudinal tears while others are obtained at right angles causing radial or horizontal tears (Fig. 5.4). Chronic instability of the knee due to cruciate or collateral ligamentous laxity can allow the menisci to migrate underneath the femoral condyle in a physiologically abnormal position, increasing the risk of tears. Acute anterior cruciate ligament (ACL) tears are associated with a high incidence of lateral meniscus tears; however, chronic ACL instability is associated more with medial meniscus tears.[22–25] Occasionally, meniscal tears can occur at the capsular ligamentous junction rather than in the substance of the meniscus. In contrast to the intersubstance tears, these capsular meniscal tears are associated with spontaneous healing because of the close proximity of an adequate blood supply and the intensity of the inflammatory response.

Normal aging is associated with texture changes in the meniscus from firm and resilient to hard and brittle. Histologic studies have demonstrated color changes from normal white or opaque to yellow or brown, indicative of degeneration of meniscal tissue.[26,27] Occa-

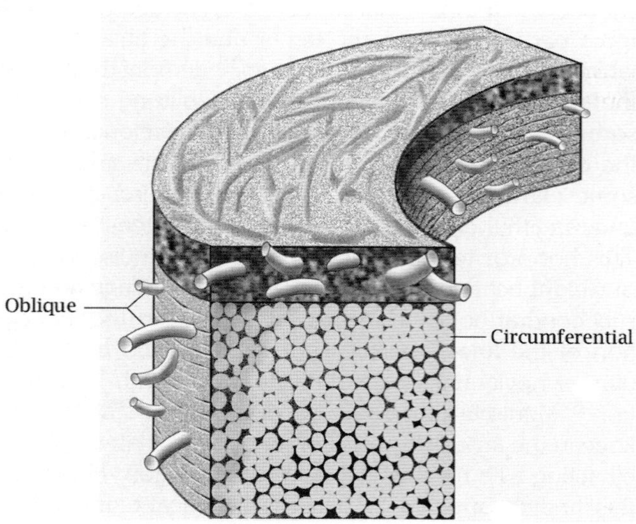

Figure 5.2. The majority of the collagen fibers are oriented along the long axis of the meniscus (i.e., following the natural curve), with a small number of fibers oriented obliquely, radially, and vertically.

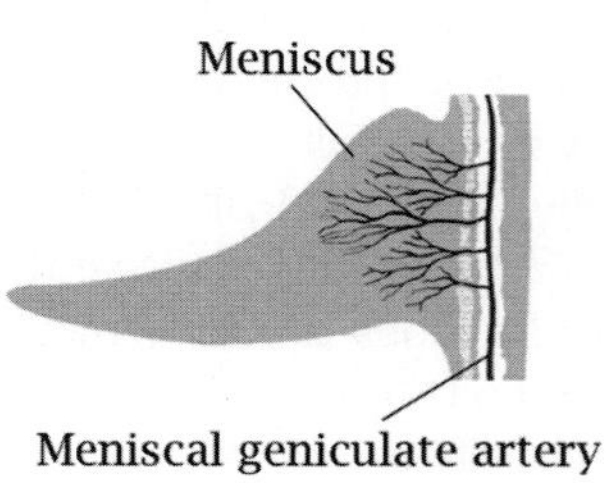

Figure 5.3. The peripheral 10% to 30% of the meniscal tissues is vascularized by synovial branches of the genicular arteries.

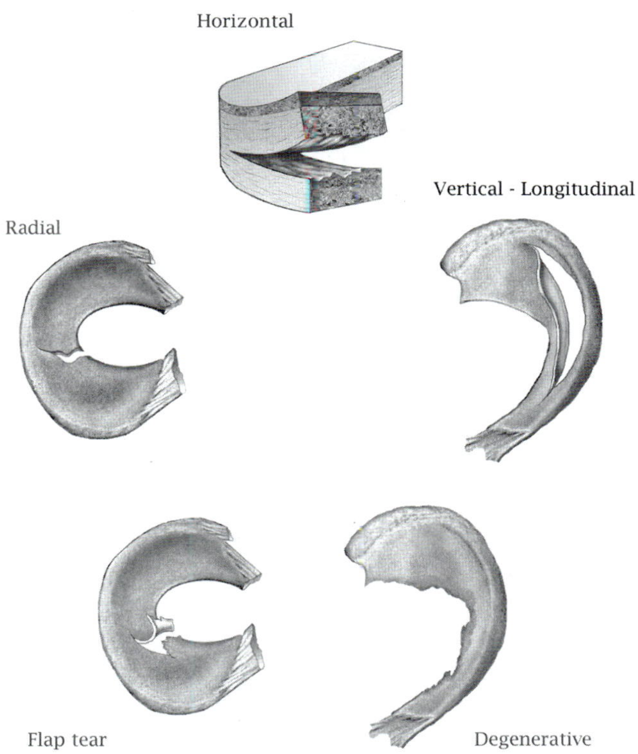

Figure 5.4. Three types of lateral discoid menisci are described by Wantanabe: complete, incomplete, and Wrisberg type.

sionally, crystals (calcium pyrophosphate dihydrate [CPPD], uric acid) may precipitate on the surface and create a crust over the meniscus. These aging changes may be associated with fraying of the free meniscal edge, hydroxyapatite in the peripheral synovial blood vessels, and eosinophilic necrosis of collagen within the substance of the meniscus.[28] Older subjects have nonhomogeneous areas within the substance of the meniscus that correlate to altered magnetic resonance imaging (MRI) signals and can be correlated with biopsy-proven degeneration. These structurally altered menisci are inferior and do not absorb compressive loads as effectively. Necropsy studies indicate that the fibrocartilage of the adult meniscus is susceptible to a focal process of matrix fraying and splitting. These degenerative meniscal changes are not associated with increased risk of causing degenerative arthrosis of the hyaline cartilage of the knee.[29–31]

Meniscal healing occurs by fibrin clot and scaffold formation, invasion by undifferentiated mesenchymal cells, and maturation of this fibrovascular scar into fibrocartilage. The vascular portion of the meniscus is capable of this fibroangioblastic response: however, isolated meniscal tears in the central 70% to 90% rarely heal because there is inadequate vascular supply to support this process. Some meniscal tears associated with acute ACL injuries have been shown to completely or partially heal, most likely due to the hemarthrosis associated with cruciate ligament injuries.[32,33] Many small meniscal tears that are stable are asymptomatic. Stable tears include radial tears less than 3 mm in length, partial-thickness tears (less than 50% of vertical height), and horizontal and vertical tears less than 1 cm that do not allow the meniscus tissue to herniate into the central portion of the joint.[34]

Clinically significant tears are most frequently associated with mechanical catching or locking, recurrent effusions, and localized joint-line pain. Locking with an inability to extend after rising from a crouched position is suggestive of a flap or bucket-handle tear. On physical examination, joint-line tenderness is present between 77% and 86% of the time with symptomatic tears. A meniscal tear is found only 58% of the time when there is a positive McMurray's test.[35,36] Congenital abnormal discoid meniscal tissue is treated only if the clinical symptoms correlate with a pathologic process (tear, meniscal instability, or impingement).

ARTHROSCOPIC MENISCECTOMY

Meniscectomy was first reported in 1866 by Brad Hurst of St. George's Hospital, London. Though many authors professed total meniscectomy to be a benign procedure, Fairbanks[37] described the degenerative radiographic changes present following total meniscectomy. Initially, total meniscectomy was the treatment of choice, and unfortunately as many as 10% of the excised menisci were found to be normal.[38,39] The effect of any meniscectomy is a decrease in the tibiofemoral condyle contact areas and an increase in contact stresses, causing higher forces concentrated on a smaller area.[40] Contact stress increases directly with progression from partial to total meniscectomy. Animal studies have demonstrated degenerative changes directly proportional to the percent of meniscus resected.[41] Certain areas of the menisci are critical. Resection of 75% to 80% of the posterior horn of the medial meniscus (one-third of the meniscus) is associated with contact stresses that are close to those of a total meniscectomy.

The use of diagnostic arthroscopy prior to open partial or complete meniscectomy allowed a more accurate and thorough diagnosis, almost totally eliminating the removal of normal menisci.[13,42] Additionally, this diagnostic procedure increased selective partial open meniscectomy. As instrumentation improved and surgical experience increased, arthroscopic partial or complete meniscectomies became common. Watanabe first described arthroscopic meniscectomy in 1962. O'Connor popularized this technique in the United States in the 1970s. As reported by DeHaven,[34] Gillquist et al,[43,44] and Newman et al[45] the ideal arthroscopic meniscectomy excises the unstable fragment, leaving behind a residual meniscus rim that is intact, stable, and reasonably contoured.

Outcome evaluation of patients demonstrates good function whether the procedure is performed open or arthroscopically as long as meniscal resection is minimized and a firm rim of peripheral tissue remains.[46–50] Arthritic changes seen on radiographs are more common in subtotal or complete meniscectomies, when initial surgery is performed after age 30, and in medial partial meniscectomies with preexisting malalignment (less than 4 degrees of valgus and greater than 10 degrees of varus).[48,49] In athletes, lateral partial meniscectomy results in more abnormal radiographs over time than does medial meniscectomy.[51,52]

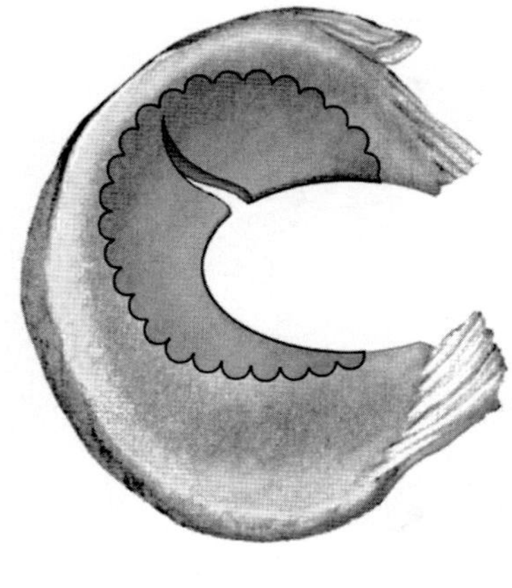

Figure 5.5. Some of the clefts created when compression or shear forces exceed the structural design of the meniscus are along the circumferential fibers of the menisci, causing vertical longitudinal tears, while others are oriented at right angles, causing radial or horizontal tears.

ADEQUATE ARTHROSCOPIC MENISCECTOMY

An arthroscopic meniscectomy is performed only after an adequate diagnostic arthroscopy identifies all pathologic problems intraarticularly.[42,53,54] The meniscus tear should then be defined visually and the extent of the tear palpated with an arthroscopic probe. A 30-degree arthroscope usually allows for a complete exam. A 70-degree arthroscope should always be available, especially if the red/red junction is difficult to visualize. The posterior compartment is best visualized through the notch. Here again, a 70-degree scope provides a more complete view around the posterior horns of both menisci. Vertical horizontal tears less than 7 mm and radial tears less than 5 mm do not require resection.[34,45,55] Partial tears, especially under surface tears, should be palpated firmly from above to ensure that the meniscus does not extrude into the joint, acting as a source of catching. When a flap tear is identified, additional time should be taken to palpate both the superior and inferior surface of the remaining meniscus to ensure that there are no remaining flaps that represent a portion of a bucket-handle tear that has been transected. The location of the tear (anterior one-third, middle one-third, posterior one-third) and the distance from the capsular attachment (peripheral one-third, middle one-third, inner one-third) should be documented. A decision to perform either a partial or total meniscectomy is based on the extent of the damage and the location of the tear.[34,42,45,55] The vast majority of the tears can be treated with partial meniscectomy (Fig. 5.5). Only when the peripheral fibers of the meniscus are violated in such a way as to completely destroy the hoop stress is a total meniscectomy indicated (Fig. 5.6).[44,56] After

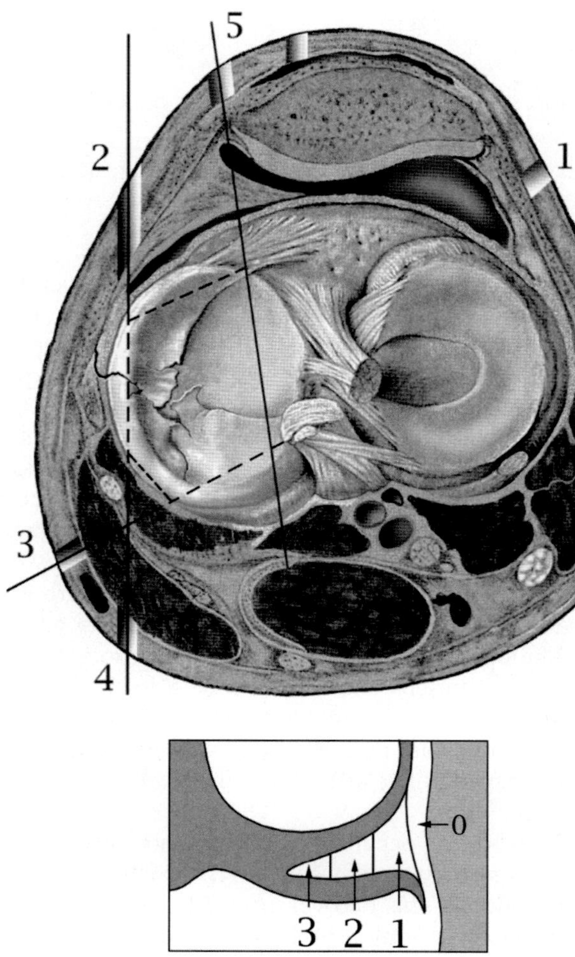

Figure 5.6. Menisci are described by type and location. The dashed lines indicate the planned resection. Note: The tear extends along and past the capsular attachment of the meniscus

the meniscus tear has been partially or totally excised, the joint surface, synovium, and ligamentous structures should be reevaluated. Partial-thickness chondral lesions require no treatment. Full-thickness chondral lesions may be treated by abrasion, abrasion and drilling, microfracture, bone grafting, or osteochondral transplant. Excessive synovial tissue should be debrided to avoid impingement. Postoperative ambulation status and use of crutches is predicated on the extent of the procedure performed interarticularly. Meniscal tears or instability in congenitally abnormal menisci (discoid, ring, double-layered, hypoplastic) are treated by partial meniscectomy, reconturing the meniscal rim to normal physiologic width, and reattachment of Wisberg-type discoid menisci to the capsule.[42,57,58]

COMPLICATIONS OF ARTHROSCOPIC MENISCECTOMY

Complications in arthroscopic meniscectomy can be categorized into either errors of judgment or technique. Errors of judgment are poor clinical decisions (issues of commission and omission) that can affect the short- and long-term outcome of patient care. Judgment errors include failure to perform a comprehensive diagnostic evaluation preoperatively and operatively, failure to adequately educate the patient, and failure to recognize the limitations of the surgeon's abilities. Technical errors are violations of standard operative procedures, usually require immediate corrective action and are frequently preventable by instituting checks and balances. Errors in technique include retained meniscal tissue, iatrogenic damage, broken instruments, formation of portal fistula, complications of treatment of discoid meniscus, and complications of total meniscectomy.

FAILURE OF DIAGNOSTIC AND THERAPEUTIC ACUMEN

Preoperatively the orthopedist should take a thorough history and perform a physical examination along with appropriate diagnostic studies.[42,53,59] Decreased range of motion, synovitis, or significant joint line narrowing will herald difficulty during routine arthroscopic procedures in passing instruments and visualization of underlying pathology. Limited range of motion and x-ray evidence of osteopenia should alert the orthopedist that excessive valgus or varus stress may be associated with iatrogenic ligamentous rupture. The presence of loose bodies, the condition of synovium and articular cartilage, and the ligamentous stability of the knee all affect the outcome of the simple arthroscopic meniscectomy. When the decision is made to excise the damaged meniscus DeHaven,[34] Gillquist et al,[44] Newman et al,[45] and others agree that the goals are to resect the torn portion that is herniating into the central part of the joint, to balance the rim to avoid catching, and to preserve of the capsular attachments of the meniscus.[34,44,45]

INADEQUATE PATIENT EDUCATION

The initial part of an uneventful meniscectomy and successful surgical outcome is patient education. The physician must understand the patient's expectations and the ultimate planned activity level. Frequently, this level of activity exceeds the potential of even the most gifted surgeons. This education process continues following the procedure. The extent of the tear and the extent of nonmeniscal pathology in the knee must be explained to the patient in such a way that postoperatively appropriate attention is paid to strengthening and reestablishing the correct level of activity for the best long-term results. In a follow-up study, Rockburn and Gillquist[49] demonstrated radiographic signs of arthrosis four times more often in knees with partial menisectomies and seven times more often in knees after subtotal meniscectomies as compared to controls. Burks et al[46] have shown in a 15-year follow-up of arthroscopic partial meniscectomy patients that there were 88% good and excellent results in ACL stable knees. In the process of educating the patient preoperatively and postoperatively, the physician may discover that the patient has litigation factors that may negatively affect the outcome of care and the procedure.

KNOWING YOUR SURGICAL ABILITY

Arthroscopic meniscectomies should not be an unpleasant experience for the patient and the surgeon. This procedure should be performed in one tourniquet time (usually less than 60 minutes, but most definitely less than 120 minutes). Surgeons should not attempt knee arthroscopy unless they are prepared to perform an arthrotomy to finish difficult cases. Complete arthroscopic diagnosis requires a working knowledge of all anterior and posterior portals (Fig. 5.7).[60–63] If there is long-standing varus alignment, medial capsule constriction, or ACL ligamentous damage, valgus stress might not open the joint adequately to pass instruments. If the area of the meniscal pathology cannot be reached easily with a spinal needle, it is unlikely that a surgical instrument can be passed interarticularly without significant damage to the joint cartilage. Gradual application of valgus or varus stress held for a prolonged period of time will take advantage of viscoelastic properties of the ligamentous and capsule structures, resulting in improved visualization. Repositioning of the extremity in

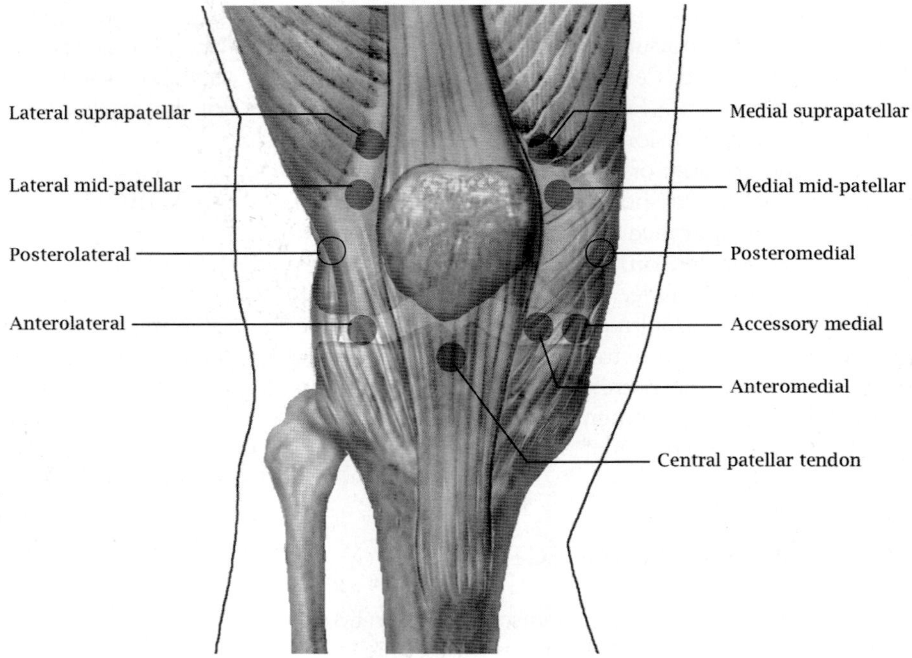

Figure 5.7. Location of all anterior and posterior portals.

the leg holder may increase the mechanical force, allowing for better visualization of the knee. Debride all obstructing soft tissue including the attachment of the ligamentous mucosum prior to operative excision. As the art of arthroscopy is learned, the operative surgeon should not look upon arthrotomy and "old-fashioned" open partial meniscectomy as a failure in capability. The "never give up" attitude of athletic competition should not be applied blindly to arthroscopy. Increased surgical time in tough arthroscopic cases has been associated with increased complication rates, especially in regard to neurovascular damage, compartment syndrome, and infection. A partial or complete meniscectomy performed well through a mini-arthrotomy following diagnostic arthroscopy is more beneficial to a patient than an inadequate meniscectomy performed arthroscopically.

TECHNICAL ERRORS

Missed Meniscal Tears

A thorough and systemic arthroscopic examination of both menisci is the best way to avoid missing a meniscal tear. In most cases clear and complete visualization of the superior and inferior surfaces of the menisci can be completed by arthroscopic visualization and probing for meniscal stability via standard anterior portals. The best view of the posterior horn of the medial meniscus from the anterior portal is obtained with the knee in full extension with the application of a valgus force. Careful probing of both meniscal surfaces provides tactile feedback regarding the structural properties of the menisci. One should not hesitate to view both menisci through the notch. This view, with either a 30- or 70-degree scope provides further assurance of the status of the posterior horns and the meniscal-capsular junction.

Auxiliary posteromedial and posterolateral portals can be used for placement of a spinal needle or probe to palpate the structures visualized in the posterior compartment. Care needs to be taken when placing these portals so as to protect the integrity of the nearby neurovascular structures; a knife is used only to incise the skin. If cannula placement is needed posteriorly, several dilation sets are available to help the arthroscopist serially and bluntly enlarge the soft tissue tracks and help avoid neurologic injury. Routine visualization of the posterior knee compartments through the notch helps increase the surgeon's confidence and makes this a less daunting task.

Retained Meniscal Fragment

Loss of a significant portion of the excised meniscus inside the joint can prolong anesthesia and frustrate the surgeons.

Immediate action: If the meniscal fragment becomes free in the joint, stop all inflow and outflow. Next, perform a complete diagnostic arthroscopy with special attention to the posterior compartment, the popliteal hiatus, the undersurface of both menisci, and the suprapatella fossa. The fragment most likely will move in the direction of flow (especially if the fluid is running through the scope) and toward the outflow cannula. If the meniscal fragment is located, attempt to prevent further migration by squiring it with an 18-gauge needle. Once the fragment is secure, grasp it with routine arthroscopic equipment and remove it through the most convenient portal. If the fragment cannot be found, evidence indicates that it can attach to synovial tissue and become asymptomatic.[64] When using basket forceps and morcelizing torn meniscal tissue, care should also be taken to remove the majority of these small fragments because they may incite a significant inflammatory response.

Prevention: To prevent large meniscal fragments from being dislodged in the joint, ensure that you leave a portion of a bucket-handle tear or large flap tear partially attached. After securely grasping the free end of the tissue with a grasping forceps, rotate the forceps 360 degrees repetitively until the tissue is freed with only a light tug. It will already be in the jaws of the grasping forceps, minimizing the potential for free migration. Consider using a proximal suprapatella lateral portal to remove large fragments.

The capsule and skin in this region are thin, there is no fat pad to trap the meniscus, and the portal is easily dilated, facilitating passage. Always observe the fragment exiting the joint. If you are performing removal by morcellation of the meniscal tear, pass the motorized shaver or other suction devices into the joint on a frequent basis to remove the smaller fragments. Occasionally the meniscus fragment can be lost between the capsule and the skin. There is a report in the literature of a meniscus fragment becoming lodged in the prepatella bursa requiring bursectomy and excision secondary to symptoms developing many weeks after the initial arthroscopy.[65]

Immediate action: If the meniscus becomes lost between the capsule and the skin, stop all inflow and outflow. Look inside the joint to ensure that the meniscus is not still partially lodged in the portal. Also make sure that the meniscus has not been dropped on the drapes, on the surgeon's gown, or on the floor prior to any further steps. Enlarge the opening of the portal and slowly dissect the soft tissue in and around the region. Rarely is a large arthrotomy required.

Prevention: Securely grasp the meniscus to be removed and hold it in such a way that the long axis parallels the long axis of the grasping instrument. This maneuver minimizes the potential of the meniscus becoming dislodged or fragmented as it passes through the portal. Always dilate the arthroscopic portal that the meniscus fragment is to be passed through prior to passage. If necessary, make a larger incision prior to passing the meniscal fragment.

Instrument Breakage

Arthroscopic instrument breakage is not infrequent during meniscal surgery.[66,67] Occasionally, meniscal tissue can calcify and even normal basket forceps can inadvertently bite into this rock-like material and snap.[68,69]

Immediate action: Stop all inflow and outflow. Prepare to put suction on the arthroscope and inflow through a secondary cannula. Never begin an arthroscopic procedure without a magnetized retrieving device available. Depending on the size of the metallic fragment, a grasping instrument may be all that is necessary initially. If, however, the fragment cannot be located or it is located in an area that is not easily accessible by standard grasping forceps, a magnetized suction device can be utilized to attract the fragment to the tip of the device and transport it to a more accessible area within the knee. An accessory portal may be necessary to secure the free fragment. Use of fluoroscopy can be beneficial. Minimize the use of inflow and outflow during this process to avoid turbulent flow that will jettison the metallic fragments throughout the knee.

Prevention: Check preoperative radiographs and identify any evidence that there are ossicles in the knee. Always check surgical instruments prior to placing them in the knee. Establish a routine for inspecting the arthroscopic instruments and ensure that this maintenance is performed. Know the limitations of your delicate hand instruments and avoid biting into rock-hard substances. Use an arthroscopic probe to define the texture and quality of the tissue to be removed. Motorized cutting instruments can break off part of the blades if the sheath or arthroscope is touched. Avoid approaching the tip of the scope with the motorized blades turning.

IATROGENIC INJURIES TO THE KNEE

Capsular Ligamentous Injuries of the Knee

Excessive valgus stress may cause ligamentous tears of the medial collateral ligament especially when using a leg holder.[70] Lateral collateral ligament injury is rare because the visualization of the lateral compartment is less of a problem due to the posterior sloping of the tibial plateau and the decreased strain in the lateral collateral ligament associated with knee flexion.

Immediate action: No immediate action is necessary other than to define the extent of the injury. Avoid excessive valgus stress if medial collateral ligament injury is suspected. Enjoy the improved visualization and finish the procedure while gently maintaining the joint opening. Check the condition of the ACL, posterior cruciate ligament (PCL) and meniscal attachments to the medial collateral ligament during your thorough evaluation. Postoperatively the patient should be treated with protective weight bearing and appropriate bracing depending on the extent of the soft tissue injury.

Prevention: Preoperative physical examination and radiographs should alert the surgeon to anticipate tightly contracted knees at risk. Injury to the medial collateral ligament is most frequently seen in elderly patients with lateral joint narrowing. Visibility of the medial compartment is best obtained with the knee flexed 15 to 20 degrees and the foot externally rotated. Lateral compartment openings are obtained by internally rotating the foot and placing the knee in flexion from 15 to 90 degrees while applying a varus stress.

Vascular Injuries

The popliteal artery and vein are located just posteriorly and slightly lateral to the posterior tip of the lateral meniscus. Popliteal artery injury is extremely rare but five cases have been reported in the literature.[71] Arthroscopically, pulsatile bleeding from a large lumen may indicate a large vessel tear.

Immediate action: Obtain an immediate vascular surgery consultation in the operating room. Heparinize the patient and inflate the tourniquet. Prepare to roll the patient over for a posterior exposure by the vascular surgery consultant. Appropriate compartment release may be necessary.

Prevention: Visualize the action end of all cutting instruments. Be especially mindful when in the region of the PCL and the posterior lateral meniscus.

Pseudoaneurysms have been reported following arthroscopy.[72] The patient may present in the clinic with a symptomatic mass associated with a palpable thrill or occasionally there is unilateral swelling in the extremity.

Immediate action: Vascular consultation will most likely indicate elective bypass grafting or excision.

Prevention: Avoid inadvertent capsular penetration by cutting instrumentation, especially in the posterior lateral or posterior medial regions.

Nerve Injuries

Nerve injuries have been reported in association with meniscectomy to the infrapatellar branch of the saphenous nerve (Fig. 5.8). The nerve is most frequently injured by portal incisions.[70,73] The sartorial branch of the saphenous nerve can also be injured with posteromedial portal placement.

Immediate action: No action is required. Many of these injuries resolve with time. Documentation by electrodiagnostic study is recommended. These sensory nerve injuries may serve as a source of causalgia and appropriate neurectomy may be necessary.

Prevention: The infrapatella branch of the saphenous nerve is palpable at the joint line and is nearly horizontal in the region of the anteromedial portal. Careful portal placement utilizing topographic anatomy, digital palpation, and transillumination will prevent in-

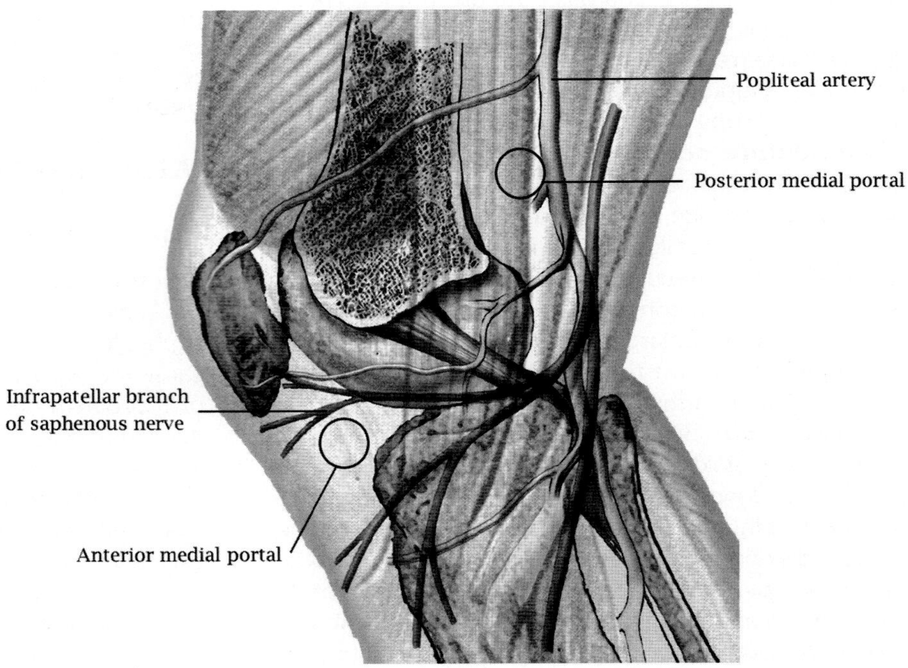

Figure 5.8. When the decision is made to excise the damaged meniscus, the goals are to resect the torn portion that is herniating into the central part of the joint to balance the rim and avoid catching, to preserve the capsular attachments of the meniscus.

juries not only to the saphenous nerve but also to other nerves in and around the knee. Knee position maintained during arthroscopy can prevent neurovascular injury. Flexion of the knee during diagnostic arthroscopy will cause the peroneal nerve to translate inferiorly to the biceps tendon away from the joint line and will also allow the tibial nerve to migrate posteriorly away from the capsule.[70] Any injury to a large motor nerve should be treated as an orthopedic emergency and urgent treatment is recommended (exploration and repair).

Articular Cartilage Damage

Articular cartilage damage is caused by poor arthroscopic instrument technique and may be partial (5 mm or less) or complete (greater than 5 mm with exposed bone) injuries. Only the complete injury should be treated.[70]

Immediate action: Complete chondral injuries with exposed bone greater than 5 mm should be treated. These lesions may be treated by abrasion chondroplasty, drilling, microfracture, or osteochondral transplant.

Prevention: Articular cartilage damage is most frequently caused by passing instruments into a tight compartment. This complication can be avoided by gradual stretching, with valgus and varus stress applied in a slow and steady fashion to the leg while the knee and thigh are held in a leg holder. In addition, elective release of the medial collateral ligament and tight capsule structures can be performed if visualization is still difficult. Instruments should be inspected regularly for sharp or rough edges. These damaged instruments should be repaired or replaced immediately.

Occasionally the meniscus in a tight knee cannot be well visualized. Moving the meniscus to the central portion of the joint will minimize the potential of chondral damage. By palpating the meniscus along the joint line with your digit it can be forcibly translated into the central portion of the compartment. A spinal needle passed into the body of the meniscus can be utilized to translate the meniscus into a more central position accessible to partial meniscectomy.[42]

Anterior and Posterior Cruciate Ligament Damage

The ACL, PCL, and meniscal femoral ligaments can become damaged by passing sharp or cutting instruments in the intercondylar notch. Care must be taken while resecting impinging synovial tissue or the ligamentous mucosum in the intercondylar notch.

Immediate action: Determine the extent of the damage to the vital structures by probing and physical examination. Rarely is there enough cruciate ligament removed to create instability. Partial tears may be treated with restricted activity for 3 to 4 months.

Prevention: Always pass sharp or cutting instruments in protective sheaths. Be especially careful with arthroscopic knives and, as always, visualize the action end of these instruments.

Portal Fistula

The reported incidences of synovial fistula is 6.1 per thousand arthroscopic procedures.[74]

Immediate action: Immobilize the extremity and take appropriate cultures to rule out any infection. Compression over the site of the open portal associated with immobilization allows gradual resolution over several days. Range of motion can be resumed as soon as the portal is closed. If there is evidence of infection, immediate excision of the portal tract, appropriate treatment with intravenous antibiotics, and serial arthroscopies and debridement are appropriate.

Prevention: Be aware that there is a higher incidence of portal fistula from posterior portals, especially in knees associated degenerative arthrosis. Consider deep and superficial sutures in these cases. There is a higher incidence of portal fistula from posterior portals especially in knees with associated degenerative arthrosis.

OTHER COMPLICATIONS

Complications of Discoid Meniscus Surgery

Symptomatic discoid menisci are best treated with partial meniscectomy and reattachment of the meniscus (Wrisberg type) to the capsule in those cases that are hypermobile. Balancing the rim of the meniscus minimizes the potential of residual symptoms of catching and locking. Discoid meniscus tissue is more frequently seen laterally than medially and as such the lateral neurovascular structures posteriorly are at risk during surgical procedures. After the meniscal tissue has been resected, methodical probing of the periphery will ensure that the meniscus is not unstable. Meniscal reattachment to the capsule can be performed arthroscopically or open.[42,57]

Complete Meniscectomies

Complete meniscectomies/subtotal meniscectomies are associated with loss of hoop stress in severe degenerative tears. Any time a complete or subtotal meniscectomy is being considered, care must be taken to avoid the genicular arteries, especially laterally, where they are in intimate contact with the meniscal tissue. The most common complication from complete or subtotal meniscectomy is early degenerative arthrosis. Gillquist et al[44,49] have demonstrated that the long-term follow-up of complete or subtotal meniscectomies performed arthroscopically, although having significant evidence of radiographic degenerative arthritis, have an acceptable functional level of activity.

Immediate action: Educate the patient about low-impact training. Follow these patients closely and intervene early if degenerative arthrosis occurs. If a complete or subtotal meniscectomy is performed in a young, active person, consideration could be given for meniscal allograft if pain develops postoperatively. However, the long-term success of this procedure has not been verified at this time.

References

1. Wan AC, Felle P. The menisco-femoral ligaments. *Clin Anat* 1995;8(5):323–326.
2. Yamamoto M, Hirohata K. Anatomical study on the menisco-femoral ligaments of the knee. *Kobe J Med Sci* 1991;37(4–5):209–226.
3. Simonian P, Sussman PS, Van Trommel M et al. Popliteomeniscal fasciculi and the unstable lateral meniscus: clinical correlation and magnetic resonance diagnosis. *Arthroscoy* 1997;13(5):590–596.
4. Thompson WO, Thaete FL, Fu F, et al. Tibial meniscal dynamics using three-dimensional reconstruction of magnetic resonance images. *Am J Sports Med* 1991;19(3): 210–215; discussion 215–216.
5. Bylski-Austrow DI, Ciarelli MJ, Kayner DC, et al. Displacements of the menisci under joint load: an in vitro study in human knees. *J Biomech* 1994;27(4):421–431.
6. Fithian DC, Kelly MA, Mow VC. Material properties and structure-function relationships in the menisci. *Clin Orthop* 1990;252:19–31.
7. Arnoczky SP, Warren RF. Microvasculature of the human meniscus. *Am J Sports Med* 1982;10(2):90–95.
8. Soren A. On the etiology of congenital malformation of the meniscus. *Arch Orthop Trauma Surg* 1985;104(5): 283–288.
9. Suzuki S, Mita F, Ogishima H. Double-layered lateral meniscus: a newly found anomaly. *Arthroscopy* 1991; 7(3):267–271.
10. Kim SJ, Kim HK. Reliability of the anterior drawer test, the pivot shift test, and the Lachman test. *Clin Orthop* 1995;317:237–242.
11. Lima D, Copp SN, Colwell CW Jr. Isolated lateral ring meniscus. Case report. *Am J Knee Surg* 1995;8(3): 117–118.
12. Ohana N, Plotquin D, Atar D. Bilateral hypoplastic lateral meniscus. *Arthroscopy* 1995;11(6):740–742.
13. Ikeuchi H. Meniscus surgery using the Watanabe arthroscope. *Orthop Clin North Am* 1979;10(3):629–642.
14. Ghosh P, Taylor TK. The knee joint meniscus. A fibrocartilage of some distinction. *Clin Orthop* 1987;224: 52–63.
15. Renström P, Johnson RJ. Anatomy and biomechanics of the menisci. *Clin Sports Med* 1990;9(3):523–538.
16. Levy IM, Torzilli PA, Warren RF. The effect of medial meniscectomy on anterior-posterior motion of the knee. *J Bone Joint Surg* 1982;64A(6):883–888.
17. Levy IM, et al. The effect of lateral meniscectomy on motion of the knee. *J Bone Joint Surg* 1989;71A(3): 401–406.
18. Radin EL, de Lamotte F, Maquet P. Role of the menisci in the distribution of stress in the knee. *Clin Orthop* 1984;185:290–294.
19. McBridge ID, Reid JG. Biomechanical considerations of the menisci of the knee. *Can J Sport Sci* 1988; 13(4):175–187.
20. Hoshino A, Wallace WA. Impact-absorbing properties of the human knee. *J Bone Joint Surg* 1987;69B(5): 807–811.
21. Walker PS, Erkman MJ. The role of the menisci in force transmission across the knee. *Clin Orthop* 1975;109: 184–192.
22. Wickiewicz TL. Meniscal injuries in the cruciate-deficient knee. *Clin Sports Med* 1990;9(3):681–694.
23. Thompson WO, Fu FH. The meniscus in the cruciate-deficient knee. *Clin Sports Med* 1993;12(4):771–796.
24. Bellabarba C, Bush-Joseph CA, Bach BR Jr. Patterns of meniscal injury in the anterior cruciate-deficient knee: a review of the literature. *Am J Orthop* 1997;26(1):18–23.
25. Rosenberg LS, Sherman MF. Meniscal injury in the anterior cruciate-deficient knee. A rationale for clinical decision-making. *Sports Med* 1992;13(6):423–432.
26. Meachim G. The state of knee meniscal fibrocartilage in Liverpool necropsies. *J Pathol* 1976;119(3):167–173.
27. Kulkarni VV, Chand K. Pathological anatomy of the aging meniscus. *Acta Orthop Scand* 1975;46(1):135–140.
28. Ogilvie-Harris DJ, Fitsialos DP. Arthroscopic management of the degenerative knee. *Arthroscopy* 1991;7(2): 151–157.
29. Casscells SW. The torn or degenerated meniscus and its relationship to degeneration of the weight-bearing areas of the femur and tibia. *Clin Orthop* 1978;132:196–200.
30. Cassells SW. The torn meniscus, the torn anterior cruciate ligament, and their relationship to degenerative joint disease. *Arthroscopy* 1985;1(1):28–32.
31. Lewandrowski KU, Muller J, Schollmeier G. Concomitant meniscal and articular cartilage lesions in the femorotibial joint. *Am J Sports Med* 1997;25(4):486–494.

32. Hede A, Hempel-Poulsen S, Jensen JS. Symptoms and level of sports activity in patients awaiting arthroscopy for meniscal lesions of the knee. *J Bone Joint Surg* 1990; 72A(4):550–552.

33. Ihara H, et al. Acute torn meniscus combined with acute cruciate ligament injury. Second look arthroscopy after 3-month conservative treatment. *Clin Orthop* 1994;307: 146–154.

34. DeHaven KE. Decision-making factors in the treatment of meniscus lesions. *Clin Orthip* 1990;252:49–54.

35. Kim SJ, Choi CH. Bilateral complete discoid medial menisci combined with anomalous insertion and cyst formation. *Arthroscopy* 1996;12(1):112–115.

36. Corea JR, Moussa M, al Orthman A. McMurray's test tested. *Knee Surg Sports Traumatol Arthrosc* 1994; 2(2):70–72.

37. Fairbanks TJ. Knee changes after meniscectomy. *J Bone Joint Surg* 1948;30B:664.

38. Noble J, Erat K. In defence of the meniscus. A prospective study of 200 meniscectomy patients. *J Bone Joint Surg* 1980;62B(1):7–11.

39. Noble J, Turner PG. The function, pathology, and surgery of the meniscus. *Clin Orthop* 1986;210:62–68.

40. Henning CE, Lynch MA. Current concepts of meniscal function and pathology. *Clin Sports Med* 1985;4(2): 259–265.

41. Cox J, Nye C, Schaefer W. The degenerative effects of partial and total resection of the medial meniscus in dog knees. *Clin Orthop* 1975;109:178–183.

42. Johnson L. *Arthroscopic Surgery: Principles and Practices,* 3rd ed, vol 2. St. Louis: CV Mosby, 1986.

43. Gillquist J, Boeryd B. Endoscopic total one-piece medial meniscectomy: its effect on the medial collateral ligament. *Acta Orthop Scand* 1982;53(4):619–623.

44. Gillquist J, Hamberg P, Lysholm J. Endoscopic partial and total meniscectomy. A comparative study with a short term follow up. *Acta Orthop Scand* 1982;53(6):975–979.

45. Newman AP, Daniels AU, Burks RT. Principles and decision making in meniscal surgery. *Arthroscopy* 1993; 9(1):33–51.

46. Burks RT, Metcalf MH, Metcalf RW. Fifteen-year follow-up of arthroscpic partial meniscectomy. *Arthroscopy* 1997;13(6):673–679.

47. Hede A, Larsen E, Sandberg H. The long term outcome of open total and partial meniscectomy related to the quantity and site of the meniscus removed. *Int Orthop* 1992;16(2):122–125.

48. Faun P, Nielsen AB. Arthroscopic partial meniscectomy: a long-term follow-up. *Arthroscopy* 1992;8(3):345–349.

49. Rockborn P, Gillquist J. Long-term results after arthroscopic meniscectomy. The role of preexisting cartilage fibrillation in a 13 year follow-up of 60 patients. *Int J Sports Med* 1996;17(8):608–613.

50. Whipple TL, Caspari RB, Meyers JF. Arthroscopic meniscectomy. An interim report at three to four years after operation. *Clin Orthop* 1984;183:105–114.

51. Jaureguito JW, et al. The effects of arthroscopic partial lateral meniscectomy in an otherwise normal knee: a retrospective review of functional, clinical, and radiographic results. *Arthroscopy* 1995;11(1):29–36.

52. Jurgensen U, et al. Long-term follow-up of meniscectomy in athletes. A prospective longitudinal study. *J Bone Joint Surg* 1987;69B(1):80–83.

53. Gillies H, Seligson D. Precision in the diagnosis of meniscal lesions: a comparison of clinical evaluation, arthrography, and arthroscopy. *J Bone Joint Surg* 1979;61A(3): 343–346.

54. Gillquist J. Operative arthroscopy. *Endoscopy* 1980; 12(6):281–287.

55. Del Pizzo W, Fox JM. Results of arthroscopic meniscectomy. *Clin Sports Med* 1990;9(3):633–639.

56. Hamberg P, Gillquist J. Knee function after arthroscopic meniscectomy. A prospective study. *Acta Orthop Scand* 1984;55(2):172–175.

57. Ikeuchi H. Arthroscopic treatment of the discoid meniscus. Technique and long-term results. *Clin Orthop* 1982;167:19–28.

58. Dimakopoulos P, Patel D. Partial excision of discoid meniscus. Arthroscopic operation of 10 patients. *Acta Orthop Scand* 1990;61(1):40–41.

59. Johnson LL, et al. Is it possible to make an accurate diagnosis based only on a medical history? A pilot study on women's knee joints. *Arthroscopy* 1996;12(6):709–714.

60. Tolin BS, Sapega AA. Arthroscopic visual field mapping at the periphery of the medial meniscus: a comparison of different portal approaches. *Arthroscopy* 1993;9(3): 265–271.

61. Patel D. Proximal approaches to arthroscopic surgery of the knee. *Am J Sports Med* 1981;9(5):296–303.

62. Gold DL, Schaner PJ, Sapega AA. The posteromedial portal in knee arthroscopy: an analysis of diagnostic and surgical utility. *Arthroscopy* 1995;11(2):139–145.

63. Goldner RD, Kulund DN, McCue FCD. The "blind side" of the medial meniscus. *Am J Sports Med* 1980; 8(5):337–341.

64. Mohr M, Henche HR. The morbidity associated with lost or irretrievable resected meniscal fragments. *Arthroscopy* 1992;8(1):84–88.

65. Janecki CJ, Hechtman KS. Prepatella bursitis: a complication of arthroscopic surgery of the knee due to a lost meniscus fragment. *Arthroscopy* 1989;5(4):342–343.

66. Small NC. Complications in arthroscopic surgery performed by experienced arthroscopists. *Arthroscopy* 1988;4(3):215–221.

67. Small NC. Complications in arthroscopic meniscal surgery. *Clin Sports Med* 1990;9(3):609–617.

68. Conforty B, Lotem M. Ossicles in human menisci: report of two cases. *Clin Orthop* 1979;144:272–275.

69. Liu SH, et al. Meniscal ossicles: two case reports and a review of the literature. *Arthroscopy* 1994;10(3):296–298.

70. Sprague N III. Minor and soft tissue complications. In: Sprague N III, ed. *Complications in Arthroscopy*. New York: Raven Press, 1989:125–142.

71. Tawes RL Jr, et al. Popliteal artery injury complicating arthroscopic menisectomy. *Am J Surg* 1988;156(2):136–138.

72. Ritt MJ, et al. Popliteal pseudoaneurysm after arthroscopic menisectomy. A report of two cases. *Clin Orthop* 1993;295:198–200.

73. Mochida H, Kukuchi S. Injury to the infrapatella branch of the saphenous nerve in arthroscopic knee surgery. *Clin Orthop* 1995;320:88–94.

74. Proffer DS, Drez DJ, Daus GP. Synovial fistula of the knee: a complication of arthroscopy. *Arthroscopy* 1991;7(1):98–100.

Chapter 6

Complications and Pitfalls in Arthroscopic Meniscus Repair

James S. Mulhollan

Repair of knee menisci was championed and popularized by DeHaven[1] as an open procedure in the early 1980s. Coincidentally, arthroscopic surgery, which was introduced at about the same time, was found to provide reduced morbidity and improved results for much of the pathology of the knee joint. Naturally, arthroscopic concepts were applied to the problem of meniscus repair. Numerous surgeons contributed to developing arthroscopic meniscus repair techniques including Henning,[2] Stone and Miller,[3] Cannon,[4] Rosenberg et al,[5] Warren,[6] Morgan and Casscells,[7] and others. Although complications occurred from the beginning, the frequency of complications became apparent when the Arthroscopic Association of North America's (AANA) complication committee reported its retrospective analysis of 395,566 arthroscopies in 1986.[8] Complications occurred along with meniscus repair in 2.4% of cases, almost five times the background complication rate of 0.56% in all arthroscopic cases.

A review of Table 6.1 from the AANA report provides insight into the spectrum of complications that occurred with early efforts at meniscus repair. Significant sophistication of repair techniques, coupled with the experience of arthroscopists, quickly made arthroscopic meniscus repair less hazardous. In the earliest efforts at meniscus repair, sutures were often tied over an external bolster. An unacceptable level of skin sloughs, as well as superficial and deep infections, caused this practice to be abandoned. By tying knots within incisions over fascial layers, instead of externally, infection became no more likely than with other arthroscopic procedures.

Chairman Small's[9] follow-up report from AANA's complication committee in 1988 on 10,262 procedures, performed by experienced arthroscopists, studied prospectively, revealed that meniscus repair was no more dangerous than the procedure of arthroscopy itself. Many of the possible complications of arthroscopic meniscus repair are no more likely than with the alternative treatment of arthroscopic menisectomy, these complications include hemarthrosis, thrombophlebitis and embolism, instrument breakage, anesthesia accidents, allergic reactions, fracture, ligament injury, and adhesions.

There is, however, a unique set of complications specific to arthroscopic meniscus repair, along with numerous pitfalls that even without complications interfere with efficacy and reduce application of the procedure. These pitfalls may lead to an increased rate of reoperation and probably increased cost. Selection of certain diagnostic and repair techniques potentially lessens the impact of these factors. Adequate performance of diagnostic techniques and realistic patient selection are the most important variables.

ANATOMIC CONSIDERATIONS

The work of Arnoczky and Warren[10] established that menisci heal by fibrovascular proliferation. Meniscus tears with the potential for healing are located in the posterior and peripheral aspects of the joint. Posteromedially, the saphenous vein and nerves are subject to injury. Posterolaterally, the peroneal nerve is at risk. The popliteal neurovascular bundle, though lateral to the midline, can be injured with both lateral and medial meniscus repair, just as it can be injured during routine arthroscopy.[8,11]

Table 6.1. Arthroscopic Association of North America 1986 meniscus repair complications: 3,034 cases studied retrospectively (8)

Complication	*Occurrences*
Saphenous nerve injuries	30
Deep infections	11
Superficial infections over button or bolster	11
Peroneal nerve injuries	6
Vascular injuries	3
Phlebitis	3
Pulmonary embolism (fatal)	1
Equipment failure	1
Skin slough	1
Other complications	6
Total	73

Posteromedial Structures at Risk

The saphenous nerve and vein course together across the posteromedial knee, deep and closely associated with the pes anserine tendon group. Their exact location varies from moment to moment along with the flexion position of the knee joint. In extension, the structures are anterior to the posteromedial corner of the joint and with the knee in flexion they move posterior to the corner. Because patients are recumbent on an operating table, the nerve and vein lie below the level of the joint line and almost parallel to it with the knee flexed 90 degrees. In full extension, the structures are drawn upward under greater tension and lie above the posteromedial corner perpendicular to the meniscus.

Posteromedial incisions, both for entrance into the knee (for open repair[1]) or for protection of the structures during inside-out meniscus repair, are placed anterior to the pes tendon group and the neurovascular structures. A retractor easily displaces the nerve and vein posteriorly in positions of knee flexion but tends to put tension on these structures with the knee closer to full extension. Maximum visualization of the posterior part of the medial meniscus demands an extended, or at least a slightly flexed, knee stressed against a leg holder.

When inside-out meniscus repair was performed without a protective posteromedial incision, the saphenous nerve was sometimes included within tied sutures. Although this is prevented with the protective incision, stretch injuries still occur. In the mid-1980s, Stone et al[12] reported a 10% transient saphenous nerve neuropraxia with medial inside-out repair and Barber[13] reported 22% neuropraxia. Although most saphenous neuropraxia caused by a stretch mechanism appears to be transient, the risk of injury to the saphenous nerve is potentially very harmful. Poehling[14] reported that 100% of 35 patients with reflex sympathetic dystrophy of the knee region demonstrated historical or physical evidence of having an insult to the infrapatellar branch of the saphenous nerve. Early symptoms of saphenous injury include hypersthesia, numbness, and a positive Tinel's sign. Pain is a rare complaint.

Warren[6] and Morgan and Casscells[7] have described meniscus repair from outside into the knee interior, the outside-in repair. Because the popliteal neurovascular bundle is lateral to the midline, and because full knee extension displaces the saphenous vein and nerve anterior to the posteromedial corner, a relative safe zone allows for the posterior one-third of the meniscus to be instrumented directly using a spinal needle without a protective incision. Morgan[15] reported only one saphenous nerve injury in 350 outside-in meniscus repairs.

The risk of saphenous nerve injury, coupled with the morbidity of posteromedial incisions, led to the author's enthusiasm for the all-inside type of meniscus repair. The technique is described by Morgan[15] and uses special instrumentation (Spectrum Soft Tissue Repair, Linvatec, Largo, FL). On the medial side of the knee, a posteromedial puncture is made by this technique; a 70-degree arthroscope views the posteromedial compartment. If room lights are dimmed, the arthroscopic light is transilluminated to reveal the optimal location for placement of a posteromedial puncture and often reveals the saphenous vein lying at the lower and posterior margin of the lighted spot. Through almost 100 of these repairs dating from 1989, there have been no neurovascular injuries in the author's series. Morgan[16] has a similar experience. Complications from posterior portals have been reported by Ogilvie-Harris et al.[17] In 179 posteromedial punctures they report three saphenous nerve injuries, including one neuroma and two saphenous vein lacerations, both detected intraoperatively. I have previously described the specific technique for passage of an arthroscope through the intercondylar notch.[18] This technique is necessary to provide transillumination.

Meniscus repair from anterior approaches using biodegradable implants such as the meniscus repair dart (Bionix, Blue Bell, PA) or the T-Fix (Acufex, Newton, MA), do not place posteromedial structures at risk, which might represent an advantage of these techniques.

Posterolateral Structures at Risk

The peroneal nerve passes the knee joint closely associated with the posteromedial corner of the biceps tendon. It crosses the lateral head of the gastrocnemius to curve around the upper fibula and enter the anterolateral compartment. Unlike with the saphenous nerve, peroneal injury frequently causes motor loss, even foot-drop. An injury to this structure has greater consequence than does neurologic injury medially.

Jurist et al[19] report a very instructive case regarding the potential of injury to the peroneal nerve. An incision was made anterior to the biceps and behind the lateral collateral ligament for insertion of a retractor to protect the peroneal nerve. Despite knee flexion and the retractor, inside-out sutures entrapped the peroneal nerve. The patient had severe pain and loss of peroneal function. Jurist et al explored the nerve and found one stitch encircling the structure and another putting traction on it. The report suggests that recovery is possible in this situation; pain resolved and nerve function returned at 6 months (even though the nerve did not function at 3 months). Jurist et al concluded that a posterolateral incision has to be developed deep to the lateral head of the gastrocnemius, not just anterior to the biceps.

I am unable to find any report suggesting that peroneal injury occurs with any significant frequency, and it certainly occurs much less often than saphenous nerve injury. This is no doubt due to the fact that a flexion knee position is necessary to view the lateral meniscus well enough to perform a repair; the flexion position allows the peroneal nerve to move posteriorly with reduced tension, out of harm's way.

When a posterolateral portal is made using transillumination for the all-inside meniscus repair, the patient is recumbent and the knee flexed 90 degrees. The transilluminated spot is above the biceps and above the nerve. This location is nerve free.

Popliteal Structures at Risk

The popliteal neurovascular bundle is located lateral to the midline and very close to the most posterocentral end of the lateral meniscus. While knee extension draws the entire neurovascular bundle against the posterior capsule, flexion allows the bundle to move away from the posterior knee, more at levels proximal to the knee than below the level of the menisci. This is because the structures enter the calf musculature and are held closely against the proximal tibia.

AANA's retrospective study of 1986 included nine popliteal artery injuries in the approximate 375,000 cases reported.[8] There were none in the 8,741 cases of arthroscopy by experienced arthroscopists reported in 1988.[9] Furie et al[20] suggest that conditions altering normal anatomy are most likely to lead to popliteal artery injury.

TECHNIQUE-RELATED COMPLICATIONS

Certain complications are specifically related to the technique of meniscus repair. In most cases the frequency of these problems cannot be exactly tabulated.

Inside-Out Technique

The possibility and probability of posteromedial and posterolateral neurologic complications are considered above. I have had one case of a synovial cyst created by tying inside-out sutures over the fascia. It required open excision of the cyst and the associated polypropylene suture. The nonabsorbable suture may have been the cause of this problem.

Outside-In Technique

Morgan[16] describes entrapment of the posterior capsule as a complication of the outside-in method. Theoretically, this problem could also occur with the inside-out method as well. Permanent restriction of extension by this mechanism would seem unlikely.

All-Inside Technique

It is occasionally necessary to combine this technique with one of the above methods, such as when the tear extends too far anterior to instrument from within the posterior compartments, or when the tear is not peripheral enough to turn the repair needle under the overlying condyle. These problems represent limitations of the procedure rather than complications. I have had to abandon efforts to repair menisci by the all-inside method in cases where tissue is too hard to penetrate with the repair needles, where visibility is limited due to fluid extravasation, and where space is limited due to the patient's anatomy. These factors impact inside-out repairs to a lesser extent.

Meniscus Darts

Bionix (Blue Bell, PA) introduced bioabsorbable polylactic acid repair darts to the American market in 1995. I am unaware of any untoward reaction to the dart itself, which is left inside the joint to be eventually absorbed. A local complication can occur with excessive implant length. I placed a 13-mm dart at the posteromedial corner of a meniscus in a thin patient for the purpose of supplementing a direct all-inside repair of the patient's posterior one-third tear. At 18 months, the tip of the dart was readily palpable, but symptoms did not warrant removal. Absorption of these darts is quite slow; I have found darts still visible after almost 2 years. Their slow absorption might cause them to act as stress risers.

On several occasions, I have broken darts during insertion. This happens when the repair cannula skids before the repair arrow is fully inserted. The straight repair cannula has a side arm through which a small pin is placed to stabilize cannula position. It is unfortunate that this feature is not available in curved cannula configurations.

TECHNICAL CONSIDERATIONS

Numerous technical factors influence the application and success of meniscus repair. Of specific concern is the quality of the diagnostic exam that is an integral part of the treatment of every patient. Other considerations include knot tying, coincidental treatment of ligament injuries, rehabilitation protocol, and patient selection.

The Recognition of Repairable Tears

Quin and Brown[21] discussed nine apparent false-positive meniscus tear diagnoses established with magnetic resonance imaging (MRI) examination of 254 cases. They concluded that the posterior compartments in these patients were not adequately visualized arthroscopically and that the tears present were probably missed. Gillquist et al[22] noted that in 39 of 68 cases, the posteriomedial compartment could not be visualized from an anterolateral arthroscope insertion site. Gillguest et al and Mulhollan[18] advocate insertion of the arthroscope in the midline through the patellar tendon. In almost every case the arthroscope can be passed through the intercondylar notch, and the posterior attachment of the meniscus can be viewed directly with the 70-degree arthroscope. Johnson[23] described a direct puncture into the posterior compartments for arthroscope placement in 1977, and Gold et al[24] in 1995 described the use of a flexible nylon guide rod (Smith & Nephew Dyonics, Andover, MA) like a switching stick to establish posteromedial arthroscope placement. All of these techniques allow recognition of the tears that are the most peripheral, most vascular, and most likely to heal if repaired. The Gillquist-Mulhollan technique allows application of the all-inside repair technique.

I have performed MRIs on all cases of anterior cruciate ligament (ACL) injury for the last 2 years. In almost 20% of cases there was a peripheral meniscal detachment undetected by the MRI. Complete arthroscopy is the only technique with which all the repairable tears occurring in ligament cases can be recognized. It is impossible to guess at the frequency of arthroscopy that is performed without posterior compartment visualization. Representatives of arthroscopy instrumentation companies, many of whom have watched thousands of procedures, have estimated (in personal communication with the author) that the posterior compartment is examined in less than one-third of cases, and that 70-degree arthroscopy is utilized in less than one in five cases.

Knot Tying

I initially patented a knot-tying device and a method of sewing inside a body cavity in 1986 as part of early efforts to perform an all-inside meniscus repair (U.S. Patent no. 4,602,635, July 29, 1986, Mulhollan and Starr). Although this technique of knot tying was described in 1989 in product literature (Baxter, Santa Ana, CA; more recently, Linvatec, Largo, FL), it had not yet been applied. I finally performed all-inside meniscus repair in 1989, and continue to utilize the technique. Recently the quality of tied knots has been considered in significant detail (Figure 6.1). The knot configuration on the left is the knot that I have used since 1986. Rimmer et al[26] demonstrated that vertical stitches have twice the pullout strength as horizontal stitches. Berry knots and meniscus darts have pullout resistance about equal to horizontal sutures.[27–29] There is an advantage to the all-inside technique in that the stitches placed by this technique are vertical.

A significant advantage exists when a placed suture slides through the tissue that is being tied. Several described repair techniques yield placed sutures that will not slide. Berry knots and the T-Fix devise are examples.[30] The knots in Fig. 6.1 require sliding sutures. Without sliding, tension is hard to maintain even with knot tying devices. Outside the knee, an incision long enough to admit the fingertip is necessary. If tension is established with a slip knot, an incision no longer than what is necessary to admit a knot pusher is needed. Without a sliding stitch, I have found significant difficulty in maintaining enough tension to adequately establish repair apposition.

Suture Material

I sewed many mensci, using open techniques, between 1980 and 1989, without performing intraarticular stabilization; that was generally not possible during that era. There was a rather high recurrent tear rate, approaching 15%. In the overwhelming majority of these cases, the new tear was completely inside the original tear plane. In two of these cases, the tear occurred at the suture line.

Some authors have advocated the use of absorbable sutures, which might lessen the possibility that a nonabsorbable suture might act as a "stress riser." I feel that there is a beneficial effect of permanent marking, that is, the use of nonabsorbable sutures (in my experience, Prolene, manufactured by Ethicon, Somerville, NJ), for academic evaluation of failed repairs. It also has the beneficial side effect of being quite slippery and, therefore, easy to use for tying a knot intraarticularly.

Coincident Treatment of Ligament Injuries

Numerous reports demonstrate enhanced success when meniscus repair is performed at the same time as ligament reconstruction. Barber and Click[31] reported 92% success when the two procedures were performed to-

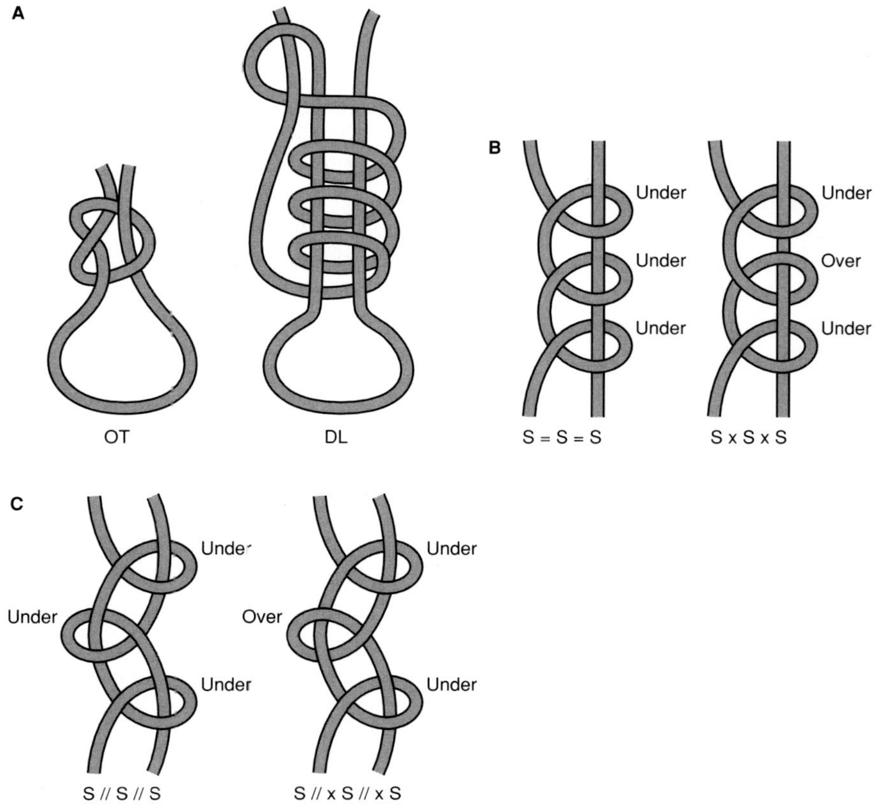

Figure 6.1. **A:** The slip knot configurations shown here were used initially to remove slack from the suture loop. The OT configuration designates the complex Duncan Loop configuration. **B:** The half-hitch configurations shown represent two combinations that do not incorporate post switching. The labels *Under* and *Over* indicate the direction for the initial pass around the post when making each half-hitch loop. Note that the directions of the half-hitch loops are reversed for the S × S × S configuration. **C:** The half-hitch configurations shown represent two combinations that incorporate post switching and reversal of the loop direction. Note that the S// × S// × S configuration combines post switching and loop direction reversal.

gether. Without reconstruction the success rate was only 67%, equal to that of repair in stable knees. Presumably the hemarthrosis associated with ligament repair bathes the repair site with fibrin. No doubt reduced movement between the femur and tibia is a contributing factor. Meniscus avulsion, the best situation for repair, is found almost exclusively in ACL cases. Jensen et al[32] reported improved results with concurrent reconstruction and meniscus repair, as did Asahina et al.[33] They found age insignificant, an observation shared by Barber and the author. Cannon and Vittor[34] achieved good results in older patients and better results laterally. I believe that many lateral tears in cruciate ligament cases heal spontaneously.[35] Asahina had better results with peripheral tears, which of course occur with much greater frequency in ligament cases.[36]

Rehabilitation Protocol

Barber[36] reported that accelerated rehabilitation did not compromise outcome. When it became apparent that early movement and restoration of function enhanced the outcome of cruciate reconstruction, I abandoned any restrictions with meniscus repair cases. Success at healing in my ACL cases equals that of Barber. I believe that successful meniscus repair in cruciate ligament cases enhances the result of reconstruction. Despite increased operating room time and costs and the small risk of complications, meniscus repair in the treatment of the unstable knee is easily justified.

Patient Selection

Elsewhere I describe a detailed consideration of meniscus tear patterns and the selection of patients.[35] I believe that meniscus repair is appropriately reserved for the traumatic injury to normal healthy tissue. These injuries occur in almost one-fourth of ligament injury cases and healing occurs with high reliability. By contrast, Schimmer et al[37] observed that favorable outcomes decreased from 90% to 63% when meniscus repair was performed in patients with joint surface pathology, that is, early degeneration. In many patients, especially those with stable knees, squatting occupations, and increased age, meniscal tissue fragments and tears are due to attrition, often with trivial trauma.

Burks and Metcalf[38] tabulated Robert W. Metcalf's patients available for follow-up; 88% of menisectomy patients had good or excellent results at 15 years. In view of this outcome, it is difficult to subject stable knee patients to meniscus repair, especially in view of increased costs and the frequency of failure to heal, leading to reoperation; this might occur in 30% to 40% of cases.

SUCCESS OF MENISCUS REPAIR

Arnoczky et al[39] reported that the MRI did not conclusively prove that meniscus repair had been successful. Neither can the clinical status of the patient, since it is impossible to conclude whether patients, presently asymptomatic, will continue to remain so. I have observed meniscus repair failure as late as 12 years. Haribe et al,[40] who examined meniscus repair patients arthroscopically, reported excellent results in 56%, good in 28%, and poor in 16%, a lesser success rate than Metcalf's arthroscopic menisectomy results described above.

CONCLUSION

Saphenous nerve neuropraxia is the most frequent complication of arthroscopic meniscus repair and is potentially serious. The occurrence of this complication is probably reduced with the outside-in and all-inside repair techniques, as well as with procedures performed by anterior approaches such as the meniscus dart.

The success of meniscus repair is high in ACL patients when the procedure is performed along with ACL reconstruction. It is less reliable in stable knees if performed as an isolated procedure or if utilized in patients with joint surface pathology. Its application in these cases is costly and may lead to eventual reoperation. Similarly, overapplication of the meniscus repair concept may lead to unnecessary reoperation and added costs. Burks and Metcalf[38] made the following observation: "The result of partial menisectomy in a stable knee is good enough that the morbidity of heroic measures to save complex tears of the meniscus may need close scrutiny."

It is probable that incomplete arthroscopy, meaning failure to examine the posterior compartments, is the most frequent pitfall affecting eventual outcome. Without examination of the posterior compartments, the best tears for repair are probably missed.

References

1. DeHaven KE. Peripheral meniscus repair an alternative to meniscectomy. *J Bone Joint Surg* 1981;63B:463.
2. Henning CE. Arthroscopic repair of meniscus tears. *Orthopedics* 1983;6 1130–1132.
3. Stone RG, Miller GA. A technique of arthroscopic suture of torn menisci. *Arthroscopy* 1985;1:226–232.
4. Cannon WD. Meniscal repair, combined open/closed techniques and results. Paper presented at the fall meeting of the Arthroscopy Association of North America, Pine Mt., GA. *Arthroscopic Meniscus Repair* Sept 1986: 14–17.
5. Rosenberg TD, Scott S, Paulos L. Arthroscopic surgery: repair of peripheral detachment of the meniscus. *Contemp Orthop* 1985;10:43–50.
6. Warren RF. Meniscus repair: outside-in technique and results. Paper presented at the fall meeting of the Arthroscopy Association of North America, 1986; Pine Mountain, GA.
7. Morgan CD, Casscells, SW. Arthroscopic meniscus repair: a safe approach to the posterior horns. *Arthroscopy* 1986;2:3–12.
8. Small NC. Complications in arthroscopy: the knee and other joints. Committee on Complications of the Arthroscopy Associaton of North America. *Arthroscopy* 1986; 2:253.
9. Small NC. Complications in arthroscopy performed by experienced arthroscopists. *Arthroscopy* 1988;4:215.
10. Arnoczky SP, Warren RP. Microvasculature of the human meniscus. *Am J Sports Med* 1982;10(2):90–95.
11. Furie E, Yerys P, Cutcliffe D. Risk factors for arthroscopic popliteal artery laceration. *Arthroscopy* 1995;11(3): 324–327.
12. Stone RG, Frewin PR, Gonzales S. Long term assessment of arthroscopic meniscus repair: a two to six year follow-up study. *Arthroscopy* 1990;6:73–78.
13. Barber FA. Meniscus repair: results of arthroscopic technique. *Arthroscopy* 1987;3:25–30.
14. Poehling GG, Pollock FE Jr., Koman LA. Reflex sympathetic dystrophy of the knee after sensory nerve injury. *Arthroscopy* 1988;4(1):31–35.
15. Morgan CD. Technical note. The "all-inside" meniscus repair. *Oper Tech Sports Med* 1994;2:201.
16. Morgan CD, Meniscus repair-the all-inside arthroscopic technique. In: Jackson DW, ed. *Reconstructive Knee Surgery—Master's Techniques in Orthopaedic Surgery*. New York: Raven Press, 1995:87–97.
17. Ogilvie-Harris DJ, Biggs DJ, Mackay M, et al. Posterior portals for arthroscopic surgery of the knee. *Arthroscopy* 1994;10(6):608–613.
18. Muhollan JS. Swedish arthroscopic approach. *Orthop Clin North Am* 1982;13:349–362.
19. Jurist KA, Greene PW 3d, Shirkhoda A. Peroneal nerve dysfunction as a complication of lateral meniscus repair: a case report and anatomic dissection. *Arthroscopy* 1989;5(2):141–147.
20. Furie E, Yerys P, Cutcliffe D, et al. Risk factors for arthroscopic popliteal artery laceration. *Arthroscopy* 1995; 11(3):324–327.
21. Quin SP, Brown, TF. Meniscus tears diagnosed with MR imaging versus arthroscopy: how reliable a standard is arthroscopy? *Radiology* 1991;181:843–847.
22. Gillquist J, Hagberg G, Oretorp N. Arthroscopic visualization of the posteromedial compartment of the knee joint. *Orthop Clin North Am* 1979;10:545–547.

23. Johnson LL. *Comprehensive Arthroscopic Examination of the Knee*. St. Louis: CV Mosby, 1977:50–53.
24. Gold DL, Schaner PJ, Sapega AA. The posteromedial portal in knee arthroscopy: an analysis of diagnostic and surgical utility. *Arthroscopy* 1995;11(2):139–145.
25. Loutzenheiser TD, Harryman DT 2nd, Yung SW, et al. Optimizing arthroscopic knots. *Arthroscopy* 1995;11(2): 199–206.
26. Rimmer MG, Nawana NS, Keene GC. Failure strengths of different meniscal suturing techniques. *Arthroscopy* 1995;11(2):146–150.
27. Post WR, Akers SR, Kish V. Load to failure of common meniscal repair techniques: effects of suture technique and suture material. *Arthroscopy* 1997;13(6):731–736.
28. Dervin GF, Downing KJ, Keene GG, et al. Failure strength of suture versus biodegradable arrow for meniscal repair: an in vitro study. *Arthroscopy* 1997;13(3): 296–300.
29. Albrecht-Olsen P, Lind T, Kristensen G, et al. Failure strength of a new meniscus arrow repair technique: biomechanical comparison with horizontal suture. *Arthroscopy* 1997;13(2):183–187.
30. Barrett GR, et al. T-Fix endoscopic meniscus repair: technique and approach to different types of tears. *Arthroscopy* 1995;11(2):245–251.
31. Barber FA, Click DMA. Meniscus repair rehabilitation with concurrent anterior cruciate reconstruction. *Arthroscopy* 1997;13(4):433–437.
32. Jensen NC, Rils J, Robertsen K, et al. Arthroscopic repair of the ruptured meniscus: one to 6.3 years follow-up. *Arthroscopy* 1994;10(2):211–214.
33. Asahina S, Muneta T, Yamamoto H. Arthroscopic meniscal repair in conjunction with anterior cruciate ligament reconstruction: factors affecting the healing rate. *Arthroscopy* 1996;12(5):541–545.
34. Cannon WD, Vittor JM. The incidence of healing in arthroscopic meniscus repairs in anterior cruciate ligament–reconstructed knees versus stable knees. *Am J Sports Med* 1992;20:176–181.
35. Mulhollan JS. Arthroscopic meniscus repair: indications and techniques. In: Chow JCY, ed. *Advanced Arthroscopy*. New York: Springer-Verlag, 1999: in press.
36. Barber FA. Accelerated rehabilitation for meniscus repair. *Arthroscopy* 1994;10(2):211–214.
37. Schimmer RC, Brulhart KB, Duff C, et al. Arthroscopic partial meniscectory: a 12 year follow-up and two step evaluation of the long term course. *Arthroscopy* 1998; 14(2):136–142.
38. Burks RT, Metcalf, MH. Fifteen year follow-up of arthroscopic partial meniscectomy. *Arthroscopy* 1997;13(6): 673–679.
39. Arnoczky SP, Cooper TG, Stadelmaier DM, et al. Magnetic resonance siginals in healing menisci: an expermental study in dogs. *Arthroscopy* 1994;10(5): 552–557.
40. Haribe S, et al. Results of isolated meniscal repair evaluated by second-look arthroscopy. *Arthroscopy* 1996; 12(2):150–155.

Chapter 7

COMPLICATIONS AND PITFALLS IN MENISCAL TRANSPLANTATION

Jeff C. Brand, Jr. and Darren L. Johnson

The loss of meniscal cartilage is a tragedy for the knee joint.[1] Meniscal transplantation has evolved because of this simple fact. Meniscal transplantation is a recent development, and the first one was performed in Europe in 1984. Improvements in allograft choices, patient selection, choice of concomitant procedures, and appropriate preparation make this surgery safe and effective.

PROCESSING

Of the choices the surgeon makes preoperatively, patient selection is arguably the most important, rivaled primarily by the choice of allograft tissue and choice of concomitant procedure. Meniscal allografts vary on the method of preparation and secondary sterilization.

Fresh Meniscal Allografts

Some of the best results in the literature come from using fresh meniscal allografts.[2,3] Fresh implants are harvested under sterile conditions and used shortly thereafter, usually within 6 days.[2] During this period of time, they are maintained in cell culture. The advantages are cell viability and mechanical integrity.[4] Siegel and Roberts[5] note that fresh allografts had comparatively good results, which suggests that a viable meniscal chondrocyte population may have a beneficial effect on the long-term survival and function of the graft. But basic science research on this topic disputes this assertion. In a goat study using deoxyribonucleic acid (DNA) probes, all the cells in a transplanted meniscus were replaced with recipient cells by 4 weeks after implantation.[6] Presently, it is unclear what advantage donor cells offer in the first 4 weeks after transplantation.

Unfortunately, there are a plethora of disadvantages, both theoretical and practical. Fresh allografts are limited to hospitals that have an active transplant harvesting program. These tissues are difficult to handle and to maintain their sterility. Sizing is difficult and patients have to be implanted on an urgent basis.[7] Disease transmission is a greater concern, as prevention rests on donor screening (Table 7.1). Because a window of time exists between contraction of the human immunodeficiency virus (HIV) particle and seroconversion, it is possible, although unlikely, to implant a meniscus with the acquired immunodeficiency syndrome (AIDS) virus. These allografts can be gamma sterilized; however, present science suggests that the dose required to inactivate the AIDS virus unfavorably alters the mechanical properties.[8,9] The dose of gamma irradiation necessary to kill the HIV particle is 3.0 Mrad by polymerase chain reaction (PCR) testing.[8] Freezing alters the antigenicity of the meniscus allograft, so if there were to be an immune reaction in transplantation, it is more likely in a fresh allograft. Garrett[2,3] has two reported series with fresh allografts. The first series reported in 1991 consisted of six patients, of whom four had second-look arthroscopy and all four appeared to be healed. In the second series published in 1993, 16 patients had fresh transplants; 13 second-look arthroscopies were performed and 12 patients had healed.

Cryopreserved Grafts

After harvesting the allograft, it is placed in a medium such as glycerol to maintain cell viability, and it is sequentially and slowly frozen and maintained at −130°C. The grafts undergo a form of secondary sterilization, usually gamma irradiation.[10] The advantage of this tech-

Table 7.1. Screening of donors

Investigation	*Exclusion Critieria*
Social history	Intravenous drug abusers
	Prostitutes
	Homosexuals
	Runaways
Medical history	Infection
	Neoplasia
Blood tests	Syphilis
	Hepatitis B/C
	HIV
Allograft cultures	Bacterial/fungal infection
Autopsy	Lymph node involvement

(From ref. 64, with permission.)

nique is that cell viability ranges from 10% to 40%, depending on the study.[11,12] Again, the role of cell viability is unsupported in basic science at this time. This is an expensive and technically difficult technique.[4] Garrett,[3] in his 1993 report, included 27 patients with cryopreserved transplants, and there were 15 second-look arthroscopies. Eight patients appeared healed, and seven had loss of a major portion of the meniscus or failure to heal at the periphery. The other 12 transplants were not studied by second-look arthroscopy and were considered "silent," that is, without clinical symptoms.

Fresh Frozen Grafts

After sterile harvest of the meniscus, it is frozen to −70° to −130°C for storage. The tissue is maintained at this temperature until it is thawed for clinical use. The meniscus is easily transported and stored. This relatively simple technique of preservation denatures the histocompatibility antigens, decreasing the probability of an immune response.[13] Fresh freezing destroys donor cells. The meniscus appears to repopulate with host synovial cells, but this is in the periphery, and the central core may remain acellular.[14,15] The collagen framework of the meniscus is largely maintained in the animal studies to date,[13] although Arnoczky et al[14,15] have noted alteration in the superficial layer of the collagen structure with some subsequent remodeling. Fresh freezing may decrease graft "incorporation,"[16] and the grafts have been noted to shrink with time.[10]

Freeze Drying (Lyophilization)

In addition to freezing, the tissue is dehydrated as it is stored. The advantage is that tissue can be stored at room temperature, greatly simplifying handling. Also, the tissue can be stored indefinitely. When the meniscus is utilized, it is rehydrated. Because the meniscus size varies with dehydration and rehydration, the tissues are more difficult to size.[5] Shrinkage in vivo is more of a problem as well.[10] Wirth et al,[17] reporting their series of freeze-dried meniscal transplants, noted three of 17 menisci had shrunk to a meniscal remnant, seven of 17 were one-third of their normal size, and six of 17 had shrunk to two-thirds of their normal size. While the HIV particle is not destroyed by the process, the risk of transmission is diminished.[18] Milachowski et al[19] in 1989 noted better results in their series of frozen meniscal transplants compared to lyophilized transplants, specifically less shrinkage and less cartilage damage (Table 7.2).

COMPLICATIONS

The majority of adverse outcomes in meniscal transplantation are caused by poor patient selection, technical errors, and biologic failures. Meniscal transplantation as presently practiced has markedly improved with respect to safety and efficacy.

Arthroscopic placement of the meniscus may be preferable to placing the transplant through an open in-

Table 7.2. Meniscal transplantation shrinkage

Author and series	*Description*	*Normal*	*Smaller*	*One-third smaller*	*Two-thirds smaller*	*Destroyed*
Garrett[3] Second-look arthroscopy	Bone plugs, fresh, cryo	27/28		1/28		
Kohn and Wirth[26] Second-look arthroscopy	Suture, deep frozen	3/5	1/5	1/5		
	Suture, lyophilized			4/13	5/13	1/13
Milachowski et al[19] Second-look arthroscopy	Suture, deep frozen	3/5	1/5		1/5	
	Suture lyophilized			4/10	4/10	1/10

cision. In addition to the usual advantages of arthroscopy, the corresponding collateral ligament needs to be released when the transplantation is performed open as opposed to arthroscopic assisted.[10] Although arthroscopy is thought of as "no big deal" by both patients and surgeons, that is not necessarily the case. Small,[20] writing in 1988, noted a 1.5% rate of complications in arthroscopic surgery, including the following: 7% superficial cellulitis, 2% phlebitis, and 38% saphenous neuropathy. All of these complications were transient. As meniscus replacement is a lengthy operation, tourniquet time and subsequent palsy is a concern.

The usual complications in knee surgery have been found in meniscal transplantation, that is, infection, suture, and hardware complications. Zukor et al[21] noted two of 26 patients required transfusion for postoperative anemia. In this series, both the meniscus and tibial plateau were transplanted together, which is different from the other series discussed. Shelton and Dukes[22] noted one of 20 patients had a postoperative hemarthrosis. Also, Zukor et al[21] had to evacuate one postoperative knee hemarthrosis in 26 patients. Goble and Wilcox[23] had to remove wire that had been used for fixation and displaced after a motor vehicle accident (MVA). Suture granuloma has been reported. Van Arkel and deBoer[24] had five of 23 patients with suture granuloma around nonabsorbable suture. Their recommendation is to use absorbable suture.

Infection has been uncommonly reported in meniscus transplantation. Milachowski et al[19] in 1989 had two of 22 patients develop a postoperative infection, one of whom was culture positive for *Staphylcoccus aureus*. At least two authors have had to remove the meniscus in the course of treating the infection; Shelton and Dukes[22] had one of 20 treated in this manner and Goble and Wilcox[23] also removed a transplant. Veltri et al[25] reported in 1994 a stitch abscess.

As in all allograft surgery, disease transmission remains an issue. Although there have been no reported cases of HIV transmission with soft tissue grafts,[26] it has occurred in bone transplantation.[27] Former U.S. Surgeon General C. Everett Koop[28] estimated that by the year 2000 there will be 100 million people worldwide with the AIDS virus, barring a medical breakthrough of a way to control this epidemic. Buck et al[29] estimated the probability of contracting the AIDS virus from a bone or soft tissue implant to range from one in 161 to one in 1,667,600 using a mathematical model. The probability of HIV of one in 161 assumes no other precautions other than testing the donor for the HIV antibody; one in 1,667,600 assumes all precautions including testing for the HIV antigen, which is not universally performed. Certainly, the hepatitis viruses are a risk, but they are not fatal without exception, as the AIDS virus is. Freezing may diminish the probability of disease transmission.[30]

Technical Failures

Sizing

In "isotropic transplantation," a right medial meniscus is substituted for a right medial meniscus.[4] The contralateral, matched meniscus may be used to size the meniscus as the two appear to be mirror images of each other.[25] Magnetic resonance imaging (MRI) at present is not consistently accurate in estimating the meniscus size; it generally tends to underestimate the size,[1] although it has also erred in the opposite direction.[25] As MRI software and technique improves it is likely accuracy will improve as well. Computed Tomography (CT) has been touted as more accurate in the sizing of meniscal transplants,[1] however it can either underestimate or overestimate.[25] X-rays have been most commonly used, as they are accurate and easy to use. Garrett and Stevensen[2] found that an AP radiograph estimated the meniscus size to within 5%. Also, L'Insalata et al[31] measured the AP articular length on lateral radiographs with a mean error of 2.4% for the medial meniscus and 3.0% for the lateral articular surface. Both the interobserver and intraobserver reliabilities were found to be excellent. If one is to err, a larger implant can be sized to fit.[25]

Bone Plug Fracture

Although, bone plug fracture occurs rarely, when it does occur it usually is recoverable. A technique of graft passage to minimize the probability of fracture is presented below (see Prevention). When the bone plug fractures, it can be salvaged with suture fixation or by securing a fractured bone bridge with the periosteum closure.

Patient Selection

Young donors and young patients are preferred, younger patients are are less likely to have significant degenerative joint disease (DJD) and conversely are more likely to develop osteoarthrosis after menisectomy.[10,32] Meniscal transplantation may prevent degenerative changes from developing. Younger donors, because of age related changes to the meniscal cartilage, are superior.[7,26] Cryolife, Inc. (Marietta, GA) limits donors to age 40.[33]

Two other important factors in patient selection are the amount of articular surface change and alignment of the involved limb. It is impossible at this time to separate the adverse influence of each, as these two are interrelated factors. For instance, a patient with significant chondral changes likely has concomitant malalignment. Many of the meniscal allograft patients reported also have an osteotomy during or near the time of the transplantation. The allograft or the osteotomy or both could have been responsible for the improvement in the patient's symptoms.

The most reliable pain relief and best longevity of the implanted meniscus have been in patients who have less extensive chondral changes. What is an acceptable amount of chondral change is not clear. The traditional thinking was that patients with Outerbridge grade III or IV changes did not fare as well as those with grade I or II changes. Rodeo et al[34] noted a "significant negative correlation between the Outerbridge score at the time of insertion and the magnitude of improvement in the International Knee Documentation Committee (IKDC) Activity Score" in their 41 patients. In Garrett's[3] series, patients with grade IV changes did more poorly than other patients. In 11 patients with grade IV changes, only two were a success; six were failures, and three did not have second-look arthroscopy. In Noyes'[32] series of 68 meniscal transplants in 57 patients, most had "arthroscopic evidence of advanced femoral, tibial cartilage changes." Many had anterior cruciate ligament (ACL) surgery at the same time. Also, many patients had significant varus angulation. Second-look arthroscopy on 45 patients showed that 18 were failures. Cryolife, Inc., which maintains a registry of meniscal allografts, noted in a personal communication to Goble and Kane that 13 of 15 menisci that had to be removed had grade III or greater changes, and 15 of 23 that had removal of a part of the transplant had "high-grade" arthritis at the time of transplantation.[35] In Shelton and Dukes'[22] series of 18 meniscal transplants, in nine of the 10 compartments that had minimal or no chondral changes, the patients had excellent pain relief. However, two of the four patients who had grade III or IV chondral changes had fair pain relief and two had poor pain relief. The two patients with poor pain relief were noted on second-look arthroscopy to have meniscal tears corresponding to the areas of articular damage, usually located over the posterior horn on the meniscus (Table 7.3). Finally, in an MRI study, Rodeo et al[36] noted more meniscal fragmentation over areas of chondral degeneration (Fig. 7.1).

However, there is evidence that meniscal transplantation can be effective in patients with grade III or IV chondral changes. Dowdy et al,[37] in a series of 20 meniscal transplants, found that 18 patients had grade II or greater changes, but only one patient had grade IV changes. Their results were gratifying, with 15 of 17 patients (88%) having significant improvement. There were two late partial menisectomies with healing rims at 6 and 7 months after surgery. Goble and Wilcox[23] reported in 1995 on 47 patients with 49 transplants, all with grade III and IV changes that were treated with cryopreserved transplants; 94% of the patients had improvement in pain and functional abilities. In a case report from 1991, a patient with significant lateral compartment arthritis had pain relief and meniscus healing on second-look arthroscopy.[38] Most recently, Cameron and Saha[40] reported a series of 67 patients with "unicompartmental arthritis" and a meniscal transplant; 34 patients had an osteotomy with their transplant, five had concomitant ACL reconstruction, and 21 had an isolated meniscal allograft. The knee score improved from a mean of 37 to a mean of 80, with three patients having a failure of the allograft due to gross nonhealing.

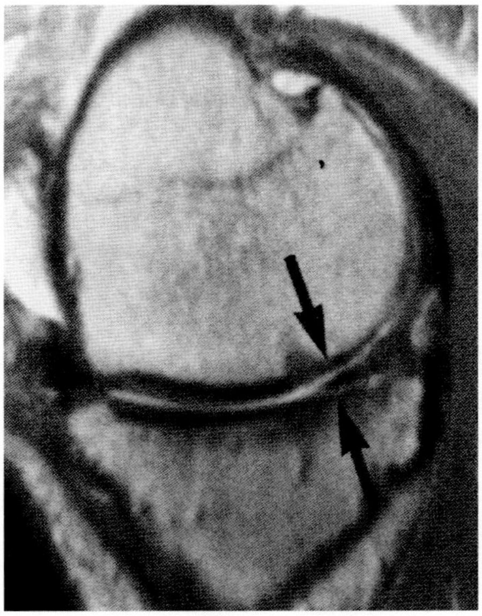

Figure 7.1. Magnetic resonance imaging (MRI) of a meniscal allograft. Sagittal images obtained 5 months postoperatively demonstrate high signal intensity at the attachment of the posterior horn, indicative of intrameniscal degeneration, which was confirmed at subsequent biopsy and histologic examination. Note the thinning of the cartilage (arrows). (From ref. 64, with permission.)

Although malalignment has not been studied as rigorously as gonarthritis, it is agreed in the literature that alignment is an important preoperative consideration. Failure of the meniscal allograft has been attributed to poor alignment.[24] If the preoperative alignment is not within the normal range for gender, an osteotomy should be considered as a simultaneous or separate procedure.[26,40–42] As noted, Van Arkle and deBoer[24] attributed their three failures to poor nutrition from malalignment. Their malaligned group of patients had a Lysholm knee mean score of 65 compared to a mean of 81 in the group that was well aligned.

Ligamentous laxity should be addressed either prior to or at the time of the transplant. The meniscus repair literature is in agreement that ligament reconstruction markedly improves the results of meniscus repair. The meniscus is a secondary restraint in the ACL-deficient knee and experiences forces that the meniscus with an intact ACL does not. Simultaneous ACL reconstruction with meniscus repair is rarely associated with failure to heal the meniscus tear. In meniscal reconstruction, Garrett[3] noted that ACL reconstruction did not adversely affect the result. Thirteen of his patients had second-look arthroscopy, and 12 were considered a success.

Biologic Failures

It has already been noted that malalignment may play a role in meniscal healing. Degenerative chondral changes articulating against an allograft meniscus may play an adverse role in incorporation of the meniscus. Ligamentous laxity interferes with healing of a rim of an autogenous meniscus with intact horns, so it is logical that it would interfere with healing of an allograft with grafted horns. Incorporation of the body of the allograft meniscus is related to horn incorporation. For the purpose of this discussion, these topics are divided into failure of meniscal body incorporation, failure of horn incorporation, shrinkage, rejection, and synovitis.

Meniscal Body Incorporation

Both animal and human studies have found differences between the native meniscus and transplanted menisci. In a canine study in which dogs' native meniscus was removed and reimplanted, the majority (86%) had abnormal collagen organization and had cleavage planes at the meniscosynovial junction.[43] In a histologic study on human transplants performed with a bone plug on the posterior horn and soft tissue fixation on the anterior horn, there was delayed and limited cellular repopulation.[32] The central core and surfaces remained acellular. There was peripheral vascular invasion, and the peripheral mensicus repopulated with fibrocytes, not fibrochondrocytes. It was uncommon to have failure of the horn or periphery, although clefts and tears in the body of the meniscus were not unusual. These changes were usually located at the posterior horn of the meniscus. The author concluded that normal meniscal cellular histology and the unique meniscus collagen architecture were not restored. Collagen architecture of the meniscus may be dependent on the restoration of the normal "hoop stresses" in the meniscus, and structure is a reflection of function. The soft tissue fixation of the meniscus at the anterior horn may alter the weight bearing of the meniscus and subsequent histologic remodeling.

Second-look arthroscopy, considered the best objective measure of transplant success, has been used extensively to assess the results of meniscus transplantation. Veltri et al[25] noted that two of seven second-look arthroscopy menisci had partial "healing" and one had fraying and degeneration. Van Arkle and de Boer[24] noted three of 23 transplants had failure of body incorporation, although two of three appeared to be healed when reexamined. In one of these three, the authors attempted to reattach the meniscus. Goble and Wilcox[23] performed 17 second-look arthroscopies in 18 transplants; four of these menisci had degenerative changes in the body, and small tears were noted at the edge of the meniscus. Garrett[3] in his 1993 study had eight menisci with loss of a major portion, failure of healing of the periphery, and fragmentation of the substance of the meniscus. In another study of two specimens with advanced chondral changes, the implanted menisci were fragmented over the area of the chondral changes.[22] Finally, in an MRI study, there was noted to be a high incidence of fragmentation on MRI.[36] These changes were more common over areas of articular cartilage degeneration (Fig. 7.1).

Horn Incorporation

The use of bone plugs or a bone bridge between the horns of the meniscus transplant may be the most important factor in the incorporation of the meniscal horns (Fig. 7.2). Techniques that suture the horns to the remaining mensical horns by soft tissue fixation have been, in most reports, less reliable. In a study with goats, when the meniscal horns were sutured with a soft tissue technique there was mensical extrusion, so the technique was changed to one utilizing bone plugs.[7] Meniscal extrusion in a human MRI study has been associated with poorer clinical results[36] (Fig. 7.3). In the case report by Keene et al[44] from 1987, both horns failed to unite and a suture technique was used. Cryolife, Inc., in a personal communication to Goble and Kane, reported there had been no horn fixation failures when using bone plugs evaluated by second-look arthroscopy. When using soft tissue suture techniques, fixation was "incomplete" in 5% and "poor" in 1%. In another report, Cryolife noted that there was a 20% increase in graft survival if bone fixation is included in the meniscal implant procedure.[35] There were two menisci with nonhealing or detachment of the horns in 22 implanted menisci with suture fixation in Milachowski et al's[19] series from 1989.

Failure of incorporation of the bone plug has been reported. Goble and Wilcox[23] and Shelton and Dukes[22] had failures of fixation when using bone plugs. Although failures have occurred with both techniques, use of bone plugs or a bone bridge is favored because of the consistent bone-to-bone healing.

Shrinkage

The evidence to date suggests that shrinkage may be related to the type of fixation of the meniscal horn and type of processing of the allograft. Lyophilized menisci

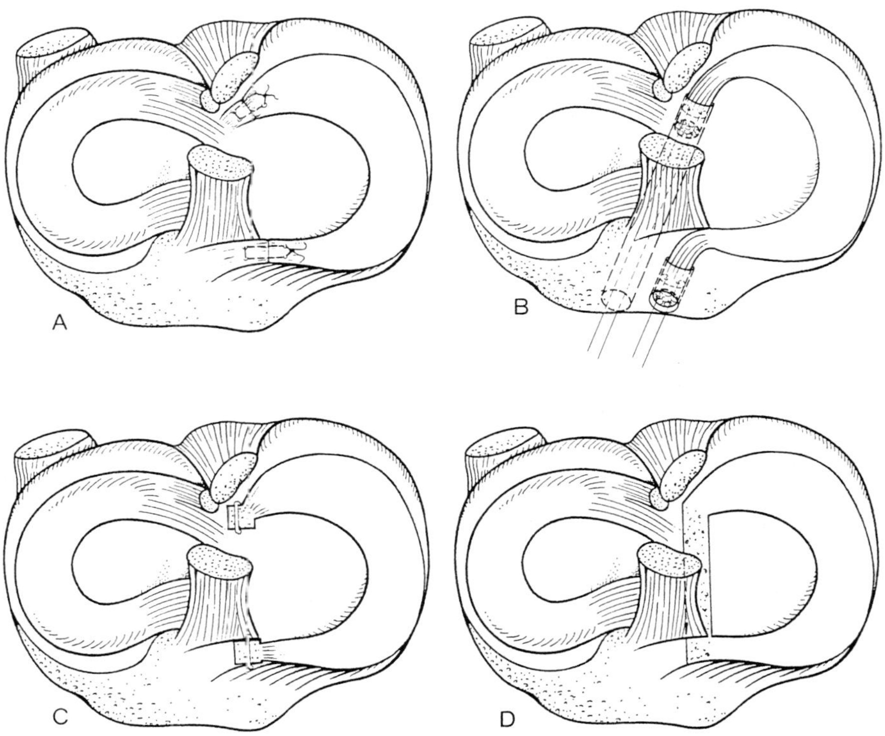

Figure 7.2. Different techniques of allograft medial meniscus replacement. **A:** The allograft is sutured to the anterior and posterior remnants of the genuine meniscus. **B:** The anterior and posterior ends of the allografts are tagged. The tag sutures are brought anterior through drill holes. **C:** Allograft bone plugs are "press-fit" at the meniscal insertions. **D:** An allograft bone bridge is fit into a tunnel, used in the keyhole technique. (From ref. 17, with permission.)

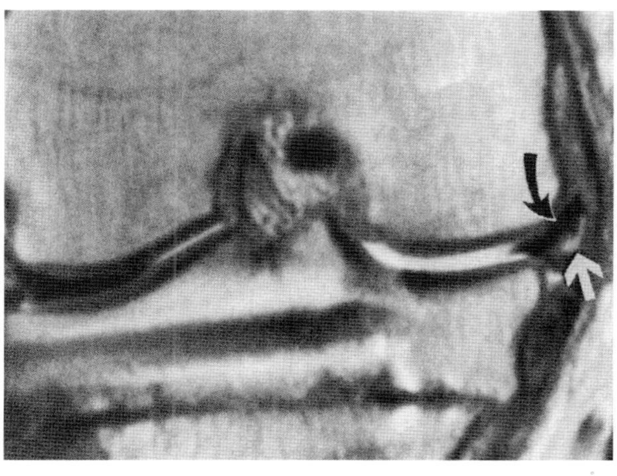

Figure 7.3. MRI after high tibial osteotomy and mensical allograft. Coronal image 4 months postoperatively demonstrates peripheral displacement of the body of the meniscal allograft relative to the axis of the femorotibial joint (curved arrow). There is biopsy-proved intrameniscal degeneration, as manifested by high signal intensity within the substance of the meniscus (straight arrow). (From ref. 64, with permission.)

have had more shrinkage than other types of processing. Garrett[3] in his 1993 series in which bone plugs were used noted shrinkage on second-look arthroscopy of only one meniscus. Both fresh and cryopreserved menisci were used in this series. In a personal communication from Cryolife to Goble and Kane,[35] 12 of 267 patients had shrinkage, five of whom were inadequately fixed at the meniscal horns. There are two series in the literature that reported significant shrinkage; both used suture techniques on the horns of the menisci. Kohn and Wirth[26] had five deep-frozen menisci that had second-look arthroscopy; three were of normal size, one was smaller, and one was a third of normal size. Their 13 lyophilized second-look arthroscopies had one meniscus that was destroyed altogether; four were reduced in size by a third of normal, and five were reduced in size by two-thirds. Similarly, Milachowski et al[19] had a series of both deep-frozen and lyophilized menisci transplants. Five deep-frozen transplants underwent second-look arthroscopy; three were normal sized, and two had some shrinkage, one of which was two-thirds smaller. Ten lyophilized menisci had second-look arthroscopy; only one patient had a normal-sized meniscus, five were reduced by one-third, four by two-thirds, and one was completely destroyed. However, only two patients were dissatisfied, one with chronic synovitis and a normal-appearing graft, and one with residual instability (Table 7.2). In conclusion, two factors have been associated in the literature with graft shrinkage: suture fixation of the horns and a lyophilized meniscus graft.

Rejection

Collagen carries little antigen, whereas the cellular component, bone, and bone marrow components carry the major histocompatibility antigens.[7,16,45,46] The size of the bone bridge may be important in any immune response.[16] Freezing destroys cellular components, and therefore would be expected to alter the immune response.[7] Cryopreservation, because of the low temperatures, denatures the histocompatibility antigens and should diminish the immune response.[7] When fresh and frozen groups are compared, the difference in incorporation occurs in the first 40 days; after this period of time biologic incorporation is similar.[7] Khoury et al[47] also noted the effects of freezing on the human leukocyte antigens (HLAs). It eliminated or reduced HLA expression by fibrochondrocytes, but had little impact on antigen expression by synovial cells and endothelial cells. Also, menisci that are harvested from a younger donor may present a larger antigen challenge than do those from an older donor. The authors concluded that tissue matching may be of benefit in meniscal transplantation. Until recently, there hadn't been a documented case of immune-mediated failure of meniscal transplantation.[23] Hamlet et al[48] reported a case of a 33-year-old man with a profound synovitis after a cryopreserved transplant. Microscopically the round cell infiltrate resembled a host-versus-graft reaction. The meniscus was removed because of the extent of the reaction. However, no tissue typing of the donor or recipient was performed. At this point, the case of acute rejection has been made on clinical grounds and review of pathology. However, failure of transplantation in other instances that have been reported is thought to be related to cell death rather than to immune-mediated response.[7]

Synovitis

Synovitis has been noted in clinical series that do not utilize glutaraldehyde or ethylene oxide in the treatment of the allografts. Milachowski et al[19] noted effusion or synovitis with four of the six deep-frozen allografts, none of which had significant antibody levels. An intense synovitis was noted in the case that was attributed to acute rejection. No tissue typing was performed; however, the clinical course and pathology resembled a host-versus-graft reaction.[48]

Late Problems

As with most procedures on the knee, persistent pain and arthrofibrosis have been reported.[49–52] Goble and Wilcox[23] have removed one meniscus because of persistent pain. Arthrofibrosis is not commonly reported. When meniscal transplants are combined with other procedures, such as ACL reconstruction, the risk of arthrofibrosis is higher.[37,53]

PREVENTION

Because there is no salvage for many of the problems that have been discussed, prevention of meniscal transplantation complications and pitfalls is critical. Much of the prevention rests in preoperative planning, and the majority of crucial decisions in meniscal transplantation are made prior to entering the operating room. Meniscus transplantation is extremely technically demanding with a steep learning curve; therefore, attention to detail is required.

Technical Factors

Although we did not identify any nerve injuries reported in the literature, they could be considered as a risk in the meniscal allograft transplantation procedure. Austin[53] has recommended performing meniscus repairs on the lateral side with the knee in 90 degrees of flexion to avoid the peroneal nerve. Most authors recommend 10 to 30 degrees of knee flexion for medial meniscus repair.[54–59]

Graft Selection

Unless one practices in a location that has an active organ transplantation program, fresh meniscal tissue simply is not an option. If fresh tissue is available, sterility and disease are more of a concern than with the variety of frozen alternatives. Two series in the literature have reported more shrinkage with lyophilized tissue than with deep-frozen tissue[19,26] (Table 7.2). For most surgeons, that leaves cryopreserved and deep frozen tissue. The primary difference is a viable cell population. Cryopreserved tissue has a population of viable cells, although small, that could aid in graft incorporation by manufacturing components needed for the meniscus.[11,12] The role of a viable cell population is unsettled at this point. Although gamma irradiation likely alters the mechanical properties of the meniscus in a dose dependent manner,[9] this is the process of choice for secondary sterilization.

Sizing

At this time plain radiograghs appear to be as accurate as, or even more accurate than, MRI or CT.[2,31] Furthermore, x-rays are less expensive, less time-consuming, and technically easier. If one is uncertain as to the correct size, a larger meniscus can be sized by removing peripheral tissue from the meniscus allograft.[25]

Bone Plug Fracture

Bone plug fracture may occur during insertion of the graft into the knee. A technique has been devised to minimize this possibility. A counterincision is made over the appropriate posterior corner of the knee similar to the incision for inside-out meniscus repair. The graft is passed through this incision. The posterior horn is inserted first by passing the sutures that are attached to the bone plug into the posterior tunnel with a suture passer or a malleable looped wire. The anterior horn sutures are passed through the ipsilateral anterior portal, thus decreasing the chance of anterior bone plug fracture. Once the anterior bone plug is in the knee, a suture passer or a malleable wire is passed through the anterior tunnel and out the portal where the sutures are retrieved. The sutures are passed out the tunnel and the bone plug is seated in the anterior tunnel[60] (Fig. 7.4).

Patient Selection

This is a difficult patient population, as all of these patients have had previous knee surgery. The most common complaint is pain. Only a small number of these patients may potentially benefit from this procedure. Patient selection is critical to success. Complications or effects from previous surgery such as reflex sympathetic dystrophy (RSD), quadriceps atrophy, decreased patellar mobility, decreased range of motion, and deconditioning are routine. Many patients have concomitant problems such as ligamentous laxity, DJD, and malalignment. It is not uncommon for these patients to be on oral narcotics or pain-management treatment of chronic knee pain. Social dysfunction is common. Many of these patients are unable or unwilling to work and have been out of work for prolonged periods of time. Often there is some degree of marital discord related to the patient's disability. Anger at the medical system is not unusual, as these patients have often seen many physicians and have few objective findings such as swelling or x-ray findings. Usually these patients have been told there is little that can be done for them. The amount of success that has been achieved in this population by meniscus transplantation is remarkable, in the senior author's experience. After meniscus transplantation, there has been a cessation of, or significant reduction in, narcotics use.

Chondral or articular cartilage changes are beyond the control of the surgeon. One can only select the appropriate procedure to address the amount of articular disease that is present in the patient. The most reliable results have been in patients with Outerbridge grade I and II articular damage (Cryolife, personal communication to Goble and Kane).[3,26,35] However, there have

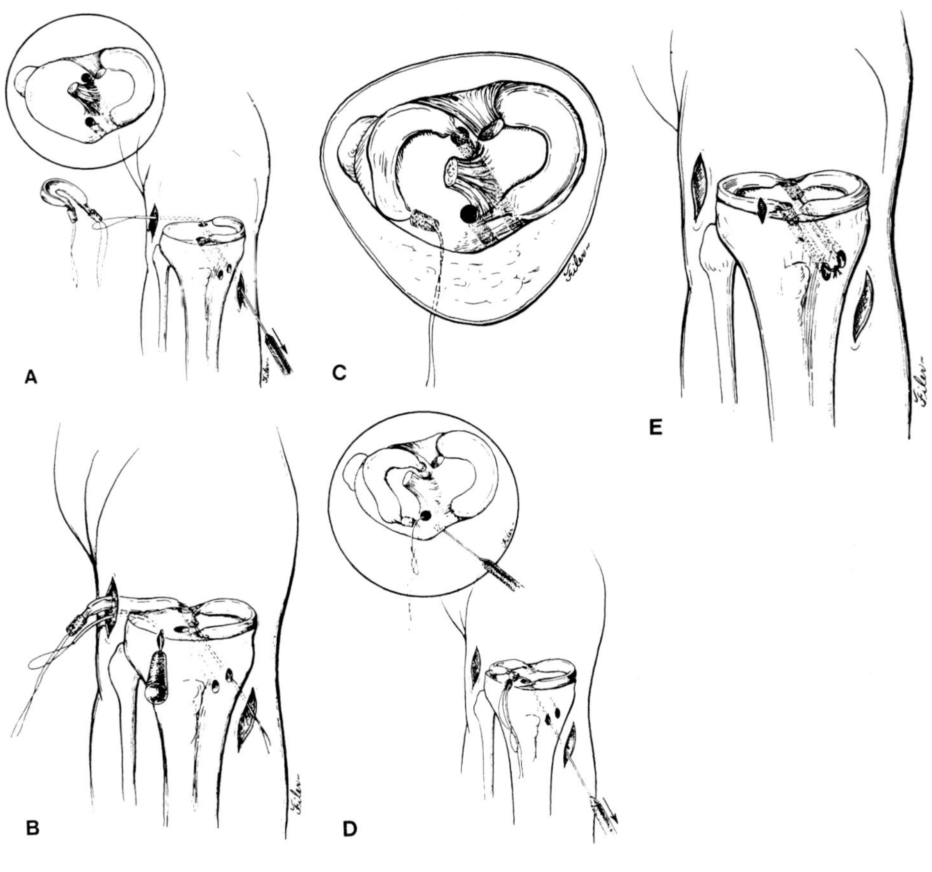

Figure 7.4. Schematic drawing showing insertion, passage, and seating of a lateral meniscal allograft.

Table 7.3. Relationship of chondral changes to the results from meniscal transplantation

	Grade I or II Outerbridge "minimal or no change"		Grade III or IV Outerbridge "advanced chondral changes"	
Author and Series	*Success*	*Failure*	*Success*	*Failure*
Garrett[3] Second-look arthroscopy			2/9	6/9
Noyes[33] Second-look arthroscopy			27/45	18/45
Shelton and Dukes[22] 8/14 Second-look arthroscopy	9/10	1/10	2/4	2/4
Goble and Wilcox[23] No second-look arthroscopy			46/49	3/49

been good results reported in advanced tibial femoral articular changes[23,40] (Table 7.3). All efforts should be made to address ligamentous laxity either at the time of the transplant or as a separate procedure. Similarly, malalignment should be addressed by an osteotomy either simultaneously or as a staged procedure.[25,40–42]

Horn Incorporation

As highlighted in the previous discussion on horn incorporation, use of bone plugs is important not only to ensure horn incorporation, but also to improve chances of meniscal body survival.[45] The precise tunnel placement and pertinent anatomy have been described.[61] The anterior horn of the medial meniscus is bounded by the anterior border of the ACL tibial insertion, articular margin of the anteromedial plateau, and anterior intercondylar fossa. The posterior horn of the medial meniscus is defined by the posterior cruciate ligament (PCL), the medial tibial spine, and the articular margin of the posterior medial tibial plateau. The anterior horn of the lateral meniscus is posterior to the anterior horn of the medial meniscus, and the posterior horn of the lateral meniscus is anterior to the posterior horn of the medial meniscus. In fact the anterior and posterior horns of the lateral meniscus very nearly touch and the lateral meniscus is O-shaped when viewed from above. The anterior horn of the lateral meniscus is at the level of the anterior half of the ACL tibial insertion, and placed adjacent to the articular margin of the anterior lateral tibial plateau. The posterior horn of the lateral meniscus is at the posterior border of the ACL tibial insertion, lateral tibial insertion, and the articular margin of the posterolateral tibial plateau[61] (Table 7.4; Figs. 7.5 through 7.11).

Table 7.4. Arthroscopic portals and landmarks for each meniscal horn bony insertion site

	Portal for arthroscope	*Port for endoscopic guide*	*Arthroscopic landmarks*
Anterior horn medial meniscus	Anteromedial	Anterolateral	1. Anterior border ACL tibial insertion 2. Articular margin of anteromedial tibial plateau 3. Anterior intercondylar fossa
Posterior horn medial meniscus	Posteromedial	Anterolateral	1. PCL 2. Medial tibial spine 3. Articular margin posteromedial tibial plateau
Anterior horn lateral meniscus	Anterolateral	Anteromedial	1. Anterior half of ACL tibial insertion 2. Lateral tibial spine 3. Articular margin of anterolateral tibial plateau
Posterior horn lateral meniscus	Anterolateral	Anteromedial	1. Posterior border ACL tibial insertion 2. Lateral tibial spine 3. Articular margin posterolateral tibial plateau

ACL, anterior cruciate ligament; PCL, posterior cruciate ligament.

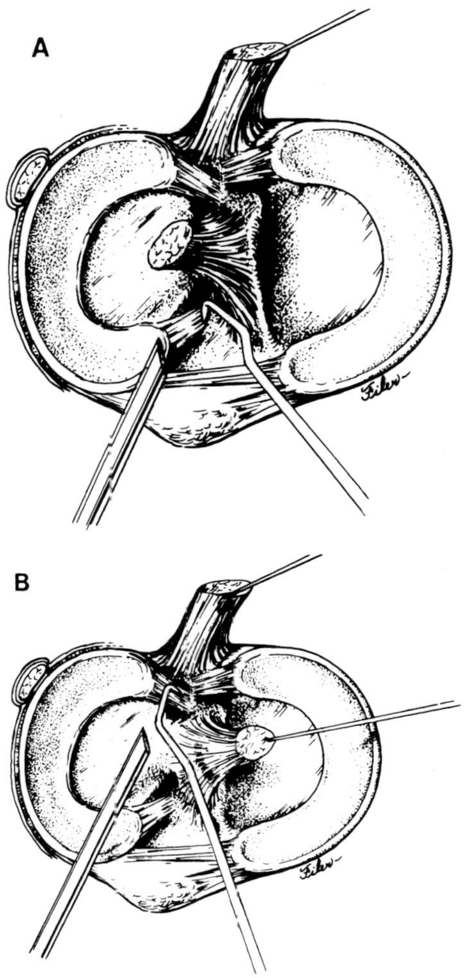

Figure 7.5. Arthroscopic visualization and arthroscopic drill guide placement for a lateral mensicus. The arthroscope is placed in the anterolateral portal and the drill guide is placed in the anteromedial portal. **A:** Positioning of the arthroscope and drill guide for the anterior horn tunnel. **B:** Instrument positioning to drill the posterior tunnel for the lateral meniscus. (From ref. 61, with permission.)

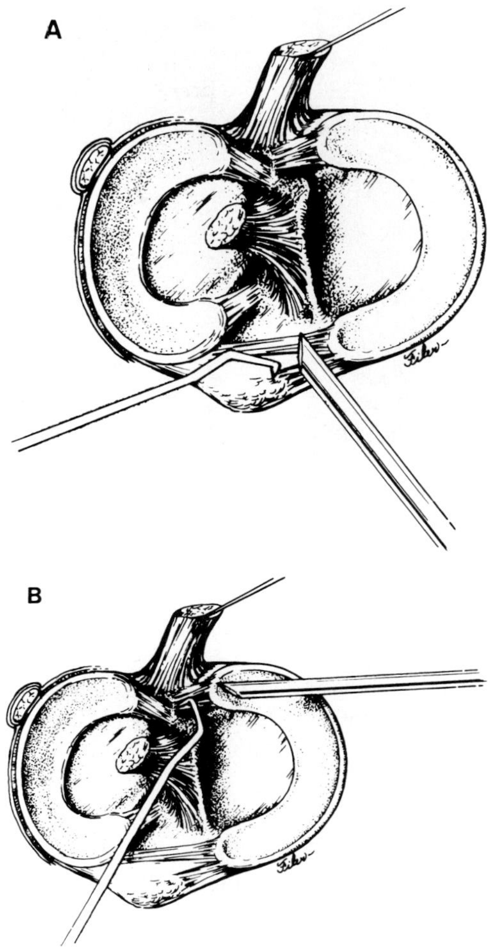

Figure 7.6. Arthroscopic visualization and drill-guide placement for the medial meniscus. **A:** For the anterior horn, the arthroscope is placed in the anteromedial portal with the arthroscopic drill guide in the anterolateral portal. **B:** For the posterior horn, the arthroscope is placed in the posteromedial portal with the arthroscopic drill guide again placed in the anterolateral portal. (From ref. 61, with permission.)

Placing the tunnels in a divergent fashion has been recommended to minimize the possibility of fracturing between the tunnels.[62] A minimum of 1 cm between the tunnels protects against this complication[60] (Fig. 7.4).

Shrinkage

The method of preservation is the factor most associated in the literature with this undesirable result. Garrett,[2,3] who used fresh and cryopreserved mensci in his two series, had no shrinkage in his first series of six patients and only one in his second series of 43 patients. In two similar series by separate authors, both of which consisted of deep-frozen grafts and lyophilized grafts, the lyophilized groups had more shrinkage than the deep-frozen groups.[19,26] The other factor that has been implicated is the use of suture on the horns. Both the Milachowski et al[19] and Kohn and Wirth[26] series used suture to fix the horns. Cryolife, Inc. has related shrinkage of the graft to inadequate horn fixation (Fig. 7.12).[35] There appear to be two factors responsible for shrinkage; unfortunately, both were present in the two reported series with significant shrinkage. So it is uncertain which factor is most important and linked directly to the shrinkage. Horn fixation with suture fixation has not been favored, for other reasons (Table 7.2).

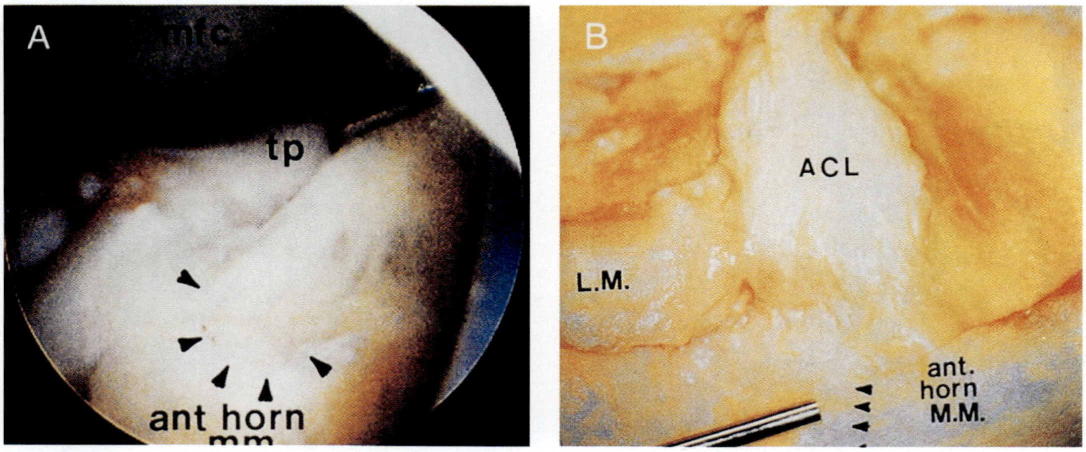

Figure 7.7. Bony insertion site for the anterior horn of the medial meniscus. **A:** Arthroscopic view. **B:** Gross dissection. Arrows indicate bony insertion site. ACL, anterior cruciate ligament; MFC, medial femoral condyle; TS, tibial spine; tp, tibial plateau; L.M., lateral meniscus. (From ref. 61, with permission.)

Synovitis

Although there have been reports of unexplained synovitis, the preventable causes of synovitis have been ethylene oxide[20,21,23] and glutaraldehyde.[52]

Late Problems

The prevention of persistent pain after surgery is at this point a matter of wishful thinking. The primary protection against this rare but agonizing problem is adequate screening of patients preoperatively. Patient selection may also be helpful in avoiding arthrofibrosis. These patients have all had at least one operation, so it is possible to gauge how the patient reacts to surgery, the amount of postoperative pain, compliance, and progression after surgery. The usual precautions in knee surgery apply here: achieve motion before surgery and early motion postoperatively[53]; emphasize full, early extension[53]; presribe physiotherapy; and stage multiple surgeries.

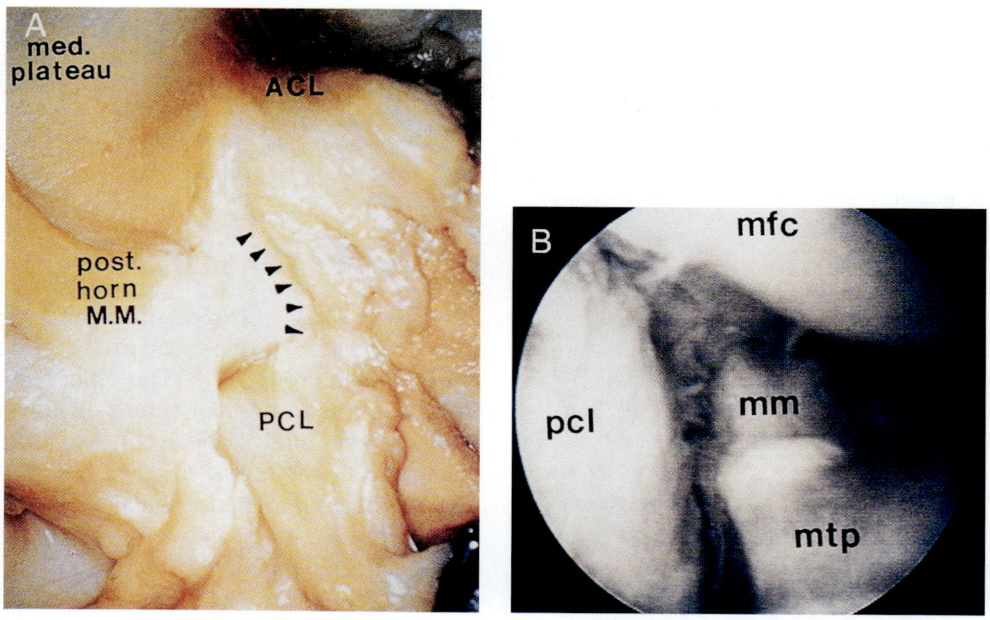

Figure 7.8. Bony insertion site for the posterior horn of the medial meniscus. **A:** Gross dissection. Arrows indicate bony insertion site. **B:** Arthroscopic view. (From ref. 61, with permission.)

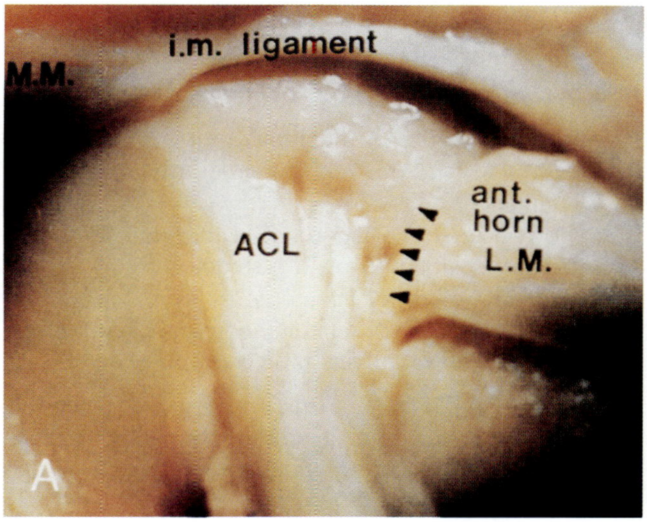

Figure 7.9. Bony insertion site for the anterior horn of the lateral meniscus. Gross dissection. Arrows indicate bony insertion site. I. M., intermeniscal ligament. (From ref. 61, with permission.)

SALVAGE

Bone plug fracture is usually a problem that is easily salvaged. The part of the bone plug that fractures is usually the portion at the tip, because the tip is smaller and more easily fractured. If not already done, through a small arthrotomy a second suture is looped through the horn attachment of the meniscus into bone. This suture can then be used to guide the remaining bone plug and

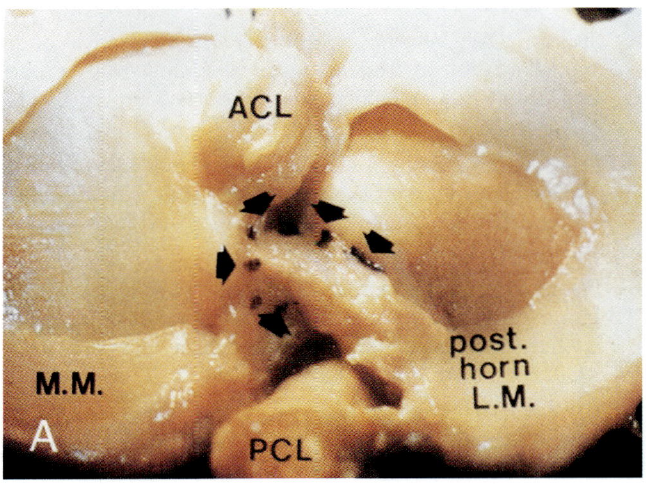

Figure 7.10. Bony insertion site for the posterior horn of the lateral meniscus. Gross dissection. Arrows indicate bony insertion site. (From ref. 61, with permission.)

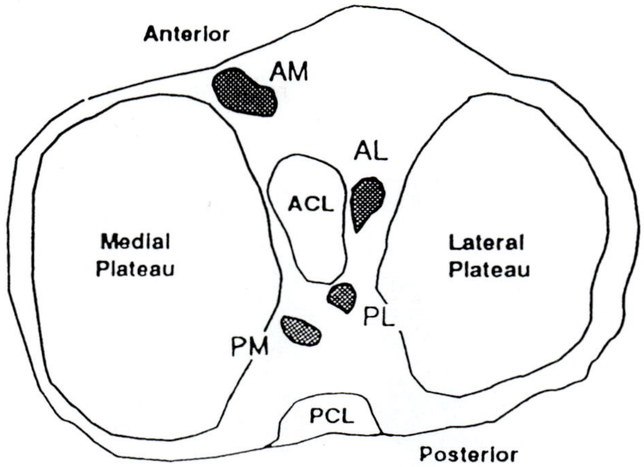

Figure 7.11. Diagram of an axial view of a right tibial plateau meniscal horn insertions. Note the intimate association of the lateral meniscal horn insertions with that of the ACL and also their close proximity to one another. (From ref. 61, with permission.)

horn insertion into the bone tunnel. The sutures can be tied in the customary fashion over the bone bridge.

Other than bone plug fracture, salvage in meniscal allograft is limited to a few options: partial or complete menisectomy,[23,39] reattachment of the meniscal horns, reattachment of the meniscal body,[24] surgical application of residual ligamentous laxity, and osteotomy for malalignment. There have been reports in the literature of reattaching a detached meniscal body with suture.[24] In the series reported by Milachowski et al,[19] a portion of a meniscus was removed and the remainder repaired after an injury. The patient remained asymptomatic after the secondary procedure. However, the majority of times the failure of meniscal body incorporation is away from the healed periphery of the meniscus and lends itself more readily to partial menisectomy.[23,39]

Infection has been salvaged with the usual measures, including irrigation, debridement, and antibiotics.[19] At least two menisci have been removed in the course of treating infection. Both Shelton and Dukes[22] and Goble and Wilcox[23] have each removed a meniscal allograft to clear infection.

In the reported case of possible acute rejection, the meniscus was removed as a salvage procedure.[48]

When stiffness is unpreventable, it has been salvaged with manipulation under anesthesia. Dowdy et al[37] manipulated one of his 20 patients for persistent stiffness. The patient had both menisci transplanted and the ACL reconstructed.

Malalignment can be salvaged post-meniscus transplant with an osteotomy after surgery if the extent of the patient's deformity is not appreciated before surgery.

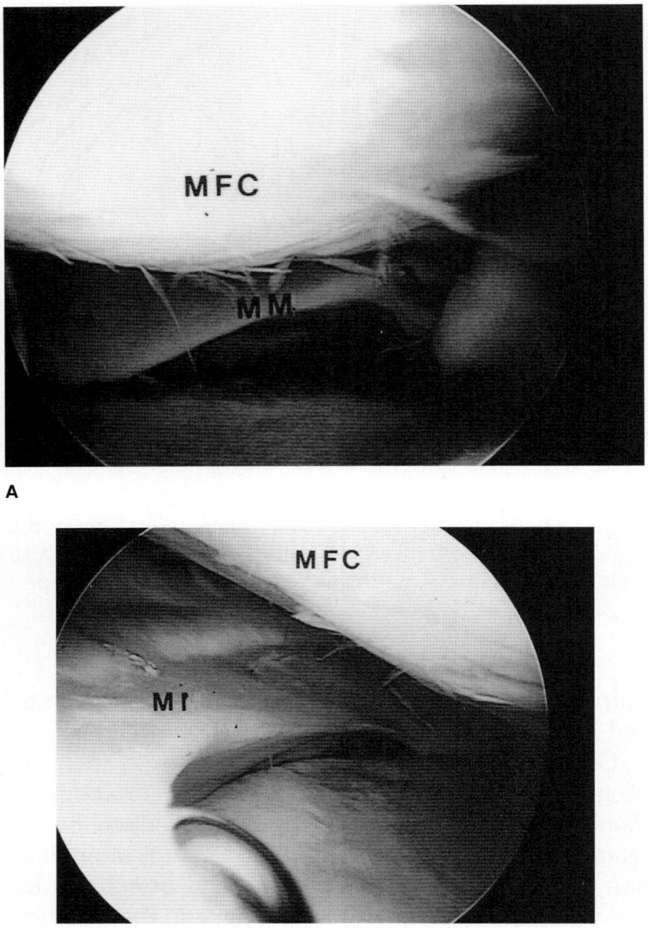

Figure 7.12. Second-look arthroscopy. 39 yowm who is s/p 3 months from a medial meniscal allograft. **A:** View of the posterior horn of the medial meniscal allograft, performed with bone plug fixation of the meniscal horn. **B:** The periphery of meniscus shows synovial proliferation.

CONCLUSIONS

1. Because salvage options are limited, prevention of problems in meniscal transplantation is the key to success.
2. Fresh frozen or cryopreserved tissue is preferred over freeze dried. The clinically reported results of fresh tissue have been among the best in the literature; however, it is of limited availability and the practical matters of storage and disease transmission are difficult to manage.
3. Plain radiographs are the most cost-efficient method of preoperative sizing.
4. Patient selection is of critical importance.
   - The best results of meniscus transplantation have been with patients with minimal articular surface changes.
   - Correct knee malalignment at the time of meniscus transplantation or in a staged fashion.
   - Surgically address ligamentous laxity before the transplantation or simultaneously. Ligamentous laxity adversely affects graft incorporation.
5. Use of bone plugs or a bone bridge will improve the clinical results of transplantation, increase the probability of meniscus body incorporation, may decrease shrinkage, and may reduce extrusion.
6. The results of currently reported series have been encouraging in a difficult patient population.

References

1. Carpenter JE, Wojtys EM, Huston LJ. Pre-operative sizing of meniscal replacements. *Arthroscopy* 1993;9:344.
2. Garrett JC, Stevensen RN. Meniscal transplantation in the human knee: a preliminary report. *Arthroscopy* 1991; 7:57–62.
3. Garrett JC. Meniscal transplantation: a review of 43 cases with 2 to 7 year follow-up. *Sports Med Arthrosc Rev* 1993;1:164–167.
4. Kuhn JE, Wojtys EM. Allograft meniscus transplantation. *Clin Sports Med* 1996;15:537–555.
5. Siegel MG, Roberts CS. Meniscal allografts. *Clin Sports Med* 1993;12:59–80.
6. Jackson DW, Whelan J, Simon TM. Cell survival after transplantation of fresh meniscal allografts: DNA probe analysis in a goat model. *Am J Sports Med* 1993;21: 540.
7. Jackson DW, Simon T. Biology of meniscal allograft. In: Mow VC, Arnoczky SP, Jackson DW, eds. *Knee Meniscus: Basic and Clinical Foundations.* New York: Raven Press, 1992:141–152.
8. Fideler BM, Vangsness CT Jr, Moore T, et al. Effects of gamma irradiation on the human immunodeficiency virus: a study in frozen human bone–patellar ligament–bone grafts obtained from infected cadavera. *J Bone Joint Surg* 1994;76A:1032.
9. Bright RW, Burchardt H. The biomechanical properties of preserved bone grafts. In: Friedlaender GE, Mankin HJ, Sell KW, eds. *Osteochondral Allografts: Biology, Banking and Clinical Applications.* Boston: Little, Brown, 1983:241–247.

10. Harner CD. Arthroscopic meniscal transplantation. Paper presented at the American Academy of Orthopaedic Surgery, Arthroscopic Surgery, Nashville, TN, March 1993.
11. Arnoczky SP, Milachowski KA. Meniscal allografts: Where do we stand? In: Ewing JW, ed. *Articular Cartilage and Knee Joint Function: Basic Science and Arthroscopy*. New York: Raven Press, 1990:129.
12. Goble EM. Meniscal allograft reconstruction (Abstract). Paper presented at the 59th annual meeting of the American Academy of Orthopaedic Surgeons, Washington, DC, February 1992.
13. Graham WC, Smith DA, McGuire MP. The use of frozen stored tendons for grafting: an experimental study. *J Bone Joint Surg* 1955;37A:624.
14. Arnoczky SP, O'Brien S, DiCarlo E, et al. Cellular repopulation of deep frozen meniscal allograft: experimental study in the dog. *Transact Orthop Res Soc* 1988;34:145.
15. Arnoczky SP, DiCarlo EF, O'Brien SJ, et al. Cellular repopulation of deep-frozen meniscal autografts: an experimental study in the dog. *Arthroscopy* 1992;8:428–436.
16. Bos GD, Goldberg VM, Powell AE, et al. The long term fate of fresh and frozen orthotopic bone allografts in genetically defined rats. *Clin Orthop* 1985;197:245.
17. Wirth CJ, Kohn D. Meniscal transplantation and replacement. In: Fu FH, Harner CD, Vince KG, eds. *Knee Surgery*. Baltimore: Williams & Wilkins, 1994:631–641.
18. Evensen SA, Ulstrup J, Skaug K, et al. HIV infection in Norwegian haemophiliacs: the prevalence of antibodies against HIV in haemophiliacs treated with lyophilized cryoprecipitate from volunteer donors. *Efr J Haematol* 1987;39:44–48.
19. Milachowski KA, Weismer K, Wirth CJ. Homologous meniscus transplantation: experimental and clinical results. *Int Orthop* 1989;13:1–11.
20. Small NC. Complications in arthroscopic surgery performed by experienced arthroscopists. *Arthroscopy* 1988;4:215–221.
21. Zukor DJ, Cameron JC, Brooks PJ, et al. The fate of human meniscal allografts. In: Ewing JW, ed. *Articular Cartilage and Knee Joint Function: Basic Science and Arthroscopy* New York: Raven Press, 1990:147–152.
22. Shelton WR, Dukes AD. Meniscal allotransplantation: a follow-up of twenty patients. Paper presented at the 19th annual meeting of the American Association of Tissue Banks, Atlanta GA, August 1995.
23. Goble EM, Wilcox TR. Meniscal allograft transplantation: 2 to 5 year follow-up. Paper presented at the 19th annual meeting of the American Association of Tissue Banks, Atlanta, GA, August 1995.
24. van Arkle ERA, de Boer HH. Human meniscal transplantation: preliminary results at 2 to 5 year follow-up. *J Bone Joint Surg* 1994;77B:589–595.
25. Veltri DM, Warren RF, Wickiewicz TL, et al. Current status of allograft meniscal transplantation. *Clin Orthop Rel Res* 1994;303:44–55.
26. Kohn D, Wirth CJ. Meniscal transplantation: the Hannover experience. In: Czitrom AA, Winkler H, eds. *Orthopaedic Allograft Surgery*. Vienna: Springer-Verlag, 1996:253–259.
27. Centers for Disease Control. Transmission of HIV through bone transplantation: case report and public health recommendations. *MMWR* 1988;37:597–599.
28. Koop CE. The aids epidemic. *Los Angeles Times* 1989 (November 19:2).
29. Buck BE, Malinin TI, Brown MD. Bone transplantation and human immunodeficiency virus. *Clin Orthop Rel Res* 1989;240:129–136.
30. Buck BE, Resmick L, Shah SM, Malinin TI. Human immunodeficiency virus cultures from bone: implications in transmission. *Clin Orthop Rel Res* 1990;251:249–253.
31. L'Insalata JC, Klatt B, Caravaggio H, Fu FH, Harner CD. Accuracy and reliability of office techniques for meniscal allograft sizing. Paper presented at the annual meeting of the Meniscal Transplantation Study Group, Atlanta, GA, February 1996.
32. Noyes FR. Current concepts: meniscus allografts. Paper presented at the American Orthopaedic Society for Sports Medicine, Sun Valley, ID, July 1993.
33. Mack DD, Fronk DM, McNally RT. Cryopreserved meniscal allograft reconstruction. Paper presented at the Cartilage Study Group meeting, San Francisco, February 1997.
34. Rodeo SA, Berkowitz M, Sultan P, et al. Clinical evaluation of meniscal allograft transplantation at minimum two-year follow-up. Paper presented at the Cartilage Transplantation Study Group meeting, San Francisco, February 1997.
35. Goble EM, Kane SM. Meniscal allografts. In: Czitrom AA, Winkler H, eds. *Orthopaedic Allograft Surgery*. Vienna: Springer-Verlag, 1996:243–252.
36. Rodeo SA, Potter HG, Wickiewicz, et al. Magnetic resonance imaging of meniscal allografts: correlation with early outcome. Paper presented at the Arthoscopic Association of North America, San Francisco, May 1995.
37. Dowdy P, Yoldas E, Navarro R, et al. Meniscal transplantation using non-irradiated fresh frozen allografts. Paper presented at the Meniscus and Articular Cartilage Transplantation Study Group 1997, San Francisco, February 1997.
38. DeBoer HH, Koudstaal J. The fate of meniscus cartilage after transplantation of cryopreserved nontissue-antigen-matched allograft: a case report. *Clin Orthop Rel Res* 1991;266:145–151.
39. Cameron JC, Saha S. Meniscal allograft transplantation for unicompartmental arthritis of the knee. *Clin Orthop Rel Res* 1997;337:164–171.

40. Noyes FR. A histological study of failed human meniscal allografts. Paper presented at specialty day, Arthroscopy Asssociation of North America, Orlando, February 1995.

41. DeBoer HH, Koudstaal J. Failed meniscus transplantation: a report of three cases. *Clin Orthop Rel Res* 1994; 306:155–162.

42. Wilcox TR, Goble EM. Indications for meniscal allograft reconstruction. *Am J Knee Surg* 1996;9:35–36.

43. Stone KR, Rodkey WG, McKinney LA, et al. Autogenous replacement of the meniscus cartilage: analysis of results and mechanisms of failure. *Arthroscopy* 1995;11:395–400.

44. Keene GCR, Paterson RS, Teague DC. Advances in arthroscopic surgery. *Clin Orthop Rel Res* 1987;224: 64–70.

45. McNally RT, Mack DD, Fronk DM. Cryopreserved meniscal allograft reconstruction. Paper presented at the annual meeting of the Cartilage Transplantation Study Group, San Francisco, February 1997.

46. Minami A, Ishii S, Ogino T, et al. Effect of the immunological antigenicity of the allogenic tendons of tendon grafting. *Hand* 1982;14:11–19.

47. Khoury M, El-Farou SM, Goldberg VM, et al. Fresh, frozen and twice-frozen human menisci express HLA-ABC and HLA-DR antigens. Paper presented at the 39th annual meeting, Orthopaedic Research Society, San Francisco, February 1993.

48. Hamlet W, Liu SH, Yang R. Destruction of a cryopreserved meniscal allograft: a case for acute rejection. *Arthroscopy* 1997;13:517–521.

49. Curtis RJ, DeLee JC, Drez DJ. Reconstruction of the anterior cruciate ligament with freeze dried fascia lata allografts in dogs. *Am J Sports Med* 1985;13:108–114.

50. Jackson DW, Windler GE, Simon TM. Intra-articular reaction associated with the use of freeze dried, ethylene oxide–sterilized bone-patella-bone allografts in the reconstruction of the anterior cruciate ligament. *Am J Sports Med* 1990;18:1–11.

51. Heidt RS, Holladay B, Karns D, et al. Allografts. In: Griffin L, ed. Orthopaedic Knowledge Update: Sports Medicine. American Academy of Orthopaedic Surgeons 1994:38.

52. Canham W, Stanish W. A study of the biological behavior of the meniscus as a transplant in the medial compartment of a dog's knee. *Am J Sports Med* 1986; 14:376–379.

53. Austin KS. Complications of arthroscopic meniscal repair. *Clin Sports Med* 1996;15:613–619.

54. Barber FA. Meniscus repair: an arthroscopic technique. *Arthroscopy* 1987;3:25–30.

55. Morgan CK, Casscells SW. Arthroscopic meniscus repair: a sage approach to the posterior horns. *Arthroscopy* 1986;2:3–12.

56. Rosenberg TD, Scott SM, Coward DB. Arthroscopic meniscal repair evaluated with repeat arthroscopy. *Arthroscopy* 1986;2:14–20.

57. Ryu RK, Dunbar WH. Arthroscopic meniscal repair with two year follow-up. *Arthroscopy* 1988;4:168–173.

58. Scott GA, Jolly BL, Henning CE. Combined posterior incision and arthroscopic intraarticular repair of the meniscus. *J Bone Joint Surg* 1986;68A:847–861.

59. Warren RF. Menisectomy and repair in the anterior cruciate ligament-deficient patient. *Clin Orthop Rel Res* 1990;252:55–63.

60. Johnson DL, Swenson TM, Harner CD. Meniscal reconstruction using allograft tissue: an arthroscopic technique. *Oper Tech Sports Med* 1994;2:223–231.

61. Johnson DL, Swenson TM, Livesay GA, et al. Insertion-site anatomy of the human menisci: gross, arthroscopic, and topographical anatomy as a basis for meniscal transplantation. *Arthroscopy* 1995;11:386–394.

62. Stone KR, Rosenberg T. Surgical technique of meniscal replacement. *Arthroscopy* 1993;9:234–237.

63. Kohn D. Meniscus transplantation. *Ad in Oper Ortho* 1994;2:49–76.

64. Potter HG, Rodeo SA, Wickiewicz TL, Warren RF. MR imaging of meniscal allografts: correlation with clinical and arthroscopic outcomes. *Radiology* 1996;198:509–514.

Section III

Complications and Pitfalls in Reconstruction of Cruciate Ligaments

Chapter 8

Complications and Pitfalls in Anterior Cruciate Ligament Reconstruction with Hamstring Tendons

Roger V. Larson

It has become generally accepted that hamstring tendon autografts are an effective graft for replacement of the anterior cruciate ligament (ACL).[1–6] They offer several advantages over other commonly used autografts, such as patellar tendons. Hamstring tendons, when doubled and combined, provide strong grafts with stiffness characteristics similar to a normal ACL.[7] They have a large surface area for revascularization and their precise positioning is facilitated by not having a bone block attached.

When the semitendinosus and gracilis tendons are both doubled or if the semitendinosus tendon is quadrupled and utilized as an ACL graft, a large-diameter, strong ACL substitute is created. This construct has a significantly greater cross-sectional area of collagen than a 10-mm-wide patellar tendon graft. The collagen cross-sectional area is numerically represented in Fig. 8.1. Not only is the cross-sectional area of collagen greater with hamstring tendon grafts, but the ability to precisely place the graft is enhanced over that of patellar tendon grafts in that both tunnels can be created in the desired locations and can then be completely filled with collagen. When the patellar tendon with an associated bone block is utilized as a graft, it is necessary to drill bone tunnels larger than those needed for the collagen portion of the graft, and the precise position of the collagen can then be distorted by the position of the bone blocks and fixation devices (Fig. 8.2). It is often not possible to place both bone blocks at the entrance into the intraarticular space due to the variable length of the collagen portion of the grafts. This necessitates recessing one or both bone blocks, allowing a loose fit of the collagen in the overdrilled tunnel. With hamstring tendon grafts, tunnels can be created so that the graft fits tightly within the tunnel. The ability of a multistranded graft to obtain nutrition either by diffusion or by vascular ingrowth is enhanced over that of a solid graft due to the increased surface area and smaller depth of penetration needed for either revascularization or nutrient diffusion to each strand of the graft.

Hamstring tendon autografts, when used as ACL substitutes, produce a graft with stiffness charactertistics more similar to normal ACL than patellar tendon autografts.[7] Since hamstring tendon grafts are not overly stiff, they allow more leeway when tensioning the reconstruction, making overconstraint of the joint less likely. Studies by Steiner et al[8] and Rowden et al[9] have demonstrated that when hamstring tendon grafts are fixed by appropriate techniques, the initial fixation strength of the construct is greater than that of bone blocks fixed with interference fit screws. A study by Rodeo et al[10] has documented the process of tendon healing in bone tunnels and has demonstrated that biologic fixation in this situation occurs relatively early. Lane et al[11] have studied the histology and biochemistry of semitendinosus tendon grafts 4 years after implantation. This study showed changes in the collagen crimp pattern, cell type, glucosaminoglycan composition, and collagen cross-linking, suggesting a structural change toward that of a normal ACL.

Probably the most compelling advantage of the use of hamstring tendon autografts for ACL reconstruction is the apparent decreased surgical morbidity associated with this procedure. Postoperative problems with motion and patellofemoral irritation appear to be rare following ACL reconstruction with hamstring tendons. A study by Hormel et al[5] has shown a success rate when utilizing hamstring tendons for ACL reconstruction comparable to published results using patellar tendon autografts. Their study showed satisfactory results in both

CROSS-SECTIONAL AREA
OF GRAFTS
RECTANGULAR GRAFT (H 3 × W)
PATELLAR TENDON
10 mm × 3 mm = 30 mm^2
CIRCULAR GRAFT (Πr^2)
TUNNEL DIAMETER: AREA
6 mm = 28 mm^2
7 mm = 38 mm^2
8 mm = 50 mm^2
9 mm = 64 mm^2
10 mm = 79 mm^2

Figure 8.1. The cross-sectional area of collagen available to serve as an anterior cruciate ligament (ACL) replacement is significantly greater when utilizing multiple strands of hamstring tendons than that provided by a patellar tendon graft.

acute and chronic situations and showed that knees stable at 1 year remained stable at 3 years. O'Neill[12] published similar results demonstrating no significant difference in results when comparing ACL reconstructions with patellar tendon or hamstring tendons either acutely or chronically. Feagin and coworkers[13] also demonstrated no significant difference in results when comparing ACL reconstructions with hamstrings to those with patellar tendons. They also showed no deterioration of results between 2 and 10 years postoperation in either group.

Although complications with the use of hamstring tendons in ACL reconstruction are rare, they can arise and can be classified into categories as follows: (1) complications associated with graft harvest, (2) complications of graft placement, (3) complications of graft fixation, (4) postoperative complications at the donor site, and (5) complications with the implanted graft. The following sections discuss in detail the potential complications in each category and make suggestions for avoiding them or dealing with them should they occur.

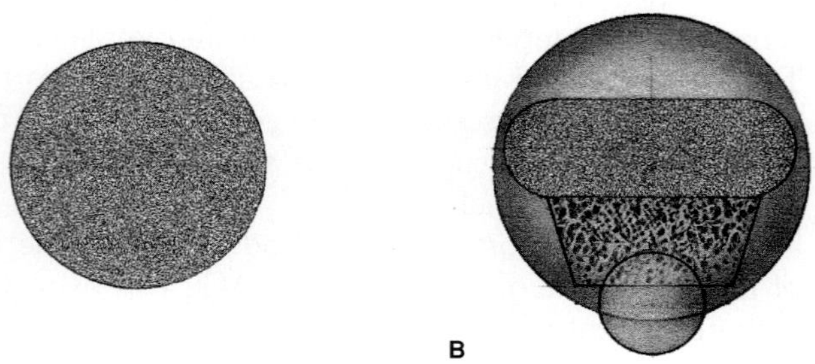

Figure 8.2. The location of the collagen portion of the graft (cross-hatched) is better controlled when the tunnel is completely filled with a soft tissue graft (**A**) than when a bone block and fixation device also are placed within the tunnel. (**B**) A snug fit of the collagen within the tunnel is also better accomplished with soft tissue grafts.

COMPLICATIONS ASSOCIATED WITH HARVEST OF HAMSTRING TENDON AUTOGRAFTS

A potential disadvantage of the use of hamstring tendon autografts is inconsistency in the grafts obtained. Inconsistency can be due to anatomically small tendons, short tendons, or to difficulties with the harvest technique that result in suboptimal graft length. The technical difficulty occasionally encountered with hamstring tendon harvest is one of the primary disadvantages to the use of these tendons. Less commonly, saphenous nerve injuries can occur and harvest-site hematomas can accumulate.

Insufficient tendon length can usually be avoided by strict attention to detail during the tendon harvesting. Also, newer endoscopic techniques of fixation require a shorter graft for reconstruction, thus decreasing the risk of inadequate graft length.

In the past, an open incision in the posterior thigh was frequently utilized to obtain hamstring tendon grafts. It is now generally accepted that superior grafts with reduced morbidity can be obtained with the use of a tendon stripper. To successfully harvest the maximal amount of graft available, however, it is imperative to pay strict attention to the anatomy and the potential variations. It is especially important to clearly identify and separate the semitendinosus and gracilis tendons and to then identify and section all extraneous bands that might deflect a tendon stripper. This can usually be done by exposing the pes anserinus, incising the superficial tissue layer, and then identifying the combined insertion of both the semitendinosus and gracilis tendons. The two tendons are usually fused together near their point of insertion into the tibia, but can be clearly separated a few centimeters proximal to their insertion. If the two tendons are identifed and then traced to the tibia and released together, they can usually be separated by inverting them. From the undersurface it is much easier to identify the separation between the two. Once each tendon has been isolated, all extraneous insertions need to be identified and sectioned. There are consistent bands that run from both tendons to the medial head of gastrocnemius muscle (Fig. 8.3). These bands are frequently multiple. They can best be identified by pulling hard upon each tendon individually. This

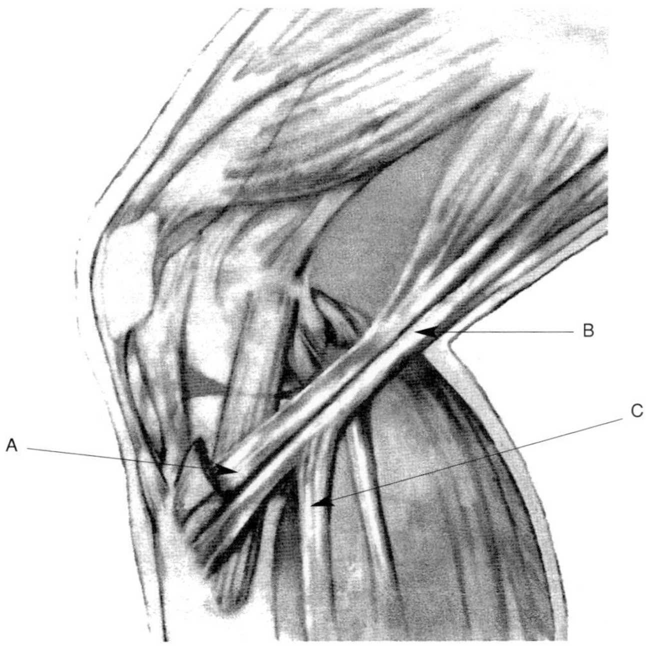

Figure 8.3. The semitendinosus (**A**) and gracilis (**B**) tendons must be isolated and separated prior to harvesting. Extraneous bands of tissue that consistently run from both tendons to the medial head of the gastrocnemius (**C**) must be identified and released prior to passing a tendon stripper to avoid deflecting the stripper and cutting the tendon short of the desired length.

breaks up small adhesions and often delivers the extraneous bands into a positon where they can be well visualized and sectioned.

It is usually possible to pass a finger up to the muscle belly to be certain that all bands have been sectioned. If this precaution is not taken, it is possible for the tendon stripper to follow an aberrant pathway and sever the tendon far short of maximal length. This often results in a graft that is too short to be used in a double-loop fashion.

In general, grafts of 28 to 30 cm in length are obtained when harvested with a tendon stripper. Most often the two tendons are of nearly equal length. For most endoscopic techniques, a graft length of 22 to 24 cm in length is sufficient. Therefore, with endoscopic techniques the most robust portion of each tendon can be utilized, and tapered ends can be debrided from the grafts.

If one or both tendons are of insufficient length to be doubled and fixed at both ends in a standard fashion, length can be added to the tendons by utilizing a Mercilene or Dacron tape. When a two-incision technique is utilized, a Mercilene or Dacron loop allows the graft to recess into the femoral tunnel, providing added length for direct fixation on the tibia. The tape is fixed at the entrance to the femoral tunnel. With endoscopic fixation on the femur, less graft is needed on the femoral side of the joint; therefore, shorter grafts can be utilized effectively.

Neuropraxia of a portion of the intrapatellar branch of the saphenous nerve is not uncommon following hamstring tendon harvest, and occasionally neuropraxia in the major distribution of the saphenous nerve occurs. This results in numbness in a portion of the nerve distribution (Fig. 8.4). The sensation in this sensory nerve distribution usually returns; however, it may take several months, and it is advisable to alert patients to this possibility before surgery. Neuromas of the saphenous nerve do not appear to be a problem in hamstring tendon harvest with tendon strippers. Bleeding is rarely a problem at the harvest site, but if, after the tourniquet is deflated, bleeding is more than expected, extension of the incision may be required to identify and cauterize the source. If bleeding is not well controlled, a drain at the harvest site should be considered.

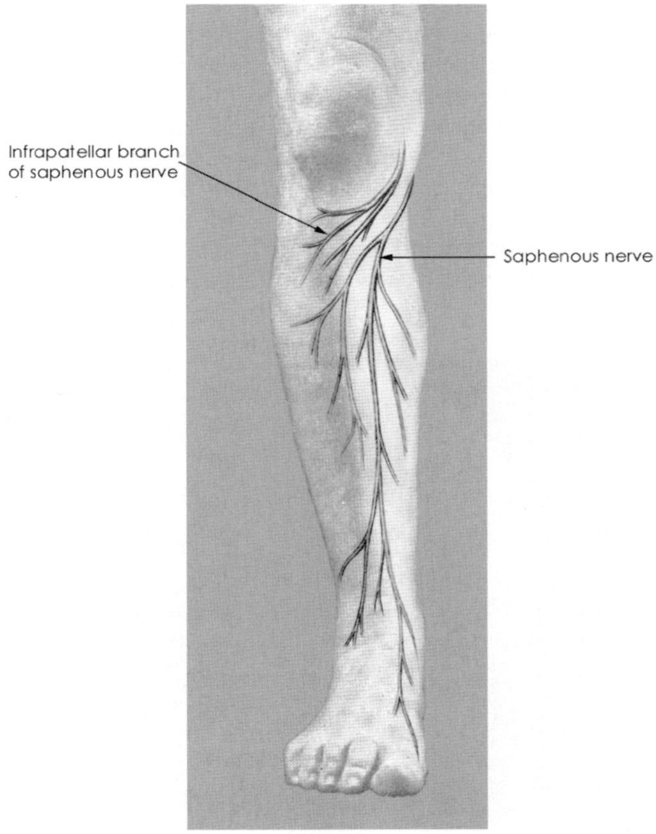

Figure 8.4. Postoperative numbness can occur in the saphenous nerve distribution or intrapatellar branch. Incisions, swelling, or hamstring graft harvest can contribute to this phenomenon. Patients should be warned of the possibility of numbness in the distribution of these sensory nerves.

COMPLICATIONS OF GRAFT PLACEMENT

For an ACL reconstruction with hamstring tendons or any other graft to be successful, the graft must be placed so that it is not overstrained as the knee passes through a full range of motion and so that it does not impinge against the bony anatomy of the intercondylar notch, particularly at terminal extension. A study by Sidles et al[14] has shown that this can usually be accomplished by placing the tibial tunnel in a central positon and the femoral tunnel high and to the extreme back of the intercondylar notch. This study was performed utilizing interactive computer graphics and digitized normal knee anatomy. It also utilized normal knee motion patterns controlled by intact ligaments. The study demonstrated that femoral attachment points depend upon tibial attachment points. To maximize the acceptable complementary area on the femur and to avoid terminal extension notch impingement, a central tibial tunnel was most appropriate. A central tibial tunnel is defined as a tunnel centered at the anatomic center of the ACL tibial attachment site. It can be found arthroscopically by placing a guide pin and then observing it as the knee is extended. The guide pin should be directly adjacent to the posterior cruciate ligament (PCL) (Fig. 8.5A), and as the knee is extended it should move toward the apex of the notch. At full extension the pin should avoid the roof of the notch by at least the radius of the tunnel to be drilled (Fig. 8.5B). This will allow the graft to be unimpinged at terminal extension. If notch impingement occurs at terminal extension, premature graft failure is likely, as demonstrated by Howell and Taylor.[15] If the initial guide pin is less than optimal, the position can be fine-tuned with the use of a guide that will allow a second pin to be placed parallel to the first. The adequacy of lateral notch clearance can also be checked by this method.

Relative to a central tibial attachment site the length changes to the femur are demonstrated in Fig. 8.6. This diagram demonstrates that there is an area on the femur relative to a central tibial attachment site that undergoes less than 5% strain and is located high and to the extreme back of the intercondylar notch. This area extends to the "over-the-top" area. To consistently create the femoral tunnel in the appropriate position, the tunnel should be centered at either the 11 o'clock or 1 o'clock position and the center of the tunnel should be no further than 5 mm from the over-the-top area. This area can be conveniently reached with a two-incision technique and a "rear-entry" guide. The area can also be reached through an appropriately placed tibial tunnel utilizing an over-the-top referencing guide with a 5-mm offset. By creating the femoral tunnel endoscopically, a straighter pathway can be maintained for the graft through the tibial tunnel and to its fixation point in the femoral tunnel. This avoids the excessive angle that the graft must bend in the frontal plane when utilizing the two-incision technique and outside-in drilling on the femur.

The use of an isometer offers no advantage in obtaining the correct position of the femoral tunnel. Bony landmarks are all that are necessary to consistently place

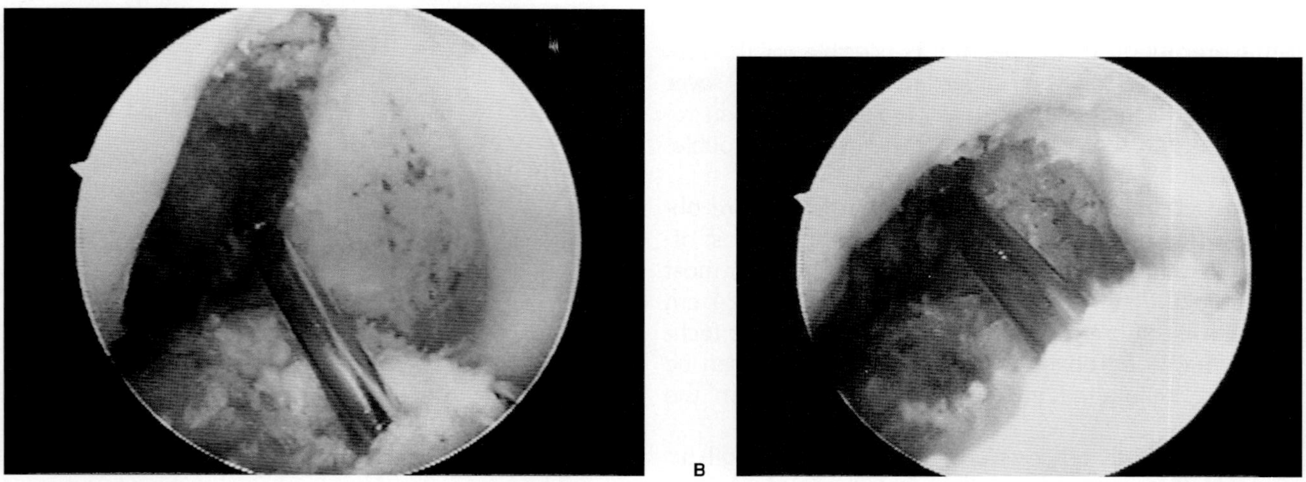

A B

Figure 8.5. A guide pin should be placed in the proposed position of the tibial tunnel to verify the desired location prior to overdrilling. The initial placement of the pin should be in the center of the anatomic footprint and adjacent to the posterior cruciate ligament (PCL) (**A**). The knee should then be extended and the guide pin should move directly toward the apex of the notch, and at the terminal extension the guide pin should be short of touching the superior notch by at least the radius of the tunnel to be drilled (**B**).

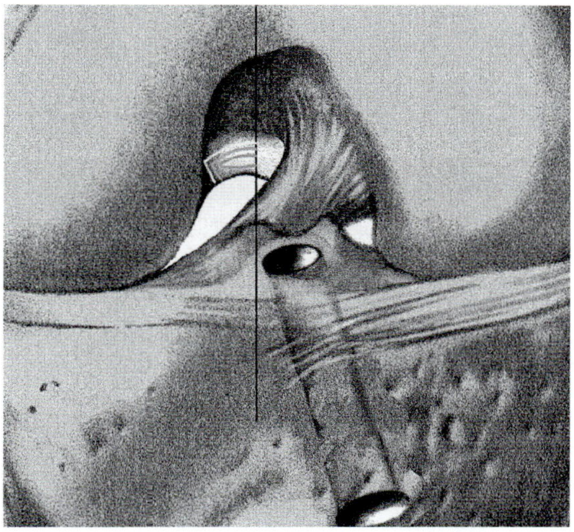

Figure 8.6. This "isometry map" shows the length changes on the femur relative to a central tibial attachment site, demonstrating that the areas of least strain are high and to the extreme back of the intercondylar notch.

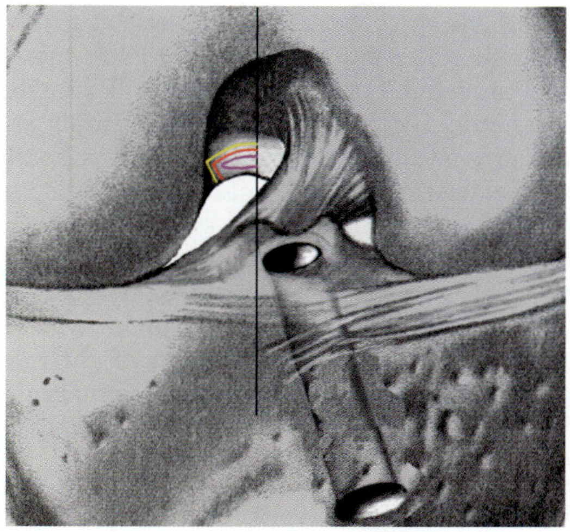

Figure 8.7. With proper tibial tunnel placement the femoral tunnel can be drilled through the tibial tunnel in a straight line as noted. The femoral placement should be to the extreme back of the intercondylar notch, and the medial edge should extend to the 12 o'clock position as shown

the tunnels accurately. When testing for isometry with an isometer, there is no guarantee that the motion patterns that the knee is being placed through are the desired motion pattern, since the knee is ACL deficient. Also, if the isometry testing is performed correctly, it would lead to a point on the femur of least strain for a single fiber. This is not the position where a drill hole should be centered. If that position, which is approximately 1 cm from the back of the intercondylar notch, were utilized as the center of a drill hole, the forwardmost part of the drill hole would be in an area of unacceptable strain. It would be further moved forward by chamfering at the tunnel edge. The appropriate tunnel can be placed by knowing where the extreme back of the intercondylar notch is located and where the 11 o'clock or 1 o'clock position is in the notch. The proper positions of the tibial and femoral tunnels are demonstrated in Fig. 8.7.

COMPLICATIONS OF FIXATION

Many options are now available for fixation of hamstring tendons when used for ACL reconstruction. When properly fixed, early loosening of hamstring tendon grafts should not be a problem. The recent studies by Steiner et al[8] and Rowden[9] demonstrate that when properly fixed, the initial pullout strength of hamstring tendon grafts exceeds that of patellar tendon bone blocks fixed with interference fit screws. Tensile strength to failure, however, is not the only important factor related to graft fixation. Construct elongation prior to failure is also a critical factor as it relates to the function of an ACL graft. The effective length of the construct is also an important consideration as it can effect eventual elongation.

Many systems are available for fixing hamstring tendon grafts, and they fall into several broad categories as follows: (1) sutures tied to a post or over buttons, (2) screws and washers, (3) staples, (4) interference fit screws, and (5) cross-pin techniques. Many suggested fixation techniques involve combinations of the above methods. In this section the basic principles of fixation and tensioning are discussed, and then each suggested technique for fixation is discussed, along with its relative advantages, relative disadvantages, potential complications, and methods for avoiding complications.

To take maximal advantage of a four-bundled graft, it is necessary to create nearly equal tension in all limbs of the grafts. The strength of the graft is nearly proportional to the individual strengths of each bundle added, as shown by Brown et al.[16] Most techniques therefore utilize initial fixation on the femur, with secondary tensioning and fixation to the tibia. To facilitate tendon healing in a bone tunnel, it is important to create the smallest tunnels possible so that the grafts fit snuggly within them. Fixation devices that require overdrilling of tunnels have the potential to compromise tendon healing within the tunnel. Some suggested fixation methods include bone grafting of overdrilled tunnels. When grafts need to share the tunnel with interference fit fixation devices, the potential exists to change the position of the graft within the tunnel and to interfere with full-radius healing of the graft to the tunnel. To limit motion within bone tunnels and to best assure desired isometry, it is preferable to fix the grafts as close to their entry into the intraarticular space as possible.[17] All fixation devices should be easily retrieved so as not to compromise possible revision surgery.

From the above it is obvious that no fixation technique is ideal in all aspects. Fortunately, most commonly used techniques provide adequate fixation when properly utilized. Following is a discussion of each general catergory of fixation and the potential complications of each. Tips for avoiding complications will be addressed.

Fixation with Sutures and Buttons or Posts

The weak link in any technique utilizing sutures is the suture material itself and the inherent creep in knots that are utilized. When utilized properly, however, this technique has been shown to be effective in fixing hamstring tendon grafts used for ACL reconstruction. It is imperative to use a suture technique that does not slip within the tendon tissue and to extend it beyond the tapered ends into robust healthy tendon. Either a Bunnell or Krakow[18] stitch should be utilized to improve fixation of the suture material to the tendon, and the suture material should be of sufficient stiffness. Square knots should be utilized when securing sutures so as to minimize slippage. It is advisable to apply tension to the construct for a period of time prior to final fixation to remove creep from the system. Fixation of hamstring tendon grafts with suture is much more problematic than the fixation of bone blocks with suture where a considerable amount of interference fit of the bone blocks in the tunnels helps faciliate the initial strength. The advantage of suture fixation is that suture material is inexpensive and readily available. The disadvantage of this technique is that it is the weakest of the commonly utilized methods for graft fixation, and there is the potential for considerable creep in the system if meticulous attention is not paid to suture technique, knot tying, and preconditioning of the construct.

The Endobutton (Fig. 8.8) is a commonly utilized form of femoral fixation that is an extension of the suture and button fixation technique. This technique utilizes an endoscopically placed button on the anterolateral femoral cortex, and the button is attached to the graft with tape or with sutures. This technique has the advantage of tightly placing the graft within the femoral tunnel. The disadvantage is that the tape or suture connection between the graft and Endobutton has the same inherent risk of other suture techniques, that is, the tendency to have creep within the system. In an attempt to eliminate the knot as a source of potential construct elongation, a newer version of the Endobutton has been developed that has preattached tapes of various lengths, avoiding the need to tie a knot.

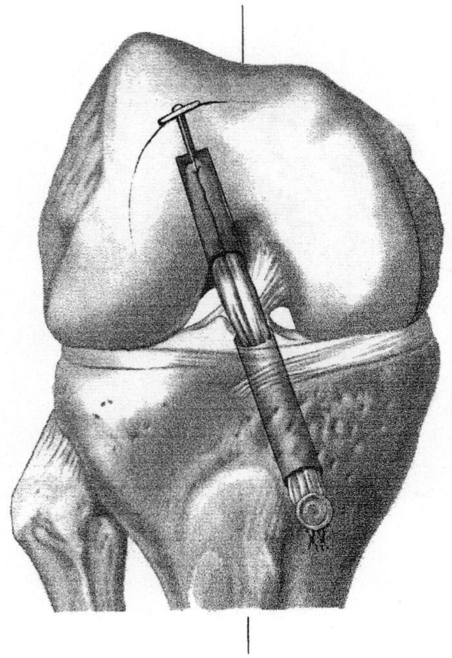

Figure 8.8. The Endobutton can be utilized to endoscopically fix the hamstring tendon grafts to the femur; a tape of variable length connects the Endobutton to the graft.

Another potential complication with the use of the Endobutton occurs when placing the Endobutton within the soft tissues rather than against the anterior femoral cortex. Simonian et al[19] have shown that this complication can be avoided by drilling the femoral socket no more than 10 mm deeper than the desired depth of graft penetration. It is necessary to drill the femoral tunnel 6 mm deeper than graft penetration to allow flipping of the Endobutton on the anterior cortex. The additional 4 mm helps facilitate this, but it is not so deep as to allow the Endobutton to enter the overlying soft tissues. The stiffness of a construct utilizing an Endobutton is equal to the stiffness of the tapes connecting the Endobutton to the hamstring tendon grafts. To obtain sufficient stiffness, it is necessary to use a stiff tape or to double the tape to increase stiffness.

Fixation with Screws and Washers

The use of screws and washers has been shown to be an effective way of fixing soft tissue grafts. The fixation strength of a washer is proportional to the contact between the washer and the graft. Therefore, washers of larger diameters are more effective than washers of smaller diameters. Steiner et al[8] have shown that the use of two screws and washers greatly increases the fixation strength over the use of a single screw and washer. The use of a suture technique as well as screw and washer fixation also strengthens the construct by extending the fixation into the robust portion of a graft and making slippage of the graft under the washer less likely. Washers have the potential for pressure necrosis of the graft and should have steps or posts to limit their penetration. The major disadvantage of utilizing screws and washers for graft fixation is that fixation must usually be done outside the tunnels and at a distance from the tunnel entrance points into the joint. This creates a greater length of the construct between fixation points, which may be of minimal importance if the grafts fit snuggly within the tunnels. Washers also occasionally cause irritation to the overlying skin and need to be removed. Occasionally a bursa or ganglion will develop over a washer and must be treated by screw and washer removal.

Fixation with Staples

Staples are still utilized on occasion for the fixation of hamstring tendon grafts. They offer the advantage of being relatively inexpensive and available. However, they have been shown to provide some of the least secure fixation, particularly if only one staple is used to secure the tendon. If two staples are utilized to provide a "belt-buckle" technique of fixation, much greater pull-out strength can be obtained. However, this technique produces a fairly bulky effect often requiring staple removal. Staple removal is also quite difficult when compared to removing a screw and washer. The use of a staple also has a high potential of traumatizing the graft at the point of fixation. Staples also are generally used outside of the bone tunnels; therefore, they have the same problem of "fixation at a distance" as do screws and washers. They do, however, allow for a tight fit of the grafts within the tunnels.

Fixation with Interference Fit Screws

Interference fit screws have recently become a fairly common way of fixing hamstring tendon grafts (Fig. 8.9). Both metallic and bioabsorbable screws have been used. The bioabsorbable screws have the advantage of eventually dissolving and allowing full-radius healing of the graft, and have been shown to provide greater initial fixation strength than comparably sized metallic screws. The bioabsorbable screws also have less of a chance of damaging the grafts during insertion. Interference fit screws have the advantage of fixing the graft near its entrance into the intraarticular space, thus shortening the length of the construct and improving stiffness. They have the disadvantages of distorting the position of the graft within the tunnel and damaging the graft during insertion, and they make it more difficult to equally tension all bands of a multiply stranded graft. Since a tibial interference fit screw is usually inserted from outside in, it also is being inserted in the opposite direction to that in which tension is being applied to the graft, again adding a degree of uncertainty to the tension obtained. With bioabsorbable screws there is also a question of how long the device remains and what replaces the device when it is removed. There is some recent evidence that these devices are replaced by bone relatively quickly. To obtain maximum fixation benefit from an interference fit screw, it must also be placed parallel to the tunnel between the graft wall and the graft. The ability to properly place an interference fit screw is in some cases facilitated by utilizing a cannulated screw over a guide pin. It has also been shown that to obtain the best initial pull-out strength from an interference fit screw, a screw should be used that is at least as large as the size of the tunnel drilled.

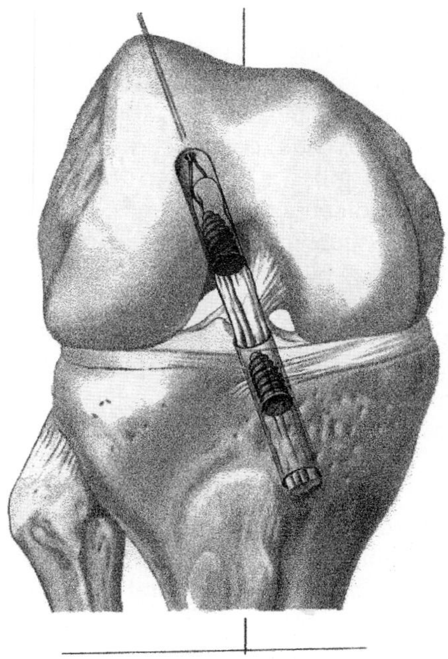

Figure 8.9. Either metallic or bioabsorbable interference fit screws can be utilized to fix hamstring tendon grafts on both the femur and tibia. They work by compressing the graft material into the adjacent cancellous bone. They can distort the position of the collagen, and their placement must take this into consideration.

Fixation by Cross-Pin Techniques

The most rigid form of femoral fixation is to utilize a cross pin. This can be done with a two-tunnel technique by looping the grafts around a screw and washer as they exit the femoral tunnel (Fig. 8.10), or it can be done endoscopically (Fig. 8.11), utilizing several commercially available techniques. Since a cross pin directly fixes the graft, this is a very rigid construct, avoiding the potential creep that is present in systems utilizing tapes and sutures. It has potential disadvantages, however, in that it is sometimes technically difficult to be sure that the cross pin is looped by both tendons. Devices to help ensure that this complication does not occur necessitate overdrilling the femoral tunnel, thus making graft fit against the tunnel walls less tight than desirable. Some cross-pinning techniques therefore utilize bone grafting techniques to help tighten the grafts in the tunnels.

Although each method of femoral fixation of the hamstring tendon grafts has its own potential complications and shortcomings, if attention is paid to detail most will provide adequate femoral fixation. A bigger problem in fixing hamstring tendons appears to be fixation on the tibia. Because the direction of the tunnel is in line with applied forces through the more functional ranges of knee motion, tibial fixation is even more critical than femoral fixation. Most of the previously described techniques of fixation have been utilized on the tibia, including sutures over buttons, staples, screw and washer fixation, interference fit screws, and cross-pin techniques. The most secure fixation on the tibia utilizes a suture technique as well as screw and washer direct fixation of the grafts. Although this is an effective way to fix the graft, the fixation is distant from the entry into the joint, and screws and washers are often prominent and require removal. To move the fixation closer to the entry point into the joint, screws and washers within the tibia tunnel have been utilized, as have interference fit screws. Interference fit screws have been used alone or as a means of augmenting other techniques. The ability to properly tension the graft is facilitated by the use of sutures and the screw and washer, and it is suggested that this technique be maintained with the possible addition of an interference fit screw to stabilize the graft at its entry into the joint.

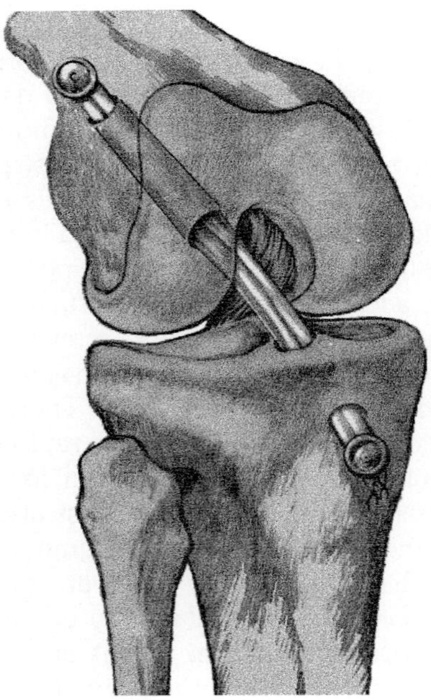

Figure 8.10. Optimal femoral fixation is obtained by directly looping the grafts around a screw (post) and washer on the femur. Fixing the tendons outside of the tunnel, however, requires a thigh incision and wastes a significant portion of the graft in the femoral tunnel. This can on occasion complicate tibial fixation.

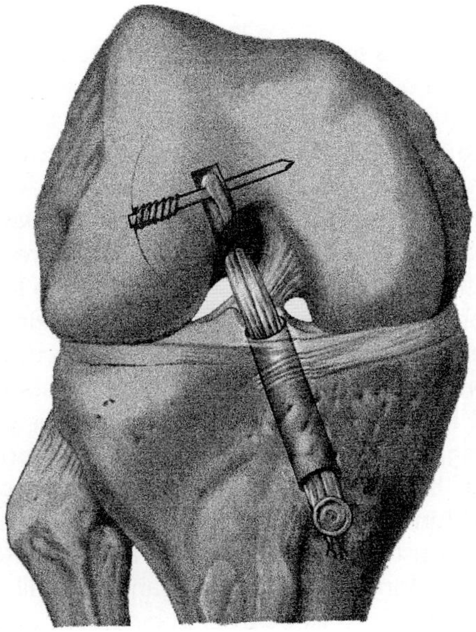

Figure 8.11. Cross-pin techniques can also be utilized within the femoral tunnel, avoiding the additional femoral incision and shortening the amount of graft needed within the femur.

POSTOPERATIVE COMPLICATIONS AT THE DONOR SITE

Significant complications related to the harvest of hamstring tendon autografts are rare. Minor complications are more common and include potential weakness due to the loss of the semitendinosus and gracilis muscle tendon units, sensory changes in the saphenous nerve distribution, and adhesions in the posterior thigh.

Knee flexion strength following the harvest of semitendinosus and gracilis tendons is a concern that has been addressed by several investigators. Lipscomb et al,[20] Aglietti et al,[21] and Karlson et al[22] have evaluated patients at 2 years or more following surgery and found no loss of knee flexion strength. Marder and colleagues[4] and Kramer and associates[23] demonstrated statistically significant decreases in hamstring strength following harvest of the semitendinosus and gracilis tendons. Hormel et al[5] evaluated patients 3 years postoperatively following the harvest of both semitendinosus and gracilis tendons for ACL reconstruction. They found an average of 90% of knee flexion strength on the operated side when compared to the nonoperative side. Their study included several patients who had regained 100% of their knee flexion strength relative to the nonoperative side, suggesting that the results appear to be dependent on on the amount of rehabilitation the patient participates in. Yasuda et al[24] looked at the isolated effects of graft harvest by studying patients who had hamstring tendon grafts harvested from the limb contralateral to the side being reconstructed. An initial loss of hamstring strength was noted; however, this was fully restored by 3 months postoperation. There is the potential to regain full knee flexion strength following the harvest of hamstring tendons for ACL reconstruction.

Adhesions in the posterior thigh creating a "bunching" effect were fairly common when open techniques were utilized to harvest the semitendinosus and gracilis tendons. After an open posterior thigh approach, scarring of the skin and subcutaneous fascia to the muscle belly was frequent and it appears to be the common cause of the skin retraction with knee flexion. This problem has been almost completely eliminated by avoiding the posterior thigh incision and harvesting the tendon grafts with a tendon stripper. When the tendons are harvested with a tendon stripper, asymmetry of the posterior thigh musculature is usually imperceptable. It was initially thought that retraction of the semitendinosus and gracilis tendon muscle bellies would be considerable, but this has not been observed in the usual case. Neither visual posterior thigh inspection nor magnetic resonance imaging (MRI) has confirmed significant muscle belly retraction to occur routinely. Studies reported by Cross and colleagues[25] showed a reformation of the semitendinosus and gracilis tendons demonstrable by palpation during resisted flexion, MRI, and electromyogram (EMG) studies. Simonian et al[26] have also investigated this phenomenon with MRI studies and have shown that tissue does indeed regenerate along the course of the semitendinosus and gracilis tendons. This tissue, however, is likely not functional. Simonian et al also demonstrated a slight proximal translation of the semitendinosus and gracilis muscle bellies but not to the extent that would be expected with complete distal detachment. This finding is probably due to the extensive origin of the muscles and attachments to surrounding structures. Although fortunately rare, occasionally adhesions or proximal muscle migration will occur, causing a cosmetic deformity as demonstrated in Fig. 8.12.

COMPLICATIONS WITH THE IMPLANTED GRAFTS

Several studies in the literature compare hamstring tendons with patellar tendon autografts in ACL reconstruction. Older reports favor the long-term results with patellar tendons, but few of these reports used double loops of both semitendinosus and gracilis tendons or applied the principles of graft placement and fixation that have been more recently appreciated. Several recent investigations including those by Aglietti and coworkers,[22] Marder and colleagues,[4] and Feagin and colleagues[13] have shown no appreciable difference in the results

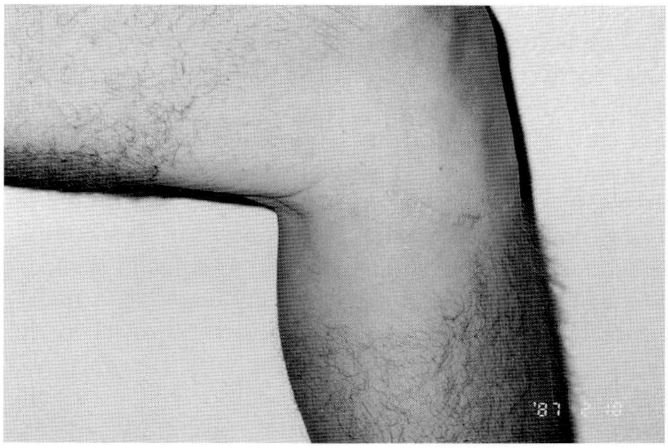

A

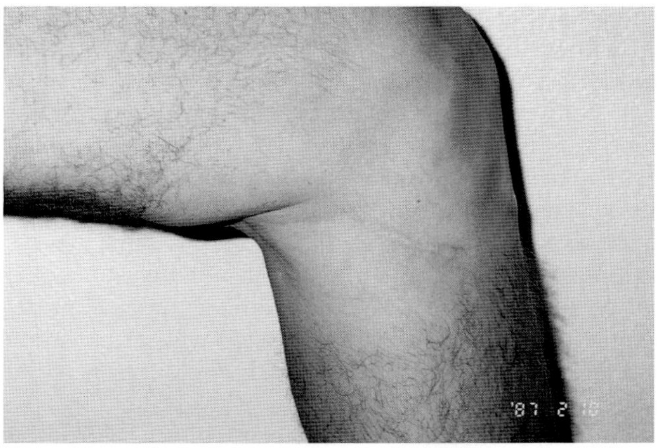

B

Figure 8.12. On rare occasions adhesions may occur after hamstring harvest, causing skin retraction with hamstring contracture. **A:** Thigh relaxed. **B:** Hamstring contraction.

with hamstring tendon autografts versus patellar tendon grafts. Studies such as those of Sgaglione et al[27] have reported long-term results with hamstring tendons for acute reconstructions that compare well with the results for patellar tendon reconstructions, yet patients with hamstring tendon reconstructions for chronic ACL deficiency showed a greater tendency for increased laxity at follow-up.

Other researchers have suggested that hamstring tendons loosen over time. A 3-year follow-up study by Hormel et al[5] of ACL reconstructions with double loops of semitendinosus and gracilis tendons demonstrated, with arthrometry testing, laxity results equal to published data on patellar tendon ACL reconstructions. Their study also noted no interval change in arthrometry data between 1 year and 3 years following surgery and no difference between those patients reconstructed acutely or chronically. This study collaborates the study of Feagin et al,[13] which showed no deterioration of results over time, and that of O'Neill,[12] which showed saisfactory results in both acute and chronic cases.

On occasion notch impingement can develop following the implantation of hamstring tendon autografts, as it can following the implantation of patellar tendon autografts. The development of notch impingement occurs despite carefully ensuring it did not exist at the time of graft implantation. The development of this complication occurs when either the graft enlarges in size during healing or the prepared notch becomes smaller. When the impingement develops, it may result in the failure of some of the anterior fibers of the graft, and these fibers may ball up in the anterior portion of the notch, blocking terminal extension by creating a "cyclops" lesion[28] (Fig. 8.13). This complication is often accompanied by fairly coarse crepitus near the terminal extension. The complication appears to be more prevalent when a notchplasty has been performed. For this reason it is advisable to avoid a notchplasty when it is at all possible. It is more appropriate to adjust graft position to fit the anatomic notch than to enlarge the notch creating bleeding cancellous surfaces. The original notch size is likely to return; therefore, all attempts should be made to fit the graft to it (Fig. 8.14). It is not always possible to avoid a notchplasty, but notchplasty should not be routinely practiced. When this complication develops, it is usually effectively treated with arthroscopy and debridement followed by repeat enlargement of the intracondylar notch.

The complication of arthrofibrosis can occur following ACL reconstruction with hamstring tendons as it can following any other intraarticular procedure of the joint. With proper graft placement and fixation allowing early range of motion and quadriceps exercise, this problem occurs much less often than it had in earlier years. A study by Howell and Taylor[29] has shown that patients treated with ACL hamstring reconstructions followed by an aggressive rehabilitation protocol showed no increased failure rates when compared to more conservative rehab regimens. By avoiding the extensor mechanism, arthrofibrosis following the use of hamstring tendons is less common than that noted following the use of the patellar tendon autografts. Should arthrofibrosis be encountered, it should be treated in routine ways.

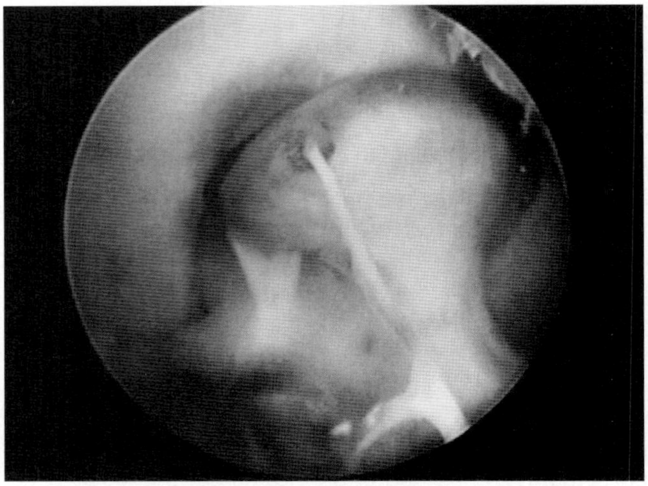

Figure 8.13. If the tibial tunnel is placed too anteriorly or if a superior notch reforms, anterior graft fibers may break and coalesce forming a "cyclops" lesion as shown.

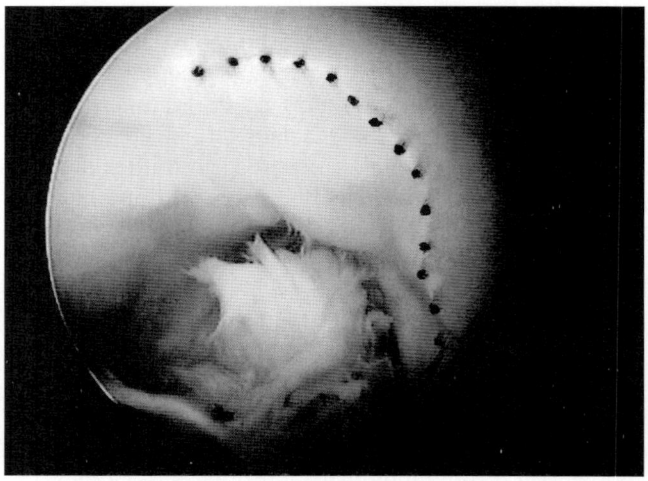

Figure 8.14. It is advisable to fit an ACL graft substitute to the anatomic notch when possible, particularly in acute situations, to avoid the need for a notchplasty. Notchplasties, which are done to fit a graft, often reform and begin to traumatize the graft causing fiber failure. (Broken line demarcates notchplasty.)

DISCUSSION

Anterior cruciate ligament insufficiency can be treated effectively with either patellar tendon autografts or hamstring tendon autografts. When procedures are performed correctly, utilizing proper tunnel placement, avoidance of bony impingement, and appropriate fixation, and are followed by appropriate rehabilitation, a good result can be expected from either technique. The primary advantage to the use of hamstring tendons is the reduced harvest-site morbidity relative to that seen with the use of patellar tendon autogafts. Pain in the patellofemoral joint seems to be considerably less when hamstring tendons are utilized for ACL reconstruction, and complications such as patellar fracture and infrapatellar contraction syndrome are essentially nonexistent. Although these problems are also rare with the use of patellar tendon autografts, when they occur they generally preclude a good result.

The importance of adhering to technical detail in performing ACL reconstructive surgery cannot be overemphasized. Attention to graft harvest and preparation, tunnel placement, fixation, and rehabilitation are much more important factors to the successful reconstruction of the ACL than is the origin of the autogenous graft. The use of hamstring tendon grafts is possible in almost all patients with ACL insufficiency, but it is particularly applicable to those patients in whom patellar tendon ACL reconstruction has failed, or in those with preexisting patellofemoral disease, or in any other situation where avoidance of the extensor mechanism is desirable. Complications from the use of hamstring tendons are rare and can usually be avoided. This chapter has presented potential pitfalls with the use of hamstring tendon grafts and has suggested ways of avoiding them when possible and dealing with them should they occur.

References

1. Cho KO. Reconstruction of the anterior cruciate ligament by semitendinosus tenodesis. *J Bone Joint Surg* 1975; 57A:608–612.
2. Mott HW. Semitendinosus anatomic reconstruction for cruciate ligament insufficiency. *Clin Orthop* 1983;172: 90–92.
3. Gomes JLE, Marczyk LRS. Anterior cruciate ligament reconstruction with a loop or double thickness of senitendinosus tendon. *Am J Sports Med* 1984;12:199–203.
4. Marder RA, Raskin JR, Carroll M. Prospective evaluation of arthroscopically assisted anterior cruciate ligament reconstruction: patellar tendon versus semitendinosus and gracilis tendons. *Am J Sports Med* 1991;19(5):478–484.
5. Hormel S, Larson RV, Larry I. *ACL reconstruction with double loops of semitendinosus and gracilis tendons: 3 year follow-up*. Paper presented at the annual meeting of the American Academy of Orthopaedic Surgeons, Orlando, FL, February 1995.
6. Brown CH, Steiner ME, Carson EW. The use of hamstring tendons for anterior cruciate ligament reconstruction: technique and results. *Clin Sports Med* 1993;12(4): 723–753.
7. Noyes, FR, Butler DL, Grood ES, Zernicke RF, Hefzy MS. Biomechanical analysis of human ligament grafts used in knee ligament repairs and reconstructions. *J Bone Joint Surg* 1984;66A:344–352.
8. Steiner ME, Hecker AT, Brown CH, Hanes WC. Anterior cruciate ligament graft fixation: comparison of hamstring and patellar tendon grafts. *Am J Sports Med* 1994;22:240–247.
9. Rowden NJ, Sher D, Rogers GH, et al. Anterior cruciate ligament graft fixation: initial comparison of patellar tendon and semitendinosus autografts in young fresh cadavers. *Am J Sports Med* 1997;25(4):472–477.
10. Rodeo SA, Arnoczky SP, Torzilli PA. Tendon-healing in a bone tunnel: a biomechanical and histological study in the dog. *J Bone Joint Surg* 1993;75A:1795–1803.
11. Lane LG, McFadden P, Bowden L, Amiel D. The ligamentization process: a four year case study following ACL reconstruction with a semitendinosus graft. *J Arthro Rec Surg* 1993;9(2):149–153.
12. O'Neill DB. Arthroscopically assisted reconstruction of the anterior cruciate ligament: a prospective randomized analysis of three techniques. *J Bone Joint Surg* 1996; 78A:803–813.
13. Feagin JA, Wills RP, Lambert KL. Anterior cruicate ligament reconstruction: bone–patella tendon–bone versus semitendinosus anatomic reconstruction. *Clin Orthop* 1997;341:69–72.
14. Sidles JA, Larson RV, Garbini JL, et al. Ligament length relationships in the moving knee. *J Orthop Res* 1988; 6:593–610.
15. Howell SM, Taylor MA. Failure of reconstruction of the anterior cruciate ligament due to impingement by the intercondylar roof. *J Bone Joint Surg* 1993;75A:1044–1055.
16. Brown C, Hammer D, Hecker A, et al. Biomechanics of semitendinosus and gracilis tendon grafts. In: *Proceedings of Sports Medicine 2000*. Stockholm, Sweden: 1995.
17. Morgan C, Kalman V, Grawl D. Isometry testing for anterior cruciate ligament reconstruction revisited. *Arthroscopy* 1995;11:647–659.
18. Krakow KA, Thomas SC, Jones LC. A new stitch for ligament tendon fixation. Brief note. *J Bone Joint Surg* 1986;68A(5):764–766.
19. Simonian PT, Behr CT, Stechschulte DJ. Potential pitfall of the Endobutton. *Arthroscopy* 1998;14(1):66–69.

20. Lipscomb AB, Johnston RK, Snyder RB, Warburton MS, Gilbert PP. Evaluation of hamstring strength following the use of semitendinosus and gracilis tendons to reconstruct the anterior cruciate ligament. *Am J Sports Med* 1982;10:340–342.

21. Aglietti P, Buzzi R, Zaccherotti G, DeBiase P. Patellar tendon versus doubled semitendinosus and gracilis tendons for anterior cruciate ligament reconstruction. *Am J Sports Med* 1994;22:211–218.

22. Karlson JA, Steiner ME, Brown CH, Johnson J. Anterior cruciate ligament reconstruction using gracilis and semitendinosus tendons. Comparison of through the condyle and over the top graft placements. *Am J Sports Med* 1994;22(5):659–666.

23. Kramer J, Nusca D, Fowler P, Webster-Bogaert S. Knee flexor and extensor strength during concentric and eccentric muscle actions after anterior cruciate ligament reconstruction using the semitendinosus tendon and ligament augmentation device. *Am J Sports Med* 1993; 21(2):285–291.

24. Yasuda K, Tsujino J, Yasumitsu O, et al. Graft site morbidity with autogenous semitendinosus and gracilis tendons. *Am J Sports Med* 1995;23(6):706–714.

25. Cross MJ, Anderson I, Roger G. Regeneration of the tendons of semitendinosus and gracilis following their transection for repair of the anterior cruciate ligament. *Am J Sports Med* 1989;17:709.

26. Simonian PT, Harrison SD, Cooley VJ, et al. Assessment of morbidity of semitendinosus and gracilis tendon harvest for ACL reconstruction. *Am J Knee Surg* 1997; 10(2):54–59.

27. Sgaglione NA, Del Pizzo W, Fox JM, Friedman MS. Arthroscopically assisted anterior cruciate ligament reconstruction with the pes anserine tendons. Comparison of results in acute and chronic ligament deficiency. *Am J Sports Med* 1993;21(2):249–256.

28. Jackson DW, Schaefer RK. Cyclops syndrome: loss of extension following intraarticular anterior cruciate ligament reconstruction. *Arthroscopy* 1990;6:171–178.

29. Howell SM, Taylor MA. Brace-free rehabilitation, with early return to activity for knees reconstructed with a double-looped semitendinosus and gracilis graft. *J Bone Joint Surg* 1996;78A(6):814–825.

Chapter 9

Complications and Pitfalls in Anterior Cruciate Ligament Reconstruction Using Bone–Patellar Tendon–Bone Autograft

Laurence D. Higgins, Mark Clatworthy, and Christopher D. Harner

Bone–patellar tendon–bone autograft (BPTB) has served as the gold standard for anterior cruciate ligament (ACL) reconstruction. Although alternate graft options have recently gained popularity, BPTB autograft is by far the most common technique employed for ACL reconstruction.[1] With an estimated 150,000 ACL reconstructions performed annually, this graft choice may account for up to 80% of all such procedures. With follow-up studies evaluating patients for up to 10 years, the complication profile of this technique has been well documented. While the overall serious complication rate is low, there are potential risks that the orthopedic surgeon must be cognizant of in order to minimize their occurrence and optimize patient outcome.

Many potential ACL reconstruction complications are independent of graft choice. Those complications that are generic to ACL reconstruction are not addressed in this chapter. Rather, the discussion focuses on complications intrinsic to ACL reconstruction with autograft BPTB and on strategies to avoid their occurrence. This chapter discusses the nature of each complication, complication prevention, and management of the complication once it has developed.

PATELLAR FRACTURES

Patellar fractures are rare complications following ACL harvest with BPTB autograft. Although no formal determination of the incidence of patellar fractures has been published to our knowledge, this is a major intra- or perioperative complication. To date only 28 reported fractures have appeared in the literature, mainly as case reports or technical notes, documenting these fracture occurrences and fixation techniques.[2–11] Christen and Jakob,[12] in a retrospective review, documented nine patellar fractures out of a total of 490 cases, yielding an incidence of 1.8%.

Most patellar fractures noted intraoperatively are nondisplaced fractures that are vertical in nature and result from harvesting an excessively long patellar bone plug.[4,10,13] The use of an osteotome to lever a BPTB ACL graft is often the inciting event, and a fissure or a frank fracture plane may be immediately visualized. These fractures are often simple in nature and should be addressed when visualized; however, it should be noted that Christen and Jakob have treated three of six of these nondisplaced fractures nonoperatively with good results. To proceed with aggressive rehabilitation, fixation at the time of the event is recommended (Fig. 9.1A,B).

Transverse patellar fractures are usually encountered in the postoperative period. These fractures most likely occur from low-energy injuries or violent quadriceps contraction to prevent a fall, resulting in this particular fracture pattern. The presence of stress risers at the site of harvest is the proximate cause of such injuries. The fracture usually occurs at the proximal extent of the bone plug with wide displacement of the fracture fragments and loss of a competent extensor mechanism. These fractures are often simple, without comminution (Fig. 9.2A–C). Transverse patellar fractures must be aggressively treated to allow appropriate postoperative ACL rehabilitation in order to obtain a successful ACL reconstruction.[5,7,10,14–18]

Prevention of Complications

Meticulous attention should be directed to harvesting the patellar tendon. To minimize the risk of fracture, no

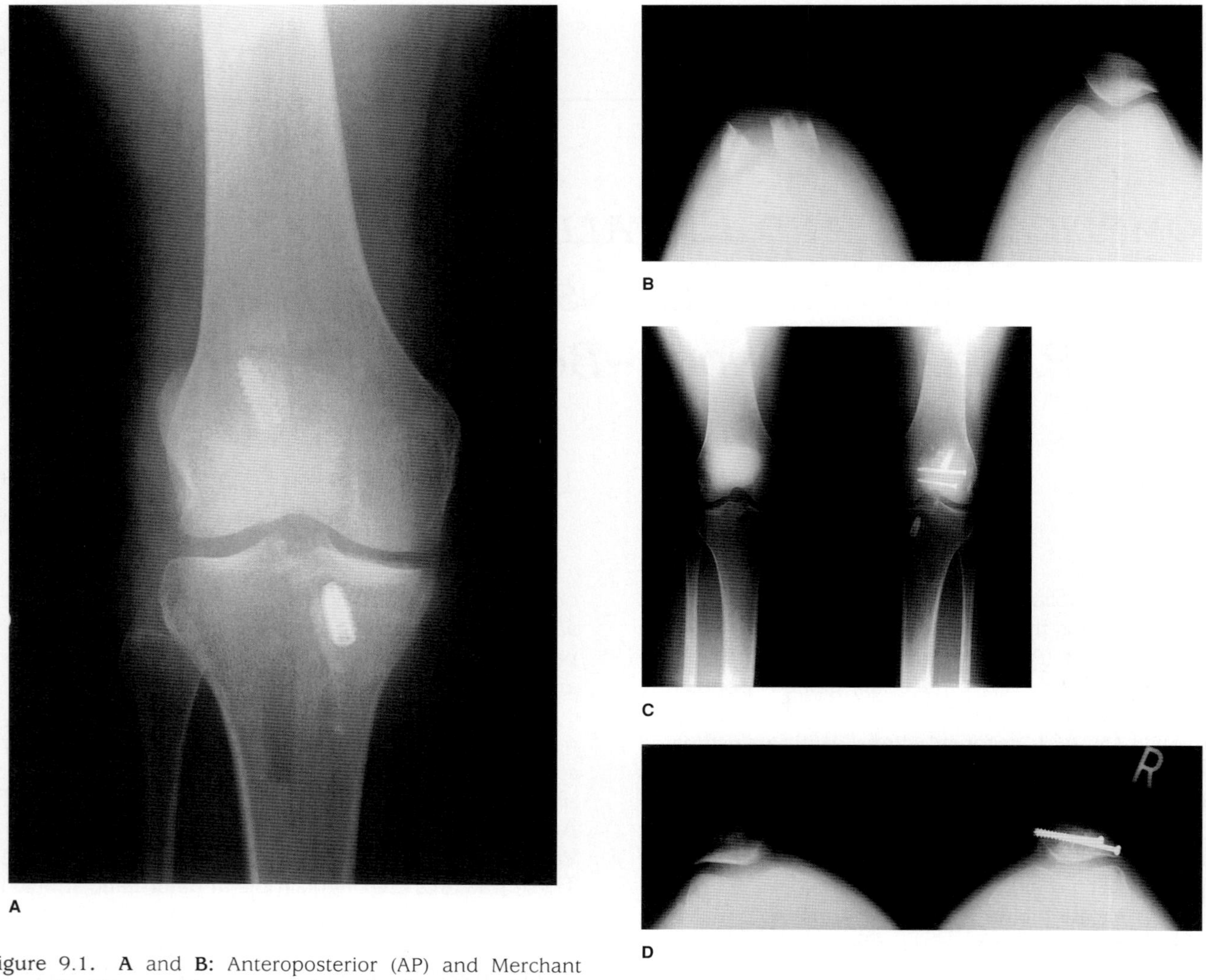

Figure 9.1. **A** and **B:** Anteroposterior (AP) and Merchant views of a 23-year-old woman 8 days after bone–patellar tendon–bone (BPTB) anterior cruciate ligament (ACL) reconstruction. The patient fell directly onto her knee. **C** and **D:** AP and lateral views 6 months after horizontal Association Osteosynthese (AO) screws fixation with excellent functional result.

more than 25 to 30 mm of the length of the patella and no more than 10 mm of width should be harvested. Additionally, using less than one-third of the preoperatively measured patellar depth for harvesting has been proposed as a measure to diminish the risk of fracture.[16] As the cortical bone of the patella is thicker and more dense, harvesting the patellar graft is technically more difficult. Ideally, the bony cuts should be performed with an oscillating saw and not with an osteotome. It is of critical importance to complete the bony cuts, particularly at the corners of the graft, to minimize the force necessary to deliver the graft. Excessive prying with an osteotome may endanger both the patella and graft itself.

Management

Vertical fissure fractures that are noticed at the time of surgery are best treated prophylactically to ensure and maintain appropriate postoperative rehabilitation. Several techniques have been described including an anterior tension band over horizontally directed Kirschner wires (K-wires).[19] The application of a tension band device may not be necessary, as tensile forces are not experienced by this fracture pattern. Berg[16] has described nonlagged bicortical screw fixation with excellent results. Berg similarly recommended against overdrilling and lagging the fracture, which may cause hinging at the intact

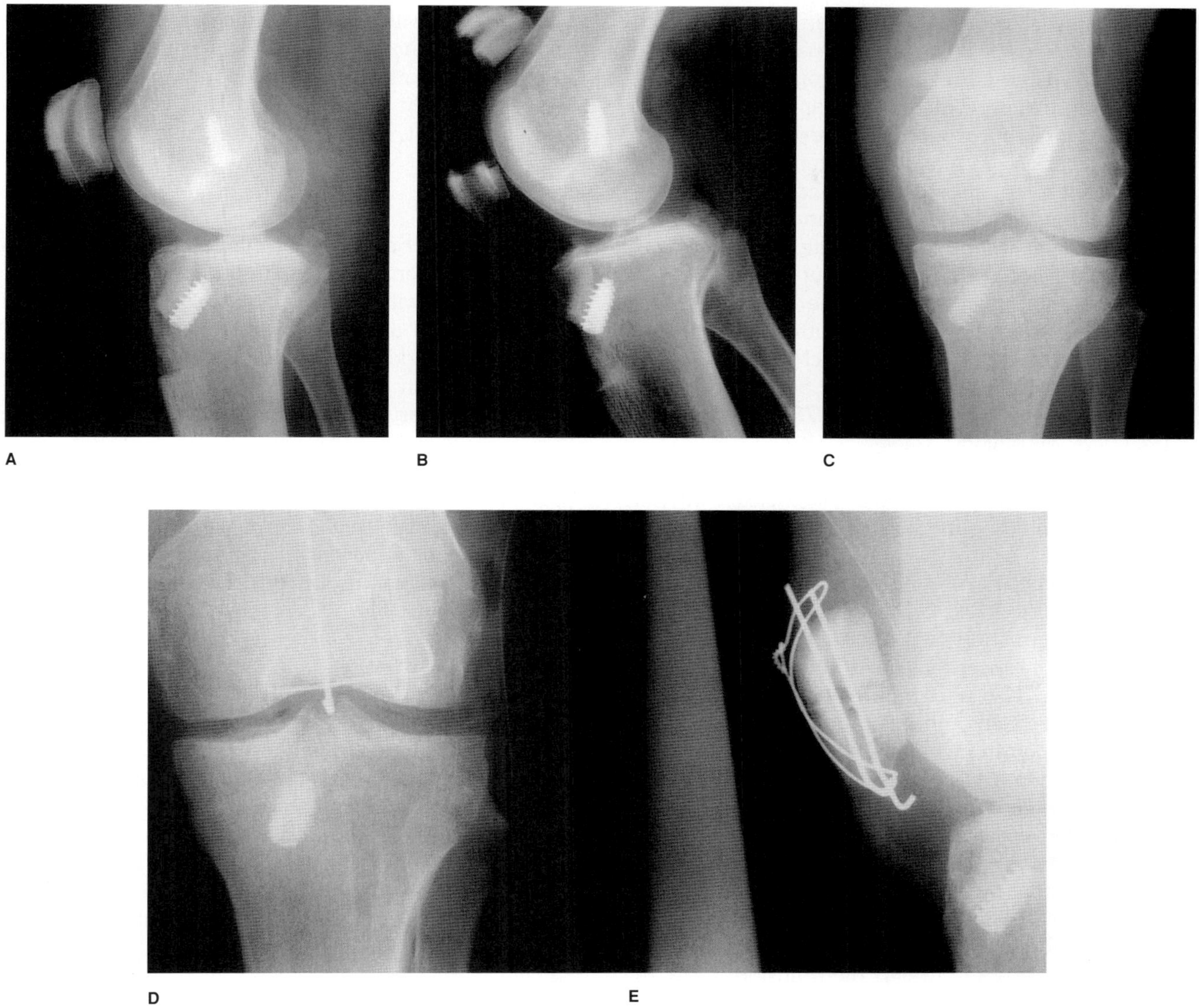

Figure 9.2. **A:** Lateral radiograph 8 days after ACL reconstruction. **B** and **C:** Lateral and AP radiographs 3 months later after fall. **D** and **E:** Open reduction with internal fixation (ORIF) with AO technique for displaced transverse fracture.

articular surface and may displace these often nondisplaced fractures (Fig. 9.1C,D).

Transverse fractures of the patella disrupt the extensor mechanism and require acute fixation. These fractures are best treated using Association Osteosynthere (AO) technique with tension band wiring through cannulated screws. By employing an 18-gauge wire, a rigid fixation construct can be obtained, permitting rehabilitation to continue with little deleterious effect. Berg[16] noted that there was no discernible difference in outcome of the ACL reconstruction at 1 year when treated with AO principles (Fig. 9.2D,E).

PATELLAR TENDON RUPTURE

Patellar tendon rupture following middle-third patellar tendon ACL reconstruction is a rare complication. There are seven reports of 12 ruptures in the literature.[5,20–25] The majority of cases occurred in the first 10 months, with six cases occurring after a Marshall/MacIntosh ACL reconstruction.[26] Two cases from one report document late ruptures at 3 years and 6 years.[20] In most cases, the rupture occurs following minor trauma. Direct impact, hyperflexion, or forceful quadriceps contractions were elicited as the mechanism of rupture. Eight of the

12 ruptures were proximal avulsions. No report documents grossly abnormal tissue in the patellar tendon defect and there is no correlation with opening or closing the defect and rupture of the patellar tendon. Several etiologies have been proposed including devascularization of the tendon, an alteration of tendon healing, remodeling of the remaining tendon, and injury to the remaining tendon at the time of graft harvest. No definitive etiology has been accepted, and to date, pathologic evaluation has not been performed to our knowledge.

The remaining two-thirds of the patellar tendon should have adequate strength to withstand significant quadriceps muscle contractions. McMaster[27] showed that a tendon must be compromised 50% before it will rupture under significant loads or by 75% before failure occurs under physiologic loads.

Animal studies have shown that the remaining patellar tendon is biomechanically and histologically inferior. Burks et al,[28] in a dog model, showed that the stiffness was 30%, failure load 40%, and tensile modulus 67% at 6 months. They also found no difference in strength if the defect was closed or not. Kamps et al[29] found similar results at a short evaluation time of 3 months in the rabbit. They report that the stiffness was 72% and tensile modulus 34% at 3 months. Jackson et al[30] reported a 50% reduction in failure load in the goat at 6 months. Histology from these studies shows that if the defect is left open it fills in with collagenous tissue that does not resemble normal tendon. Burks et al[28] report poorly oriented collagen fibers; however, the scar formation is exuberant throughout the whole tendon, with the cross-sectional area increasing 460%.

Closure of the defect is controversial. Closer apposition of the tendon should reduce the amount of poorly organized scar tissue; however, high tension in the defect closure may result in tendon necrosis.[22] There is also concern that closing the defect shortens the patellar tendon, which may be associated with poor clinical outcome.[31–33] Van Eijden et al[34] have used a mathematical model to show that a 25% decrease in patellar tendon length can result in a 17% increase in anteroposterior shear force at its insertion. A randomized prospective trial comparing defect closure and bone grafting of the patellar donor site vs. leaving the defect open and no bone grafting showed no difference in clinical outcome.[35]

Prevention of Complications

Patellar tendon rupture is an uncommon event after ACL reconstruction and its etiology is not completely elucidated. Care while harvesting the patellar tendon must be exercised to avoid iatrogenic injury. The use of an ACL knife with a 10-mm distance between the scalpel blades to minimize the risk of injury is preferred by some surgeons. Unfortunately, postoperative patellar tendon rupture is likely to represent a rare complication that may be difficult, if not impossible, to prevent.

Management

The diagnosis of rupture of the patellar tendon is critical and time sensitive. Ideally, the repair of the tendon should occur within 1 week of the injury as abundant scar formation and tissue retractions occur rapidly. As such, a high index of suspicion is necessary in order not to miss such an injury.

Acute primary repair of the patellar tendon after rupture has yielded excellent clinical results. In one series, two patients with delayed rupture both made full recovery.[26] The technique employed direct suture repair of the tendon with excellent results at 3-year follow-up. In fact, to our knowledge, no case report exists documenting a reconstruction of a chronic patellar tendon rupture after BPTB ACL reconstruction.

GRAFT CONTAMINATION

Intraoperative contamination of the ACL graft, usually by dropping the graft, is a dreaded complication. To date, only one study has analyzed the effect of graft contamination and a variety of methods to eradicate graft contamination. Cooper et al[36] dropped 10 BTPB grafts on a clean operating room floor for 3 minutes and obtained cultures. Six grafts (60%) were culture-positive at the end of 1 week. The authors subsequently evaluated several sterilization procedures with bacterial-sensitive antibiotic soak with lavage, and, despite this aggressive protocol, 30% of the grafts remained culture-positive. Although this complication is not unique to BPTB autograft, no similar study on the effects of dropping alternative graft material exists to our knowledge.

Prevention of Complications

Meticulous attention must be paid to harvesting the graft at all times. Dropping the graft is far more likely when passing the graft to the table for preparation or passing it back for delivery into the knee. Ideally, one individual handles the graft at all times, and passage from one individual to another is avoided. Finally, during preparation, the graft should be well secured if drilling of the bone plugs for suture passage is performed. This may be accomplished by having an assistant secure the graft while drilling is performed.

Management

Cooper et al[37] demonstrated a 30% infection rate after aggressive lavage with antibiotic solution that was sensitive to the cultured bacteria. As such, simple lavage is inadequate, and the graft must be assumed to be contaminated. If the graft is contaminated, there are several options: (1) proceed to harvest an alternate graft material (i.e., hamstrings or quadriceps tendon) and continue the procedure; (2) aggressively lavage the graft, obtain multiple cultures from the graft, and delay the reconstruction until negative culture results are obtained; (3) harvest graft material from the contralateral knee; or (4) use allograft tissue for reconstruction. It is not recommended at any time to proceed with reconstruction with the potentially contaminated graft until multiple negative culture results have been obtained. Even with these findings, serious consideration should be given to the aforementioned graft alternatives.

INTRAOPERATIVE COMPLICATIONS

Injury to the graft itself during harvest, preparation, passage, and screw placement has been reported. During graft harvest and preparation, injury to the bone block can occur and, if severe, may compromise fixation. Particular care should be exercised when using compaction-type pliers for graft shaping, as their use may result in cortical fracture. Injury to the bone block itself, however, is most likely to occur during graft passage, particularly when excessive force is used. Subsequent fracture of the bone plug may occur and impede interference screw fixation. Furthermore, laceration of the graft itself may occur while placing interference screws, particularly when a sheath is not used. Although transection of the tendinous portion of the graft is unlikely, significant injury and near transection may occur.[38,39]

As a corollary to graft injury discussed above, bone retraction into the joint may be encountered when fixation on the femoral side is inadequate. This may be a result of graft injury, screw divergence, improper femoral tunnel placement, or poor bone quality.[38] Bone plug comminution with loss of fixation has been reported in the literature.[40] Finally, the posterior cruciate ligament (PCL) (primarily the anterolateral bundle) is at risk during tibial and/or femoral drilling. The PCL may become entwined within the tibial drill during passage of the bit into the joint. Similarly, the drill may engage the PCL during femoral tunnel drilling if it is not protected.[41–43]

Prevention of Complications

Intraoperative complications are infrequent and easily avoidable. Meticulous attention must be directed to graft harvest and preparation. Once adequate exposure has been obtained, direct measurements must be made of the proposed tendon width and size of the bone blocks. These measurements are critical for obtaining appropriately sized blocks for fixation as well as for preventing donor site complications including patellar fracture or injury to the patellar tendon. Shaping of the bone block must be done with extreme care, particularly when compaction-type pliers (Instrument Makar, Inc., Okemos, MI, and Arthrex, Inc., Naples, FL) are used. If excessive force is applied to the pliers with weak bone or to a graft that is not close to the ideal size, cortical fracture may occur.

Graft passage may also be fraught with danger. The use of graft sizing blocks, which are widely available, is highly recommended. These devices allow passage of the graft through predetermined tunnel diameters to appropriately fashion the graft and the risk of injury. The graft should slide easily through the tunnels without undue force. Placing large holes for suture passage may also create stress risers and is unnecessary. Furthermore, there may be some theoretical benefit to placing the drill holes for suture passage in different planes to minimize fracture risk. Currently, the use of a small K-wire (0.045 inch or less) is recommended to create tunnels for suture passage.

Injury to the PCL and the graft is a potential complication of femoral fixation using an arthroscopic approach. Protection of the PCL during tibial drilling is an important component of ACL reconstruction using any graft choice, and may be easily accomplished with a curette over the guide pin or a small elevator in the joint. The synovial lining on the PCL should be left intact to prevent adhesions between it and the ACL. Finally, injury to the PCL may occur with placement of femoral fixation using interference screws. While securing fixation, the screw threads may injure the most lateral PCL fibers within the notch. This complication is easily avoided with a sheathed screw with a blunt tip, which shields the PCL from the interference screw.

Bone plug retraction into the joint may occur for a variety of reasons, causing inadequate femoral fixation. If posterior bone deficiency occurs, poor bone quality is encountered, or nonlinear screw placement results from attempts at femoral fixation, the potential for both bone plug migration and loose hardware in the joint exists. The use of commercially available offset femoral aiming guides is highly encouraged. Furthermore, the proposed tunnel may be reamed for 3 to 5 mm to impart the "footprint" of the reamer. If the posterior cortex is violated, the guide pin is translated anteriorly. Finally, to diminish the likelihood of posterior cortical breakthrough with the endoscopic technique, the knee should be maintained at a minimum of 70 degrees of flexion. If fixation is not deemed adequate at the time of surgery, it must be revised to prevent complications and to allow ACL rehabilitation.

Management

If a loose bone plug is encountered with interference screw fixation, a larger interference screw may salvage the fixation if the posterior bone is adequate.[44] However, if the posterior bone has been fractured, it must be carefully evaluated. This situation may be encountered with a excessively posterior femoral tunnel or with screw divergence and posterior bone deficiency. When the fracture extends more than approximately 5 mm proximally, fixation may be inadequate with interference screw fixation. Therefore, when this extent of posterior bone deficiency is present, alternate fixation methods may be the most appropriate solution. Fixation may be accomplished with any number of techniques including rear-entry fixation, "over-the-top" passage with a screw and post, or using an Endobutton device (Smith and Nephew Richard, Inc., Memphis, TN), which would obtain fixation in the presence of a posterior wall fracture.

Additionally, screw divergence may compromise fixation and result in graft slippage. While this is not problematic with a two-incision technique,[45] studies indicate that screw divergence of greater than 15 degrees may be associated with a diminishing ultimate strength of failure.[46,47] Several options exist to minimize divergence. Interference screw fixation inserted over a guidewire will minimize divergence of the screw, and several commercially available devices have been designed to allow femoral screw fixation to be performed through the tibial tunnel. Finally, if confirmation of screw position is needed, an intraoperative radiograph may be requested. If screw divergence is noted, femoral fixation may be compromised if the screw is replaced. In this instance, a larger screw may be necessary to obtain fixation once the misdirected screw is removed.

ANTERIOR KNEE PAIN

Patellofemoral or anterior knee pain is often cited as a major complication of ACL reconstruction using BPTB autograft. Reports in the literature have ranged from less than 5%[48–51] to 55%[52,53] during the first year following ACL reconstruction. While the pathophysiology of patellar tendinitis is poorly understood, a high incidence (58%) of anterior knee pain has been encountered in acute reconstruction of the knee.[54] Furthermore, the severity of symptoms ranges from a mild nuisance to inability to perform activities of daily living. Suspected etiologies include premorbid degeneration of articular cartilage, poor patellar alignment and incongruity, notchplasty, nonanatomic graft position, damage during graft harvest, donor-site morbidity, excessive scarring, and inadequate rehabilitation.

The occurrence of patellofemoral complaints in females may be related to subtle degrees of patellar maltracking. The presence of a positive congruence angle on the Merchant view has been associated with an increased risk of anterior knee pain in females).[55–57] Several studies have concurred that such a proclivity may increase the incidence of anterior knee pain after ACL reconstruction.[55–58] In acute ACL reconstructions, evidence supports an increased incidence of patellofemoral problems.[58–60] This may be due to a higher incidence of arthrofibrosis, which is more frequent with acute ACL reconstruction, particularly when preoperative range of motion is not obtained.[61–67] However, the development of arthrofibrosis is certainly multifactorial, with potential etiologies including concomitant medial collateral ligament and meniscal injury, gender, reflex sympathetic dystrophy, preoperative range of motion, postoperative immobilization, and infection.[19,61,68–72]

Sachs et al[71] first proposed the association between anterior knee pain with postoperative flexion contracture and quadriceps weakness. Later Fisher and Shelbourne[73] documented their series of arthroscopic scar resection and restoration of full knee hyperextension in a group of patients with symptomatic flexion contractures after ACL reconstruction. After restoration of extension, patients exhibited significant improvement in anterior knee symptoms. These findings have contributed to the widespread acceptance of the importance of obtaining full extension postoperatively after ACL reconstruction to diminish anterior knee pain.

The possibility that harvesting the BPTB itself may be responsible for anterior knee pain was addressed in a recent study. Rubinstein and Shelbourne[52] performed 20 ACL reconstructions with BPTB grafts to isolate the incidence of and nature of donor-site morbidity. Using the accelerated rehabilitation protocol to obtain full symmetric hyperextension rapidly, patients were followed for a minimum of 1 year after reconstruction and were evaluated both subjectively and objectively. Eleven on the 20 patients (55%) had symptoms of patellar tendinitis at times within the first year of follow-up. The symptoms were not related to the presence of patellofemoral crepitus or with lower isokinetic strength as determined by Cybex testing (Lumex, Inc., Ronkonkoma, NY). The authors concluded that anterior knee pain after ACL reconstruction primarily comes from two sources. One component is the lack of full hyperextension, creating a "mismatch" between the graft and the intercondylar notch. The second component arises from postoperative rehabilitation attempting to restore the integrity and functionality of the extensor mechanism in the early (i.e., up to 6 months) period.

Despite a concerted effort to obtain full preoperative range of motion, to accurately place the ACL graft intraoperatively, and to enroll the patient in aggressive postoperative rehabilitation, the incidence of symptomatic loss of extension is at least 4%.[73] To date, a prospective randomized study evaluating the incidence of anterior knee pain and the severity of donor-site morbidity with a variety of ACL reconstruction techniques has not been performed. Only with this kind of study will it be possible to distill out the direct morbidity of harvesting the BPTB graft for ACL reconstruction.

Prevention of Complications

Until the contribution of harvesting the BPTB graft to anterior knee pain is understood, and the interplay of the many etiologies that play a part in this problem can be delineated, prevention is the key. Thus, achieving symmetric hyperextension is an important and early goal of rehabilitation. The early return of quadriceps function and vigilant commitment to rehabilitation by the patient, therapist, and physician are necessary to reduce the likelihood and severity of anterior knee pain. ACL reconstruction should be delayed until the knee is not inflamed and has recovered its full preoperative range of motion. At the time of surgery, accurate graft position and tensioning with rigid fixation pemits appropriate and timely postoperative rehabilitation. Finally, in the postoperative period, early full extension is facilitated by early quadriceps contraction, prone heel hangs, extension exercises, and judicious use of commercially available extension boards (Instrument Makar, Inc., Okemos, MI, and Indiana Brace Company, Indianapolis, IN) to obtain symmetric hyperextension. It is clear that it is significantly more difficult to obtain a full range of motion postoperatively when it was not present preoperatively.

Management

Although a thorough discourse of the treatment of arthrofibrosis is beyond the scope of this chapter, several tenets should be addressed. When conservative measures fail, operative intervention to restore full extension, improve quadriceps function, and alleviate symptoms may take the form of arthrotomy or arthroscopy.[19,72,74–76] Paulos et al[76] documented an improvement from a 17-degree flexion contracture to a 5-degree contracture at follow-up of 3 months to 4 years with an open arthrotomy and debridement. This procedure often involved removing any impinging tissue and excising a portion of the anterior fat pad. Patients were placed in an aggressive therapy program to encourage full extension. Fisher and Shelbourne[73] noted a 12-

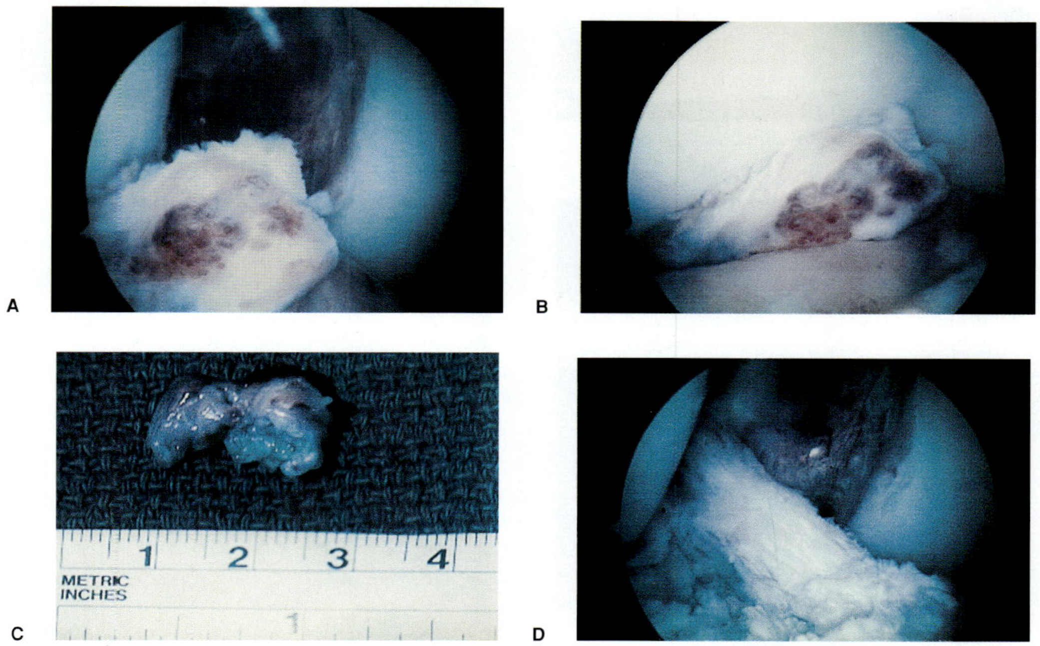

Figure 9.3. **A** and **B**: Arthroscopic view 4 months after ACL reconstruction with BPTB autograft. The patient had an extension block with a 9-degree flexion loss. Note impingement of Cyclops lesion in full extension. **C**: Cyclops lesion after excision. D: Appearance of intercondylar notch after excision.

degree improvement from neutral at a minimum of 3 months follow-up. This was obtained with arthroscopic debridement, and a similar postoperative rehabilitation program. Similarly, Jackson and Schaefer[77] had similar results after arthroscopic excision of the "Cyclops" lesion, a fibrous tissue proliferation at the base of the tibial attachment of the ACL graft (Fig. 9.3A–C). The authors noted further improvement in extension after removal of impinging tissue and an expanded notchplasty.

At the time of surgery, a thorough exam under anesthesia is performed. If full symmetric extension is not present, an arthroscopy is performed and the ACL graft is inspected. A thorough, systematic evaluation of the remainder of the knee is performed, searching for other potential causes for extension loss (e.g., meniscal pathology). If a Cyclops lesion is found, it is excised often in conjunction with partial excision of the anterior fat pad (Fig. 9.4A,B). Particular attention is directed at the intercondylar notch, and resection of additional bone here is performed as necessary. The knee is brought into full extension and impingement is excluded. At this point, extension contractures are addressed by gentle manipulation into flexion, after the arthroscope is removed. The patient is placed in a well-padded extension cast for 2 to 3 days, and thereafter is enrolled in an aggressive rehabilitation program stressing full extension. Close follow-up is necessary and the use of electrical stimulation on the quads as well as extension boards are employed as needed (Fig. 9.4C,D).

QUADRICEPS STRENGTH

The effect on quadriceps muscle strength of using the central third of the patellar tendon as a graft for ACL reconstruction has been a cause for debate. Stud-

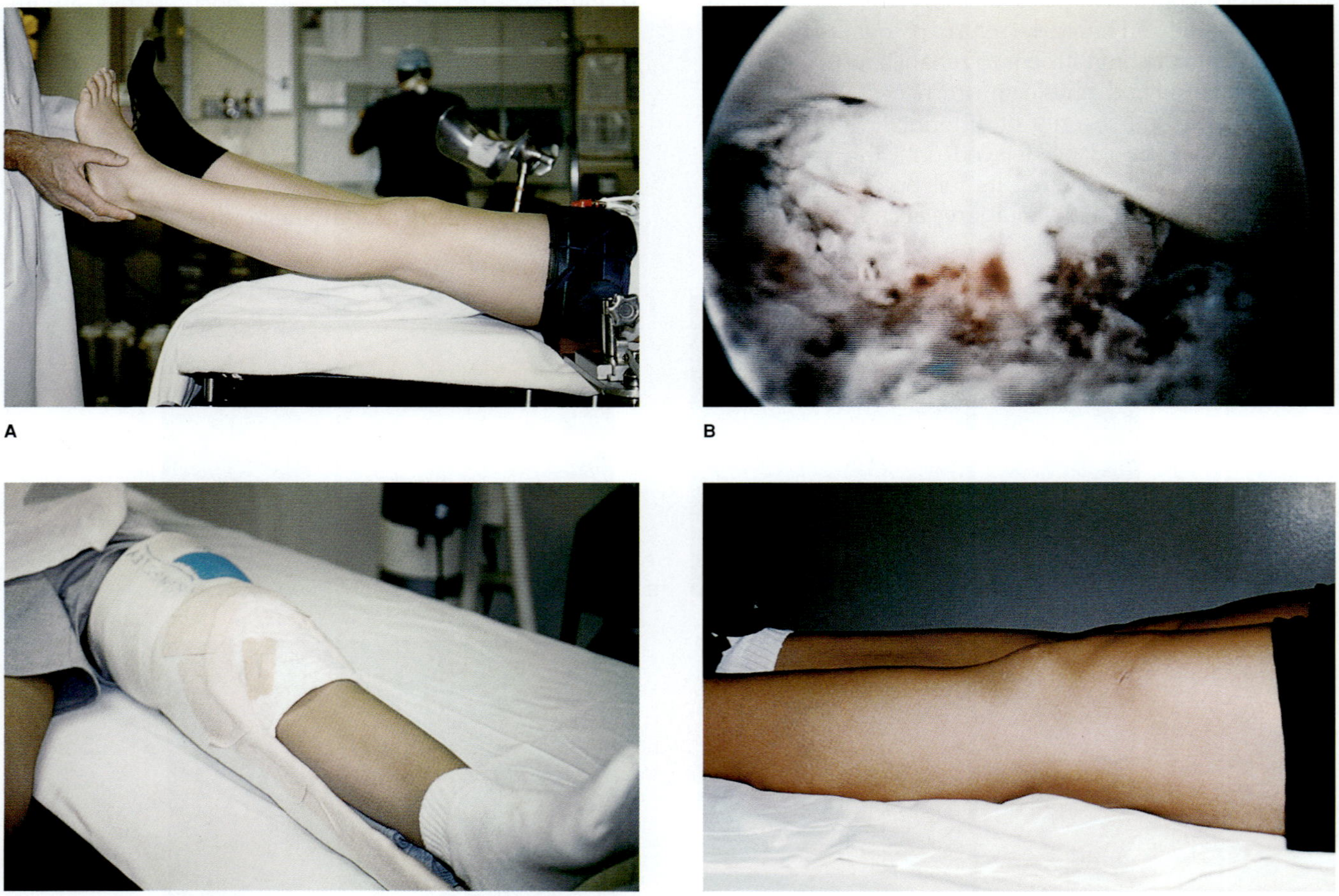

A B C D

Figure 9.4. **A:** 23-year-old patient with 10-degree flexion contracture after BPTB ACL reconstruction. **B:** A Cyclops lesion was excised arthroscopically. **C:** Extension block cast applied for 3 days. Note towels under posterior calf to increase extension. **D:** Full symmetric extension was obtained with excellent functional result. Appearance of leg 3 months postoperatively.

ies that evaluated the strength of postoperative knees consistently showed significant deficits in quadriceps strength.[78–84] The degree of quadriceps deficit varied markedly from 6%[78] to 33%.[84] The patients with the biggest deficits were from older series where patients had combined intra- and extraarticular procedures and the knee was immobilized for up to 6 weeks. The smallest deficits occurred in Shelbourne and Gray's[78] patients who underwent an aggressive postoperative rehabilitation program. Shelbourne et al[85] further documented that ultimate quadriceps strength was unrelated to the tendon width remaining at a minimum of 6 months follow-up.

To determine whether the quadriceps deficit is due to the knee injury itself or to the graft harvest, studies have compared quadriceps strength following allograft and autograft bone-patella-bone reconstruction. Three studies have been performed, and all three document relative quadriceps weakness consistent with no difference between allograft and autograft.[86–88] Lephart et al[86] compared 15 autograft with 18 allograft patients. All patients were young and active. At 18 months there were no differences in peak torque (strength), torque acceleration energy (power), or functional strength testing. Stringham et al[87] compared 47 autograft with 31 allografts at 34 months. They showed no difference in isokinetic muscle strength; however, there was a trend toward a higher concentric peak extension torque at 60 degrees/sec in allograft reconstruction. Saddemi et al[88] compared 31 autograft with 19 allografts at 2 years. The authors documented no difference in isometric quadriceps strength between the two groups.

No difference in quadriceps strength is also reported when hamstring grafts are compared with patellar tendon grafts.[79,89] Marder et al[79] compared patellar tendon with hamstring grafts and showed no difference in isokinetic muscle testing at 60 degrees/sec. Clatworthy et al[89] evaluated isokinetic quadriceps muscle strength at 60, 180, and 350 degrees/sec. They similarly showed no difference in strength in a well-matched series.

Further insight is gained when the data on conservatively treated ACL-deficient knees are evaluated. Wojtys and Huston[90] compared 40 normal knees with 100 cruciate-deficient knees. They reported a 21.4% deficit in males and a 33.5% deficit in females. Lorentzon et al[91] evaluated 18 patients and found a 13% to 29% deficit in the injured limb.

CONCLUSION

There is a persistent deficit in quadriceps strength following ACL injury. It appears to be independent of surgery and graft choice. Thus, there is no significant deficit in quadriceps strength attributable to harvesting the central third of the patellar tendon.

References

1. Garth WPJ. Current concepts regarding the anterior cruciate ligament. *Orthop Rev* 1992;21:565–575.
2. Benson ER, Barnett PR. A delayed transverse avulsion fracture of the superior pole of the patella after anterior cruciate ligament reconstruction. *Arthroscopy* 1998;14:85–88.
3. Brownstein B, Bronner S. Patella fractures associated with accelerated ACL rehabilitation in patients with autogenous patella tendon reconstructions. *J Orthop Sports Phys Ther* 1997;26:168–172.
4. Berg EE. Management of patella fractures associated with central third bone- patella tendon–bone autograft ACL reconstructions. *Arthroscopy* 1996;12:756–759.
5. Bonatus TJ, Alexander AH. Patellar fracture and avulsion of the patellar ligament complicating arthroscopic anterior cruciate ligament reconstruction. *Orthop Rev* 1991;20:770–774.
6. Delzell PB, Schils JP, Recht MP. Subtle fractures about the knee: innocuous-appearing yet indicative of significant internal derangement. *AJR* 1996;167:699–703.
7. Delee JC, Craviotto DF. Rupture of the quadriceps tendon after a central third patellar tendon anterior cruciate ligament reconstruction. *Am J Sports Med* 1991;19:415–416.
8. Daluga D, Johnson C, Bach BR, Jr. Primary bone grafting following graft procurement for anterior cruciate ligament insufficiency. *Arthroscopy* 1990;6:205–208.
9. Small NC. Complications in arthroscopic surgery of the knee and shoulder. *Orthopedics* 1993;16:985–988.
10. Christen B, Jakob RP. Fractures associated with patellar ligament grafts in cruciate ligament surgery [see comments]. *J Bone Joint Surg* 1992;74B:617–619.
11. Graf B, Uhr F. Complications of intra-articular anterior cruciate reconstruction. *Clin Sports Med* 1988;7:835–848.
12. Friis EA, Cooke FW, McQueen DA, Henning CE. Effect of bone block removal and patellar prosthesis on stresses in the human patella. *Am J Sports Med* 1994;22:696–701.
13. McCarroll JR, Shelbourne KD, Porter DA, Rettig AC, Murray S. Patellar tendon graft reconstruction for midsubstance anterior cruciate ligament rupture in junior high school athletes. An algorithm for management. *Am J Sports Med* 1994;22:478–484.
14. Blevins FT, Hecker AT, Bigler GT, Boland AL, Hayes WC. The effects of donor age and strain rate on the biomechanical properties of bone-patellar tendon-bone allografts. *Am J Sports Med* 1994;22:328–333.

15. Marumoto JM, Mitsunaga MM, Richardson AB, Medoff RJ, Mayfield GW. Late patellar tendon ruptures after removal of the central third for anterior cruciate ligament reconstruction. A report of two cases. *Am J Sports Med* 1996;24:698–701.

16. Wallenbock E. [Rupture of the patellar ligament—a late complication after removal of a bone-tendon-bone transplant as cruciate ligament replacement]. *Langenbecks Arch Chir* 1993;378:339–340.

17. Bonamo JJ, Krinick RM, Sporn AA. Rupture of the patellar ligament after use of its central third for anterior cruciate reconstruction. A report of two cases. *J Bone Joint Surg* 1984;66A:1294–1297.

18. Langan P, Fontanetta AP. Rupture of the patellar tendon after use of its central third. *Orthop Rev* 1987;16:317–321.

19. Daniel DM, Woodward EP, Loose G. *The Marshall/MacIntosh anterior cruciate ligament reconstruction with the Kennedy ligament augmentation device: Report of the United States clinical trials.* Philadelphia: WB Saunders Co, 1988.

20. Hardin GT, Bach BRJ. Distal rupture of the infrapatellar tendon after use of its central third for anterior cruciate ligament reconstruction. *Am J Knee Surg* 1992;5:140–143.

21. McMaster PE. Tendon and muscle ruptures: clinical and experimental studies on the causes and location of ruptures. *J Bone Joint Surg* 1933;15A:705–722.

22. Burks RT, Haut RC, Lancaster RL. Biomechanical and histological observations of the dog patellar tendon after removal of its central one-third. *Am J Sports Med* 1990;18:146–153.

23. Kamps BS, Linder LH, DeCamp CE, Haut RC. The influence of immobilization versus exercise on scar formation in the rabbit patellar tendon after excision of the central third. *Am J Sports Med* 1994;22:803–811.

24. Jackson DW, Grood ES, Goldstein JD, et al. A comparison of patellar tendon autograft and allograft used for anterior cruciate ligament reconstruction in the goat model. *Am J Sports Med* 1993;21:176–185.

25. O'Brien SJ, Warren RF, Pavlov H, Panariello R, Wickiewicz TL. Reconstruction of the chronically insufficient anterior cruciate ligament with the central third of the patellar ligament. *J Bone Joint Surg* 1991;73A:278–286.

26. Paulos LE, Rosenberg TD, Drawbert J, Manning J, Abbott P. Infrapatellar contracture syndrome. An unrecognized cause of knee stiffness with patella entrapment and patella infera. *Am J Sports Med* 1987;15:331–341.

27. van Eijden TM, Kouwenhoven E, Weijs WA. Mechanics of the patellar articulation. Effects of patellar ligament length studied with a mathematical model. *Acta Orthop Scand* 1987;58:560–566.

28. Brandsson S, Faxen E, Eriksson BI, Kalebo P, et al. Closing patellar tendon defects after anterior cruciate ligament reconstruction: absence of any benefit. *Knee Surg Sports Traumatol Arthrosc* 1998;6:82–87.

29. Cooper DE, Arnoczky SP, Warren RF. Contaminated patellar tendon grafts: incidence of positive cultures and efficacy of an antibiotic solution soak—an in vitro study. *Arthroscopy* 1991;7:272–274.

30. Malek MM, Kunkle KL, Knable KR. Intraoperative complications of arthroscopically assisted ACL reconstruction using patellar tendon autograft. *Instr Course Lect* 1996;45:297–302.

31. Berg EE. Lateral femoral condyle fracture after endoscopic anterior cruciate ligament reconstruction. *Arthroscopy* 1994;10:693–695.

32. Berg EE. Autograft bone-patella tendon-bone plug comminution with loss of ligament fixation and stability [see comments]. *Arthroscopy* 1996;12:232–235.

33. Matthews LS, Soffer SR. Pitfalls in the use of interference screws for anterior cruciate ligament reconstruction: brief report. *Arthroscopy* 1989;5:225–226.

34. Butler JC, Branch TP, Hutton WC. Optimal graft fixation—the effect of gap size and screw size on bone plug fixation in ACL reconstruction. *Arthroscopy* 1994;10:524–529.

35. Lemos MJ, Albert J, Simon T, Jackson DW. Radiographic analysis of femoral interference screw placement during ACL reconstruction: endoscopic versus open technique. *Arthroscopy* 1993;9:154–158.

36. Lemos MJ, Jackson DW, Lee TQ, Simon TM. Assessment of initial fixation of endoscopic interference femoral screws with divergent and parallel placement. *Arthroscopy* 1995;11:37–41.

37. Jomha NM, Raso VJ, Leung P. Effect of varying angles on the pullout strength of interference screw fixation. *Arthroscopy* 1993;9:580–583.

38. Jackson DW, Jennings LD. Arthroscopically assisted reconstruction of the anterior cruciate ligament using a patella tendon bone autograft. *Clin Sports Med* 1988;7:785–800.

39. Ray JM. A proposed natural history of symptomatic anterior cruciate ligament injuries of the knee. *Clin Sports Med* 1988;7:697–713.

40. Wainer RA, Clarke TJ, Poehling GG. Arthroscopic reconstruction of the anterior cruciate ligament using allograft tendon. *Arthroscopy* 1988;4:199–205.

41. Clancy WG, Jr., Nelson DA, Reider B, Narechania RG. Anterior cruciate ligament reconstruction using one-third of the patellar ligament, augmented by extra-articular tendon transfers. *J Bone Joint Surg* 1982;64A:352–359.

42. Rubinstein RA, Jr., Shelbourne KD, VanMeter CD, McCarroll JC, Rettig AC. Isolated autogenous bone-patellar tendon-bone graft site morbidity. *Am J Sports Med* 1994;22:324–327.

43. Arendt EA, Hunter RE, Schneider WT. Vascularized patella tendon anterior cruciate ligament reconstruction. *Clin Orthop* 1989;222–232.

44. Kaplan N, Wickiewicz TL, Warren RF. Primary surgical treatment of anterior cruciate ligament ruptures. A long-term follow-up study. *Am J Sports Med* 1990;18:354–358.

45. Aglietti P, Insall JN, Cerulli G. Patellar pain and incongruence. I: Measurements of incongruence. *Clin Orthop* 1983;176:217–224.

46. Insall JN, Aglietti P, Tria AJJ. Patellar pain and incongruence. II: Clinical application. *Clin Orthop*. 1983;176:225–232.

47. Laurin CA, Dussault R, Levesque HP. The tangential x-ray investigation of the patellofemoral joint: x-ray technique, diagnostic criteria and their interpretation. *Clin Orthop* 1979;144:16–26.

48. Aglietti P, Buzzi R, D'Andria S, Zaccherotti G. Patellofemoral problems after intraarticular anterior cruciate ligament reconstruction. *Clin Orthop* 1993;288:195–204.

49. Shelbourne KD, Gray T. Anterior cruciate ligament reconstruction with autogenous patellar tendon graft followed by accelerated rehabilitation. A two- to nine- year followup. *Am J Sports Med* 1997;25:786–795.

50. Shelbourne KD, Patel DV. Prevention of complications after autogenous bone-patellar tendon-bone ACL reconstruction. *Instr Course Lect* 1996;45:253–262.

51. Shelbourne KD, Wilckens JH, Mollabashy A, DeCarlo M. Arthrofibrosis in acute anterior cruciate ligament reconstruction. The effect of timing of reconstruction and rehabilitation. *Am J Sports Med* 1991;19:332–336.

52. Wasilewski SA, Covall DJ, Cohen S. Effect of surgical timing on recovery and associated injuries after anterior cruciate ligament reconstruction. *Am J Sports Med* 1993;21:338–342.

53. Fisher SE, Shelbourne KD. Arthroscopic treatment of symptomatic extension block complicating anterior cruciate ligament reconstruction. *Am J Sports Med* 1993;21:558–564.

54. Cosgarea AJ, DeHaven KE, Lovelock JE. The surgical treatment of arthrofibrosis of the knee. *Am J Sports Med* 1994;22:184–191.

55. Cosgarea AJ, Sebastianelli WJ, DeHaven KE. Prevention of arthrofibrosis after anterior cruciate ligament reconstruction using the central third patellar tendon autograft. *Am J Sports Med* 1995;23:87–92.

56. Aglietti P, Buzzi R, D'Andria S, Zaccherotti G. Long-term study of anterior cruciate ligament reconstruction for chronic instability using the central one-third patellar tendon and a lateral extraarticular tenodesis. *Am J Sports Med* 1992;20:38–45.

57. Engebretsen L, Benum P, Fasting O, Molster A, Strand T. A prospective, randomized study of three surgical techniques for treatment of acute ruptures of the anterior cruciate ligament. *Am J Sports Med* 1990;18:585–590.

58. Sachs RA, Daniel DM, Stone ML, Garfein RF. Patellofemoral problems after anterior cruciate ligament reconstruction. *Am J Sports Med* 1989;17:760–765.

59. Mohtadi NG, Webster-Bogaert S, Fowler PJ. Limitation of motion following anterior cruciate ligament reconstruction. A case-control study. *Am J Sports Med* 1991;19:620–624.

60. Dodds JA, Keene JS, Graf BK, Lange RH. Results of knee manipulations after anterior cruciate ligament reconstructions. *Am J Sports Med* 1991;19:283–287.

61. Meyers JF, St.Pierre RK, Sutter JS, Caspari RB, Whipple TL. Arthroscopic evaluation of anterior cruciate ligament reconstructions. *Arthroscopy* 1986;2:155–161.

62. Jackson DW, Schaefer RK. Cyclops syndrome: loss of extension following intra-articular anterior cruciate ligament reconstruction. *Arthroscopy* 1990;6:171–178.

63. Marder RA, Raskind JR, Carroll M. Prospective evaluation of arthroscopically assisted anterior cruciate ligament reconstruction. Patellar tendon versus semitendinosus and gracilis tendons. *Am J Sports Med* 1991;19:478–484.

64. Rosenberg TD, Franklin JL, Baldwin GN, Nelson KA. Extensor mechanism function after patellar tendon graft harvest for anterior cruciate ligament reconstruction. *Am J Sports Med* 1992;20:519–525.

65. Yasuda K, Ohkoshi Y, Tanabe Y, Kaneda K. Quantitative evaluation of knee instability and muscle strength after anterior cruciate ligament reconstruction using patellar and quadriceps tendon. *Am J Sports Med* 1992;20:471–475.

66. Tibone JE, Antich TJ. A biomechanical analysis of anterior cruciate ligament reconstruction with the patellar tendon. A two year followup [see comments]. *Am J Sports Med* 1988;16:332–335.

67. Gerber C, Hoppeler H, Claassen H, Robotti G, Zehnder R, Jakob RP. The lower-extremity musculature in chronic symptomatic instability of the anterior cruciate ligament. *J Bone Joint Surg* 1985;67A:1034–1043.

68. Seto JL, Orofino AS, Morrissey MC, Medeiros JM, Mason WJ. Assessment of quadriceps/hamstring strength, knee ligament stability, functional and sports activity levels five years after anterior cruciate ligament reconstruction. *Am J Sports Med* 1988;16:170–180.

69. Shelbourne KD, Rubinstein RAJ, VanMeter CD, McCarroll JR, Rettig AC. Correlation of remaining patellar tendon width with quadriceps strength after autogenous bone-patellar tendon-bone anterior cruciate ligament reconstruction. *Am J Sports Med* 1994;22:774–777.

70. Lephart SM, Kocher MS, Harner CD, Fu FH. Quadriceps strength and functional capacity after anterior cruciate ligament reconstruction. Patellar tendon autograft versus allograft. *Am J Sports Med* 1993;21:738–743.

71. Stringham DR, Pelmas CJ, Burks RT, Newman AP, Marcus RL. Comparison of anterior cruciate ligament reconstructions using patellar tendon autograft or allograft. *Arthroscopy* 1996;12:414–421.

72. Saddemi SR, Frogameni AD, Fenton PJ, Hartman J, Hartman W. Comparison of perioperative morbidity of anterior cruciate ligament autografts versus allografts. *Arthroscopy* 1993;9:519–524.

73. Clatworthy, M. G Annear P, B¸low J-U, and Bartlett RJ. Isokinetic muscle strength following ACL reconstruction: Hamstrings vs patella tendon grafts. 1998. (GENERIC) (Unpublished Work)

74. Wojtys EM, Huston LJ. Neuromuscular performance in normal and anterior cruciate ligament- deficient lower extremities. *Am J Sports Med* 1994;22:89–104.

75. Lorentzon R, Elmqvist LG, Sjostrom M, Fagerlund M, Fuglmeyer AR. Thigh musculature in relation to chronic anterior cruciate ligament tear: muscle size, morphology, and mechanical output before reconstruction. *Am J Sports Med* 1989;17:423–429.

Chapter 10

Complications and Pitfalls in Anterior Cruciate Ligament Reconstruction with Allograft

Michael T. Havig and Lonnie E. Paulos

Anterior cruciate ligament (ACL) reconstruction has become a relatively common orthopedic procedure as a result of a better understanding of ACL function and the natural history of the unstable knee in an athletic individual. There has also been an increased awareness of ACL injuries and their diagnosis by physicians and their patients, as well as improvements in reconstructive techniques. As increasing numbers of ACL reconstructions are performed, subsequent complications will also arise. This chapter discusses complications associated with allograft ACL reconstructions, their avoidance, and their treatment. Most of the complications of autograft ACL reconstruction (see Chapter 9) apply to allografts as well. This chapter focuses on complications arising specifically from the selection of allograft tissue for ACL reconstruction.

COMPLICATIONS AND BASIC SCIENCE

Graft Selection

The goals of ACL reconstruction are to restore stability to the injured knee and return the patient to preinjury activity levels. These goals are achieved by a surgery that provides adequate graft strength, fixation, and isometry, which allow early rehabilitation, healing and return to sports. One important factor in a successful reconstruction is the selection of graft material. Options include autografts, allografts, and synthetics. The ideal graft should have adequate strength, low donor-site morbidity, and no risk of disease transmission; it should be readily available and cost-effective; it should have the ability to heal in a timely fashion; and it should duplicate ACL physiology.

Numerous studies have examined the ultimate load and stiffness of the human femur-ACL-tibia complex (FATC). Noyes and colleagues[1,2] have shown an ultimate load of 1725 ± 269 N, and stiffness of 182 ± 33 N/mm for the FATC in young specimens with lower values in older specimens (734 ± 266 N, 129 ± 39N/mm). Woo and colleagues[3] also examined properties of the human FATC in various age groups. Ultimate loads and stiffness of 2160 ± 157 N and 242 ± 28 N/mm were noted in the younger specimens with load applied along the axis of the ACL. When load was applied along the axis of the tibia, lower values were noted 1602 ± 167 N and 218 ± 27 N/mm. These values decreased significantly with donor age.[3,4]

Ideally, a healed ACL graft should duplicate the strength and stiffness of the native FATC. Biomechanical studies have examined the initial properties of graft materials.[2,5] Numerous studies have demonstrated that autograft and allograft ACL reconstructions lose significant strength during early remodeling, which slowly increases over time.[6–11] Therefore, an ACL graft must be initially stronger than the native FATC to duplicate its function when healed.

Patellar Tendon Autografts

Middle one-third patellar tendon autograft has been the "gold standard" for ACL reconstruction. Ultimate loads and stiffness have been reported as 2900 ± 260 N and 685 ± 85.6 N/mm for a 14-mm graft.[2] The graft also provides for bone plugs for excellent fixation and bone-to-bone healing.[12,13] Unfortunately, complications associated with its use have been reported. These include tendonitis, patellar chondrosis, quadriceps weakness, tendon rupture, patellar fracture, patellar entrapment, and patella infera.[14–19] These complications have led surgeons to seek other graft choices including hamstring autografts, synthetics, and various allograft tissues.

Hamstring Autografts

Semitendinosus (ST) and gracilis (G) autografts have gained popularity in ACL reconstruction. They are harvested through a smaller incision, with minimal morbidity.[20,21] One concern with these grafts was their initial strengths. Ultimate loads of the single-stranded gracilis and semitendinosus, 838 ± 30 N and 1216 ± 50 N, respectively, are lower than that of the FATC.[2] However, multiple-stranded grafts such as quadrupled semitendinosus or doubled semitendinosus and gracilis are currently used. Quadrupling the graft (double ST/G) gives an ultimate load approximately two times that of the FATC.[22] Additionally, Simonian and colleagues[23] have recently demonstrated no difference in strain, stress, or modulus between cyclically loaded quadrupled hamstring and patellar tendon grafts of similar cross-sectional area.[23]

Another concern with hamstring grafts in the past has been fixation strength. Newer fixation devices, however, give initial fixation strengths equal to or higher than that of patellar tendon/interference screw fixation.[24–26] Recent reports have shown excellent results using these grafts with up to 5-year follow-up.[27–30]

Quadriceps Tendon Autografts

Like middle one-third patellar tendon, quadriceps tendon grafts have the advantage of bone block fixation. Biomechanical studies have shown similar strength compared to that of patellar tendon grafts.[31] Disadvantages are also similar to those of the patellar tendon and include risks of anterior knee pain and quadricep weakness. There has been limited use of this graft, and more follow-up studies need to be done prior to its widespread acceptance.

Synthetics

In an attempt to avoid problems associated with autografts and allografts, synthetic materials such as carbon fiber, woven polyester, and braided polytetrafluoroethylene (Gore-Tex, W.L. Gore and Associates, Flagstaff, AZ) have been used for ACL grafts.[32] These generally have had unacceptable rates of failure and are no longer marketed.[33]

Allografts

Because of the donor-site morbidity seen with autografts and failures with synthetics, allograft tissue gained popularity as a graft choice for ACL reconstruction. One of the first clinical reports of allograft use for ACL reconstruction in humans utilized Achilles tendon, tibialis anterior, and flexor tendons, with good results.[34] Subsequently, fascia lata was used but has been abandoned, in part because of low initial ultimate load (628 ± 35 N).[2] Patellar tendon is now the most commonly used allograft for ACL reconstructions. It offers advantages of good strength, bone-to-bone fixation, and the ability to fill revision tunnels with large bone plugs. Achilles tendon can also be used and has the advantages of a large graft and bone block. We employ Achilles allografts more frequently for posterior cruciate ligament reconstructions. Hamstring allografts are less frequently used, but work well to augment small hamstring autografts.

Advantages

There are numerous advantages to allograft use in ACL reconstructions (Table 10.1). Perhaps most important is the lack of donor-site morbidity, which is especially appealing in patients with a history of patellofemoral complaints. A smaller incision is used, which improves cosmesis, and with no graft harvest operative time is decreased. A large graft can be utilized, which is helpful in patients with small autogenous tissues. This is also beneficial in revisions, as autogenous tissue has often been used, and bone blocks can be tailored to fit tunnels. Our primary indication for the use of allograft tissues is multiligament reconstructions where there is limited availability of autogenous grafts.

Disadvantages and Complications

Unfortunately, there are numerous disadvantages and complications associated with allograft use (Table 10.1). These include risk of disease transmission and infection transmitted by the graft,[35–37] as well as potential weakening of the graft by sterilization and storage techniques.[38,39] Allografts exhibit slower healing and remodeling compared to autografts,[8,40] and there are reports of immune responses to allograft tissue.[8,9,41] Allografts add significant expense to the procedure, and their availability may be limited. Additionally, some studies have shown no difference between patellofemoral problems in groups of autograft and allograft middle

Table 10.1. Advantages and disadvantages of allograft use

Advantages	*Disadvantages*
No donor-site morbidity	Risk of disease transmission
Smaller incision	Slower healing
Decreased operative time	Expensive
Larger graft size	Increased laxity and late failures
Use in multiligament reconstructions	Tunnel enlargement/cyst formation
Use in revisions	Variable graft quality
	Immunologic reactions/effusions

one-third patellar tendon reconstructions.[42–45] Other reported complications include cyst formation, bone tunnel enlargement, graft variability with physical defects in the graft, and effusions.[46–49]

Disease Transmission. Perhaps the complication of greatest concern associated with allograft ACL reconstruction is disease transmission. Despite extremely low risk, transmission of the human immunodeficiency virus (HIV) is the primary concern in patients undergoing allograft procedures. There has been one reported case of HIV transmission from allograft tissues that were harvested in 1985.[37] The donor was seronegative for antibodies and had no know risk factors for HIV other than a traumatic death (gunshot wound). Of 41 identified tissue recipients tested for HIV, all three who received fresh frozen bone and four who received organs were infected. Interestingly, three patients who received freeze-dried soft tissue and one who received marrow-evacuated fresh frozen bone tested negative. Buck and colleagues[35] have estimated the risk of obtaining a graft from an HIV-positive allograft donor at 1 in 1,667,600. This estimate assumes adequate screening and testing of donors and allows for an 8-week window between HIV infection and detectable antibodies. It is possible that this risk could be higher today, as a larger percentage of the population is HIV positive. However, many tissue banks now use polymerase chain reaction (PCR) testing, which directly detects viral antigens, decreasing the window of undetectable HIV infection.[50]

Hepatitis transmission is another concern and has been documented by Conrad et al.[36] In this study two of nine graft recipients from one donor acquired hepatitis C. Six of 12 patients who received gamma-irradiated tissue from another hepatitis C–positive donor were also tested and none was positive. This suggests that 17 krad of gamma irradiation may inactivate hepatitis C virus.

Transmission of bacterial infection in allograft tissue is another potential problem. In a review of 134 small grafts, of which 21 were tendon grafts and the others bone, there were no bacterial infections.[51] All grafts were collected according to guidelines of the American Association of Tissue Banks,[52] under sterile techniques, and were fresh frozen, indicating that proper collection and screening adequately prevents bacterial transmission from small allografts. In a series of 2,500 ACL reconstructions, Williams and colleagues[53] report only seven intraarticular infections. All of these were autograft reconstructions with six of the seven undergoing concurrent open procedures, none of which used allografts. The number of allografts in the series was not reported.

Sterilization: Efficacy and Biomechanical Consequences. In an attempt to avoid the problem of disease transmission, many methods of graft sterilization have been developed. Unfortunately, there is often a compromise between sterilizing the graft and altering the mechanical properties in an unfavorable manner.[38] Therefore, the best method of preventing disease transmission is maintaining appropriate donor screening and testing, as well as sterile harvest and storage techniques.

Many sterilization techniques have been used for allografts including ethylene oxide, alcohol and gamma irradiation, and antibiotic soaks. The latter two methods are currently used. Ideally, grafts are harvested and processed under sterile conditions, eliminating the need for sterilization.

Secondary sterilization techniques such as gamma irradiation are often used if the graft is harvested or processed in a clean rather than sterile manner. Investigators have evaluated the efficacy of various doses of gamma irradiation in eliminating HIV from allografts. Fideler and colleagues[54] used PCR to assess the presence of HIV deoxyribonucleic acid (DNA) in fresh frozen patellar tendon/bone grafts treated with either 2, 2.5, 3, or 4 megarads (Mrad) of gamma irradiation. They concluded that 3 and 4 Mrad effectively eliminated viral DNA, which was still detectable at doses less than 3 Mrad. In a similar study, Conway et al[55] concluded that 1.5 Mrad would not reliably eliminate HIV from tissues. Most tissue banks employ doses of 1.5 to 2.5 Mrad to sterilize grafts, which do not eliminate HIV.[56]

Higher doses of gamma rays are not used as they have been shown to have detrimental effects on graft material properties. Our lab investigated effects of 2.5 to 3.5 Mrad on freeze-dried patellar tendon grafts and found decreased ultimate strength.[38] Similarly, 4.0 Mrad shortens the graft and significantly decreases strength.[57] Gibbons et al[58] showed decreased material properties of goat patellar tendon after 3, but not 2, Mrad of gamma irradiation. A related clinical study from the same lab examined 2 Mrad–irradiated grafts in the goat model at 6 months and found no significant biomechanical differences between irradiated and fresh frozen grafts.[59] Another clinical study has shown no significant biomechanical differences between 2.5 Mrad–irradiated and fresh frozen grafts in the dog model at 12 months.[60]

In summary, it appears that gamma irradiation treatment of less than 2.5 Mrad has little affect on biomechanical graft properties. While this amount of exposure is effective in eliminating some bacteria and viruses, it is not sufficient to eradicate HIV from tissues.

Ethylene oxide (ETO) sterilization is no longer used for sterilization of ligament allografts. Early studies showed no detrimental biomechanical effects on initial graft strength.[38,61] Many patients with ETO-treated grafts, however, developed persistent intraarticular reactions, which resolved with graft removal.[49] Also, higher failure rates have been noted in groups of patients treated with ETO-sterilized grafts.[62,63] Residual ETO in the grafts and its residues, ethylene chlorhydrin and ethylene glycol, have been implicated in the reaction.[49,64]

Antibiotic soaks and screening with cultures have been fairly effective in eliminating bacteria from ligament allografts.[51] Most tissue banks soak grafts in antibiotic solutions during processing. We also reconstitute our freeze-dried grafts, and soak our fresh frozen grafts in antibiotic solution prior to implantation.

Storage. Most ligament grafts are stored and transported either fresh frozen or freeze-dried. Fresh frozen grafts can be stored at −70° to −80°C for up to 5 years, and can be stored at −20°C for up to 6 months.[65] No deleterious biomechanical effects of freezing have been noted.[66] Freeze-dried grafts are processed by desiccating the frozen graft in a vacuum to less than 5% water content. They can be stored at room temperature for up to 5 years.[65] Numerous studies show no adverse biomechanical changes in tissues after freeze-drying, and adequate clinical results have been demonstrated using freeze-dried tissue.[6,7,67,68] Indelicato et al,[69] however, reported better results for fresh frozen versus freeze-dried grafts with significant differences in three of 21 categories including pivot shift and symptomatic giving way. However, the freeze-dried group contained patients with revision intraarticular procedures, had small numbers compared to the other group, and were up to 1 year further postoperation at the time of follow-up than the fresh frozen group.

At our institution we use primarily fresh frozen bone-tendon-bone (BTB) for allograft ACL reconstructions. We have noted some weakness at the bone-tendon junction in freeze-dried BTB tissues and have had failures while tensioning the grafts. Freeze-dried soft tissue grafts are frequently used for extraarticular reconstructions and to augment autografts.

Interestingly, in the case of HIV transmission, discussed above, recipients of freeze-dried grafts did not seroconvert.[37] This may lead one to believe that freezing or lyophilization may sterilize the grafts. It should be stressed, however, that neither deep freezing nor freeze-drying of grafts reliably eliminate viral transmission.[70,71]

Allograft Healing. Both autografts and allografts go through similar stages of healing with synovialization, ischemic necrosis, revascularization, cellular proliferation, and remodeling.[13] One concern with allografts, however, is slow or incomplete healing resulting in a weaker graft and higher incidence of late failure (Fig. 10.1). Early animal studies showed good results with allografts.[6,7,10,11,72,73] In early tendon studies, however, Cordrey and colleagues[74] observed that autografts appeared to reach viability sooner than allografts. Subse-

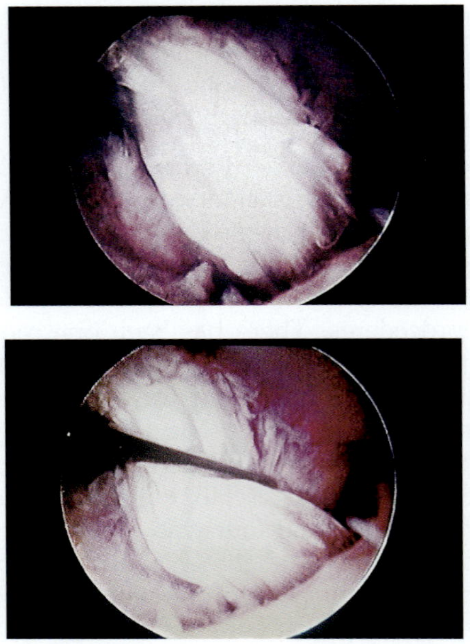

A

B

Figure 10.1. Allograft anterior cruciate ligament reconstruction at 6 months. Note the laxity and avascular appearance.

quent studies have confirmed prolonged healing of allograft compared to autograft.[8,9] Histologic studies of allograft superficial biopsy specimens have demonstrated immature portions at 18 and 20 months postoperatively.[75,76] Our lab examined deep biopsy samples of allograft ACL reconstructions ranging from 2 to 52 months postoperatively and found acellular and avascular central portions in all grafts, indicating incomplete healing at over 4 years.[40]

Many early follow-up studies (approximately 24 months) report good results with allograft ACL reconstructions.[44,45,77] Careful analysis of these studies reveal trends toward greater laxity in the allografts compared to the autografts, though these are not significant. Stringham et al[45] report significantly increased traumatic ruptures in the allograft group, and Indelicato et al[77] report three of 41 patients sustained graft rupture in the first 2 years.

Our experience with allografts revealed similar trends toward increased laxity in the allograft group with short-term follow-up, but no statistical significance.[78] This encouraged us to examine a group of allografts at an average of 44 months postoperatively. Increased laxity (KT 1000 >5 mm difference, grade 2 and 3 Lachman) in the chronic allograft compared to chronic autograft group was noted. Additionally, more failures were seen in both acute and chronic allograft reconstructions compared to autografts.[78] Malek and DeLuca[79] also reported deterioration of allograft results at late follow-up. Conversely, Noyes and Barber-Westin[80,81] demonstrated good long-term results in acute reconstructions with allograft, but high rates of allograft failures in chronic reconstruction.

In summary, allograft tissue appears to mature slowly and incompletely compared to autograft tissue used in ACL reconstruction. This may explain the trends toward increased laxity and failure compared to autograft, especially in chronic reconstructions, though a few series report good allograft results with long-term follow-up.[67,80]

Immunogenicity of Allografts. Immune responses to soft tissue allografts may be responsible for their delayed maturation. Work with osteochondral allografts has shown deep-freezing and lyophilization reduce immunogenicity from histocompatibility antigens.[82] Similarly, Arnoczky et al[72] demonstrated decreased immunogenicity in deep-frozen versus fresh allografts. Many studies have used fresh frozen or freeze-dried tissue and have not demonstrated an immune response.[6,10,72,73] Others have noted immune reactions. Vasseur and colleagues[9] observed antibodies to donor antigens in all frozen allograft reconstructions and no autograft reconstructions. Jackson et al[8] demonstrated persistent inflammation in allograft goat knees compared to autograft. Both of these studies demonstrated delayed allograft healing.

Immunogenicity of allografts has not been examined in many human clinical studies. ETO-sterilized grafts have shown marked immunogenic responses.[41,49] Synovial fluid analysis on allograft recipients has demonstrated intraarticular humoral response 6 months postoperatively.[83] The significance of these immune responses is not known, but they may contribute to delayed allograft maturation.

Expense. Another disadvantage of allograft reconstruction is the expense of the grafts. At most institutions a single allograft adds approximately $1,000 to the cost of the procedure. Some of this is offset by decreased surgical time; however, insurance companies may refuse to pay for the allograft if autogenous tissues can be used.

Tunnel Widening. Graft tunnel widening has been reported in association with allograft ACL reconstructions[47,80,84] (Fig. 10.2). No correlation between tunnel widening and failure was noted in any of these studies. The reason for tunnel widening is unknown but may be secondary to immune response at the bone plugs. In the case of soft tissue fixation, it may be unrelated to the allograft and the result of distant cortical fixation. A similar phenomenon has been observed with some hamstring autografts.

Cysts. Anterior tibial cysts associated with allograft ACL reconstructions have been described. Their formation is likely secondary to graft necrosis and incomplete tunnel incorporation, which allows leakage of synovial fluid to the pretibial region.[46]

A

B

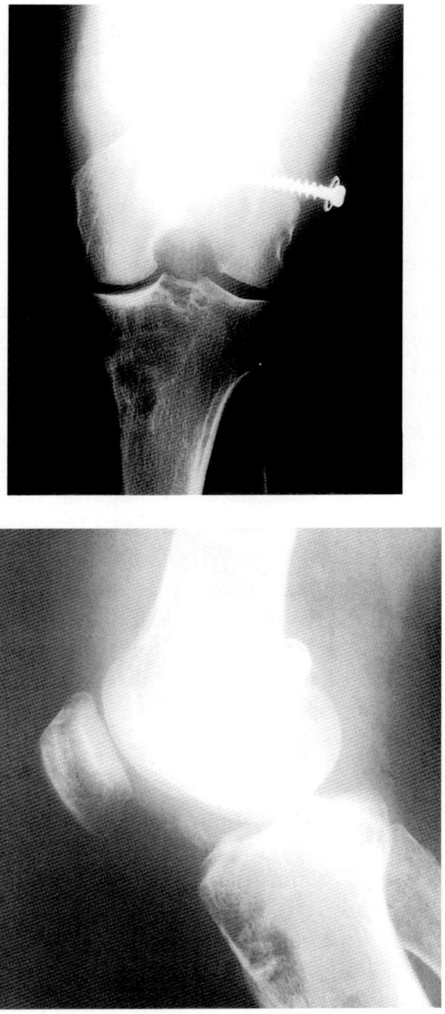

Figure 10.2. Anteroposterior **(A)** and lateral **(B)** views demonstrating tibial tunnel widening in an Achilles allograft reconstruction.

Allograft Variability. Allografts may be inadequate for ACL reconstruction because of intrinsic damage or defects, inadequate size, and lack of strength.[48] Age has been shown to affect strength of human patellar tendon grafts,[2] and a large amount of variability in graft strength has been demonstrated.[5]

AVOIDANCE OF COMPLICATIONS IN ALLOGRAFT ACL RECONSTRUCTION

The complications described in the previous section are the result of selecting allograft tissue for reconstruction of the ACL. The obvious way to prevent these complications is to use autograft rather than allograft. We currently recommend autograft use for ACL reconstruction for this reason. However, occasions arise when allograft is necessary or advantageous (multiligament reconstructions and some revisions). In these cases steps can be taken to avoid the previously described problems.

Disease Transmission

The best prevention of allograft disease transmission is appropriate graft procurement, testing, and storage, as outlined by the American Association of Tissue Banks.[52] Graft procurement starts with careful donor screening, which includes medical and social history, and physical examination. Table 10.2 lists exclusionary criteria. Laboratory testing includes screening for HIV antibodies, hepatitis B surface antigen, hepatitis C antibody (second-generation test), human T-cell lymphotropic virus type 1 antibody, blood cultures, and syphilis, with positive results eliminating the donor. Additional recommended testing includes PCR testing for HIV, which decreases the window for undetectable HIV-infected donors compared to antibody testing.

Sterilization

Sterile harvest and storage techniques are important in preventing bacterial infections. If secondary sterilization is necessary, gamma irradiation is recommended at doses less than 2.5 Mrad to avoid biomechanical compromise of the graft. It should be stressed that this dose is not adequate to eliminate HIV.

Soaking the graft in antibiotic solution does decrease bacterial counts in grafts and is recommended while thawing or reconstituting grafts. ETO sterilization of soft tissue grafts is contraindicated.

Storage

Both fresh frozen and freeze-dried allografts are used at our institution. The obvious advantage of freeze-dried tissue is the ability to store it at room temperature. However, we have had problems with weak bone-tendon attachments in freeze-dried preparations. To prevent avulsion of the tendon from the bone block, we use fresh frozen patellar tendon and Achilles grafts. Freeze-dried soft tissue grafts (hamstrings) work well for extraarticular reconstructions and autograft augmentation.

Grafts must be thawed slowly at temperatures no higher than 40°C. Higher temperatures may weaken the graft by denaturing collagen.[85] Once fresh frozen tissue has been thawed it must be used or discarded.

Freeze-dried tissue is reconstituted by soaking in antibiotic solution for at least 1 hour. Preferably this takes place over a longer period of time, which allows uniform hydration of the tissues. Many tissue banks recommend overnight reconstitution, which is often difficult, and may put the graft at risk for contamination.

Graft Healing

One advantage of allografts is their large size; however, this may limit their ability to revascularize and remodel. Surgeons should therefore be cautious when considering placement of larger grafts, and perhaps consider a double-tunnel technique to provide more surface area for bone tunnel healing.

Delayed healing of allografts should also be considered in rehabilitation. Initially allografts were thought to be advantageous for faster recovery and return to activities. Prolonged maturation times, however, dictate that allografts need to be protected longer than autograft reconstructions. Return to sport prior to graft maturation may be one factor responsible for the increased late laxity and failures. We allow our autograft reconstruction patients to return to sports at 6 months if they have met rehabilitation criteria. We generally do not return allograft reconstruction patients to cutting, jumping, and pivoting sports for 8 to 12 months. Most of these are revisions, as we have stopped performing primary allograft reconstructions with few exceptions.

The reason we perform few primary allografts is we have embraced the quadrupled hamstring technique. As noted previously quadrupled hamstring grafts are approximately two times stronger than the FATC, giving adequate initial strength, and, for a given cross-sectional area, they have similar material characteristics to the patellar tendon.[5,23] Newer techniques provide comparable fixation to the interference screw/bone block construct, and allow for early range of motion and aggres-

Table 10.2. American Association of Tissue Banks' history exclusion criteria for graft donors

Homosexual activity	Intravenous drug use
Hemophilia or related clotting disorders	Prostitution
Known HIV-positive sexual partner	Inmate of correctional system

From ref. 52.

sive rehabilitation. We have found our results to be comparable to our patellar tendon autografts without the associated problems. In summary, we feel hamstring autografts offer all of the advantages of allografts without the aforementioned complications.

It should be stressed that graft choice is one small portion of a successful reconstruction. Techniques that apply to a successful autograft reconstruction also apply to allografts. Graft healing is enhanced by isometric placement, adequate notchplasty to prevent impingement, and adequate fixation to encourage tunnel healing, followed by appropriate rehabilitation.

Allograft Variability

Intrinsic problems with grafts can be avoided by careful selection by the surgeon. Exclusion criteria should be placed on graft requests. It is the responsibility of the surgeon to specify an age range for tissue. Most studies have shown a negative correlation between age and graft strength.[2,4,68] Blevins and colleagues,[86] however, have shown no correlation between age and graft strength in specimens from donors 17 to 57 years old. Nevertheless, we recommend obtaining grafts from donors 40 years of age or younger to ensure optimal graft strength.

Tunnel Widening and Cysts

As tunnel widening and cysts are relatively infrequent complications of allograft reconstruction, they are difficult to anticipate and avoid. They are thought to result from poor graft healing in the tunnel, with necrosis and inflamation leading to destruction of the surrounding bone. Presumably avoiding oversized grafts with resultant necrosis of the avascular portions may decrease this complication.

SALVAGE OF COMPLICATIONS IN ALLOGRAFT ACL RECONSTRUCTION

Complications associated with allograft ACL reconstructions usually present complex management decisions to the treating surgeon. The previously described shortcomings can be divided into three main treatment categories: disease transmission/infection, complications without frank graft failure, and failure of the reconstruction.

Disease Transmission/Infection

As noted previously, transmission of viral and bacterial infections in allograft tissue is of paramount concern to both the surgeon and the patient. The treatment of viral infections such as hepatitis and HIV are beyond the scope of this chapter, and fortunately viral transmission is quite rare.

Bacterial infections after allograft reconstruction also occur infrequently with apparently no higher incidence than with autografts.[51,53] If infection does occur, aggressive treatment is required, including cultures with sensitivities before administration of antibiotics, surgical lavage and debridement (usually arthroscopic), and treatment with broad-spectrum antibiotics that are tailored to culture results.

The question of whether to remove the graft fixation hardware is difficult. We usually leave the graft intact if it appears viable and functional without obvious signs of intrasubstance necrosis. If the graft is left in place, any devitalized or fibrous tissue surrounding the graft needs to be removed, which occasionally includes a small portion of the graft. If the graft is preserved, and the infection does not resolve on appropriate antibiotics after the first or subsequent debridements, the graft should be removed.[53] Because of avascularity and slow maturation of allografts, we tend to be more aggressive in their debridement.

Fixation hardware should generally be removed, especially intraarticular interference screws. It is usually advisable to remove extraarticular hardware as well. Occasionally, extraarticular fixation may be left in place in an acute situation prior to complete graft healing. However, hardware should be removed immediately if there is any indication of infection at the fixation site, or if symptoms persist after the first debridement and appropriate antibiotics.

After the infection has stabilized, we recommend a minimum of 6 weeks of intravenous antibiotic therapy. If the patient remains symptom free with no evidence of infection (negative clinical, laboratory, and radiographic studies), revision may be carried out, if indicated, after 1 year.

Complications without Frank Graft Failure

As discussed previously, tunnel widening, tibial cysts, and graft laxity occur with allograft ACL reconstructions. Cysts and tunnel widening often occur without failure of the graft.[46,47,80,84] Generally, tunnel widening is asymptomatic and no surgical treatment is necessary. We recommend close follow-up and educating the patient concerning the possibility of graft failure or cyst formation. We have successfully treated tibial cysts with hardware removal, debridement, and freeze-dried cancellous allograft bone grafting.[46] Infection should be ruled out at the time of debridement as well. Despite graft necrosis in the tunnel, most of these patients remain stable after this treatment.

Laxity has been observed in late follow-up of ACL

allografts. Presumably this occurs because of slow graft incorporation and must be treated on an individual basis. Frequently, mild objective laxity on physical exam or arthrometer testing is clinically asymptomatic. Minimally symptomatic patients often respond to quadriceps and hamstring strengthening exercises and bracing. If significant symptomatic laxity is present and does not respond to rehabilitation and activity modification, revision surgery is often necessary, as outlined below.

Failure of the Reconstruction

Unfortunately, many of the shortcomings described above result in graft failure, and revision must be considered. Prior to undertaking an ACL revision, the surgeon and patient must consider both nonoperative and operative treatment options and discuss what goals can be accomplished with an ACL revision. Often years have passed between the initial surgery and subsequent failure, and changes in patients' lifestyle may allow them to tolerate an ACL-deficient knee. Patients must also understand that revisions usually require longer periods for healing, a prolonged rehabilitation, and perhaps inferior results compared with their index procedure. Patients should also realize that two procedures may be necessary for a successful reconstruction, which will further prolong their rehabilitation and return to activities.

Preoperative planning for revision surgery includes careful analysis of what caused the graft failure. Grafts generally fail because of technical or diagnostic reasons, biologic reasons, or traumatic rupture in a technically sound reconstruction.[87] Of these, technical flaws are the most common reasons for failure and include errors in tunnel placement, fixation, graft selection, notch impingement, and failure to treat associated laxities. Biologic failures occur with any graft tissue, but in our experience are more commonly seen with allografts. We see significantly more traumatic ruptures of allografts than autografts though these are likely biologic failures. They are frequently seen at approximately 5 years post operatively, and occasionally occur with relatively minor trauma.

Treatment of these allograft failures depends primarily on previous tunnel placement and fixation technique. Femoral tunnel placement and whether the hardware is intraarticular or extraarticular usually dictates whether a one- or two-stage procedure will be performed. The tibial and femoral tunnels in the failed reconstruction may be too anterior, in the correct position, or too posterior. Generally, an anteriorly placed femoral tunnel is frequently encountered in revision surgery, and results in a graft that is overloaded in flexion.[88] Failures are also frequently seen with anteriorly placed tibial tunnels, which result in graft impingement at the notch.[89] It is crucial to avoid compromising revision tunnel placement because of previously placed tunnels and hardware.

Hardware is usually removed, but if it does not interfere with visualization or drilling of the proper revision tunnel, it may be left in place. We have found extraarticular hardware to be more amenable to one-stage revision than interference screw fixation. Removal of endoscopically placed femoral interference screws often results in an unacceptably large defect requiring bone grafting. Frequently, interference screws placed with a two-incision technique and rear-entry guide are less problematic, as an endoscopic revision will place the femoral tunnel more vertically, often avoiding the existing hardware.

Our approach to revision of failed allografts is as follows. Initially hardware is removed if necessary, followed by graft debridement. As noted previously, allograft tunnels are often widened with bone loss secondary to graft necrosis and inflammation. It is crucial to clean the existing tunnels of all graft material and inflammatory tissues to provide an environment that will encourage graft healing. This is accomplished by placing a guide pin up the existing tibial tunnel and hand reaming, starting with a reamer approximately 1 mm smaller than the existing tunnel and proceeding until healthy cancellous bone is exposed. In the event a previous bone block construct has been used and there is a well-healed tunnel, debridement is not necessary if a new tunnel can be placed without significant overlap. The femoral tunnel is addressed in a similar manner.

If the revision tunnel has no overlap with the primary, a one-stage revision can be carried out with bone grafting of the primary tunnel if necessary (Table 10.3). If there is minimal overlap, a larger bone block or soft tissue graft with bone block interposition to fill the tunnel

Table 10.3. One-versus two-stage revision of allograft ACL reconstructions

One-stage revision	*Two-stage revision with bone grafting*
Primary tunnels in acceptable position	Tunnels malpositioned with significant overlap
Minimal bone loss with removal of hardware (often extraarticular)	Significant bone loss (often endoscopically placed interference screw)
No tunnel widening/cyst formation	Tunnel widening with significant bone loss

can be utilized. Unfortunately, with allograft revisions the tunnels are frequently widened and unacceptably large for a one-stage procedure. In this setting we recommend bone grafting of the existing tunnels with freeze-dried cancellous allograft or iliac crest autograft bone. We allow 3 months for bone healing and then treat the revision as we would a primary ACL reconstruction.

Graft choices for allograft revisions are the same as with a primary reconstruction, as no autogenous tissue has been used. Repeat allograft reconstruction is one option, and is often advantageous as large bone blocks can be used to fill existing defects. Noyes et al[90] reported a 33% failure rate in allograft revisions, related to both instability and functional limitations, which correlated with chondral lesions. Harner and colleagues,[91] however, have reported good results using allograft in revision surgery. We recommend use of autogenous tissue whenever possible in treating allograft failures. We feel the autogenous tissue has better healing potential and may avoid biologic issues, which may have predisposed the original allograft to failure. Patellar tendon has advantages of bone blocks and can be used to fill defects. Quadriceps tendon also provides a bone block, but we prefer other graft sources. We have had good results with quadrupled semitendinosus and gracilis grafts. Good fixation can be obtained with newer fixation devices. If necessary, bone can be incorporated into these grafts to help fill large tunnels.

CONCLUSIONS

We currently feel the complications associated with allograft ACL reconstruction outweigh the advantages. While short-term follow-up studies report good results, there is a trend toward increased laxity and failure in allograft reconstruction compared to autograft. Additional long-term studies are necessary to elucidate the fate of ACL allografts. If at all possible, autogenous tissues are recommended for primary and revision ACL reconstruction. Many of the indications for allograft reconstruction (patellofemoral problems, previous patellar tendon graft use) can be addressed with the use of hamstring grafts. Use of these grafts has virtually eliminated our allograft use in primary ACL reconstruction. Additionally, more aggressive rehabilitation programs seem to be decreasing the incidence of complications associated with middle one-third patellar tendon autograft use. This will likely decrease the use of allografts among surgeons who routinely use patellar tendons.

Fortunately, allografts do provide a reliable graft source if autogenous tissues are not available. If autograft tissue is available, it is our first choice for primary and revision ACL reconstruction. We currently use allografts only in multiligament reconstructions and in revisions where autogenous tissue have been used.

References

1. Noyes FR, Grood ES. The strength of the ACL in humans and rhesus monkeys. *J Bone Joint Surg* 1976; 58A(12):1074–1082.
2. Noyes FR, Butler DL, Grood ES, et al. Biomechanical analysis of human ligament grafts used in knee-ligament repairs and reconstructions. *J Bone Joint Surg* 1984; 66A(3):344–352.
3. Woo S, Hollis JM, Adams DJ, Lyon RM, Takai S. Tensile properties of the human femur-anterior cruciate ligament-tibia complex: the effects of specimen age and orientation. *Am J Sports Med* 1991;19(3):217–225.
4. Woo S, Adams DJ. The tensile properties of human anterior cruciate ligament (ACL) and ACL graft tissues. In: Dale MD, WH Akesan, JJ O'Connor, eds. *Knee Ligaments: Structure, Function, Injury, and Repair*. New York: Raven Press. 1990:279–289.
5. McKernan DJ, Wiess JA, Deffner KT, et al. Tensile properties of gracilis, semitendinosus, and patellar tendons from the same donor. Paper presented at the 41st annual meeting of the Orthopaedic Research Society, 1995, Orlando, FL.
6. Curtis R, Delee J, Drez D Jr. Reconstruction of the anterior cruciate ligament with freeze dried fascia lata allografts in dogs. *Am J Sports Med* 1985;13(6):408–414.
7. Drez DJ, DeLee J, Holden JP, Arnoczky S, Noyes FR, Roberts TS. Anterior cruciate ligament reconstruction using bone–patellar tendon–bone allografts: a biological and biomechanical evaluation in goats. *Am J Sports Med* 1991;19(3):256–263.
8. Jackson D, Grood ES, Goldstein JD, et al. A comparison of patellar tendon autograft and allograft used for anterior cruciate ligament reconstruction in the goat model. *Am J Sports Med* 1993;21(2):176–185.
9. Vasseur P, Rodrigo J, Stevenson S, Clark G, Sharkey N. Replacement of the anterior cruciate ligament with a bone-ligament-bone anterior cruciate ligament allograft in dogs. *Clin Orthop Rel Res* 1987;219:268–277.
10. Shino K, Kawasaki T, Hirose H, et al. Reconstructions of the ACL by allogenic tendon graft: An experimental study in the dog. *J Bone Joint Surg* 1984;66B:672–681.
11. Paulos LE, Rosenberg TD, Gurley WD. ACL allografts. In: Friedman M, Ferkel R, eds. Prosthetic Ligament Reconstruction of the Knee. Philadelphia: WB Saunders, 1988:186–192.
12. Kurosaka M, Yoshiya S, Andrish JT. A biomechanical comparison of different surgical techniques of graft fixation in ACL reconstruction. *Am J Sports Med* 1987; 15:225–229.

13. Arnoczky SP. Biology of ACL reconstructions: what happens to the graft? In: Pritchard D, ed. *Instr Course Lect* 1996;45:229–233.

14. Bonamo J, Krinick RM, Sporn AA. Rupture of the patellar ligament after use of its central third for ACL reconstruction. *J Bone Joint Surg* 1984;66A:1294–1297.

15. Christen B, Jakob RP. Fractures associated with patellar ligament grafts in cruciate ligament surgery. *J Bone Joint Surg* 1992;74B:617–619.

16. Paulos L, Rosenberg T, Drawbert J, Manning J, Abbott P. Infrapatellar contracture syndrome: an unrecognized cause of knee stiffness with patella entrapment and patella infera. *Am J Sports Med* 1987;15(4):331–341.

17. Rosenberg T, Franklin JL, Baldwin GN, Nelson KA. Extensor mechanism function after patellar tendon graft harvest for anterior cruciate ligament reconstruction. *Am J Sports Med* 1992;20(5):519–526.

17a. Shino K, Nakagawa S, Inoue M, Horibe S, Yoneda M. Deterioration of patellofemoral articular surfaces after anterior cruciate ligament reconstruction. *Am J Sports Med* 1993;21(2):206–211.

18. Sachs RA, Daniel DM, Stone ML, Garfein RF. Patellofemoral problems after anterior cruciate ligament reconstruction. *Am J Sports Med* 1989;17(6):760–765.

19. Shino K, Nakata K, Horibe S, Inoue M, Nakagawa S. Quantitative evaluation after arthroscopic anterior cruciate ligament reconstruction. *Am J Sports Med* 1993; 21(4):609–616.

20. Lipscomb AB, Johnston RK, Snyder RB, et al. Evaluation of hamstring strength following use of semitendinous and gracilis tendons to reconstruct the ACL. *Am J Sports Med* 1982;10(6):340–342.

21. Pagnani M, Warner J, O'Brien S, Warren R. Anatomic considerations in harvesting the semitendinosus and gracilis tendons and a technique of harvest. *Am J Sports Med* 1993;21(4):565–571.

22. Friedman MJ. Patellar tendon versus hamstring ACL reconstruction. Paper presented at Arthroscopy Association of North America Specialty Day, 1997, San Francisco.

23. Simonian PT, Williams RJ, Deng XH, et al. Hamstring and patellar tendon graft response to cyclical loading. *Am J Knee Surg* 1998;2:101–105.

24. Barrett GR, Papendick L, Miller C. Endobutton fixation technique in ACL reconstruction. *Arthroscopy* 1995;3: 340–343.

25. Clark R, Olsen RE, Larson BJ, et al. Cross-pin femoral fixation: a new technique for hamstring ACL reconstruction of the knee. *Arthroscopy* 1998;143:258–267.

26. Ellis BJ, Weiss JA. Final report: in vitro evaluation of initial pullout strength of the innovasive devices LinX HT hamstring fastener in cancellous bone. Performed at the Orthopaedic Biomechanics Institute, 1997. Submitted.

27. Pinczewski LA. The use of RCI screw for endoscopic fixation of quadruple strand hamstring tendon autograft in ACL reconstruction. Paper presented at AANA Specialty Day, 1997, San Francisco.

28. Rosenberg TD, Deffner KT, Cooley VJ. Quadrupled semitendinosus ACL reconstructions 5 year results in patients without meniscus loss. Paper presented at the AANA 16th annual meeting, April 1997, San Diego, CA, and at 1998 AAOS, New Orleans, LA.

29. Brown CH, Steiner ME, Carson EW. The use of hamstring tendons for ACL reconstruction. Techniques and results. *Clin Sports Med* 1993;12(4):723–756.

30. Howell S, Taylor M. Brace-free rehabilitation with early return to activity for knees reconstructed with a double-looped semitendinosus and gracilis graft. *J Bone Joint Surg* 1996;78A:814.

31. Harris NL, Smith DA, Lamoreaux L, et al. Central quadriceps tendon for ACL reconstruction. *Am J Sports Med* 1997;25:23–28.

32. Jackson D, Heinrich J, Simon T. Biologic and synthetic implants to replace anterior cruciate ligament. *Arthroscopy* 1994;10(4):442–452.

33. Paulos L, Rosenberg T, Grewe S, Tearse D, Beck C. The Gore-Tex anterior cruciate ligament prosthesis. *Am J Sports Med* 1992;20(3):246–252.

34. Shino K, Kimura T, Hirose H, Inoue M, Ono K. Reconstruction of the anterior cruciate ligament by allogeneic tendon graft: an operation for chronic ligamentous insufficiency. *J Bone Joint Surg* 1986;68B(5):739–746.

35. Buck BE, Malinin TI, Brown MD. Bone transplantation and human immunodeficiency virus: an estimate of risk of acquired immunodeficiency syndrome (AIDS). *Clin Orthop Rel Res* 1989;240:129–136.

36. Conrad EU, Gretch DR, Obermeyer KR, et al. Transmission of the hepatitis C virus by tissue transplantation. *J Bone Joint Surg* 1995;77A:214–224.

37. Simonds RJ, Holmberg SD, Hurwitz RL, et al. Transmission of HIV-1 from a seronegative organ and tissue donor. *N Eng J Med* 1992;326:726–732.

38. France EP, Paulos L, Rosenberg T, Harner C. The biomechanics of anterior cruciate allografts. In: Friedman M, Ferkel R, eds. *Prosthetic Ligament Reconstruction of the Knee*. Philadelphia: WB Saunders, 1988:180–185.

39. France EP, Weiss J, Paulos L. Allograft ligament reconstruction: biomechanical issues and testing. *Sports Med Arthrosc Rev* 1993;1:47–60.

40. Cooper JL, Beck CL, Paulos LE. Allograft ACL remodeling: histologic evaluation. Paper presented at the American Academy of Orthopaedic Surgeons annual meeting, 1994, New Orleans, LA.

41. Pinkowski JL, Reiman PR, Chen SL. Human lymphocyte reaction to freeze-dried allograft and xenograft ligamentous tissue. *Am J Sports Med* 1989;17(5):595–600.

42. Lephart S, Kocher M, Harner C, Fu F. Quadriceps strength and funtional capacity after anterior cruciate ligament reconstruction. *Am J Sports Med* 1992;21(5): 738–743.

43. Saddemi SR, Frogameni AD, Fenton PJ, Hartman J, Hartman W. Comparison of perioperative morbidity of anterior cruciate ligament autografts versus allografts. *Arthroscopy* 1993;9(5):519–524.

44. Shelton WR, Papendick L, Dukes AD. Autograft versus allograft anterior cruciate ligament reconstruction. *Arthroscopy* 1997;13(4):446–449.

45. Stringham D, Pelmas C, Burks R, Newman A, Marcus R. Comparison of anterior cruciate ligament reconstructions using patellar tendon autograft or allograft. *Arthroscopy* 1996;12(4):414–421.

46. Victoroff B, Paulos L, Beck C, Goodfellow D. Subcutaneous pretibial cyst formation associated with anterior cruciate ligament allografts: a report of four cases and literature review. *Arthroscopy* 1995;11(4):486–494.

47. Fahey M, Indelicato PA. Bone tunnel enlargement after anterior cruciate ligament replacement. *Am J Sports Med* 1994;22(3):410–414.

48. Tarandy D, Williams J Jr, Bacj B. An unusual intrinsic complication of a patellar tendon allograft and recommendations for tissue banking. *Arthroscopy* 1995;11(4): 475–477.

49. Jackson D, Windler GE, Simon TM. Intraarticular reaction associated with the use of freeze-dried, ethylene oxide–sterilized bone–patella tendon–bone allografts in the reconsruction of the anterior cruciate ligament. *Am J Sports Med* 1990;18(1):1–11.

50. Shelton WR, Treacy SH, Dukes AD, et al. Use of allografts in knee reconstruction: I. Basic science aspects and current status. *J AAOS* 1998;6(3):165–168.

51. Tomford WW, Thongphasuk J, Mankin HJ, Ferraro MJ. Frozen musculoskeletal allografts: a study of the clinical incidence and causes of infection associated with their use. *J Bone Joint Surg* 1990;72A(8):1137–1143.

52. American Association of Tissue Banks. Standards for Tissue Banking. Arlington, VA: American Association of Tissue Banks, 1993.

53. Williams RJ, Laurencin CT, Warren RF, et al. Septic arthritis after arthroscopic ACL reconstruction: diagnosis and management. *Am J Sports Med* 1997;25(2): 261–267.

54. Fideler BM, Vangsness CT, Moore T, et al. Effects of gamma irradiation on the human immunodeficiency virus. *J Bone Joint Surg* 1994;76A(7):1032–1035.

55. Conway B, Tomford WW, Hirsch MS, et al. Effects of gamma irradiaion on HIV-1 in a bone allograft model. *Trans Orthop Res Soc* 1990;15:225.

56. Jackson DW. Use of allografts for ACL reconstructions. *Am Acad Orthop Surg Bull* 1992;40:10–11.

57. Rasmussen T, Feder S, Butler D, Noyes F. The effects of 4 Mrad of irridation on the initial mechanical properties of bone–patellar tendon–bone grafts. *Arthroscopy* 1994; 10(2):188–197.

58. Gibbons MJ, Butler DL, Grood ES, Bylski-Austrow DI, Levy MS, Noyes FR. Effects of gamma irradiation on the initial mechanical and material properties of goat bone–patellar tendon–bone allografts. *J Orthop Res* 1991;9: 209–218.

59. Butler DL, Oster DM, Feder SM, et al. Effects of gamma irradiation on the biomechanics of patellar tendon allografts of the ACL in the goat. *Trans Orthop Res Soc* 1991;16:205.

60. Goertzen MJ, Clahsen H, Burrig KF, Schulitz KP. Sterilisation of canine anterior cruciate allografts by gamma irradiation in argon: mechanical and neurohistological properties retained one year after transplantation. *J Bone Joint Surg* 1995;77B(2):205–212.

61. Jackson D, Grood ES, Wilcox P, Butler DL, Simon TM, Holden JP. The effects of processing techniques on the mechanical properties of bone–anterior cruciate ligament–bone allografts. *Am J Sports Med* 1988;16(2): 101–105.

62. Roberts T, Drez D Jr, McCarthy W, Paine R. Anterior cruciate ligament reconstruction using freeze-dried, ethylene oxide-sterilized, bone–patellar tendon–bone allografts. *Am J Sports Med* 1991;19(1):35–41.

63. Sterling JC, Meyers MC, Calvo RD. Allograft failure in cruciate ligament reconstruction. *Am J Sports Med* 1995;23(2):173–178.

64. Silvaggio V, Fu F, Georgescu H, Evans C. The induction of IL-1 by freeze-dried ethylene oxide–treated bone–patellar tendon–bone allograft wear particles: an in vitro study. *Arthroscopy* 1993;9(1):82–86.

65. Schrock KB, Jackson DW. Allograft reconstruction of the ACL: basic science. *Oper Tech Sports Med* 1995;3(3): 139–147.

66. Jackson DW, Grood ES, Cohn BT, Arnozcky SP, Simon TM, Cummings JF. The effects of *in situ* freezing on the anterior cruciate ligament. *J Bone Joint Surg* 1991; 73A(2):201–213.

67. Pritchard J, Drez D Jr, Moss M, and Heck S. Long-term followup of anterior cruciate ligament reconstructions using freeze-dried fascia lata allografts. *Am J Sports Med* 1995;23(5):593–596.

68. Paulos LE, France EP, Rosenberg TD, et al. Comparative material properties of allograft tissues for ligament replacement: effects of type, age, sterilization, and preservation. *Trans Orthop Res Soc* 1987;12:129.

69. Indelicato PA, Bittar ES, Prevot TJ, Woods GA, Branch TP, Huegel M. Clinical comparison of freeze-dried and fresh frozen patellar tendon allografts for anterior cruciate ligament reconstruction of the knee. *Am J Sports Med* 1990;18(4):335–342.

70. Buck BE, Resnick L, Shah SM, Malinin TI. Human immunodeficiency virus cultured from bone: implications for transplantation. *Clin Orthop Rel Res* 1990;251:249–253.

71. Nemzek JA, Arnocxky SP, Swenson CL. Retroviral transmission by the transplantation of connective-tissue allografts. *J Bone Joint Surg* 1994;76A(7):1036–1041.

72. Arnoczky SP, Warren RF, Ashlock MA. Replacement of the anterior cruciate ligament using a patellar tendon allograft. *J Bone Joint Surg* 1986;68A(3):376–385.

73. Nikolaou PK, Seaber AV, Glisson RR, Ribbeck BM, Bassett FH III. Anterior cruciate ligament allograft transplantation: long-term function, histology, revascularization, and operative technique. *Am J Sports Med* 1986; 14(5):348–360.

74. Cordrey LJ, McCorkle H, Hilton E. A comparative study of fresh autogenous and preserved homogenous tendon grafts in rabbits. *J Bone Joint Surg* 1963;45B(1): 182–195.

75. Horstman JK, Ahmadu-Suka F, Norrdin RW. Anterior cruciate ligament fascia lata allograft reconstruction: progressive histologic changes toward maturity. *Arthroscopy* 1993;9(5):509–518.

76. Shino K, Inoue M, Horibe S, Nagano J, Ono K. Maturation of allograft tendons transplanted into the knee: an arthroscopic and histological study. *J Bone Joint Surg* 1988;70B(4):556–560.

77. Indelicato PA, Linton R, Huegel M. The results of fresh-frozen patellar tendon allografts for chronic anterior cruciate ligament deficiency of the knee. *Am J Sports Med* 1992;20(2):118–121.

78. Cooper JL, Paulos LE, Beck CL, et al. A prospective and retrospective long-term analysis comparing allograft and autograft tissue for ACL reconstruction. Paper presented at AOSSM 20th annual meeting, 1994, Palm Desert, CA.

79. Malek MM, DeLuca JV. Freeze-dried Achilles tendon allograft in ACL reconstruction; two and five year follow-up comparison. Paper presented at the AAOS 60th annual meeting, San Francisco, 1993.

80. Noyes F, Barber-Westin S. Reconstruction of the ACL with human allograft: comparison of early and late results. *J Bone Joint Surg* 1996;78A(4):524–537.

81. Noyes F, Barber S. The effect of a ligament-augmentation device on allograft reconstructions for chronic ruptures of the anterior cruciate ligament. *J Bone Joint Surg* 1992;74A(7):960–973.

82. Friedlander GE. Immune responses to osteochondral allografts: current knowledge and future directions. *Clin Orthop Rel Res* 1983;174:58–68.

83. Harner C, Thompson W, Jamison J, et al. The immunologic response to fresh-frozen patellar tendon allograft ACL reconstruction. Paper presented at 1994 AAOS annual meeting, New Orleans.

84. Linn RM, Fischer DA, Smith JP, et al. Achilles tendon allograft reconstruction of the ACL deficient knee. *Am J Sports Med* 1993;21:825–831.

85. Olson EJ, Harner CD, Fu FH, Silbey MB. Clinical use of fresh, frozen soft tissue allografts. *Orthopedics* 1992; 15(10):1225–1232.

86. Blevins FT, Hecker AT, Bigler GT, Boland AL, Hayes WC. The effects of donor age and strain rate on the biomechanical properties of bone–patellar tendon–bone allografts. *Am J Sports Med* 1994;22(3):328–333.

87. Jaureguito JW, Paulos LE. Why grafts fail. *Clin Orthop* 1996;325:25–41.

88. Maday MG, Harner CD, Fu F. Revision ACL surgery: evaluation and treatment. In: Feagin JA, ed. *The Crucial Ligaments*. New York: Churchill Livingstone, 1994:711–723.

89. Howell SM, Taylor MA. Failure of reconstruction of the ACL due to impingement by the intercondylar roof. *J Bone Joint Surg* 1993;75A:1044–1055.

90. Noyes F, Barber-Westin S, Roberts CS. Use of allografts after failed treatment of rupture of the anterior cruciate ligament. *J Bone Joint Surg* 1994;76A(7):1019–1031.

91. Harner CD, Jamison JP, Thompson W, et al. Revision ACL reconstruction using fresh-frozen allograft tissue. Classification, indications, techniques, results, and controversies. Paper presented at the annual meeting of the American Academy of Orthopaedic Surgeons, 1994, New Orleans, LA.

Chapter 11

Complications and Pitfalls in Anterior Cruciate Ligament Reconstruction with Synthetic Grafts

Mark H. Getelman and Marc J. Friedman

Anterior cruciate ligament (ACL) reconstruction is now widely accepted and routinely performed. It is estimated that 60,000 to 75,000 surgical procedures are performed annually in the United States.

Several graft sources have been employed since the development of current reconstruction techniques in the 1980s. Ligament substitutes included autogenous tissue, allografts, and synthetic materials. Initially, synthetic devices were popular. Early results appeared promising and the concerns of graft-site morbidity and disease transmission were nonexistent. However, as long-term follow-up became available, there were unacceptably high failure rates from synthetic reconstructions, with many associated problems. Subsequently, many patients have had additional surgery including revision ACL reconstruction or simply graft removal.

At the present time in the United States, synthetic substitutes have been removed from the market and are no longer indicated for use in primary ACL reconstruction. However, several patients still have synthetic ligaments and these patients may require additional treatment. This chapter discusses the various synthetic ligaments that may be encountered, and a treatment plan and technique for revision.

HISTORY

In 1914, Corner[1] presented one of the earliest descriptions of prosthetic ACL reconstruction. He replaced the torn ACL of a football player with a loop of silver wire. This description predated Hey-Groves[2] by 3 years; in 1917, he gave what is felt to be the first true description of an ACL reconstruction.

Since then there have been many advances in ACL surgery, and multiple synthetic substitutes have been introduced and subsequently removed from the market. History has shown many potential problems related to prosthetic ligaments. Problems from early breakage due to repetitive loading, to fixation failures, and to reactions of the synovial host tissue to the implant have all occurred.

SYNTHETIC LIGAMENT CLASSIFICATION

Prosthetic ligaments are designed to function in one of three ways. Permanent ligaments, such as the Gore-Tex and Stryker Dacron ligaments, are designed with high strength and are built to resist fatigue failure. They rely on inherent mechanical properties to resist load over a prolonged period of time. They receive no contribution from the host tissue or new tissue growth.

The second type of prosthesis is designed to augment the strength of the autogenous intraarticular graft tissue. These augmentation devices or stents improve the security of fixation and provide greater strength during the early healing and rehabilitation phase. The autogenous tissue increases its strength over time and the augmentation device becomes less important.

The final type of prosthetic ligament is a scaffold or ingrowth type of device. These ligaments rely on the host s collagen derived from the fibroblasts present in the knee. The collagen may fill in spaces within the existing graft, as with the Leeds-Keio, or may actually replace the scaffold as it is degraded over time as in a carbon fiber ligament. Theoretically, the newly developed tissue can last indefinitely without fatigue failure.

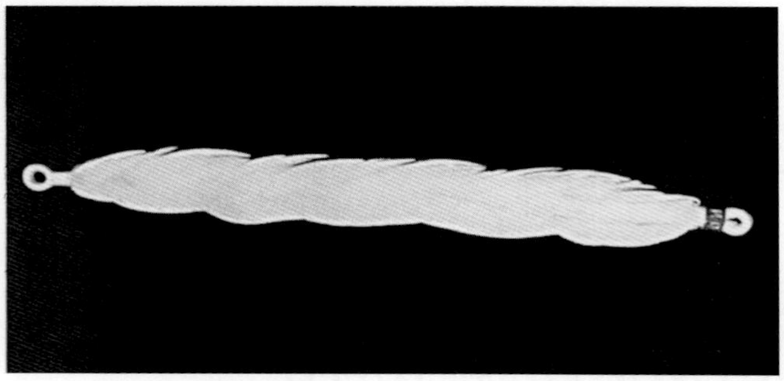

Figure 11.1. Gore-Tex ligament is composed of polytetrafluoroethylene (PTFE). The prosthesis is constructed from a single strand of material wound into multiple loops.

Permanent Grafts

Gore-Tex

The Gore-Tex ligament graft was one of the most popular grafts used in the United States. The ligament is composed of polytetrafluoroethylene (PTFE). The prosthesis is constructed from a single strand of the material wound into multiple loops. The strands are then woven into a three-bundle braid with fixation at each end (Fig. 11.1). Permanent fixation is thought to occur by tissue ingrowth into the strands of the graft within the bony tunnels over a period of 6 months. The ultimate strength of the graft is 5,300 N, which is roughly 2½ times that of the native ACL. It is also much stiffer than the ACL, with only 2% to 5% strain at failure compared to 25% for the ACL.[3]

The graft was approved by the Food and Drug Administration (FDA) in October 1986 for general use in patients with failed previous ACL reconstructions . The early reports on this ligament were promising. Indelicato et al[4] presented a satisfactory outcome in 87% of his patients at 2 year follow-up, and a study from our institution looking at 61 patients showed improved subjective and objective criteria.[5] However, there were still problems. Indelicato et al had nine patients with effusions, and on a follow-up study at 36 months they noted 11 failures.[6] In our study there were five complete ruptures, three infections, and 16 sterile effusions, five of which became chronic.

Paulos et al[7] found less than 50% improvement in subjective and objective factors in his series of 188 patients followed for 4 years. They had a total complication rate of 76% in those patients who had had a previous intraarticular ACL reconstruction. Sledge et al[8] found a 29% failure rate in their 5-year follow-up and recommended that the graft no longer be used.[8]

The ligament was removed from the market by its manufacturer in 1993. The Gore-Tex CD, the second-generation ligament, which was still in multicenter trials, was similarly removed at the same time.[3]

Stryker Dacron

The Stryker Dacron prosthetic ligament was a composite of four Dacron tapes surrounded by a Dacron velour sleeve. It was originally designed as an augmentation device for use with the iliotibial band. However, the ligament had an ultimate tensile strength of 3,600 N and it became commonly used as a permanent prosthesis.[9] When used in this fashion, no significant ingrowth was noted intraarticularly.

The graft, too, appeared promising in the early results and short-term follow-up. However, long-term studies again identified problems. Wilk and Richmond[10] reported a failure rate of 35.7% at 5 years in 84 patients. This was a dramatic increase from the 20% failure rate they saw at 2 years.[10] Gillquist and Odensten[11] prospectively followed 70 patients for 5 years and reported good to excellent results in only 56%, and a 23% graft rupture rate. In 1997, they presented long-term follow-up of the same patients. The overall rupture rate increased to 44%, 29% had undergone second reconstructions, and five had third reconstructions; 83% had radiographic arthritic changes and only 14% had acceptable knee stability and function.[12]

Stryker discontinued this product in 1994.

Scaffold Prostheses

Leeds-Keio

The Leeds-Keio (LK) graft is popular internationally. It was designed in a collaboration between Leeds University in England and Keio University in Japan. It is a polyester fiber graft woven to form a mesh structure (Fig. 11.2). The open weave was designed to promote ingrowth. The graft is secured with two bone plugs in a press-fit application. Without ingrowth, the ultimate

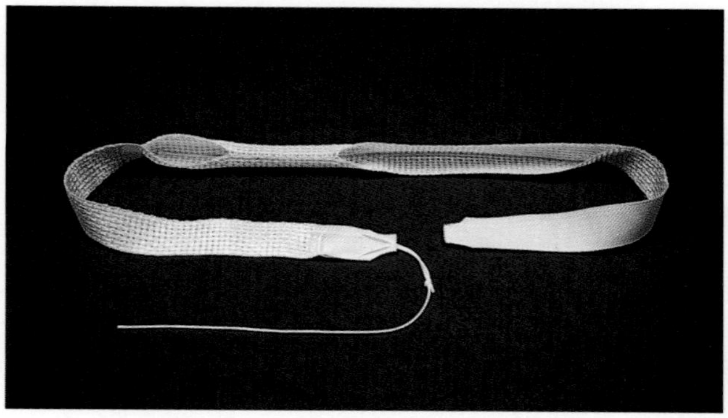

Figure 11.2. Leeds-Keio ligament is a polyester fiber graft woven to form a mesh structure.

strength is roughly 850 N; however, with fibrous tissue ingrowth the strength had been shown to be in excess of 2,000 N.[9]

Over 14,000 grafts have been implanted around the world, but the graft has not been approved for use in the United States. Denti et al[13] presented their results at 33 months follow-up on 26 patients. They found improvements in both objective and subjective factors and had two reported ruptures. Fujikawa,[14] one of the designers at Keio, reviewed 152 patients who had greater than 4 years follow-up. Postoperatively, 90.1% had negative Lachman tests and 82.2% had negative anterior drawer tests. No patients had chronic effusions, synovitis, or infections. Arthroscopy was performed on 42 cases. At 3 to 4 months postoperation, the implant was covered with newly formed immature fibrous tissue. At 6 to 7 months there was decreased surface vascularity, and at 1 year the graft appeared mature, with an appearance resembling the native ACL in both shape and thickness. Rupture occurred in only 3.3% of cases. However, Engstrom et al[15] compared the LK graft to autogenous patellar tendon (PT) in a prospective randomized study. There were 26 PT and 29 LK patients. Those patients in the LK group had significantly higher instrumented anterior laxity testing and greater pivot shift. The authors concluded that at 28-month mean follow-up the LK graft did not meet satisfactory criteria for ACL reconstruction.

Augmentation Devices

Ligament Augmentation Device (LAD)

The LAD was introduced in 1979 by Dr. John Kennedy[16] working with the 3M company. This device was a flat braid of high-strength polypropylene (Fig. 11.3). It had an ultimate strength of 1,500 N and 3% creep, with dynamic loading of 500 N. This profile was much lower than the other permanent prosthetic ligaments, and if used alone early failure would certainly be expected. It was developed as a load-sharing device, designed to deflect some of the force on the autogenous graft during the early healing process.

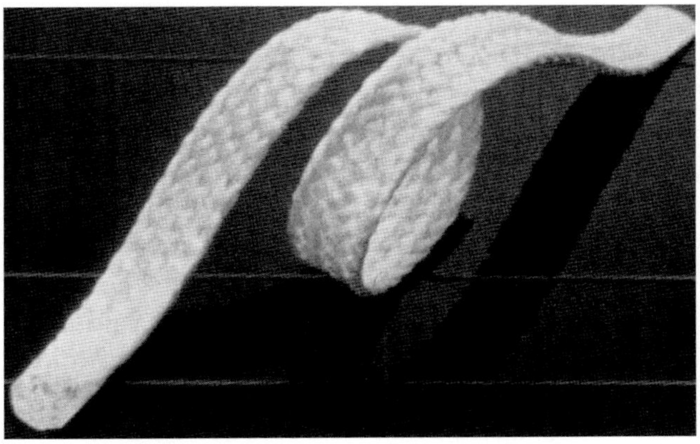

Figure 11.3. LAD (Ligament Augmentation Device) is a flat braid of high-strength polypropylene introduced in 1979 by Dr. John Kennedy.

The LAD was secured to the autogenous graft at only one end. If fixed at both ends, then stress shielding would result in the autogenous graft and thus the LAD would be acting as a permanent ligament rather than a stent. Thus, the load-sharing concept was essential to the success. The stent would protect the graft from excessive stress while the graft was weak. As revascularization occurred, the strength and stiffness improved and the autogenous graft carried a greater proportion of the load.

Animal and early human studies appeared promising. The initial studies by Roth et al[17] evaluated the results with a Marshall-McIntosh technique reinforced with the LAD. They found significant improvements in terms of functional stability and laxity. Del Pizzo[18] evaluated his patients with a 3-year minimum follow-up; 95% had a 0 to 1+ pivot shift and 72% had less than 3-mm laxity with arthrometer testing. The infection rate was 0.7%; 1% had sterile effusions and 1.4% had graft rupture. In 1996, Thuresson et al[19] compared patients with and without LAD augmentation of autogenous patellar tendon ACL reconstructions. The outcome was good in both groups. There was no significant difference in the Lysholm knee function scores.

COMPLICATIONS

Several commonly encountered complications of prosthetic ACL grafts are now accepted, and consequently these devices are no longer routinely used in the United States. That does not mean, however, that the problems will no longer be encountered. There are still many patients who have prosthetic ligaments, and there remains the possibility that these patients will still present with problems and possible need for revision surgery.

Rupture, synovitis and chronic effusions, and osteolysis are the problems that may still be encountered. Additionally, there was a higher risk of postoperative infection. The reported incidence of infection was as high as 2% to 3%.[3] While disastrous, this is more likely to occur in the perioperative period and is thus not very likely to be encountered. Like most other postoperative infections, the findings can be quite dramatic, and usually the graft must be removed.

Rupture

Despite ultimate strengths much higher than the native ACL, rupture of permanent prosthetic grafts occurred frequently. Ruptures have been associated with abrasion within the osseous tunnels, improper positioning leading to poor stress distribution or abrasion, and primary fatigue failure related to the repetitive cyclical loading.[3,20]

While primary failures occur from cyclical loading, the majority of ruptures appear to begin with abrasion. Abrasion can occur within the osseous tunnel, from inadequate notchplasty, or from improper tunnel positioning. The graft can be abraded where the tunnel enters the joint. It is important to avoid steep angles, and the tunnel edges should be chamfered to avoid sharp bony surfaces that can lead to graft fraying with repetitive cycling.

Proper notchplasty is also imperative. If the notch is not wide and deep enough to allow for the prosthesis, then there will be abrasion with repetitive cycling, which can lead to failure. The amount of bone resection is mandated by the prosthesis used, the size of the notch, and the position of the tunnels. With anatomically correct tunnel positions, often only a very limited notchplasty needs to be performed. However, the graft must be tested to be sure that full extension can be achieved without any impingement. Howell and Taylor[21] have carefully documented the effects of graft impingement, particularly as to how it affects an anteriorly placed graft.

Improper femoral placement anteriorly often results in failure. During terminal extension the graft will be impinged by the roof of the notch, which can lead to loss of extension, graft abrasion, and eventual graft failure. Additionally, the anteriorly placed graft will tighten as the knee is flexed, thereby capturing the joint resulting in increased graft tension and loss of flexion. Conversely, a posteriorly positioned graft will have excessive tension in extension and will be lax in flexion.

Synovitis and Chronic Effusions

Synovitis is commonly encountered in patients who have prosthetic ligaments within the knee. It has been reported to occur with a permanent prosthesis as well as the LAD. The synovitis is most commonly due to particulate debris within the joint, which results in synovial irritation that manifests as an effusion with swelling and pain. There may also be associated warmth and leukocytosis despite the absence of infection. If transient, this can be treated with aspiration, nonsteroidal antiinflammatory drugs (NSAIDs), and joint rest. However, when related to abrasion and prosthetic wear, the knee may develop chronic effusions and may often require graft removal.

The effect of particulate debris has been carefully studied using animal models at the University of Pittsburgh. Olson et al[22] examined the effect of seven different prosthetic ligaments on synovial cells both in vitro and in vivo. All ligaments induced significantly elevated enzyme levels including interleukin-1, collagenase, and gelatinase, which are all detrimental to the joint. The foreign body response resulted in synovial hypertrophy and giant cell and macrophage accumulations about the wear particles. The extent of the foreign body reaction was based on the type of ligament and amount of particulate debris. Xenografts and carbon fiber grafts had the most enzyme production.

Osteolysis

Osseous tunnel changes can also be seen. Osteolysis has been reported by Seeman and Steadman[23] following the use of Gore-Tex grafts. The authors noted progressive widening of the tunnel over time, which often resulted in late failure, as the tunnel widening causes functional incompetency of the graft. The precise mechanism of osteolysis has not been elucidated. However, it has been hypothesized that this is an enzyme-mediated problem as well. The interleukin-1 that is released in response to the wear debris is felt to gravitate to the tibial tunnel via the intraarticular opening, where it stimulates a foreign body response, resulting in bone resorption.[3,23]

The osteolysis can often be seen on plain radiographs. There is widening about the osseous tunnel, with sclerosis along the margins. If there is a question as to the extent of the lysis, then either a computed tomography (CT) scan or magnetic resonance imaging (MRI) should be done to better demonstrate the extent of the changes. Either can be quite useful for preoperative consideration when contemplating a revision. In those cases where the defect is quite large, the revision can be staged. The graft is first removed, and the tunnel is bone grafted. The revision is then performed several weeks later, after the graft has incorporated.

Lymphadenopathy

A more recent complication of the Gore-Tex graft has been reported. Wilson et al[24] identified two patients who developed inguinal lymphadenopathy. Both patients had Gore-Tex CD ligaments in place at the time the lymphadenopathy developed. The patients developed chronic knee effusions and subsequently underwent graft removal 1 year after the lymphadenopathy was first noted. The patients both had superficial inguinal lymph nodes excised at the time of surgery.

Microbiologic and histologic examinations were performed including electron microscopy. The findings were consistent with acute lymphadenitis, with Gore-Tex particulate debris identified within the lymph node. Thus, there may be effects distant from the knee as well.

TECHNICAL CONSIDERATIONS

Preoperative Evaluation

The preoperative evaluation of patients with failed prosthetic ACL reconstructions is important for many reasons. It is at this time that the surgeon must counsel the patient. The patient must have realistic expectations. Results following revision ACL reconstruction do not compare favorably with primary procedures. It is important to emphasize that the surgery is a salvage procedure. The goal is to allow patients to perform their activities of daily living without instability, and patients must understand that they may not be able to return to sports. False expectations can lead to a subjective failure despite a technically successful procedure.[25]

Once a decision is made to proceed with revision reconstruction, several details must be addressed prior to surgery. A careful history should be obtained. The surgeon should address aspects of the primary procedure as well as the postoperative rehabilitation, return to activity, and time frame of the sensation that the surgery has failed. Instability rather than pain should be identified in patients considering revision. A painful knee that demonstrates some laxity on examination is quite different from a knee demonstrating recurrent instability. Pain can be due to several factors often unrelated to the laxity, and such patients often will not improve even if their ACL reconstruction is revised.

The physical examination should be comprehensive. Other causes of pain should be sought. Range of motion and crepitus should be noted. Any sign of sepsis must be noted and fully investigated . The patient s gait, alignment, and stability are evaluated. The physician must carefully address the secondary restraints in addition to the anterior instability. Unrecognized laxity may be the difference between success and failure of the revision reconstruction.

Radiographs are also recommended. Weight-bearing anteroposterior and 45-degree posteroanterior x-rays are helpful in determining alignment and articular wear. Lateral radiographs in full extension allow evaluation of the tunnel position and size. Patella axial views and long-standing films (i.e., standing weight-bearing films on long films or cassettes) are also useful. If there is concern about significant tunnel osteolysis on the x-rays, then CT or MRI can be done to gain better understanding of the defect. While the CT scan allows better bony definition, the MRI provides greater information with regard to meniscal injury and the status of the articular surfaces.

The previous records should be obtained, as they may provide valuable information that can dictate prognosis and facilitate the procedure. The original operative report can be quite helpful. The status of the knee at that time can be determined. Attention should be directed to the condition of the menisci and the articular surfaces. The type of prosthetic graft and technique should be gleaned. The exact hardware should be noted so that the necessary equipment can be obtained for future removal.

Staging

If there is significant tunnel enlargement, then staged reconstruction should be considered. The first procedure would involve graft removal, tunnel curettage, and bone grafting. The revision can then be performed 6 to 12 weeks later, once the graft has incorporated. Furthermore, if patients have significant loss of motion, lacking greater than 5 degrees extension or 20 degrees flexion, then the first goal becomes restoration of motion, and the revision procedure may need to be staged.[26]

Skin Incisions

Skin incisions should be carefully planned to avoid complications. Whenever possible, previous incisions should be reused if they will allow access to proper tunnel placement and allow hardware removal. Skin bridges of less than 7 cm should be avoided. Periosteum should be handled gently and closed when possible to avoid complications. Allografts usually require smaller incisions and should be considered if the skin is of particular concern.

Hardware Removal

With present ACL fixation techniques, there is a myriad of different types of hardware. Occasionally, the hardware does not interfere with the revision procedure. In those cases, it can be left alone. However, in most prosthetic ligament revisions, the fixation will need to be removed. If the exact type of hardware can be determined, then the proper equipment can be made available. But actual removal can be difficult. Soft tissue or bone often obscures the device. To successfully remove interference screws, the proper screwdriver must be completely seated, and thus the knee flexion angle of screw insertion must be duplicated. Thus, it may be necessary to remove the overlying tissue, and curettes, a burr, or coring reamers may be required. If the screw is stripped, it can be drilled out. But often, excessive bone will also be removed, necessitating a staged procedure. If staples are used, then the appropriate extractor or osteotome should be used.

The surgeon should be capable of doing different techniques for revision. Often changing from an endoscopic to two-incision technique, or vice versa, can avoid the need for hardware removal. This may allow preservation of bone stock and reduce operative time.

Prosthetic Ligament Removal

The prosthetic ligament must be removed at the time of revision. It is ideal to remove the prosthesis en bloc. A gouge can be used to loosen the bony attachments prior to removal. It is necessary to remove the bony attachments circumferentially so that the entire graft is removed. If particulate debris is left behind, there is the potential for a marked inflammatory response, with possible bone tunnel and cartilage destruction. The arthroscope can be inserted into the intraosseous tunnels to confirm that the entire prosthesis has been removed. If the synthetic ligament demonstrates intraarticular damage, then it may be necessary to perform a concomitant synovectomy to eliminate the particulate debris. Two-staged reconstructions are often necessary in cases where there is marked tunnel osteolysis from the synthetic ligament.

Revision Notchplasty

Most revision cases require repeat notchplasty. There can be natural regrowth of up to 1 cm following an ACL reconstruction. In cases where failure was due to graft impingement, revision notchplasty is imperative. The roof and lateral wall can both cause graft impingement and must be addressed at the time of revision. It is necessary to remove enough bone to prevent impingement and to allow visualization for proper tunnel placement. The over-the-top position and the previous tunnels must be visualized prior to creating any new tunnels. Excessive bone removal must be avoided, however, to ensure adequate bone stock is maintained for proper graft fixation.

Bone Tunnel Placement

Proper bone tunnel placement is the most important and challenging aspect of a revision ACL reconstruction. When the original tunnels are placed improperly, new tunnels must be created.

On the femoral side, the most common situation reveals the original tunnel is placed too far anteriorly. In this case, often a new tunnel can be drilled posterior to the original one and existing hardware need not be removed. If the tunnel is only slightly anterior, there are several options. First, the tunnel can be expanded posteriorly, and a larger graft bone plug (allograft) can be used. For autograft use, alternative fixation techniques, such as stacked interference screws, may be required in these cases. Alternatively, a two-incision technique can be used to move the tunnel more posteriorly and allow fixation within the tunnel. Rosenberg[27] advocates a bisocket technique, which allows the creation of two small tunnels posterior to the malpositioned tunnel. A hamstring graft is divided in half and each half is placed into a 6-mm tunnel and fixed with separate Endobuttons.

When the existing tunnel is placed too far posteriorly, the posterior wall is often deficient, which will require converting to a two-incision or over-the-top technique. In those cases where a Gore-Tex ligament was used, the femoral tunnel is positioned over the top and thus a new femoral tunnel can be created in a standard fashion. Finally, when the intraarticular position is adequate, changing from a two-incision to endoscopic technique can facilitate graft placement and fixation.

It is possible to apply similar principles to the tibial tunnel. If placed too anteriorly, the graft will impinge and fail. Often the existing tunnel and hardware can be ignored and a new tunnel can be created more posteriorly. If the tunnel is slightly malpositioned so that the existing tunnel must be incorporated, then the tunnel is expanded anteriorly or posteriorly and a larger bone block is used as in the femur. For large capacious tunnels, the surgeon can either use bone graft simultaneously with the new ACL graft or stage the reconstruction. Most commonly, capacious tunnels are encountered with failed synthetic or allograft reconstructions.

Graduated tunnel expanders can be rather helpful when fashioning these new tunnels (Instrument Makar, Okemos, MI). They are available commercially and allow the surgeon to create a small-diameter hole initially, which can then be enlarged in a controlled progressive manner. Thus, there is less risk of cortical perforation. Additionally, the expanders allow compacting of bone, which can aid in better graft fixation.

Graft Selection

Graft selection is important when considering revision ACL reconstruction. The decision to be made is between autograft and allograft. Both have advantages and disadvantages and there are advocates for both graft sources. Autografts include bone–patellar tendon–bone, hamstrings, quadriceps-patella, and iliotibial band. These grafts offer shortened incorporation times without the potential for disease transmission or immunologic reaction. However, there is associated morbidity, and in the revision situation availability may prevent or limit the use of autologous tissue. Contralateral bone–tendon–bone (BTB) grafts have been used by Shelbourne's group[28] with no significant complications reported. Repeated ipsilateral BTB harvesting has been reported and is more commonly used in Europe. MRI studies have documented reconstitution of the central one-third of the BTB donor site at 1 year.[20,29] Karns et al[30] reported a revision case that used a reharvested patellar tendon 4 years after the primary reconstruction. While this sounds enticing, there are no biomechanical studies documenting the mechanical properties and tensile strength of the reharvested graft. Furthermore, Hang et al[31] have shown that there is no longer the same histologic composition at the tendon-bone interface of the reconstituted ligament, and suggest that this is scar tissue rather than actual reconstituted ligament. Thus, at the present time we cannot recommend the routine use of this graft.

Allografts include bone–patellar tendon–bone, calcaneus–Achilles tendon, and iliotibial band. These grafts have been used successfully for both primary and revision ACL reconstructions. There are several advantages to their use: shorter operative times, smaller incisions, and no potential for donor-site morbidity. Furthermore, there is relatively no size limitation. In the revision case, there may be need for larger tunnel diameters, which can more easily be accommodated with larger allograft bone plugs. However, there are disadvantages inherent in the use of allograft tissue: potentially longer incorporation times, theoretical immunologic reactions, and the inherent cost. But the greatest risk is the potential for viral disease transmission. It is presently estimated that the risk of disease transmission with allograft use is less than 1 per 1,000,000 uses, assuming the present American Association of Tissue Banks (AATB) guidelines are rigidly followed. With the present AATB protocol, there has never been a reported case of viral transmission from allograft connective tissue.[32] Unfortunately, freezing does not eradicate the virus. Radiation, however, will kill the virus, but the necessary dosage will also alter the collagen and reduce the graft strength.[33]

Thus, graft selection needs to be individualized. The only absolute requirement is that the chosen graft have adequate strength to provide long-term stability. Beyond that, the ultimate decision is between the patient and the treating physician.

Graft Fixation

Graft fixation is critical in the early postoperative period following revision ACL reconstruction. If the tunnels are created without difficulty or significant bone loss, then routine fixation techniques can be employed. However, if there is any concern about fixation strength using these methods, then secondary techniques should be employed. Post and washer and staple fixation can easily be added and used as secondary fixation. Furthermore, there are always new techniques being developed for fixation, and it is recommended that the treating surgeon become familiar with the different options.

Associated Patholaxities

Patients with chronic ACL insufficiency can develop laxity in their secondary restraints. Failure to address the associated instability will ultimately result in failure of the revision ACL reconstruction. Several structures can be responsible for these problems. Bony alignment, meniscal loss, and rotatory instability patterns are commonly implicated. The surgeon must identify these problems preoperatively and address them at the time of reconstruction.

In cases of anteromedial rotatory instability (AMRI), the posteromedial corner needs to be addressed. Often this instability can be treated by reefing the lax tissues. However, if there is significant AMRI and the patient has had a previous medial meniscectomy, then a medial meniscal transplant should also be considered. This allows the "break-stop mechanism" of the posterior medial meniscal horn to be restored.[25]

Chronic posterolateral rotary instability (PLRI) is more difficult to control. Several treatment options are available, and the selected method is determined by the extent of the instability. For severe laxity, reconstruction with autograft or allograft is often required. Patients with long-standing ACL insufficiency and PLRI can further develop marked varus alignment of the lower extremity. In these cases it is also necessary to perform a valgus osteotomy to correct the alignment and limit tension on the reconstructed posterolateral corner. An osteotomy is also considered in those patients with advanced articular cartilage changes and malalignment coexistent with the instability.

REHABILITATION

Rehabilitation following revision ACL reconstruction is rather different from the aggressive protocols used for primary ACL reconstruction. The general plan is much more conservative. The patients must be reminded that the results are less predictable and thus they must not exceed the limits placed upon them. Each rehabilitation protocol is individualized and is based on the type of reconstruction, strength of fixation, and any associated reconstructions that were performed. Weight bearing is protected for up to 6 weeks, and return to activities is delayed. Patients should be advised that the return to sports cannot be guaranteed and will take at least 1 year to accomplish.

References

1. Corner EM. Notes of a case illustrative of an artificial anterior crucial ligament, demonstrating the action of the ligament. *Proc R Soc Med* 1914;7:120–121.
2. Hey-Groves EW. Operation for the repair of crucial ligaments. *Lancet* 1917;2:674–675.
3. Steadman JR, Seemann MD, Hutton KS. Revision liga-

ment reconstruction of failed prosthetic anterior cruciate ligaments. *Inst Course Lect* 1995;44:417–429.

4. Indelicato PA, Pascale MS, Huegel MO. Early experience with the Gore-Tex polytetrafluoroethylene anterior cruciate ligament prosthesis. *Am J Sports Med* 1989;17: 55–62.
5. Karzel RP, Diefendorf DR, Fox JM, et al. Four year experience with the Gore-Tex prosthetic ligament in anterior cruciate deficient knees. *Orthop Trans* 1990;14: 618.
6. Woods GA, Indelicato PA, Prevot TJ. The Gore-Tex anterior cruciate ligament prosthesis: two versus three year results. *Am J Sports Med* 1991;19:48–55.
7. Paulos LE, Rosenberg TD, Grewe SR, et al. The Gore-Tex anterior cruciate ligament prosthesis: a long term follow-up. *Am J Sports Med* 1992;20:246–252.
8. Sledge SL, Steadman JR, Silliman JF, et al. Five-year results with the Gore-Tex anterior cruciate ligament prosthesis. *Am J Knee Surg* 1992;5:65–70.
9. Friedman MJ. Prosthetic anterior cruciate ligament. *Clin Sports Med* 1991;10:499–513.
10. Wilk RM, Richmond JC. Dacron ligament reconstruction for chronic anterior cruciate ligament insufficiency. *Am J Sports Med* 1993;21:374–380.
11. Gilquist J, Odensten M. Reconstruction of old anterior cruciate ligament tears with a Dacron prosthesis: a prospective study. *Am J Sports Med* 1993;21:358–366.
12. Maletius W, Gilquist J. Long-term results of anterior cruciate ligament reconstruction with a Dacron prosthesis. The frequency of osteoarthritis after seven to eleven years. *Am J Sports Med* 1997;25:288–293.
13. Denti M, Arosio A, Monteleone M, et al. Preliminary assessment of anterior cruciate ligament reconstruction with the Leeds-Keio artificial ligament. *Am J Knee Surg* 1990; 3:181–186.
14. Fujikawa K. Clinical study of anterior cruciate ligament reconstruction with the Leeds-Keio artificial ligament. In: Friedman MJ, Ferkel RD, eds. *Prosthetic Ligament Reconstruction of the Knee*. Philadelphia: WB Saunders, 1988:132–139.
15. Engstrom B, Wredmark T, Westblad P. Patellar tendon or Leeds-Keio graft in the surgical treatment of anterior cruciate ligament ruptures. Intermediate results. *Clin Orthop* 1993;295:190–197.
16. Kennedy JC. Application of prosthetics to anterior cruciate ligament reconstruction and repair. *Clin Orthop* 1983;172:125–128.
17. Roth JH, Kennedy JC, Lockstadt H, et al. Polypropylene braid augmented and nonaugmented intraarticular anterior cruciate ligament reconstruction. *Am J Sports Med* 1985;13:321–336.
18. Del Pizzo W. U.S. Kennedy LAD clinical experience. Paper presented at the Sixth International Symposium on Advances in Cruciate Ligament Reconstruction of the Knee, March 1989, Los Angeles.
19. Thuresson P, Sandberg R, Johansson O, Balkfors B, Westlin N. Anterior cruciate ligament reconstruction with the patellar tendon—augmentation or not? A 2-year follow-up of 82 patients. *Scand J Med Sci Sports* 1996; 6:247–254.
20. Greis PE Steadman JR. Revision of failed prosthetic anterior cruciate ligament reconstruction. *Clin Orthop* 1996;325:78–90.
21. Howell SM, Taylor MA. Failure of reconstruction of the anterior cruciate ligament due to impingement by the intercondylar roof. *J Bone Joint Surg* 1993;75A:1044–1055.
22. Olson EJ, Kang JD, Fu FH, et al. The biochemical and histological effects of artificial ligament wear particles: in vivo and in vitro studies. *Am J Sports Med* 1988;16: 558–570.
23. Seeman MD, Steadman JR. Tibial osteolysis associated with Gore-Tex grafts. *Am J Knee Surg* 1993;6:31–38.
24. Wilson AG, Plessas SJ, Gray T, Forster IW. Lymphadenopathy after Gore-Tex anterior cruciate ligament reconstruction. *Am J Sports Med* 1998;26:133–135.
25. Safran MR, Harner CD. Technical considerations of revision anterior cruciate ligament surgery. *Clin Orthop* 1996;323:50–64.
26. Wetzler MJ, Bartolozzi AR, Gillespie MJ, Rubenstein DL, Cacatua MG, Miller LS. Revision anterior cruciate ligament reconstruction. *Oper Tech Orthop* 1996;6:181–189.
27. Rosenberg. Paper presented at the annual meeting of the American Academy of Orthopaedic Surgeons, 1995.
28. Rubinstein RA, Shelbourne KD, VanMeter CD, McCarroll JD, Rettig AC. Isolated autogenous bone–patellar tendon–bone graft site morbidity. *Am J Sports Med* 1994;22:324–327.
29. Johnson DL, Harner CD, Maday MG. Revision ACL surgery. In: Fu FH, Harner CD, Vince KG, eds. *Knee Surgery*. Baltimore: Williams & Wilkins, 1994:877–895.
30. Karns DJ, Heidt RS Jr, Holladay BR, Colosimo AJ. Case report: revision anterior cruciate ligament reconstruction. *Arthroscopy* 1994;10:148–151.
31. Hang DW, Lui S, Gentili A, et al. MRI characteristics of patellar donor site following graft harvest for anterior cruciate ligament reconstruction. Paper presented at the Annual meeting of the Arthroscopy Association of North America, Washington, DC, 1996.
32. Ritchie JR, Parker RD. Graft selection in anterior cruciate ligament revision surgery. *Clin Orthop* 1996;325: 65–77.
33. Gibbons MJ, Butler DL, Grood ES, Bylski-Austrow DI, Levy MS, Noyes FR. Effects of gamma irradiation on the initial mechanical and material properties of goat bone-patellar tendon-bone allografts. *J Orthop Res* 1991;9: 209–218.

Chapter 12

Complications and Pitfalls in Posterior Cruciate Ligament Reconstruction

Gregory C. Fanelli and Timothy J. Monahan

Anterior cruciate ligament (ACL) surgery is a frequently performed orthopedic surgical procedure in the United States. Posterior cruciate ligament (PCL) injuries occur less frequently in this country, and the experience of the orthopedic surgeon is correspondingly less for PCL examination, diagnosis, and surgical reconstructive procedures. Studies indicate that acute PCL injuries are related to geographic region, frequency of blunt trauma, and the population density of orthopedic surgeons.[1,2] Fanelli[1,2] reports a 38% incidence of PCL tears in acute knee injuries at his tertiary care regional referral center. The frequency of PCL-related injuries in this study is 38.3% (85 cases) of acute knee injuries in a study population of 222 knees; 48 of the PCL injuries, (56.5%) were multiple trauma related, while 28 (32.9%) were sports related. There were only three isolated PCL injuries (3.5%), and 82 (96.5%) PCL combined with one or more injured ligaments. The most frequently encountered PCL/combined knee ligament injuries were PCL/posterolateral corner (35/85, 41.2%) and combined ACL/PCL tears (39/85, 45.9%).

It is estimated that relatively few orthopedic surgeons perform PCL surgery when compared to ACL surgery, and complications may result from lack of experience in diagnosis, surgical techniques, and postoperative care.

This chapter discusses the nature and type of each complication related to PCL surgery, how the particular complication could have been prevented, and how to treat, manage, or salvage the problem. Our goal is to provide practical solutions to problems that may arise in conjunction with PCL surgery. Table 12.1 summarizes the complications associated with PCL surgery.

ASSOCIATED LIGAMENT INJURIES

Failure to recognize associated ligament injuries is possibly the most common reason for poor results following PCL surgery. Studies have shown that the isolated PCL tear is an uncommon injury, and combined PCL/posterolateral, and combined ACL/PCL instabilities are the most common injury patterns involving the PCL.[1,2] Failure to recognize posterolateral instability that is combined with PCL instability is a common error, and is the most likely reason for poor results following PCL reconstruction. PCL reconstruction without addressing or achieving good static posterolateral stability will yield poor results. Failure to correct the posterolateral laxity results in excessive external rotation at both 30 and 90 degrees of knee flexion. This causes the posterior tibial insertion of the PCL to rotate medially and anteriorly, shortening the distance to its insertion on the medial femoral condyle, producing a functionally lax PCL.[3]

The best way to determine if there are associated ligament injuries in addition to the PCL injury is with careful history and physical examination, magnetic resonance imaging (MRI) studies in selected cases, and examination under anesthesia and diagnostic arthroscopy.[4] Physical examination findings suggestive of multiple ligament injuries include opening on varus/valgus stress on full extension, grade 3 posterior drawer test, negative tibial step-off test, positive dial test, increased external rotation thigh foot angle test of 10 degrees greater than the normal side, and a positive posterolateral drawer test.[4] If the integrity of other ligaments or capsular structures is in doubt based on physical examination, appropriate diagnostic studies should be performed. Examination under anesthesia and diagnostic arthroscopy are our pre-

Table 12.1. Complications associated with posterior cruciate ligament surgery

Failure to recognize associated ligament injuries
Neurovascular complications
Persistent posterior sag
Osteonecrosis
Knee motion loss
Anterior knee pain
Fractures

ferred methods for accurate evaluation; however, MRI may be useful if the above are impractical. The most predictable way to salvage knees with multiple ligament injuries is with the correct preoperative diagnosis, and appropriate treatment of all injured ligaments.

NEUROVASCULAR COMPLICATIONS

The neurovascular structures most at risk during PCL reconstruction are the popliteal artery and the tibial nerve. The neurovascular bundle is located posterior to the posterior horn of the lateral meniscus, with the posterior capsule of the knee joint interposed between the two structures[5] (Fig. 12.1).

Reconstruction of the PCL using the transtibial tunnel technique involves passing a guidewire from anterior to posterior through the proximal tibia. The guidewire emerges at the inferior lateral aspect of the PCL fossa-tibial ridge area. The tunnel is subsequently created by reaming over the guidewire with a cannulated reamer. Arterial and/or nerve injury can occur with overpenetration of the guidewire during placement, or with inadvertent guidewire advancement during tibial tunnel reaming. It is also possible to cause neurovascular injury with the drill bit during reaming, either by direct contact of the drill bit or by "winding up" of the neurovascular structures (Fig. 12.2).

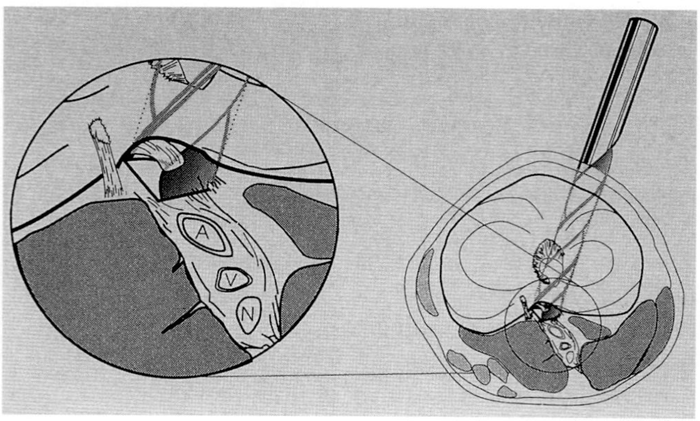

Figure 12.1. Axial section at the level of the posterior cruciate ligament insertion demonstrating the relationship of the neurovascular structures and their proximity to the exit point of the drill bit. (From ref. 6, with permission.)

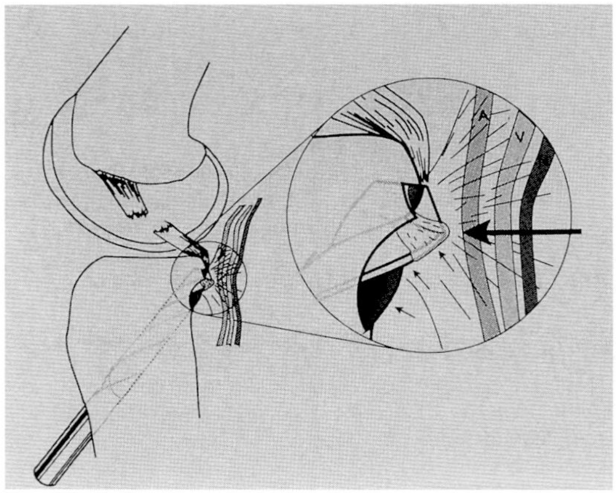

Figure 12.2. Sagittal section demonstrating the relationship of the neurovascular structures to the drill bit that has prematurely exited the posterior cortex. (From ref. 6, with permission.)

There are several methods to make transtibial tunnel creation safer. The use of a spade-tip guidewire instead of a trochar-tip guidewire, the use of an oscillating drill, and the use of a tapered instead of a square drill bit will reduce the likelihood of penetration, or winding up the neurovascular structures.[6]

Intraoperative radiographs and image intensification/fluoroscopy help to confirm guidewire placement and to monitor guidewire and reamer position during drilling. The use of intraoperative C-arm image intensifier is cumbersome, and care must be taken not to compromise the sterile field.

The best method of neurovascular injury prevention during transtibial drilling is the use of a posteromedial safety incision[4,7,8] (Fig. 12.3). The posteromedial safety incision is a 2-cm incision made just inferior to the posterior medial joint line. The crural fascia is carefully incised, and the interval is developed between the posterior capsule of the tibiofemoral joint anteriorly and the medial head of the gastrocnemius muscle and the neurovascular structures posteriorly. The surgeon can then place his finger in this extracapsular position to monitor the position of tools, guidewires, reamers, and drill bits in the posterior aspect of the knee, thus protecting the neurovascular structures.

Two additional advantages of the posteromedial safety incision are to provide better guidewire placement in the medial-lateral and superior-inferior planes, and to allow an escape pathway for extravasating arthroscopic irrigation fluid if a capsular tear occurs. This posteromedial safety incision will reduce or eliminate the likeli-

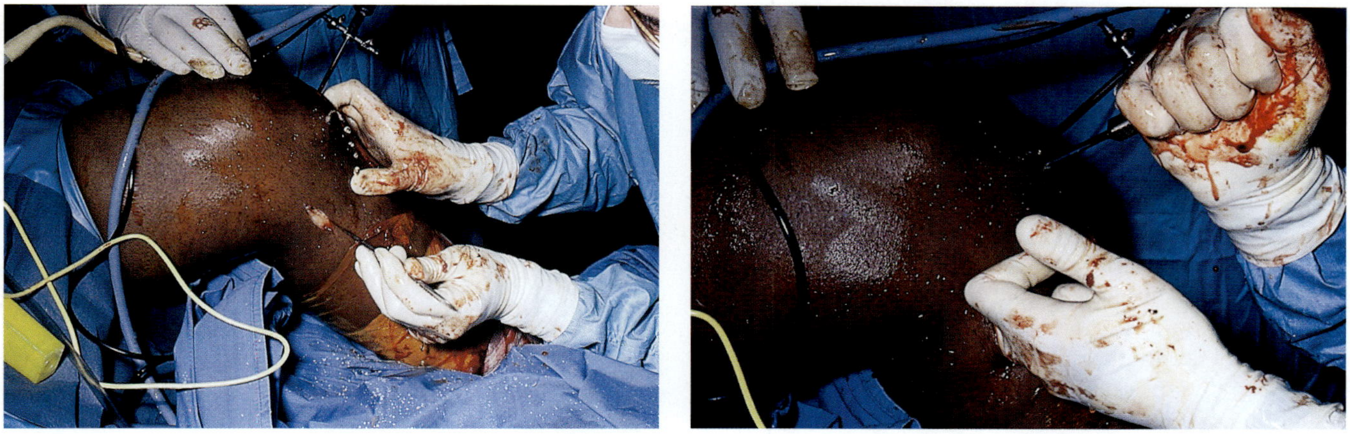

A B

Figure 12.3. The posteromedial safety incision is made on the posteromedial aspect of the proximal tibia area just inferior to the medial joint line. This allows the surgeon's gloved finger to assume an extraarticular position posterior to the capsule of the tibiofemoral joint, and anterior to the neurovascular structures. This facilitates guidewire placement and correct tibial tunnel positioning, and protects the neurovascular structures.

hood of a posterior calf compartment syndrome due to arthroscopic irrigation fluid extravasation. We have reported our results in 21 arthroscopically assisted combined PCL/posterolateral complex reconstructions, and 20 arthroscopically assisted combined ACL/PCL reconstructions,[7,8] and have performed a total of 107 PCL reconstructions using the transtibial tunnel technique. Spade-tip guidewires, tapered reamers, and the posteromedial safety incision were used in each case, and no neurovascular injuries or compartment syndromes occurred.

Particular caution should be exercised in the case of previously PCL operated knees with posterior scarring due to the prior surgical procedures. In these cases it is possible to have aberrant positions of the neurovascular structures. Inadvertent damage may occur during routine PCL surgery due to the transposed neurovascular bundle (Fig. 12.4). Arthroscopic application of vascular clips and immediate vascular repair are required.

The only salvage procedure of an intraoperative vascular injury is recognition of the injury and arterial repair by a vascular surgeon. The orthopedic surgeon

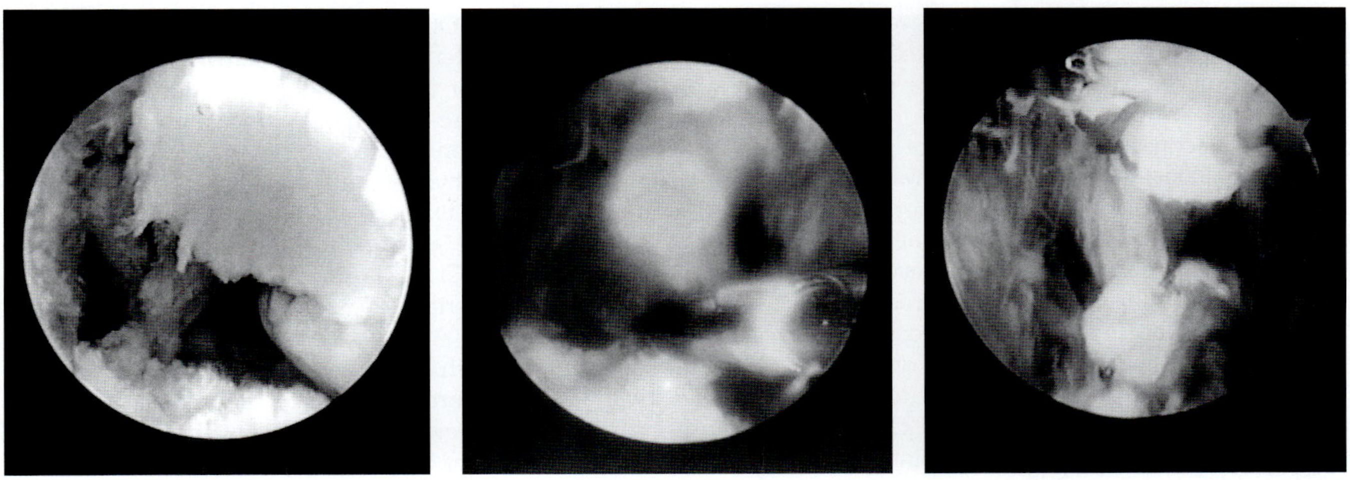

A B C

Figure 12.4. A: Posterior view of the capsule demonstrating a septum-like structure that is actually the popliteal artery transposed after prior PCL surgery. B: Lacerated popliteal artery from arthroscopic shaver. C: Arthroscopically applied vascular clamps applied to the popliteal artery before arterial repair. (Photographs courtesy of M.M. Malek, M.D.)

should always have a safety-first attitude with PCL surgery.

PERSISTENT POSTERIOR SAG

Persistent posterior sag following PCL surgery produces a suboptimal result of PCL reconstruction. Factors contributing to persistent posterior sag include failure to address posterolateral or posteromedial instability, early weight bearing in flexion, PCL substitute of insufficient mechanical strength, improper graft placement, improper graft tensioning, poor graft fixation, and early initiation of open chain hamstring strengthening during rehabilitation.[9–14]

Failure to recognize associated ligament injuries is possible the most common reason for poor results following PCL surgery. We have shown that the isolated PCL tear is an uncommon injury, and that combined PCL/posterolateral and combined ACL/PCL instabilities are the most common injury patterns involving the PCL.[1,2] The best way to determine if there are associated ligament injuries in addition to the PCL injury is by taking a careful history and doing a physical examination, with MRI studies in selected cases and examination under anesthesia and diagnostic arthroscopy.[4] The most predictable way to salvage this situation is with the correct preoperative diagnosis and appropriate treatment of all injured ligaments.

The correct diagnosis of ligament injuries occurring in association with the PCL injury is critical, and plans must be developed to treat these associated injuries. While it is preferable to address these acute knee injuries within a 3- to 6-week time period of the index injury, this may be impossible in severe multisystem-injured patients. We have reported excellent results with delayed surgery provided the knee is protected in the preoperative period.[7–9]

Technical considerations to prevent persistent posterior sag include the use of strong graft tissue, correct tunnel placement, correct graft tensioning, and secure graft fixation. Regardless of graft material chosen, incorrect tunnel placement will doom even the strongest graft material to failure. The most predictable PCL reconstructive procedures occur with reconstruction of the anterior lateral fiber bundle region of the PCL. The femoral tunnel should be positioned to reproduce the anterolateral band of the PCL (Fig. 12.5). This is distal and anterior to the PCL isometric point, and allows the graft to tighten in flexion.[11]

The ideal placement for the tibial tunnel is to have it emerge inferior to the apex of the tibial ridge in the lateral aspect of the PCL anatomic insertion site. This will allow the PCL substitute to turn a series of gentle 45-degree turns around the posterior proximal tibia with no acute 90-degree angle turns that may compromise graft integrity.[7,8]

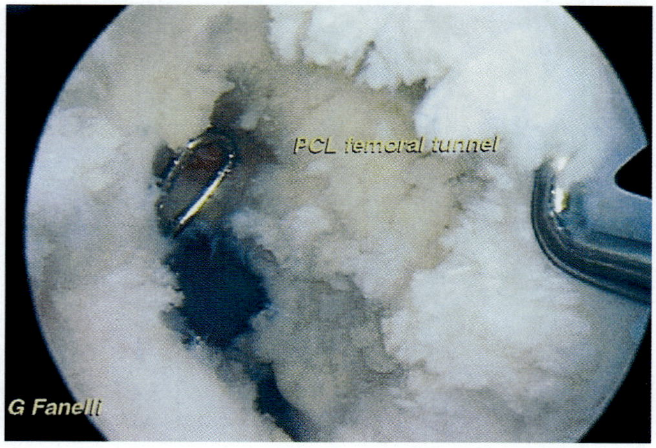

Figure 12.5. The femoral tunnel in posterior cruciate ligament reconstruction is optimally placed in the center of the stump of the anterolateral fiber bundle region of the native PCL. This provides the most successful and reproducible results.

Given proper tunnel placement, graft tensioning should be performed in 70 to 90 degrees of knee flexion.[11] This allows for achievement of the tibial step-off without restricting range of motion into flexion. Tensioning of the PCL substitute in full extension causes excessive graft tension, as the knee progresses into flexion with subsequent graft rupture or range of motion loss in flexion.[11]

Secure graft fixation is critical to the success of PCL reconstruction. Direct fixation of the graft material to bone with interference fixation, screw and spiked ligament washer, or a combination of fixation methods is preferable. Suture fixation of grafts to a post and washer assembly is a very successful method of fixation; however, postoperative care must be modified by the security of the graft fixation.

Inappropriate postoperative rehabilitation can adversely affect PCL reconstruction results and lead to a persistent posterior sag.[12–14] The PCL sees higher forces than the ACL does, so a slower postoperative course than with ACL postoperative rehabilitation is warranted. Recurrence of the posterior tibial sag will occur with early weight bearing in flexion, or open chain hamstring activity, which will increase forces in the PCL. Postoperative immobilization should be in full extension for a period of 4 to 6 weeks. This allows for preliminary biologic fixation of the graft material in the tunnels to occur. If early mobilization is utilized, the proximal tibia must be supported.

OSTEONECROSIS

Avascular necrosis of the medial femoral condyle has been reported by Athanasian et al[15] as a complication of PCL reconstructive surgery. Patients present with medial knee pain and tenderness over the medial femoral condyle. Radiographic findings include a flattened articular surface of the medial femoral condyle and radiolucency. The osteonecrosis is thought to occur from increased pressure in the bone causing vascular insufficiency. Etiologic factors include drilling the femoral tunnel too close to the articular surface, which may disturb the single nutrient vessel providing the intraosseus blood supply to the medial femoral condyle,[16] and extensive soft tissue dissection over the medial femoral condyle during surgery, which may compromise the vascular supply to the medial femoral condyle.

Prevention of this complication is accomplished with accurate femoral tunnel placement, leaving an adequate bone bridge between the femoral tunnel and the medial femoral condyle articular surface. Our preferred method for femoral tunnel creation is the outside-in method using an ACL/PCL drill guide[4,7,8,17] (Fig. 12.6). The knee is flexed 90 degrees, and the guidewire is positioned externally with the help of the ACL/PCL drill guide at a point halfway between the medial femoral epicondyle and the articular surface of the medial femoral condyle at the level of the superior one-third of the patella with the knee in 90 degrees of flexion.[17] The guidewire emerges through the center of the femoral insertion of the anterior lateral bundle of the PCL. These guidelines result in accurate and reproducible PCL femoral tunnel placement. Our series had no complications of osteonecrosis.[7,8] When an Achilles tendon allograft is used for PCL reconstruction, we prefer to contour the calcaneal bone plug into the shape of a wedge, and to press fit this portion of the Achilles tendon allograft into the femoral tunnel. This technique bone grafts the femoral tunnel and provides secure fixation for the Achilles tendon allograft in PCL reconstruction.

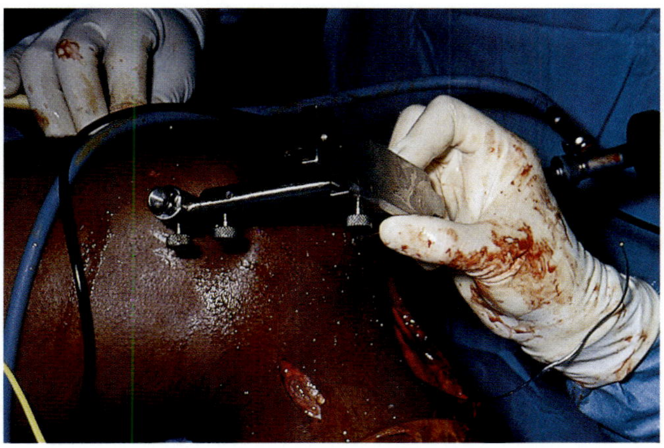

Figure 12.6. ACL/PCL drill guide positioned for creation of femoral tunnel.

Salvage of this complication lies in early detection of the osteonecrosis. A high index of suspicion should be maintained in a postoperative patient with persistent medial femoral condylar pain. Clinical examination and imaging studies will confirm the diagnosis. Non–weight bearing and bone grafting of the tunnel defect may salvage the problem.[15]

MOTION LOSS

Motion loss may occur after PCL reconstruction, and may present as loss of extension or loss of flexion.[18] Loss of flexion appears to be more common after PCL reconstructive surgery that loss of extension, and may become a functional problem when knee flexion fails to exceed 110 degrees. Causes of knee flexion loss include suprapatellar pouch adhesions, improper femoral tunnel placement, improper position of graft tensioning, and multiple concurrent ligament procedures.

Suprapatellar pouch adhesions may occur following an arthrotomy, or after harvesting a bone-quadriceps tendon graft.[7,8,10] Any surgery that induces scarring in the suprapatellar pouch area predisposes to flexion loss. Methods to minimize the incidence of this complication include the use of arthroscopically assisted procedures instead of an arthrotomy to minimize scarring. When a quadriceps tendon graft is harvested, care should be taken to preserve the integrity of the suprapatellar pouch. When loss of flexion occurs due to suprapatellar pouch adhesions, arthroscopic lysis of adhesions and gentle manipulation is a successful method of treatment.[7,8]

Femoral tunnel placement anterior and distal in the PCL stump to reproduce the anterolateral fiber region of the PCL is the desired position for the PCL substitute. This nonisometric positioning will cause the graft to shorten as the knee is brought into flexion. When the knee is in 70 degrees of flexion as the graft is tensioned, this tightening of the graft eliminates the posterior drawer and maintains the normal tibial step-off, while allowing near full range of motion into flexion.[7,8,11] When the graft is tensioned in full extension, excessive tension occurs in the PCL substitute as flexion progresses, resulting in flexion range of motion loss, or graft failure through tension overload.

Medial collateral ligament repair combined with PCL reconstruction may be associated with loss of motion. The large surgical dissection required, combined with plication types of procedures, increases the risk of postoperative motion loss. Direct anatomic repair is preferable to plication procedures in acute cases. When augmentation grafts are used, they must reproduce anatomic structures. This is preferred to capsular plication procedures, which may be nonanatomic and nonisometric.

It should be noted that some loss of terminal flexion is to be expected with PCL reconstruction surgery. This is due to the nonisometric nature of PCL reconstructions and their failure to reproduce the complex PCL fiber bundle regions. Our series demonstrated a mean 10-degree terminal flexion range of motion loss.[7,8] This has not proven to be a functional problem for these patients. Rapid return of full flexion after PCL reconstructive surgery should be avoided as it may compromise the graft integrity and lead to persistent posterior sag.

Graft rupture, or failure through elongation may be related to surgical technique, graft material, fixation, and postoperative activity level.[10,19,20] Artificial ligaments have been associated with failure due to abrasion of the graft around tunnel edges. Technical considerations that may reduce or eliminate this complication include smooth, well-chamfered tunnel edges and anatomic positioning of the PCL reconstruction tunnels so that the graft material does not make any acute angle turns or experience severe tension overloads.

The area that has the most acute bend for the graft is the proximal portion of the tibial tunnel in the transtibial reconstructive technique. The technique to avoid this problem is to have the guidewire exit inferior to the apex of the tibial ridge in the lateral aspect of the PCL anatomic insertion site. This allows the PCL substitute to make two 45-degree turns, instead of a 90-degree bend on the posterior aspect of the proximal tibia. This applies to autograft, allograft, and synthetic ligament PCL surgical reconstructive techniques.

Another technique to avoid acute angle graft bending at the proximal tibial tunnel edge is to position the bone plug tendon interface at the edge of the tunnel opening.[21] This will allow the graft's soft tissue portion to hinge on its own anatomic insertion into the bone plug, and not the tunnel edge. The tibial inlay technique of PCL reconstruction is performed with direct posterior exposure of the proximal tibia, and fixation of a bone–patellar tendon–bone graft in a posterior tibial trough.[22] This eliminates acute graft bending around the corner of a tibial tunnel.

ANTERIOR KNEE PAIN

Anterior knee pain following PCL reconstruction may occur as a result of persistent posterior sag with resultant patella baja and increased patellofemoral forces.[13] This increased patellofemoral force may cause patellofemoral degenerative joint disease in long-term follow-up.[3] The solution for this problem is a technically sound PCL reconstruction with strong graft material to restore the anatomic tibial step-off and return patellofemoral forces to a more normal level.

Other causes of anterior knee pain are prominent hardware, graft harvest site pain, and postoperative synovitis. Painful hardware can be removed in the postoperative period; however, low profile fixation devices may reduce the need for this second procedure. Anterior knee pain associated with the harvest of an autogenous bone–patellar tendon–bone graft may be reduced with the following technical considerations.[23] The harvested bone–tendon–bone (BTB) autograft should be no wider than one-third the width of the patellar tendon measured at the tibial tubercle insertion. Harvesting the patellar bone plug should be done with an oscillating saw, not with osteotomes. This minimizes concussive effects to the articular cartilage. The depth of the patella bone plug harvest should not exceed one-third the thickness of the patella at the median ridge, usually about 8 mm. The superior one-third of the anterior cortex of the patella should be left intact. This will reduce stress riser effects to the patella. Bone grafting of the patella harvest defect may decrease the stress riser effect, but we have found no difference in the incidence of anterior knee pain with or without bone grafting of the patella donor defect.[23]

Tibial fracture has been reported as an intraoperative complication during PCL reconstruction.[24] It can occur as a result of large-diameter tunnels in the femur and tibia, as well as the convergence of two tibial tunnels in combined ACL/PCL reconstruction.[8] During combined ACL/PCL reconstructions, the ACL and PCL tibial tunnels must diverge to prevent proximal tibial fracture. Tibial fracture has also been associated with hammering staples into the tibia for graft fixation. Our recommendation is to use screws and spiked ligament washers or interference screws for graft fixation. If staples are to be used, predrilling the holes may avoid tibial fractures associated with hammering. As mentioned earlier, femoral tunnels should be positioned to allow adequate bone stock between the femoral tunnel, and the medial femoral condyle articular surface. This will decrease the likelihood of subchondral bone collapse and/or osteonecrosis as outlined above.

FANELLI SPORTS INJURY CLINIC EXPERIENCE

We have performed 92 PCL reconstructions at our center from August 1990 through March 1998. These reconstructions have included ACL/PCL reconstructions,

PCL/posterolateral corner reconstructions, ACL/PCL/posterolateral reconstructions, ACL/PCL/medial collateral ligament (MCL) reconstructions, and PCL/MCL reconstructions. Our complications include loss of flexion requiring arthroscopic lysis of adhesions and manipulation (five cases), removal of painful prominent hardware used for graft fixation (21 cases), and superficial suture abscess (one case). We have had no incidence of nerve injuries, vascular injuries, deep infections, fractures, osteonecrosis, or skin slough complications. Our clinical results evaluated with Lysholm, Tegner, and Hospital for Special Surgery knee ligament rating scales and the KT-1000 arthrometer have been previously published.[7,8]

Analysis of our patients with loss of flexion requiring arthroscopic lysis of adhesions and manipulation is as follows. The first patient had ACL, PCL, MCL, posterolateral complex tears, and an acutely dislocated patella. Repair/reconstruction of all four ligaments and extensor mechanism repair were performed as an open procedure. Adhesions developed requiring arthroscopic adhesolysis and manipulation.

The second patient had right knee ACL/PCL/MCL tears and an ipsilateral tibial shaft fracture. The tibial shaft fracture was treated with open reduction and internal fixation using plate and screws. The MCL was treated in a brace for 6 weeks, and it healed with normal valgus stability. Arthroscopic combined ACL/PCL reconstruction was then performed using double-loop semitendinosus/gracilis hamstring autograft, and bone–patellar tendon–bone autograft. The patient developed suprapatellar pouch adhesions postoperatively, requiring arthroscopic adhesolysis and manipulation.

The third patient was a 20-year-old with a right PCL/posterolateral complex tear combined with a hip fracture and multiple fractures of the foot. The fractures were addressed with open reduction and internal fixation, followed by arthroscopic PCL/posterolateral complex reconstruction with bone–patellar tendon–bone autograft and biceps tendon transfer. The patient developed postoperative suprapatellar pouch adhesions that responded well to arthroscopic lysis of adhesions and manipulation.

Patients four and five were females ages 15 and 22 with PCL/posterolateral complex tears (one acute, one chronic) who underwent arthroscopic PCL/posterolateral reconstruction with Achilles tendon allograft and Clancy biceps tendon tenodesis in one case, and bone–patellar tendon–bone autograft and split biceps tendon transfer in the second case. Both patients developed suprapatellar pouch adhesions postoperatively, requiring arthroscopic lysis of adhesions and manipulation. Both patients returned to full unrestricted activity with stable knees.

We were not able to develop any trends to predict which patients may develop motion loss postoperatively with the exception of arthrotomy versus arthroscopy. Arthrotomy seems more likely to have postoperative range of motion problems. Only five patients of 92 (5.4%) developed motion loss requiring surgical intervention and manipulation, indicating a low rate of this complication.

We attribute our low rate of complications in our series of PCL reconstructions to our accurate preoperative evaluations, surgical technique, and postoperative rehabilitation.

Procedure

All but one patient in our series of 92 PCL reconstructions underwent the reconstruction as an arthroscopically assisted procedure. In the acute cases the reconstruction was performed approximately 3 to 6 weeks postinjury to allow for restoration of motion and for other injuries to stabilize. In the chronic case the surgery was performed from 6 months to 16 years postinjury. Our surgical technique has been described elsewhere.[4,7,8] We describe here specific technical aspects of arthroscopically assisted PCL/posterior lateral corner reconstruction.

When allograft tissue is selected, it is prepared prior to bringing the patient into the operating room. When autograft tissue is used, it is harvested and prepared at the beginning of the surgical procedure. The arthroscopic instruments are then inserted into the knee through the standard portals, and gravity inflow is used.

An extracapsular posterior medial safety incision is made that allows the surgeon's gloved finger to be positioned between the posterior capsule and the neurovascular structures. This allows the surgeon to feel through the capsule all instruments working in the back of the knee joint. The PCL stumps are debrided, and the posterior capsule is elevated from the posterior tibial ridge with the special PCL curved instruments.

The PCL tibial and femoral tunnels are then drilled with the help of an ACL/PCL drill guide, and the PCL graft is positioned. The PCL graft is anchored on the femoral side first, and left free on the tibial side. The posterolateral reconstruction is then performed. We used the biceps femoris tendon tenodesis described by Clancy[3] in our reported series.[7]

The posterolateral reconstruction is tensioned with the knee in 30 degrees of flexion. With the knee in 70 degrees of flexion, an anterior drawer force is applied to the proximal tibia to restore the normal tibial step-off, and the PCL graft is then secured on the tibial side. Restoration of the normal tibial step-off at 70 degrees of flexion has provided the most reproducible method of establishing the appropriate tibia-femoral relationship in our experience. Wound closure is performed in the standard fashion, and the knee is immobilized in full extension.

The knee is kept in full extension for 5 to 6 weeks, with progressive weight bearing using crutches. Progressive range of motion occurs after week 6. The brace is unlocked at the end of 6 weeks, and the crutches are discontinued. Progressive closed kinetic chain strength training and continued motion exercises are performed. The brace is discontinued after the 10th postoperative week. Return to sports and heavy labor occurs after the ninth postoperative month, when sufficient strength and range of motion have returned.

CONCLUSION

Posterior cruciate ligament reconstruction is technically demanding surgery. Complications encountered with this surgical procedure include failure to recognize associated ligament injuries, neurovascular complications, persistent posterior sag, osteonecrosis, knee motion loss, anterior knee pain, and fractures. A comprehensive preoperative evaluation, including an accurate diagnosis, a well-planned and carefully executed surgical procedure, and a supervised postoperative rehabilitation program will help to reduce the incidence of these complications.

References

1. Fanelli GC. PCL injuries in trauma patients. *Arthroscopy* 1993;9(3):291–294.
2. Fanelli GC, Edson CJ. PCL injuries in trauma patients. Part II. *Arthroscopy* 1995;11:526–529.
3. Clancy WG. Repair and reconstruction of the posterior cruciate ligament. In: Chapman M, ed. *Operative Orthopaedics.* Philadelphia: JB Lippincott, 1988:1651–1665.
4. Fanelli GC, Giannotti BF, Edson CJ. Current concepts review. The posterior cruciate ligament arthroscopic evaluation and treatment. *Arthroscopy* 1994;10(6):673–688.
5. Muller W. *The knee: Form, Function, and Ligamentous Reconstruction.* New York: Springer-Verlag, 1983.
6. Jackson DW, Proctor CS, Simon TM. Arthroscopic assisted PCL reconstruction: a technical note on potential neurovascular injury related to drill bit configuration. *Arthroscopy* 1993;9(2):224–227.
7. Fanelli GC, Giannotti BF, Edson CJ. Arthroscopically assisted combined posterior cruciate ligament/posterior lateral complex reconstruction. *Arthroscopy* 1996;12(5): 521–530.
8. Fanelli GC, Giannotti BF, Edson CJ. Arthroscopically assisted combined anterior and posterior cruciate ligament reconstruction. *Arthroscopy* 1996;12(1):5–14.
9. Thomann YR, Gaechter A. Dorsal approach for reconstruction of the PCL. *Arch Orthop Trauma Surg* 1994;113:142–148.
10. Noyes FR, Barber-Westin SD. Posterior cruciate ligament allograft reconstruction with and without a ligament augmentation device. *Arthroscopy* 1994;10(4):371–382.
11. Burns WC, Draganich LF, Pyevich M, Reider B. The effect of femoral tunnel position and graft tensioning technique on posterior laxity of the posterior ligament–reconstructed knee. *Am J Sports Med* 1995;23(4);424–430.
12. Ogata K. Posterior cruciate ligament reconstruction: a comparative study of two different methods. *Bull Hosp J Dis Orthop Inst* 1991;5(2):186–198.
13. Paulos LE, Wnorowski DC, Beck CL. Rehabilitation following knee surgery. Recommendations. *Sports Med* 1991;11(4):257–275.
14. Ogata K, McCarthy JA. Measurements of length and tension patterns during reconstruction of the posterior cruciate ligament. *Am J Sports Med* 1992;20(3):351–355.
15. Athanasian EA, Wickiewicz TL, Warren RF. Osteonecrosis of the femoral condyle after arthroscopic reconstruction of a cruciate ligament. *J Bone Joint Surg* 1995;77A(9):1418–1422.
16. Reddy AS, Frederick RW. Evaluation of the intraosseous and extraosseous blood supply to the distal femoral condyles. *Am J Sports Med* 1998;26(3):415–419.
17. Rosenberg TD, Paulos LE, Abbot PJ. Arthroscopic cruciate repair and reconstruction: an overview and description of technique. In: Feagin JA, ed. *The Crucial Ligaments.* New York: Churchill Livingstone, 1988:409–423.
18. Irrgang JJ, Harner CD. Loss of motion following knee ligament reconstruction. *Sports Med* 1995;19(2):150–159.
19. Bosch U, Kasperczyk WJ. Healing of the patellar tendon autograft after posterior cruciate ligament reconstruction—a process of ligamentization? An experimental study in a sheep model. *Am J Sports Med* 1992;20(5): 558–566.
20. Sterling JC, Meyers MC, Calvo RD. Allograft failure in cruciate ligament reconstruction. *Am J Sports Med* 1995;23(2):173–178.
21. Miller MD, Harner CD, Koshwaguchi S. Acute posterior cruciate ligament injuries. In: Fu FH, Harner CD, Vince KG, eds. *Knee Surgery.* Baltimore: Williams & Wilkins, 1994:749–767.
22. Berg EE. Posterior cruciate ligament tibial inlay reconstruction. *Arthroscopy* 1995;11(1):69–76.
23. Fanelli GC, Desai BM, Cummings PD, Hanks GA, Kalenak A. Divergent alignment of the femoral interference screw in single incision endoscopic reconstruction of the anterior cruciate ligament. *Contemp Orthop* 1994;28(1): 21–25.
24. Malek MM, Fanelli GC. Technique of arthroscopically assisted posterior cruciate ligament reconstruction. *Orthopaedics* 1993;16(9):961–966.

Chapter 13

Complications and Pitfalls in Extraarticular Knee Surgery

Glenn C. Terry and Grant L. Jones

Restoration of the physiologic joint after an injury is the perceived goal of any applied treatment. The physiologic joint consists of the long bones, the articular cartilage, the menisci, the cruciates, the extraarticular ligaments, the musculotendinous units, the peripheral nerves, and the soft tissues of both intraarticular and extraarticular areas. All of these structures contribute to the normal health and function of the physiologic joint. Our goal in treatment, as Iver Palmer[1] indicated, is restoration of the physiologic joint.

There is much apparent confusion regarding treatment of the extraarticular components, but we believe the confusion is actually a difference in applied logic rather than a right versus wrong approach. The classic logic approach suggests that a four-bar link system defines the anterior-posterior translation limits of the joint, while the Burmester curve defines the instant center of motion of the periphery of the joint in flexion and extension in coordination with the four-bar link system (Fig. 13.1).[2] Also, this logic suggests that a single clinical test can define a single-ligament injury, and repair of that single ligament can restore the normal kinematics and normal function.

The quantum logic approach suggests that the four-bar link system is a principle used to define the anterior translation relationships, but the anterior-posterior cruciates have elastic limits, and therefore the four-bar link system is a philosophy. The Burmester curve also has elastic limits and functions in harmony with the four-bar link system of the cruciates to position the femur and tibia.[3] But the menisci, the joint surfaces, and the musculotendinous units fine-tune the joint apposition to refine the instant center of rotation. At the extremes of tibial rotation, ligaments are tensed and experience load sharing with each other to achieve stability of the joint. These functional parameters are guided and further stabilized and stress protected by the musculotendinous units.[4–6] Also, the meniscus position is maintained dynamically by hamstrings and the popliteus to increase the tibiofemoral contact area in order to decrease joint stress. All of these factors contribute their individual components to form a very highly developed and complex machine that allows the individual to function at high levels of lower-extremity agility during activity.

Abnormal states, such as those produced by injury, disrupt the machine's kinematics in a variable way. If the ligaments have been injured and loosened, when the patient tries to do a complex activity requiring lower extremity agility the abnormal kinematics will allow joint motion that is too excessive for musculotendinous recovery or stability. The menisci and the joint are not in optimal apposition. Thus, the menisci can tear, joint stress may be increased, and, as a consequence of shear force to the joint, a plowing effect can occur, which can injure articular cartilage.[7–14] Nonequal load sharing of the ligaments that have been previously uninjured jeopardizes their ability to sustain the new loads, thus causing them either to be injured or to stretch, creating a more complex instability pattern and causing poor function as well as joint wear.[15,16]

In some cases, the terminology "too loose" can also apply to the extensor mechanism as a result of an acute knee injury that disrupts the stabilizing ligaments of the extensor mechanism. This can result in dynamic instability of the extensor mechanism as well as tibiofemoral instability.[17]

The loss of menisci in the presence of physiologic abnormal joint looseness can certainly result in adaptive

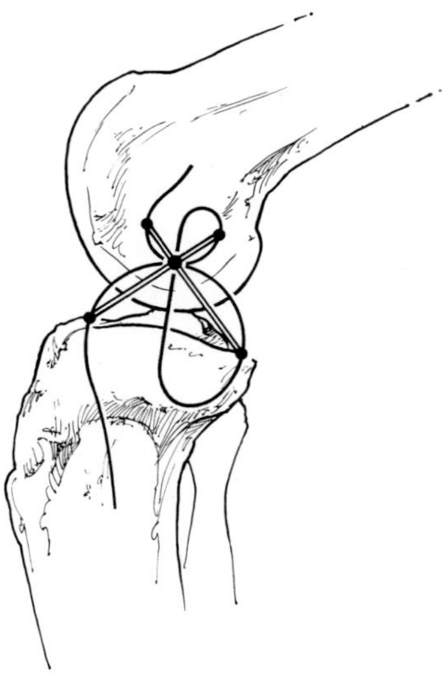

Figure 13.1. The Burmester curve (solid line), which is roughly a figure-of-eight curve consisting of two third-order curves: the "vertex cubic" (the tibia) and the "pivot cubic" (the femur). A ligament's origin that is on the pivot cubic will be isometric if it passes through the instant center of knee rotation and inserts on a corresponding point on the vertex cubic. The double line represents the crossed four-bar linkage system. The cruciate ligaments form the crossed bars that intersect at the instant center of knee rotation. The crossed bars represent the neutral fibers of each of the cruciates.

bone changes as the knee attempts to stabilize itself. This is presumably the cause of Fairbank's[18] radiographic changes.

The opposite circumstance can occur in which the joint is too tight after treatment. The overconstraining ligament may create a kinematic ankylosis situation. This produces abnormal kinematics with nonequal loads on the ligaments as a consequence of the overconstraint of the repaired ligaments. This abnormal effect can lead to the joint developing a kinematic ankylosis via the abnormal restraint of the repaired ligaments.[19] This increases the joint stress, decreases function, and can aggravate the tendency to develop arthritis. Function is decreased as a consequence of all of these factors. This decrease can also occur as a consequence of overconstraint of the capsular ligaments or as the result of an arthrofibrosis, with the extensor mechanism being tethered inappropriately due to abnormal anterior cruciate ligament positioning. Arthritic changes can occur as a consequence of the increased joint compression loads.[20] Articular cartilage withstands normal compressive loads quite well, but excessive loads are not tolerated any better than the shear forces that can occur as a consequence of a joint that is too loose.

It is important to understand the mechanism of injury and its effect on our ability to diagnose the anatomic injury. Since the joint is positioned in different degrees of flexion and extension, abduction and adduction, and compression and distraction at the time of load application to produce an injury, and since the forces that are applied to the individual are complex, a variable ligament injury can occur to the same joint with a similar-appearing mechanism of injury.

The confirmation of anatomic injury by the motion limit testing is predictive of the anatomic injury that surgery might correct. It is important to realize that clinically, multiple ligaments share the load when complex forces are applied. After an injury produced by a single force, a different ligament will take up the load once displacement of the knee occurs, which can cause injury to more than one ligament. This then necessitates the development of a clinical diagnostic system to provide predictive information concerning the anatomic injury based on a clinical examination test sequence. Thus, an appropriate clinical diagnosis by classification of the injury is imperative and is the first step in avoiding the most serious complication in the treatment of these complex problems, which is an oversimplified misdiagnosis.

It is also very important to realize that, with any ligament injury, there is a significant probability that musculotendinous injury has also occurred, as in the case of a severe anteromedial or posterolateral instability.

Treating only one component of a complex problem does not provide good long-term results. This is demonstrated by the poor long-term results of the Slocum[21] pes transfer for the treatment of medial ligament instability, where the dynamic transfer of the pes tendons was inadequate without the retensioning of medial ligaments, a deficiency that was corrected in Slocum and Larson's[22] later writings. Also, the tethering of rerouted musculotendinous units in combination with the abnormal tensioning of the ligaments produced a kinematic condition that was doomed to failure in the long term as evidenced by the poor results in Nicholas's[23] 5-in-1 medial ligament reconstruction.

Thus, to successfully repair or reconstruct an unstable knee, the procedure of choice must restore the appropriate tension in the anatomic structures injured and restore appropriate joint kinematics, both passively and actively. This is accomplished by restoring the ligament tension to the injury state of load sharing and the musculotendinous units to their normal functional position and tension. This philosophy is certainly not new, as both Palmer[1] and Hughston[15] have recommended anatomic restoration of these complex injuries.

Avoiding complications was emphasized by Hippocrates, who said that the physician should first do no harm. Hughston[15] also emphasized avoidance of complications when he stated that there was no knee injury that could not be made worse by inappropriate surgical treatment.

HISTORY

Surgeons today stand taller than our predecessors because we stand on our mentors' shoulders.

Hey-Groves[24] initially reconstructed the anterior cruciate with a strip of iliotibial tract. Smith[25] modified the procedure by adding a capsular ligament reinforcement as well, which improved the results. This adaptation was later adopted by Hey-Groves because of its potential to improve his outcomes as well. This combined procedure marks the initial philosophic view that restoration of all the injured structures is appropriate in a complex knee injury.

The extraarticular repairs can be divided into medial, anterolateral, and posterolateral categories. The contributors to our understanding of medial injuries include Bosworth,[26] Milch,[27] Campbell,[28,29] Mauk,[30] Slocum[21] (pes transfer), Hughston and Eilus[31] (posterior oblique and semimembranosus), Slocum and Larson[22] (pes and capsular reefing), and Nicholas (5-in-1).[23] Ian Smillie[32] also contributed to our understanding of the treatment of the torn meniscus and the effects of meniscectomy, as did Hughston[33] (simple meniscectomy).

Lateral extraarticular treatment was discussed by Bruiser,[34] and the treatment of chronic anterolateral instability was presented by MacIntosh and Darby,[35] Kennedy et al,[36,37] Ellison,[38] Lemaire[39] (iliotibial tract tenodesis), Muller[2] (screw tenodesis), Losee et al[40] (deepest iliotibial tract repair), DeHaven[41] (screw tenodesis), Draganich et al[42,43] (screw tenodesis), Andrews and Sanders[44] (iliotibial tract tenodesis and suture), and a consensus group.

The evolution of treatment for posterolateral instability can be traced to Mayer[45] (strip of iliotibial tract and biceps in the paralytic knee), Muller[2] (iliotibial tract substitution for the popliteus), Bousquet et al[46] (popliteal recession), Casey (personal communication; Bondi Junction, Australia) (bone-tendon-bone substitution for the fibular collateral), Hughston and Jacobson[16] (arcuate complex advancement), Clancy et al[47] (biceps tenodesis), Jakob et al[3,48] (strip of biceps tendon to substitute for the fibular collateral, as well as the popliteus tendon), and Kentsch (personal communication; Stuttgart, Germany) (fibular head osteotomy with advancement). Understanding of anatomy, acute repairs, and delayed primary repairs can lead to good outcomes.

TREATMENT COMPLICATIONS

The success of any treatment for chronic instability must address the anatomic injuries that have occurred, both as a consequence of the injury and the reinjury effects from chronic instability. The treatment must allow adequate rehabilitation and restore the four-bar link system, the Burmester curve, the meniscus function, and the musculotendinous units. Failure to address any of these issues can result in harm to the patient by causing failure of functional restoration.

The largest group of failures in extraarticular surgery can be categorized as technical and may be separated into two groups. In the first group, the treatment was inadequate to restore the normal tension in the ligaments. As a result, the reconstruction is too loose, which leads to poor kinematics, which in turn contributes to poor function. In the second group, the kinematics are altered because the ligament reconstruction is too tight. This kinematic ankylosis may create a stable knee, but does not allow normal range of motion. Because of the increased stress on the joint caused by tight knee reconstruction, arthritis may develop over time.

Failure to restore the musculotendinous unit can be associated with a surgical procedure that may provide initial ligament stability but, over time, will stretch out because of the lack of musculotendinous support, particularly of the posterior third capsular ligament–semimembranosus complex on the medial side. On the lateral side, the posterolateral complex stability provided by the biceps will be lost over time if this important dynamic stabilizer is not retensioned at the time of surgical reconstruction of the ligaments for posterolateral instability.

In addition to inappropriate capsular ligament tension, which creates a kinematic ankylosis, frank ankylosis of the knee can occur. Fat pad and synovial fold fibrosis with retinacular adhesions can be caused by the surgical procedure and by sutures in the repaired ligaments that are not placed on the Burmester curve.

Attention must be paid at all times to avoid injury to the fat pad, which can lead to fibrosis. Fibrosis may, in turn, create patella baja or infera, which can result in profound dysfunction of the knee.

An ill-placed scar from medial ligament repair can also create a deeper scar in the synovial fold, which can irritate the edge of the medial femoral condyle with flexion and extension. Over time, it can cause a chronically painful knee. All attempts should be made to keep the surgical scars from crossing movable joint edges to prevent this phenomenon from occurring. The "tent-pole" effect of a capsular incision adjacent to the patella can keep the synovial scar from abrading the edge of the medial femoral condyle. Similarly, posteromedial arthrotomy access is safe because it is on the flat of the joint and not over a bone edge.

The use of heavy, large suture and metal fixation devices can create a suture granuloma or metal bursitis, necessitating removal of the offending material. These strong, high-stress–producing materials can also produce tissue necrosis of the very tissue that the surgeon is attempting to repair. Tissue necrosis can result in loosening, and thus failure, of the repair.

Painful neuromas can occur as a consequence of poor surgical technique, and all efforts should be made to reduce the chance of this complication. Small sensory nerve division by itself does not usually cause functional difficulty if the nerve is divided sharply as close to its termination as possible. Attention to surgical detail is critical to avoid painful neuroma formation, which can create a functionally limiting condition.

Infection is always a risk in any reconstructive surgical procedure. Attention to technical detail, asepsis, and postoperative wound management, and the use of prophylactic antibiotics minimize this risk.

A coordinated team approach to these complex surgical problems is important in achieving a successful outcome. It is better to prevent complications than to have to deal with them.

AUTHORS' PREFERRED TREATMENT

Medial Ligaments

A curved incision is placed on the medial side of the knee, with the proximal portion of the incision parallel to the medial intermuscular septum of the femur, turning distally parallel to the tibia between the anterior tibial tuberosity and the midlateral line parallel to the longitudinal axis of the tibia that bisects the medial femoral epicondyle. This incision is deepened through the subcutaneous tissue to the fascia layer. Once the fascia layer is encountered, a subcutaneous flap is developed posteriorly, which should lift the branches of the infrapatellar saphenous nerve off the fascia layer with the subcutaneous layer, leaving only the fascial investments. The posterior extent of this incision is just posterior to the adductor tubercle, which avoids injury to the main saphenous nerve. There is a 30% to 40% chance of an area of anesthesia over the anterior aspect of the knee, which frequently cannot be avoided with incisions for the medial ligament repair because of the numerous small infrapatellar branches of the saphenous nerve. The sartorius fascia is then identified, and the medial epicondyle and adductor tubercle are palpated with the knee in 60 degrees of flexion and the hip externally rotated and slightly abducted.

A longitudinal incision is made parallel to the longitudinal axis of the tibia, from the proximal extent in the interval between the adductor tubercle and the epicondyle. This incision separates the sartorius layer from the underlying capsule and tibial collateral ligament. An incision posterior to the tibial collateral ligament that splits the mid-third capsular ligament and posterior oblique ligament is made in this posteromedial interval. The tibial collateral ligament, the mid-third capsular ligament, and the three portions of the posterior oblique ligament can all be inspected in this fashion, and the fascial investments of the semimembranosus can be investigated (Fig. 13.2). Surgical repair can follow if the

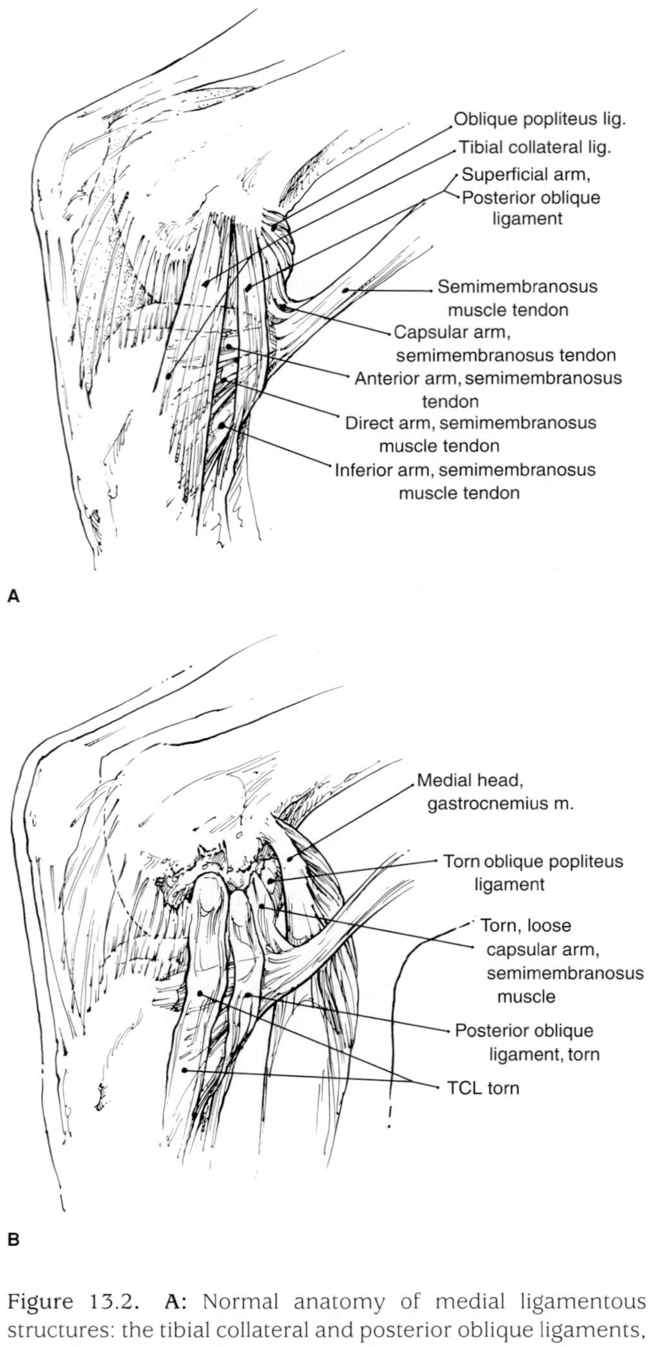

Figure 13.2. **A:** Normal anatomy of medial ligamentous structures: the tibial collateral and posterior oblique ligaments, and the semimembranosus tendon and its attachments. **B:** Tear of the femoral attachments of the tibial collateral ligament, the posterior oblique ligament, and the capsular arm of the semimembranosus tendon.

injury is acute, or surgical reconstruction can be accomplished if the injury is chronic.

The interior of the joint can be inspected arthroscopically before or after this portion of the procedure. Using arthroscopy after the surgical exposure facilitates identification of the tissue planes in a more thorough way and allows easier assessment of a chronic injury. However, fluid extravasation is a problem.

A guiding principle for any reconstructive procedure to this portion of the joint is that the suture lines need to follow the Burmester curve. If they are well off the curve, they will be under too much strain with flexion and extension of the knee and will fail.

The proper technique is to create a stable post of the tibial collateral and mid-third capsular ligaments. This is accomplished by direct suture repair with advancement of the mid-third capsular and tibial collateral ligaments proximally to the epicondylar area of the femur. The tibial attachment of the tibial collateral ligament is also checked, and, if torn or loose, is repaired. The tibial attachment of the mid-third capsular ligament can be evaluated and repaired under the tibial collateral ligament. Once a stable post of the tibial collateral and mid-third capsular ligaments is created, the posterior oblique ligament is then advanced, moving the femoral attachment anteriorly and proximally. The tibial attachment of the posterior oblique ligament is advanced distally and anteriorly, thus tensioning both ends of the posterior oblique ligament (Fig. 13.3).

The central portion of the posterior oblique ligament is then advanced in a "bowstring" fashion over the top of the tibial collateral ligament, further tightening the midportion of the posterior oblique ligament. The proximal posterior oblique ligament advancement needs to incorporate the capsular arm of the posterior oblique ligament in the repair to make sure that this portion is retensioned.

The final portion of the medial ligament reconstruction is the dynamic reconstruction. Sutures are placed in the capsular arm and the oblique popliteal portion of the semimembranosus tendon, which allows tightening of the posterior capsule behind the medial femoral condyle (Fig. 13.4). This is a very important portion of the procedure because this area has a significant risk of injury. Because the semimembranosus keeps the posterior oblique ligament tensioned in flexion, any marked looseness of the semimembranosus must be corrected. At the completion of this portion of the procedure, the sartorius fascia is repaired, followed by the subcutaneous tissue and the skin.

A protective brace is used for approximately 4 weeks, with the knee in approximately 60 degrees of flexion. The motion limits of the brace can be modified to protect the knee ligaments from strain, but to allow the motion gained in therapy for that week.

Extraarticular Approach for Anterior Lateral Instability

A curved incision is placed on the lateral side of the knee, with the proximal portion of the incision parallel to the lateral intermuscular septum and the distal portion curving distally between Gerdy's tubercle and the fibular head. A subcutaneous flap is developed anteri-

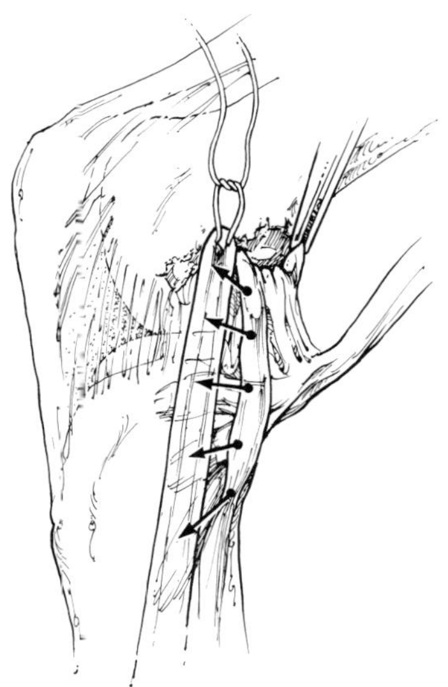

Figure 13.3. A stable post is created by advancing and repairing the tibial collateral and underlying mid-third capsular ligaments to the epicondylar area of the femur. The posterior oblique ligament is then advanced to this stable post.

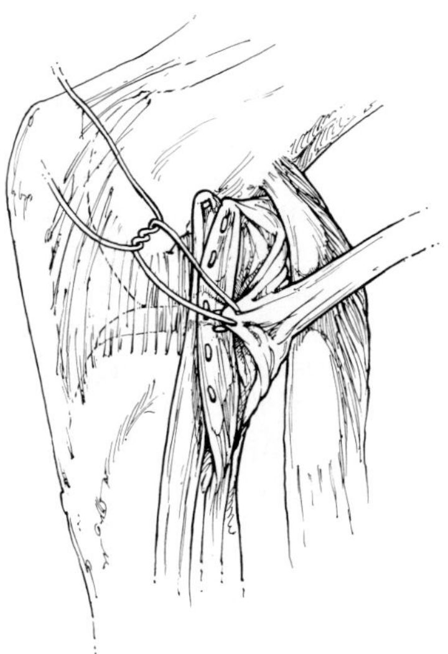

Figure 13.4. The capsular arm of the semimembranosus tendon and the oblique popliteal ligament are advanced to the posterior oblique ligament.

orly and posteriorly so that the area of the biceps muscle can be identified, as well as the distal, middle, and proximal portions of the iliotibial tract.

In the case of an acute injury, edema in the iliotibial tract can guide the surgeon to the area of injury. Depending on the site of injury, one, two, or three splitting incisions may be used.[49] These include (1) splitting the iliotibial tract in line with its fibers, (2) incising below and parallel to the lateral intermuscular septum through the fascia of the short head of the biceps muscle, and (3) developing an interval between the peroneal nerve and the posterior edge of the biceps tendon (which provides access to the long tendon of the biceps and allows for protection of the peroneal nerve).

In most cases, the iliotibial tract splitting incision is used. As the incision is carried proximally, one can determine the site of injury to the iliotibial tract. Fifty percent of iliotibial tract injuries will occur in the deep layer, which is found in the area of the lateral intermuscular septum. Twenty-five percent of these injuries are in the midportion of the iliotibial tract at the biceps capsulo-osseous confluence. The remaining 25% are distal at the tibial attachment of the capsulo-osseous iliotibial tract, either with or without a bone fragment (Segond fracture). Also, the capsular arm of the biceps is commonly injured, as is the capsulo-osseous confluence, and these injured structures must be inspected and repaired.

A capsular splitting incision can be used. With the knee in approximately 60 degrees of flexion, an incision is made parallel to the longitudinal axis of the tibia in the midlateral plane. The starting point of this incision is in line with the anterior margin of the fibular head. The incision then crosses the lateral capsule between the retracted halves of the iliotibial tract. Care must be taken at the proximal portion of this incision not to cut the popliteus tendon, which crosses the lateral capsule in this region. Also, because the incision crosses the edge of the lateral meniscus, the lateral geniculate artery must be protected from injury. If it is cut, suture ligatures must be placed through the artery to avoid formation of a hematoma postoperatively.

Through this combined exposure of the splitting incision of the iliotibial tract and the capsular incision, the entire joint can be inspected, along with the different components of the mid-third capsular ligament, iliotibial tract, and biceps complex, which are commonly injured in anterolateral instability. Direct repair can be accomplished through imbrication of the capsule. Peripheral meniscal repair, iliotibial tract reconstruction, and biceps tendon repair and reconstruction can all be accomplished through these incisions.

If a chronic injury to the iliotibial tract cannot be identified, then an imbrication of the capsulo-osseous iliotibial tract under the lateral intermuscular septum should be accomplished. This ensures that the iliotibial tract has a more medial attachment under the septum, as well as sagittal tensioning under the lateral intermuscular septum. The procedure is done with the knee in acute flexion, and, as the sutures are tied, the iliotibial tract is compressed into the area of the lateral intermuscular septum to ensure that it can be tensioned as tightly as practical. Once this is accomplished, the splitting incision of the iliotibial tract is repaired, taking care not to capture the deeper layer with the repair of the iliotibial tract. The two are not normally connected and connecting them could create an ankylosis. Finally, the subcutaneous tissue and skin are repaired, and the patient is placed in a flexed knee brace in approximately 60 degrees of flexion for about 4 weeks. After that time, the joint can gradually be mobilized in physical therapy. The motion limits are adjusted to protect the ligament repair while accommodating the motion obtained each week in therapy.

Posterolateral Repair and Reconstruction

The patient's knee is placed in 60 degrees of flexion. The same curved incision that is used for anterolateral repair can be used for posterolateral repair. Anyone of the same three fascial incisions may be used to identify the pathology and to provide access for the repair.[49] The peroneal nerve must be freed to allow access to the various components of the posterolateral complex and to protect the peroneal nerve from injury.

The best results are obtained with an acute repair, and anatomic principles are very important in obtaining good results. Thus, the various layers need to be repaired in a meticulous way. A single-layer repair is not as good as a repair that establishes continuity of each respective layer of the posterolateral complex and the biceps complex.

Again, edema guides the surgeon in selecting the appropriate fascial-splitting incision for repair in the acute injury. Therefore, all three fascial incisions may not be necessary in the acute injury. In the chronic injury, one must be prepared to use all three fascial incisions to identify the area of pathology. It is also important to realize that the lateral, the fibular, and the posterior portions of the posterolateral complex and biceps complex are commonly injured simultaneously. Therefore, reconstructive procedures need to be directed toward restoration of stability in all three areas for a chronic injury.

The issue of which reconstruction should be used depends on the site of pathology. If it can be identified as proximal, the authors' preferred technique is Hughston and Jacobson's[16] arcuate complex advancement (Fig. 13.5). The bone block that is harvested carries with it the femoral attachment of the arcuate complex, which includes the fibular collateral ligament, the popliteus tendon, the lateral ligament biceps expansion, and a por-

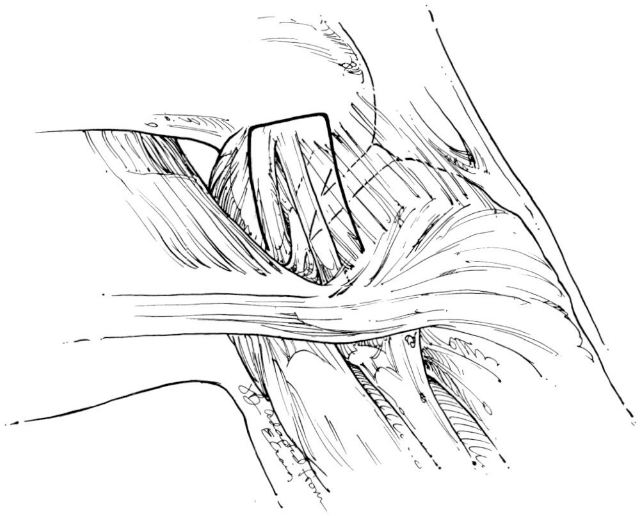

Figure 13.5. An incision is made around the arcuate complex.[16] (Redrawn from Hughston, JC, Jacobson, KE. Chronic posterolateral rotary instability of the knee. *Journal of Bone and Joint Surgery* 1982;67A:351–359. With permission.

tion of the tendon of the lateral gastrocnemius (Fig. 13.6). The posterior incision for this bone block advancement, if continued distally, would split the medial and lateral limbs of the arcuate arch. As such, it is very effective in the repair of a proximal injury because as the bone block is advanced to its site of placement on the femur, the sutures are placed in the posterior portion to imbricate the medial arcuate limb and posterior capsule and the soft tissue attached to the lateral complex and lateral arcuate limb. This procedure retensions the posterior portion of the capsule as well as the fibular components of the capsule.

Another technical hint for providing good results is that as the bone block is advanced parallel to the fibular collateral ligament (which is distally and anteriorly with the knee in 60 degrees of flexion), it is rotated in a clockwise fashion for a right knee and in a counterclockwise fashion for a left knee. The rotation of the bone block then allows for the fibular collateral to be in the same orientation as before the advancement and allows for retensioning of the lateral ligaments (Fig. 13.7).

The bone block is then seated with a Puddu staple (Fig. 13.8). The sutures, which have been placed before

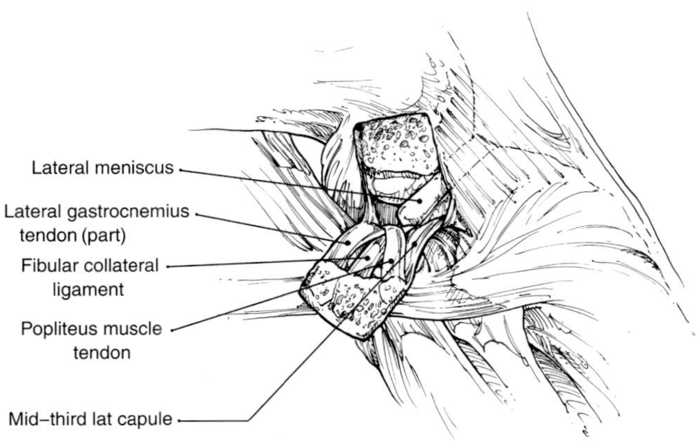

Figure 13.6. A bone block with femoral attachments of the arcuate complex is harvested from the lateral epicondylar area.

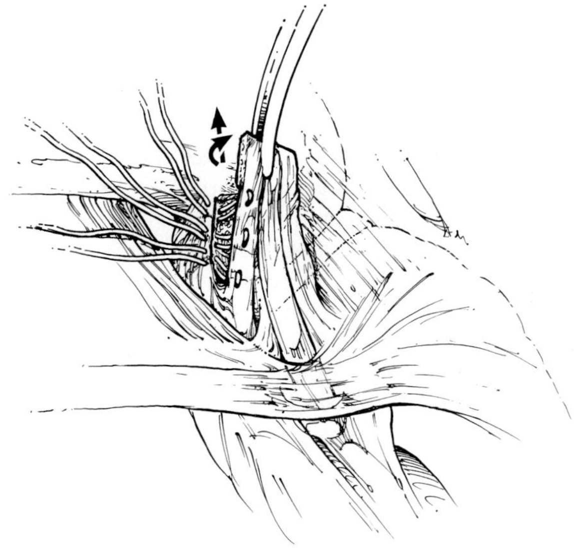

Figure 13.7. The bone block is advanced parallel to the fibular collateral ligament (anteriorly and distally with the knee in 60 degrees of flexion) and is rotated in a clockwise direction for a right knee and a counterclockwise direction for a left knee. Before seating the bone block, the posterior capsule is imbricated with sutures.

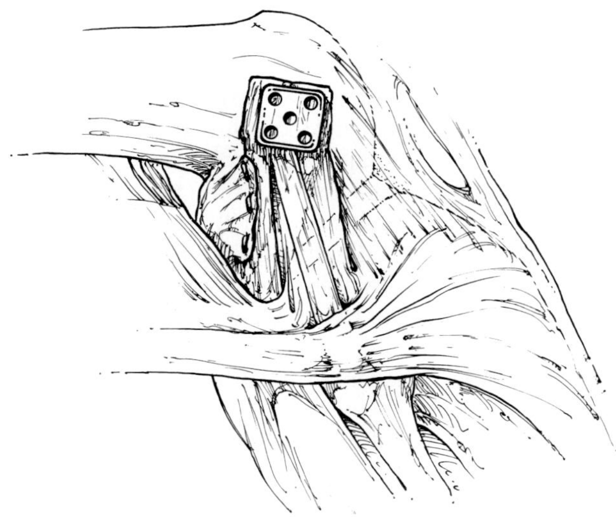

Figure 13.8. The bone block is seated with a Puddu staple.

the bone block advancement for the purposes of imbrication, are then tied. The midlateral incision is also repaired with an imbrication technique that further tightens the lateral soft tissues. The biceps complex is specifically assessed to make sure that its tension is restored. It may be necessary to repair the capsular arm of the biceps muscle and the capsulo-osseous biceps confluence or the fibular attachments. Closure of the fascial incisions is accomplished; the nerve is left free without repair of the fascial incision overlying the nerve. The subcutaneous tissue skin is repaired, and a long-leg brace with a pelvic band to prevent femoral external rotation is applied. The brace is kept in place for approximately 6 weeks, even though knee motion can be allowed by 4 weeks. Protection against femoral external rotation is continued for at least 6 to 8 weeks to allow connective tissue to mature, so it will not stretch out in the recovery phase. Once the knee has enough extension that the patient need not put the knee in a figure-four position while recumbent, the pelvic band can be discontinued.

If the injury to the posterolateral complex is distal, then a distal advancement is accomplished, either by acute repair or by delayed primary advancement in the chronic condition. Delayed primary repair requires an intimate understanding of the anatomic structures that are normally present and how the ligamentous and dynamic structures interact. After the reconstruction, postoperative protection is continued in a similar fashion to that described previously.

In the case of a tissue-depleted individual who has had previous surgery, an imbrication procedure for the posterior complex can be used, and restoration of the biceps tendon is required for success. The fibular collateral ligament can be repaired with a bone–patellar tendon–graft, with care being taken to reestablish the biceps' relationship to the fibular collateral at the completion of the repair.

The popliteus tendon can be restored with a long strip of the biceps tendon that is routed medial to the fibular styloid and then through the soft tissues along the course of the normal popliteus. It enters a drill hole at the normal site of attachment of the popliteus on the femur and is fixed to the area of the lateral intermuscular septum through a suture-over-post arrangement. This technique provides an isometric repair of the popliteus tendon and, if the tissue is harvested carefully, the biceps complex will not be harmed. Postoperative protection is accomplished in a similar fashion as previously described.

Avoidance of hematomas postoperatively is very important in every repair and reconstruction, both anterolateral and posterolateral. If a tourniquet is used, one should release the tourniquet before the ligament imbrication or before the sutures are tied. One obtains hemostasis with either Bovie cautery or with suture ligatures and then completes the reconstruction without the use of a tourniquet to avoid a postoperative hematoma. Also, the use of a secure compressive dressing will prevent swelling of the skin flaps and eliminate the need for postoperative drains.

References

1. Palmer I. On the injuries to the ligaments of the knee joint. A clinical study. *Acta Chir Scand*, Suppl 53 1938; 81:3–282.
2. Muller W. *The knee—Form, Function, and Ligament Reconstruction*. Berlin/Heidelberg: Springer-Verlag, 1983.
3. Jakob RP, Staubli HU. *The Knee and the Cruciate Ligaments—Anatomy, Biomechanics, Clinical Aspects, Reconstruction, Complications, and Rehabilitation*. Berlin/Heidelberg: Springer-Verlag, 1992.
4. Hughston JC. The importance of the posterior oblique ligament in repairs of acute tears of the medial ligaments in knees with and without an associated rupture of the anterior cruciate ligament. *J Bone Joint Surg* 1994; 76A:1328–1344.
5. Terry GC, Hughston JC, Norwood LA. The anatomy of the iliopatellar band and iliotibial tract. *Am J Sports Med* 1986;14:39–45.
6. Terry GC, LaPrade RF. The biceps femoris muscle complex at the knee. *Am J Sports Med* 1996;24:2–8.
7. Cox JS, Nye CE, Schaefer WW, et al. The degenerative effects of partial and total resection of the medial meniscus in dogs' knees. *Clin Orthop* 1975;109:178–183.
8. Johnson RJ, Kettelkamp DB, Clark W, et al. Factors affecting late results after meniscectomy. *J Bone Joint Surg* 1974;56A:719–729.
9. King D. The function of semilunar cartilage. *J Bone Joint Surg* 1936;18A:1069–1076.
10. Krause WR, Pope MH, Johnson RJ, et al. Mechanical changes in the knee after meniscectomy. *J Bone Joint Surg* 1976;58A:599–604.
11. Levy IM, Torzilli PA, Warren RF. The effect of medial meniscectomy on anteroposterior knee motion. *J Bone Joint Surg* 1982;64A:883–888.
12. Terry GC, Hughston JC. Associated joint pathology in the anterior cruciate ligament–deficient knee with emphasis on a classification system and injuries to the meniscocapsular ligament-musculotendinous unit complex. *Orthop Clin North Am* 1985;16(1):29–39.
13. Walker PS, Erkman MJ. The role of the menisci in force transmission across the knee. *Clin Orthop* 1975;109: 184–192.
14. Warren RF, Levy IM. Meniscal lesions associated with anterior cruciate ligament injury. *Clin Orthop* 1983;172: 32–37.

15. Hughston JC. The absent posterior drawer test in some acute posterior cruciate ligament tears of the knee. *Am J Sports Med* 1988;16:39–43.
16. Hughston JC, Jacobson KE. Chronic posterolateral rotatory instability of the knee. *J Bone Joint Surg* 1982;67A: 351–359.
17. Terry GC. The anatomy of the extensor mechanism. *Clin Sport Med* 1989;8(2):163–177.
18. Fairbank TJ. Knee joint changes after meniscectomy. *J Bone Joint Surg* 1948;30B:664–670.
19. Harner CD, Irrgang JJ, Paul J, et al. Loss of motion after anterior ligament reconstruction. *Am J Sports Med* 1992;20:499–506.
20. Daniel DM, Stone ML, Dobson BE, et al. Fate of the ACL-injured patient: a prospective outcome study. *Am J Sports Med* 1994;22:632–644.
21. Slocum DB. Pes anserinus transplantation. *J Bone Joint Surg* 1968;50A;226–242.
22. Slocum DB, Larson RL. Late reconstruction of ligamentous injuries of the medial compartment of the knee. *Clin Orthop* 1974;100:23–55.
23. Nicholas JA. The five-one reconstruction for anteromedial instability of the knee. *J Bone Joint Surg* 1973; 55A:899–922.
24. Hey-Groves EW. The cruciate ligaments of the knee joint. Their function, rupture, and the operative treatment of the same. *Br J Surg* 1919;7:505–515.
25. Smith A. The diagnosis and treatment of injuries to the crucial ligaments. *Br J Surg* 1918;6:176.
26. Bosworth DM. Transplantation of the semitendinosus for repair of laceration of medial collateral ligament of the knee. *J Bone Joint Surg* 1952;34A:196–201.
27. Milch H. Injuries to the crucial ligaments. *Arch Surg* 1935;30:805–819.
28. Campbell WC. Repair of the ligaments of the knee. *Surg Gynecol Obstet* 1936;62:964–968.
29. Campbell WC Reconstruction of the ligaments of the knee. *Am J Sports Med* 1939;43:473–480.
30. Mauk HP. A new operative approach for instability of the knee. *J Bone Joint Surg* 1936;18A:984–990.
31. Hughston JC, Eilus AF. The role of the posterior oblique ligament in repairs of acute medial ligament tears of the knee. *J Bone Joint Surg* 1973;55A:923–940.
32. Smillie IS. *Injuries of the Knee Joint*, 4th ed. Baltimore: Williams & Wilkins, 1970.
33. Hughston JC. A single meniscectomy. *J Sports Med* 1975;3:179–187.
34. Bruiser DM. A direct lateral approach to the lateral compartment of the knee joint. *J Bone Joint Surg* 1960; 42B:348–351.
35. MacIntosh DL, Darby TA. Lateral substitution reconstruction. *J Bone Joint Surg* 1976;58B:142.
36. Kennedy JC, Swan WJ. Lateral instability of the knee following lateral compartment injury. *J Bone Joint Surg* 1972;54B:763.
37. Kennedy JC, Stewart R, Walker DM. Anterolateral instability of the knee joint: an early analysis of the Ellison procedure. *J Bone Joint Surg* 1978;60A:1031–1039.
38. Ellison AE. Distal iliotibial-band transfer for anterolateral rotatory instability of the knee. *J Bone Joint Surg* 1979; 61A:330–337.
39. Lemaire M. Instabilite chronique du genore. *J Chir* (Paris) 1975;110:281–294.
40. Losee RE, Johnson TR, Southwick WO. Anterior subluxation of the lateral tibial plateau: a diagnostic test and operative repair. *J Bone Joint Surg* 1978;60A:1015–1030.
41. DeHaven KE. Classification and Diagnosis of Knee Instabilities. Symposium on Reconstructive Surgery of the Knee. St. Louis: Mosby, 1978.
42. Draganich LF, Andriacchi TP, Andersson GB. Interaction between intrinsic knee mechanics and the knee extensor mechanism. *J Orthop Res* 1987;5:539–547.
43. Draganich LF, Reider B, Miller PR. An in vitro study of the Muller anterolateral femorotibial ligament tenodesis in the anterior cruciate ligament deficient knee. *Am J Sports Med* 1989;17:357–362.
44. Andrews JR, Sanders R. A "mini-reconstruction" technique in treating anterolateral rotatory instability (ALRI). *Clin Orthop* 1983;172:93–96.
45. Mayer L. An operation for the cure of paralytic genu recurvatum. *J Bone Joint Surg* 1930;12A:845–852.
46. Bousquet G, Charmion L, Passot JP, et al. Stabilisation du condyle exterme du genoudans les laxite anterieures chroniques importance du muscle poplite. *Rev Chir Orthop Reparatrice Appar Mot* 1986;72:427–434.
47. Clancy WG, Meister K, Craythrone CB. Posterolateral corner collateral ligament reconstruction. In: Jackson DW, ed. *Reconstructive Knee Surgery*. New York: Raven Press, 1995:143–159.
48. Jakob RP, Hanlin H, Staubli HU. Observations on rotatory instability of the lateral compartment of the knee. *Acta Orthop Scand* 1981;(suppl):191.
49. Terry GC, LaPrade RF. The posterolateral aspect of the knee: anatomy and surgical approach. *Am J Sports Med* 1996;24:732–739.

Chapter 14

Complications and Pitfalls in Anterior Cruciate Ligament Revision Reconstruction

Deryk G. Jones, Mark Galland, and Freddie H. Fu

There has been a clear increase in the number of anterior cruciate ligament (ACL) reconstructions performed over the last 15 years. Indications for reconstruction of ACL-deficient knee have broadened, increasing the number of operative cases per year. Further, there are more surgeons performing this procedure who are adequately trained in current arthroscopic techniques. Both factors have accounted for the overall increase. With this increase in total number of cases, there has also been an increase in the number of successful reconstructions. However, as with any procedure, unsatisfactory outcomes can occur. There are numerous causes for these failures. Certainly, the patient with untreated and/or unrecognized chondral or osteochondral damage, meniscal injury, associated ligamentous laxity, or other intraarticular pathology can have continued pain postoperatively as well.

O'Donoghue et al's[1] classic article was often quoted and formed the basis for a large volume of basic science and clinical practices in the 1970s and 1980s.[2–4] Orthopedists justified their reconstructive procedures based on their antiarthritic benefits. Dale Daniel et al's[5] article on a large group of postoperative reconstructed patients demonstrating significant rates of osteoarthritis placed a great deal of literature and clinical practices into question. More recently, there are an increasing number of studies both at the basic science and clinical level supporting reconstruction of the ACL in patients at high risk for or suffering from recurrent instability.[6,7] There is clearly a relationship between chondral defects and meniscal pathology and recurrent episodes of instability. The degree of associated damage to these structures should have a significant impact on the overall outcome following stabilization procedures. This chapter outlines the causes of failure in ACL reconstructive surgery and details how these factors influence preoperative planning, intraoperative surgical decisions, and technical factors, as well as postoperative rehabilitation in revision ACL surgery.

ETIOLOGY OF GRAFT FAILURE

Categorizing the cause of an unsuccessful outcome is an important step in treating this patient population. Previous articles have divided the primary etiology for failure into three categories: graft failure, technical error(s), and traumatic events.[8,9] An article by Johnson and Coen[10] described four main categories for ACL surgery to fail:

1. traumatic arthritis
2. arthrofibrosis
3. extensor mechanism dysfunction
4. recurrent patholaxity.

Surgical Technique

Surgical technique is a common source of graft failure and usually involves incorrect tunnel position or poor fixation.[10–12] The surgeon should be aware of several key tenets in ACL reconstruction to avoid these errors. Tunnels should reproduce the "normal" attachment site of the ACL. Poorly positioned femoral or tibial tunnels result in excessive length changes of the graft as the knee is brought through a physiologic range of motion (ROM). Clinically, this is manifest as either restricted ROM or as increased laxity of the joint. Tunnel placement that minimizes graft elongation during motion is desirable.[13–15]

Previously, emphasis was placed on restoring the "isometry" of the native ligament during ACL reconstruction. Woo et al[16] have shown that load distribution between the separate anatomic regions of the ACL changes with knee motion. As the best location for a graft may change according to the position of the joint and the type of external loading, the concept of isometry should give way to a more functional definition of placement.[16,17]

Many authors have studied the importance of femoral tunnel position. It has been well established that the femoral attachment site is the most important determinant of graft length change during knee motion.[13,14] Insertions that are too anterior on the femur lead to graft lengthening with knee flexion. If very anterior, there is increased tension in both flexion and extension. Posterior insertions result in decreased length and increased laxity of the graft as the knee is flexed. If too vertical there will be decreased resistance to anterior tibial translation. A medial or lateral femoral position will result in graft impingement, abrasion, and subsequent failure.[10–12]

As most surgeons have become aware of the importance of proper femoral tunnel positioning and have become more consistent in femoral tunnel placement, the problems associated with incorrect tibial tunnel placement have become apparent. A tibial tunnel placed too anterior is associated with roof impingement. In addition, endoscopic placement of the femoral tunnel will be more difficult, and the tunnel will tend to be malpositioned if the "over-the-top" guide is placed anterior to its desired position on the roof. The posterior cruciate ligament (PCL) may be damaged during tunnel reaming if the tibial tunnel is too posterior. Posterior placement of the tibial tunnel is also associated with extensor lag. Excessive lateral placement of the tunnel may result in damage to the anterior horn of the lateral meniscus or impingement against the medial portion of the lateral femoral condyle. Excessive medial placement may result in damage to the articular cartilage of the medial plateau during reaming and difficulty in passing the graft past the PCL (Fig. 14 1). The ACL graft should just touch the lateral aspect of the PCL and not be deflected by this structure.[15,18]

Jackson and Gasser[15] have described a method for reproducible selection of the central point of the tibial tunnel using four consistent anatomic landmarks. They note that choosing the center of the anatomic footprint of the ACL stump will position the graft too anteriorly in relation to the intercondylar roof. The anatomic consistency of these structures has an embryologic basis. These landmarks are the anterior horn of the lateral meniscus, the medial tibial spine, the PCL, and the ACL stump. The anteroposterior center of the tibial tunnel is in line with the inner edge of the anterior horn of the lateral meniscus. Intersection of this point with a point 7 mm anterior to the anterior border of the PCL should correspond with a depression just medial to the midportion of the medial tibial spine. Use of these landmarks places the center of the tibial tunnel in the posterior half of the ACL footprint. This is more posterior than previously recommended,[19] a fact that will undoubtedly simplify tunnel placement in the revision setting.

Improper tensioning of the graft is a potential cause of graft failure. The most common error in technique is excessive tensioning of the graft, resulting in graft elongation and restriction of flexion. Both the anatomic position of the graft and the type of fixation are factors that affect tension. Overtensioning not only can result in a loss of knee motion, but has been noted in experimental models to result in delayed vascularization and myxoid degeneration of graft fibers.[20] Inadequate tension will result in persistent instability due to a nonfunctioning graft. There is still debate over the ideal graft tension. Interestingly, Yoshiya et al[20] noted adverse effects of excessive tension on graft tissue at a magnitude of 39 N. These undesirable effects were not seen in grafts tensioned at 1 N. Surprisingly, the authors found no difference in knee laxity between the groups at 3 months, despite differences noted in the immediate postoperative period. Similarly, Gertel et al[21] found graft force and joint motion to be unaffected by the magnitude of the tensioning force. Further, they found that current methods of graft tensioning produced a posteriorly and externally rotated tibial configuration compared with normal. They suggested that excessive graft forces might be avoided by applying tension distally (from the tibial side) with the knee in extension. If a more physiologic joint configuration is desired, they recommend that tension be applied proximally (via the femoral side of the graft). Others recommend more reproducible techniques. Richmond's group[22] advocates the "maximum one-handed pull," defined as the maximum force that could be sustained by the surgeon for a 1- to 2-minute period with one hand. This technique is readily reproducible, and because it is performed with the knee in full extension, ensures that full extension is possible. Also, frictional forces between the bone block and tibial tunnel are lessened and it is unlikely that graft tension will be lost during screw placement.

Fixation

Many authors agree that graft fixation is the weak link in ACL reconstruction, representing the initial limiting factor in the immediate postoperative period.[23–25] Fixation must be secure enough to prevent changes in graft

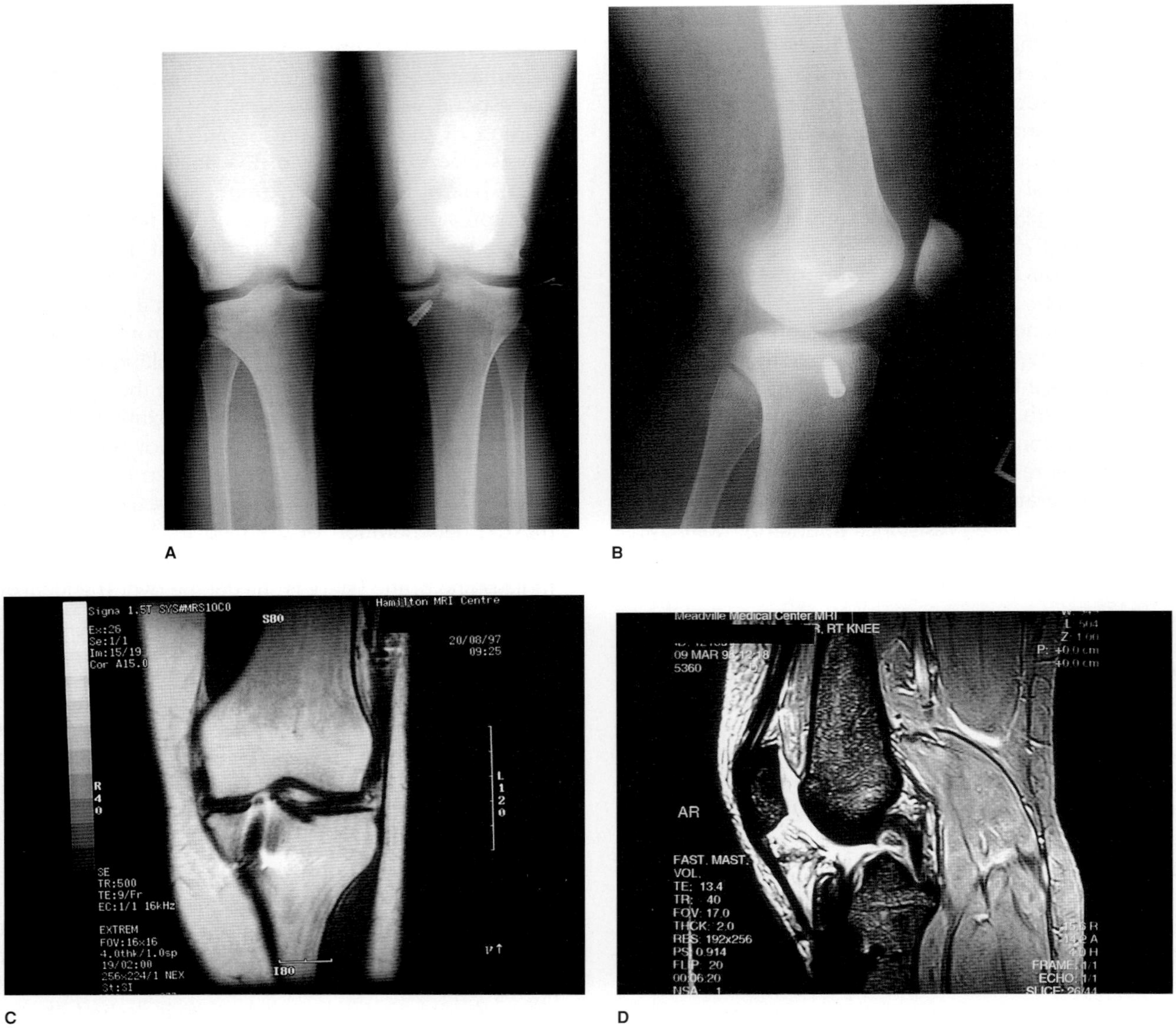

Figure 14.1. **A:** Posteroanterior (PA) weight-bearing view after two-incision anterior cruciate ligament (ACL) reconstruction demonstrating extreme medial placement of the tibial tunnel and hardware (left knee). **B:** Lateral radiograph (same patient) demonstrating extreme anterior femoral interference screw placement and posterior placement of the tibial interference screw. **C:** Coronal T1-weighted magnetic resonance imaging (MRI) image demonstrating interference screw penetration of medial tibial plateau caused by improper tibial tunnel placement. **D:** Sagittal T1-weighted MRI demonstrating tibial tunnel penetration of medial plateau. Note the remaining graft tissue within the tunnel.

position while graft incorporation occurs. No in vivo measurements of functional forces on the ACL graft have been performed, yet various authors have estimated these forces to be approximately 500 N.[25,26] Kurosaka et al[23] determined that for a bone-tendon-bone graft, interference screw fixation with a 9-mm screw provides the strongest pullout strength when compared with staple fixation and suture techniques. Notably, this method provided nearly twice the maximum tensile strength achieved with a 6.5-mm screw.

Other factors influence the stability of the bone–screw interface, including the diameter of the screw as well as the size and shape of the bone plug. Recent evidence suggests that fixation may be enhanced with the creation of circular (rather than trapezoidal) bone plugs.[27] Butler et al[28] introduced the concept of "gap size" as an important variable in fixation strength. Using a porcine model, the authors determined that for gap sizes of 1 to 4 mm, a 9-mm interference screw provided the highest resistance to pullout force. They noted that for gaps of 1 to 2 mm, a 7-mm interference screw was acceptable. While gaps greater than 4 mm were not specifically tested, by extrapolating data the authors suggested the use of suture/post fixation combined with the use of a 9-mm interference screw for gaps larger than 4 mm. Additionally, it seems that the use of circular bone plugs would help to decrease gap size, thereby enhancing fixation strength.

It is generally accepted that the interference screw should be placed adjacent to the cancellous surface of the bone plug. Among the reasons in favor of this position is the decreased likelihood of damage to the collagenous portion of the graft. Interestingly, Rupp et al[29] found that while the mode of fixation failure was dependent on the position of the screw relative to the bone plug, initial fixation strength was not affected.

Ishibashi et al[30] have shown the site of tibial graft fixation to be of significant importance in the immediate postoperative period. They assessed the stability of knees following ACL reconstruction with different sites of tibial graft fixation: proximal, central, and distal. They reported that in the immediate postoperative period, proximal graft fixation provided the greatest resistance to anterior tibial translation and graft forces more closely resembling those of the normal ligament. The method is purported to entail decreased functional length and decreased "windshield wiper effect" as well as increased graft stiffness.

Robertson et al[31] experimentally evaluated immediate fixation strengths for various soft tissue to bone fixation methods. These techniques included the use of staples, sutures, or screws with a spiked soft tissue plate or plastic spiked washer. The authors reported the most secure method of soft tissue fixation to bone occurred with a screw and spiked washer or spiked soft tissue plate. They also noted that increased resistance to pullout could be obtained by placing the screw directly through the graft via a stab incision or by wrapping the graft around the screw. Similarly, Steiner et al[25] reported the strongest fixation technique for a hamstring graft is one in which the semitendinosus and gracilis are doubled. The free ends of the graft are fixed to the femur in a figure-of-eight weave around two 4.5-mm bicortical screws and two spiked washers. The looped ends of the graft are fixed to the tibia by three number-5 nonabsorbable sutures passed through the loop and tied around a 6.5-mm cancellous screw with a metal washer.[32] Notably, Steiner et al reported all hamstring grafts secured with suture fixation failed with prolonged pullouts, either by complete suture-graft disruption or by graft stretching. They concluded that the washer technique is superior to the suture technique in achieving ACL reconstruction with closer-to-normal strength and stiffness.

Many studies comparing the fixation strength of bioabsorbable interference screws with that of metal screws have yielded inconsistent results. Pena et al[33] have shown the bioabsorbable models fail by a bone block pullout mechanism at lower loads than that seen for the metal screws. A significantly lower pullout strength in the bioabsorbable group was reported, but when the failure strength was corrected for patient age and bone density, the failure loads were nearly 700 N and comparable to those noted in the metal screw group. Although the average load before failure in the bioabsorbable group was greater than 500 N, compared to just over 400 N in the metal group, Johnson and VanDyk[34] reported no statistical difference between the groups. However, the studies do not agree on the significance of these findings. At the current time, since there has been no overwhelming number of fixation failures with the bioabsorbable screw seen clinically, perhaps the estimated loads for activities of daily living are too high. Additionally, pullout testing is generally performed with the load in line with the longitudinal axis of the ligament, a situation not representative of physiologic loads seen with the graft. Certainly, this is an issue that warrants further investigation.

Graft Incorporation

Autograft and allograft tissues undergo a similar sequence of biologic remodeling and incorporation.[35,36] These stages include ischemic necrosis, revascularization, cellular repopulation/proliferation, and collagen remodeling.[37] The process, in which these tissues undergo biologic and histologic transformation, adopting features characteristic of ligamentous tissues, has been termed "ligamentization" by Amiel et al.[38] While recent studies confirm that the grafts do undergo a transformation, the collagen ultrastructural pattern is characteristic of organized scar repair tissue rather than of the native ligament.[39] As current techniques and tissues cannot reproduce the exact physiology of the ACL, this transformed scar tissue serves as a check to anterior translation, rather than a physiologic duplicate of the native ACL. Thus, while the function of the knee is improved, the reconstructed knee does not truly duplicate the original knee biomechanics.

The mechanisms that lead to failure of graft incorporation are poorly understood. Authors who have performed second-look arthroscopies after ACL surgery report that functional grafts appear taut and revascularized.[39] In addition, biopsy of these specimens reveal normal cellularity and well-arranged collagen bundles. Conversely, in nonfunctioning grafts there is no evidence of revascularization. These grafts are often seen in association with obvious technical error.[39,40] The work of Yoshiya et al[20] and Corsetti and Jackson[35] supports this finding, and implicates the importance of both the biomechanical and histochemical factors in the determination of the functional characteristics and performance of the graft. Furthermore, Corsetti and Jackson suggest that the loss of strength of grafts during the remodeling process is more related to the inability, intraoperatively, to produce physiologic tension and position.

Resorption surrounding bony tunnels is a rare manifestation of failure of graft incorporation. Some authors postulate an immune-mediated reaction as the etiology.[41,42] While this may be a reasonable explanation for cases involving allograft tissue, it fails to account for those failures involving autograft tissue.

Trauma

Failure of ACL reconstruction can result from the application of excessive load to the graft prior to graft maturation. All biologic grafts undergo a period of ligamentization characterized by an initial decline in mechanical strength followed by a gradual return to full strength.[38] This period may last as long as 1 year. Any of the factors previously mentioned may contribute to either early or late reconstruction failure.

Early failure occurs prior to complete incorporation of the graft and prior to the completion of the rehabilitation program. It may be related to overzealous rehabilitation or to premature return to full activity. In either instance, the graft is exposed to excessive forces prior to completion of the maturation process.

Late failure occurs after completion of a rehabilitation program and after full activity has been resumed. Significant trauma to the knee is usually involved, and in these cases there is an assumption that a functioning ligament was damaged by a sufficient force that would have torn a normal, physiologic ACL.

Late failure may also be the consequence of uncorrected associated ligament injuries, such as posterolateral rotatory instability or valgus laxity. Under these circumstances, in addition to the forces to which the ACL is typically exposed, the graft is also exposed to forces that would normally be borne by other static restraints to knee motion.

Preoperative Evaluation

Preoperative evaluation begins by obtaining information on the nature and timing of the primary injury as well as the number of recurrent episodes of instability. The patient's current symptoms are important as well. Symptoms associated with articular, ligamentous, and meniscal pathology should be sought, which include pain, grinding, swelling, locking, or giving way. The level of activity prior to and after the initial reconstruction and after the most recent injury is important as well. Not to be overlooked are the patient's expectations, as a return to high levels of vigorous physical activity may not be a realistic expectation following revision ACL surgery.

Details regarding the primary procedure may be obtained from the operative report. Of note are the technique (two-incision, endoscopic, extraarticular), fixation method, and graft selection. Additionally, information regarding the condition of the articular surface, menisci, PCL, posterolateral corner, collateral ligaments, alignment, and patellofemoral tracking must be noted.

Physical examination should begin with analysis of the patient's gait. Berchuck et al[43] noted a decreased magnitude of flexion moment in the ACL-deficient knee. This was interpreted as the patient's effort to reduce or to avoid contraction of the quadriceps, minimizing the anterior tibial translation that normally occurs as the quadriceps contracts and the knee approaches full extension. This abnormal gait pattern has been termed the "quadriceps avoidance gait." Timoney et al[44] noted a tendency toward gait normalization after ACL reconstruction and a disappearance of the quadriceps avoidance mechanism.

Examination of the skin to determine the location of previous surgical incisions is invaluable. Previous incisions should be used when possible. When additional incisions are required, inadequate skin bridges should be avoided. Next, muscle bulk and tone should be assessed. The presence of atrophy of the quadriceps, particularly the vastus medialis oblique (VMO), is often overlooked but can be a significant source of knee pain and effusion. In the presence of significant atrophy and weakness, a trial of rehabilitation should be completed prior to revision reconstruction of the ACL.

Evaluation of range of motion is crucial prior to performing a revision procedure. Flexion is evaluated in the supine position. Extension, if limited in the supine position, should be evaluated in the prone position with the knees hanging over the side of the table. Disparity between supine and prone extension suggests an extensor lag with associated quadriceps atrophy. Loss of extension is more detrimental than loss of flexion and is associated with the development of patellofemoral pain.[45] The etiologies of a flexion contracture include roof impingement, improper tunnel placement, and soft tissue impingement such as a "cyclops lesion"[46] (Fig. 14.2). Loss of motion should be addressed before revision surgery. In some cases a staged procedure may be necessary to regain motion, followed by ACL revision at a later date.[45]

An assessment to determine the presence of associated ligamentous injuries should be performed. Most commonly, this involves posterolateral rotatory instability with or without valgus laxity, but the integrity of the

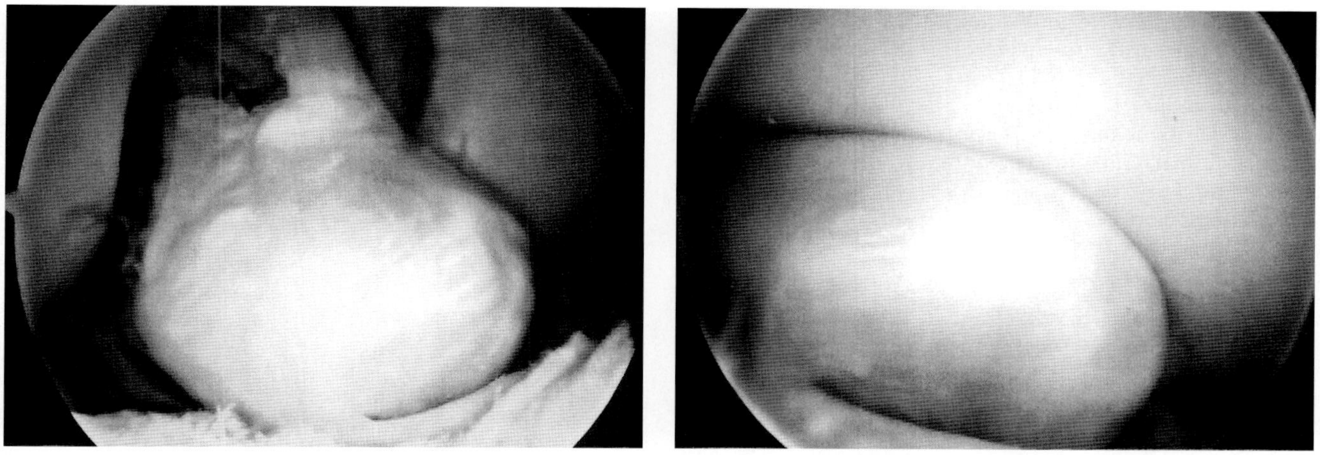

A B

Figure 14.2. A: Arthroscopic view of a failed ACL reconstruction with a resultant "cyclops lesion" (90-degree knee flexion). B: With attempted extension the lesion blocks terminal motion by impinging on the anterosuperior surface of the intercondylar notch.

PCL and other ligamentous structures should also be determined. In the case of a hemarthrosis, acute ligamentous injury should be expected.

Attention should then be directed to the patellofemoral joint. Crepitus, fibrosis, or subluxation should be noted. Particularly in those patients who have previously undergone a bone–patellar tendon–bone autograft, examination for patella alta or baja should be sought. An effusion may alert the clinician to the presence of associated articular or meniscal pathology, and the examination concludes with an assessment of meniscal and chondral structures. Palpation along the joint line should be performed, but specific palpation along the condyles medially and laterally should be performed at varying flexion angles and the degree of flexion in which pain can be elicited should be noted.

Once this information has been obtained, the failure may be one of four types as described by Marder.[18] A patient who remains symptomatic despite a stable knee and has complaints consistent with a nongraft condition can be expected to respond favorably to directed rehabilitation program and activity modification within the first 2 years. These conditions include chondromalacia, quadriceps atrophy, and mild flexion contracture. Flexion contracture of >5 degrees, meniscal tears, or patellofemoral arthrosis cannot be expected to be improved by nonoperative treatment. Revision notchplasty and debridement of scar tissue may improve extensor lag. Mensical pathology may respond to debridement.

Patients with an isolated ACL injury should be considered candidates for a revision reconstruction. Those patients with ACL laxity in combination with other ligamentous laxity should be considered for revision reconstruction and reconstruction of associated ligamentous pathology. The presence of early arthrosis should not be a contraindication to these procedures. More significant chondral lesions and meniscal pathology should be addressed at the time of reconstruction or treated in a staged fashion.

RADIOGRAPHIC EVALUATION

Radiographic evaluation begins with anteroposterior and lateral radiographs, from which the surgeon may obtain information regarding tunnel location, type and position of hardware, and surgical technique (Fig. 14.3). In addition, bone density can be assessed, and osteolysis may be noted. Patellar height may be measured, and the presence of alta or baja recorded. Two other important radiographic views include the Merchant and 45-degree posteroanterior (PA) flexion weight-bearing views. The former radiograph assesses the degree of patellofemoral arthrosis or patellar subluxation. An assessment of the patellar defect from previous graft harvest is also possible. The latter view evaluates the joint space narrowing and degenerative changes in the 45-degree flexion zone. This radiograph demonstrates subtle chondral degeneration and is especially sensitive to postmenisectomy compartment changes. This view also gives an excellent demonstration of the intercondylar notch and can evaluate early stenosis from osteophyte formation.

If there is a concern about the patient's overall alignment, long-leg standing films should be obtained. The mechanical axis (the line from the center of the femoral head to the center of the ankle joint) and femoral-tibial

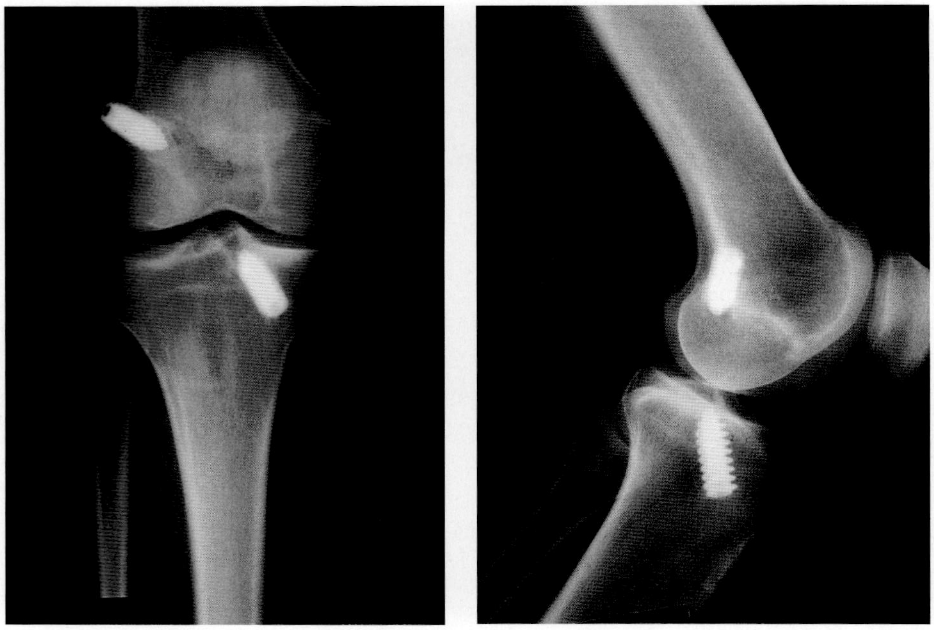

A B

Figure 14.3. **A:** PA weight-bearing radiograph demonstrating failure of femoral interference screw fixation resulting from improper insertion and minimal screw thread contact with the graft. **B:** Lateral radiograph demonstrating improper tunnel position and failure of fixation following a two-incision ACL reconstruction.

angles (center femoral diaphysis to center tibial diaphysis) should be obtained. These radiographs are particularly important in the setting of an observed lateral thrust or excessive valgus alignment with associated medial collateral ligament instability.

Other radiographic modalities useful in preoperative planning include computed tomography (CT) scan and magnetic resonance imaging (MRI). If concerned about tunnel expansion and/or bony loss as well as bone density, the CT scan is an excellent analytic modality. MRI, while certainly not a mandatory preoperative aid, can be of valuable assistance in the diagnosis and assessment of associated meniscal, articular, and ligamentous pathology (Fig. 14.4). In addition, it has proven accurate in evaluation of the integrity of the ACL graft itself.

Graft Selection

There are currently three graft sources available: autograft, allograft, and synthetic. There are three broad categories of prosthetic ligaments that have been used in the past: permanent, scaffold, and augmentation-type devices.[47] These devices have the theoretical advantages of eliminating graft harvest morbidity, unlimited availability, no risk of disease transmission, strength exceeding normal tissue, and facilitating early return to sports.

Permanent grafts exhibit high ultimate strength and stiffness acting as permanent ACL replacements. The two most commonly used in North America in the 1980s were the Gore-Tex (Gore and Co., Flagstaff, AZ) and Stryker Dacron (Stryker Endoscopy Co., Sunnyvale, CA).

The Gore-Tex device is a triple-helical, multifilament strand composed of polytetrafluoroethylene (PTFE) with loops on each end. Fixation was achieved by placing screws through these loops. Biomechanically the device demonstrated an ultimate strength of 5,300 N and strain at yield of 2% to 5% versus 25% for the normal ACL.[48] Due to increasing failure rates, Gore-Tex designed a compact diameter cruciate ligament (CDCL) with a 40% reduction in diameter with improved results. Despite these improvements, the company discontinued all prosthetic implants in 1993.[49]

The Dacron (Stryker) prosthesis is composed of a core of four strands of Dacron tape surrounded by a knitted Dacron velour tube. This device has an ultimate strength of 3,613 N and is less stiff than the normal ACL at 42 N/mm.[48] Multiple studies have demonstrated extremely high failure rates at 2 years with this device.[50–54]

As one can see, despite excellent theoretical advantages, in clinical practice these implants have been associated with early ruptures, progressive prosthetic stretching at 4 to 5 years, cystic ganglion formation, and recurrent sterile effusions.[50,55] Scaffold implants were developed in response to the failures with the above permanent devices.

The Leeds-Keio prosthesis has been used extensively outside the United States.[47] This implant is a polyester with an open-weave tube. It was designed to promote

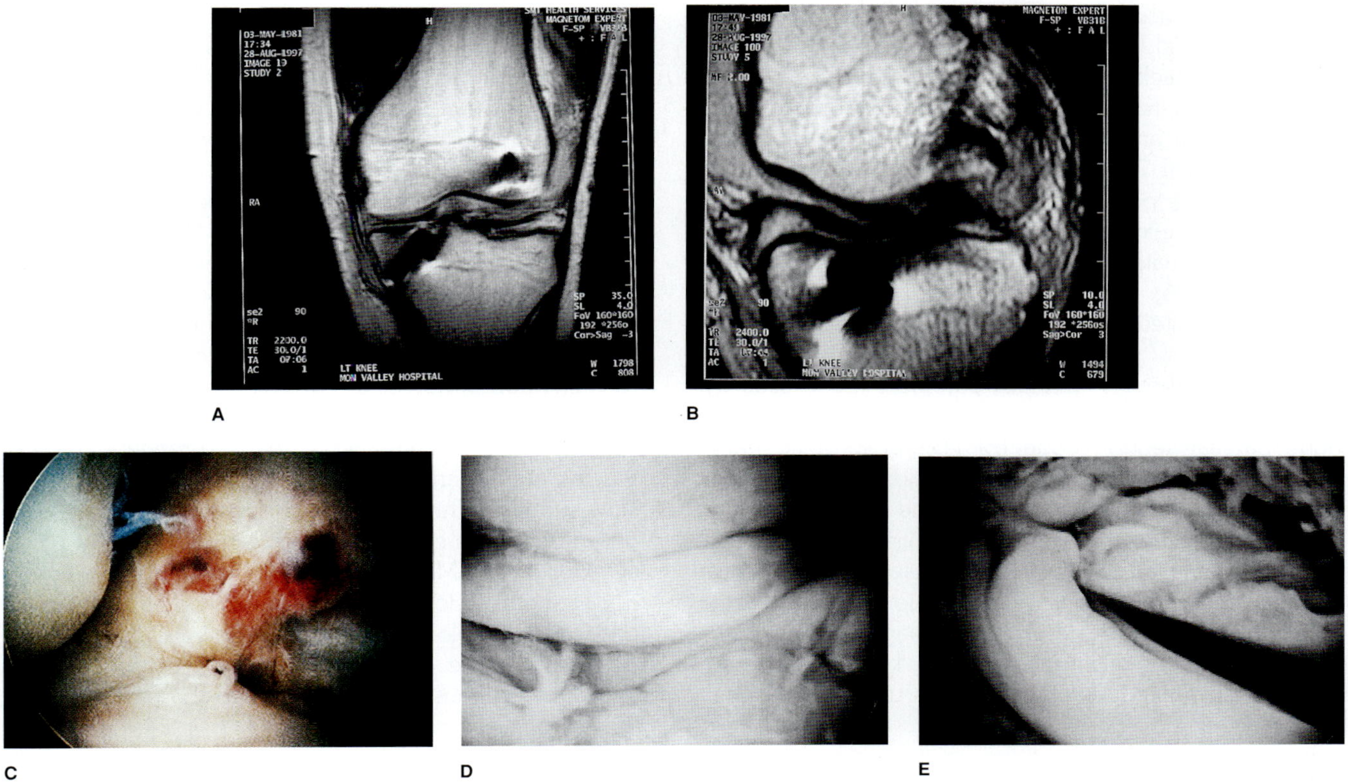

Figure 14.4. A: Coronal T1-weighted MRI demonstrating penetration of the subchondral bone of the medial tibial plateau by hardware secondary to improper (posteromedial) tibial tunnel placement. Note the patient also has a displaced bucket-handle tear of the medial meniscus. B: Corresponding sagittal T1-weighted image demonstrating penetration of subchondral bone of the medial tibial plateau by hardware, tibial tunnel widening, and a bucket-handle meniscal tear. C: Arthroscopic view (anterolateral) at revision in the same patient, revealing hemorrhage and inflammation, in an abraded, elongated, and failed graft. D: Arthroscopic view (anterolateral) of the displaced bucket-handle medial meniscal tear. Note the damage to the medial tibial plateau caused by previous drill and graft passage through this region. E: Arthroscopic view (anterolateral) during attempted reduction of the medial meniscal tear. Note the severe articular cartilage damage along the medial tibial plateau. (Top: femoral condyle. Bottom: tibial plateau. Views correspond with radiographs and MR images in Fig. 14.1).

fibrous ingrowth. Femoral fixation is achieved by placement of a tubular bone graft in a loop on the end of the prosthesis that is then press fit into place. Distal fixation is achieved by placing a similar bone graft along the flat end of the graft distally. Initial recommendations were for 4 to 6 weeks of immobilization allowing for fibrous ingrowth. Biomechanical testing demonstrated an ultimate strength of 340 to 870 N, which theoretically increased to 2,000 N with fibrous ingrowth.[56–59] Two separate studies demonstrated low failure rates and few complications 4 years postoperatively.[56,57] Fujikawa and Iseki[57] on second-look arthroscopy reported new random tissue with rich vascularity at 3 months. At 12 months a mature ligament resembling the normal ACL was observed. While these results are promising, long-term follow-up is required to reach more definitive conclusions, and the technique does have questionable initial fixation that requires prolonged postoperative immobilization.

Carbon fiber implants have been used in knee ligament surgery as well.[60,61] These devices were strong and theoretically bioinert and demonstrated a propensity to induce fibrous ingrowth.[62–64] Unfortunately, if not surrounded by autogenous tissue such as fascia lata, carbon fiber particle formation created a synovitic response and minimal neotendon formation was seen.[60,64,65] Follow-up of patients treated with these implants has demonstrated persistent pain, effusion, and synovial thickening, most likely attributable to particle formation.[66]

J.C. Kennedy[67] designed the ligament augmentation device (LAD), which is a permanent, woven prosthesis composed of braided polypropylene with an ultimate strength of 1,500 to 1,730 N.[68] The implant and autogenous tissue are tubularized around one another and secured with nonabsorbable suture. The LAD is attached at only one end (i.e., femur or tibia) to prevent subsequent stress-shielding and graft elongation or rupture that has been reported with device fixation on both ends.[68] Fowler and Capra[68] reported 91% good to excellent results at 7.5-year mean follow-up of augmented reconstructions performed using the modified Marshall Macintosh technique. Roth et al[69] noted improved functional stability with augmentation with low complication rates as well. As a result, synthetic grafts are currently used on a limited basis for augmentation purposes by select surgeons.[70]

There are three sources of autograft tissue used by most surgeons at the current time: central one-third bone–patellar tendon–bone (BPTB), quadrupled hamstring tendon (gracilis and semitendinosus), and quadriceps tendon. Although popular in the past, use of the fascia lata (proximal fascia or distal iliotibial band) has fallen out of favor due to the decreased tensile and ultimate strengths demonstrated by biomechanical testing.[26] The advantages and disadvantages of the three main tissue types are listed in Table 14.1. In the revision setting the patient typically has undergone either BPTB or hamstring ACL reconstruction. Typically, this leaves the alternate tissue available for autogenous ACL reconstruction. In addition, the use of quadriceps tendon (anterior one-half tendon with attached bone block) is gaining popularity in these situations.[71] As opposed to using allograft tissue when no autogenous source is available, some surgeons prefer to use contralateral autogenous tissue (usually BPTB).[72,73] While having the advantages provided by an autogenous tissue source (described below), there is obviously a risk of potential damage and postoperative morbidity associated with these techniques. Further, there may be a more complicated rehabilitation period as the patient is concerned with recovery in both knees rather than one knee.

Some surgeons have recommended repeat harvest of the ipsilateral central patellar tendon graft during revision surgery. Three significant histologic studies have raised questions concerning this clinical practice. Liu et al[74] performed MRI analysis on 16 patients and further donor-site biopsies on four patients who had previously undergone autologous patellar tendon ACL reconstruction an average of 7 years prior to the study. MRI showed tendinous reconstitution into the patellar defect

Table 14.1. Advantages and disadvantages of the three types of autograft tissue

Central bone patellar tendon–bone (BPTB)		*Quadrupled semitendinosus/gracilis*		*Quadriceps tendon*	
Advantages	*Disadvantages*	*Advantages*	*Disadvantages*	*Advantages*	*Disadvantages*
High tensile/ ultimate: Strength Stiffness	↑ Potential donor-site morbidity[a]	High tensile/ ultimate: Strength	Stiffness—femur-tendon-tibia complex[e]	Highest stiffness/ strength measured	potentially bulky graft
Bone-to-bone healing	Persistent anterior knee pain[b]	Lower % persistent anterior knee pain[b]			
High initial fixation strength	Long-term deficit quadriceps strength[c]	No long-term deficit hamstring function	Lower initial fixation strength		Lower initial distal fixation strength
	Smaller tendon diameter than native ACL (1 cm)	Larger cross-sectional area (cylindrical)[d]	Inability to fill large bony defects (bone grafting)		Limited North American experience
		↓ Potential donor-site morbidity			

[a]Patellar fractures, patellar tendon ruptures.[95,96]
[b]Patellofemoral pain, ↓ patellofemoral mobility, tendinitis.[97,98]
[c]Controversial (some studies have demonstrated postoperative quadriceps deficits while others have not).[99–102]
[d]Estimated need for 15.9-mm wide/4-mm thick BPTB graft to equal 9-mm wide hamstring graft.[32]
[e]Despite similar initial fixation strengths, hamstring elongation at failure is double BPTB.[25]
ACL, anterior cruciate ligament.

Table 14.2. Advantages and disadvantages of autograft and allograft tissue

Autograft		*Allograft*	
Advantages	*Disadvantages*	*Advantages*	*Disadvantages*
No disease transmission	Increased operative time	Decreased operative time	Risk viral transmission
No immune reaction	Potential donor-site morbidity	No donor-site morbidity	Possible immune reaction[c]
Faster fibroblast repopulation	Exacerbate preexisting condition/process	No effect on underlying conditions	Slower fibroblast repopulation
Faster revascularization	Increased postoperative pain	Greater freedom in choice graft size	Slower revascularization
	Potentially unavailable[a]	Readily available[b]	Need reliable tissue bank
			Tissue processing: potential damage collagen/tensile strength

[a]Previous graft harvest, prior donor-site trauma, congenital dysplasia.
[b]Assumes tissue bank availability and adequate tissue quality.
[c]No clinical significance demonstrated at current time.

with no evidence of bone formation. Histology showed an indirect insertion pattern with absence of the normal fibrocartilage zone. Two other histologic studies revealed 50% to 60% reductions in the average load to failure, ultimate stress, and Young's modulus.[75,76] These same two studies also demonstrated decreases of 67% to 73% in the energy to failure of the reharvested tissue at 6 and 12 months in comparison to controls. The stiffness of the tissue was decreased by 27% but was not statistically significant. Clearly, based on these studies the reconstituted tissue is not satisfactory for revision surgery.

At the current time, there are two types of allograft tissues that most surgeons are using on a regular basis: Achilles tendon and patellar tendon with attached patella and tibial bone.[70] Manning et al[77] reported on the use of fascia lata allograft to reconstruct the ACL with 78% good to excellent results in 50 patients. This last tissue type is no longer under standard use due to the biomechanical findings described above. Most tissue-bank facilities are using fresh frozen tissue as opposed to freeze-dried or irradiated tissues. Radiation, while killing the human immunodeficiency and hepatitis viruses, has been shown to damage the collagen structure, weakening the tensile strength.[78] Currently the American Association of Tissue Banks has recommended a dose of 2.5 megarad (Mrad) of gamma irradiation. Fideler et al[79] demonstrated that a dose of 3 Mrad was needed to completely kill human immunodeficiency virus in human cadaveric specimens with known positive histories. Conway et al[80] demonstrated similar findings. Rasmussen et al[81] reported no difference in initial tensile strength between tissues irradiated with 4 Mrad and controls. Obviously, effective screening programs are required to prevent disease transmission. At the current time, using strict guidelines, the American Association of Tissue Banks estimates the risk of disease transmission to be less than 1 per 1,000,000.[82] Since the implementation of these screening criteria, there has not been a documented case of disease transmission from allograft tissue. The advantages and disadvantages of autogenous and allograft tissues are listed in Table 14.2.

SURGICAL TECHNIQUE

As described previously, careful preoperative assessment for etiology, history, and prior surgical procedures is the most important initial step in revision ACL surgery. Previous incisions, muscle atrophy, limited range of motion, retained hardware, bony loss, and concomitant ligamentous instability must be addressed both preoperatively and during the initial examination under anesthesia.

Examination Under Anesthesia

This is a crucial part of the procedure and should always be performed. Ideally, all findings during this step will have already been anticipated based on the preoperative evaluation in the office.

Range of Motion

Loss of extension suggesting possible arthrofibrosis should be addressed with a manipulation and application of a "drop-out" cast (Fig. 14.5). This cast contains a circumferential thigh component proximal to the superior pole of the patella and an additional posterior

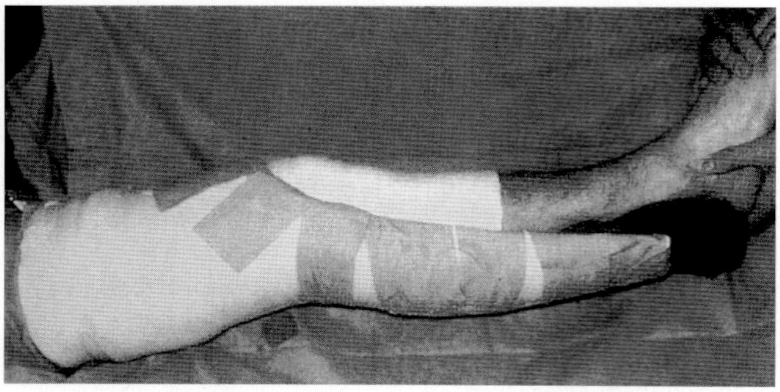

Figure 14.5. "Drop-out" cast producing a hyperextension force. The cast is removed the next day (18 hours postoperatively) and range of motion initiated. Significant pressure can be applied to the posterior calf and Achilles region. These regions should be observed closely for the development of skin and soft tissue necrosis.

component (posterior one-half) distally. Extra padding is applied at the most proximal posterior portion and suprapatellar pouch regions. The knee is sequentially forced into hyperextension by the addition of surgical towels between the distal calf, Achilles tendon and heel, and the inner surface of the distal cast. The patient is maintained in the hospital overnight as there can be significant pain as well as the possibility of posterior skin necrosis. The amount of hyperextension applied is easily modified through the number of towels distally. The cast is removed after approximately 18 hours and range of motion therapy initiated as well as application of a $3 \times 10 = 0$" brace (Instrument Makar, Inc., Okemos, MI) and/or dynamic splint as needed. The former brace applies a hyperextension force three times per day for 10 minutes each time. The latter splints work over longer periods of time and would be required for more significant flexion contractures. Terminal flexion is easier to maintain. Loss of motion (side to side extension disparity >5 degrees and flexion disparity >20 degrees) is a contraindication to revision reconstruction, and treatment for these problems should be performed as a separate operative procedure. Once motion has been returned and adequate muscular strengthening has been performed, the actual reconstructive procedure can be performed.

Associated Ligamentous Injuries

If full range of motion is obtained, examination should proceed to assessment for ligamentous damage. Standard examination includes the Lachman's maneuver, pivot-shift test, anterior/posterior drawer testing at 90 degrees, evaluation of medial femoral condyle to tibial plateau step-off at 90 degrees, and assessment for rotational stability at 30 degrees and 90 degrees of flexion. Care should be taken to reduce the tibia anteriorly if underlying posterior tibial subluxation is suspected. Posterior tibial subluxation can mask posterolateral corner instability. These associated ligamentous findings should be addressed either as a staged procedure or simultaneously at the time of ACL reconstruction.

Skin Incisions

The final portion of the examination under anesthesia should be to check the skin and note the previous operative incisions. These will have to be incorporated into the planned approach if the incisions are within 5 to 7 cm of the area of concern. Avoidance of narrow skin bridges prevents subsequent tissue necrosis.

Technical Considerations

Hardware Removal

Preoperative radiographs and the previous operative note(s) should be assessed. The appropriate instrumentation for hardware removal should be available. Tibial screws are typically more accessible and may be removed through a small portion of the prior incision. Femoral interference screws placed arthroscopically with an anatomic tunnel location should be removed if possible (Fig. 14.6). In some circumstances the hardware can be maintained in place and the tunnel placed adjacent to the metal (Fig. 14.7). For example, if a two-incision technique was used for femoral fixation during the prior operative procedure, or if the previous tunnels were placed incorrectly, or if it is deemed possible to miss the previous screw(s), consideration can be given to retaining the hardware. The graft can be placed adjacent to the hardware in this situation, avoiding a large bony defect and the need for bone grafting.[83] As with any hardware removal, care should be taken to clear all bone and soft tissue from around the implant. When removing screws specifically, it is imperative that the screwdriver is embedded firmly within the screw head to prevent metal stripping. One helpful technique is to gently tap the end of the screwdriver with a mallet while simultaneously twisting the screwdriver. This maintains screwdriver-to-screw contact while also loosening the screw from its bony fixation. Metal stripping prevents removal of the screw without associated removal of bone producing large defects requiring bone grafting.

Prosthetic Ligament Removal

These ACL failures should be viewed as a separate group with a complete host of important, unique preoperative considerations. The type of synthetic ligament as well as operative technique should be clearly understood. Operative details may be difficult to find. As these ligaments have demonstrated widespread failure, the techniques associated with their use have become obsolete.

Permanent implants (Gore-Tex or Dacron [Stryker]) and carbon fiber implants should be removed en bloc, avoiding piecemeal removal due to the potential risk of

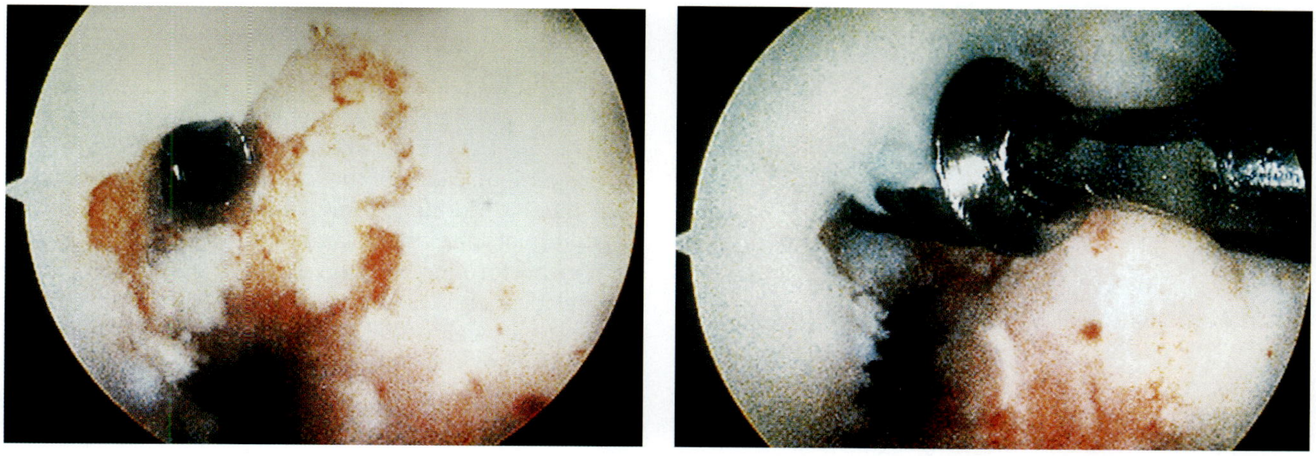

A B

Figure 14.6. **A:** Arthroscopic view (anterolateral portal) of a femoral interference screw in place during a revision procedure and **(B)** during removal. In this case the screw was near the desired tunnel position and would interfere with the revision procedure if retained. (Orientation: the femoral surface at the posterior aspect of the intercondylar notch is at the top of the arthroscopic view.)

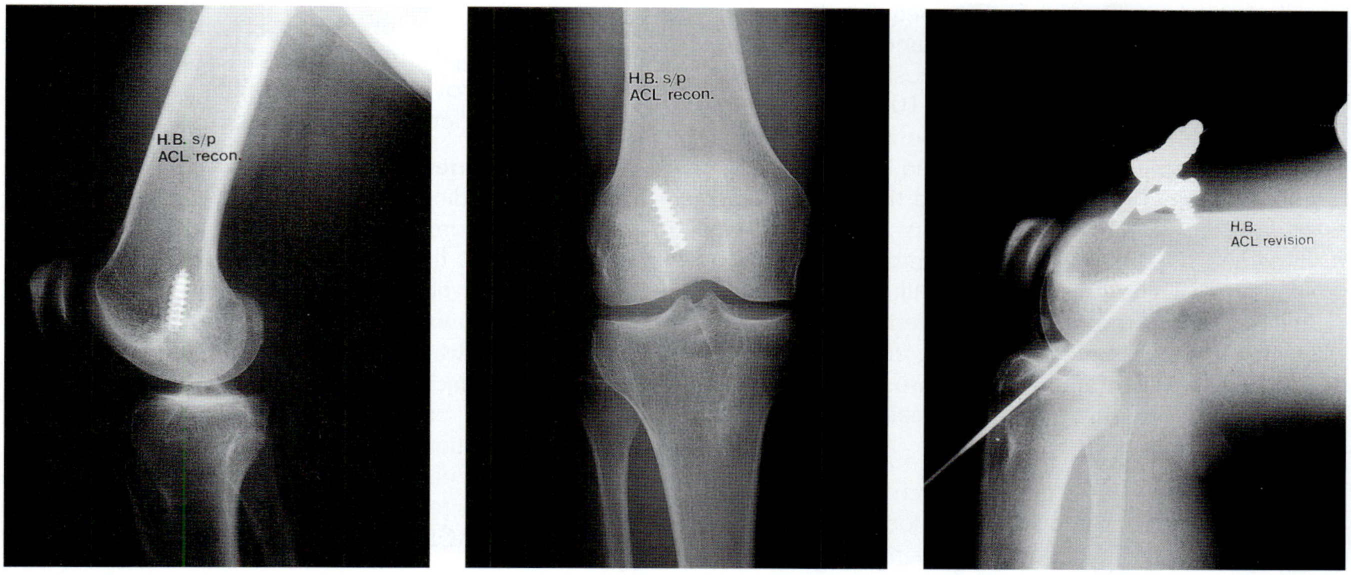

A B C

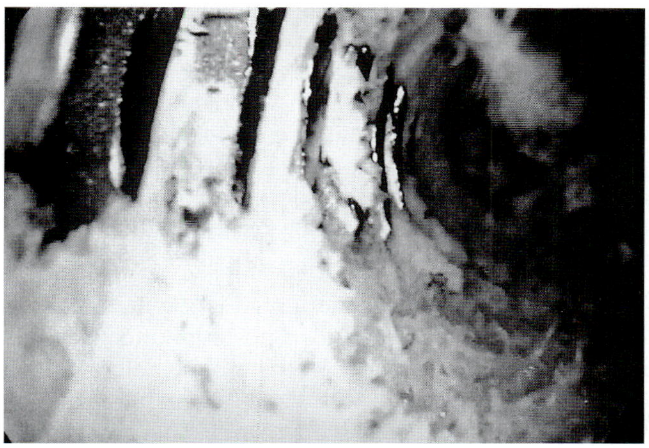

D

Figure 14.7. **A:** Lateral radiograph demonstrating anterior femoral tunnel placement. **B:** On the corresponding anteroposterior (AP) view the interference screw appears to be in the appropriate position. **C:** Intraoperative lateral radiograph during revision surgery. The femoral tunnel guide pin was easily placed posterior to the previous interference screw. Note the knee is at about 85 degrees flexion, causing a slight curvature in the guide pin. **D:** Intraoperative view of a bone tunnel using the arthroscope. In this case it was possible to retain the hardware, placing the tunnel adjacent to the previous interference screw.

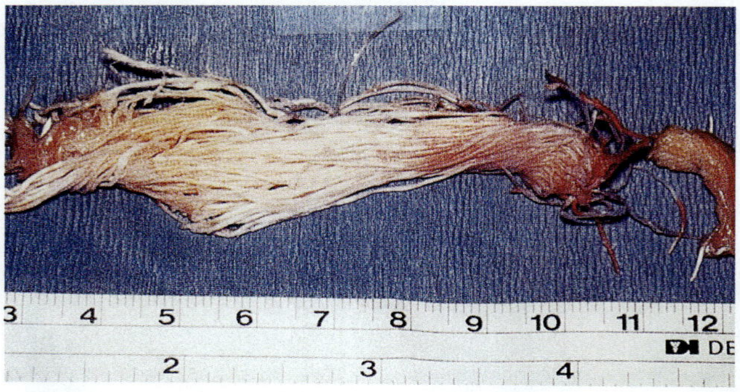

Figure 14.8. The appearance of a failed Gore-Tex ACL graft retrieved at the time of revision ACL reconstruction. Note that the graft has been removed en bloc, avoiding particle formation that can lead to synovitis, sterile effusions, and possible articular cartilage degeneration. (From ref. 103, with permission.)

particle formation (Fig. 14.8). This requires the avoidance of drills and arthroscopic knives and punches. Usually the extraarticular portion of the prosthesis is grasped with a Kocher clamp and a gouge (8–10 mm) is inserted into the tunnel. This serves to release the fibers at the tunnel wall/ligament interface.[7,16] The ligament is then removed by winding the graft around the clamp in circular fashion. Additional material is removed using curettes and a pituitary grasper as needed. As stated previously, LADs are fixed at one end, and the details of the operative report are important to determine where fixation occurred. Once again, en bloc resection should be performed and use of arthroscopic resectors avoided, producing minimal debridement.

Revision Notchplasty

The importance of intercondylar notch size and shape as well as its relationship to tunnel location has been clearly delineated.[13,84,85] An MRI obtained prior to graft failure will demonstrate signal change anteriorly as the knee is moved into extension. This finding represents impingement on the anterosuperior notch.[86–89] It is important to obtain a lateral radiograph in maximal knee extension to determine whether graft impingement on the intercondylar notch led to the reconstructive failure.[90] Howell and Taylor[90] clearly demonstrated that increased failure rates occur when any portion of the tibial tunnel is located anterior to the slope of the intercondylar roof. Abnormal tunnel location and subsequent notchplasty to remove the impinging bone may lead to later notch regrowth or overgrowth followed by impingement and failure.

Knowledge of potential sites of graft impingement is important when performing a notchplasty. The graft can impinge at the anterosuperior roof and the medial wall of the lateral femoral condyle. In addition, the anterior aspect of the femoral tunnel, posterior aspects of the tibial tunnel, and tibial spines are potential sites of graft impingement. Many of the standard anatomic landmarks are missing during revision surgery, leading to abnormal tunnel placement and excessive bone removal. When performing revision ACL surgery, correct tibial tunnel location should be carefully planned, the specifics of which are delineated in the next section. Olson et al[91] demonstrated the importance of tibial tunnel location. Following tibial tunnel placement, the "impingement test" should be performed with tunnel expanders (Instrument Makar, Inc., Okemos, MI); this is a helpful way to assess for potential graft impingement (Fig. 14.9).[92]

One additional benefit of an adequate notchplasty, particularly during revision ACL surgery, is improved visualization of the posterior arch of the intercondylar notch or the "over-the-top" position. It is important to clearly define the junction between the posterior bone of the notch and the fascia on the posterior surface of the femur. A probe or curette can be used to verify the "over-the-top" position (Fig. 14.10A). Notchplasty should also improve visualization of the previous femoral tunnel and interference screw locations (Fig. 14.10B).

Tunnel Placement

Preoperative radiographs and other imaging modalities provide vital information for tunnel placement. As outlined previously, these studies should alert the surgeon to the potential need for bone grafting as well as the most suitable tunnel location. Once again, if previous tunnel and hardware were in an extremely abnormal location simply placing the tunnels in a more ideal location will suffice. Similarly, revision of two-incision-type ACL reconstructions using a one-incision technique can take advantage of the different femoral tunnel angles created by each technique.[12] The femoral tunnel from a two-incision ACL enters the intercondylar notch at a more acute angle. There is such a large disparity in tunnel location between the two techniques that there is typically no need to remove the hardware or tissue from the failed reconstruction.

Commonly the previous reconstruction was performed through a one-incision technique and the tunnel location is nearly anatomic or anatomic. Tunnel placement in these cases can be difficult. The decision in these circumstances should center on whether the tunnel is at the optimal position or just anterior or posterior to this position.

Tibial Tunnel. If the tibial tunnel is slightly anterior, the tunnel should be expanded posteriorly to the optimal position. This typically leaves a bony defect anteriorly, which can be filled with either a separate block of bone graft or impacted with bone graft. The graft is then

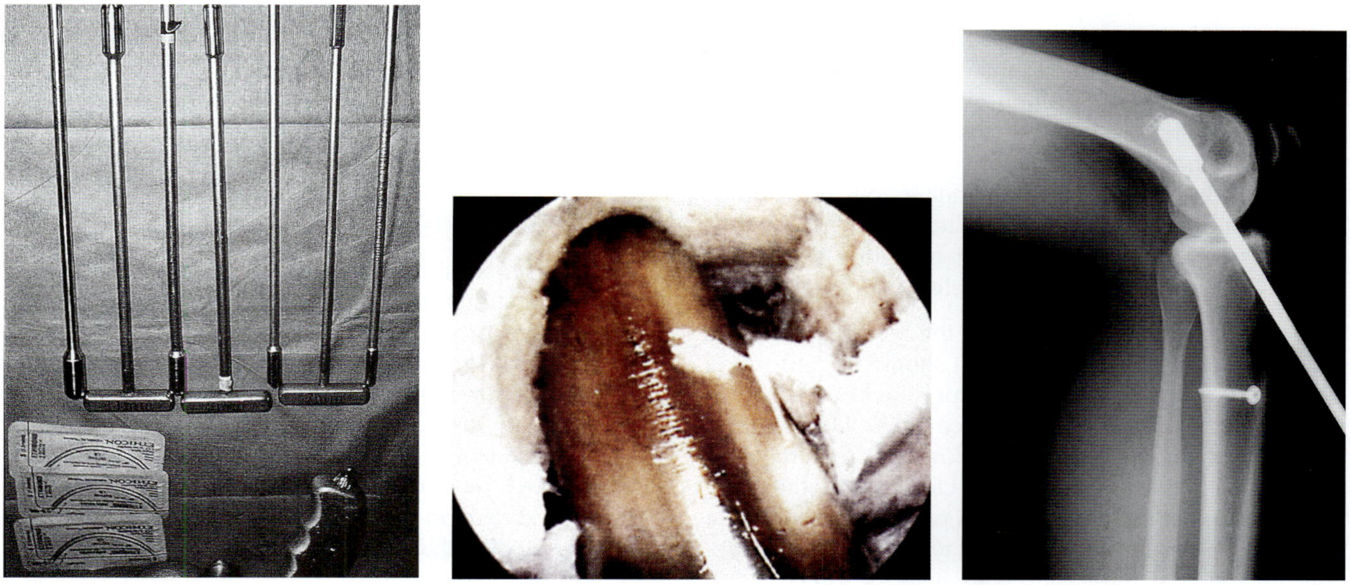

A B C

Figure 14.9. **A:** Lanny Johnson tunnel dilator set (Instrument Makar, Inc., Okemos, MI). A wide variety of sizes are available with either a smooth or serrated tip. These implants allow removal of previous graft tissue while maintaining bone. **B:** Arthroscopic view (anterolateral portal) demonstrating placement of tunnel dilator into femoral tunnel (orientation: top of dilator at entrance to femoral tunnel). **C:** Intraoperative lateral radiograph verifying proper tunnel position using a tunnel dilator with the knee flexed at 90 degrees. Note: Previous hardware (Endobutton, Acufex Inc., Mansfield, OH, and distal post) used in primary ACL with hamstring tendon graft). (From ref. 103, with permission.)

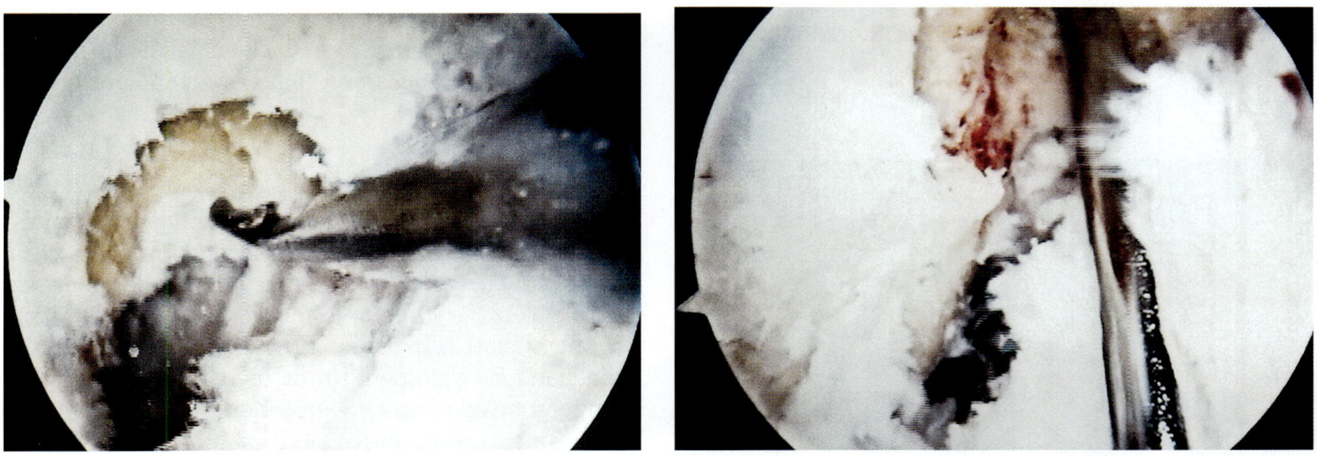

A B

Figure 14.10. **A:** Arthroscopic view (anterolateral portal) demonstrating a curette at the "over-the-top" position (posterior intercondylar notch). Note the fascial layer on the posterior surface of the bone, an excellent landmark to verify proper tunnel position. The original graft (which was malpositioned) is superolateral to the curette. **B:** Same case. Femoral guidewire has been placed through the previously created starting point at the posterior aspect of the intercondylar notch (1 o'clock position).

placed in the desired position. If the tunnel is slightly posterior, the reverse can be performed. Large, capacious defects encountered at the optimal position should be treated with bone grafting and a staged procedure under most circumstances. If the defect is larger than desired but the overall diameter is about 12 to 14 mm, consideration can be given to simultaneous bone grafting and placement of the graft. Alternatively, if allograft BPTB tissue is used, an appropriately sized tibial bone block can be created to fill the defect.

Femoral Tunnel. As above, if the femoral tunnel is slightly anterior, tunnel expansion should be performed posteriorly (Fig. 14.7). An attempt should be made to use a larger ACL bone block. Once again there are size limitations, and excessive bone loss will require bone grafting, which can be difficult. Unlike with the tibial tunnel, if the femoral tunnel is too posterior, a complete loss of all posterior tunnel continuity, or a "blowout" occurs. In the past these situations have been converted to a standard two-incision reconstructive procedure or an over-the-top technique. Alternatively, the Endobutton System (Acufex, Mansfield, OH) can be utilized to provide femoral fixation in the case of poor fixation or a violated posterior femoral cortex.

Bone Loss

Bone resorption or tunnel expansion should be addressed preoperatively with radiographs and either MRI or CT scan (Fig. 14.11). These studies should give the surgeon an idea as to the extent of bone loss and the type of tissue within the tunnel. Significant defects and/or large, capacious tunnels encountered intraoperatively should be treated with autologous bone grafting (Fig. 14.12). The actual reconstruction should be performed following radiographic demonstration of graft incorporation within the tunnel, which usually occurs at about 12 to 16 weeks (Fig. 14.13). Clearly, appropriate preoperative patient education of the possible need for a staged treatment plan is necessary. The preoperative imaging studies are helpful in this regard.

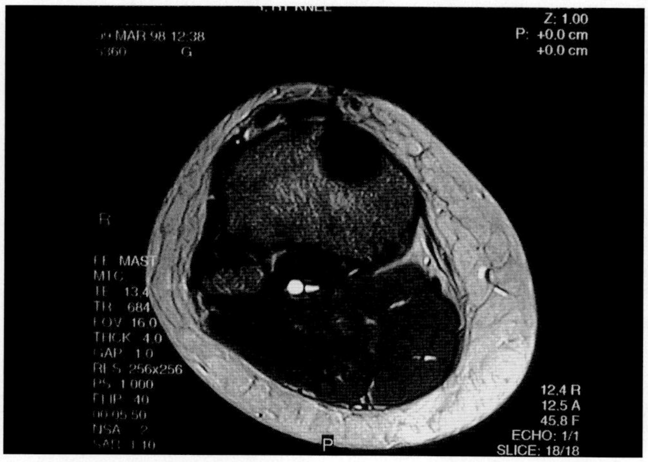

Figure 14.11. Transverse T1-weighted MR image demonstrating tunnel widening and bony resorption.

Graft Fixation

Fixation is most important during the initial 6 to 8 weeks after reconstruction and represents the weak link in reconstructive procedures during the immediate postoperative period. Fixation strength is dependent on contact surface area with the graft, bone quality (graft and tunnel bone), tissue type, and the fixation device (Fig. 14.3). Reliance on one particular method of graft fixation should be avoided. Flexibility in operative techniques and fixation devices is a must during these cases. Despite studies that demonstrate a clear superiority of interference screw fixation over suture techniques, there will be scenarios where interference screw fixation is compromised (Fig. 14.14). Alternative fixation methods include staple fixation into a bony trough (BPTB) or directly onto the soft tissue (Achilles, quadriceps, or hamstring tendon), suturing over a post, screw and spiked washer, and Hughston button or Endobutton. The use of bioscrew fixation is becoming popular but should be used when good tunnel and graft bone quality is present. In some instances multiple interference screws can be used to fill bony defects and supplement fixation. Bioscrews may be a helpful adjunct to fixation in these cases, avoiding the later problem of multiple retained metal interference screws. Once again, it is imperative that the primary surgeon be well acquainted with these alternative techniques and that the equipment be readily available.

Secondary Restraints

As stated previously, concern for secondary restraints is critical to a successful outcome in revision surgery. The preoperative workup and examination under anesthesia should alert the surgeon to these issues. Appropriate instrumentation and tissues should be available to allow simultaneous treatment of the associated pathology, or the surgeon can stage the procedures appropriately. The decision should be based on the surgeon's experience, operative staff availability, and individual patient issues such as age, activity level, job status and type, family support, and financial constraints.

Varus instability, if present, is usually associated with posterolateral rotatory instability. If a true lateral thrust is demonstrated preoperatively by the patient, consideration should be given to performance of a high tibial osteotomy (opening or closing wedge). This can be per-

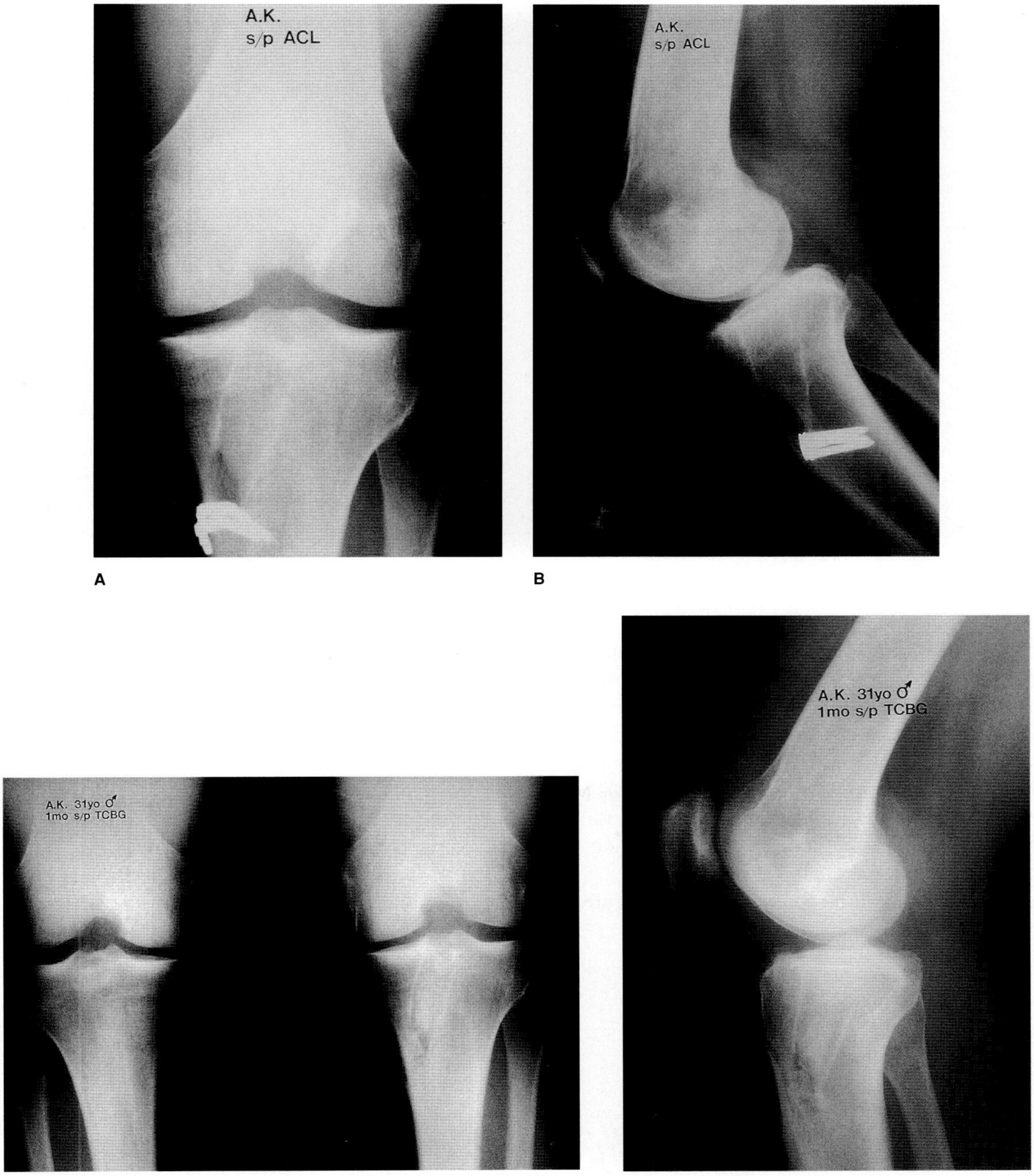

Figure 14.12. The 45-degree PA weight-bearing view **(A)** and lateral radiograph **(B)** demonstrating bony resorption and tibial tunnel widening after a primary ACL reconstruction (BPTB). Bilateral 45° PA weight-bearing view **(C)** and lateral radiograph **(D)** 1 month following curettage and bone grafting to a large tibial tunnel defect.

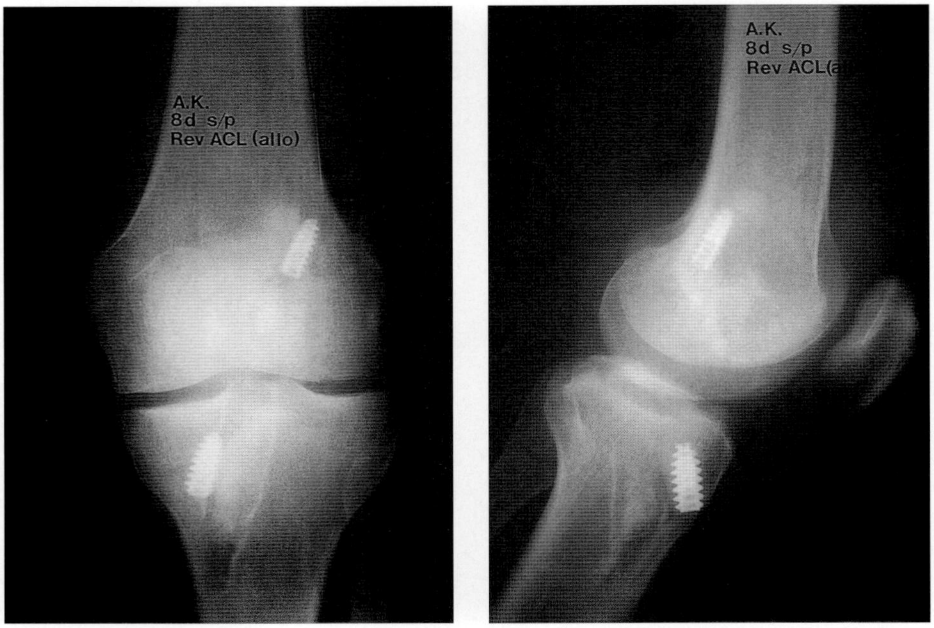

Figure 14.13. AP (A) and lateral (B) radiographs 8 days after a staged revision ACL reconstruction. Note that bone grafting the previous tibial tunnel has allowed for complete healing of the bony defect. The new tibial bone block and interference screw have been placed anteromedial to the bone grafted region.

formed as part of a staged reconstruction or simultaneously using allograft tissue for ACL reconstruction. Numerous techniques have been devised for posterolateral corner reconstruction, including reefing and/or autograft or allograft reconstructive procedures. Concomitant lateral collateral ligament injury should be treated along with the posterolateral corner reconstruction, if identified, but it usually occurs following a true knee dislocation from a significant traumatic event.

Valgus instability should be determined preoperatively as well, and can be associated with an isolated medial collateral ligament injury or with prior menisectomy. The stabilizing role of the medial meniscus should not be overlooked. If anteromedial rotatory instability is present, it should be addressed with a simultaneous or staged medial meniscus reconstruction. Most medial collateral ligament or posterior oblique ligament injuries are chronic at the time of revision surgery and can be treated with a reefing procedure, insertional advancement, or, rarely, allograft vs. autograft reconstruction.

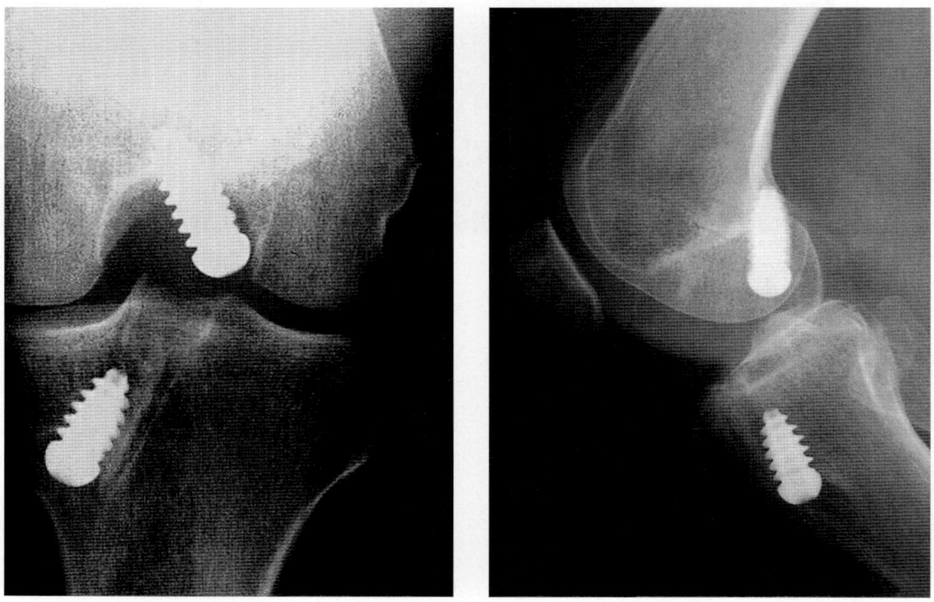

Figure 14.14. AP (A) and lateral (B) radiographs demonstrating loss of fixation in femoral tunnel that occurred during the initial postoperative period. The screw has fallen inferiorly into the posterior aspect of the intercondylar notch. During the revision procedure it was noted that the bone graft had displaced inferiorly as well.

Chondral damage can also contribute to operative failure and, if large enough, to instability. These problems have to be addressed. Depending on the technique used and the size of the lesion, this pathology can be treated either simultaneously or in a staged fashion. Similarly, meniscal tears should be repaired at all costs, avoiding the destabilizing effect of total or subtotal menisectomy. Alternatively, the menisectomy and reconstruction can be performed, and the patient told of the potential problems and observed for the development of symptoms. Once again, the meniscal reconstruction can be performed at a later time.

Rehabilitation

In contrast to the primary ACL reconstruction, revision cases should be customized based on surgical and patient variables. In other words, the patient should not be rehabilitated according to a standard protocol.

Important surgical factors that determine the postoperative rehabilitative regimen include graft source (autograft or allograft); graft type (BPTB, Achilles, hamstring, or quadriceps tendon); fixation technique and strength; and alignment and concomitant pathology, which includes treated and untreated conditions. The patient variables are equally if not more important than the above factors and include age, activity level, elasticity, weight, work demands, reliability, and motivation. Both sets of variables should determine postoperative weight-bearing status, bracing (type and length of time), range of motion (degrees, timing, active, active-assisted and passive), and time to return to full activity.

CONCLUSION

As more surgeons become skilled at performing primary ACL reconstructions, there will be an increase in the total number of reconstructions. A subsequent increase in the number of failures has been, and will be, the natural progression.

The surgeon should perform a thorough history and examination as well as order the appropriate imaging studies to delineate the true etiology of the failure. The surgeon should also have the experience, comfort, and ability to perform the appropriate procedures required to treat all secondary restraint and associated pathology that can lead to recurrent surgical failures. Further, as more surgeons become skilled at the one-incision, arthroscopic-assisted ACL, flexibility in treating the failed reconstruction will be required. Many of the bridges used to perform a primary ACL reconstruction will have been "burned." Preoperative and intraoperative decisions will be required that lead to the use of alternative techniques, fixation methods, and rehabilitative protocols. Finally, before embarking on these challenging cases, it will be important to decide whether simultaneous or staged procedures will be performed. Once again, surgical and patient-related issues specific to each case should determine this decision.

Recent follow-up studies have demonstrated improved objective and subjective criteria following revision ACL surgery.[93,94] However, the overall outcome using the International Knee Documentation Committee guidelines is less than that for primary ACL reconstructions, and this fact should be related to the patient preoperatively. Many factors probably account for this finding. The most significant factor may be the associated articular and meniscal cartilage injuries as well as patholaxity commonly seen in this patient population. The patient, if adequately warned preoperatively, will have a higher level of satisfaction. These operative failures are challenging but can be quite interesting. As with all surgical procedures, if correct preoperative planning and patient education occurs followed by a technically sound operation, a successful outcome can be achieved.

References

1. O'Donoghue DH, Frank GR, Jeter GL, et al. Repair and reconstruction of the anterior cruciate ligament in dogs. Factors influencing long-term results. *J Bone Joint Surg* 1971;53A:710–718.
2. Dejour H, Walch G, Deschamps G, et al. Arthrosis of the knee in chronic anterior laxity. *Rev Chir Orthop* 1987;73:157–170.
3. Funk FJJ. Osteoarthritis of the knee following ligamentous injury. *Clin Orthop* 1983;172:154–157.
4. Kannus P, Jarvinen M. Posttraumatic anterior cruciate ligament insufficiency as a cause of osteoarthritis in a knee joint. *Clin Rheumatol* 1989;8:251–260.
5. Daniel DM, Stone ML, Dobson BE, et al. Fate of the ACL injured patient: a prospective outcome study. Paper presented at the 19th Annual American Orthopaedic Society for Sports Medicine meeting, 1993, Sun Valley, ID.
6. Brandt KD, Braunstein EM, Visco DM, et al. Anterior (cranial) cruciate ligament transection in the dog: a bona fide model of osteoarthritis, not merely of cartilage injury and repair. *J Rheumatol* 1991;18:436–446.
7. Clatworthy M, Amendola A. The anterior cruciate ligament and arthritis. *Clin Sports Med* 1999;18:173–198, vii.
8. Greis PE, Johnson DL, Fu FH. Revision anterior cruciate ligament surgery: causes of graft failure and technical considerations of revision surgery. *Clin Sports Med* 1993;12:839–852.
9. Greis PE, Steadman JR. Revision of failed prosthetic anterior cruciate ligament reconstruction. *Clin Orthop* 1996;325:78–90.
10. Johnson DL, Coen MJ. Revision ACL surgery. Etiology,

indications, techniques, and results. *Am J Knee Surg* 1995;8:155–167.

11. Carson EW, Simonian PT, Wickiewicz TL, et al. Revision anterior cruciate ligament reconstruction. *Instr Course Lect* 1998;47:361–368.
12. Safran MR, Harner CD. Technical considerations of revision anterior cruciate ligament surgery. *Clin Orthop* 1996;325:50–64.
13. Hefzy MS, Grood ES. Sensitivity of insertion locations on length patterns of anterior cruciate ligament fibers. *J Biomech Eng* 1986;108:73–82.
14. Henning CE, Lynch MA, Glick KRJ. An in vivo strain gage study of elongation of the anterior cruciate ligament. *Am J Sports Med* 1985;13:22–26.
15. Jackson DW, Gasser SI. Tibial tunnel placement in ACL reconstruction. *Arthroscopy* 1994;10:124–131.
16. Woo SL, Livesay GA, Engle C. Biomechanics of the human anterior cruciate ligament. ACL structure and role in knee motion. Orthop Rev 1992;21:835–842.
17. Livesay GA, Rudy TW, Woo SL, et al. Evaluation of the effect of joint constraints on the in situ force distribution in the anterior cruciate ligament. *J Orthop Res* 1997; 15:278–284.
18. Marder RA. The failed ACL reconstruction. In: Zarins B, Marder RA, eds. *Revision of Failed Arthroscopic and Ligament Surgery*. Malden, MA: Blackwell Science, 1998:1–15.
19. Clancy WGJ, Nelson DA, Reider B, et al. Anterior cruciate ligament reconstruction using one-third of the patellar ligament, augmented by extra-articular tendon transfers. *J Bone Joint Surg* 1982;64:352–359.
20. Yoshiya S, Andrish JT, Manley MT, et al. Graft tension in anterior cruciate ligament reconstruction. An in vivo study in dogs. *Am J Sports Med* 1987;15:464–470.
21. Gertel TH, Lew WD, Lewis JL, et al. Effect of anterior cruciate ligament graft tensioning direction, magnitude, and flexion angle on knee biomechanics. *Am J Sports Med* 1993;21:572–581.
22. Nabors ED, Richmond JC, Vannah WM, et al. Anterior cruciate ligament graft tensioning in full extension. *Am J Sports Med* 1995;23:488–492.
23. Kurosaka M, Yoshiya S, Andrish JT. A biomechanical comparison of different surgical techniques of graft fixation in anterior cruciate ligament reconstruction. *Am J Sports Med* 1987;15:225–229.
24. Matthews LS, Lawrence SJ, Yahiro MA, et al. Fixation strengths of patellar tendon–bone grafts. *Arthroscopy* 1993;9:76–81.
25. Steiner ME, Hecker AT, Brown CH Jr, et al. Anterior cruciate ligament graft fixation. Comparison of hamstring and patellar tendon grafts. *Am J Sports Med* 1994;22:240–246.
26. Noyes FR, Butler DL, Grood ES, et al. Biomechanical analysis of human ligament grafts used in knee-ligament repairs and reconstructions. *J Bone Joint Surg* 1984; 66A:344–352.
27. Shapiro JD, Cohn BT, Jackson DW, et al. The biomechanical effects of geometric configuration of bone-tendon-bone autografts in anterior cruciate ligament reconstruction. *Arthroscopy* 1992;8:453–458.
28. Butler JC, Branch TP, Hutton WC. Optimal graft fixation—the effect of gap size and screw size on bone plug fixation in ACL reconstruction. *Arthroscopy* 1994;10: 524–529.
29. Rupp S, Seil R, Krauss PW, et al. Cortical versus cancellous interference fixation for bone–patellar tendon–bone grafts. *Arthroscopy* 1998;14:484–488.
30. Ishibashi Y, Rudy TW, Livesay GA, et al. The effect of anterior cruciate ligament graft fixation site at the tibia on knee stability: evaluation using a robotic testing system. *Arthroscopy* 1997;13:177–182.
31. Robertson DB, Daniel DM, Biden E. Soft tissue fixation to bone. *Am J Sports Med* 1986;14:398–403.
32. Brown CHJ, Steiner ME, Carson EW. The use of hamstring tendons for anterior cruciate ligament reconstruction. Technique and results. *Clin Sports Med* 1993;12: 723–756.
33. Pena F, Grontvedt T, Brown GA, et al. Comparison of failure strength between metallic and absorbable interference screws. Influence of insertion torque, tunnel-bone block gap, bone mineral density, and interference. *Am J Sports Med* 1996;24:329–334.
34. Johnson LL, vanDyk GE. Metal and biodegradable interference screws: comparison of failure strength. *Arthroscopy* 1996;12:452–456.
35. Corsetti JR, Jackson DW. Failure of anterior cruciate ligament reconstruction: the biologic basis. *Clin Orthop* 1996;325:42–49.
36. Jackson DW, Grood ES, Cohn BT, et al. The effects of in situ freezing on the anterior cruciate ligament. An experimental study in goats. *J Bone Joint Surg* 1991; 73A:201–213.
37. Arnoczky SP, Tarvin GB, Marshall JL. Anterior cruciate ligament replacement using patellar tendon. An evaluation of graft revascularization in the dog. *J Bone Joint Surg* 1982;64A:217–224.
38. Amiel D, Kleiner JB, Roux RD, et al. The phenomenon of "ligamentization": anterior cruciate ligament reconstruction with autogenous patellar tendon. *J Orthop Res* 1986;4:162–172.
39. Oakes BW. Collagen structure in the normal ACL and in ACL graft. In: Jackson DW, Arnoczky SP, eds. *The Anterior Cruciate Ligament: Current and Future Concepts*. New York: Raven Press, 1993:209.
40. Jaureguito JW, Paulos LE. Why grafts fail. *Clin Orthop* 1996;325:25–41.
41. Fahey M, Indelicato PA. Bone tunnel enlargement after anterior cruciate ligament replacement. *Am J Sports Med* 1994;22:410–414.
42. Shino K, Inoue M, Horibe S, et al. Surface blood flow and histology of human anterior cruciate ligament allografts. *Arthroscopy* 1991;7:171–176.

43. Berchuck M, Andriacchi TP, Bach BR, et al. Gait adaptations by patients who have a deficient anterior cruciate ligament. J Bone Joint Surg 1990;72A:871–877.

44. Timoney JM, Inman WS, Quesada PM, et al. Return of normal gait patterns after anterior cruciate ligament reconstruction. *Am J Sports Med* 1993;21(6):887–889.

45. Shelbourne KD, Johnson GE. Outpatient surgical management of arthrofibrosis after anterior cruciate ligament surgery. *Am J Sports Med* 1994;22:192–197.

46. Jackson DW, Schaefer RK. Cyclops syndrome: loss of extension following intra-articular anterior cruciate ligament reconstruction. *Arthroscopy* 1990;6:171–178.

47. Friedman MJ. Prosthetic anterior cruciate ligament. *Clin Sports Med* 1991;10:499–513.

48. McCarthy DM. Prosthetic replacement for the anterior cruciate ligament. In: Jackson DW, Arnoczky SP, Woo SL, eds. *The Anterior Cruciate Ligament: Current and Future Concepts.* New York: Raven Press, 1993:343.

49. Steadman JR, Seemann MD, Hutton KS. Revision ligament reconstruction of failed prosthetic anterior cruciate ligaments. *Instr Course Lect* 1995;44:417–429.

50. Gillquist J, Odensten M. Reconstruction of old anterior cruciate ligament tears with a Dacron prosthesis. A prospective study. *Am J Sports Med* 1993;21:358–366.

51. Lopez-Vazquez E, Juan JA, Vila E, et al. Reconstruction of the anterior cruciate ligament with a Dacron prosthesis. *J Bone Joint Surg* 1991;73A:1294–1300.

52. Lukianov AV, Richmond JC, Barrett GR, et al. A multicenter study on the results of anterior cruciate ligament reconstruction using a Dacron ligament prosthesis in "salvage" cases. *Am J Sports Med* 1989;17:380–385.

53. Richmond JC, Manseau CJ, Patz R, et al. Anterior cruciate reconstruction using a Dacron ligament prosthesis. A long-term study. *Am J Sports Med* 1992;20:24–28.

54. Wilk RM, Richmond JC. Dacron ligament reconstruction for chronic anterior cruciate ligament insufficiency. *Am J Sports Med* 1993;21:374–379.

55. Paulos LE, Rosenberg TD, Grewe SR, et al. The Gore-Tex anterior cruciate ligament prosthesis. A long-term followup. *Am J Sports Med* 1992;20:246–252.

56. Denti M, Bigoni M, Dodaro G, et al. Long-term results of the Leeds-Keio anterior cruciate ligament reconstruction. *Knee Surg Sports Traumatol Arthrosc* 1995;3:75–77.

57. Fujikawa K, Iseki F, Seedhom BB. Arthroscopy after anterior cruciate reconstruction with the Leeds-Keio ligament. *J Bone Joint Surg* 1989;71B:566–570.

58. Fujikawa K, Iseki F. Anterior cruciate ligament reconstruction with the Leeds-Keio artificial ligament. *Bull Hosp Jt Dis Orthop Inst* 1991;51:140–154.

59. Schinchelm K, Rogers GJ, Milthorpe BK, et al. Autograft and Leeds-Keio reconstructions of the ovine anterior cruciate ligament. *Clin Orthop* 1991;267:278–293.

60. Strover AE, Firer P. The use of carbon fiber implants in anterior cruciate ligament surgery. *Clin Orthop* 1985;196:88–98.

61. Weiss AB, Blazina ME, Goldstein AR, et al. Ligament replacement with an absorbable copolymer carbon fiber scaffold—early clinical experience. *Clin Orthop* 1985;196:77–85.

62. Goodship AE, Wilcock SA, Shah JS. The development of tissue around various prosthetic implants used as replacements for ligaments and tendons. *Clin Orthop* 1985;196:61–68.

63. Howard CB, Tayton KJ, Gibbs A. The response of human tissues to carbon reinforced epoxy resin. *J Bone Joint Surg* 1985;67B:656–658.

64. Parsons JR, Bhayani S, Alexander H, et al. Carbon fiber debris within the synovial joint. A time-dependent mechanical and histologic study. *Clin Orthop* 1985;196:69–76.

65. Mendes DG, Soudry M, Angel D, et al. Carbon reconstruction in the anterior cruciate deficient knee. *Orthopedics* 1985;8:1244–1248.

66. Rushton N, Dandy DJ, Naylor CP. The clinical, arthroscopic and histological findings after replacement of the anterior cruciate ligament with carbon-fibre. *J Bone Joint Surg* 1983;65B:308–309.

67. Kennedy JC. Application of prosthetics to anterior cruciate ligament reconstruction and repair. *Clin Orthop* 1983;172:125–128.

68. Fowler PJ, Capra SW Jr. Anterior cruciate ligament reconstruction with the Kennedy ligament augmentation device. In: Scott WN, ed. *Ligament and Extensor Mechanism Injuries of the Knee: Diagnosis and Treatment* St. Louis: Mosby Year Book, 1991:301.

69. Roth JH, Kennedy JC, Lockstadt H, et al. Polypropylene braid augmented and nonaugmented intraarticular anterior cruciate ligament reconstruction. *Am J Sports Med* 1985;13:321–336.

70. Ritchie JR, Parker RD. Graft selection in anterior cruciate ligament revision surgery. *Clin Orthop* 1996;325:65–77.

71. Wirth CJ, Kohn D. Revision anterior cruciate ligament surgery: experience from Germany. *Clin Orthop* 1996;325:110–115.

72. Kartus J, Stener S, Lindahl S, et al. Ipsi- or contralateral patellar tendon graft in anterior cruciate ligament revision surgery. A comparison of two methods. *Am J Sports Med* 1998;26:499–504.

73. Uribe JW, Hechtman KS, Zvijac JE, et al. Revision anterior cruciate ligament surgery: experience from Miami. *Clin Orthop* 1996;91–99.

74. Liu SH, Hang DW, Gentili A, et al. MRI and morphology of the insertion of the patellar tendon after graft harvesting. *J Bone Joint Surg* 1996;78B:823–826.

75. LaPrade RF, Hamilton CD, Montgomery RD, et al. The reharvested central third of the patellar tendon. A histologic and biomechanical analysis. *Am J Sports Med* 1997;25:779–785.

76. Proctor CS, Jackson DW, Simon TM. Characterization of the repair tissue after removal of the central one-third of the patellar ligament. An experimental study in a goat model. *J Bone Joint Surg* 1997;79A:997–1006.

77. Manning JB, Meyers JF, Caspari RB, et al. Arthroscopic intraarticular reconstruction of the anterior cruciate ligament using lyophilized allograft ligament stabilizers. Paper presented at the annual meeting of the American Academy of Orthopaedic Surgeons, 1989, Las Vegas.

78. Gibbons MJ, Butler DL, Grood ES, et al. Effects of gamma irradiation on the initial mechanical and material properties of goat bone-patellar tendon-bone allografts. *J Orthop Res* 1991;9:209–218.

79. Fideler BM, Vangsness CTJ, Moore T, et al. Effects of gamma irradiation on the human immunodeficiency virus. A study in frozen human bone–patellar ligament–bone grafts obtained from infected cadavera. *J Bone Joint Surg* 1994;76A:1032–1035.

80. Conway B, Tomford WW, Hirsch MS, et al. Effect of gamma irradiation on HIV-1 in a bone allograft model. *Trans Orthop Res Soc* 1990;15:225(abst).

81. Rasmussen TJ, Feder SM, Butler DL, et al. The effects of 4 Mrad of gamma irradiation on the initial mechanical properties of bone–patellar tendon–bone grafts. *Arthroscopy* 1994;10:188–197.

82. Buck BE, Malinin TI, Brown MD. Bone transplantation and human immunodeficiency virus. An estimate of risk of acquired immunodeficiency syndrome (AIDS). *Clin Orthop* 1989;240:129–136.

83. Miller MD. Revision cruciate ligament surgery with retention of femoral interference screws. *Arthroscopy* 1998;14:111–114.

84. Howell SM. Arthroscopic roofplasty: a method for correcting an extension deficit caused by roof impingement of an anterior cruciate ligament graft. *Arthroscopy* 1992;8:375–379.

85. Howell SM, Clark JA. Tibial tunnel placement in anterior cruciate ligament reconstructions and graft impingement. *Clin Orthop* 1992;283:187–195.

86. Howell SM, Berns GS, Farley TE. Unimpinged and impinged anterior cruciate ligament grafts: MR signal intensity measurements. *Radiology* 1991;179:639–643.

87. Howell SM, Clark JA, Farley TE. A rationale for predicting anterior cruciate graft impingement by the intercondylar roof. A magnetic resonance imaging study. *Am J Sports Med* 1991;19:276–282.

88. Howell SM, Clark JA, Blasier RD. Serial magnetic resonance imaging of hamstring anterior cruciate ligament autografts during the first year of implantation. A preliminary study. *Am J Sports Med* 1991;19:42–47.

89. Howell SM, Clark JA, Farley TE. Serial magnetic resonance study assessing the effects of impingement on the MR image of the patellar tendon graft. *Arthroscopy* 1992;8:350–358.

90. Howell SM, Taylor MA. Failure of reconstruction of the anterior cruciate ligament due to impingement by the intercondylar roof. *J Bone Joint Surg* 1993;75A:1044–1055.

91. Olson EJ, Fu FH, Harner CD, et al. Towards optimal tibial tunnel placement in endoscopic anterior cruciate ligament reconstruction. Presented at the American Academy of Orthopaedic Surgeons, 1993, San Francisco.

92. Johnson DL, Miller MD, Fu FH. The arthroscopic "impingement test" during anterior cruciate ligament reconstruction. *Arthroscopy* 1993;9:714–717.

93. Johnson DL, Swenson TM, Irrgang JJ, et al. Revision anterior cruciate ligament surgery: experience from Pittsburgh. *Clin Orthop* 1996;325:100–109.

94. Noyes FR, Barber-Westin SD, Roberts CS. Use of allografts after failed treatment of rupture of the anterior cruciate ligament [see comments]. *J Bone Joint Surg* 1994;76A:1019–1031.

95. Langan P, Fontanetta AP. Rupture of the patellar tendon after use of its central third. *Orthop Rev* 1987;16:317–321.

96. McCarroll JR. Fracture of the patella during a golf swing following reconstruction of the anterior cruciate ligament. A case report. *Am J Sports Med* 1983;11:26–27.

97. Buss DD, Warren RF, Wickiewicz TL, et al. Arthroscopically assisted reconstruction of the anterior cruciate ligament with use of autogenous patellar-ligament grafts. Results after twenty-four to forty-two months. *J Bone Joint Surg* 1993;75A:1346–1355.

98. Lipscomb AB, Johnston RK, Snyder RB. The technique of cruciate ligament reconstruction. *Am J Sports Med* 1981;9:77–81.

99. Indelicato PA, Linton RC, Huegel M. The results of fresh-frozen patellar tendon allografts for chronic anterior cruciate ligament deficiency of the knee. *Am J Sports Med* 1992;20:118–121.

100. Lephart SM, Kocher MS, Harner CD, et al. Quadriceps strength and functional capacity after anterior cruciate ligament reconstruction. Patellar tendon autograft versus allograft. *Am J Sports Med* 1993;21:738–743.

101. Rosenberg TD, Franklin JL, Baldwin GN, et al. Extensor mechanism function after patellar tendon graft harvest for anterior cruciate ligament reconstruction. *Am J Sports Med* 1992;20:519–525.

102. Saddemi SR, Frogameni AD, Fenton PJ, et al. Comparison of perioperative morbidity of anterior cruciate ligament autografts versus allografts. *Arthroscopy* 1993;9:519–524.

103. Johnson DL, Harner CD, Maday MG, et al. Revision anterior cruciate ligament surgery. In: Fu FH, Harner CD, Vince KG eds. *Knee Surgery*. Baltimore: Williams and Wilkins, 1994;889–892.

Section IV

Complications and Pitfalls of Patellofemoral Surgery

Chapter 15

Complications and Pitfalls in Lateral Retinacular Release

Kevin L. Kunkle and M. Mike Malek

This chapter discusses arthroscopy's most complication-fraught procedure—the lateral retinacular release. In 1970, Willner[1] described the use of an isolated lateral retinacular release for recurrent patellar dislocation, and this was subsequently followed by a report by Merchant and Mercer[2] in 1974. Since then, numerous methods of lateral retinacular release have been proposed, including open, closed, percutaneous, arthroscopic, and combined open/arthroscopic. Results with this procedure, given the proper indications, have been good, ranging from 14% to 100%,[2–22] with two-thirds of the studies reporting more than 70% satisfactory results. Much of the confusion in the literature about results following lateral retinacular release arises from the different indications for release used, and the criteria used for a successful result. No matter how it is performed, the success of a lateral release depends more on proper patient selection than on technique.[23]

While arthroscopic knee surgery is one of the most common orthopedic surgical procedures performed today, with an overall complication rate of 1.7%, the procedure with the highest complication rate of 7.2% is the lateral retinacular release.[24] Hemarthrosis is the most commonly reported complication, not only for lateral retinacular release, but for all arthroscopic surgical procedures combined, which accounts for 60% of all complications, and is nearly five times more common than infection, the second most common complication. Thus, lateral retinacular release is not a benign procedure no matter how it is performed, and it should not be performed randomly or haphazardly. Whether the procedure is performed open, closed, or arthroscopically, attention to detail in terms of patient selection, indications for the procedure, and meticulous surgical technique are crucial.

INDICATIONS FOR RELEASE

When is a lateral retinacular release indicated? The literature is replete with articles offering different criteria for release, and there seems to be little general consensus.[1–16,18–23,25–57] Poor indications and improper technique of release may initially yield early satisfactory results in 70% to 85% of patients, but their results tend to worsen with time.[11,20,45] Reports have indicated that a positive apprehension sign with patellar subluxation, an increased Q angle,[21,57] or anterior knee pain[37] are indications for lateral retinacular release. While the efficacy of lateral release in the treatment of resistant patellar pain without instability has been questioned,[9] other studies have reported favorable results.[10,11,21,47,51,57] Patients that displayed increased malalignment responded less favorably to lateral retinacular release alone.[57] Gecha and Torg[36] found that symptom evaluation, clinical diagnosis of recurrent subluxation or dislocation, and radiographic evaluation to be of no benefit in predicting the success of lateral retinacular release.

Dzioba[15] did not find the Q angle to be a significant predictor of surgical outcome, whereas peripatellar pain upon knee extension, pain upon resisted flexion, a positive apprehension sign, a positive lateral overhang noted on arthroscopic evaluation, and toughened lateral retinacular structures on surgical sectioning were good predictors of outcome. He believed that the single best predictor of success following lateral retinacular release was the finding of the patella reduced in the sulcus on the postoperative Merchant view x-ray.

Kolowich et al[40] looked for factors involved in patients with failed lateral release and determined specific objective criteria that would yield predictable, consistent results. They found that a lateral patellar tilt of less than

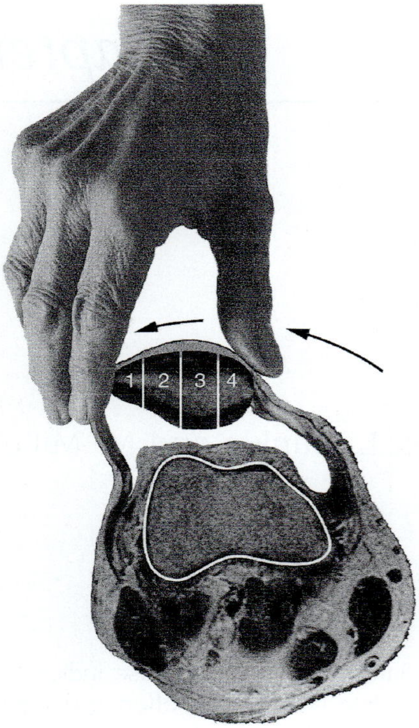

Figure 15.1. Lateral displacement of the patella by two quadrants (excessive lateral overhang).

5 degrees, patellar glides of less than two quadrants (Figs. 15.1 and 15.2) in either medial or lateral direction, and an tubercle sulcus angle of less than 5 degrees predicted a more favorable result. They also found that patients who demonstrated patellar instability tended to do worse, and that the congruence angle as measured on x-ray does not reliably predict a successful outcome.

HEMARTHROSIS

Hemarthrosis is the most common complication of lateral release, regardless of the technique,[2–4,6–9,11,13,15,16,18–20,22,23,25–27,29–32,35,40–42,47,52,57–60] and is most likely due to arterial bleeding from the lateral superior genicular artery or its branches, but can also occur from the lateral inferior genicular artery. While the patella does have a richly anastomotic venous system, these vessels are rarely the cause of hemarthrosis.

Patients usually present with a significant amount of swelling, redness, shiny skin, loss of motion and severe pain. Often the amount of pain is proportional to the amount of blood present in the joint. Attempts at aspiration, even with a large-bore needle, are often futile if the blood has coagulated. In severe cases, operative evacuation of the hematoma, or possible exploration and coagulation of the bleeding vessel, if it is discovered early in the postoperative period, should be performed.

With regard to final functional results, Busch and DeHaven[27] reported that in none of their cases did a hemarthrosis or subcutaneous hematoma appear to be related to a long-term poor result. However, a significant hemarthrosis can lead to subsequent motion loss, reflex sympathetic dystrophy, or an infrapatellar contracture syndrome. In addition, its presence can inhibit the ability of the quadriceps, especially the vastus medialis obliquus, to generate a forceful contraction, therefore significantly altering the ability to rehabilitate the patient.[15] Although hemarthrosis is usually thought of as having only immediate postoperative morbidity, it has been shown to produce long-term sequelae and compromise the final functional result by promoting synovitis and scar tissue formation.[18,47]

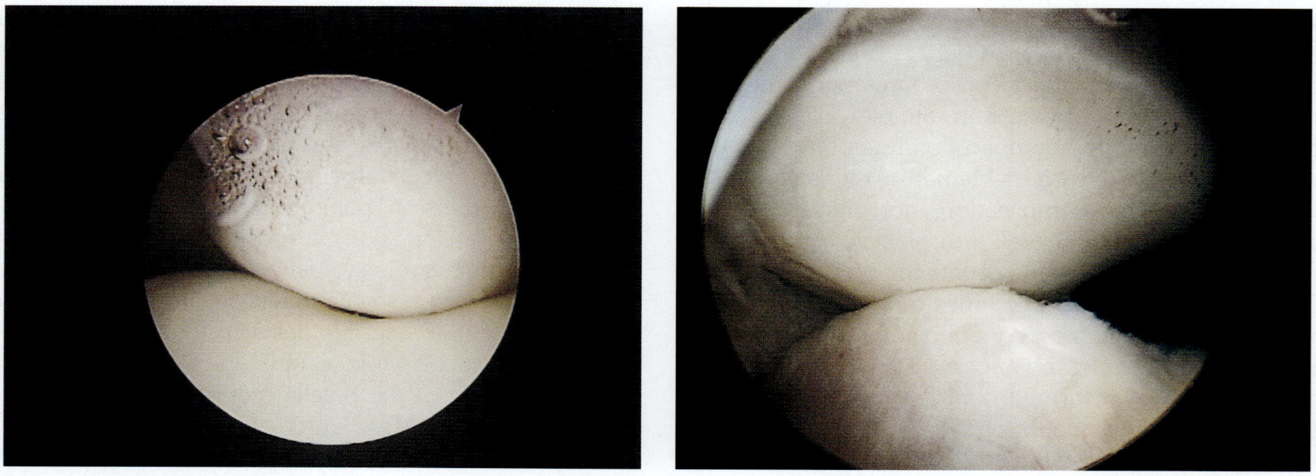

A B

Figure 15.2. **A:** Arthroscopic view of patella femoral relationship in a normal knee. **B:** Center of the patella rests over the lateral femoral condyle. Glide test of two quadrants in a chronic subluxating patella.

Postoperative hemarthrosis has been listed as a complication of lateral retinacular release, with frequency between 7% and 42%,[7,18,20] and Bray et al[3] found that release was always associated with some degree of hemarthrosis. No patient required aspiration, and the presence of hemarthrosis did not prevent early mobilization or physical therapy. They also found that hemarthrosis did not lead to significant scarring or fibrosis of the incised retinaculum, and did not affect the final outcome.

Small,[59] in his prospective study, found that the use of a tourniquet was associated with a higher incidence of hemarthrosis. The complication rate when a tourniquet was used was found to be 9.2%; without a tourniquet it was 3.3%. This difference was statistically significant ($p = .037$). He offers as a possible explanation for this the inability to visualize many of the small retinacular vessels and the lateral superior genicular artery when the tourniquet is inflated. Coupens and Yates[46] also found a higher complication rate when tourniquet control was utilized.

Performing the release subcutaneously under arthroscopic control, as opposed to using a purely arthroscopic method, is associated with an increased incidence of complications. The hemarthrosis rate is twice as high. The difference may be a result of the improved visualization of the incised retinacular vessels when performed arthroscopically as compared to the subcutaneous method.

The use of electrocautery to perform the release did not appear to lower the incidence of hemarthrosis (Figs. 15.3 and 15.4). The complication rate when electrocautery was used to release the retinaculum was 8.6%; when some other instrument was used (knife, scissors, etc.) the complication rate was 6.3%. However, this difference was not statistically significant.[59]

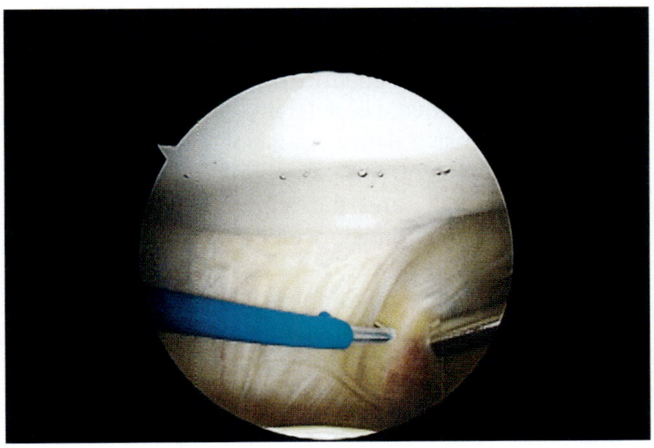

Figure 15.3. Usage of electrocautery in performing arthroscopic lateral retinacular release in the right knee. Point of start is at the junction of the oblique fibers of the vastus lateralis and vertical fibers of the retinaculum.

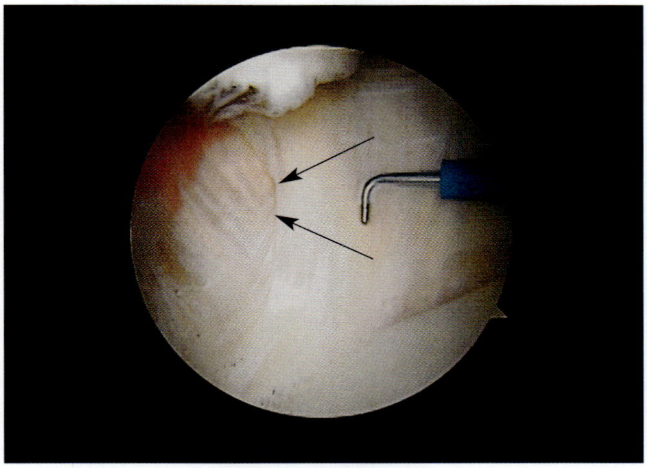

Figure 15.4. Another arthroscopic view of the lateral retinaculum of the left knee. Note the different orientation of the vastus lateralis fibers of the retinaculum. Arrows point to junction.

The use of a postoperative suction drain for more than 24 hours was associated with a significantly higher incidence of hemarthrosis. Use of a drain for more than 24 hours had a 13.4% complication rate, but if no drain was used, or it was used for less than 24 hours, the rate dropped to 2.4%. A possible explanation for this is that the pressure of the drain does not allow the bleeding vessels to tamponade off as the intraarticular pressure rises.[59]

Recommendations to minimize hemarthrosis following lateral retinacular release arthroscopically involve performing the procedure with attention to detail and ensuring that all bleeding vessels are cauterized at the end of the procedure. If the procedure is being performed under tourniquet control, at some point the tourniquet should be deflated and the borders of the release should be explored for evidence of bleeding.

INFRAPATELLAR CONTRACTURE SYNDROME/PATELLA BAJA

Infrapatellar contracture syndrome (IPCS) is a condition similar to arthrofibrosis. This condition may occur as a result of scar tissue or adhesion formation between the patellar tendon and the tibia, causing shortening of the patellar tendon and increased force being applied to the patellofemoral joint. It occurs most commonly after harvesting the patellar tendon for autograft for ligament reconstructions, but can occur following lateral release[61,62] (Fig. 15.5). Another possible mechanism may be as a result of aggressive release, especially if this

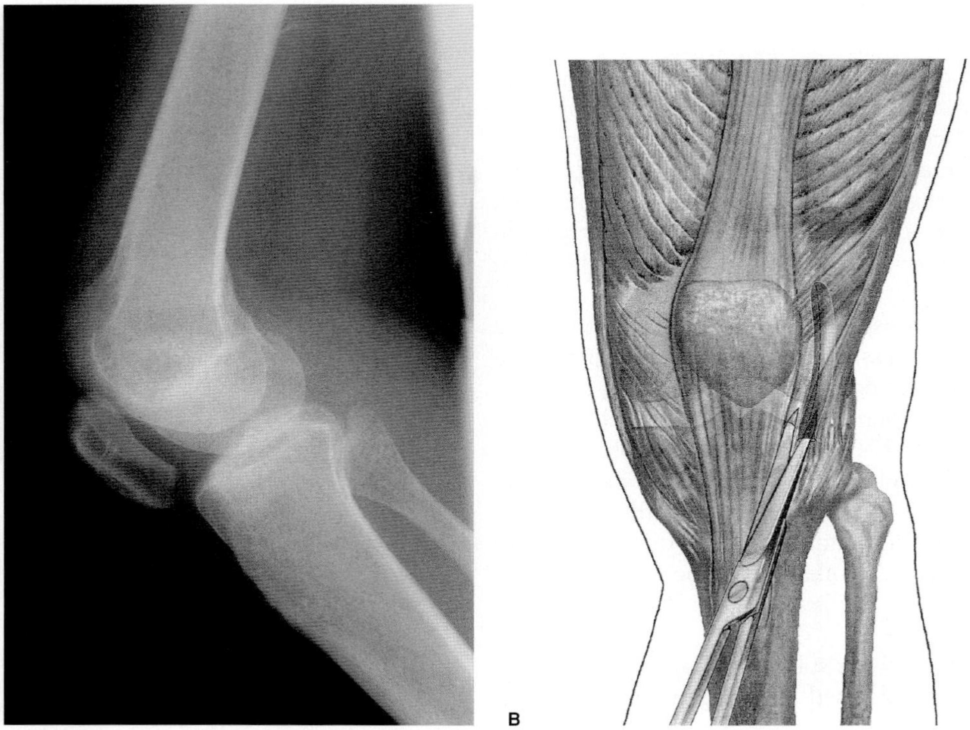

A B

Figure 15.5. **A:** Infrapatellar contracture syndrome may develop after an aggressive release, which may include fibers of the vastus and around the superior pole of the patella. **B:** Drawing a line of reference (cut should end at the junction of the lateral retinacular and fibers of the vastus lateralis; beyond that would be aggressive release). This junction can easily be seen arthroscopically. (See Figs. 15.7 and 15.8.)

release curves around the patella superiorly. Because of force imbalance, aggressive release may cause the patella to rotate distally and toward the lateral side, causing both incongruity of the patella in the trochlea and increased pressure. Postoperative tearing of the central quadriceps fibers due to trauma may also result in this deformity, with resulting weakness and loss of flexion. On exam the patient will exhibit diminished patellar mobility, decreased patellar tilt, decreased quadriceps strength and range of motion, distal patellar migration, and possible significant crepitus. Their diminished range of motion is due to a combination of loss of extension greater than 10 degrees, and loss of flexion greater than 25 degrees.

The "shelf sign," as described by Paulos et al,[61] is demonstrated in patients with IPCS who have induration that results in prominent anterior patellar structures. This syndrome is composed of three stages. Stage I is the prodromal stage, which is manifested by diffuse edema, diminished patellar mobility, and the patient's failure to progress with rehabilitation. This occurs in the first 2 to 8 weeks. Treatment involves early range of motion, patellar mobilization, nonsteroidal antiinflammatory drugs (NSAIDs), analgesics, and the judicious use of a drop-out cast. It is imperative that the patient regain good voluntary quadriceps contractions. Stage II is the active stage, presenting with significant quadriceps atrophy, worsening patellar mobility, and a positive shelf sign. This occurs at 6 to 20 weeks postoperation. Treatment is usually surgical, with the main goal being achievement of terminal extension. Surgical intervention may need to be delayed until the inflammation is decreased and voluntary quadriceps contraction is demonstrated. Surgery involves a lateral arthrotomy and release, and extensive debridement of the hypertrophied tissues and all the intraarticular adhesions from the lateral gutters, notch, and the suprapatellar pouch. Arthroscopy and manipulation alone may give good results as long as there are no extraarticular adhesions. Otherwise, open debridement is indicated. Postoperative treatment involves aggressive physical therapy to attain voluntary quadriceps contraction, continuous passive motion machine, and nighttime use of a drop-out cast. As reported, the average amount of improvement of range of motion is 45 degrees.[61,62] Most patients will be left with some residual patellofemoral arthrosis. Stage III is the residual stage, in which the patient demonstrates patella baja and significant patellofemoral arthrosis. It may be necessary to perform salvage procedures such as a Maquet procedure, proximal tibial tubercle advancement, total knee arthroplasty, or patellectomy.

Prevention of IPCS is possible with early weight bearing, early aggressive range of motion (especially extension), patellar mobilization exercises, and a functional closed-chain rehabilitation program.

Treatment of this complication may be difficult or impossible to correct,[50,61,62] as secondary contracting of the infrapatellar tendon often results following debridement. If the deformity is a result of excessive release or subsequent trauma of the quadriceps, the defect should be repaired.

QUADRICEPS TENDON RUPTURE

The extent and direction of the lateral release proximally can predispose the patient to complications.[52] Many techniques recommend releasing the vastus lateralis insertion, which necessitates extending the release proximally for 6 to 8 cm along the medial border of the musculotendinous junction.[16,20,54] As a result, the patient can experience patellar hypermobility, medial patellar subluxation, significant quadriceps weakness, and quadriceps tendon rupture.[25,37,40,55,58,63,64] Blaiser and Ciullo[63] reported on a case in which the patient sustained a quadriceps tendon rupture following an arthroscopic lateral release in which incidental injury occurred to the extensor mechanism proximal to the patella.

Complete detachment of the vastus lateralis may result in significant quadriceps weakness and medial patellar subluxation.[25,37] In a study looking at 54 patients who failed to improve following lateral retinacular release and whose symptoms worsened, Hughston and Deese[37] found that 50% of the knees exhibited medial subluxation with retraction of the vastus lateralis, significant atrophy, and a visible void at the patellar insertion site. Computed tomography (CT) scans confirmed this.

QUADRICEPS INSUFFICIENCY

Quadriceps insufficiency or weakness can occur as a result of excessive release of the vastus lateralis.[40,44,50,58] This can be a serious complication, as the patients often feel that the leg is worse off than before the release. They may present with complaints of persistent weakness, which may manifest as buckling or giving way, and anterior knee pain. On examination, they may display a defect in the vastus lateralis extending proximal to the patella or curving around the superior pole of the patella toward the midline. Hughston and Deese[37] have reported on findings of atrophy and retraction of the vastus lateralis muscle on examination. On passive patellar tilt, patients demonstrate a tilt of greater than 90 degrees. They have significant quadriceps weakness, especially with eccentric contractions, and may be resistant to improvement with rehabilitation.

Treatment for this difficult problem may require repair or reconstruction of the vastus lateralis tendon. In a retrospective study, Kolowich et al[40] reported on 16 knees that required vastus lateralis repair for excessive release of the lateral structures. All patients displayed persistent quadriceps weakness with associated patellar pain. Metcalf[20] reported that residual quadriceps weakness was the most important factor in those patients who had a fair or poor result. Simpson and Barrett[18] reported on 26 of 55 knees that underwent lateral release and demonstrated quadriceps strength of only poor to fair at 24 to 56 months postoperation. They attributed this finding to incomplete rehabilitation. It was suggested by Marumoto et al[58] that the real cause of the poor quadriceps function may have been a "surgically defuctionalized vastus lateralis muscle."

MEDIAL SUBLUXATION

This complication can also occur following overly aggressive or extensive lateral release (Fig. 15.6), but more commonly occurs with improper patient selection. The patient in whom this complication would occur exhibits mild lateral subluxation on x-ray, but has hypermobility or patella alta on physical exam. This complication should be avoidable by close attention to detail with the physical examination.

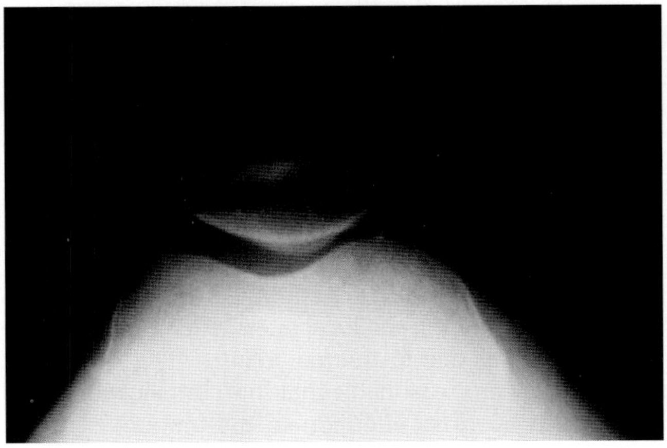

Figure 15.6. Post-lateral release medialization of the patella. This condition should be recognized quickly and treated promptly to prevent medial patellar facet arthrosis development.

When the complication does occur, patients often present with quadriceps weakness, complaints of medial sided patellar pain, and a feeling of instability.[53] They may even dislocate medially. Kolowich et al[40] reported on three patients who had quadriceps weakness and experienced recurrent medial dislocation. In a larger group, most of 16 patients who went on to require vastus lateralis repair demonstrated medial subluxation at examination, with increased patellar tilt of 80 degrees or more. Normally the Merchant view x-ray confirms medialization of the patella (Fig. 15.6). Upon recognition of this problem, surgical repair of the quadriceps defect may restore function and rectify the problem. However, if it is not treated quickly, significant medial patellofemoral facet arthrosis may occur.

Using kinematic magnetic resonance imaging, Shellock et al[55] demonstrated medial subluxation in 63% of patients studied for persistent symptoms following lateral release. Hypermobility of the patella following lateral release has been demonstrated, with both medial and lateral subluxation and even dislocation occurring.[37,55,64,65] This results following release of the lateral patellofemoral restraints in a patient who already demonstrates absent medial restraints. Preoperative assessment should prevent this complication from occurring. A patient who has an increased patellar glide or a hypermobile patella will be predisposed to this complication, and surgical treatment should be avoided, if at all possible. If it is necessary, the patient will probably also require a medial plication, and possibly even a distal realignment procedure, if examination warrants.

THERMAL INJURY

Lord et al[66] reported on three cases in which a skin burn occurred following lateral retinacular release performed using an intraarticular approach and electrocautery. In their analysis they were unable to determine whether the thermal injuries were caused by technical error or were inherent to the use of electrocautery. In another report, McGuire[67] discussed two patients who had arthroscopic lateral retinacular releases performed by electrocautery, who subsequently developed peeling of the skin in the overlying area. Whereas he attributed this complication to the epinephrine in the local anesthetic, it is quite possible that it was due to thermal injury.

It would seem reasonable that this complication could be avoided by close attention to the amount of tissue being incised and the depth of the cautery tip during the lateral release. Only the synovium and lateral retinaculum should be transected (Figs. 15.7 and 15.8). Avoid cutting into the adipose layer, as this can lead to either partial- or full-thickness burns.[49] Also, caution must be exercised when releasing inferiorly in the region of the lateral infrapatellar portal, so as to avoid thermal injury there, because the thickness of the retinaculum and overlying adipose tissue decreases. Other means of avoiding this injury include using nonconductive fluid such as glycine or glycerol, using an impedance-matched isolated current generator, using a capacitive-coupled dispersive grounding pad, using an electrocautery instrument that is insulated except for the

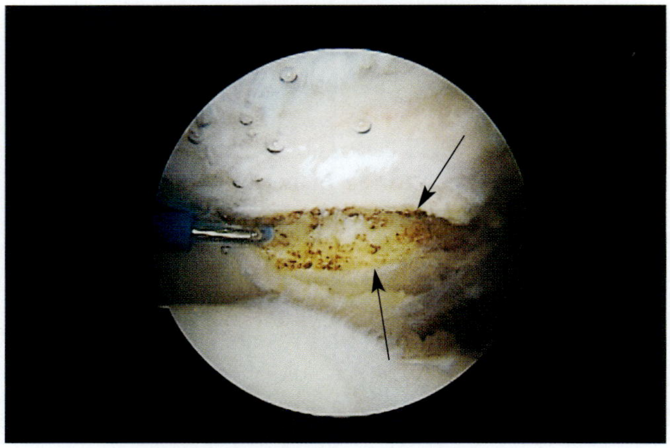

Figure 15.7. Usage of electrocautery in lateral retinacular release should be done carefully and release should be performed layer by layer and include only the synovium and the retinacular fibers. Subcutaneous tissues should not be violated. Note the thickness of the retinacular fibers and synovium layers (arrows). Subcutaneous tissues are at the depth of the opening (small arrow).

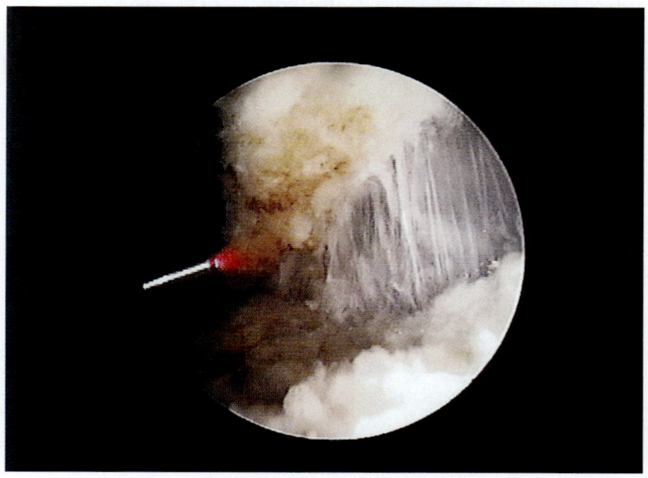

Figure 15.8. Use of holmium laser in performing the lateral retinacular release. Advantage is reduction of postoperative bleeding/hemarthrosis and disadvantage is deep penetration and formation of postoperative soft tissue hemarthrosis.

very tip, and using the lowest setting on the generator necessary to effectively transect the tissue.

INFECTION

This is a potential complication that can occur with any surgical procedure, and its sequelae can be devastating. Fortunately, this complication does not occur often and should be easily avoided by adhering to sterile technique, even without the use of prophylactic antibiotics. The surgeon should always maintain a high level of suspicion for a postoperative infection. If the patient presents with swelling, erythema, increased warmth, pain, or fever, the joint should be immediately aspirated and the fluid sent for Gram stain, culture, and sensitivity. At the same time, a complete blood count with differential and Westergren erythrocyte sedimentation rate should be obtained. Following aspiration, antibiotic therapy should be started. If the cultures come back positive, early irrigation and debridement of the joint by either arthroscopic or open methods is indicated, followed by a full course of parenteral antibiotics.

PULMONARY EMBOLUS/DEEP VENOUS THROMBOSIS

Deep venous thrombosis following lateral retinacular release is a known complication.[3,7,11,18,27,41,59] As with any type of surgery, one must maintain a high level of suspicion for this problem and treat it promptly. With treatment, further significant sequelae can usually be avoided. In a study by Bray et al,[3] in which they reported a 4% complication rate in 50 knees following lateral retinacular release, they had one patient present at 5 days postoperation with a pulmonary embolus and signs of deep venous thrombosis.

Busch and DeHaven[27] reported on 80 knees that underwent lateral retinacular release; two developed superficial thrombophlebitis, and one developed deep venous thrombosis.

REFLEX SYMPATHETIC DYSTROPHY

Reflex sympathetic dystrophy (RSD) can be a devastating problem after any type of injury or surgical procedure, not just following lateral retinacular release. Fortunately, it is an infrequent complication of knee surgery[3,4,23,27,32,68,69] but it has been especially noted to occur following patellofemoral surgery. In a series of 14 patients who developed RSD, 11 had surgery on the patellofemoral joint as the precipitating factor (lateral release, realignment procedure, chondral shaving).[68] In another series of patients who developed RSD, 64% had surgery or injury to the patellofemoral joint.[69] These patients usually complain of pain out of proportion to their injury or surgical procedure. Following lateral release, the pain, which is persistent and sometimes burning in quality, may be localized to the anterior aspect of the knee or it may radiate throughout the leg. In the early stages, the skin temperature may be increased, with erythema that blanches to the touch. The skin is often shiny and dry (hyperhidrosis). Range of motion may be impaired, and the patient will frequently be unable to bear weight. In RSD's early stages, a triple-phase bone scan may be helpful to collaborate the diagnosis. In the later stages, diffuse osteopenia may be noted on x-ray. Clinical response to sympathetic lumbar blockade may also help to confirm the diagnosis.[68,69] To give maximally effective treatment, it is imperative to start early. Treatment for this complication should involve a pain management team using a multifactorial approach to the problem. Analgesics and sympatholytic medications, liberal use of NSAIDs, aggressive early supervised physical therapy for mobilization of the joint, and the possible use of epidural or sympathetic nerve blocks are the mainstays of treatment. Good results have been reported with the use of continuous epidural anesthesia in conjunction with manipulation, continuous passive motion machines, and electrical stimulation. Occasionally, surgical sympathectomy may be indicated.

When clinical findings suggest RSD of the knee and symptoms have been present for less than 6 weeks, it has been recommended that a trial of NSAIDs, gentle pain-free physical therapy to increase motion and modalities, and progressive weight bearing be tried. If there is no relief of pain or no increase in motion, or if symptoms suggesting RSD have clearly been present for more than 6 weeks and are progressing, then diagnostic sympathetic block is recommended.[68]

Epidural blockade has several advantages over sympathetic blockade. While a sympathetic block may relieve the pain initially, when the stiff joint is aggressively mobilized the pain usually returns, and the pain cycle is reconstituted. Epidural blockade allows pain-free mobilization because it blocks sympathetic pain fibers as well as somatic pain fibers.[68] Also, a continuous in-dwelling epidural catheter can be used. Patients who have early diagnosis and prompt treatment should have a better chance of successful outcome.

FLUID EXTRAVASATION AND COMPARTMENT SYNDROME

While this complication is not unique to arthroscopic lateral retinacular release, it can occur with any arthroscopic procedure and could conceivably occur with greater frequency considering the large capsular defect created by transecting the retinaculum. Interestingly enough, compartment syndrome was not even mentioned as a complication in the articles written by Small[24,59,60,70] that reported on complications of arthroscopic procedures. Evans and Paulos[52] reported this complication only in conjunction with a distal realignment procedure in patellofemoral joint surgery. Therefore, it seems reasonable to assume that this is a rare entity. One possible explanation for this is that when lateral retinacular release is performed in conjunction with other arthroscopic procedures, it is usually the last procedure performed, followed by obtaining hemostasis, and then the surgery is terminated. Therefore, the capsular defect is not subjected to increased hydrostatic pressures for any significant amount of time.[43]

In the literature, there have been reports of compartment syndrome developing following simple knee arthroscopy. In a cadaveric animal study, Peek and Haynes[71] they documented that the presence of a capsular defect caused compartment pressures to be elevated 80 mm above normal. In the normal limb without a capsular defect, the pressure elevation caused by saline extravasation returned to normal levels within 15 minutes of releasing the tourniquet. However, in the limbs with the capsular defect, this compartment pressure remained above 40 mm Hg for at least 8 hours following release of the tourniquet, with resultant muscular death as noted on histologic studies. Their results indicate that extravasations of fluid in the face of a capsular tear can cause a compartment syndrome and tissue death.

Noyes and Spievack[72] reported on fluid dissection that occurred following flexion of the knee, which was distended for the purpose of arthroscopy. This condition was noted clinically on four occasions in 300 cases. There was rapid resolution of the condition following release of the tourniquet. They reported that intraarticular fluid can dissect via the path of the semimembranosus bursa, beneath the pes anserinus, and into the calf muscles, even with an intact knee capsule.

Prevention of this complication involves having a high level of clinical suspicion and monitoring the size and amount of swelling in the limb both intraoperatively and postoperatively. If the condition is suspected, the proper course of action includes immediate termination of the procedure and discontinuation of fluid inflow, followed by the evacuation of as much fluid from the joint as possible. If a tourniquet is being used, it should be deflated. This will normally result in decrease of the compartment pressure. If it does not and the muscular compartment remains firm, compartment pressure measurements should be performed, followed by fasciotomy when indicated.

ARTHROFIBROSIS AND JOINT STIFFNESS

Of 43 failed lateral retinacular releases, Kolowich et al[40] reported on four patients who developed arthrofibrosis and required manipulation under anesthesia. This complication can be associated with RSD.[27] Sherman et al[8] reported on a patient in their series who required a second arthroscopic procedure following lateral retinacular release for lysis of adhesions that had formed in the lateral gutter and the suprapatellar pouch. They reported no loss of motion at follow-up.

CHRONIC SYNOVIAL SINUS AND WOUND HEALING

Kolowich et al[40] reported on 43 patients who failed lateral retinacular release, one of whom required excision of a chronic sinus tract. Many patients can develop a significant and persistent effusion following lateral retinacular release, which can facilitate formation of a chronic draining synovial sinus if they encounter problems with wound healing.

CONCLUSION

To avoid complications in performing lateral retinacular release, patient selection, meticulous attention to detail, and disciplined postoperative care and rehabilitation are necessary.

References

1. Wilner P. Recurrent dislocation of the patella. *Clin Orthop* 1970;69:213–215.
2. Merchant AC, Mercer ND. Lateral release of the patella, a preliminary report. *Clin Orthop* 1974;103:40–45.
3. Bray RC, Roth JH, Jacobsen RP. Arthroscopic lateral release for anterior knee pain: a study comparing patients who are claiming worker's compensation with those who are not. *Arthroscopy* 1987;3:237–247.
4. Henry JH, Goletz TH, Williamson B. Lateral retinacular release in patellofemoral subluxation: indications, results, and comparison to open patellofemoral reconstruction. *Am J Sports Med* 1986;14:121–129.
5. Jackson RW, Kunkel SS, Taylor GJ. Lateral retinacular release for patellofemoral pain in the older patient. *Arthroscopy* 1991;7:283–286.
6. Lankenner PA, Micheli LJ, Clancy R, et al. Arthroscopic

percutaneous lateral patellar retinacular release. *Am J Sports Med* 1986;14:267–269.

7. McGinty JB, McCarthy JC. Endoscopic lateral retinacular release. A preliminary report. *Clin Orthop* 1981;158: 120–125.
8. Sherman OH, Fox JM, Sperling H, et al. Patellar instability: treatment by arthroscopic electrosurgical lateral release. *Arthroscopy* 1987;3:152–160.
9. Schonholtz GJ, Zahn MG, Magee CM. Lateral retinacular release of the patella. *Arthroscopy* 1987;3:269–272.
10. Larson RL, Cabaud HE, Slocum DB, et al. The patellar compression syndrome: surgical treatment by lateral retinacular release. *Clin Orthop* 1978;134:158–167.
11. Ceder LC, Larson RL. Z-Plasty lateral retinacular release for the treatment of patellar compression syndrome. *Clin Orthop* 1979;144:110–113.
12. Dandy DJ, Griffiths D. Lateral release for recurrent dislocation of the patella. *J Bone Joint Surg* 1989;71B: 121–125.
13. Ogilvie-Harris DJ, Jackson RW. The arthroscopic treatment of chondromalacia patellae. *J Bone Joint Surg* 1984;66B:660–665.
14. Chen SC, Ramanathan EBS. The treatment of patellar instability by lateral release. *J Bone Joint Surg* 1984; 66B:344–348.
15. Dzioba RB. Diagnostic arthroscopy and longitudinal open lateral release. A four year follow-up study to determine predictions of surgical outcome. *Am J Sports Med* 1990;18:343–348.
16. Aglietti P, Pisaneschi, A, Buzz, R, et al. Arthroscopic lateral release for patellar pain or instability. *Arthroscopy* 1989;5:176–182.
17. Schreiber SN. Arthroscopic lateral retinacular release using a modified superomedial portal, electrosurgery and postoperative positioning in flexion. *Orthop Rev* 1988; 17:375.
18. Simpson LA, Barrett JP. Factors associated with poor results following arthroscopic subcutaneous lateral retinacular release. *Clin Orthop* 1984;186:165–171.
19. Bigos SJ, McBride GG. The isolated lateral retinacular release in the treatment of patellofemoral disorders. *Clin Orthop* 1984;186:75–80.
20. Metcalf RW. An arthroscopic method of lateral release of the subluxating or dislocating patella. *Clin Orthop* 1982; 167:9–18.
21. Micheli LJ, Stanitski CL. Lateral patellar retinacular disease. *Am J Sports Med* 1981;9:330–336.
22. Harwin SF, Stern RE. Subcutaneous lateral retinacular release for chondromalacia patella: a preliminary report. *Clin Orthop* 1981;156:207–210.
23. Fulkerson JP. *Disorders of the Patellofemoral Joint.* Baltimore: Williams & Wilkins, 1997.
24. Small NC. Complications in arthroscopic surgery performed by experienced arthroscopists. *Arthroscopy* 1988;4:215–221.
25. Betz RR, Magill JT, Lonergan RP. The percutaneous lateral retinacular release. *Am J Sports Med* 1987;15: 477–482.
26. Brief LP. Lateral patellar instability: Treatment with a combined open-arthroscopic approach. *Arthroscopy* 1993;9:617–623.
27. Busch MT, DeHaven KE. Pitfalls of the lateral retinacular release. *Clin Sports Med* 1989;8:279–296.
28. DeLee J. Complications of arthroscopy and arthroscopic surgery: results of a national survey. *Arthroscopy* 1985; 1:214–220.
29. Fabbriciani C, Panni AS, Delcogliano A. Role of arthroscopic lateral release in the treatment of patellofemoral disorders. *Arthroscopy* 1992;8:531–536.
30. Fu FH, Maday MG. Arthroscopic lateral release and the lateral patellar compression syndrome. *Orthop Clin North Am* 1992;23:601–612.
31. Fulkerson JP. Patellofemoral pain disorders: evaluation and management. *J Am Acad Orthop Surg* 1994;2: 124–132.
32. Fulkerson JP, Kalenak A, Rosenberg TD, et al. Patellofemoral pain. *AAOS Instr Course Lect* 1992;41:57–71.
33. Fulkerson JP, Schutzer SF. After failure of conservative treatment for painful patellofemoral malalignment: lateral release or realignment? *Orthop Clin North Am* 1986; 17:283–288.
34. Fulkerson JP, Shea KP. Current concepts review: disorders of patellofemoral alignment. *J Bone Joint Surg* 1990;72(9):1424–1429.
35. Ficat RP, Hungerford DS. *Disorders of the Patellofemoral Joint.* Baltimore: Williams & Wilkins, 1977.
36. Gecha SR, Torg JS. Clinical prognosticators for the efficacy of retinacular release surgery to treat patellofemoral pain. *Clin Orthop* 1990;253:203–208.
37. Hughston JC, Deese M. Medial subluxation of the patella as a complication of lateral retinacular release. *Am J Sports Med* 1988;16:383–388.
38. Insall JN. *Surgery of the Knee.* New York: Churchill Livingstone, 1984.
39. Insall JN. Current concepts review: patellar pain. *J Bone Joint Surg* 1982;64A:147–151.
40. Kolowich PA, Paulos LE, Rosenberg TD, et al. Lateral release of the patella: indications and contraindications. *Am J Sports Med* 1990;18:359–365.
41. Malek MM. Arthroscopic lateral retinacular release: functional results in series of 67 knees. *Orthop Rev* 1985; 14:55–60.
42. Malek MM, Fanelli GC. Patellofemoral pain: an arthroscopic perspective. *Clin Sports Med* 1991;10:549–567.
43. Post WR. Lateral retinacular release: arthroscopic and open techniques. *Tech Orthop* 1997;12:145–150.

44. Scuderi GR. Surgical treatment for patellar instability. *Orthop Clin North Am* 1992;23:619–630.
45. Shea KP, Fulkerson JP. Preoperative computed tomography scanning and arthroscopy in predicting outcome after lateral retinacular release. *Arthroscopy* 1992;8:327–334.
46. Coupens SD, Yates CK. The effect of tourniquet use and hemovac drainage on postoperative hemarthrosis. *Arthroscopy* 1991;7:278–282.
47. Grana WA, Hinckley B, Hollingsworth S. Arthroscopic evaluation and treatment of patellar malignment. *Clin Orthop* 1984;186:122–128.
48. Hughston JC. Subluxation of the patella. *J Bone Joint Surg* 1968;50:1003–1026.
49. Banas MP, Ferkel RD, Friedman MJ. Arthroscopic lateral retinacular release of the patellofemoral joint. *Oper Tech Sports Med* 1994;2:291–296.
50. Rosenburg TO, Kolowich PA. Complications of lateral retinacular release. In: Sprague NF III, ed. *Complications in Arthroscopy*. New York: Raven Press, 1989:145–155.
51. Greenfield MA, Scott WN. Arthroscopic evaluation and treatment of the patellofemoral joint. *Orthop Clin North Am* 1992;23:587–600.
52. Evans IK, Paulos LF. Complications of patellofemoral joint surgery. *Orthop Clin North Am* 1992;23:697–710.
53. Holmes PF, Henry JH. The results of extensor mechanism realignment following failed lateral retinacular releases. *Clin Sports Med* 1989;8:291–296.
54. Hughston JC, Walsh WMM. Proximal and distal reconstruction of the extensor mechanism for patellar subluxation. *Clin Orthop* 1979;144:36–42.
55. Shellock FG, Mink JH, Deutsch A, et al. Evaluation of patients with persistent symptoms after lateral retinacular release by kinematic magnetic resonance imaging of the patellofemoral joint. *Arthroscopy* 1990;6:226–234.
56. Crosby EB, Insall J. Recurrent dislocation of the patella. *J Bone Joint Surg* 1976;58A:9–13.
57. Krompinger W, Fulkerson JP. Lateral retinacular release for intractable lateral retinacular pain. *Clin Orthop* 1983;179:191.
58. Marumoto JM, Jordan C, Akins R. A biomechanical comparison of lateral retinacular releases. *Am J Sports Med* 1995;23:151–155.
59. Small NC. An analysis of complications in lateral retinacular release procedures. *Arthroscopy* 1989;5:282–286.
60. Small NC. Complications in arthroscopic surgery of the knee and shoulder. *Orthopedics* 1993;16:985–988.
61. Paulos LE, Rosenburg TD, Draubach J, et al. Infrapatellar contractive syndrome: an unrecognized cause of knee stiffness with patellar entrapment and patella infera. *Am J Sports Med* 1987;15:331–341.
62. Richmond JC, Assal MA. Arthroscopic management of arthrofibrosis of the knee including infrapatellar contraction syndrome. *Arthroscopy* 1991;7:144–147.
63. Blaiser RB, Ciullo JV. Rupture of the quadriceps tendon after arthroscopic lateral release: a case report. *Arthroscopy* 1986;2:262–263.
64. Langeland N. Recurrent dislocation of the patella following lateral retinacular release: a case report. *Arch Orthop Trauma Surg* 1983;102:65–66.
65. Schreiber SN. Proximal superomedial portal in arthroscopy of the knee. *Arthroscopy* 1991;7:246–251.
66. Lord MJ, Maltry JA, Shall LM. Thermal injury resulting from arthroscopic lateral retinacular release by electrocautery: report of three cases and a review of the literature. *Arthroscopy* 1991;7:33–37.
67. McGuire DA. Lateral retinacular release with Ringer's lactate irrigating medium [letter to the editor]. *Arthroscopy* 1987;3:216–217.
68. Cooper DE, DeLee JC, Ramamurthy S. Reflex sympathetic dystrophy of the knee. *J Bone Joint Surg* 1989; 71A:365–369.
69. Katz MM, Hungerford DS. Reflex sympathetic dystrophy affecting the knee. *J Bone Joint Surg* 1987;69B: 797–803.
70. Small NC. Complications in arthroscopy—the knee and other joints. *Arthroscopy* 1986;2:253–258.
71. Peek RD, Haynes DW. Compartment syndrome as a complication of arthroscopy. A case report and study of interstitial pressures. *Am J Sports Med* 1984;12: 464–468.
72. Noyes FR, Spievack ES. Extraarticular fluid dissection in tissues during arthroscopy. A report of clinical cases and a study of intraarticular and thigh pressure in cadavers. *Am J Sports Med* 1982;10:464–468.

Chapter 16

Complications and Pitfalls in Proximal Realignment Procedures

Alexander Kalenak and Gregory A. Hanks

The complications of proximal realignment surgery for patellofemoral disorders are as follows:

1. Bleeding/hematoma
2. Skin/subcutaneous tissue (disfigurement and contracture)
3. Infection (superficial, deep, joint)
4. Pain
5. Lateral tilt
6. Lateral subluxation
7. Medial subluxation
8. Arthrofibrosis
9. Weakness/atrophy
10. Reflex sympathetic dystrophy

These complications can occur intraoperatively, perioperatively, or postoperatively.

PREVENTION AND SALVAGE/TREATMENT OF INTRAOPERATIVE COMPLICATIONS

Bleeding/Hematoma

The complication of intraoperative bleeding is best addressed by the prevention of bleeding, provided a coagulopathy does not exist that would preclude a surgical procedure. Clamping and tying or electrocoagulation of all bleeders intraoperatively and paying attention to meticulous surgical technique (dissection in avascular tissue planes), will go a long way in preventing perioperative or postoperative bleeding. Consideration should be given to not using a tourniquet at all. This helps in identifying all bleeding points intraoperatively and would, in addition, be an aid in assessing the realignment procedure in a dynamic way. An inflated tourniquet, rigid and tight and constricting, will affect the excursion of the quadriceps and hamstring mechanisms, and therefore may be an inhibiting factor in patellofemoral excursion. Regardless of the anesthesia (general or regional), this inhibiting factor may give an inaccurate picture of patellofemoral excursions proximally/distally as well as medially/laterally.

Iatrogenic Trauma

Scuffing of the articular cartilage can be minimized by attention to detail when handling the arthroscope and the operating instruments.

Patella Positioning

Undercorrection or overcorrection can be prevented by assessing the active and passive excursions of the patella preoperatively and intraoperatively. Assessment of tracking, under general anesthesia, gives an indication of patella excursions in the passive mode. A second method of assessing the excursions of the patella dynamically requires active and volitional quadriceps and hamstring activity. To have volitional control of quadriceps and hamstring activity, it is necessary to perform the surgery under epidural anesthesia, which selectively provides pain relief but permits motor activity. Following lateral retinacular release, the patient should actively flex and extend the knee. The surgeon should observe dynamically the excursion of the patella proximally/distally and medially/laterally. The same observation should be made following the vastus medialis advancement. Comparison should be made with the preoperative patella excursion to determine whether or not there is undercorrection or overcorrection.

In reality, however, it is very difficult to assess intraoperatively the accuracy of the realignment by either of the above methods. Thus, under most circumstances, one empirically does the lateral release followed by the vastus medialis obliquus (VMO) advancement and arbitrarily assesses the patella tracking. The goal is to restore appropriate soft tissue tension and anatomic patella tracking. The dynamic role of the musculature plays a crucial role in the ultimate result and may, in fact, be a more important factor in the repair or realignment itself.

Lateral Retinacular Release

Arthroscopic lateral release and open lateral release are both acceptable methods of releasing the lateral retinaculum (see Chapter 15).

Vastus Medialis Obliquus Advancement

The vastus medialis advancement is typically done by mobilizing the VMO and advancing it over the patella approximately one-third to one-half the width/length of the patella from the superior medial margin to the central one-third of the patella.[1–3] Meticulous surgical technique is required for success of the advancement. The plane between the deep fascia of the VMO and the joint capsule/synovium need not be violated in order to perform the advancement procedure. Nonabsorbable sutures (three or four are typically used to provide adequate fixation of the advanced VMO (Fig. 16.1). Large knots over the patella are sometimes symptomatic and require late surgical excision. Thus, sutures are placed so that the knots are tied into the soft tissue on the VMO side or to the periosteum at the margin of the patella. Directly over the patella, the suture should be placed in such a manner that the knot is buried between the advanced VMO and the periosteum of the patella.

The Insall VMO technique is another method of proximal realignment that has been successful and is an acceptable alternative to the VMO advancement described above[4] (Fig. 16.2).

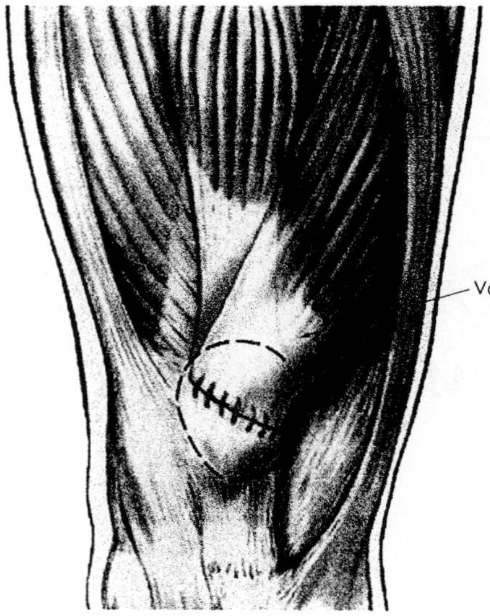

Figure 16.1. Vastus medialis obliquus (VMO) advancement at least one-half of the oblique diameter of the patella, anchoring the VMO to the medial retinaculum and to the periosteum on the anterior aspect of the patella but not to the lateral retinaculum tissue.

PREVENTION AND SALVAGE/TREATMENT OF PERIOPERATIVE COMPLICATIONS

The perioperative complications include bleeding/hematoma, infection, and swelling and pain.

Bleeding/Hematoma

The complication of bleeding is usually due to inadequate hemostasis. The use of the tourniquet prevents intraoperative bleeding but the prevention of perioperative bleeding requires adequent hemostasis during the procedure. Deflating the tourniquet, clamping and tying, or electrocoagulating all bleeding points prior to closure ensures adequate hemostatis. Continuous application of ice or the continuous use of a commercial cooling apparatus may be helpful in minimizing bleeding as well as in the alleviation of pain.

The complication of postoperative infection can be eliminated or minimized by preoperative intravenous antibiotics. One dose preoperatively and postoperatively every 8 hours for 3 doses is a typical regime.

Infection

Infection occurs as a complication most often two to five days following the date of the index surgical procedure. Administration of IV antibiotics such as Cephazolon in the intraoperative and immediate postoperative period will most often prevent infection. One gram of IV Cephazolon q 8 h during the 24 hour period immediately following the index operative procedure is usually sufficient to prevent infection at the operative site. Onset of fever, chills, and other signs of infection require that the joint be aspirated and sent for gram stain as well as culture and sensitivity. Blood cultures should be taken should the temperature spike. Confirmation of an infection in the joint requires immediate arthroscopic irrigation or open irrigation. IV antibiotic therapy often requires administration for a 6-week period.

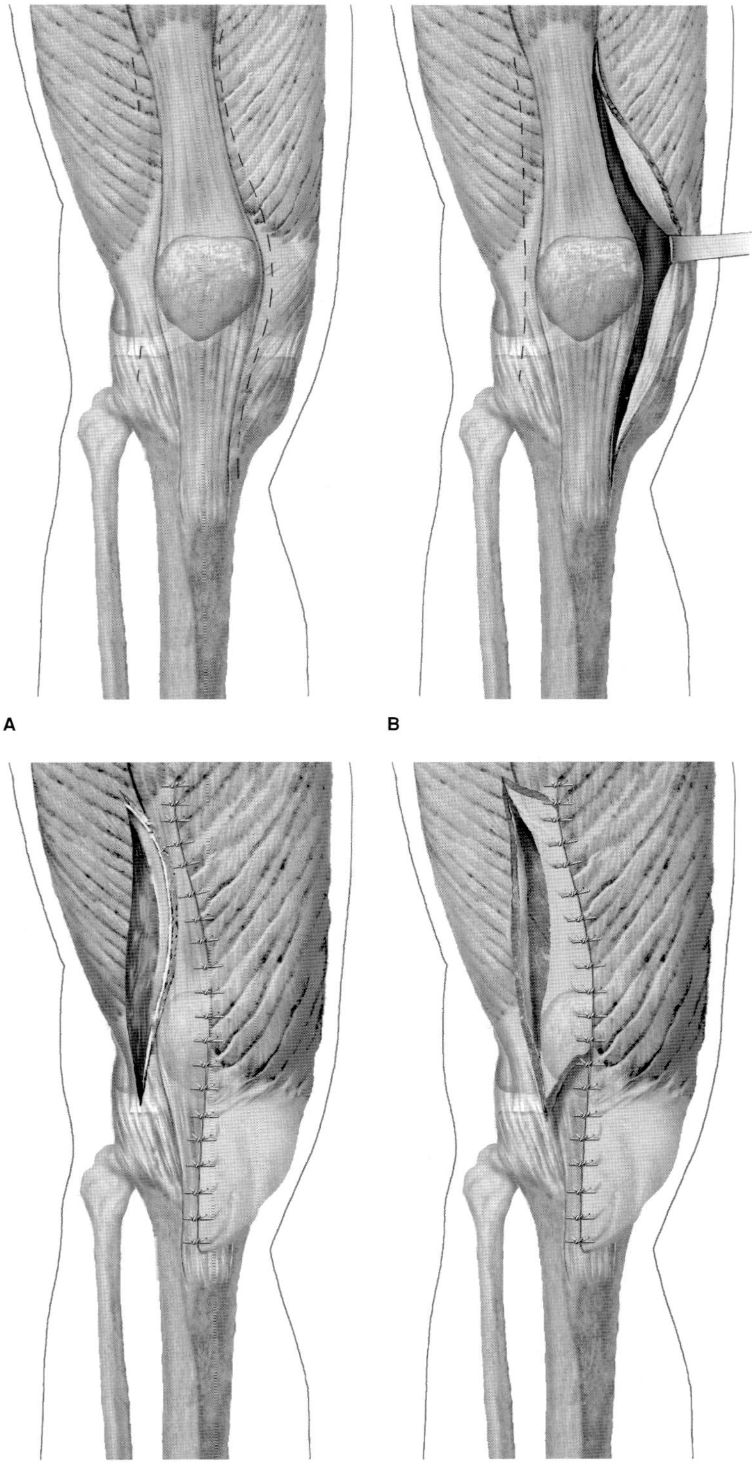

A B C D

Figure 16.2. Proximal soft tissue alignment as advocated by Insall et al.[4] **A:** A medial incision mobilizes the vastus medialis and sizes the remainder of the capsule down to the proximal tibial metaphysis adjacent to the patella tendon. A lateral retinacular release is performed well proximally into the vastus lateralis, inserting into the quadriceps mechanism. **B:** Mobilization of the medial flap of the entire length of the medial retinacular incision. **C:** Advancement of the vastus medialis obliquus and the medial capsule over the quadriceps tendon, patella, and patella tendon at least one-half the width of the patella and one-half the width of the quadriceps tendon and patella tendon. The lateral retinacular release opening is widened. **D:** The medial edge of the lateral retinacular release incision sutured to the suture line of the advanced vastus medialis obliquus and medial capsular tissue.

Signs of systemic infectious illness and local infectious processes such as fasciculitis, carbuncles, or furuncles are absolute contraindications for performing a surgical procedure.

Swelling and Pain

The swelling that eventually ensues postoperatively can be successfully treated by cryotherapy. Ice applications should be continuous rather than intermittent. Applying ice for 20 minutes every hour or every 2 hours permits bleeding and swelling to occur between ice applications. It is strongly recommended that the ice be applied continuously. The ice bag should be changed as soon as ice melts. The alternative is to use a cooling apparatus that applies continuous cold via a circulating fluid system.

Management of pain can be successfully addressed by the use of preemptive anesthesia.[5] Instillation of local anesthetic into the skin prior to the incision blocks afferent pain pathways at the skin and has been shown to be a significant factor in reducing postoperative pain.[6] Following closure, Duramorph is injected into the joint (5 mg intraarticularly). A mixture of Xylocaine/Marcaine into the incision and subcutaneous tissue after closure helps to provide postoperative analgesia. The use of Toradol intravenously in the perioperative period followed by 10 mg of Toradol four times a day postoperatively also helps to alleviate pain by reducing swelling and the inflammatory response. Oral analgesic medication in the form of Tylox or Vicodin is typically used in alleviating pain. The use of such analgesics may be minimized by the above pain-relieving regimen.

PREVENTION AND SALVAGE/TREATMENT OF LATE POSTOPERATIVE COMPLICATIONS

The complications in the late postoperative period include the following:

1. Pain
2. Patella malpositioning
3. Arthrofibrosis
4. Atrophy, paresis
5. Reflex sympathetic dystrophy
6. Patient selection

Pain

The complication of pain can generally be addressed by the previously mentioned modalities of treatment including preemptive anesthesia, ice, intraarticular Duramorph, and injections of anesthetic medication into the incision area at closure. Transcutaneous electrical nerve stimulation (TENS) applied to the skin in the operative area can help to relieve pain. Ultrasound, iontophoresis, and phonophoresis in physical therapy are modalities that can relieve pain. Nonsteroidal antiinflammatory medication, as well as intraarticular injection of steroids for the inflammatory response, may also help to relieve the pain.

Patella Malpositioning

The recurrence of lateral tilt and lateral subluxation are mechanical complications that may be prevented or minimized by early patella mobilization techniques. The patient can be taught these techniques and can start patella mobilization as early as pain will permit, optimally within 24 hours. This can be aided by the help of the physical therapist or athletic trainer. In addition to patella mobilization of almost equal importance is strengthening of the VMO, which helps to pull the patella cephalad and medially. Following the patella mobilization exercises and the strengthening of the VMO exercises, the wearing of a sleeve with a lateral buttress, which pushes the patella from the lateral to the medial direction, would also be helpful. A lateral buttress should be applied as soon as possible in the postoperative period, but soreness and swelling in the incision area and in the area of the lateral retinacular release definitely may be a hindering factor in its application in the perioperative period or late postoperative period. Prevention of contracture of the lateral retinaculum is of utmost importance in recurrence of tilt and subluxation.

It is almost self-evident that the prevention of lateral lilt and lateral subluxation first can be minimized or eliminated by observation of the tracking at surgery. Intraoperative assessment of patellofemoral excursion prior to and following the lateral release/VMO advancement is strongly suggested, in order to determine the degree of correction. It is recommended this observation be performed under selective epidural anesthesia that spares motor function but anesthetizes sensation.[7,8] Alternatively, stimulating the quadriceps mechanism (femoral nerve stimulation) while the patient is under a general anesthetic is another way of assessing the patella excursions but is probably less dynamically representative of what happens to the patellofemoral mechanism when the patient is awake and actively using the knee.

Medial subluxation is a complication that is due to excessive tightening or advancement of the VMO. Preventative measures include intraoperative observation during passive range of motion and/or active/dynamic range of motion. Salvage procedures require repeat surgical intervention to reposition the VMO or possibly a distal realignment of the patellofemoral mechanism.

Arthrofibrosis

Arthrofibrosis is an overreaction of a normal healing mechanism. It is a response of the tissues to a surgical trauma that results in an abundance of scar tissue or fibrous tissue formation within the joint especially around the patellofemoral mechanism, fat pad, and patellar tendon. Early physical therapy (within 24 hours) to include passive range of motion and patellofemoral mobilization is mandatory to preclude the detrimental effects of arthrofibrosis and can be quite successful if followed on a daily regime. Nonsteroidal antiinflammatory medication in the form of Toradol immediately postoperatively following by other nonsteroidal antiinflammatory medication is recommended. Intraarticular steroid injection is another consideration in the postoperative period. Again, applications of ice 24 hours a day immediately postoperatively and even into the late postoperative period is strongly recommended. As long as swelling exists and there is limitation of motion, it is imperative that ice be applied to minimize additional swelling and additional fibrosis formation.

Atrophy, Paresis

Quadriceps weakness and atrophy is one of the more difficult problems to prevent or treat. A portion of the etiology of the condition is frequently related to quadriceps/VMO weakness, and this is probably compounded due to the atrophy produced after surgery. Prompt initiation of isometric contractions, leg lifting exercises, and physical therapy is important for successful treatment. The patient should be counseled about the importance of the rehabilitation. Poorly motivated patients do poorly. Counseling and wisdom in preoperative patient selection is crucial to the success of patellofemoral-surgical procedures.

Reflex Sympathetic Dystrophy

Reflex sympathetic dystrophy is a dreaded complication that fortunately occurs infrequently. Pain is a prominent symptom along with other neurovascular and musculoskeletal manifestations. Active range of motion, progressive resistive exercises, and nonimpact aerobic activity are helpful in maintaining range of motion and strength. Nonsteroidal antiinflammatory medication is recommended. Nerve blocks may be helpful in the early phases of the disorder. Counseling, biofeedback, and referral to a pain management service are strongly recommended. Persistence in all the above methods and modalities of treatment is the key to coping with and overcoming this complication.

Patient Selection

Patient selection and indications are other factors in determining complications. Patients with a significant amount of arthrosis are probably not good candidates for proximal realignment, as postoperative pain is likely to persist. These patients should be considered candidates for distal tibial tubercle procedures, which elevate as well as realign the patella mechanism.[9,10]

The need for immediate cryotherapy and immediate patellofemoral mobilization in physical therapy is paramount for the success of these procedures. The patient must understand the rationale for early range of motion and patellofemoral mobilization and must cooperate for the operation to be successful. The uncooperative patient who is unwilling to participate in a strict patellofemoral rehabilitation regime and follow appropriate instructions is most likely to find the procedure a failure. Arthrofibrosis and all the above complications of the patellofemoral mechanism are more likely to occur.

References

1. Madigan R, Wissinger HA, Donaldson WF. Preliminary experience with a method of quadricepsplasty in recurrent subluxation of the patella. *J Bone Joint Surg* 1975; 57A:600.
2. Hughston JC. Subluxation of the patella. *J Bone Joint Surg* 1968;50A:1003–1026.
3. Hughston JC. Reconstruction of the extensor mechanism for subluxing patella. *Am J Sports Med* 1972;1:6–13.
4. Insall J, Bullough PG, Burstein AH. Proximal realignment of patella. *Clin Orthop* 1979;144:63.
5. Skeehan TM. The use of pre-emptive anesthesia. (Personal communication.)
6. Maliniak K. Selective epidural anesthesia as an aid in assessing patella tracking during surgical reconstruction. (Personal communication.)
7. Fulkerson J, Hungerford D. *Disorders of the Patellofemoral Joint.* Baltimore: Williams & Wilkins, 1990.
8. Maquet PGJ. *Biomechanics of the Knee with Application to the Pathogenesis and the Surgical Treatment of Osteoarthritis.* Berlin: Springer, 1976.

Chapter 17

Complications and Pitfalls in Tibial Tubercle Osteotomy Associated with Distal Extensor Mechanism Realignment

Fred Flandry and Raymond Hui

Osteotomy of the tibial tubercle is a surgical tactic that should be reserved for the treatment of symptomatic instability, arthritic deterioration of the patellofemoral articulation, or extensile exposure. This chapter primarily addresses reported complications resulting from surgery for the first two indications as components of distal extensor mechanism realignments, although there can be carryover to the third indication. Although they are technically straightforward, procedures for tubercle osteotomy demand a thorough understanding of the regional anatomy, treatment goals, precise execution of the osteotomy, and fixation for a successful outcome. An outline of problems encountered with tibial tubercle osteotomies lists complications in broad groups (Table 17.1).

SURGICAL ANATOMY

The tibial tubercle is erroneously thought of as the sole insertion point of the extensor mechanism on the proximal tibia. This misconception alone accounts for many complications. A more in-depth understanding of the anatomy of this region can help to avert many of these complications.

The term *extensor* is a misnomer. The extensor mechanism functions as an eccentric decelerator during walking, running, descending stairs or inclines, landing, or slowing of one's momentum. This fact has implications not only for surgery but for rehabilitation after injury or surgery, as well.

The extensor mechanism proper is a broad aponeurosis of connective tissue constituting the medial and lateral anterior thirds of the knee's capsular ligaments (commonly termed *retinacular ligaments* or *retinaculum*). The patella, the largest sesamoid of the body, is contained in the center of this aponeurosis. The quadriceps comprises six heads: the rectus femoris, the vastus lateralis, the vastus lateralis obliquus, the vastus medialis, the vastus medialis obliquus, and the vastus intermedius. This group of muscles furnishes a direct motor input to the patella, providing both power (all heads), positioning (vastus lateralis, vastus medialis, vastus medialis obliquus), and proprioceptive functions (rectus femoris). More proximal muscles act through the iliopatellar band along with the short head of the biceps femoris muscle laterally and semimembranosus medially to modulate the action of the quadriceps. These hamstring muscles modulate action in two ways: they serve as antagonists to the quadriceps contraction (along with other hamstring muscles that insert more directly on the tibia), and they adjust tension in the lower retinaculum. Inherent in the latter action is a likely, but as yet unproven, proprioceptive function.

The more distal region of the extensor mechanism is an area of great concern from the standpoint of surgical anatomy. Pivotal to avoiding problems in this area is the surgeon's ability to appreciate the extensor mechanism's insertion points on the tibia and their relationship to, i.e., their distance from, the tibial articular rim. The patellar tendon is a continuum of the quadriceps tendon from the patella to the tibial tubercle. This insertion is fully 2 to 3 cm distal to the articular rim. Deep to the patellar tendon is the infrapatellar bursa (Fig. 17.1) and an inferiorly projecting tongue of the infrapatellar fat pad, which is contained within the bursa. These structures separate the deep surface of the tendon from the underlying bone.[1,2] Thus, at the most anterior point the extensor mechanism attaches well distal to the articular rim. Because of this orientation, when

Table 17.1. Categorical grouping of complications associated with tibial tubercle osteotomy

Improper indications
Failure to accomplish goals
Failure to correct luxation
Failure to unload the patellofemoral articulation
Iatrogenic anatomic derangements
Infrapatellar bursa and retinaculum scarring
Patella baja
Genu recurvatum
Distal migration of the tubercle
Fat pad fibrosis
Postsurgical complications (local)
Infection
Hematoma
Failure of fixation and graft displacement
Nonunion
Patellar tendon rupture
Fracture
Skin slough
Progressive arthrosis
Osteotomy in the presence of total knee components
Donor-site morbidity
Postsurgical complications (distant)
Compartment syndrome
Reflex sympathetic dystrophy
Deep venous thrombosis
Neurovascular compromise
Rehabilitation

the quadriceps contracts, resolution of force vectors provides for some of the power of the contraction to be translated into a direct axial load. The load is dispersed over the full weight-bearing surface of the tibiofemoral joint (Fig. 17.2). This phenomenon has great relevance to tibiofemoral stability. The medial and lateral middle third capsular ligaments insert on the tibia at a point only 0.5 to 1.0 cm from the articular rim. From their most anterior edge, however, the retinacular ligaments' point of insertion follows a line from the insertion point of the patellar tendon to the insertion point of the medial middle third capsular ligaments (Fig. 17.3). Likewise, the space deep to the retinaculum is not adherent to the underlying bone.

Failure to appreciate these relationships could cause the surgeon to create incisions that generate scar tissue. Scar tissue can obliterate the bursa and cause the distal extensor mechanism to adhere to underlying bone as far proximal as the articular rim. When this occurs, the patella is pulled distally creating a patella baja, and its inferior pole tilts inward toward the femoral intercondylar notch (Fig. 17.4). The pull of the quadriceps is now exerted nearer the articular rim, focusing tibiofemoral pressures in a much smaller area along the an-

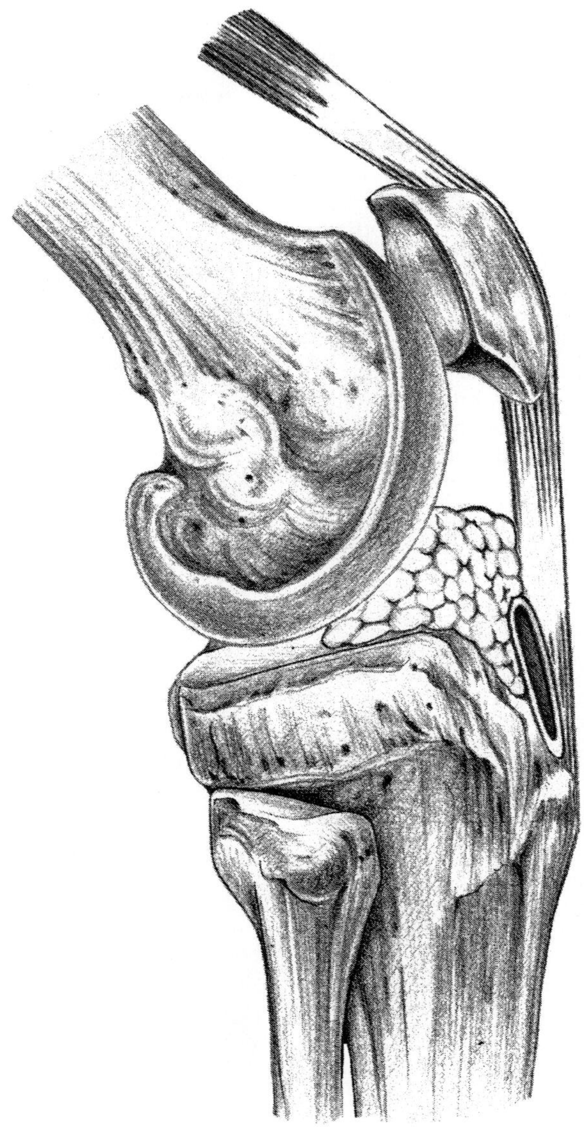

Figure 17.1. The deep infrapatellar bursa. Insertion of the patellar tendon is several centimeters distal to the articular rim. A "tongue" of the fat pad hangs down within the bursa.

terior rim. Because there is reduced surface area for contact and lubrication, greater tensile forces are generated.

Pain of multiple orgins is the usual result of these abnormal mechanics. The increased tensile forces stimulate pain fibers in the richly innervated retinaculum.[3] In addition, tension on the retinaculum that is abnormally scarred to the periosteum (proximal to the normal line of insertion) generates pain from nerve endings in the periosteum. Finally, the abnormal contact forces on the articular surfaces can eventually accelerate arthritic changes and trigger inflammatory cascades.[4]

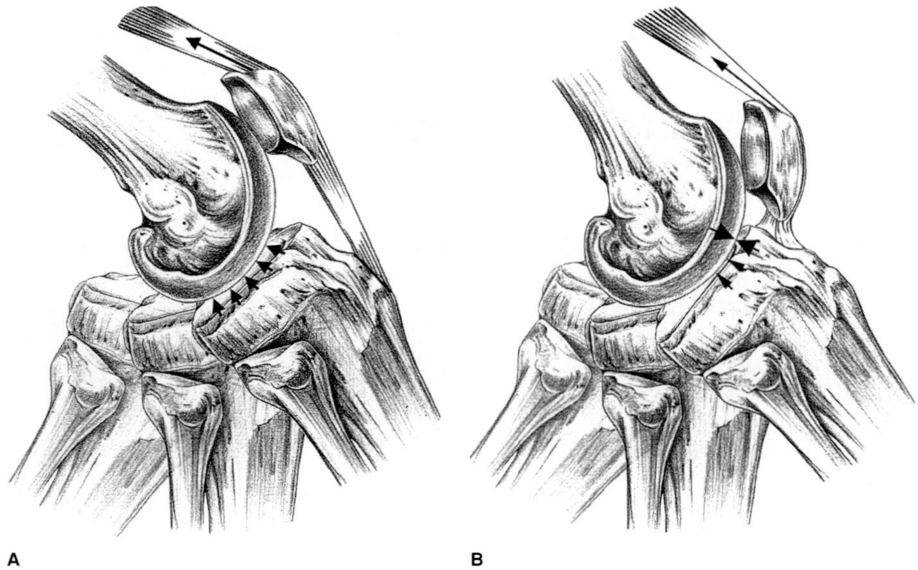

Figure 17.2. **A:** In a normal patellofemoral joint, the pull of the extensor mechanism allows the load (arrows) to be dispersed over the full surface of the joint. **B:** When the infrapatellar bursa is obliterated, the pull is shifted proximal to the articular rim, resulting in disproportionate anterior loading of the tibiofemoral joint.

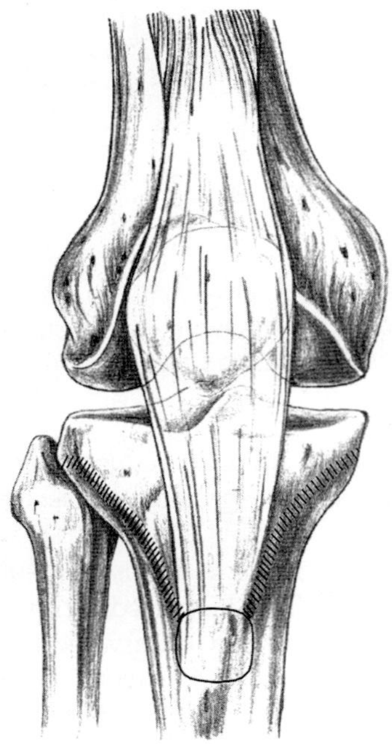

Figure 17.3. A bony ridge seen on the proximal anterior tibia is the insertion point of the capsular ligaments. Note the insertion point becomes more distal at the tibial tubercle.

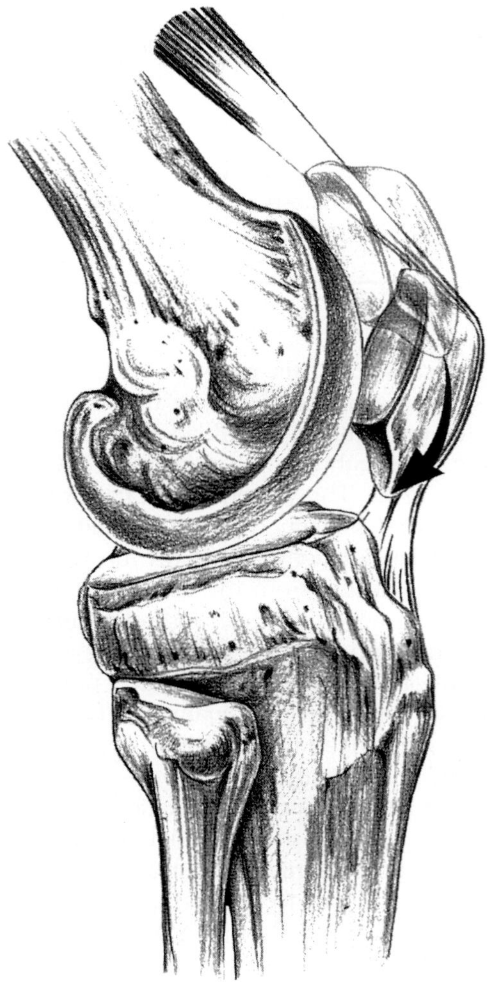

Figure 17.4. When patella baja occurs, the patella is pulled distally, and the inferior pole is drawn deep toward the intercondylar notch.

One further progression can occur. In patients who form severe scars, scarring in the bursa can involve the entire fat pad and extend through the ligamentum mucosum into the femoral intercondylar notch. A large mass of dense noncompliant scar is created in the anterocentral portion of the knee. With knee extension, the mass impinges against the intercondylar shelf, creating the so-called infrapatellar contracture syndrome[5,6] (Fig. 17.5). This tissue mass can become so large it blocks full extension.

In terms of complications related to skeletal anatomy, the issue of physeal injury is germane to our discussion. The tibial tubercle is an epiphyseal structure. Osteotomy before physeal closure carries with it the risk of deformities associated with premature closure or partial closure of the proximal tibial physis.

GOALS OF TREATMENT

In the context of this discussion, a tibial tubercle osteotomy is needed for one of three reasons: extensile exposure, stabilization of a subluxating or dislocating patella, or unloading an arthritic patellofemoral joint. There are distinctly different goals for each of these generic procedures, and these goals should guide performance of the operation.

Extensile exposure carries the most obvious goal—surgical exposure for an unrelated procedure. The considerations here are to osteotomize the tubercle in such a manner that it heals readily, to cause no marked morbidity to the extensor mechanism, and to accomplish fixation despite the possible presence of an intramedullary or extramedullary tibial implant.

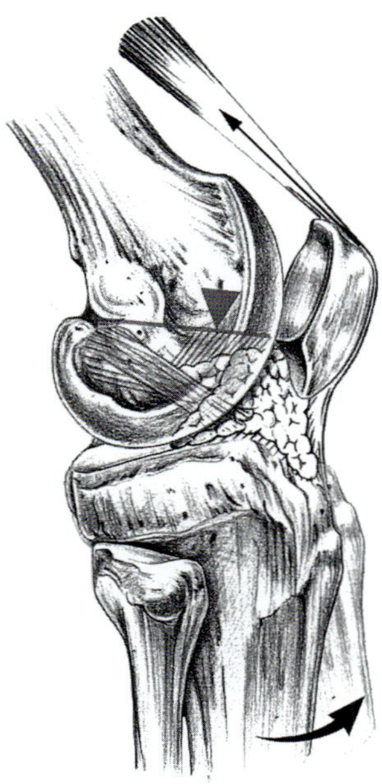

Figure 17.5. In advanced patella baja, fibrotic scarring of the fat pad bridges the anterior cruciate ligament to the patellar tendon. With attempted knee extension (arrow), this fibrotic mass impinges on the intercondylar shelf.

Osteotomy of the tubercle as a component of a patellofemoral-stabilizing procedure requires an understanding of the anatomic derangements that contribute to the instability. Beyond the focus of this discussion are the releases and muscle transfer components of the proximal realignment. Specific abnormalities that indicate the need for a distal realignment (osteotomy) are patella alta and an excessive Q angle. Although elevation of the tubercle can be done with the stabilization procedure, it is a treatment for arthrosis, not instability, and therefore should be considered separately.

Patella alta is a serious but often ignored abnormality. It can be corrected only if the tubercle fragment is completely detached so that it can be shifted distally. The goal is to bring the inferior pole of the patella to lie on Blumensaat's line when the knee is flexed 45 to 55 degrees or about 2 cm above the tibial articular surface regardless of the degree of flexion.[7]

Correction of the Q angle is designed to bring it out of the excessive range. Hughston and Walsh[7] recommend correction of values in excess of 10 degrees. Kolowich et al[8] recommend correction of a tubercle sulcus angle of greater than 5 degrees. The theory that correction should be made to attain an arbitrary "normal" value is probably flawed and difficult if not impossible to execute. Although methods have been advocated for engineering an exact correction, intraoperative execution to that degree of precision is difficult. A more attainable and functionally relevant goal is to correct the Q angle so that passive tracking is normalized after the patella alta is corrected.

In a patient with an arthritic patellofemoral articulation, the goal is to unload the joint by elevation of the tubercle. Theoretically, the Maquet osteotomy unloads the articulation evenly. The anteromedial osteotomy by its combined medial shift can unload the lateral facet a relatively greater amount than the medial facet. The implication is obvious and the application eloquent. Subchondral sclerotic changes can be used as a biologic indicator of joint loading (P. Maquet, personal communication, 1993). The goal of even unloading or selective unloading can therefore be determined by assessing patterns of sclerotic subchondral bone (coupled with other radiographic signs of arthrosis) on plain x-ray films or tomograms. By varying the angle of the osteotomy from coronal plane (Maquet) to oblique (anteromedial) the amount of medial shift relative to elevation can be varied. Thus, the lateral articulation can be selectively unloaded if lateral arthrosis predominates.

The other issue or goal regarding an elevation-type osteotomy is the degree of elevation. With such considerations as the likelihood of bleeding, compartment syndrome, and skin slough increasing with increasing amount of elevation,[9–15] the goal is to perform the minimal elevation that will produce adequate relief of symptoms. Maquet[11] recommended a minimum 2-cm elevation; however, others have shown that beyond 1.25 to 1.5 cm of elevation, the symptomatic gains decrease dramatically versus the increasing risk of complication.[10,16] Therefore, limiting the elevation to 1.5 cm is a reasonable surgical goal. Pan et al[17] argue that the combination of elevation and shingle length is the true determinant of articular unloading and advocate a 2-cm elevation with a 20-cm shingle. It is clear that controversy still exists in this area, and the surgeon's goals should be based on his or her interpretation of the current literature.

PROCEDURES OF HISTORICAL INTEREST

If viewed in terms of a generic operation, osteotomy of the tubercle can involve (1) translocation of a wafer of the tubercle containing the insertion of the patellar tendon (prototype: Elmslie-Trillat),[18] (2) elevation of the tubercle (prototype: Maquet),[19] (3) elevation combined with medial translocation of the tubercle (prototype: anteromedialization),[20] (4) medial transfer of a split lateral half of the patellar tendon (prototype: Roux-Goldthwait),[21,22] or (5) translocation of the full cortical thickness tubercle to be countersunk into a cortical window (prototype: Hauser).[23] Other so-called distal alignment procedures such as the semitendinosus transfer or Galeazzi procedure[24] do not fall into this category because they are purely soft tissue transfers that do not involve an osteotomy of the tubercle. While the Elmslie-Trillat, Maquet, and anteromedialization procedures remain in use, the Roux-Goldthwait and Hauser procedures have largely been abandoned because of associated complications.[1] Reviewing these complications illustrates their many pitfalls and helps us to avoid them.

In the Roux-Goldthwait procedure, the patellar tendon is split into medial and lateral halves. The lateral half is transferred deep to the medial half and is anchored to medial soft tissues or periosteum, or both. In terms of accomplishing goals, while the Q angle can be corrected, patella alta is unchanged. If significantly decreased, all pull would be through the transferred half. Whiteside[25] demonstrated that lateral tilt could even be accentuated when the lateral split tendon was transferred in this manner. Balancing pull through both halves of the tendon was difficult to achieve, and if it was not equally balanced the transferred half was pulled loose, ruptured, or autolysed.[1,7,26] Failure to protect the infrapatellar bursa during transfer of the split tendon resulted in the bursa and tendon scarring down to the underlying anterior tibial cortex. This had the effect of transferring extensor mechanism forces from the tibial tubercle to a more proximal location near the articular rim. Despite these drawbacks, when the operation was performed with attention to these technical details, it produced champions historically[27] and recently.[25]

With the Hauser procedure, an entire bone block containing the tubercle and tendon's insertion was translocated to and countersunk into a cortical window remote from the donor site. Probably the most lasting criticism of the procedure was the relative ease of inadvertent overcorrection resulting in a patella baja.[28] The patella baja led to pain, a dynamic external rotational tibial deformity if the bone block was also transferred too far medially (Fig. 17.6), and patellofemoral arthrosis.[29] If the location of the cortical window was not correct initially, the procedure did not allow for adjustment or correction. Severe complications such as those above, compartment syndrome,[30] or overall complication rates approaching 54%[13] caused many surgeons to abandon this procedure. One reported series of patients treated with a "modified Hauser" procedure claimed no serious complications; however, the osteotomized bone was not countersunk and the operation therefore resembled an Elmslie-Trillat more than a Hauser osteotomy.[31]

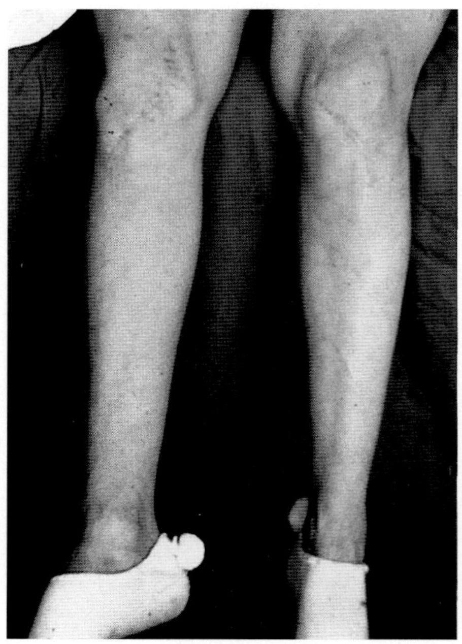

Figure 17.6. A complication of the Hauser procedure. In addition to patella baja, a dynamic external rotation torque is imposed.

DISTAL ALIGNMENT PROCEDURES IN CURRENT USE

At this time there are three tibial tubercle osteotomies that are commonly performed: the Elmslie-Trillat, or Hughston, procedure, which involves the translocation of a wafer of the tubercle containing the insertion of the patellar tendon[7,18]; the Maquet procedure, in which a shingle of tubercle is elevated[19]; and the anteromedialization, or Fulkerson, procedure, which combines an elevation with medial translocation of the tubercle.[20] We will focus only on the tubercle osteotomy technique of each procedure while acknowledging that it may be only a component of the overall procedure.

Patellar Stabilizing and Extensile Exposure Procedures

The Elmslie-Trillat, or Hughston, procedure is primarily directed at correcting instability rather than arthrosis.[32] Because it does not intentionally elevate the tubercle, unloading other than correction of abnormal loading as a consequence of the malalignment is serendipitous. Without the translocation, the surgical sequence for the osteotomy and refixation serve also as an ideal method when osteotomy for extensile exposure is indicated. As described, this is the only currently popular osteotomy that has the capacity to correct patella alta.

Medial and lateral arthrotomy incisions, components of the proximal soft tissue realignment, are extended distally along the borders of the patellar tendon to the tubercle. Care is taken to incise only the retinaculum so as not to disturb the underlying bursa or periosteum. The periosteum outlining the medial, lateral, and distal borders of the tubercle, however, is incised. With the patellar tendon gently elevated to expose the bursa and proximal border of the tubercle, an osteotome is inserted from the lateral retinacular incision deep to the tendon and is seated against the proximal edge of the tubercle at the insertion of the patellar tendon. The osteotome is oriented from superolateral toward the distal medial portion of the tubercle and just deep enough to cut a slightly more than cortical thickness wafer of bone—at least 5 mm but less than 10 mm thick (Fig. 17.7). The perimeter of the osteotomized fragment should be relatively square and should correspond to the periosteal incision described above. Sometimes it is helpful to initially make a 5-mm-deep osteotomy along the distal border of the tubercle to prevent the "wafer" from becoming a "shingle."

Care should be exercised against injudicious handling of the wafer lest it fragment. When osteotomized, it can be freely reflected superiorly, but the deep surface of the patellar tendon should not be detached from the fat

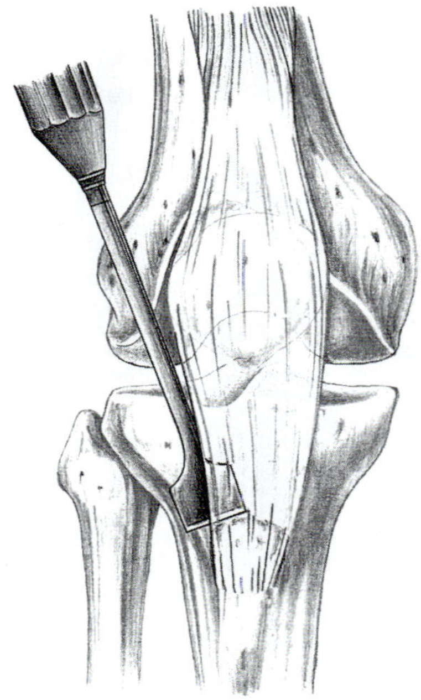

Figure 17.7. The osteotome is set gently into the bursa and rested against the superior edge of the tubercle. In this way, the bursa is protected from scarring.

pad. Fixation using a four-pronged staple with narrow tines is preferable to screw fixation because it allows adjustment by millimeters rather than by centimeters if the original position for fixation proves suboptimal after tracking is checked. The staple can be seated in the wafer fragment immediately after osteotomizing it. One sharp impact should drive the tines through the fragment. The staple and fragment can then be lifted away and a joker retractor used to press and seat the fragment fully to the base of the staple (Fig. 17.8).

Two clinical methods are available intraoperatively to determine the proper amount of distal transposition.[1,7,32,33] With the knee flexed 45 to 55 degrees, the inferior pole of the patella should just make contact with a straight instrument or probe inserted into the joint so that it lies against the intercondylar shelf (Fig. 17.9). This is a clinical representation of Blumensaat's line. The second method is not dependent on flexion angle but requires the surgeon to know the width of his or her index finger, which should be approximately 2 cm. The height of the inferior pole of the patella above the articular surface should be constant regardless of flexion angle. Therefore, with one side of the tip of the index finger resting against the articular surface, the tubercle should be transposed distally until the inferior pole just touches the other side of the tip of the finger (Fig. 17.10).

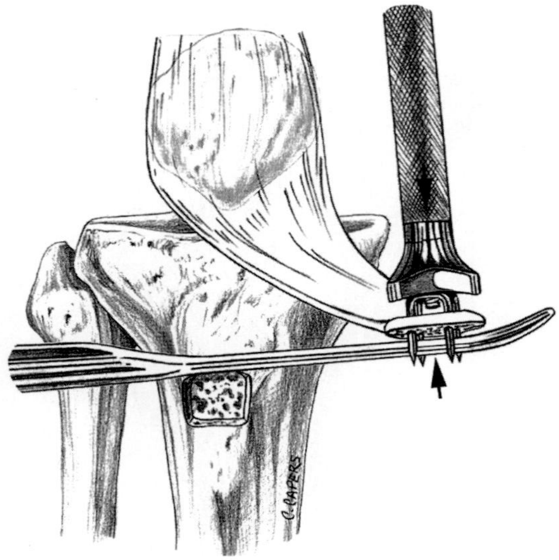

Figure 17.8. After impacting the staple partially through the tubercle bone "wafer," a joker retractor is used to push the fragment up until it is seated under the base of the staple.

Medial transposition is performed to correct the Q angle clinically and is usually about half the width of the wafer fragment of the tubercle. It averages between 5 and 10 mm. The location for fixation is estimated and the bone is fish-scaled to improve fixation. The fragment is provisionally fixed and passive tracking checked. If adequate correction has not been achieved, the fragment is repositioned. To seat the staple, the proximal edge should be levered distally so that it does not cut into the tendon (Fig. 17.10). In an osteotomy for extensile exposure, the fragment would simply be replaced in its original bed. The proximal soft tissue balancing is done, and the retinacular incisions are closed by side-to-side anastomosis to the patellar tendon. The periosteum around the tubercle is closed where possible.

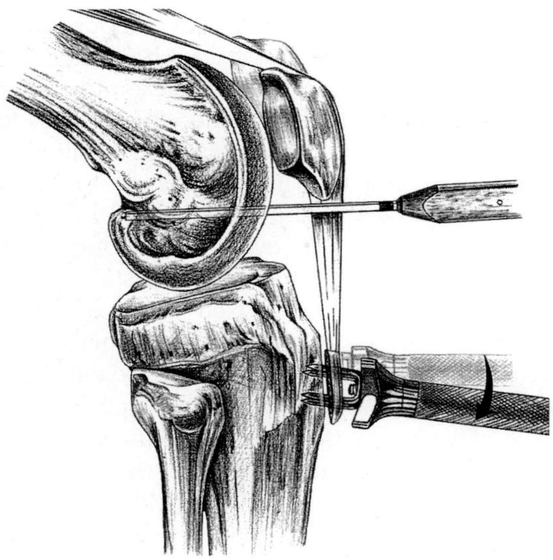

Figure 17.9. The tubercle wafer is translocated distally until the inferior pole of the patella contacts a straight instrument lying against the intercondylar shelf. The knee must be flexed to between 45 and 55 degrees for this measurement to be accurate. Angling the impactor slightly distalward prevents the superior edge of the staple from cutting into the tendon.

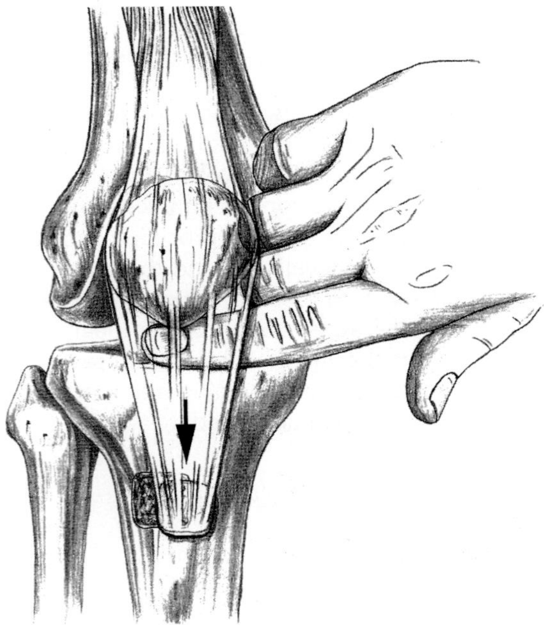

Figure 17.10. An average-sized index finger (2 cm) rests on the articular surface. The tubercle is translocated distally until the inferior pole of the patella contacts the opposite side of the finger. This method is independent of knee flexion angle.

Patellofemoral Unloading Procedures

Two procedures are designated as patellofemoral unloading osteotomies. They are indicated for the treatment of symptomatic patellofemoral arthrosis. The Maquet osteotomy uniformly unloads the patellofemoral joint, while the anteromedialization more selectively unloads the lateral half of the articulation and improves the Q angle. Neither procedure, as described, corrects patella alta and neither is appropriate for extensile exposure.

In the classic Maquet[34] osteotomy, the tubercle is shingled but left attached at a point approximately 12 cm distal. Maquet made his approach through a longitudinal incision just medial to the tibial crest. Multiple drill holes were made 7 to 8 mm posterior to the anterior crest and connected with a thin osteotome. Care was taken to keep the distal crest intact, thus creating a tongue of bone about 2.5 cm wide and 11.5 cm long. The osteotomy was done from the medial side attempting to keep the periosteum on the lateral face of the tibia intact. A block of iliac crest 2 to 3 cm thick was placed deep to the tubercle's position on the crest, thus elevating the "tongue" or shingle. Maquet originally advocated a 2 cm elevation; however, more contemporary researchers continue to argue the ideal amount.[9,10,12–14,16,35] The bony dead space created by elevation of the shingle was filled with morselized cancellous bone graft. If stable, the shingle was not fixed. Maquet also described a medial shift of the shingle if needed in patients with relatively excessive lateral patellofemoral contact pressures.[34,36] After early reports of skin problems, modifications to the skin incision[10,15] or closure have been recommended.

Many variations of this osteotomy have been described.[10,13,35–38] These variations involve shingle length and height of elevation primarily, but they also involve exposure, creation, and fixation of the osteotomy. Controversy continues regarding the fine details of the technique, and surgeons who use the procedure should be familiar with the current literature.

The anteromedialization procedure is approached similarly by a logitudinal incision through the lateral retinaculum. It extends distally just lateral to the crest of the tibia.[20] A 10- to 12-cm periosteal incision is made just on the medial border of the crest of the tibia and extends from the tubercle distally. Subperiosteal dissection is carried out to expose the lateral face of the tibia down to the posterolateral angle. Multiple drill holes made from just off the medial edge of the crest are directed posterolaterally so they exit on the lateral face of the tibia. Care is taken that the drills or osteotomy do not penetrate at the posterolateral angle, where the anterior tibial artery and deep peroneal nerve are vulnerable, or at the posterior face, where the posterior tibial artery and nerve are vulnerable. Varying the obliquity of the angled osteotomy allows a relatively greater medialization (shallow angle) or anteriorization (steep angle) (Fig. 17.11). The osteotomy is turned to exit the anterior cortex proximally just superior to the patellar tendon insertion. It extends distally for 5 to 8 cm distal to the tubercle. The cuts are completed with a reciprocating saw and osteotomes. The shingle is mobilized to slide anteromedially while the surgeon attempts to maintain the distal hinge intact. Unlike the Maquet osteotomy, no dead space is created, so bone grafting is unnecessary. Fulkerson's goal was a 1.0- to 1.5-cm anterior displacement. Internal fixation is by a cortical lag screw through the posterior face of the tibia or by a cancellous lag screw.

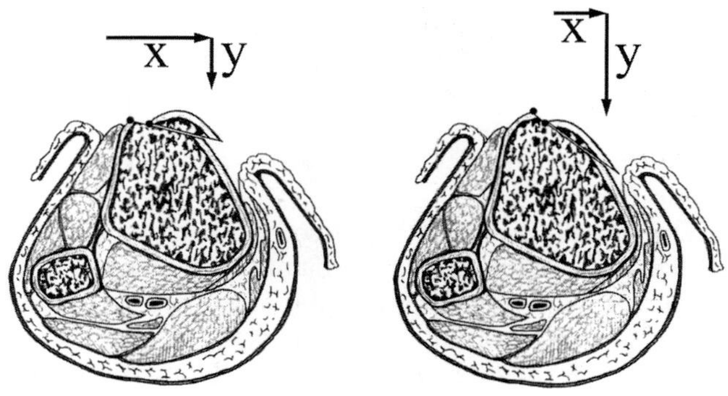

Figure 17.11. Varying the obliquity of the osteotomy allows the "shelf" to be shifted relatively more medial (shallow osteotomy) (left), or anterior (steep osteotomy) (right).

COMPLICATIONS AND SOLUTION STRATEGIES

Improper Indications

The first and only indication for reconstructive surgery on the extensor mechanism is for symptomatic instability or arthrosis. This cannot be emphasized enough. The mere presence of excessive clinical measurements (Q angle, sulcus angle, patella alta) or abnormal radiographic measurements or signs (Merchant angle, tilt, sclerosis, loss of joint space, osteophytes, etc.) without significant symptoms is not an indication for surgery.

Perhaps the most critical steps in performing a tubercle osteotomy occur before the skin incision is made. A clear vision should exist as to whether the tubercle osteotomy is being performed for (1) patellar stabilization; (2) unloading the patellofemoral articulation; (3) extensile exposure for an unrelated procedure, such as an arthroplasty or a fracture reduction; or (4) some combination of the above. Specifically, stabilization-type procedures should be carried out more for instability than for pain and unloading procedures, more for arthritic pain than for instability. However, tibial tubercle osteotomies have no place in the management of anterior knee pain in the absence of arthrosis or instability.[1,39] Failure to observe proper indications has been correlated to suboptimal outcomes.[40]

Timing of the procedure may appropriately be considered along with indications. Even with proper indications and goals, Cox[41] reported a decreased range of motion when the procedure was done too soon after an acute patellar dislocation.

Solution Strategies

Always approach a tubercle osteotomy with clear indications based on the goals of the correction. For patellar stabilizing procedures, the indications are correction of excessive patella alta and excessive Q angle with the ultimate goal of restoring stability. For patellofemoral unloading procedures, the indication is excessive patellofemoral contact pressures and arthrosis and the ultimate goal is decreasing contact pressures and relieving discomfort.

Developing an algorithm based on the preoperative clinical and radiographic examination is helpful. If instability is present, the osteotomy along with other elements of proximal soft tissue balancing should correct anatomic derangements contributing to the instability. If patella alta is present, distal transposition is indicated. Conti et al [42] recommend distal transposition if the Insall-Burstein index is greater than 1.3, and Hughston and associates[7,32,33] recommend the procedure if the inferior pole of the patella sits proximal to Blumensaat's line with the knee flexed 45 to 55 degrees. If the Q angle is excessive or the limb extremely valgus, medialization may be indicated. If arthrosis is present, pure elevation is indicated. If arthrosis is largely in the lateral patellofemoral articulation, anteromedialization is indicated. When a combination of these factors is present, a combination of surgical tactics is appropriate. In the case of an acute patellar dislocation, surgery should be delayed for a 4- to 6-week period during which an active rehabilitation program is implemented.

Failure to Accomplish Goals

Failure to Correct Luxation

Both medial[43] and persistent lateral subluxation have been reported from either over- or undercorrection.[33,44] Molina et al[45] recommend medialization from 0.5 to 1.0 cm. Conti et al[42] advocate limiting medial transposition in an Elmslie-Trillat–type osteotomy to 10 mm, arguing that greater amounts will lead to painful medial impingement.

Solution Strategies. Reconstruction should proceed in a logical sequence. In a combined proximal-distal realignment, the distal component must be done first because proximal soft tissue balancing is based on the new position of the patellar tendon insertion. Knowledge, experience, and the intraoperative guidelines discussed above will allow an approximation of the new insertion site, but the surgeon should approach this point initially as a trial location. With provisional fixation, tracking should be checked and the position adjusted until tracking is optimized. Note that the distal position alone may not correct the instability completely; however, it should provide the optimal position on which to retension the retinaculum and the heads of the quadriceps. If the initial goals are not achieved, it is reasonable to allow time to determine if rehabilitation of the quadriceps coupled with a presumably improved albeit suboptimal realignment can produce an asymptomatic or acceptable knee. If symptoms remain despite rehabilitation efforts, revision surgery is indicated.

Failure to Unload the Patellofemoral Articulation

Adequate anterior displacement, coupled with medialization if arthrosis disproportionately affects the lateral portion of the patellofemoral articulation, is necessary to relieve symptoms.[40,45,46] Again, the exact amount is debated and is a compromise. Displacement that is sufficient to improve symptoms must be weighed against the risk of complications. For the present, this amount seems to lie somewhere between 1.0 and 2.0 cm.[9,10,12–14,16,17,34,35,40,45,46]

Solution Strategies. If the symptoms are not alleviated by the procedure, the strategy is similar to that above. Fulkerson et al[46] reported improvement in symptoms with revision osteotomy and further anterior displacement. Again, it seems wise that revision should follow an appropriate period of healing and rehabilitation.

Iatrogenic Anatomic Derangements

The most obvious tactic here is prevention. Knowledge of the anatomy and of the consequences of not appreciating and thus obliterating functionally important tissue planes is the best means of preventing this problem. Surgical tactics that protect these structures must be observed. Incisions in the retinaculum should be made along the medial or lateral edge of the patellar tendon, and care taken that the depth of that cut is sufficient only to divide the retinaculum but not to score underlying bursal tissue or bone. Retractors placed in the bursa should be dull, not sharp. Finally, the tubercle should be osteotomized from within the bursa outward to prevent the osteotomy line from extending proximally and involving the floor of the bursa.

Infrapatellar Bursa and Retinaculum Scarring

Trauma to the infrapatellar bursa results in scarring and obliteration of the bursa.[1,2] The deep surface of the patella adheres to and ultimately scars to the bursal periosteal surface of the proximal anterior tibia. In effect, this causes the tendon to insert on the tibia near or at the articular rim rather than 2 to 3 cm distally at the tibial tubercle, adversely affecting normal extensor mechanism biomechanics.

Likewise, the retinacular expanse medially and laterally can scar down to the underlying periosteum if the periosteum is disrupted.[1] This causes abnormal adherence to richly innervated periosteum and increased tension at this adherence due to the resultant abnormal extensor biomechanics.

Solution Strategies. The tactics necessary to prevent this complication are described above (see Surgical Anatomy). Dealing with the complication, when it exists, can be frustrating for removing scar tissue causes new scar tissue to form. A "normal" knee is an unrealistic goal, and patients should be so advised. They will retain some limitations particularly in kneeling and squatting. If possible, waiting until the scar tissue is mature and the healing physiology is quiescent is helpful. The surgical approach should be as atraumatic as possible. Every attempt must be made to lyse the adherence through the plane of the adhesion and to avoid incising or inadvertently stripping the periosteum. A bulky compressive dressing is maintained the first two postoperative days to minimize hematoma formation, which might itself lead to new scar formation, in the dead spaces created. The key to success, as it were, is to institute early motion (within 3 days of the operation) so that tissue planes move against each other, minimizing the likelihood of adhesion formation.

Patella Baja

Patella baja is caused by scarring of the bursa, overcorrection of the transplanted tubercle, or, rarely, from procedures done in patients with an open physis.[1,6,7,28,33,47,48] Sadly, it is almost always an iatrogenic condition, and, as if to punish the surgeon, it is rarely asymptomatic. Retropatellar pain, loss of motion, crepitation, and extensor mechanism disuse and dysfunction are common sequelae. The pathomechanics of this condition have already been described.

Solution Strategies. Nonopervative measures are not successful in resolving this problem. Therefore, early surgical intervention has been advocated.[23] The tubercle must be reosteotomized. Adhesions in the infrapatellar bursa area must be lysed until pull on the quadriceps tendon freely moves the patellar tendon and adjacent retinaculum independently of the tibia. A methodology such as that described by Hughston and Walsh[7] and discussed above is critical for determing the proper level for refixation of the tubercle. If the surgeon is in doubt on clinical grounds alone, intraoperative radiographs should be obtained.

Genu Recurvatum

Failure to delay osteotomy procedures about the tibial tubercle until a time at or near physeal closure puts the patient at risk of complete or, more likely partial growth arrest and resultant growth deformities, such as hyperextension, varus, valgus, external tibial torsion, or distal migration of the tubercle.[5,6,7,29,41,47,49–53] The most likely deformity is the anterior hemiepiphyseal arrest that causes an apparent genu recurvatum over time. The prominence of the tubercle disappears, and the visible deformity has much the same appearance and has been mistaken for the posterior sag of a posterior cruciate ligament injury. In severe cases, the extensor mechanism is functionally unloaded as the patient is biomechanically habituated to walk with a "recurvatum gait" because the quadriceps is not used as a momentum dissipater. Severe quadriceps atrophy, pes anserine bursitis, and peroneal neuritis can be further sequelae.

Solution Strategies. The most obvious solution is to not perform a tubercle osteotomy until after physeal closure. When a distal realignment procedure is needed and cannot be delayed, one of the distal soft tissue procedures such as the Galeazzi transfer can function effectively.[24]

If the deformity has occurred, it is characterized by a reversal in the normal 10-degree anterior to posterior slope of the articular surface of the proximal tibia. The most appropriate but technically demanding solution is to perform an anterior opening wedge osteotomy just proximal to the insertion of the patellar tendon while maintaining the continuity of the posterior cortex. This can be accomplished either in a one-stage procedure with bone grafting (although the risk of scarring in the infrapatellar bursa is greater with this option), or by the use of Ilizarov techniques, which allow an anterior hemicorticotomy to be performed at the same level with a gradual distraction using an external fixator with an anterior self-centering hinge oriented in the sagittal plane. With this method, much less dissection is required and much less scarring ensues.

Distal Migration of the Tubercle

If the tubercle is transplanted distal to the physis while it is still open, an abnormally distal insertion of the patellar tendon can result (a severe patella baja). Although less common than genu recurvatum, it has been reported.[6]

Solution Strategies. Again, avoid tubercle osteotomy before physeal closure. To correct a migrated tubercle, the tubercle should be osteotomized and transplanted using methodology as described for the Elmslie-Trillat type osteotomy. The goal should be to move the tubercle proximally until the inferior pole of the patella is positioned on Blumensaat's line when the knee is flexed from 45 to 55 degrees. In severe, long-standing cases, soft tissue releases in the infrapatellar tendon bursa may be necessary, as well. The prognosis in these cases is not as favorable. Ideally, this salvage procedure should be delayed until at or near physeal closure to avoid multiple revisions.

Fat Pad Fibrosis

The infrapatellar fat pad can be damaged by incisions placed too deeply through the retinaculum or into the infrapatellar bursa. The fat pad forms a supporting conduit for a rich vascular anastomotic plexus connecting inferomedial and inferolateral geniculate arteries with vessels supplying the anterior cruciate ligament.[54] If completely severed by a deep incision, these vessels may go into spasm for several hours and thus go unrecognized during closure. If bleeding occurs after the fat pad is closed, the hematoma is usually contained within the fat pad and will eventually organize and fibrose. A large fibrotic nodule in the fat pad is painful and blocks full extension and flexion.

Solution Strategies. Two strategies are aimed at preventing this problem. If the tourniquet is used, it should be released immediately after initial dissection to allow the arteries sufficient time to relax, bleed, and thus be detected before closure. Even without detectable bleeding, hemostatic absorbable sutures should be placed in the fat pad to ligate any arteries that are at risk of being severed by an incision into the fat pad.

If an organized fibrotic nodule is present, it must be excised sharply and then treated as above for closure.

Postsurgical Complications (Local)

Infection

Although included primarily for completeness, a discussion of infection allows us to outline the pitfalls that lead to infection and to review appropriate strategies for dealing with them. Hematoma, which is discussed below, is a preventable cause of infection. Its presence provides a portal of entry for pathogens through gaps in suture lines and draining suture lines. Skin necrosis from hematoma provides yet another portal for contamination. Infection related to wound problems has been more commonly reported following Maquet-type osteotomies,[55] although it has been reported in Elmslie-Trillat–type procedures as well.[44] Particularly in the case of the Maquet-type osteotomy, infection can involve the bone by rapid contiguous spread if the initial wound problem is not dealt with aggressively.[13,37]

Solution Strategies. Hematomas should be prevented or evacuated if they are large. If an infection occurs, the wound should be immediately opened surgically and irrigated with an antibiotic solution. Necrotic tissue should be excised without regard for the defect created, and all foreign material, such as sutures, anchors, or implants, should be removed. The spatial relationship of the patella to the tibia can be maintained by application of a tensioned wire ring–hybrid external fixator or the more conventional half pin external fixator or by olecranization of the patella (either of the former two methods is preferable).

We have found that with a complete initial debridement, it is possible to proceed with wound closure, either primarily or with flap coverage, if a wound irrigation system is used. We use a modified double-lumen abdominal sump tube (Fig. 17.12) with large outflow fenestrations. It is connected to intravenous inflow by gravity only (to prevent compartment syndrome) and outflow to a urometer bag. In this manner, fluid flows in distending tissue away from the fenestrations of the outflow tube and thus allows drainage. This "milking" action has an advantage over older "suction-perfusion" systems. The solution used is a plain Ringer's with bacitracin and polymyxin additive. The system is maintained for several days on a decreasing inflow rate. In most

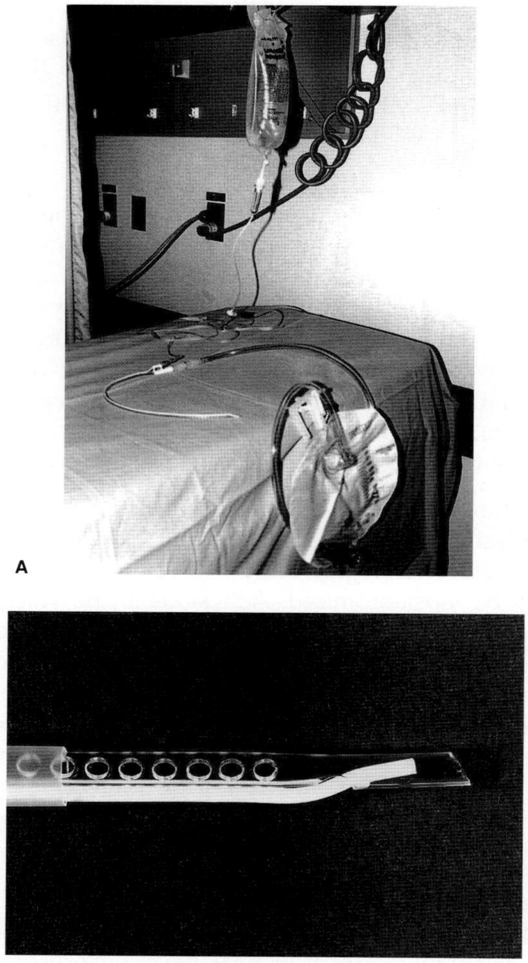

A

B

Figure 17.12. The closed wound irrigation system. **A:** An IV bag is connected to a double-lumen abdominal sump tube. The other port on the tube is connected to a GU bag. **B:** Close-up photo of the tip of the tube. Rather than using suction, which tends to draw in tissue occluding fenestration in the tube, inflow of fluid distends tissue away from the fenestrations facilitating fluid egress.

cases, with wound control and no recurrent signs of wound sepsis, a second surgical irrigation and reinsertion of fixation implants can be undertaken in approximately a week.

Hematoma

The development of a postoperative hematoma should not be thought of as just a trivial annoyance. It can result in wound problems, prolonged recovery periods, ankylosis, infection, reoperation (for evacuation),[44] compartment syndrome, or peroneal nerve palsy.[1]

Increased tension by the hematoma can cause gaps at the suture line with prolonged drainage and a portal for entry of pathogens. In cases where large skin flaps have been elevated or in cases where an alternative skin incision has been made to avoid scars from previous procedures, the collateral cutaneous circulation around the incision may be compromised, and skin viability can depend on early reestablishment of collateral circulation from deeper layers. The hematoma interposed between the subcutaneous and deeper layers can block these collaterals from forming and causing marginal wound or flap necrosis.

Similarly, the increased tension or pressure by the volume of the hematoma can cause pain or compartment syndrome (discussed below). Increased pain carries implications far beyond the need for increased analgesics. The reestablishment or maintenance of normal joint recesses and tissue planes requires early motion. Pain serves to limit a patient's compliance with rehabilitation protocols. At the least, recovery periods will be prolonged, and formation of intraarticular as well as extraarticular adhesions is possible mandating additional operative procedures.

After extensor mechanism surgery, most patients lie with the knee extended and the femur in an externally rotated position. This places the peroneal nerve in the most dependent position as it courses through a narrow sheath around the metaphyseal flair of the proximal fibula. Extravasated blood or hematoma will migrate to this area, and its accumulation has been linked to peroneal nerve neuropraxia.[56]

Solution Strategies. If a tourniquet is used, it should be released after exposure to gain hemostasis. If release is delayed until closure, some arterioles can remain in spasm long enough to escape detection as a source of bleeding. If, however, the tourniquet is deflated during the reconstruction portion of the procedure rather than afterward, the bleeding will become apparent. In procedures with a greater risk of bleeding, such as the Maquet or anteromedialization procedure, liberal use of drains is prudent.

A bulky postoperative dressing should be maintained for the first several days after surgery to provide an external tamponade to accumulation of blood or fluids in any potentially dead-tissue spaces. As dressing, we utilize, in order from the skin out, a nonadherent gauze pad, cotton gauze sponges, cotton cast padding roll, a sterile synthetic mechanics waste (pillow stuffing), cotton combine roll, wide nonelastic roll bandage, and a foam straight-knee immobilizer. Although many devices now available to provide cold compression are helpful, their advantages beyond those described above must be weighed against the additional expense.

Failure of Fixation or Graft Displacement

Although any fixation method is subject to failure and failures of fixation have been reported in extensor mechanism realignment procedures,[1,29,46,53] several aspects of fixation of a tibial tubercle osteotomy merit special mention.

The choice of a fixation device can be as important as the execution of the fixation, particularly in the Elmslie-Trillat–type procedure in which a small thin wafer of the tubercle is transferred. When adjustment in 1- to 2-mm increments is critical, the use of a 3.5- or 4.5-mm screw demands that any change in position be relocated at least 5 mm away to avoid cutting into the original drill hole. As important, the contact stress imparted by a screw through a thin bone wafer is more likely to fracture the tubercle fragment.

With concerns for skin necrosis in Maquet osteotomies, many advocate avoiding hardware fixation of the shingle if soft tissue and interference fit of the graft appear stable.[9,13,15] This practice, however, has resulted in graft displacement rates as high as 5%.[12–14]

Although not a true "failure," the subcutaneous location of any fixation device makes it prone to recurrent irritation and development of painful hardware bursitis, requiring removal.[7,44] Overly aggressive rehabilitation can also cause fixation failures (see below).

Solution Strategies. In the case of Elmslie-Trillat–type osteotomies, the use of a four-pronged table staple (Fig. 17.13) provides four points of fixation, narrow tines to allow greater flexibility in repositioning the tubercle in increments of 1 to 2 mm, and a broad surface area of contact against the fragment, which minimizes the risk of fracture.[1,7,32] This fixation is not without its potential faults. Care must be taken to adjust the angle of insertion so that it does not cut into and possibly rupture the patellar tendon.

In Maquet osteotomies, if fixation hardware is avoided, several strategies are useful. The graft should be carefully fitted gaining as much interdigitation and interference fit as possible. Maintaining the integrity of the periosteal envelope (i.e., by cutting the osteotomy from only one side) will help to interlock the graft and stabilize the shingle. Intraoperatively, the knee should

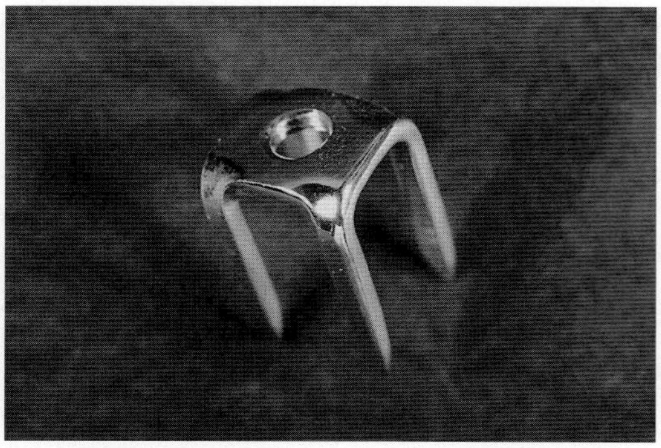

Figure 17.13. A four-pronged table staple used for tubercle fixation of Elmslie-Trillat type osteotomies. This one, designed by Puddu, has strong tines, yet allows adjustment of position within 3 mm.

be taken through a range of motion to observe for any instability of the shingle. Use of countersinking techniques and newer low profile head screws may obviate the need to avoid hardware. An unfixed shingle demands greater protection during rehabilitation and from inadvertent trauma during the early postoperative period.

Nonunion

Nonunions occur for reasons both understood and not understood. Unstable fixation allowing gross motion, interposed soft tissue, an atrophic bed, and infection are all preventable causes if they are anticipated. As just discussed, consciously avoiding fixation in Maquet osteotomies increases the risk of nonunion. Overly aggressive aftercare can also contribute. While an asymptomatic nonunion may pose no problem[37] other than the concern of late migration, most nonunions are painful and require revision.[1,36]

Solution Strategies. If nonunion or displacement of the tubercle fragment occurs, the site should be opened. All interposed fibrous tissue should be resected and raw bony beds obtained on both the tubercle fragment and tibial recipient site. This can be augmented by "fish scaling" the tibia (turning up small, thin, closely packed slivers of cortical bone) with a sharp osteotome. If the tubercle fragment is sclerotic and atrophic (i.e., with minimal punctate cortical bleeding), autologous bone grafting may be indicated as well. The cause of the original failure should be determined and adjustments made with the fixation or aftercare to prevent a recurrence.

Patellar Tendon Rupture

Although it is more common in cases of extensor mechanism realignment coupled with total knee arthroplasty,[57,58] the complication of patellar tendon rupture has been reported in pure extensor mechanism realignment procedures as well.[1,44,51] It can occur from direct damage and weakening of the insertional fibers of the patellar tendon during the osteotomy or from a fixation device, such as a staple, cutting into the tendon, as previously described. In either case, these ruptures usually take the form of sharply demarcated transverse avulsions near the insertion rather than the long interstitial failures seen with tensile loading traumatic ruptures.

Solution Strategies. By some means, the tendon must be anchored to a raw bony bed on the tibia. When some bone remains attached, this task is easier. Using a strong (no. 5) nonabsorbable suture, a double row of Bunnell-type sutures is placed in the tendon from the distal pole of the patella to the edge of the rupture. The four tails of the suture are secured by suture through bone or with some form of suture anchor (Fig. 17.14). The cortex just proximal to the point of suture should be "fish scaled" to enhance tendon-to-bone healing.

If no sound means of distal anchorage is available, a central third patellar tendon–bone graft can be harvested, reversed, and anchored to the tibia with more conventional bone-to-bone fixation methods. At that point, the tendon "tails" can be repaired with a V-Y technique (Fig. 17.15). In the most refractory situations or in long-standing cases when patellar tendon substance is lost, a complete bone–patellar tendon–bone allograft preparation can be implanted.

In either situation, optimal outcome depends on the

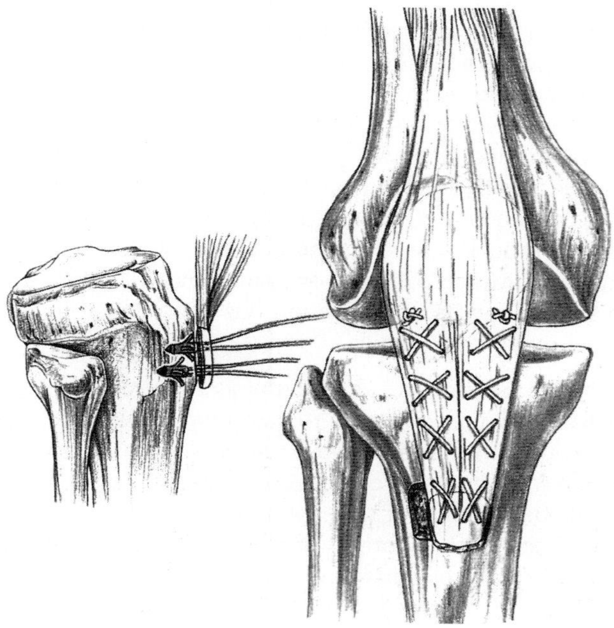

Figure 17.14. If the wafer fragments, suture techniques in the tendon combined with suture anchors in bone at the recipient site can be used to salvage fixation.

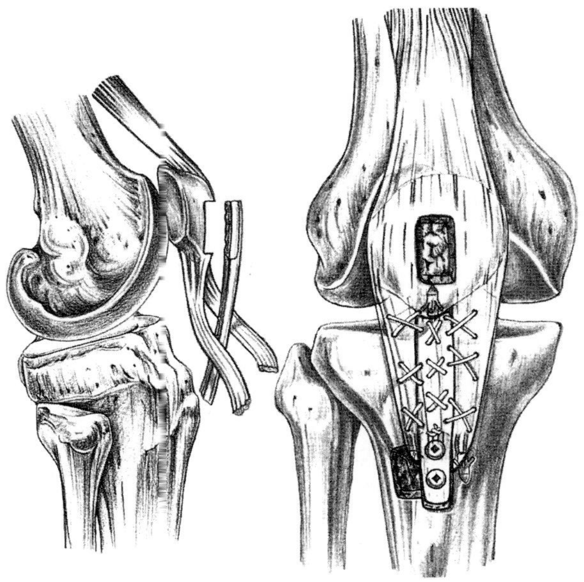

Figure 17.15. In this salvage technique, a V-Y split of the tendon is performed, and the central third is harvested with a plug of bone from the patella. Bone from a trough cut at the recipient site can be used to graft the patella. The central-third, free tendon graft is flipped, the bone is anchored in the trough with screws, and the V-Y split is repaired by suture techniques.

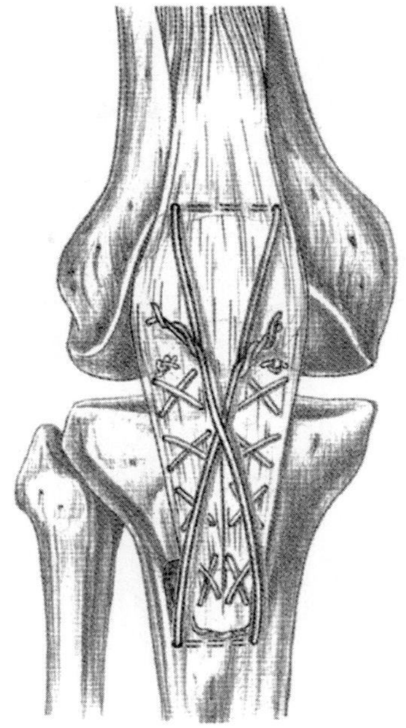

Figure 17.16. Protection of tenuous tubercle fixation. The wire is passed through the quadriceps tendon proximally and the tibial crest distally. It is adjusted just to load share between the tendon and the wire. The wire is removed 6 weeks postoperatively.

ability to initiate knee motion within several days to prevent intraarticular adhesions and adhesions in the infrapatellar bursa. To accomplish this, we create a modified tension band wire for temporary load sharing with the patellar tendon. This protects the insertional repair, yet allows motion. An 18-gauge wire is passed deep in the substance of the quadriceps tendon just on the superior pole of the patella. Next, it is brought in a figure-of-eight fashion distally on the anterior surface of the patella and the patellar tendon and anchored through a drill hole in the anterior tibial crest at the level of the tibial tubercle (Fig. 17.16). Tension on the wire should be adjusted to create as much tension as possible on the patellar tendon without compromising the repair seams. A range-of-motion arc of 0 to 90 degrees is usually satisfactory during the period that the wire is implanted. At 6 weeks, barring any problems, the repair will be at 80% of normal tensile strength and the wire can and should be removed. If retained, it will ultimately break. By 3 months, functional rehabilitation can usually be instituted.

Fracture

Fracture can be characterized as fracture of the wafer or shingle fragment or of the tibia. As would be expected, fracture of the tibia is more likely to occur in procedures where a markedly large cortical opening has been created causing a stress riser. Accordingly, reports exist of fracture complicating Hauser,[52] Maquet,[13,36,37] arthroplasty exposure,[59] and anteromedial transfer procedures,[46,60,61] and are lacking with Elmslie-Trillat procedures.

The fractures after anteromedialization involved the proximal tibia more often than the shingle as in a Maquet osteotomy, and thus were more serious in nature. Stetson et al[60] reported a series in which the overall rate of fracture of the proximal tibia was 2.6%, but in the patients who were treated with early weight bearing the rate was 9.8%.

The shingle of a Maquet osteotomy can fracture at its distal hinge compromising fixation or proximally if the graft is placed somewhat distal so as to cantilever the proximal end (Fig. 17.17).

Solution Strategies. Treatment is dictated by the fracture configuration, stability, and amount of displacement. It is more appropriate in this context to devote attention to prevention of the fracture. In osteotomies in which a stress riser in the tibia is created (i.e., the more invasive osteotomies), weight bearing should be limited in the early phases of healing.[60] The length of time a patient remains non– and partially weight bear-

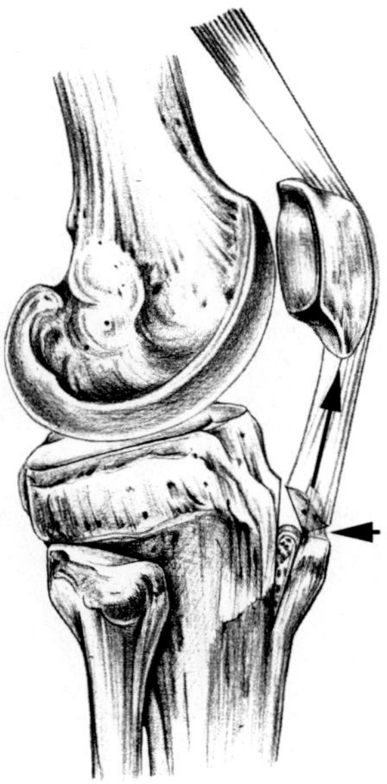

Figure 17.17. Placing the iliac graft too distally can cantilever the shingle, making it vulnerable to fracture.

ing is a decision based on the magnitude of the initial stress riser and the rate of healing.

The iliac block in a Maquet osteotomy should be placed well proximal and should be flush with the end of the shingle.[15] This placement minimizes the risk of fracture of the proximal end of the shingle. If the distal hinge of the shingle fractures, even postoperatively, internal fixation is indicated.

Skin Slough

Skin and wound problems have largely accounted for the high complication rates associated with Maquet-type osteotomies. The two are almost synonymous.[10,13,36,37,40,51] Moreover, it is not uncommon for these soft tissue problems to progress to osteomyelitis.

Solution Strategies. The complication can be prevented in several ways. Limiting the anterior translation[35] can decrease tension on the skin, but it can also compromise the effectiveness of the unloading. Ferguson et al[10] and Radin and Labosky[15] proposed modifiying the longitudinal skin incisions to more transverse or oblique ones to minimize the dissection and possibility of dehiscence. Several authors have advocated "fish mouthing" or "pie crusting" the skin to decrease tension.[11,13,15,36] However, this technique has the consequence of opening multiple portals to the deep wound—the implications of which are obvious. Siegel[62] discussed the preoperative use of tissue expanders. Mendes et al[12] described a preoperative "skin pinch test": if the skin can be pinched and pulled forward, adequate expandibility exists. Some authors have advocated avoiding fixation hardware, although this increases the risk of graft or shingle displacement.[9,13]

Skin at risk can be salvaged in some cases. Splinting the knee in extension for 1 to 3 weeks can limit tension until adequate collateral circulation is established. Dressings should not be stretched too tightly, and compressive casts over the shingle should be avoided. Experience with vasodilators or leeches has not been reported but may be an option if one is faced with impending massive skin necrosis. If other methods are unsuccessful, the wound can be reopened to release tension, dressed sterilely, and closed using a progressive wound closure device, such as Sure-Close (Life Medical Sciences, Princeton, NJ) or one of the coverage methods listed later in this chapter.

The approach to established wound sloughs must be individualized. Early wound control and coverage appears to offer the best prognosis. All devitalized and foreign material, such as fixation devices, should be debrided. Dead and infected bone should be saucerized. If in doubt, take it out! Temporizing coverage can be achieved with Silvadiene (Surewood Medical, St. Louis, MO) or Biobrane (Don Hickman Pharmaceuticals, Sugarland, TX) or equivalent synthetic skin. Definitive coverage is accomplished by a skin graft, local rotation flap,[12] local muscle flap (gastrocnemius head), or free flap.

Progressive Arthrosis

Arthrosis was reported to occur in 60% to 70% of Hauser-type distal realignments. Inherent in the Hauser procedure was a posterior rather than an anterior displacement that actually resulted in an increase in patellofemoral contact forces.[53] In a comparison of Elmslie-Trillat procedures with proximal realignments alone, Cohen et al[63] found no difference in the progression of arthritis based on type of procedure. Rather, progression correlated with age and preexisting arthritis at the time of the index procedure. Other authors reported progressive arthrosis after Maquet osteotomies when the surgical goals were not accomplished.[40,46,51]

Solution Strategies. If the procedure's original goals are not met, consideration may be given to revision realignment with limited debridement of osteophytes and synovectomy. If an unloading-type procedure was not performed initially, anterior transposition may provide relief of symptoms. This decision is highly patient-specific, based on personality, age, activity, and degree of arthrosis. Salvage options include arthroplasty and patellectomy.

Osteotomy in the Presence of Total Knee Components

Although it has been used more often in the past for extensile exposure in complex procedures,[58] authors are advocating the importance of rebalancing the extensor mechanism as a component of a total knee arthroplasty even if it involves osteotomy of the tubercle.[57] Studies of tubercle osteotomy in total knee replacement surgery report complication rates as high as 23% that were related directly to the tubercle osteotomy and failure of the method of fixation to achieve rigid fixation.[25,57] The presence of total knee components and, in particular, the stemmed cemented tibial components present added challenges because the stem and cement usually lie directly deep to the osteotomy site. In these patients, traditional fixation methods can be difficult to orient around the component or can fracture a freshly cured cement mantle. The defect from some osteotomies may serve to destabilize the tibial component.

Solution Strategies. With these thoughts in mind, special surgical tactics, such as those reported by Masini and Stulberg,[57] continue to be developed. The use of fixation staples that span rather than perforate the tubercle fragment and preserve medial and lateral soft tissue sleeves typify these approaches.

Donor-Site Morbidity

This problem is unique to the Maquet osteotomy because of the need for an iliac crest graft. The problems encountered, however, are common to those associated with any iliac crest graft—scar tenderness, hematoma, and hernia.[12,51]

Solution Strategies. Methods that preserve the inner and outer table periosteal sleeve, hemostasis using bone wax or other hemostatic agents as needed, drains, and sound closure help the surgeon to avoid these donor-site problems. Difficult herniations may require the use of mesh or other advanced hernia repair techniques to achieve success.[12]

Postsurgical Complications (Distant)

Compartment Syndrome

Compartment syndromes have been reported in Hauser procedures, although they are more likely to occur in a Maquet or an anteromedialization procedure. In these procedures, a large surface area of communication is created between the tibial intramedullary canal and anterior compartment.[30,64] The swelling and subsequent ischemia can rapidly spread to compartments in the leg. If it is unrecognized and untreated, disastrous and permanent neurovascular damage results.

Solution Strategies. A high index of suspicion must always be maintained. Intracompartmental pressure measurements should be obtained when patients report pain out of proportion to the situation, tense compartments are palpated, and pain is accentuated by passive stretching of muscles in a suspected compartment. These symptoms coupled with findings of high compartmental pressure readings constitute a surgical emergency and the need for immediate fasciotomy.[65] No good solution exists for the missed compartment syndrome.

Reflex Sympathetic Dystrophy

Although they are a rare occurrence, injuries to or surgery on the patellofemoral joint account for a large percentage of reflex sympathetic dystrophy cases in knee patients.[55,66] Functional use and meaningful rehabilitation of the extremity is largely halted until the dystrophic process can be arrested. Surgery should not be undertaken in patients with reflex sympathetic dystrophy until the dystrophy has been treated and is largely, if not completely, resolved.

Solution Strategies. Authors agree that the best prognosis comes when treatment is instituted early after the onset of reflex sympathetic dystrophy.[66,67] Narcotic analgesics must be rapidly tapered and discontinued. Detoxification measures may be required. Medications that raise the pain threshold, such as tricyclic antidepressants, nonsteroidal antiinflammatory drugs (NSAIDs), and high doses of anxiolytics are indicated, as well as psychological evaluation and support. A high priority in the early phase of treatment is to break the pain cycle and sympathetic dysfunction. Although isolated lumbar sympathetic blocks have reportedly been successful,[66] we prefer continuous epidural infusion for several days' duration. Range of motion and other physiotherapy desensitization modalities are initiated and continued as the mainstay of treatment as the epidural doses are tapered. We have seen greater success when these measures are offered as an intense inpatient program.

Deep Venous Thrombosis

Also rarely, postoperative deep venous thrombosis has been linked to osteotomies of the tubercle.[13,46,55] The use of anticoagulation in patients who have had an osteotomy (particularly the long shingle-type techniques) balances the risk of deep venous thrombosis against the risk of excessive bleeding, wound complications, infection, and compartment syndrome.

Solution Strategies. Full anticoagulation can be deferred in favor of pneumatic compression pumps, stockings, early motion, vena cava umbrellas, and delayed or subtherapeutic early anticoagulation. The exact tactic must be individualized by considering each patient's unique risk factors. A diagnosed postoperative deep venous thrombosis requires anticoagulation and activity modification.

Neurovascular Compromise
Although no major arteries or nerves are directly adjacent to the tibial tubercle, rare reports of neurovascular compromise exist. As discussed previously, the peroneal nerve is dependent when the leg rolls into slight external rotation, a normally assumed posture at rest. Blood accumulates in the nerve sheath resulting in a neuropraxic-type dysfunction.[56]

The anterior tibial artery or its branches can be vulnerable in an osteotomy that splits the lateral face in the proximal tibia. Wall[64] reported 11 such cases that resulted in occult bleeding and compartment syndrome. This vulnerability is greatest with a Maquet-type osteotomy, less with anteromedialization, and virtually absent in an Elmslie–Trillat-type osteotomy.

Solution Strategies. Awareness and prevention are the best treatment. Fortunately, peroneal neuropraxia is usually transient and resolves spontaneously. Serial nerve conduction studies that fail to show improvement can prompt exploration and neurolysis.

A high index of suspicion and awareness of the possible injury to the anterior tibial artery should be maintained when performing Maquet or anteromedial osteotomies.

Rehabilitation

Problems with rehabilitation programs have included stiffness, hardware failure, and fracture. Fulkerson and coworkers[46] report a high percentage of stiffness in patients immobilized in extension for 1 month versus those treated by immediate motion postoperatively. One patient from their original series required manipulation due to the lack of adequate rehabilitation.[20] Hardware pullout has been reported in all three types of osteotomies as a result of early aggressive rehabilitation.[1,46,51] Early full weight bearing after a large-shingle–type osteotomy carries an unacceptable risk of proximal tibial fracture.

Solution Strategies
The current consensus for a rehabilitation program that adds no additional risk of complications emphasizes early motion of 0 to 90 degrees. As the osteotomy heals, it also includes progressive strengthening consisting of high repetition, no resistance isotonic and low stress isometrics, initially, followed in 4 to 6 weeks by progressive resistance and eccentric closed-chain strengthening. Protected weight bearing is indicated for 4 to 6 weeks after surgery, especially with shingle-type osteotomies.

CONCLUSION

Surgery on the extensor mechanism of the knee challenges our ability as surgeons. In general, osteotomies are advanced procedures and should not be left to the inexperienced surgeon. It therefore follows that osteotomies involving the extensor mechanism are highly demanding and fraught with pitfalls for even the most experienced surgeon. The best way to avoid the complications associated with these surgical procedures is to prevent them. Understand the anatomy. Understand the indications. Understand the goals. Knowing how others got into trouble can be our best teacher.

References

1. Flandry F, Hughston JC. Complications of extensor mechanism surgery for patellofemoral malalignment. *Am J Orthop* 1995;24:534–543.
2. LaPrade RF. The anatomy of the deep infrapatellar bursa of the knee. *Am J Sports Med* 1998;26:129–132.
3. Fulkerson JP, Tennant R, Jaivin BS, et al. Histologic evidence of retinacular nerve injury associated with patellofemoral malalignment. *Clin Orthop* 1985;197:196–205.
4. Chrisman OD. The role of articular cartilage in patellofemoral pain. *Orthop Clin North Am* 1986;17:231–234.
5. Noyes FR, Wojtys EM, Marshall MT. The early diagnosis and treatment of developmental patella infera syndrome. *Clin Orthop* 1991;265:241–252.
6. Paulos LE, Rosenburg TD, Drawbert J, et al. Infrapatellar contracture syndrome: an unrecognized cause of knee stiffness with patella entrapment and patella infera. *Am J Sports Med* 1987;15:331–341.
7. Hughston JC, Walsh WM. Proximal and distal reconstruction of the extensor mechanism for patella subluxation. *Clin Orthop* 1979;144:36–42.
8. Kolowich PA, Paulos LE, Rosenberg TD, et al. Lateral release of the patella: indications and contraindications. *Am J Sports Med* 1990;18:359–365.
9. Besette GC, Hunter RE. The Maquet procedure: a retrospective review. *Clin Orthop* 1988;232:159–167.
10. Ferguson AB, Brown TD, Fu FH, et al. Relief of patellofemoral contact stress by anterior displacement of the tibial tubercle. *J Bone Joint Surg* 1979;61A:159–166.
11. Maquet PGJ. *Pathomechanics of Osteoarthritis of the Knee. Biomechanics of the Knee, with Application to the Pathogenesis and Surgical Treatment of Osteoarthritis*. Berlin: Springer-Verlag, 1984:107–109.
12. Mendes DG, Soudry M, Iusim M. Clinical assessment of Maquet tibial tuberosity advancement. *Clin Orthop* 1987;222:228–238.

13. Radin EL. Anterior tibial tubercle elevation in the young adult. *Orthop Clin North Am* 1986;17:297–302.
14. Radin EL. The Maquet procedure—anterior displacement of the tibial tubercle: indications, contraindications, and precautions. *Clin Orthop* 1986;213:241–248.
15. Radin EL, Labosky DA. Avoiding complications associated with the Maquet procedure. *Comp Orthop* 1989; 4:48–53.
16. Heatley FW, Allen PR, Patrick JH. Tibial tubercle advancement for anterior knee pain: a temporary or permanent solution. *Clin Orthop* 1986;208:215–224.
17. Pan HQ, Kish V, Boyd RD, et al. The Maquet procedure: effect of tibia shingle length on patellofemoral pressures. *J Orthop Res* 1993;11:199–204.
18. Trillat A, Dejour H, Couette A. Diagnostic et traitement des subluxation recidivantes de la rotule. *Rev Chir Orthop* 1964;50.
19. Maquet P. Advancement of the tibial tuberosity. *Clin Orthop* 1976;115:225–230.
20. Fulkerson JP Anteromedialization of the tibial tuberosity for patellofemoral malalignment. *Clin Orthop* 1983;177: 176–181.
21. Roux C. Recurrent dislocation of the patella: operative treatment. *Clin Orthop* 1979;144:4–8.
22. Goldthwait JE. Permanent dislocation of the patella. *Ann Surg* 1895;29:62–68.
23. Hauser EDW. Total tendon transplant for slipping patella: a new operation for recurrent dislocation of the patella. *Surg Gynecol Obstet* 1938;66:199–214.
24. Baker RH, Carroll N, Dewar FP, et al. The semitendinosus tenodesis for recurrent dislocation of the patella. *J Bone Joint Surg* 1972;54B:103–109.
25. Whiteside LA. Distal realignment of the patellar tendon to correct abnormal patellar tracking. *Clin Orthop* 1997;344:284–289.
26. Slocum DB, Larson RL, James SL. Late reconstruction of ligamentous injuries of the medial compartment of the knee. *Clin Orthop* 1974;100:23–55.
27. Chrisman OD, Snook GA, Wilson TC. A long-term prospective study of the Hauser and Roux-Goldthwait procedures for recurrent patellar dislocation. *Clin Orthop* 1979;144:27–30.
28. Blazina ME, Fox JM, Carlson GJ, et al. Patella baja. A technical consideration in evaluating results of tibial tubercle transplantation. *J Bone Joint Surg* 1975;57A: 1027.
29. Crosby EB, Insall J. Recurrent dislocation of the patella. *J Bone Joint Surg* 1976;58A:9–13.
30. Wiggins HE. The anterior tibial compartment syndrome. A complication of the Hauser procedure. *Clin Orthop* 1975;113:90–94.
31. Rantanen J, Paananen M. Modified Hauser operation for patellar instability. *Acta Orthop Scand* 1996;67:455–458.
32. Hughston JC. Reconstruction of the extensor mechanism for subluxating patella. *J Sports Med* 1972;1:6–13.
33. Hughston JC, Walsh WM., Puddu G. Patellar subluxation and dislocation. In: Sledge CB, ed. *Saunders Monographs in Clinical Orthopaedics*. Philadelphia: WB Saunders, 1984:87–128.
34. Maquet P. Consideration biomechaniques sur l'authoredu genou. Un traitment biomechanique de l'arthrose femotopate-laire. L'advancement du tendon rotulin. *Rev Rheum* 1963;30:779.
35. Bandi W. Les résultats de l'advancement de la tubérosité antérieure du tibia. *Rev Chir Orthop* 1989;66:275–278.
36. Rappoport LH, Browne MG, Wickiewicz TL. The Maquet osteotomy. *Orthop Clin North Am* 1992;23:645–656.
37. Radin EL, Pan HQ. Long-term follow-up study on the Maquet procedure with special reference to causes of failure. *Clin Orthop* 1993;290:253–258.
38. Benvenuti JF, Rakotomanana L, Leyvraz PF, et al. Displacements of the tibial tuberosity. Effects of the surgical parameters. *Clin Orthop* 1997;343:224–234.
39. Fulkerson JP. Operative management of patellofemoral pain. *Ann Chir Gynaecol* 1991;80:224–229.
40. Schmid F. The Maquet procedure in the treatment of patellofemoral osteoarthrosis. Long-term results. *Clin Orthop* 1993;294:254–258.
41. Cox JS. Evaluation of the Roux-Elmslie-Trillat procedure for knee extensor realignment. *Am J Sports Med* 1982;10:303–310.
42. Conti C, Berruto M, Bianchi M. The Elmslie-Trillat procedure for recurrent subluxation of the patella. One to five year follow-up. *Ital J Traumatol* 1992;18:341–349.
43. Chrisman OD, Snook GA, Wilson TC. A long term prospective study of the Hauser and Roux-Goldthwait procedures for recurrent patellar dislocation. *Clin Orthop* 1979;144:27–30.
44. Wootton JR, Cross MJ, Wood DG. Patellofemoral malalignment: a report of 68 cases treated by proximal and distal patellofemoral reconstruction. *Injury* 1990; 21:169–173.
45. Molina A, Ballester J, Martin C, et al. Biomechanical effects of different surgical procedures on the extensor mechanism of the patellofemoral joint. *Clin Orthop* 1995;320:168–175.
46. Fulkerson JP, Becker GJ, Meaney JA, et al. Anteromedial tibial tubercle transfer without bone graft. *Am J Sports Med* 1990;18:490–497.
47. Macnab I. Recurrent dislocation of the patella. *J Bone Joint Surg* 1952;34A:957–967.
48. Crosby EB, Insall J. Recurrent dislocation of the patella. Relation of treatment to osteoarthritis. *J Bone Joint Surg* 1976;58A:9–13.
49. Harrison MHM. The results of a realignment operation for recurrent dislocation of the patella. *J Bone Joint Surg* 1955;37B:559–567.

50. Fielding JW, Liebler WA, Tambakis A. The effect of a tibial tubercle transplant in children on the growth of the upper tibial epiphysis. *J Bone Joint Surg* 1960;42A: 1426–1434.

51. Evans IK, Paulos LE. Complications of patellofemoral joint surgery. *Orthop Clin North Am* 1992;23:697–710.

52. DeCesare W. Late results of Hauser procedure for recurrent dislocation of the patella. *Clin Orthop* 1979; 140:137–144.

53. Barbari S, Raugstad TS, Lichtenburg N. The Hauser operation for patellar dislocation: 3–32 year results in 63 knees. *Acta Orthop Scand* 1990;61:32–35.

54. Arnoczky SP. Blood supply to the anterior cruciate ligament and supporting structures. *Orthop Clin North Am* 1985;16:15–28.

55. Jenny JY, Sader Z, Henry A, et al. Elevation of the tibial tubercle for patellofemoral pain syndrome. An 8- to 15-year follow-up. *Knee Surg Sports Traumatol Arthrosc* 1996;4:92–96.

56. Garland DE, Hughston JC. Peroneal nerve paralysis: a complication of extensor reconstruction of the knee. *Clin Orthop* 1979;140:169–171.

57. Masini AM, Stulberg SD. A new surgical technique for tibial tubercle transfer in total knee arthroplasty. *J Arthroplasty* 1992;7:81–86.

58. Wolff AM, Hungerford DS, Krakow KA, et al. Osteotomy of the tibial tubercle during total knee replacement. *J Bone Joint Surg* 1989;71A:848–852.

59. Ritter MA, Carr K, Keating M, et al. Tibial shaft fracture following tibial tubercle osteotomy. *J Arthroplasty* 1996;11:117–119.

60. Stetson WB, Friedman MJ, Fulkerson JP, et al. Fracture of the proximal tibia with immediate weightbearing after a Fulkerson osteotomy. *Am J Sports Med* 1997;25: 570–574.

61. Bellemans J, Cauwenberghs F, Witvrouw E, et al. Anteromedial tibial tubercle transfer in patients with chronic anterior knee pain and a subluxation type patellar malalignment. *Am J Sports Med* 1997;25:375–381.

62. Siegel M. The Maquet osteotomy: a review of risks. *Orthopedics* 1987;10:1073–1078.

63. Cohen JL, Flandry F, Hughston JC. Late patellofemoral arthritis after extensor mechanism realignment: average 18 year follow up. *Orthop Trans* 1991;15:17–18.

64. Wall JJ. Compartment syndrome as a complication of the Hauser procedure. *J Bone Joint Surg* 1979;61A: 185–191.

65. Mubarak SJ, Owen CA. Double-incision fasciotomy of the leg for decompression in compartment syndromes. *J Bone Joint Surg* 1977;59A:184–187.

66. Katz MM, Hungerford DS. Reflex sympathetic dystrophy affecting the knee. *J Bone Joint Surg* 1987;69B:797–803.

67. Ogilvie-Harris DJ, Roscoe M. Reflex sympathetic dystrophy of the knee. *J Bone Joint Surg* 1987;69B:804–806.

Chapter 18

COMPLICATIONS AND PITFALLS IN INJURIES OF THE QUADRICEPS AND PATELLAR TENDON

M. Mike Malek

Injuries to the quadriceps and patellar tendons generally occur with rapid contraction of the quadriceps with varying degrees of flexion. In younger individuals, tears usually are midsubstance and through the tendon; in older individuals, tears generally occur at the attachment site (avulsion).

It has been reported that tendinous ruptures occur through a preexisting pathologic condition of the tendon.[1] The most frequent causes are gout, repeated microtrauma, arthritis, fatty degeneration, calcifications/calcific tendinitis, diabetes, metabolic diseases and tumors. Steroid injections into the tendon can also be a causative factor. Acute trauma is an obvious cause of injuries to the quadriceps and patellar tendon and can be in the form of a direct blow or penetrating wound/laceration (Fig. 18.1).

Presently, surgical management of quadriceps and patellar tendon ruptures is the standard of care in disruptions of these tendons. Varieties of techniques have been described in surgical repair and reconstruction of the quadriceps and patellar tendons. The goal should be to restore the anatomic and functional integrity of the extensor mechanism. There also is a demographic variation in reference to ruptures of the quadriceps and patellar tendons. Siwek and Rao[2] reported on 117 tendon ruptures of which 88% of quadriceps tendon ruptures were in patients 40 or over, while 80% of patients with patellar tendon rupture were less than 40 years of age.

CLINICAL CONSIDERATION: QUADRICEPS/PATELLAR TENDON

Generally early surgical treatment of quadriceps and patellar tendon disruptions are associated with better anatomic and functional outcome with little or no residual morbidity. Those injuries detected after 3 to 4 weeks and treated surgically may not achieve optimum results in contrast with those detected and treated early. With this in mind, it is extremely important to identify and treat these ruptures as soon as possible.

Quadriceps

It is generally agreed that a key to successful surgical treatment of quadriceps ruptures is early diagnosis and surgical repair within the first week and ideally within 72 hours of the injury. To identify this condition, the following factors are helpful:

1. A detailed history, with special attention to the mechanism of injury, is important. The mechanism of injury in quadriceps ruptures is a sudden contracture of the quadriceps and/or hyperflexion. Hyperflexion injury is quite common in weight lifting (Fig. 18.2).
2. Usually there is a loud pop, immediate severe pain, and a large joint effusion (hemarthrosis) within minutes (Fig. 18.3).
3. The patient is not able to extend the knee fully and is not able to lift the leg against gravity.
4. A palpable gap/defect above the superior pole of the patellar tendon can be palpated.
5. Extreme tenderness is present at the tear junction.
6. There are positive findings on plain radiography and magnetic resonance imaging (MRI). On plain radiography (Fig. 18.4) an anterior tilt of the superior pole of the patella is present on lateral view in acute cases. In chronic situations there may be the presence of patella baja. MRI is best for identifying tears of the quadriceps tendon, especially the partial tears.

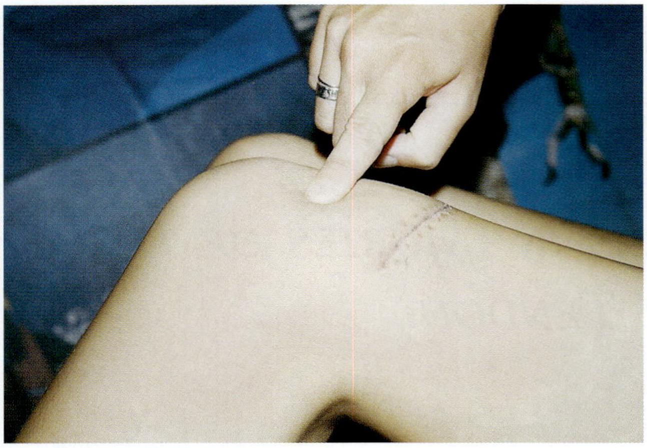

Figure 18.1. A 19-year-old woman who was involved in an automobile accident sustained a laceration on the anterolateral aspect of the knee, just above the tibial tubercle, which was primarily sutured in the emergency room. However, the complete laceration and disruption of the patellar tendon was missed. The finger points to the gap in the area of patellar tendon disruption (6 weeks postinjury).

Pitfalls

The following are the main pitfalls when dealing with acute rupture of the quadriceps tendon:

1. Not recognizing the extent of injury—partial or total.
2. In cases of total disruption, not proceeding with surgical repair within the first week and preferably within the first 72 hours.

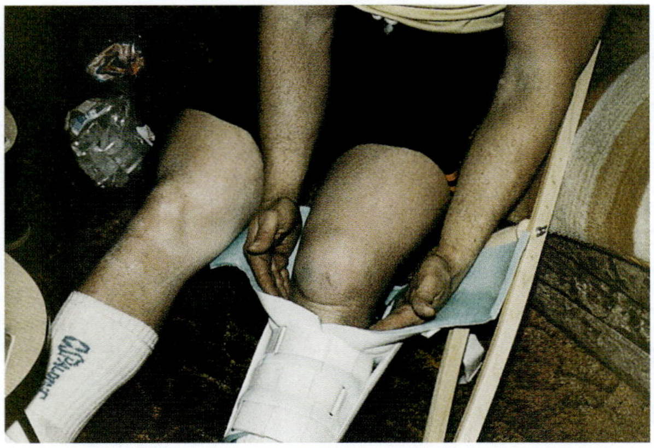

Figure 18.3. Ten minutes following acute disruption of quadriceps in another weight lifter's knee with large and intense hemarthrosis.

3. In cases of surgical repair, not performing an adequate and solid repair and augmentation, if necessary.
4. Not protecting the repair within the first 6 to 8 weeks after surgery.

Complications

The following complications are common with delayed diagnosis and inappropriate surgical repair (general complications of knee surgery are not included):

1. Quadriceps insufficiency: This condition occurs with delay in diagnosis or neglected quadriceps rupture. Most cases develop patella baja, and a palpable and

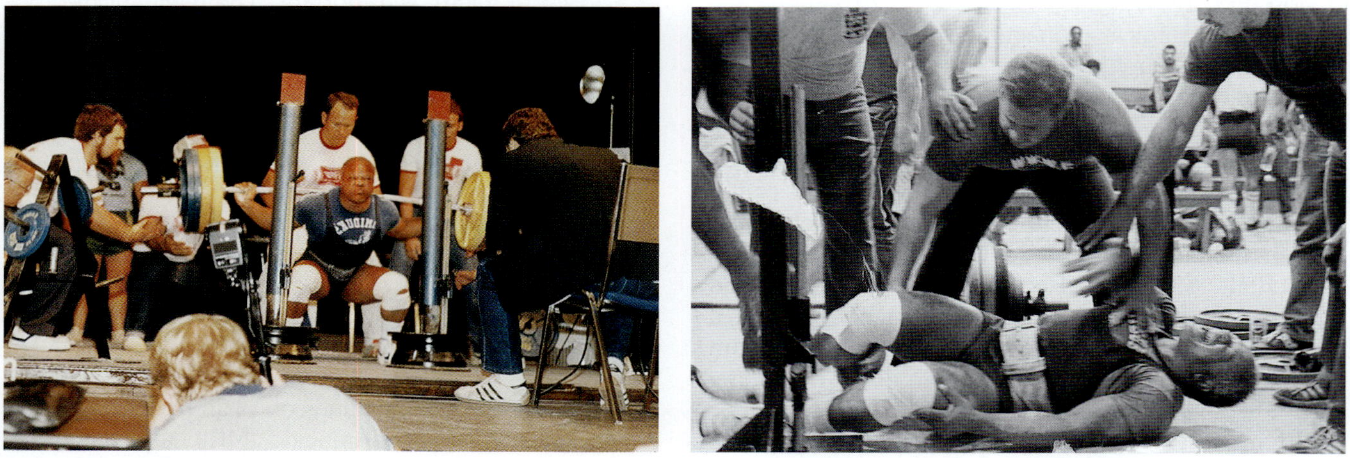

A B

Figure 18.2. **A:** A 40-year-old power lifter in the process of lifting 500 pounds. Both knees at hyperflexion are ready to contract and go to extension, lifting weights over the shoulders. **B:** Seconds later, the right quadriceps ruptures with a loud pop and excruciating pain.

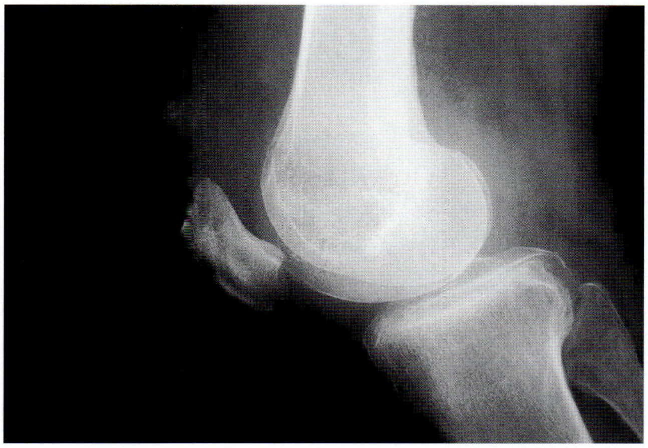

Figure 18.4. Anterior tilt of the superior pole of the patella on lateral x-ray view in the acute tear of the quadriceps tendon.

at times visible gap can be noted just above the superior pole of the patella.

2. Rerupture: In cases of inadequate repair and/or inadequate postoperative protection, tendon rerupture is common (Fig. 18.5).
3. Calcific tendinitis: This is a predisposing factor for rerupture of the tendon in cases of repeated trauma.
4. Myositis ossifications: These generally occur postsurgically and do not interfere with tendon healing at the repair site.
5. Patella baja: This condition may develop even in cases of functional quadriceps tendon (Fig. 18.6).
6. Arthrofibrosis: This condition generally is due to scarring in the suprapatellar pouch. There may be a need for arthroscopy and release of adhesions, but no earlier than at 12 weeks postoperation.
7. Patellofemoral malalignment and excessive lateral pressure syndrome: This condition develops secondary to surgical dissection and tight closure of the vastus lateralis and its extension. Arthroscopic evaluation and management are necessary in cases of continuous symptoms.

SURGICAL REPAIR/RECONSTRUCTION ACUTE QAUDRICEPS RUPTURE

In most cases quadriceps rupture occurs just above the insertion of the tendon to the superior pole of the patella with approximately ½ inch of stump attached to the patella. Numerous surgical techniques have been described for repair of acute quadriceps ruptures.

Early reports described direct repair using catgut or silk.[1–3] Gallie and Lemesurier[4] have described the use of free fascial graft. McLaughlin[5] described the traction suture technique in 1947. Scuderi[6] described in 1958 his technique of a midline incision where the ruptured tendon was repaired end to end after debridement of the edges. This was followed by reinforcement by a triangular proximal tendon flap. All these authors have reported satisfactory results with their techniques.

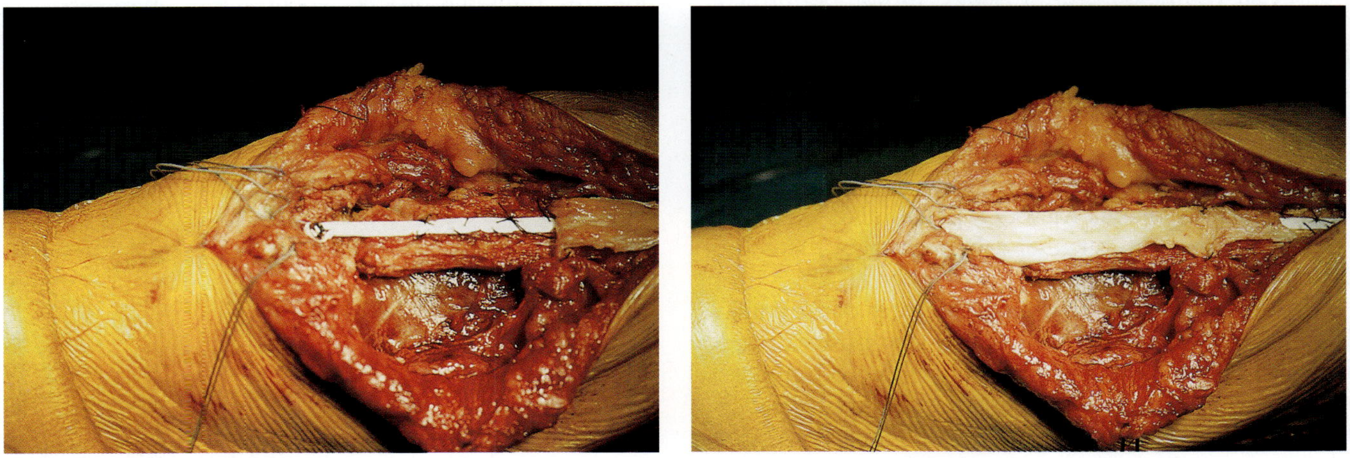

A B

Figure 18.5. A: A 40-year-old man with rerupture of quadriceps × 3. Eventually with a combination of allograft and synthetic rod the quadriceps integrity was restored and the patient returned to his original level of activity after 2 years of treatment. The synthetic rod (W.H. Gore) was removed 9 months after reconstruction. (This synthetic rod is no longer on the market in the United States. B: Once the synthetic rod is fixed in place, the quadriceps tendon is covered with a fascia lata allograft in a wraparound fashion.

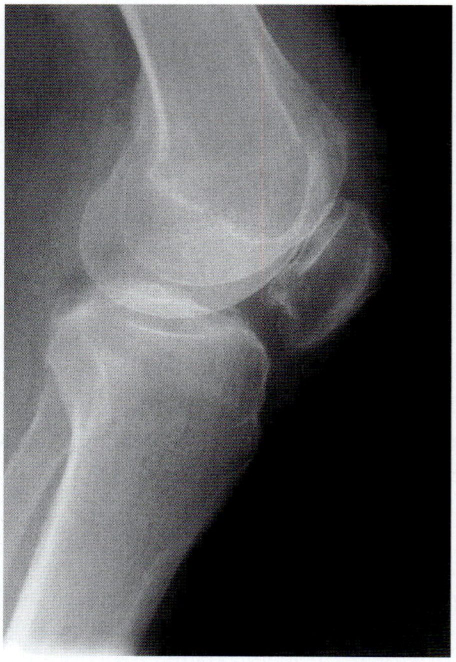

Figure 18.6. Three years following untreated quadriceps rupture in a 42-year-old male construction worker. Lateral radiograph shows distal migration of the patella. There is weakness of the quadriceps, with difficulty in knee flexion beyond 90 degrees.

Author's Preferred Technique

The knee is prepped and draped in the usual sterile fashion. Unless specifically indicated for the presence of intraarticular pathology, arthroscopy is not performed. The quadriceps rupture site is exposed through a 4- to 6-inch longitudinal midline incision. The lower end of the incision generally will be at the level of the superior pole of the patella.

The medial and lateral retinaculum is examined and the two ends of the ruptured tendon are identified. In cases of closed injuries without a penetrating wound or foreign bodies, very minimal debridement of the edges is sufficient.

The stump attached to the superior pole of the patella is vertically divided into two anterior and posterior segments, and a groove of approximately 2 to 3 mm deep and about 3 cm wide at the superior pole of the patella is created (Fig. 18.7) utilizing a dental burr. Four pairs of nonabsorbable sutures (no. 1 Ethibond, Ethicon, Somerville, NJ) are passed through the upper portion of the quadriceps tendon utilizing the Bunnell or Krackow method (Fig. 18.8). Once the sutures are passed, the proximal end of the quadriceps is brought into the previously prepared groove. This groove also has four tunnels created in it proceeding to the mid-

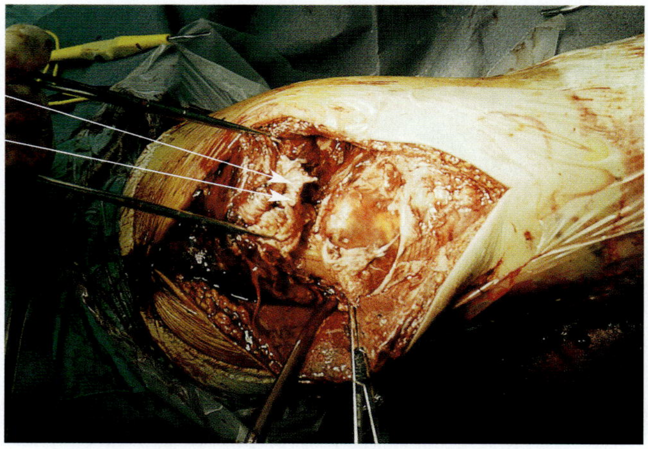

Figure 18.7. Arrows point to the superior pole of the patellar pole, where a transverse groove of 2 to 3 mm in depth will be created using a dental burr.

portion of the patella with a Kirschner wire (K-wire). Each pair of sutures is passed through its own designated tunnel, and after they all have been passed and the proximal tendon end is completely seated in the groove suture and then tied over the anterior aspect of the patella, additional repair of the medial and lateral retinaculum is performed when needed.

The anterior and posterior stump, which was previously divided, is then sutured back to the tendon for reinforcement. The recent development of suture anchors has made this reattachment technically easier and stronger. In this fashion usually four anchors are placed into the prepared groove, about 7 mm apart, and su-

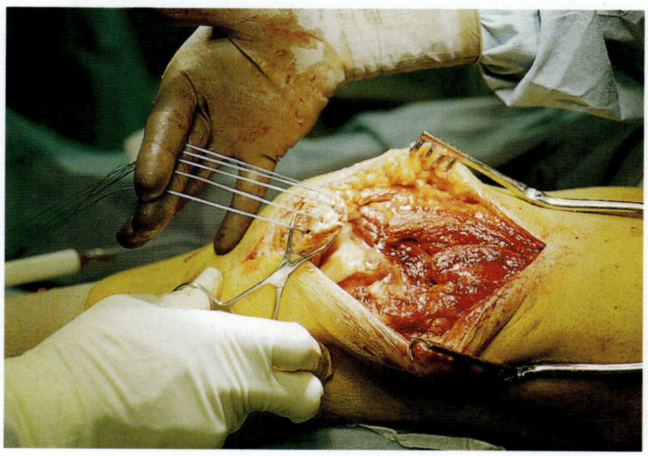

Figure 18.8. Four or five pairs of sutures are passed through the proximal quadriceps tendon and pulled down until they are seated in the prepared groove. This can be easily accomplished by the use of suture anchors.

tures are then passed through the proximal tendon segment, pulling it down into the groove (Fig. 18.8). Postoperative radiographs (Fig. 18.9) show the placement of the anchors in the anteroposterior (AP) and lateral projections following quadriceps repair. A circlage wire through the tendon above the repair site and transversely through the patella can also augment this repair. The circlage wires are then removed at 6 weeks postoperation (Fig. 18.10).

In chronic cases and in repair of reruptured quadriceps tendons where there is significant scar tissue, fibrosis, or calcifications, there may be a need for a staged procedure in which the proximal tendon needs to be stretched and the patella may need to be lifted from its contracted position. In severe cases of patella baja, this condition needs to be addressed prior to undertaking the repair of the quadriceps tendon.

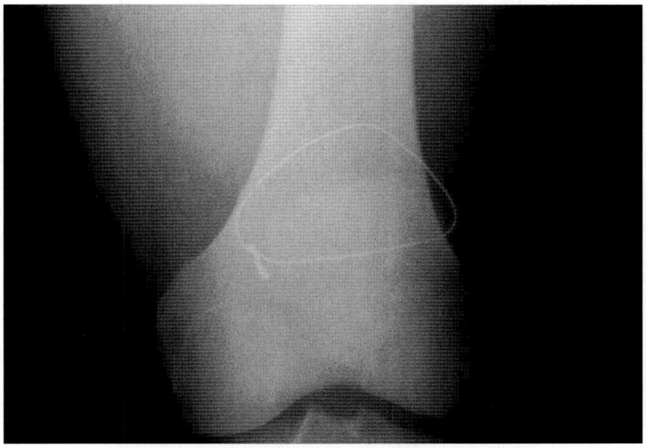

Figure 18.10. Circlage wire is utilized to reinforce the repair.

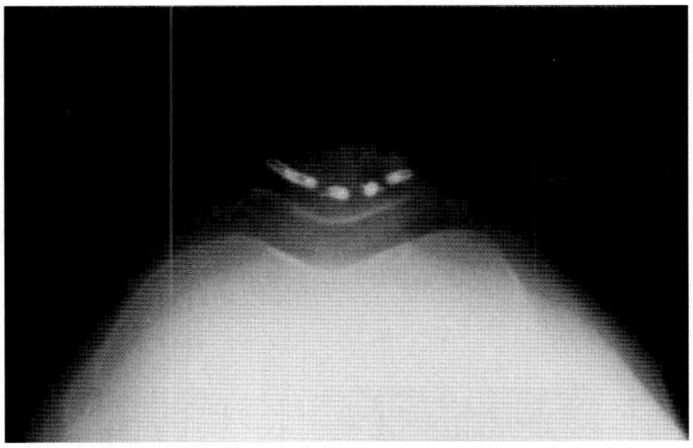

A

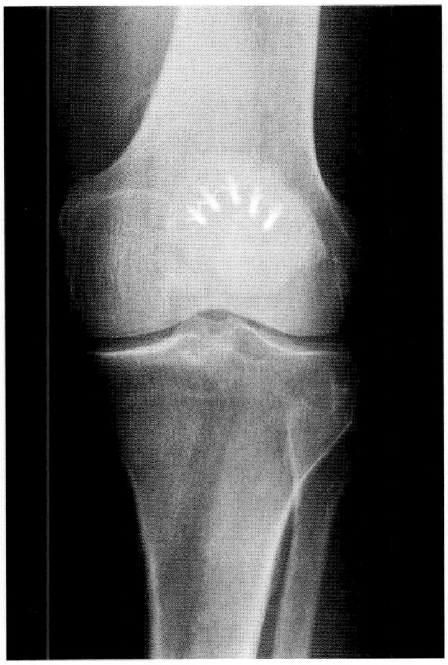

B

Figure 18.9. A,B: Five suture anchors have been utilized in reattaching the quadriceps tendon to the superior pole of the patella

Allograft also is useful in cases where there is significant gap and tissue loss. Artificial materials previously available for this technique are no longer in use in the United States (Fig. 18.5).

Postoperative Rehabilitation

Generally it is recommended to immobilize the knee for 6 weeks. At the end of this period any hardware is removed, and gradual and gentle range of active and passive motion is instituted. The quadriceps mechanism is not stressed for up to 12 weeks postoperation and isokinetic exercises are not utilized. A program of flexibility, closed chain, and pool therapy is utilized from 8 to 16 weeks postoperation, at which time the rehabilitation program is intensified until full range of motion and strength is achieved. Contact sports are not allowed for up to 9 months postoperation, nor are weight-lifting activities. The power lifter illustrated in Fig. 18.2 returned to competitive weight lifting following his quadriceps repair and won the world championship in his age category at the age of 40 by lifting 665 pounds (Fig. 18.11).

PATELLAR TENDON RUPTURES

Ruptures of the patellar tendon are less common than those of the quadriceps tendon. Patellar tendon disruptions usually occur in younger individuals. Those disruptions associated with athletic injuries usually follow a preexisting patellar tendinitis or jumper's knee condition. Traumatic patellar tendon rupture may be associated with other musculoskeletal injuries, especially in high-speed motor vehicle accidents, and may go unrecognized and thus untreated due to the severity of associated injuries (Fig. 18.1).

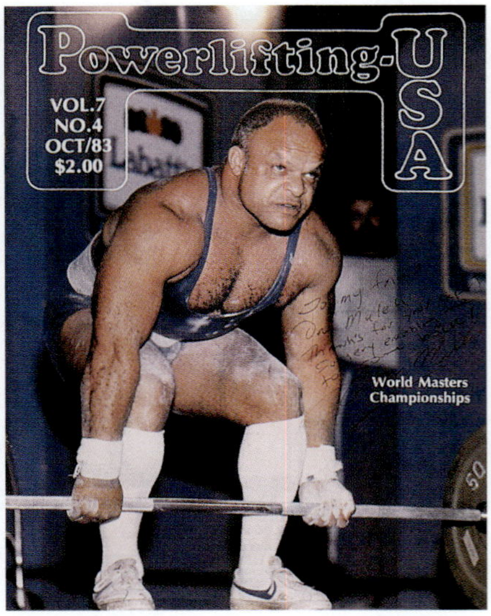

Figure 18.11. A 40-year-old power lifter 10 months after quadriceps tendon repair competing in the world championship in his age category. He won with a lift of 665 lbs.

Steroid injections into the patellar tendon have been associated with rupture of these tendons at a later date.[1] Most patellar tendon ruptures occur at or close to the insertion into the lower pole of the patella (Fig. 18.12), except those caused by a direct blow or laceration, which may be at any level.

As previously mentioned in the case of quadriceps tendon, early recognition and surgical treatment are the key to a successful outcome. The following is a list of steps necessary to make an early diagnosis:

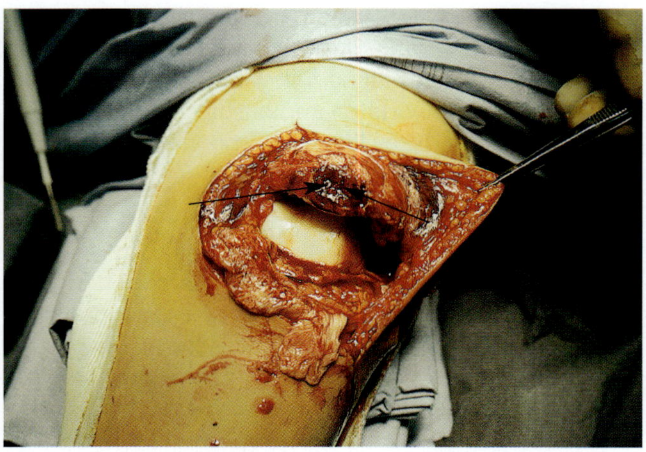

Figure 18.12. Patella tendon avulsion from the inferior pole of the patella. Arrows point to the area of avulsion.

1. A detailed history, including mechanism of injury.
2. A careful and detailed examination of the involved and uninvolved knee, including observation, palpation, and assessment of active and passive range of motion. Individuals with complete disruption of the patellar tendon are not able to lift the extremity against gravity in a straight fashion.
3. Presence of a very tender and painful gap, which is palpable in the area close to the inferior pole of the patella, especially in cases of acute ruptures.
4. Positive radiographic and MRI findings. A plain AP and lateral view of the injured and uninjured knee always should be taken for determination of patellar tendon length and assessment of patella alta. In complete patellar tendon rupture, almost always a detectable and noticeable patella alta is present compared to the opposite knee (Fig. 18.13). MRI is very helpful in partial disruptions and avulsions. In chronic cases or reruptures, MRI is helpful in preoperative assessment of the remaining tendon and appropriate surgical planning (Fig. 18.14).

Pitfalls

The following are the main pitfalls when dealing with acute ruptures of the patellar tendon:

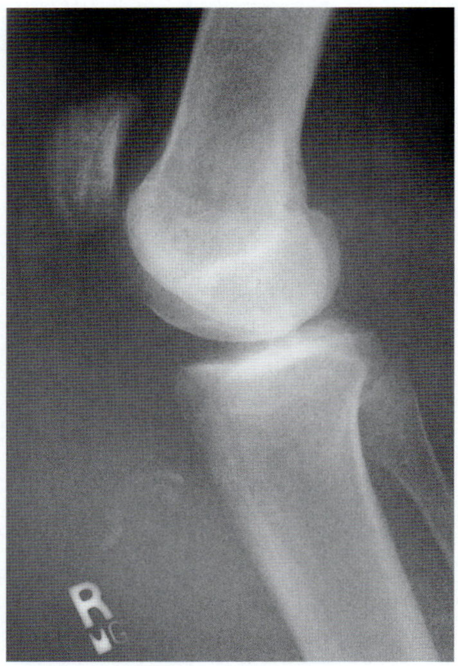

Figure 18.13. Patella alta in a chronic and untreated patella tendon rupture.

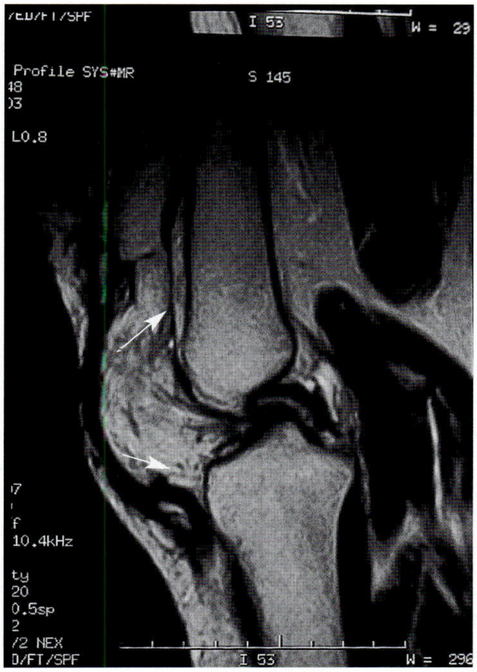

Figure 18.14. MRI of an untreated rupture of the patella tendon. The superior and inferior stump of the patellar tendon is marked by the arrows.

1. The extent of injury, partial or total, is not recognized.
2. End-to-end repair is not usually sufficient and will lead to a stretched patellar tendon and a very high riding patella (pathologic patella alta), with resulting functional difficulties and instabilities.
3. In cases of disruption close to the tibia tubercle, pulling on the upper position of the tendon with fixation to the patella will lead to development of patella baja and functional difficulties associated with it (Fig. 18.15).
4. Early motion with only end-to-end repair will lead to pathologic lengthening of the patellar tendon and patella alta.

Complications

1. Patella alta: Unrecognized and untreated patellar tendon ruptures will lead to a chronic patella alta with recurrent episodes of instability, weakness of leg extensions, and difficulty in activities of daily living.
2. Patella baja in cases of excessive traction and patella tendon reattachment (Fig. 18.16).
3. Arthrofibrosis: In the presence of arthrofibrosis with limited range of motion, arthroscopic debridement of the infrapatellar fat pad and gentle controlled manipulation is indicated after 6 weeks. Circlage wires must be removed prior to manipulation.
4. Broken and dislocated hardware.
5. Posttraumatic chondromalacia of the patella and anterior knee pain.

Surgical Management

In 1947 McLaughlin[5–7] reported the repair of the patellar tendon end to end with reinforcement by stainless steel wire anchored to a bolt inserted across the tibial tubercle. The wires are removed at 8 weeks.

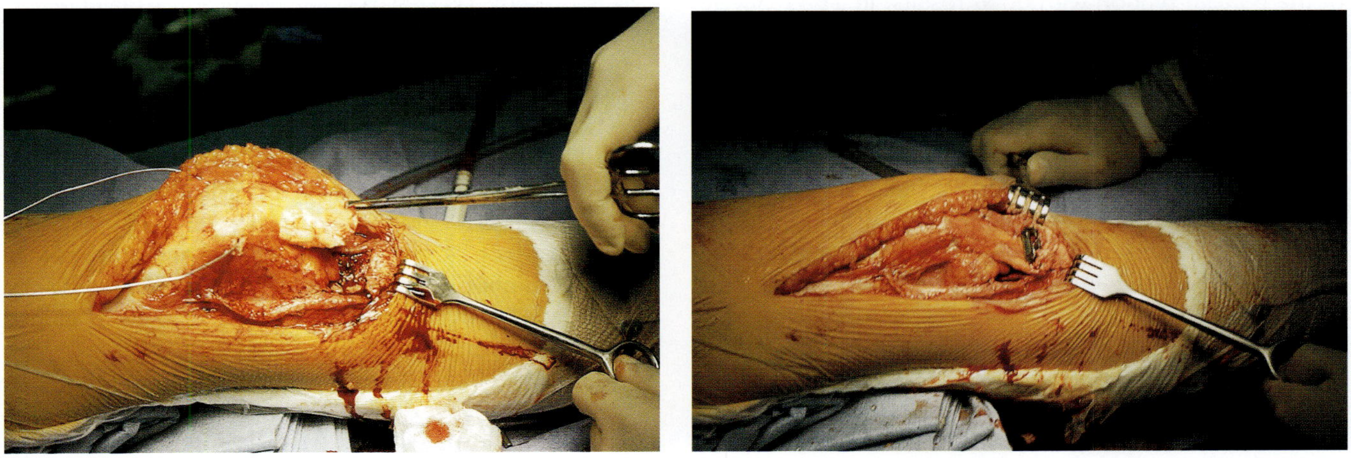

A B

Figure 18.15. A,B: Six-week status post–patella tendon rupture. The tendon is debrided and reattached by staple to the area of the tibial tubercle.

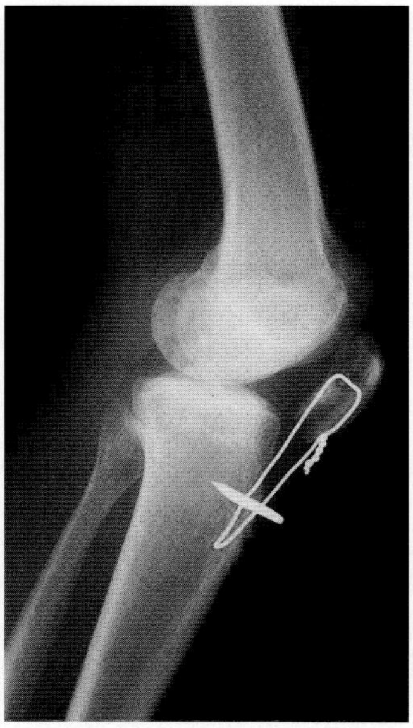

Figure 18.16. Postoperative iatrogenic patella baja.

In 1957 Kelikian et al[8] described a technique for reconstruction of the patellar tendon using the semitendinosus tendon. This procedure was used in chronic cases where a preliminary procedure had been performed utilizing traction pins to mobilize the patella prior to reconstruction with the semitendinosus. In 1979 Ecker et al[9] described using the semitendinosus and gracilis in cases of late reconstruction. In this technique preoperative traction was not required.

In 1980 Frazier and Clark[10] reported on the use of a 5-mm Dacron vascular graft to repair acute ruptures of the patellar tendon with good results. In 1981 Siwek and Rao[2] recommended reinforcement by Bunnell pullout wires tied to a Steinman pin through the tibia or through both the tibia and patella for all immediate repairs.

In 1980 Miskew et al[11] recommended the use of Mersilene (Ethicon) strips for the repair of quadriceps and patellar tendon disruptions. In 1988 Mandelbaum et al[12] described a technique in which a Z-plasty of the quadriceps tendon as well as the patellar tendon in neglected tears of the patellar tendon were performed. With this technique, the authors brought down the proximally retracted patella and shortened the stretched and nonfunctional patellar tendon.

In 1994 Falconiero and Pallis[13] reported on the use of the Achilles tendon allograft for reconstruction of a chronic patellar tendon rupture. In 1994 Hsu et al[14] reported on a primary repair with neutralization wire reinforcement, with 85% of the results rated excellent or good. No reruptures were reported in their series.

In 1995 Larsen and Simonian[15] reported on their technique of patellar tendon repair and augmentation with the semitendinosus and with immediate mobilization. Four cases were reported with excellent functional outcome. In 1998 McNally and Marcelli[16] reported on the use of Achilles tendon allograft reconstruction for a chronic patellar tendon rupture.

Author's Preferred Method

Acute Ruptures of the Patellar Tendon

If there is functional and usable tendon present at one end, midsubstance tears are carefully debrided and reapproximated with nonabsorbable suture. The position of the patella is determined radiographically. Once intraoperative lateral films are obtained and compared with preoperative views of the opposite knee, then a circlage neutralization wire is utilized for reinforcement (Fig. 18.17). This technique allows up to 45 degrees of flexion from 0 degrees in the early postoperative phase without undue tension at the repair site. Wires are then removed at 6 weeks postoperation and a careful program of physical therapy and rehabilitation is instituted.

Tears close to the inferior pole of the patella or associated with small avulsion fractures are reattached to the lower pole after excision of the avulsed fragment. This can easily be accomplished with the placement of three suture anchors into the patella and reattachment of the patellar tendon to the lower pole of the patella. With appropriate postoperative brace protection, additional circlage or neutralization wire is not necessary.

Chronic or Unrecognized Patellar Tendon Ruptures

In these cases if severe quadriceps contracture or fibrosis is present, skeletal/patellar traction is usually necessary to bring the patella down and stretch the contracted and fibrotic quadriceps. However adequate medial and lateral releases are also necessary to allow adequate mobilization of the patellar prior to repair. Again, the patellofemoral relationship should be compared to the opposite knee radiographically prior to the final repair/reconstruction.

In cases of severe patellar stretch and thus patella alta, the author's preferred method is an exchange tibial tubercle plasty rather than a double Z-plasty described by Mandelbaum et al.[12]

In this technique the tibial tubercle is osteotomized as a block, generally 2 cm by 2 cm. This is then pulled down until the patella reaches a level equal to the opposite side radiographically. The release of any fibrotic tissue and adhesions in the area of the prepatellar fat pad can easily be carried out simultaneously.

This technique can be easily accomplished by reflecting the osteotomized tibial tubercle proximally.

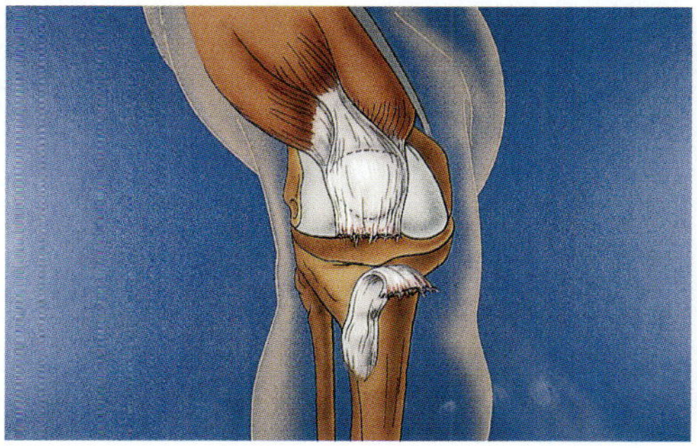

A

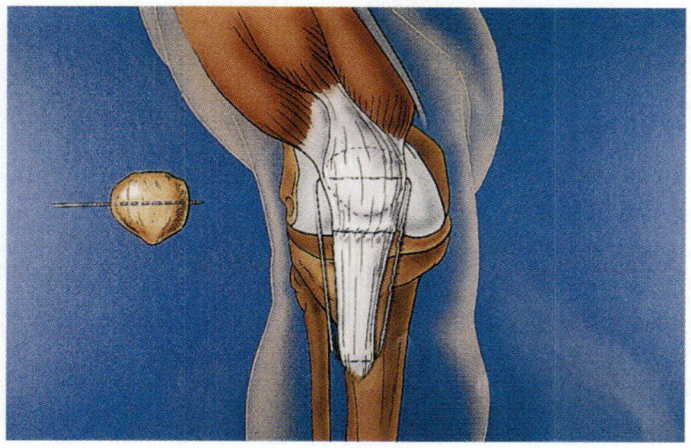

B

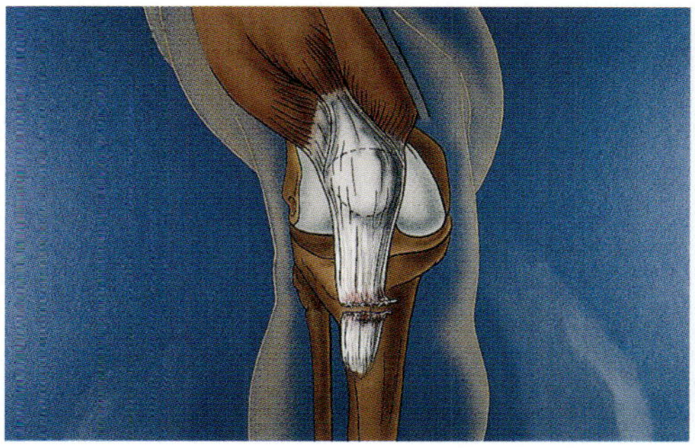

C

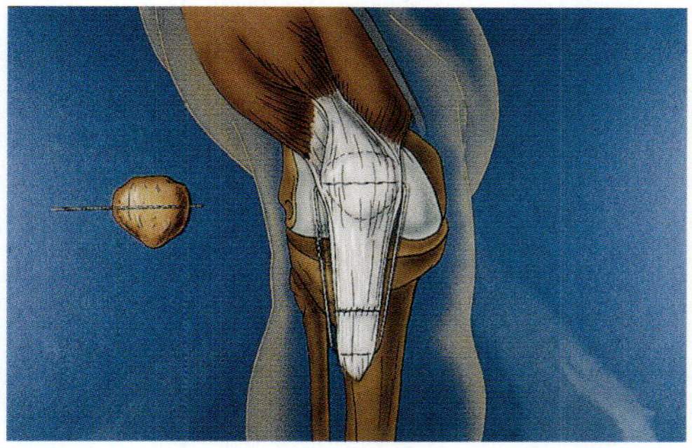

D

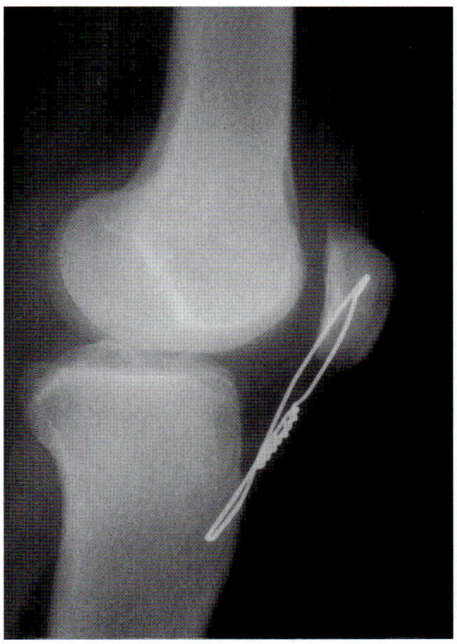

E

Figure 18.17. **A,B,C,D:** Schematic drawing of a patellar tendon rupture at different levels repaired and reinforced by circlage wire. **E:** Maintenance of patellar tendon height with circlage wire.

Once the appropriate level on the tibia is identified and marked, a block of 2 cm by 2 cm bone will be removed from this area. This block is fixed into the defect where the tibial tubercle had been osteotomized (Fig. 18A,B). Then the osteotomized tibial tubercle is seated into the new insertion site and is fixed with a bicortical screw (Fig. 18.18C), creating an elongated patellar tendon with adequate tension. Measurements are taken from the lower pole of the patella, again comparing to the preoperative lateral x-ray of the opposite knee. The elongated patellar tendon is then attached to the anterior tibia by staple or by two suture anchors 2 inches below the lower pole of the patella and above the previously reattached tibial tubercle. If it is decided to rein-

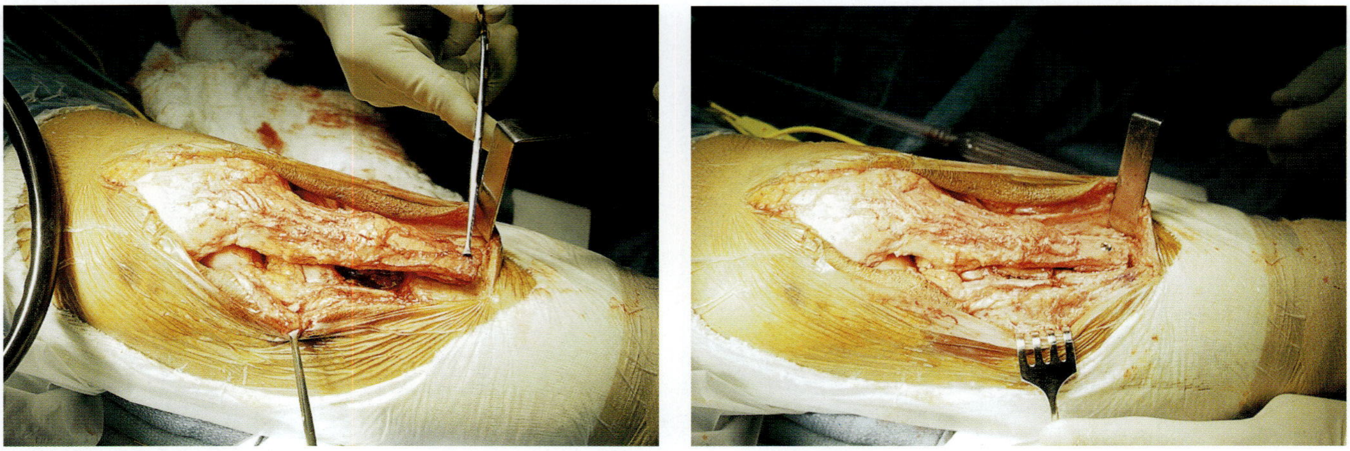

A B

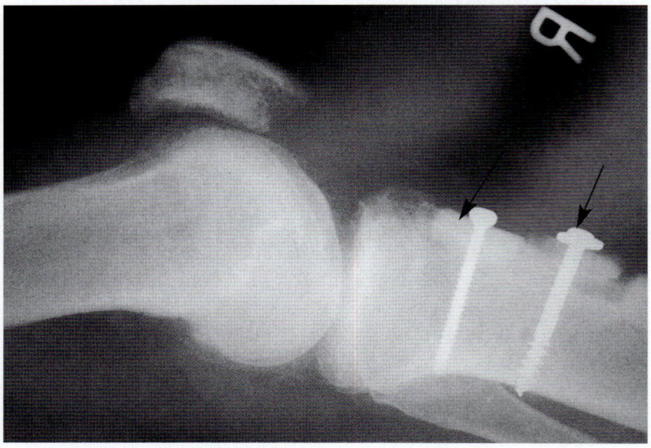

C

Figure 18.18. **A,B:** Exchange tibial tubercle plasty. **C:** New position of the patellar tendon, which is transferred distally (arrows). The block fixation to the original tibial tubercle site is shown (small arrow).

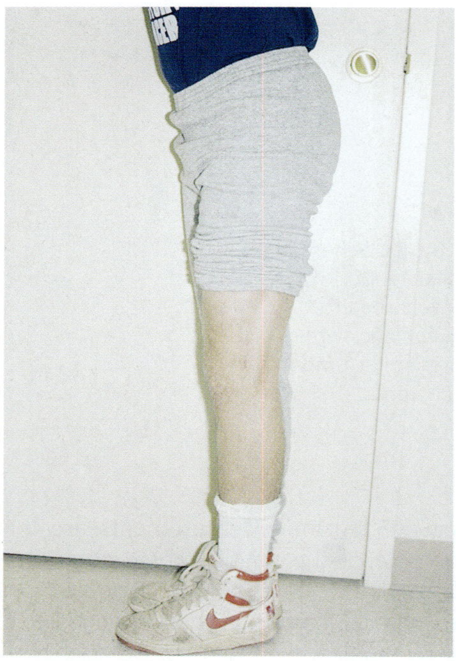

A

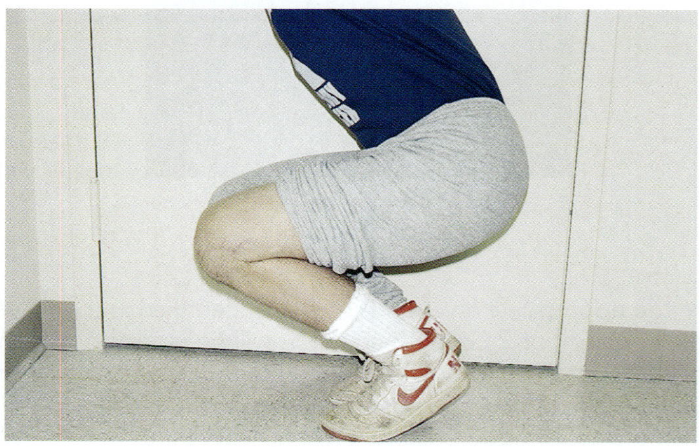

B

Figure 18.19. **A:** Postoperative range of motion in patient with exchange tibial tubercle plasty. Figure A shows full extension in standing position and figure B demonstrates full flexion, identical to the opposite side.

force the new patella ligament, this can be accomplished by using the semitendinosus or an allograft. We have not found this to be necessary with our technique.

Postoperatively, the knee is kept in a cylinder cast for 3 weeks, at which time a program of physical therapy and rehabilitation is instituted. We have performed this technique since 1982 and have experienced excellent outcomes with full range of motion, return to the preinjury level of activity, and no residual morbidity (Fig. 18.19).

CONCLUSION

Quadriceps and patellar tendon ruptures should be diagnosed immediately and treated surgically for optimum functional recovery. Partial disruptions should also be recognized with the help of MRI and protected until complete healing has taken place. Restoration of the anatomic and functional integrity of the extensor mechanism is most important for a full and complete recovery and return to the preinjury level of activity and sports.

References

1. Hohl M, Lardon R, Jones D. Disruption of the extensor mechanism In: Rockwood CA Jr, Green DP, eds. *Fractures in Adults*. Philadelphia: JB Lippincott, 1984.
2. Siwek CW, Rao JP. Ruptures of the extensor mechanism of the knee joint. *J Bone Joint Surg* 1981;63A: 932–937.
3. McBurney C. Suture of the divided ends of a ruptures quadriceps extensor tendon with perfect recovery. *Ann Surg* 1887;6:170.
4. Gallie WE, Lemessurier AB. The late repair of fractures of the patella and of rupture of the ligamentum patellar and quadriceps tendon. *J Bone Joint Surg* 1927; 9:47–54.
5. McLaughlin HL. Repair of major tendon rupture by buried removable suture. *Am J Surg* 1947;74:758–764.
6. Scuderi C. Ruptures of the quadriceps tendon: study of twenty tendon ruptures. *Am J Surg* 1958;95:626–635.
7. McLaughlin HL. Repair of ruptures through the larger tendons by removable staple suture. *Arch Surg* 1946;52: 547–556.
8. Kelikian H, Riashi E, Gleason J. Restoration of quadriceps function in neglected tear of patellar tendon. *Surg Gynecol Obstet* 1957;104:200–204.
9. Ecker ML, Lotke PA, Glazer RM. Late reconstruction of the patellar tendon. *J Bone Joint Surg* 1979;61A: 884–886.
10. Frazier CH, Clark EM. Major tender repairs with Dacron vascular graft suture. *Orthopaedics* 1980;3:323–325.
11. Miskew WBW, Pearson RL, Pankovich AM. Musilene strip suture in repair of disruptions of the quadriceps and patellar tendons. *J Trauma* 1980;20:867–872.
12. Mandelbaum B, Bartolozzi A, Carney B. A systemic approach to reconstruction of neglected tears of the patellar tendon. *Clin Orthop Rel Res* 1988;235:268–271.
13. Falconiero R, Pallis M. Chronic rupture of patellar tendon: technique for reconstruction with Achilles allograft. *Arthroscopy* 1996;12:623–626.
14. Hsu K, Wang K, Ho W, et al. Traumatic patellar tendon ruptures: a follow up study of primary repair and neutralization wire. *Trauma* 1994;36(5):658–660.
15. Larsen R, Simonian P. Semitendinosus augmentation of acute patellar tendon repair with immediate mobilization. *Am J Sports Med* 1995;23(1):82–86.
16. McNally P, Marcelli E. Achilles tendon reconstruction of a chronic patellar tendon rupture. *Arthroscopy* 1998;14: 340–344.

Section V

Complications and Pitfalls in Fractures Around the Knee

Chapter 19

FRACTURES OF THE DISTAL FEMUR

Robert E. Leggon, Daniel D. Feldmann,
and Ronald W. Lindsey

Fractures of the distal third of the femur have traditionally been and continue to be very challenging injuries for the orthopedic surgeon. Motor vehicle accidents and escalating urban violence contribute to an increasingly difficult fracture population. Due to the violent nature of these injuries, the selection of appropriate treatment may pose a significant challenge to the orthopedist. One needs to be aware of not only the fracture pattern and the best way to "put the puzzle back together," but also of the extent of soft tissue injury, contamination, and neurovascular complications. Each method of treatment for these injuries is associated with many potential complications. Early complications, such as infection, loss of reduction, compartment syndrome, and medically related problems, need to be immediately recognized and treated to prevent a poor outcome. Late complications, such as delayed union, nonunion, hardware failure, malunion, leg length discrepancy, stiffness, and degenerative joint disease, can be lessened or prevented with adequate preoperative evaluation, planning, and a thorough knowledge of the most up-to-date treatment methodology.

This chapter provides a brief historical review of the treatment of distal-third fractures of the femur, the major complications most commonly encountered, how they can be avoided, and how to salvage a poor outcome. The principles of modern management include anatomic reduction, stable fixation, and early mobilization.

HISTORICAL REVIEW

Prior to the 1900s, the treatment of supracondylar femur fractures consisted of strict splint or cast immobilization of the entire affected leg, without adequate control of limb alignment. The advent of traction pins in 1907 by Steinmann and 1909 by Kirschner enabled the physician to better resist the deforming forces at the fracture site.[1] Advances in skeletal radiography improved the physician's ability to achieve acceptable reduction of the fracture. Yet, prolonged immobilization in traction or a cast required serial x-ray follow-up and clinical adjustment, and frequently resulted in profound knee stiffness. Outcomes with closed treatment prompted most authors to eventually advocate operative treatment for all distal femur fractures.

The development of intramedullary (IM) fixation and plate devices in the 1930s provided a more stable fixation construct. Kuntscher[2] is credited with advancing the IM nail technique. Campbell[3] described the application of a plate with bolts and screws (Blount plate). Rush pin techniques were also popular in the treatment of supracondylar fractures in the 1940s and 1950s. Early attempts at open reduction and internal fixation were met with poor results secondary to problems with infection and loss of fixation.

In 1956, White and Russin[4] suggested that open reduction with internal fixation (ORIF) was the standard of care for treatment of supracondylar femur (SCF) fractures, although 25% of their patients did poorly. The Swiss Arbeitsgemeinscaft für Osteosynthesefragen (AO) was formed in 1958 and recommended anatomic reduction, preservation of blood supply, stable internal fixation, and early pain-free mobilization. Rigid internal fixation, as advocated by the Swiss AO, proved to be a more effective method of restoring early motion to the injured limb. In the 1970s, Schatzker and coworkers[5,6] promoted AO principles and techniques, and concluded that previous poor results in treating SCF fractures were due to improper implants, poor anatomic reduction, failure to achieve interfragmentary compression with lag screws, improper use of cement to facilitate screw fixation, and failure to bone graft when necessary. Chiron and coworkers[7] reported 75% good to excellent results utilizing AO technique and the condylar blade plate.

Closed treatment methods were still being considered the standard of care as late as the 1960s and 1970s. Neer and coworkers[8] followed treatment of 110 fractures of the distal 3 inches of the femur and reported that "no category of fracture at this level seemed well suited for internal fixation." They reported only 52% with satisfactory results with existing ORIF implants consisting of blade plates, Rush pins, plate and screw, or wire constructs. Other researchers also advocated closed reduction and early cast-brace ambulation.[9,10] Retrospectively, the implants of that era where inferior to those of today.

In another review of SCF fractures, Healy and Brooker[11] in 1983 compared closed versus surgical treatment (blade plate and screws) using stringent standards for normal limb function. In their series, 80% of patients treated by open measures had good functional results. Only 35% of patients achieved even satisfactory results when treated by closed methods. The superiority of open treatment was soon supported by other authors.[12–15]

The dynamic condylar screw (DCS) and side plate has generally replaced the 95-degree blade plate for acute fractures. The blade plate could be technically difficult to install if there was significant comminution. The DCS is inserted after drilling a path for the screw, which is much less traumatic than precutting the seat for the blade plate with a chisel. The insertion of the screw is safer, as it can be screwed in rather than hammered in, avoiding displacement of a previously reduced fracture. The lag screw is biomechanically advantageous, as it can compress intracondylar fracture extension. Schatzker and coworkers[16] have shown that the DCS and side plate is an excellent treatment option for fractures in the distal femur.

Other plate and screw constructs such as the condylar buttress plate have been used with varying degrees of success. The problem with this implant is that it is not as mechanically strong as the blade plate or the DCS plate because there is no fixed relationship between the screws and the plate. Often, the fracture falls into varus. To overcome this problem, adjunctive medial fixation has been recommended by some.[17] This requires additional periosteal dissection and should be avoided if the fracture can be stabilized by some other method. There has been recent interest in the use of plates with locked screws to improve fracture fixation. A new condylar plate device is being developed that allows the plate/screw construct to act as a fixed-angle device. Preliminary biomechanical data have shown significantly greater fixation stability than both a standard buttress plate and a 95-degree blade plate in a distal femoral gap osteotomy model. This device may be promising clinically in fractures with a high degree of comminution or osteoporosis.[18,19]

The last 20 years have brought improvements in intramedullary techniques.[20,21] The Zickel nail, interlocking antegrade nail, and the newer retrograde nail have been introduced. Intramedullary techniques are useful when soft tissue damage is extensive or bone quality is poor. Reasonable supracondylar fracture alignment can be obtained without further sacrificing soft tissue. Shelbourne and Brueckmann[21] demonstrated that with proper technique, Rush-pin fixation could be used successfully to treat supracondylar fractures. External splint or cast support is required and knee stiffness is a potential complication. Pin backout, loss of reduction, malunion, and the inability to address intercondylar displacement are limitations.

In an attempt to overcome some of the pitfalls of Rush pinning, the use of Ender's nails connected to cancellous screws has been described.[22] Most patients still require a cast or cast-brace for 8 weeks after surgery. Newer devices have made this technique obsolete. Zickel[23] developed an IM device designed for insertion through the condylar area to treat distal-third femur fractures. Zickel et al[24] and Marks et al[25] have shown that this device has been useful, especially in osteoporotic bone. Zickel et al stated that this device was "ideally suited for transverse supracondylar fractures" but felt that is was also able to stabilize "oblique, 'T,' and high fractures." Marks et al found the Zickel nail to be especially useful with periprosthetic fractures about the knee. Unfortunately, it does not address intercondylar extension. Because it is only semirigid, and usually requires external support, the Zickel nail can be prone to loss of reduction and cutout, does not reliably control rotation or length, and thus has lost favor.

More recently the antegrade IM nail has been used with success to treat distal-third femur fractures.[26,27] Antegrade techniques, however, are not suited for the most distal femur fractures or those with intracondylar extension. Nevertheless, in distal-third femur fractures where one can gain adequate purchase of the distal fragment, it may be advantageous to avoid violating the knee joint.

Most recently, the retrograde supracondylar locked intramedullary nail has been developed and used successfully to treat distal femur fractures, both supracondylar and supracondylar-intracondylar in nature.[28–32] Theoretical advantages to these IM devices include less soft tissue dissection, ability to insert the nail without the use of a fracture table, decreased blood loss, less operative time in the polytrauma patient, and their load-sharing biomechanical characteristics. They are somewhat limited when intercondylar displacement or comminution is severe. We favor their use in a percutaneous fashion for supracondylar fractures, and supracondylar-intercondylar fractures when the intercondylar component is minor. Nails inserted in a retrograde fashion generally have not caused knee stiffness as long as adjunct external immobilization is not needed.

External fixation, rarely used to treat fractures in the SCF, is most commonly indicated for the open supracondylar fracture with significant bone loss. Relative indications have included severe soft tissue injury, severe comminution, vascular injury, and multiple system dysfunction. Unlike tibial plateau fractures, ring fixators have a limited role acutely because the circumferential nature of the frames can be large and bulky, they can impede soft tissue access, and they can require significant expertise in application. Wires and/or half pins impale muscle and block motion. Occasionally the residual bone stock in the distal femur is too deficient for fixation solely in the femur, and pins/wires must be placed in the proximal tibia. If the fixator crosses the knee joint, immobility often leads to stiffness. In addition, pin-site infection is common, and can seed the adjacent joint or fracture. External fixation, which requires ongoing physician and patient management, may or may not be reasonable when patient compliance is poor. However, the external fixator may be the only means of fixation in the most complex fractures.[33] Table 19.1 reviews current acceptable treatment options for distal femur fractures.

Table 19.1. Implants currently used for distal femur fractures.

Implant Type	*Relative Indications*	*Relative Contraindications*	*Advantages*	*Disadvantages*
Blade plate	Noncomminuted low fractures	Intracondylar comminution, diaphyseal comminution, poor soft tissue envelope	Maintains varus/valgus alignment	Technically demanding, can displace unrecognized fracture, significant dissection
DCS/plate	Intracondylar displacement	Diaphyseal comminution, poor soft tissue envelope	Less demanding than blade plate, compresses simple intercondylar fractures, maintains varus/valgus alignment	Significant dissection
Condylar Plate	Intercondylar comminution	Loss of medial buttress, poor soft tissue envelope	Multiple distal screws	Traditional version allows motion between distal screws and plate (poor resistance to varus/valgus moments)
Dual plate	Extensive condylar comminution that requires ORIF of both condyles	Poor soft tissue envelope		Potential for "dead bone sandwich"
Antegrade nail	Shaft fractures, diaphyseal extension	Low fractures, intracondylar extension	Potential for minimal dissection	Can displace unrecognized fracture, alignment can be difficult to control, use of Fracture table
Retrograde nail	Osteoporosis, comminuted fracture, polytrauma, some supracondylar periprosthetic fractures, obesity	Significant intracondylar displacement	Potential for minimal dissection	Can displace unrecognized fracture, potential for unstable nail construct
External fixator	Extensive comminution, very low fractures, bone defects	When another device may be used	Bridging knee construct may provide stability when there is no other solution	Knee stiffness, pin-tract sepsis, may limit soft tissue access

DCS = dynamic condylar screw; ORIF = open reduction and internal fixation

COMPLICATIONS

Infection and Soft Tissue Complications

Infection is a prevalent complication of surgical intervention, and the spectrum of infection includes the following: cellulitis, a superficial stitch or wound abscess, infection of the knee joint, acute infection in an operatively stabilized fracture, chronic infection in a healed fracture, and infected nonunion (Fig. 19.1). Generally, the infection rate recently has ranged from 0% to 7%,[5,7,11,14,15,34] but historically, infection rates have been reported as high as 20%.[8,35] In the treatment of the floating knee, an infection rate of 30% has been noted.[36] Prognosis obviously depends on the extent of the infection, the nature and type of injury, and the condition of the patient.

Factors that predispose to infection include those associated with the injury, with treatment, and with the health of the patient.[37–40] Factors associated with the injury include the level of contamination and the degree of violence. Open fractures, comminution, devitalized bone, soft tissue injury, loss of tissue, compartment syndrome, and vascular injury predispose to infection. Factors associated with the treatment include inappropriate antibiotic prophylaxis, extensive surgical dissection, inadequate fixation, inadequate soft tissue management, prolonged operative time, or a delay in operative intervention. Finally, the health of the patient may significantly affect the risk for infection due to conditions such as end-stage renal disease, diabetes, chronic steroid use, polytrauma, obesity, age, and immunodeficiency syndrome.

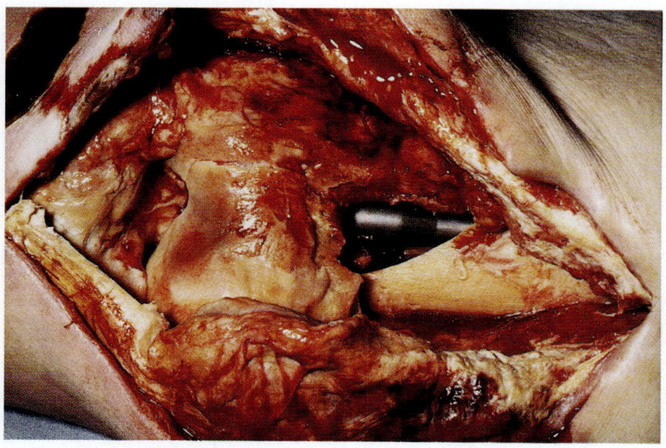

Figure 19.1. Infected nonunion. The condyles are avascular and infected with multiple organisms. Unfortunately, in this elderly patient, amputation was the result.

Nonunion and Loss of Fixation

Nonunion of the distal femur occurs less often than in the proximal femur, but more commonly than in the shaft. The current incidence is reported between 0% and 6%.[41] Factors that contribute to nonunion include bone loss, soft tissue loss, vascular stripping, fracture overdistraction, inadequate stabilization, infection, and failure to bone graft.[41] Historically, these fractures have healed following collapse and angulation. Improved techniques have maintained alignment and permitted early mobilization of the patient, but at the risk of potentially inhibiting union.

The diagnosis of nonunion is easily detected by hardware failure, loss of fixation, obvious pathologic motion, or excessive pain. Occasionally, nonunion can pose diagnostic challenge, especially following multiple procedures, in the presence of extensive hardware or when occult in nature (Fig. 19.2). We recommend high-quality anteroposterior, lateral, and oblique x-rays to assess bony healing. The clinician must frequently review sequential films, and tomograms, computed tomography (CT), or magnetic resonance imaging (MRI) may be necessary.

Malunion

Malunion has become less prevalent with the advent of improved surgical implants and techniques.[42] Malunion had been a frequent complication of closed treatment

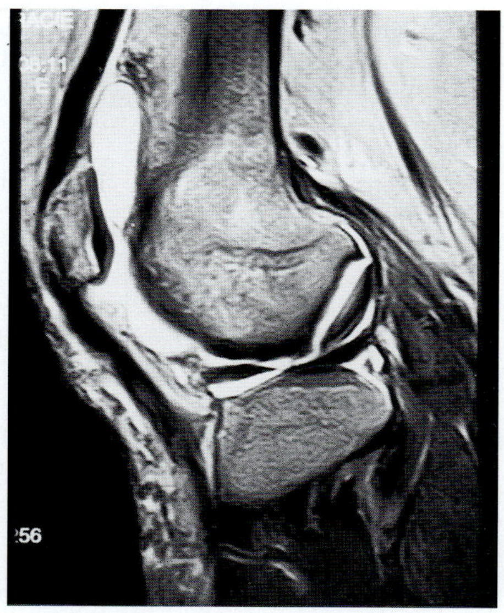

Figure 19.2. Intraarticular nonunion. Magnetic resonance imaging eventually revealed osteochondral nonunion after plain films were read as negative. Patient complained of instability despite intact ligaments and menisci.

of SCF fractures, and was a major impetus for the development of open reduction technique.[41] Any angular deformity may occur; however, the most common position of malunion is one of internal rotation, varus, and hyperextension of the distal fragment.[43] Translation of the fragments may also exist and adds yet another element of complexity to the deformity.[44]

Analyses of alignment following open reduction and internal fixation using AO techniques have demonstrated that malunion remains a problem. In a review of 59 SCF fractures, Zehntner et al[42] found that differences in alignment between limbs were within 5 degrees of varus/valgus in 74%, of ante/recurvation in 78%, and of rotation in 83%. The authors cited varus/valgus alignment as the most difficult to control, and conceded that malunion was common.

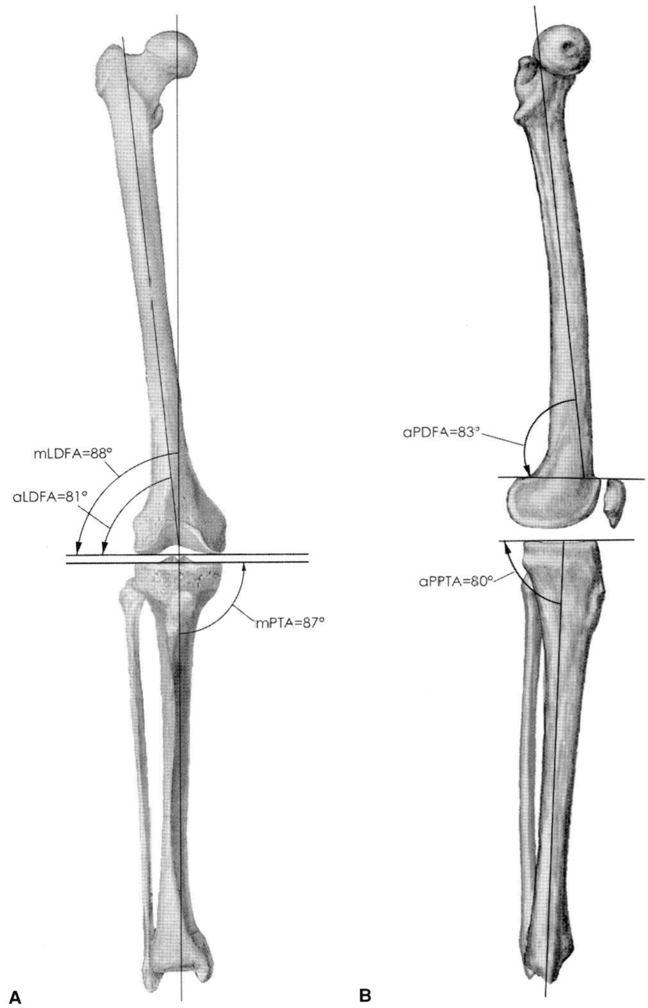

Figure 19.3. Malalignment and malunion is prevented by consideration of both the anatomic and mechanical axes.

Presently there are no absolute criteria for acceptable alignment in SCF fractures. The authors define malunion as an angular deformity of more than 5 degrees, rotational malalignment of greater than 15 degrees, leg length discrepancy of greater than 2.5 cm, and intraarticular incongruity of greater than 3 mm. The treating surgeon must be aware of the contralateral limb anatomy and adjust his reduction accordingly (Fig. 19.3).

The first key to effective treatment of the deformity is to understand the deformity, whether it is simple or complex.[45] Evaluation may be undertaken according to anatomic or mechanical axes. If one does not perform correction at the center of rotation and angulation (CORA), translation will occur. Deformity at one level is termed *uniapical*, while one at many levels is termed *multiapical*. An oblique plane deformity occurs in a plane that is not frontal or coronal. In contrast to developmental deformities that may be only angular and rotational in nature, deformity secondary to trauma may also entail translation and shortening (Fig. 19.4).

Stiffness

Decreased range of motion is the most common complication after closed or open treatment of SCF fractures, with the loss of flexion exceeding the extension loss. Functionally, even a small loss of extension (15 degrees) can be more of a functional impairment than a comparable loss of flexion. Stiffness is usually due to (1) closed treatment with prolonged immobilization; (2) external fixation, especially if bridging the knee[33]; (3) casting as a salvage procedure following unstable open reduction or loss of fixation; (4) infection; (5) delayed union and nonunion; (6) malpositioned hardware; (7) treatment requiring vascular or plastic reconstruction[46]; (8) ipsilateral fractures of the tibia, patella, or more proximal femur[36]; and (9) head injury.

Loss of motion can result from extrinsic and intrinsic causes.[47] Extrinsic infers soft tissue contracture of the capsular, ligamentous, or muscular tissue.[48] Capsular and ligamentous adhesions or heterotopic bone can occur in the medial compartment, lateral compartment, or the region of the suprapatellar pouch. Loss of elasticity and subsequent excursion of the quadriceps muscle group is more common than that of the hamstrings. Heterotopic ossification can be particularly difficult to manage in these muscles, especially in the head-injured patient.

Intrinsic contracture implies a cartilaginous or osseous origin to motion inhibition. Intraarticular adhesions may exist between the patella and femur, or between the femur and tibia. Loss of articular cartilage, with exposed subchondral bone, can accelerate this process. Rarely,

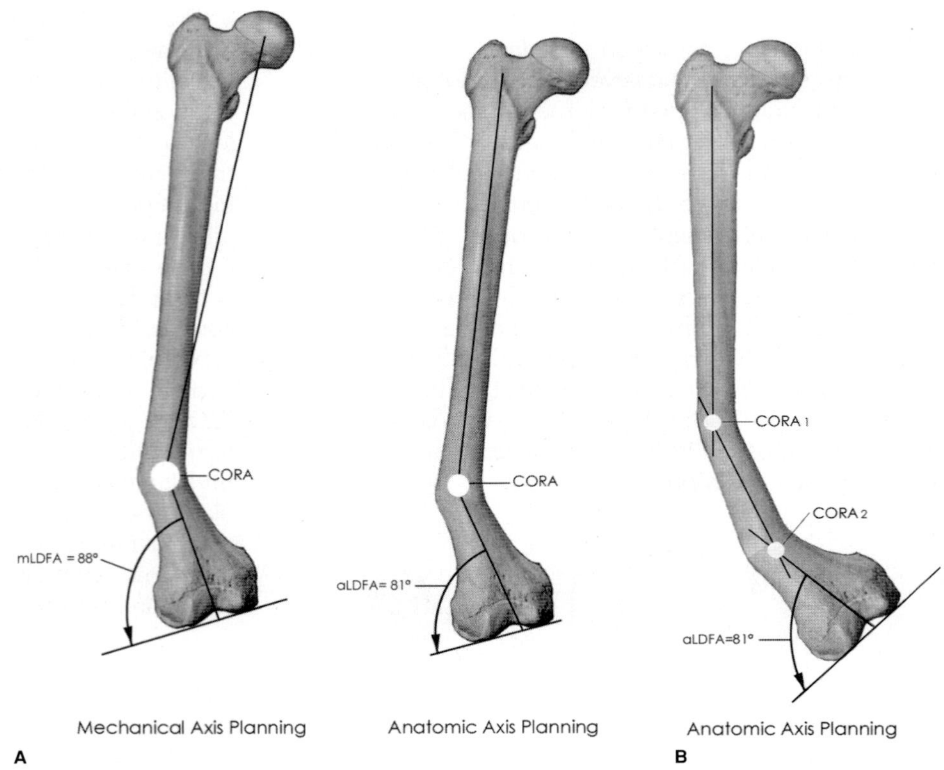

Figure 19.4. The spectrum of deformity. **A:** Uniapical deformity, anatomic and mechanical axis planning. **B:** Multiapical deformity. Oblique plane deformities and complex deformities with translation, angulation, and rotation are even more challenging,[44,45] and require considerable preoperative plannning.

union can occur between bony surfaces. Finally, intrinsic contracture can occur from gross joint incongruity, with a mechanical block to motion.

Osteoarthritis

The principal cause of posttraumatic osteoarthritis is the damage sustained by the articular cartilage at the time of injury. Blunt trauma to the cartilage even without a fracture can cause eburnation and, ultimately, ensuing arthritis. Continuous passive motion has been shown to aid in healing and remodeling of full-thickness defects in articular cartilage.[49]

The healing and remodeling of osteochondral step-offs differ substantially from cartilage defects.[50] Increased cartilage pressures are generated in the high side of the defect, and while cartilage and subchondral bone can adapt to their surface incongruities by remodeling, the surface remodeling is incomplete (Fig. 19.5). Continuous passive motion does not appear to improve healing or remodeling, particularly for large step-offs.

The fracture pattern greatly influences the risk for posttraumatic arthritis. Intercondylar extension and comminution increases this risk in all three compartments of the knee joint. A nonanatomic reduction of fractures involving the condylar surface will also lead to arthritis. In an experimental rabbit model, a 5-mm condylar defect leads to arthritic changes within 20 weeks.[51] In humans, a step-off of 3 mm has been shown to cause significant gonarthritis.[52]

Mechanical malalignment of the limb can further accentuate posttraumatic arthritis in the knee. For example, a narrowed medial joint space or a couple of millimeters of articular incongruity may be well tolerated if the overall mechanical alignment of the limb is near neutral or in a few degrees of valgus. However, the same degree of medial joint pathology can rapidly progress to joint arthrosis if the mechanical axis is in varus malalignment.

Vascular Compromise

Vascular compromise resulting from the surgical treatment of SCF fractures is extremely rare. The incidence of vascular injury in supracondylar femur fractures associated with blunt trauma is approximately 2% to 3%. This incidence is surprisingly low as the vascular bundle is tethered at the adductor hiatus. Segmental arterial defects may also occur.[46] The incidence of vascular injury associated with gun shot wounds is higher, given the penetrating nature of the trauma. Adamson and coworkers[36] report a 21% incidence of vascular injuries with floating knees.

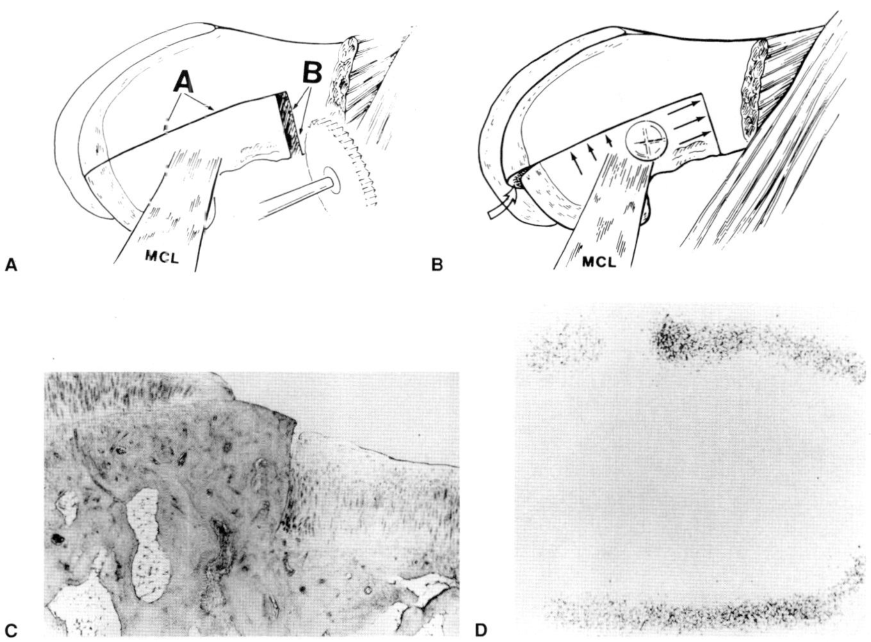

Figure 19.5. Healing and remodeling of articular incongruities in a rabbit fracture model. **A** and **B:** Osteotomy to create osteochondral step-off. **C:** Histologic slide of healed 1-mm step-off. The subchondral bone has rounded off at the rim of the lesion. There is a rounding of cartilage on the high side and an increase in thickness on the low side. **D:** Change in contact pressures generated by healed step-off. (From ref. 50, used with permission)

PREVENTION OF COMPLICATIONS

Infection and Soft Tissue Complications

Infection is an inherent complication of open reduction and internal fixation. In major trauma centers with experienced surgeons, the rate of infection should not exceed 5% in most operatively treated cases.[53] The optimal timing of surgery is essential with the open injury due to the extent of contamination or tissue devitalization. Timing may be just as important with closed injuries, considering the medical status of the patient and the extent of the soft tissue swelling. A developing compartment syndrome requires early recognition and an immediate fasciotomy.[54] A cephalosporin antibiotic should be administered preoperatively and for at least 24 hours postoperatively. The prolonged use of antibiotics for draining wounds is controversial, and the authors recommend that its use be individualized.

The extent of soft tissue trauma associated with the injury can alter the complexity of its management. The combination of bone devascularization and wound contamination significantly decreases the potential for an acceptable outcome. The current treatment recommendations by Gustilo[37,38] for grade I, II, and III open fractures include prophylactic antibiotics, early debridement, copious irrigation and often a second-look debridement at 36 to 72 hours. Although some clinicians site no increase in the incidence of deep infection with a delay of up to 24 hours to surgery,[55] the authors recommend irrigation and debridement within 6 hours of injury. Also, the fracture should be stabilized immediately,[56] as the soft tissue benefits of immediate internal fixation outweigh the risk of infection. In grade IIIB and IIIC open fractures, external fixation with delayed internal fixation may be optimal with serial debridements every 36 to 72 hours until definitive wound closure can be achieved. In grade I and II open fractures, cefazolin should be administered for 48 hours following the final debridement.

Current antibiotic recommendations for grade I and II (Gustilo classification[37,38]) open fractures include 3 days of a first-generation cephalosporin (generally cefazolin, 1g every 8 hours) intravenously, for grade III open fractures, 5 days of cefazolin and gentamicin (2 mg/kg adjusted to serum levels). Addition of penicillin, 4 million units IV every 6 hours, is recommended for wounds with gross contamination (e.g., barnyard, lake, stream) to cover anareobic organisms (including *Clostridium perfingens* and *Clostridium septicum* which can cause gas gangrene).[57] Immunization against *Clostridium tetani* also needs to be undertaken.

Green and Trafton[58] have strongly advocated open fracture wound healing by secondary intention. They experienced a greater deep infection rate when grade II or III injuries were subjected to delayed primary closure as opposed to healing by secondary intention. Furthermore, they recommend delayed bone grafting in the treatment of open fractures. In their study deep infection occurred in 3 of 4 cases when bone grafting was performed within the first 7 days.

Appropriate fixation selection can also alter the rate of infection. Soft tissue injuries secondary to high-energy trauma do poorly when fixation requires extensive additional dissection. In these cases it may be more appropriate to treat the SCF fractures with a minimally

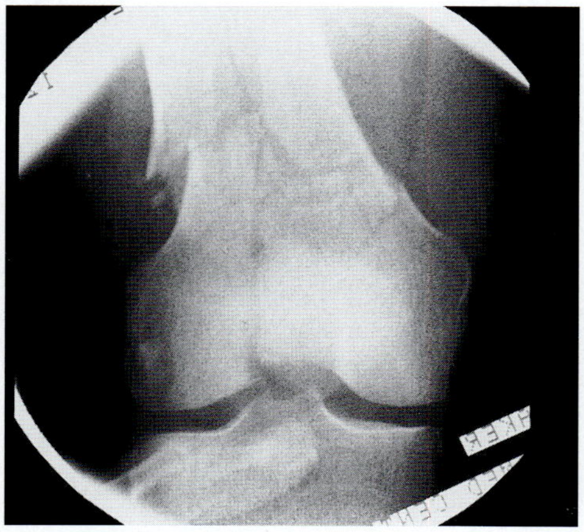

A

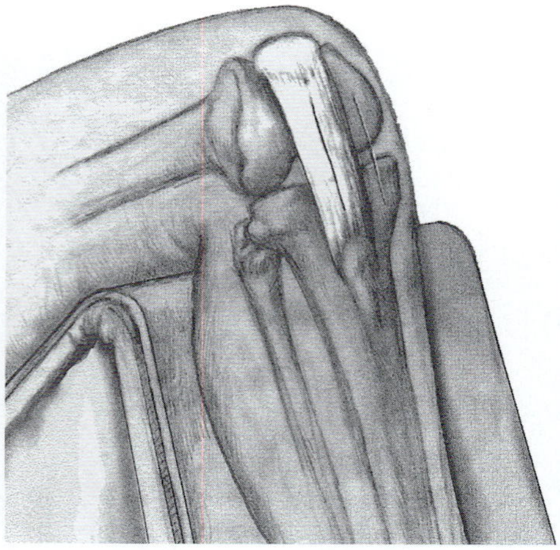

B

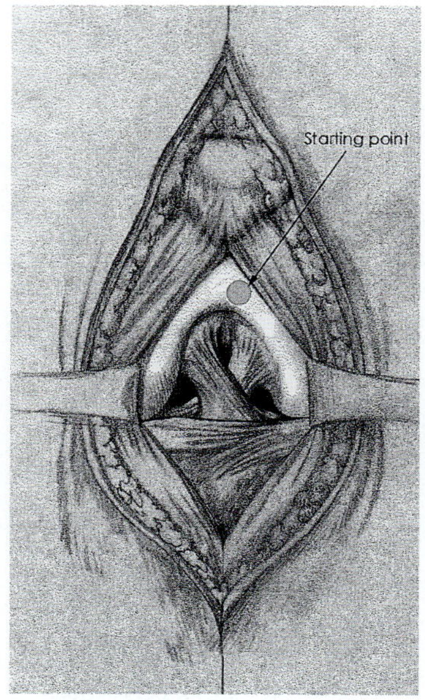

C

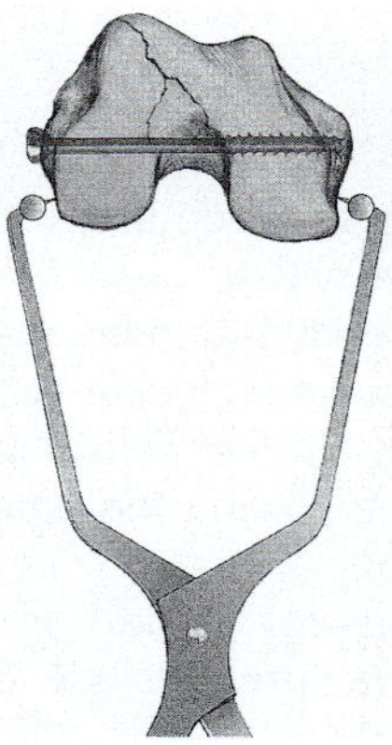

D

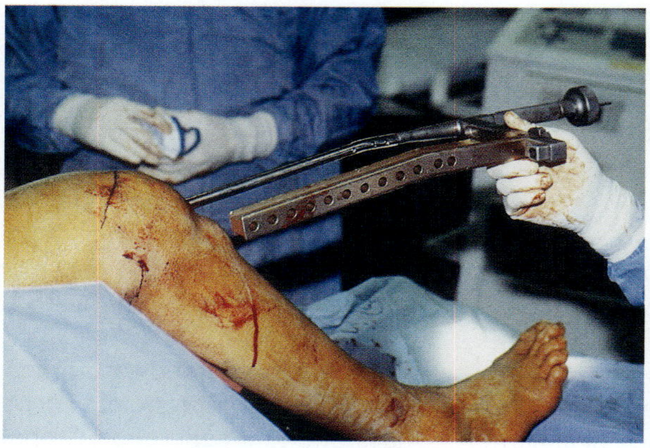

E

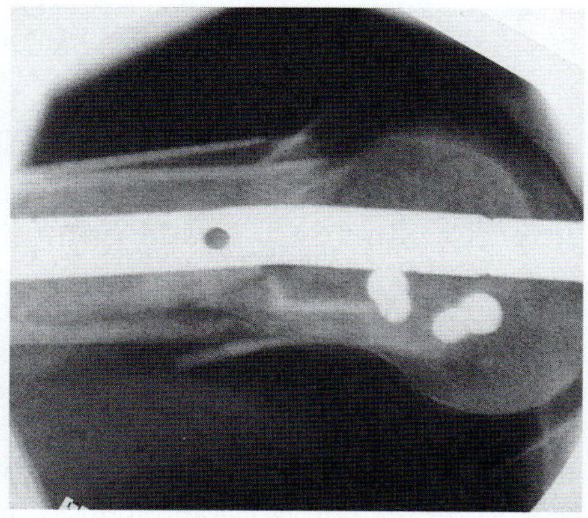

F

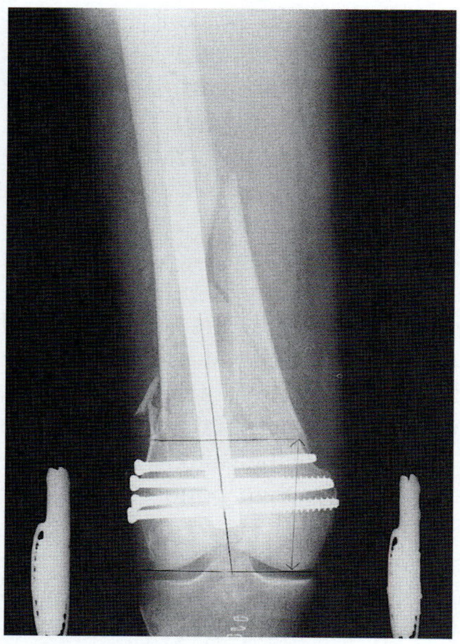

G

Figure 19.6. Technique of minimally invasive retrograde nailing for supracondylar-intracondylar distal femur fracture. **A:** A 3 to 4 mm articular step-off is visualized. This may be the limit of displacement that one can accept in attempting a percutaneous technique. **B:** Positioning with knee flexed. The use of autoclavable triangles marketed for fixation of tibia fractures can be useful in patient positioning. Insertion site may be either through the patellar tendon or just medial to it. **C:** The best entry site is determined by the specific nail; however, it is usually anterior to the attachment of the anterior cruciate ligament and just medial to the notch. Incision size often decreases as experience increases. **D:** Large pelvic reduction clamps are useful in manipulating and compressing the intracondylar fracture. Two posterior cannulated lag screws are placed prior to placement of retrograde nail to prevent further displacing the intracondylar fracture. Reaming over a guidewire is preferable to the use of a curved awl in obtaining a starting point. **E:** Percutaneous nail insertion. **F:** Nail anterior to previously inserted lag screws on lateral view. **G:** Stable nail construct and anatomic reduction of the articular surface. Note that four cortices are grasped by the distal interlocking screws of the retrograde nail. With this nail, 7.5 mm of distal femur are necessary to obtain four-cortex fixation. For proper alignment, the anatomic lateral distal femoral angle should be 81 degrees.

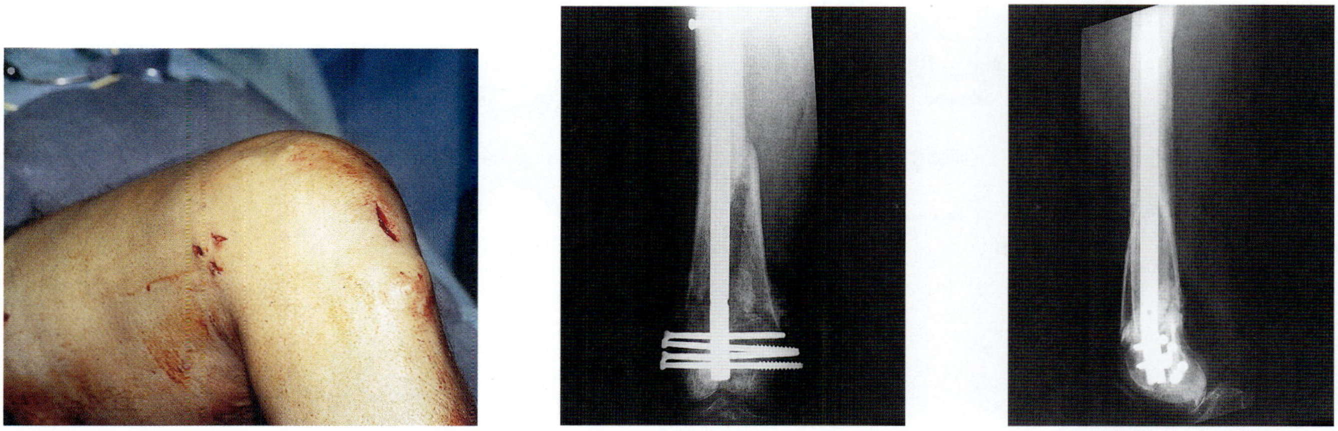

H I1 I2

Figure 19.6. (*cont.*) **H:** Minimal incision technique can often be useful in patients with a poor soft tissue envelope or in the massively obese. **I:** AP and lateral views show union at six months with 110 degrees of active motion.

invasive IM rod.[56] The IM rod is also applicable for supracondylar-intercondylar fractures when the intercondylar component is relatively minor (Fig. 19.6). When using a dynamic compression screw and side plate, "indirect fracture reduction" techniques can decrease the risks for nonunion and infection.[59] Limited provisional external fixation can be useful in select open fractures with massive soft tissue disruption. Generally, one should avoid the combination of extensive internal fixation and external fixation (Fig. 19.7).

Fractures secondary to low-velocity gunshot wounds are comparable to grade I fractures and can be managed with immediate internal fixation.[60] The authors prefer intramedullary nailing when possible to avoid additional soft tissue disruption. Limited antibiotic prophylaxis with a cephalosporin is appropriate.[61] High-velocity fractures, fortunately, are less common in civilized populations, are comparable to grade III fractures, and usually require multiple debridements. Simple, unilateral external fixation, often bridging the knee, provides effective preliminary fixation. After the wound is stable, definitive internal fixation should be performed.

Nonunion and Loss of Fixation

The AO principles of rigid internal fixation and early knee motion have established the modern standard for the treatment of these fractures and their basic tenets of fracture repair have been well detailed in many texts. The limb reconstruction using the DCS consist of reduction of the articular surface, preliminary lag screw fixation of the condyles, and final application of the plate (Fig. 19.8). Typically, the lateral approach provides adequate exposure with routine need for a tibial tubercle osteotomy,[15] as it can be a source of a nonunion. Tibial tubercle osteotomy may occasionally be used when a more generous exposure is needed, for nonunions or malunions.

The original AO approach can compromise bone of its vital blood supply. When there is extensive soft tissue disruption, as in high-energy trauma, it is imperative the surgeon not extensively strip soft tissues via a large open procedure. Recently, biologic (indirect) reduction techniques have been advocated to minimize the surgical trauma to the tissue.[62] Bone[59] describes fixating the device (blade plate) distally and applying a femoral distractor to the femur, which would allow the comminuted bony fragments to be indirectly reduced by their

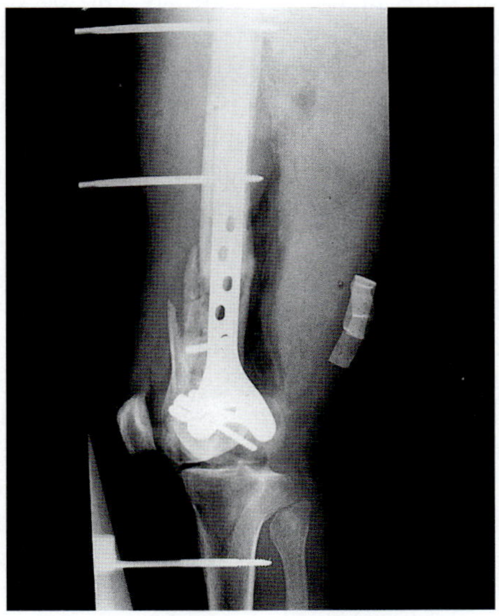

Figure 19.7. Overlapping internal and external fixation. A pin tract infection seeded this internally fixed fracture.

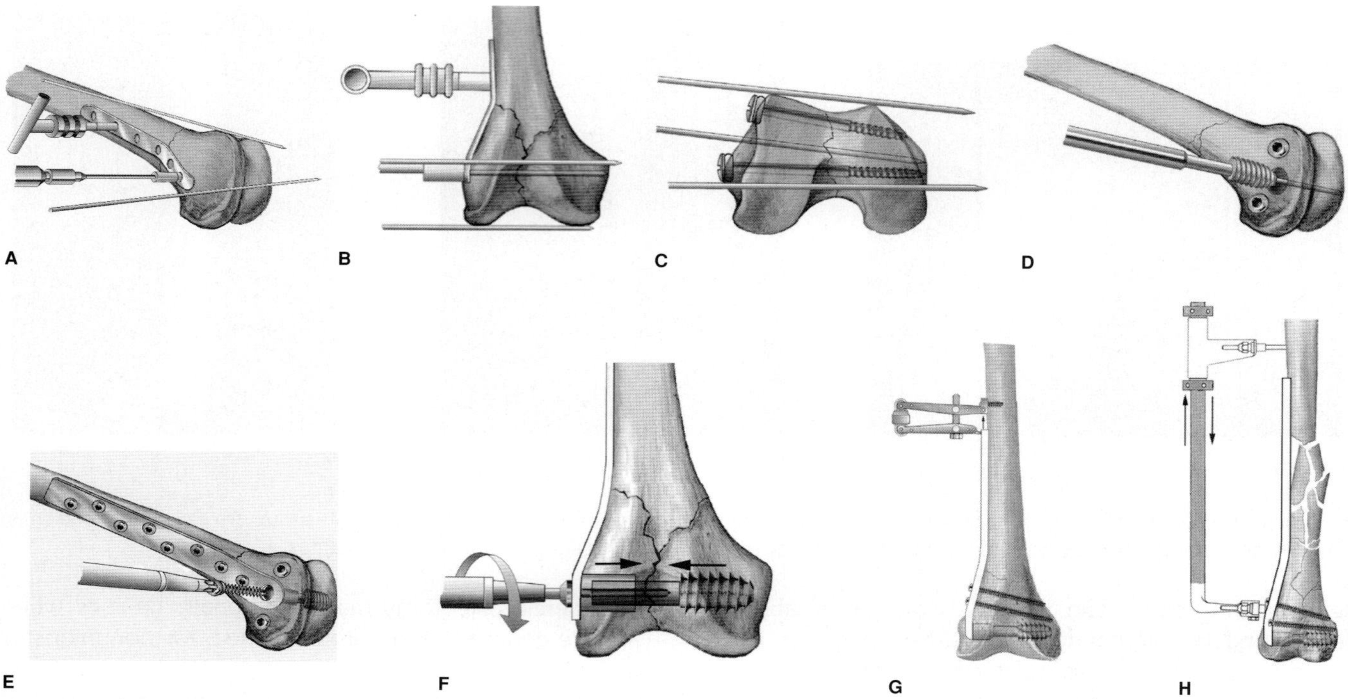

Figure 19.8. Employing the DCS and side plate. **A–F:** schematic of technique. **G:** Use of the articulating tension device to apply compression. **H:** Use of the femoral distractor to control alignment.

soft tissue attachments (Fig. 19.9). Bolhofner and coworkers[62] reported no nonunions in treating 57 distal femur fractures with a condylar blade plate or buttress plate utilizing biologic reduction techniques.

It must be emphasized that with a rigid system (plate) even small gaps at the fracture site can be dangerous and lead to nonunion. Although stability facilitates early knee motion, callus formation is inversely proportional to the rigidity of the system. Considerations to prevent nonunions include shortening of the fracture (accepting some leg length discrepancy), or bone grafting (with donor-site morbidity, and perhaps a higher incidence of infection). All treatment methods have inherent complications and the ideal treatment should be individualized to the fracture and the patient.

The indications for bone graft can be controversial. In closed fractures with significant comminution, bone should always be considered, especially if healing progresses slowly. In open fractures with bone loss, the application of bone graft should be delayed until the wound has healed without evidence of infection. When larger volumes of bone graft are required, the authors recommend harvest of graft from the posterior crest with the patient placed in a lateral or semilateral position during the procedure. The graft should not be harvested until

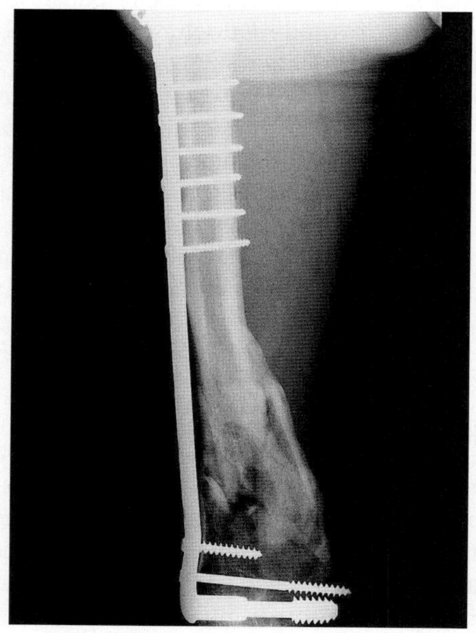

Figure 19.9. "No-touch technique" in managing extensive supracondylar comminution. Union is aided by avoiding devascularization of comminuted bone fragments.

it is clear that the nonunion site is not infected through surgical exposure (Fig. 19.10).

Appreciating the biomechanics of the fixation is crucial to maintaining stability. Simple errors such as forgetting the compression screw in the DCS/plate construct can lead to instability (Fig. 19.11). The quality of screw placement in hardware and bone may also affect the construct's strength. Tornkvist and coworkers[63] demonstrated that bending strength (gap opening and gap closing) of plated fractures was affected more by screw placement than the number of screws placed. A few screws spaced over a larger distance was stronger than multiple screws in a short distance (plate constructs). Polymethylmethacrylate can occasionally be used to augment screw purchase or lag screw purchase in osteoporotic bone.[64,65]

The length of the plate above the fracture is also important in preventing loss of fixation. The authors recommend a minimum of at least eight cortices of solid fixation. Inadequate plate length proximally may lead to proximal failure (Fig. 19.12). Ipsilateral hip or knee arthroplasties can also prevent biomechanically sound fixation. A femoral arthroplasty component will limit the number of proximal attainable cortices. In this situation, cables may be utilized to increase the fixation of the fracture construct. To prevent a stress riser between the plate and femoral stem, the two components should overlap (Fig. 19.13).

Supracondylar femur fractures above a total knee arthroplasty present a special management challenge. Nonoperative methods usually fail to control alignment and do not allow for early knee motion or stable ambulation. Fixation options include dynamic condylar plate and screws, and retrograde nails[66,67] (Fig. 19.14).

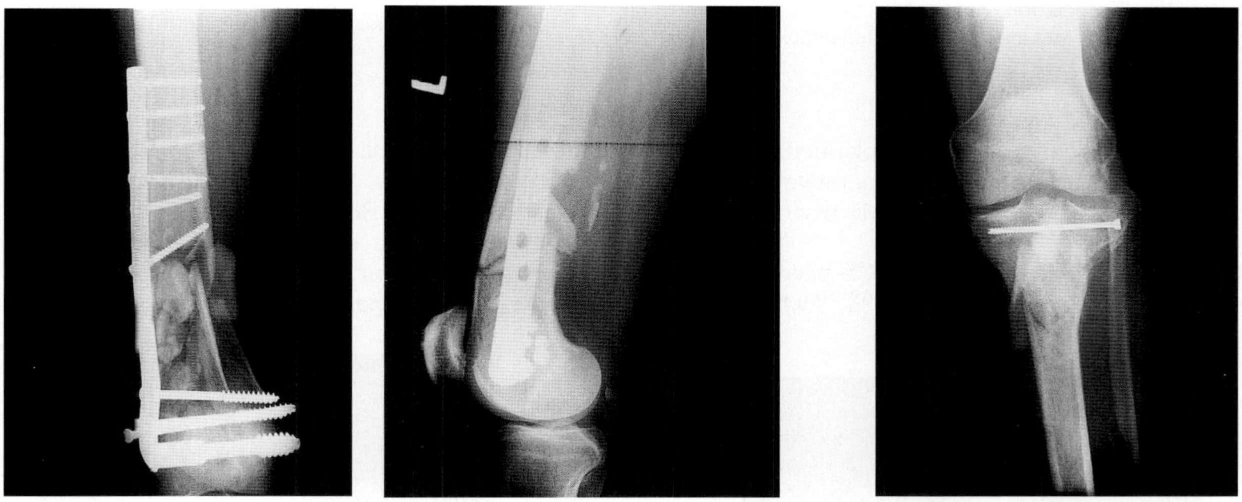

A B

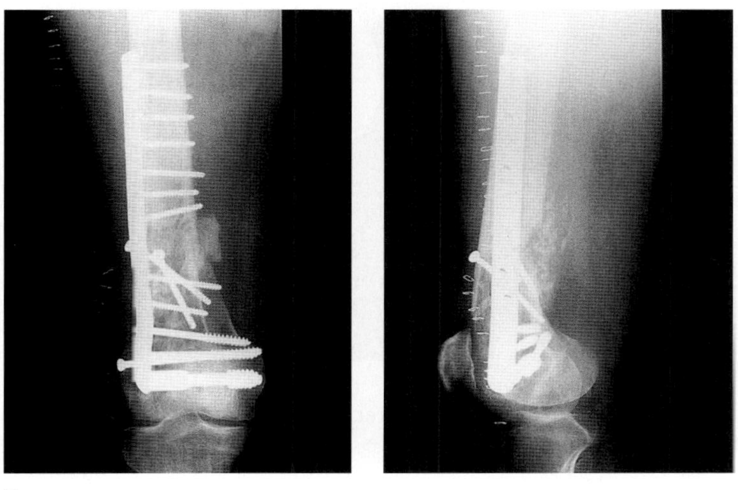

C

Figure 19.10. Bone grafting a nonunion. **A:** AP and lateral views of a nonunion. **B:** Contralateral traumatic below knee amputation. **C:** AP and lateral views after posterior iliac crest bone grafting to delayed union. Subacute shortening of the fracture was performed using the articulating tension device to decrease the fracture gap. Lag screw fixation was added to stabilize the construct. A small leg length discrepancy was inconsequential given the contralateral below knee amputation.

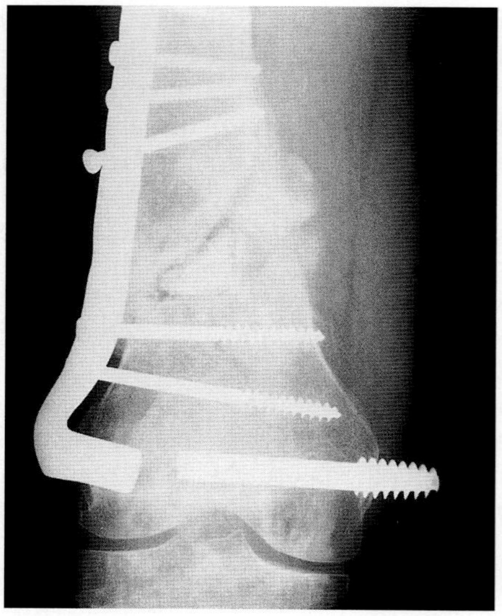

Figure 19.11. Dissociation of lag screw from dynamic condylar plate. Failure to include compression screw led to construct instability.

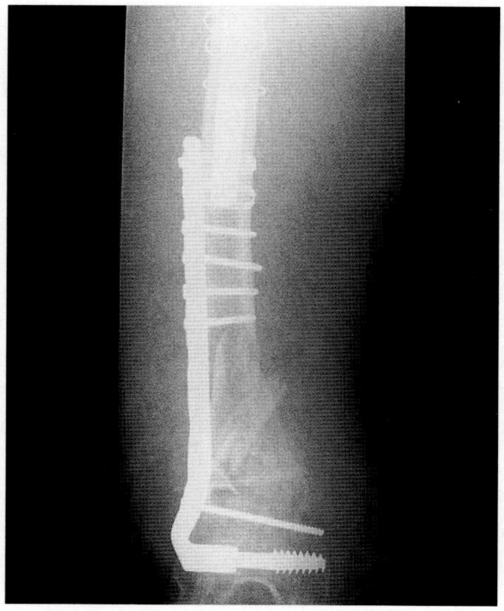

Figure 19.13. Cables can supplement proximal fixation.

If fixation with a retrograde nail is planned, the physician may need to obtain the prior operative note to assure that the femoral component will permit nail passage.

The 95-degree blade plate and DCS-plate constructs provide more rigid torsional fixation,[68–70] while IM nails are stronger in axillary loading.[68,71] However, the surgeon needs to ask, "How rigid must the fixation be for fracture healing?" Recently, IM nailing has become popular, relying more on callus formation in a semirigid load-sharing system than on primary bone healing in a very rigid load-sparing system. Reaming the intra-

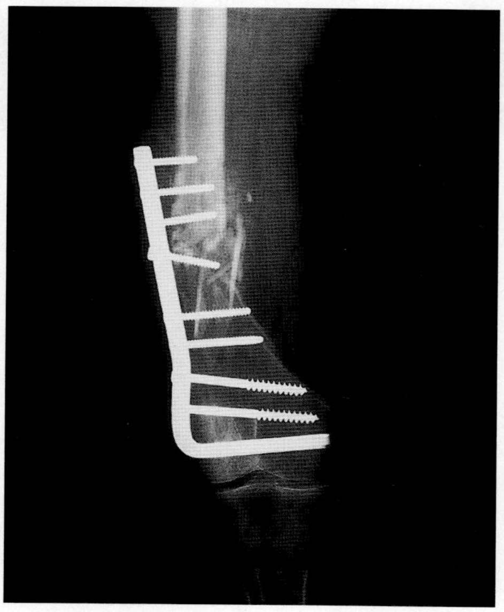

Figure 19.12. Inadequate proximal fixation. Intraoperatively, the surgeon realized long plates were not in inventory, necessitating use of an inadequate-length plate. The short plate with inadequate proximal fixation ultimately failed.

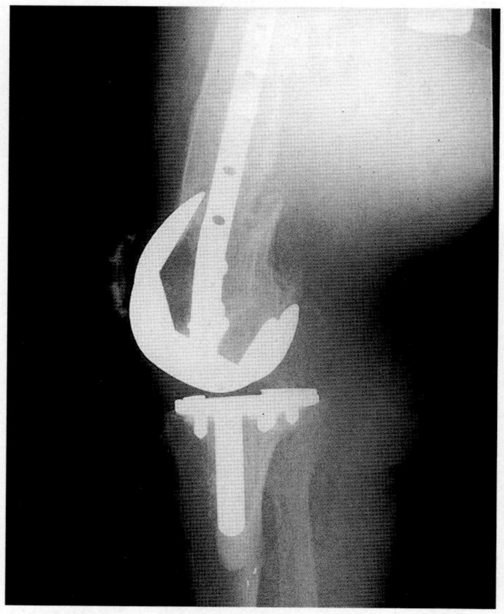

Figure 19.14. Supracondylar femur (SCF) fracture above total knee. If one elects for fixation, treatment options include DCS and side plate, or retrograde nail. Retrograde nail can be utilized only if the femoral prosthesis design allows room for nail insertion.

medullary canal prior to IM nailing has been clinically shown to aid in the healing process.[60,72,73] The technique of retrograde nailing is discussed elsewhere in this chapter (see Fig. 19.6).

The biomechanics of retrograde nailing also require clinician appreciation to avoid implant pitfalls. The authors recommend locking with proximal and distal interlocking screws to provide both rotational and axial stability to the construct. The proximal screws are technically more difficult, as targeting guides are ineffective due to nail deformation during insertion. Some systems allow for anterior to posterior proximal locking screw placement, which appears to be less demanding (using an image table). Screw placement in this region avoids the femoral artery, but branches of the femoral nerve remain at risk and warrant open blunt dissection and a cannulated tissue protector for maximum safety.[74] The authors have found it beneficial to utilize a screw clamp (similar to that used during acetabular arthroplasty) to prevent loss of the screw in the soft tissue. Single screw placement closer to an experimental osteotomy site significantly increases rotational stability.[75] David and coworkers[68] have found that if more than one screw is used, a grouped configuration with two proximal screw close to the fracture site may be more stable than a dispersed pattern (bending moments were not studied). More recently, it has been shown that multiple holes are best avoided in smaller diameter nails to prevent fatigue failure of the nail itself.[76]

Distal screws can be effectively placed utilizing the distal interlocking screw outrigger guide. Unfortunately, it is still possible to misplace the distal interlocking screws, and interoperative confirmation is essential (Fig. 19.15). The more proximal of the distal screws is frequently close to the fracture, and it is important to place the nail as distal as possible without violating the knee joint.

We have defined a stable nail construct as one that involves at least four solid cortices purchased by the screws in the distal portion of the nail. Fogler et al[77] demonstrated that a second distal interlocking screw significantly improves distal femur intramedullary fixation after antegrade nailing of distal-third fractures. The minimal distance from the notch of the femur to the fracture to allow for such a construct is probably about 7 cm. A stable construct usually allows for early knee motion without bracing. Occasionally, with more proximal fractures, early partial weight bearing is allowed.

Unstable nail constructs (two or three cortices) should always be braced and subjected to limited loads. Unstable constructs occur more frequently with the distal, comminuted, and/or osteoporotic fracture. We use this construct on occasion to avoid large wounds and periosteal stripping.

Dynamization without loss of rotational control is possible with some rod systems and is indicated in simple nonsegmental fracture patterns. Dynamization is contraindicated in the extensively comminuted fracture where axial dynamization results in limb shortening and possible rod backout.

Excessive comminution may also provide a challenge to fracture management (Fig. 19.16). Occasionally in

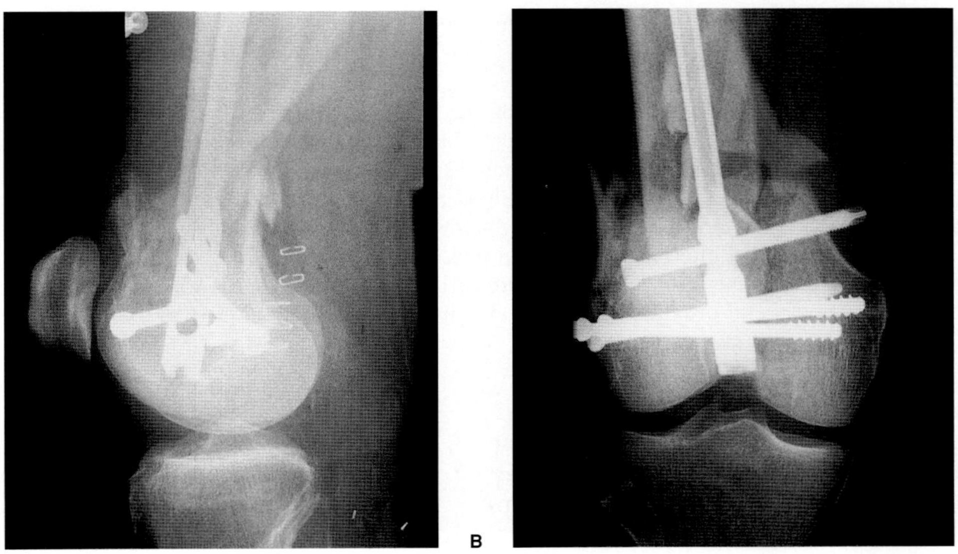

A B

Figure 19.15. Unstable nail construct. A: Lateral view shows that the distal of the two locking screws missed the nail posteriorly. B: AP view shows the more proximal screw gains purchase in only one cortex.

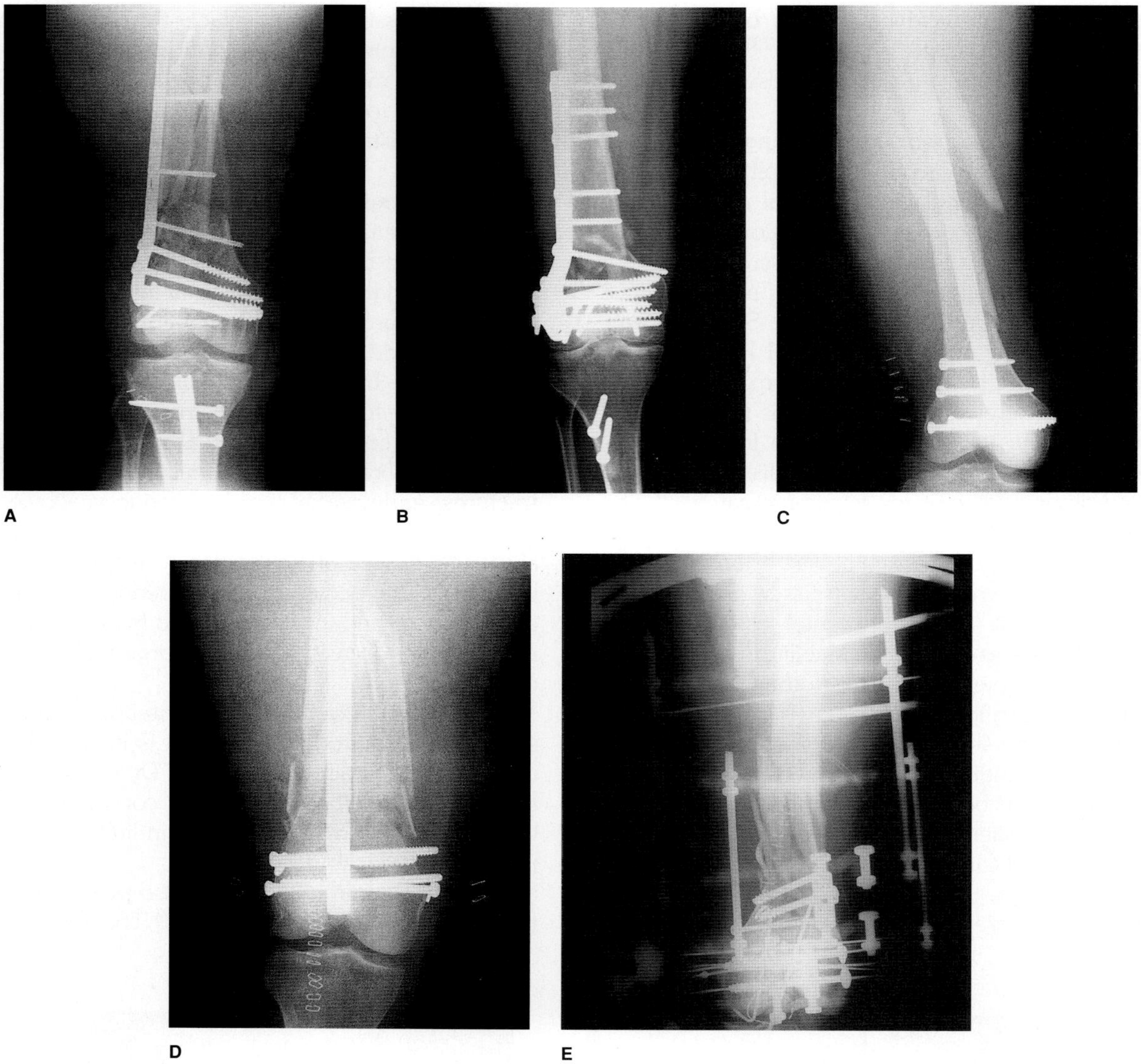

Figure 19.16. Fixation options with excessive comminution. **A:** Dynamic condylar screw and side plate for Arbeitgemeinschaft fur Osteosynthesefragen (AO) type C3 fracture. **B:** Cloverleaf plate with tibial tubercle osteotomy exposure for excessive intraarticular comminution. The standard cloverleaf plate should only be utilized when there is an appropriate medial buttress; otherwise, the fracture will collapse in varus. **C:** Antegrade nail and intracondylar lag screws chosen because of extensive diaphyseal extension. **D:** Retrograde nail and intracondylar lag screws performed with minimal dissection of the supracondylar region. Stable nail construct. **E:** Limited internal and external fixation. High-energy injury with severe comminution over the entire distal third of the femur. Ligamentous injury was severe as demonstrated by the wide lateral joint space. External fixation was also performed for the ipsilateral proximal tibia fracture. Hinges were placed between the two frames to close the lateral joint space.

very distal femur fractures one may have to avoid a plate or nail construct and opt for limited internal and external fixation that bridges the knee (Fig. 19.17). Each implant has its strengths and weaknesses.

Wound irrigation solutions have also been shown to affect fracture healing. Betadine solutions and hydrogen peroxide solutions have been shown to have a lethal effect on osteoblasts, while bacitracin solutions have been shown to be safe.[78] In severely comminuted open fractures, it may be prudent to avoid the use of toxic solutions in favor of copious volumes of normal saline. Pulse lavage is reserved for contaminated wounds.

Nonsteroidal antiinflammatory drugs (NSAIDs), which are prescribed routinely, may also contribute to non-

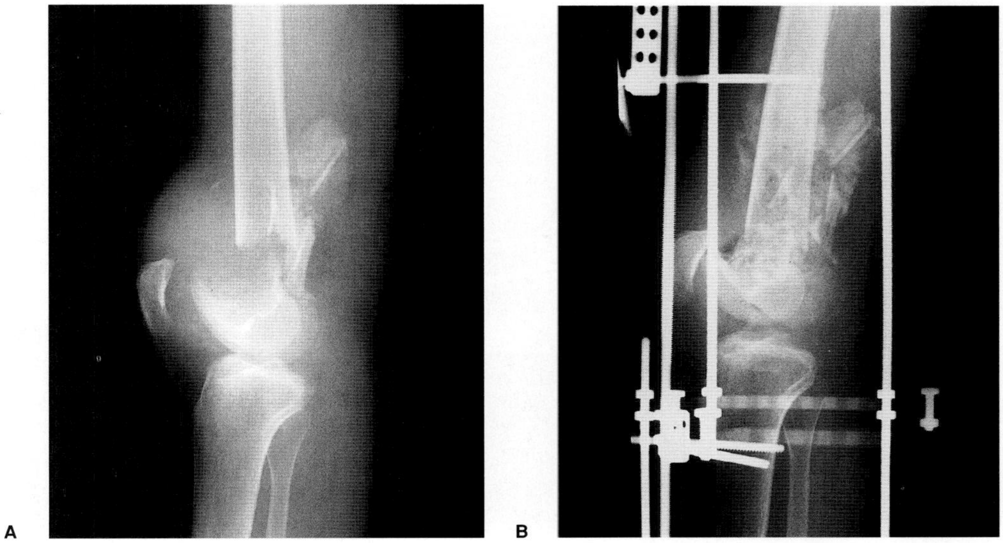

Figure 19.17. Very distal SCF fracture. **A:** To avoid loss of fixation, one should avoid a plate or nail construct. **B:** The prudent choice of multiplanar external fixation, supplemented with bone graft. Potential long-term knee stiffness may be dealt with later by utilizing a quadricepsplasty.

union. It has been demonstrated in rats that NSAIDs, specifically ibuprofen, have an inhibitory effect on fracture repair.[79] In addition, the use of tobacco products has been shown to inhibit fracture healing.[80]

Malunion

When the fracture is treated with skeletal traction, the setup requires attention to detail. Placement of the tibial pin should be in internal rotation 1 cm below the tibial tubercle. The leg is maintained in a Thomas splint with 20 to 30 degrees of flexion at the knee. A two pin technique can be employed to obtain and maintain adequate alignment at the fracture site. A second pin through the distal femur with force applied in a dorsal fashion prevents the rotation of the fragment secondary to the pull of the gastroc-soleus complex. For greater patient mobilization one can consider the traditional pins and plaster form of treatment. Sequential radiographs are vital as fracture alignment usually changes with time in nonoperatively managed cases.

When applying a DCS plate, the most crucial step is to appropriately place the guidewires under image. Wire no. 1 is inserted parallel to the knee joint axis; wire no. 2 is inserted parallel to the anterior patellofemoral articulation; wire no. 3 is the definitive guide wire for the condylar screw. Wire no. 3 should be placed at the junction of the anterior and middle thirds of the longest sagittal diameter of the lateral femoral condyle, 2 cm proximal to the joint line. This will ensure proper placement of lag screws and the condylar screw (see Fig. 19.8). Inappropriate placement for the definitive guidewire for the condylar screw will result in malunion. An inclining guidewire placement results in a valgus deformity, while a declining guidewire results in a varus deformity (Fig. 19.18). Preoperative views of the normal side can be reversed, and this mirror image used to guide reconstruction.

When utilizing an antegrade nail, it is important to control the distal fragment during guidewire placement and reaming, to avoid valgus deformity (Fig. 19.19). Manipulation of the distal fragment (with temporary Steinmann pins or by tibial manipulation) can assist alignment during placement of the nail.

Malunion may also occur with the use of a supracondylar nail. It is important to visualize the starting point for each nail on both anteroposterior and lateral images prior to insertion of the guidewire. The fracture reduction should also be optimal prior to nail insertion. Supracondylar fractures with intercondylar extension benefit from a lag screw across the condyles to prevent displacement during reaming and nail insertion (see Fig. 19.6). Alignment can be aided with longer and larger diameter nails that gain better purchase in the femur (Fig. 19.20). When treating a floating knee, it is often preferable to fix the tibia first so that the distal limb can be used as a lever arm to help reduce the distal femur fracture. A popular technique is to repair a floating knee through one incision, with a supracondylar nail placed in the femur and an intramedullary nail placed in the tibia.[81]

The lateral condylar buttress plate should be used se-

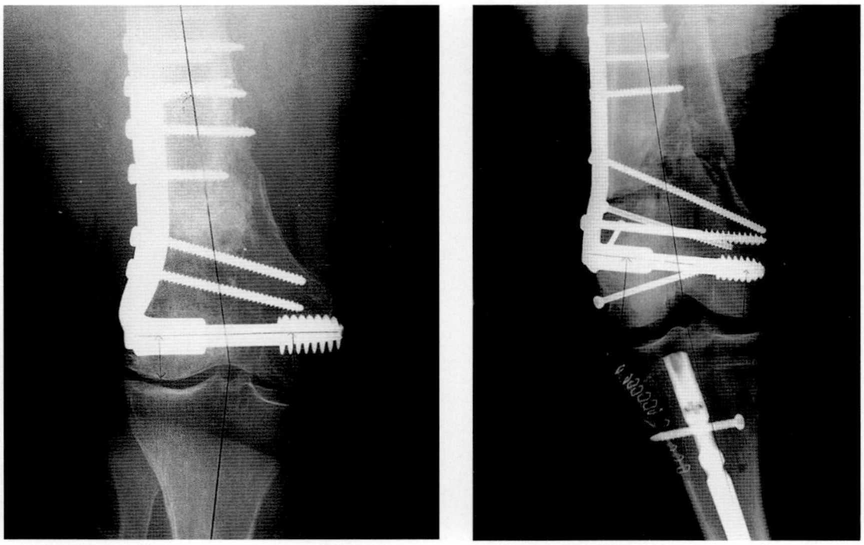

A B

Figure 19.18. Malalignment in utilization of the DCS and side plate. **A:** Inclining guidewire placement results in valgus orientation. **B:** Declining guidewire placement results in varus orientation.

lectively in the stable fracture, as it does not allow for locking between the screws and the plate. If a bony buttress does not exist medially, the fracture will invariably fall into varus when the plate is placed laterally. A dual-plating technique has been described for medial cortex comminution.[17] We recognize that the potential for extensive bone devascularization is extremely high with this technique.

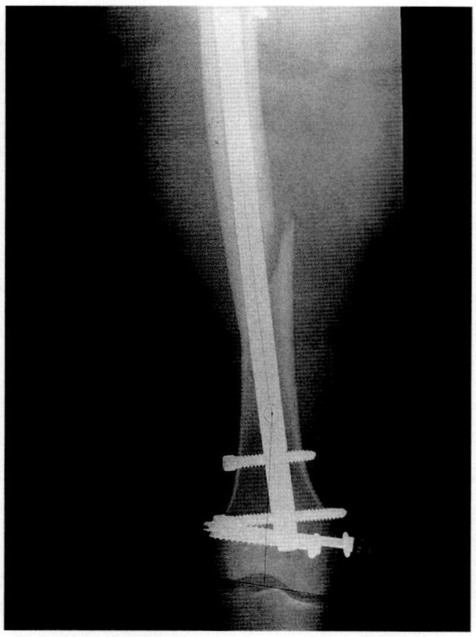

Figure 19.19. Malalignment in utilization of antegrade nail. Intercondylar component was fixed prior to insertion of antegrade nail. Failure to control the distal fragment allows this valgus deformity. Temporary Steinmann pin joysticks can aid in manipulation.

Rotational malalignment is common and is prevented by attention to anatomic landmarks. Torsional malalignment tends to be more common with closed intramedullary devices than with ORIF techniques. A bump under the hip can prevent a tendency for external rotation of the proximal fragment. Mismatch of width at a simple fracture is often a clue. Frequent image comparisons of the rotation of the hip and knee, radiographic evaluation of the fracture reduction, and clinical assessment of the limb alignment can all be helpful.

Preventing articular malunion is accomplished by obtaining and maintaining an anatomic reduction. Appropriate intraoperative visualization directly with serial x-rays or fluoroscopy is helpful. A three-dimensional (3D) understanding of the anatomy of the fracture pattern is paramount for effective reduction of the articular surface (Fig. 19.21). Preoperative CT scan, with or with out frontal/sagittal plane, or 3D reconstructions can be helpful. The sequela of intraarticular malunion is early posttraumatic arthritis.

Stiffness

Prevention of knee stiffness begins with early range-of-motion exercises following the injury. A more stable construct, anatomic reduction, and less surgical insult will also decrease the rate of arthrofibrosis. Generally, tenuous fixation is to be avoided if at all possible. Unstable plate fixation of a SCF fracture with extensive extension, comminution, or osteoporosis may incur all the risks of surgery without any of the benefits. If postoperative casting is required for more than 3 to 4 weeks, loss of flexion often ensues. In circumstances where plate fixation is going to yield an unstable construct, it

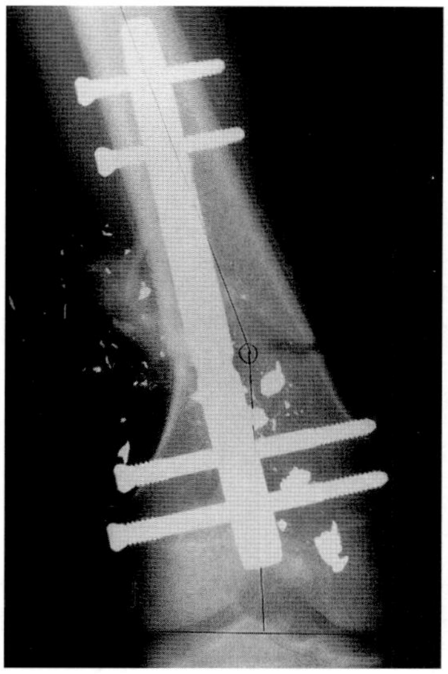

A

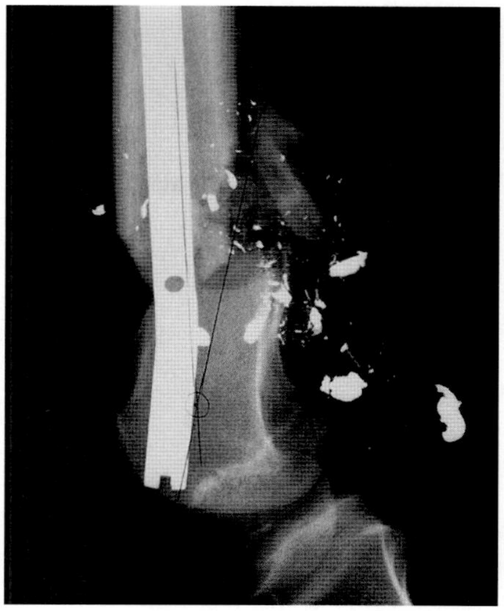

B

Figure 19.20. Malalignment in utilization of retrograde nail. **A:** Entry allowing for excessive valgus. Nail is too short and allows further collapse into valgus. **B:** Lateral view shows that the nail was placed “backward” (rotated 180 degrees), resulting in a combined deformity of angulation (apex posterior) and translation.

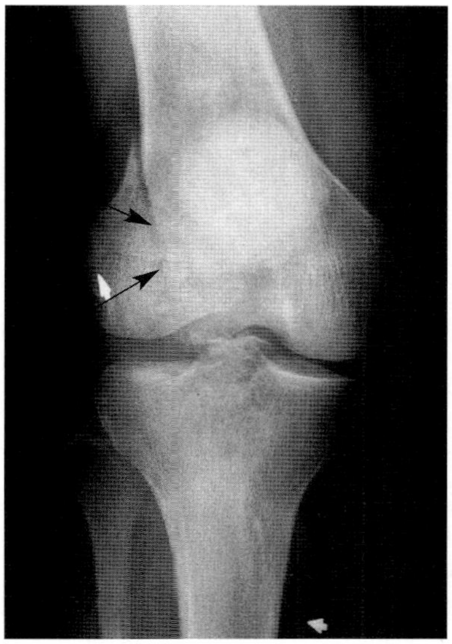

A

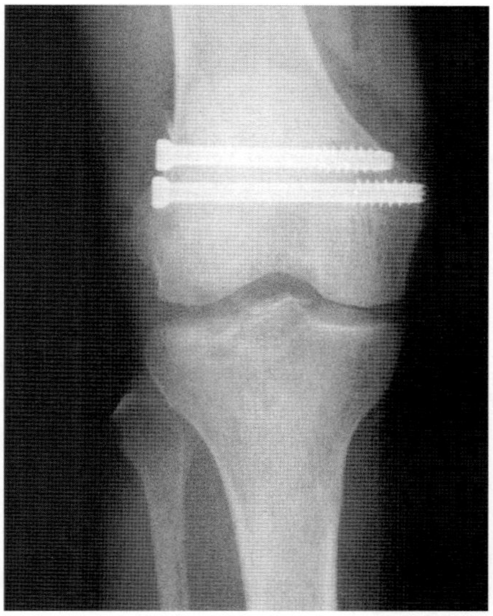

B

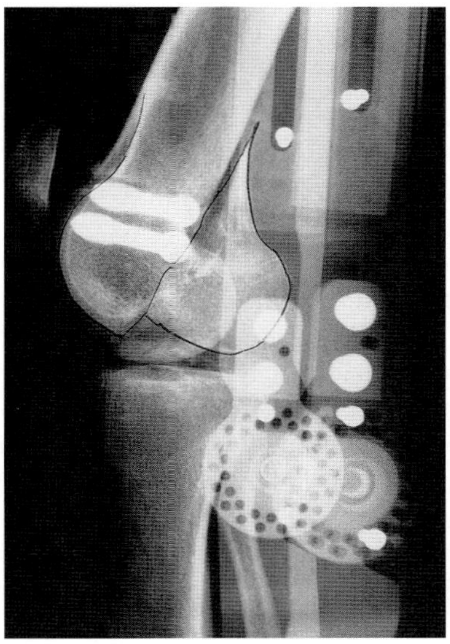

C

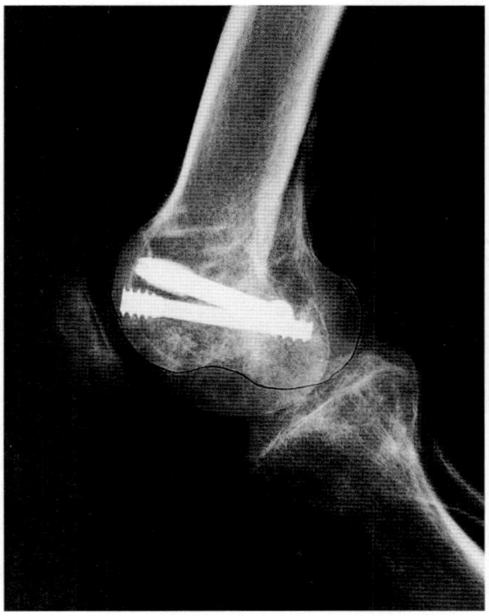

D

Figure 19.21. Intraarticular malunion. **A:** Condylar fracture caused by low-velocity missile (arrows mark entrance and exit wounds). **B:** AP view shows apparent anatomic reduction. **C:** Surgeon fails to realize the three-dimensional nature of the fracture. **D:** Despite revision surgery, intraarticular malunion results with accompanying arthrosis.

may be preferable to avoid extensive dissection with percutaneous nailing, external fixation, or traction.

With intramedullary nails, prominent distal locking screws should be avoided. In cases with severe osteopenia, slight prominence of the locking screw may be preferable for better screw purchase. It is essential that the distal end of the retrograde nail does not extend beyond the articular surface of the distal femur (Fig. 19.22). Screw removal after bone healing may still promote an increase in knee motion.

External fixation, as definitive treatment, is avoided if possible. Pins or wires placed in the vastus lateralis impede muscle excursion and predispose to joint stiffness. If a unilateral external fixator is used, the pins should be placed posterolaterally in the diaphysis between muscle groups. If wires are placed in the distal femur, the epicondylar area is the preferred site for fixation, as the combined flexion-extension excursion of the surrounding soft tissues seems least in this area. Bridging knee external fixation should be limited to circumstances in which there is no other reasonable option for stabilization. Hinge placement at the instantaneous center of rotation, to allow for controlled motion, is extremely difficult. When a static, bridging, multiplane fixator is utilized, one can occasionally remove the tibial portion before the femoral portion to try to encourage knee motion.

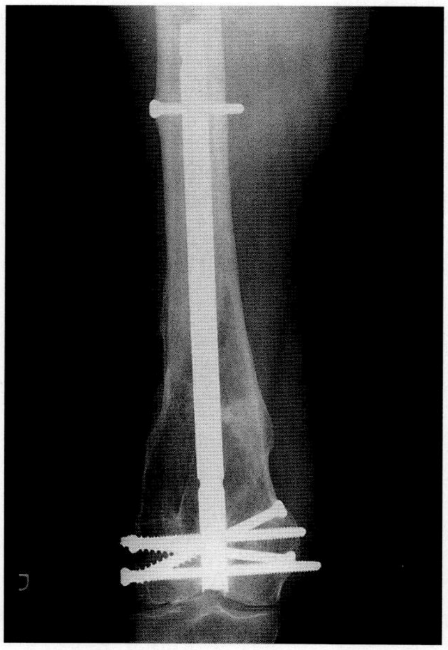

Figure 19.22. Prominent hardware in retrograde nailing. Failure to impact the nail proximal enough resulted in an intraarticular rod. The prominent nail end was burred with a Midas-Rex to avoid attempts at refixation. Prominent medial screw caused pain with knee motion.

Osteoarthritis

Within the limits of the fracture pattern, surgery should achieve the best anatomic reduction possible. This requires judicious use of image and exacting technique. The joint surface congruity and overall limb alignment both need to be addressed, as less than perfect reduction of either results in increased focal cartilage pressures leading to arthritic change (Fig. 19.21). The prevention of septic arthritis has been previously discussed.

Vascular Compromise

Absent pulses in a traumatized extremity is due to arterial injury until proven otherwise, usually by arteriography.[82] In managing vascular compromise secondary to a SCF fracture, the time frame of the sequence of events is extremely important. Irreversible changes in muscle viability occur if the ischemic time becomes greater than 6 hours.[46] Often simple reduction of the fracture can reconstitute arterial flow. A vascular surgery consult is indicated immediately upon the suspicion of a vascular injury. Arteriography can be done intraoperatively if necessary. The absence of pulses distally may be mistaken for an impending compartment syndrome,[83] and performing a fasciotomy for unrecognized arterial injury will have little therapeutic effect.

The ischemic time directs the sequence of events after documentation of a vascular injury. Ideally, bony stabilization prior to vascular surgery is preferable. Plating may be time-consuming, and the surgical exposure for fixation is different from that for vascular reconstruction. If time is limited, an external fixator may be adequate for provisional fixation. An appropriately trained surgeon can expediently apply a retrograde nail. The authors have found this method of stabilization particularly advantageous. Once the fracture is stabilized, arterial and venous repair may be undertaken.

If ischemic time is approaching 6 hours, the sequence of surgical events may need to be reversed to prevent loss of limb (Fig. 19.23). A temporary shunt can be placed prior to orthopedic fixation.[84] A vein graft can be harvested during orthopedic fixation from the contralateral limb, and definitive vascular reconstruction then follows. Intraoperative four-compartment fasciotomies (a medial and lateral incision) of the leg are important to prevent compartment syndrome (CS), which can occur during reperfusion of the limb following vascular reconstitution.

Compartment syndrome must be differentiated from a true vascular injury. CS usually occurs when there is a palpable pulse and no major arterial compromise, although bleeding from an arterial injury can be an occasional cause. Compartment syndrome occurs when the postcapillary venule pressure exceeds capillary per-

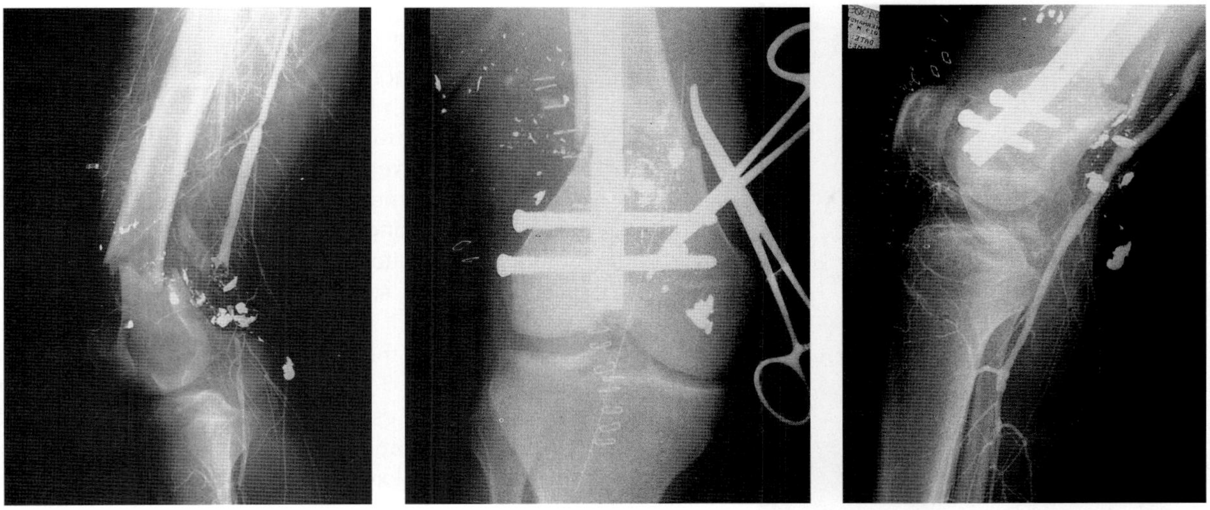

A B C

Figure 19.23. Prevention of excessive ischemic time. **A:** Low velocity missile causes SCF fracture with associated popliteal artery injury. **B:** Temporary arterial shunt placed prior to bony stabilization due to excessive ischemic time. Vein graft was harvested during orthopedic fixation. **C:** Successful reconstitution of flow after saphenous vein graft. In general, one strives for bone stabilization prior to vascular surgery, but in unusual cases, the order must be reversed.

fusion pressure. The diagnosis begins with clinical assessment of the compartment tenseness and the level of pain perceived by the patient, especially pain with passive muscle stretch. A clinical diagnosis should be reinforced by measuring intracompartmental pressures. In the case of a borderline diagnosis, or impending CS, it is safer to perform the fasciotomies. Once a CS becomes established, permanent limb compromise or amputation is often the result.[54]

TREATMENT OF COMPLICATIONS

Infection and Soft Tissue Complications

Delayed wound healing must be differentiated from infection and managed simply with local wound care and immobilization until healing is complete. Occasionally patients realize a better response to surgical debridement and wound healing by secondary intention or delayed primary closure. Split-thickness grafting or muscle flaps (pedicle or free) may also be necessary.

The management of infection depends on its nature and severity. Cellulitis postoperatively or following an open injury can be treated effectively with parenteral antibiotics. A superficial wound infection or stitch abscess warrants intravenous antibiotics, local wound care, and immobilization. Irrigation and debridement is required only if the wound fails to improve within 72 hours.

When a deep wound infection is suspected, needle aspiration through an uninvolved area can assist in determining the diagnosis. Proper treatment of deep infections depends on several variables: the stage of fracture healing, the stability of the fixation, and the degree of bony involvement. All should be treated with culture-specific antibiotics and formal irrigation and debridement. In wound infections prior to fracture healing with stable fixation and viable bone, the hardware may initially be retained and managed with irrigation and debridement in combination with either closure over drains, delayed primary closure, or healing by secondary intention. Antibiotic-impregnated methylmethacrylate beads can be placed in the wound on a temporary basis. Even so, the hardware may have to be removed to eradicate the deep infection, and external fixation may be necessary (Fig. 19.24). Serial debridements increase the likelihood that all necrotic and infected bone is removed. Large soft tissue defects require local or free muscle flaps, while smaller wounds can heal by secondary intention. One can begin to reconstitute the bony defect once the infection is controlled.

Infections that occur after fracture union are infinitely easier to manage. They can routinely be treated with hardware removal during debridement. Antibiotic beads can be applied temporarily (3 weeks) to deliver local antibiotics in combination with 6 weeks of intravenous antibiotics.

Chronic osteomyelitis or recurrence is always a risk following deep infection, and can resurface years after the initial insult. Definitive treatment begins with identification of the sequestrum as the source of the chronic

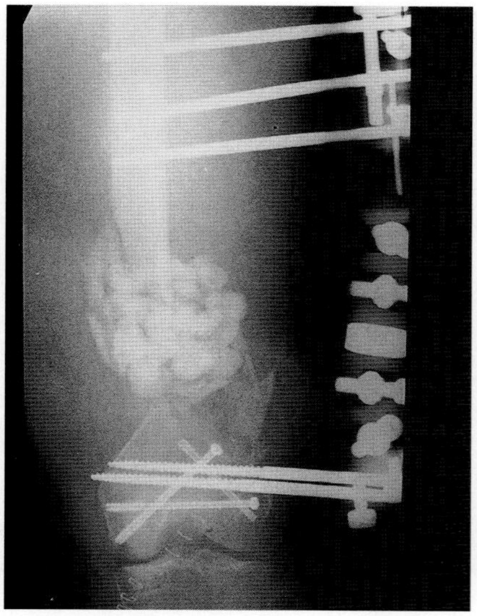

Figure 19.24. Treatment of infected supracondylar fracture with irrigation and debridement, external stabilization, and antibiotic methylmethacrylate beads.

osteomyelitis (Fig. 19.25), and then removal of all devitalized bone. Cure may be difficult, and the patient may have to choose between suppression with repeated recurrence, or sometimes radical surgery.

Arthrodesis is indicated for most cases of significant postinfectious arthritis of the knee. Multiplane external fixation is the fixation of choice. With more severe bone loss, bony defects may need to be reconstituted. Autogenous iliac crest bone graft is preferable for the smaller defects. Unfortunately, the graft may serve as a nidus if the infection is not completely eradicated. Vascularized fibular bone grafts are an option, but they are relatively small in diameter and are associated with donor-site morbidity.[85–87] The Ilizarov technique of distraction osteogenesis is especially effective for defects in these difficult circumstances (Fig. 19.26). The authors do not advocate the use of segmental allografts[88] or custom femoral replacements with persistent infection.[89]

Supracondylar femur fractures in the elderly with severe preexisting osteoarthritis can be managed effectively with total knee replacement arthroplasty, although the infection rate in these procedures is slightly higher than that for traditional fixation.[89] When infection does occur, a favorable response may occasionally be obtained with serial attempts at suppression in this population (Fig. 19.27). Prosthesis removal provides a more thorough debridement, but results in a large defect, difficult to manage in these older patients. Ancient septic arthritis can be successfully managed with total knee arthroplasty, with an acceptable infection rate, as long as the infection is truly ancient.[90]

Nonunion and Loss of Fixation

Distal femoral nonunions, although rare, are difficult to treat.[91] Once a nonunion is established, the success of subsequent operations decreases proportionately with the number of repeat operations.[92] The surgeon must approach treatment with the utmost caution and preoperative planning. To effectively treat a nonunion, the surgeon must attain apposition of fragments, adequate immobilization, soft tissue healing, and stimulation of osteogenesis.[93]

Noninvasive treatment of nonunions includes electrical stimulation[23,94] and casting. Once a pseudoarthrosis has become established, the authors have not found electrical stimulation to be effective clinically or experimentally.[95] Prolonged casting of a nonoperated delayed union can occasionally succeed by enhancing fracture stability. Casting may also complement if there is loss of fixation or implant failure in the poor candidate for revision surgery (Fig. 19.28). Rarely, however, can cast immobilization alone alter the fate of an established nonunion. Significant loss of knee motion is always a consequence of cast treatment for these problems.

Operative treatment of the nonunion is varied and depends on the "personality" of the nonunion. Intraarticular nonunions may be difficult as the fragments rarely tend to fit together perfectly in delayed presentation. Knee motion may have caused wear of the subchondral bone. A purely arthroscopic approach may be difficult (Fig. 19.29). Subsequent collapse secondary to avascularity may result.

Treatment of nonunions that have not had prior intervention may be simpler than those having undergone previous surgical manipulation. Bone stock typically is better, and risk of previous infection is usually less. The optimal method of osteosynthesis depends on the nonunion location and whether it is hypertrophic or atrophic. Hypertrophic nonunions of the distal shaft are best addressed with closed reamed antegrade femoral nailing if alignment allows.[96] Atrophic nonunions often require takedown. When it is opened for removal of fibrous tissue, or to aid realignment, we often prefer plate fixation to avoid disruption of both the endosteal and the periosteal blood supply. The dynamic condylar screw/plate or blade plate is suited for the more distal nonunion. Compression can be applied when the fracture pattern is amenable. One can utilize the articulating tension device in addition to the properties of the plate itself. Lag screws are considered for oblique fracture lines. Nonunions that are directly exposed are usually augmented with bone graft. The authors prefer autogenous bone graft, harvested from the posterior crest with the patient in a semilateral position. We avoid irrigation of the graft and try to apply it to the nonunion without a long intraoperative delay. Research in bone

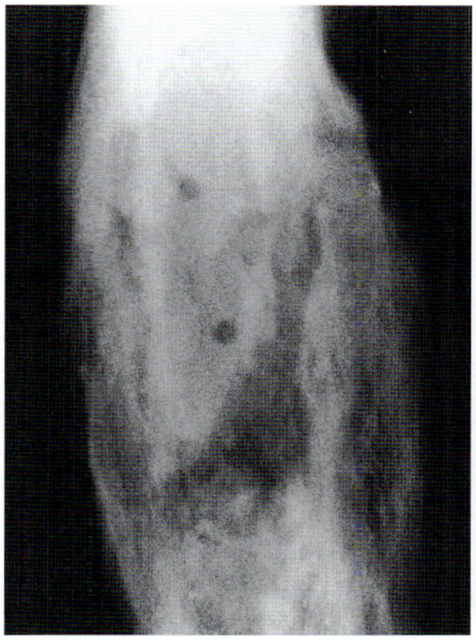

A

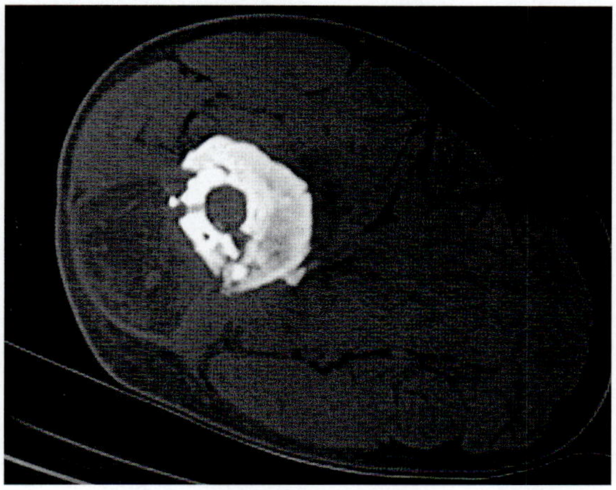

B

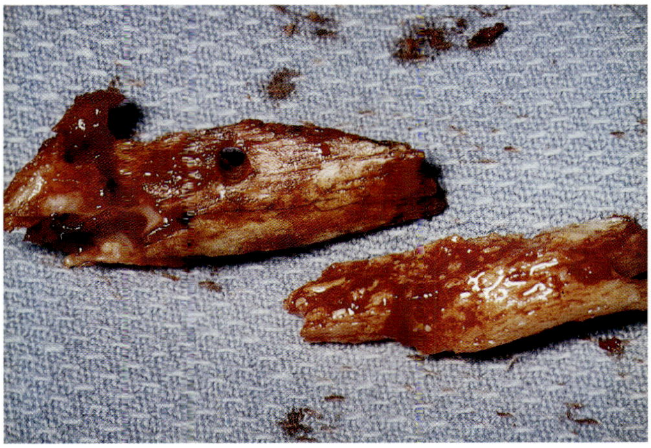

C

Figure 19.25. Sequestrum as a source of chronic osteomyelitis. **A:** Treatment of chronic osteomyelitis begins with identification of any source of devitalized bone. Infection surfaced 15 years after the patient's initial fracture and 10 years after plate removal. Unremodeled appearance of old bone fragment with original screw holes still visible. **B:** Computed tomography scan shows "bone within a bone" appearance at the level of the sequestrum and adjacent soft tissue change. **C:** Clinical appearance of the sequestrum, which grew out enterococcus.

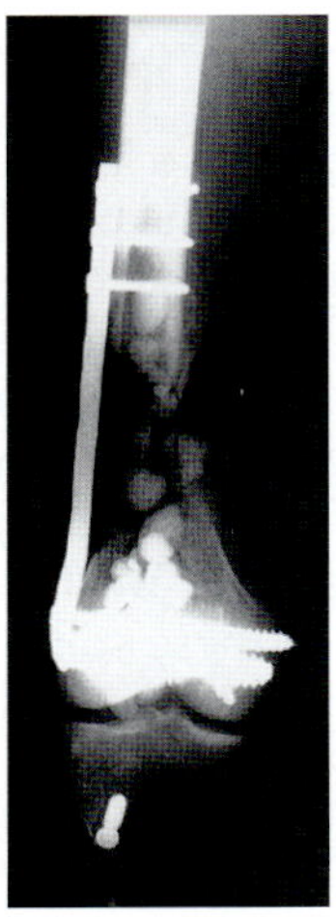

A

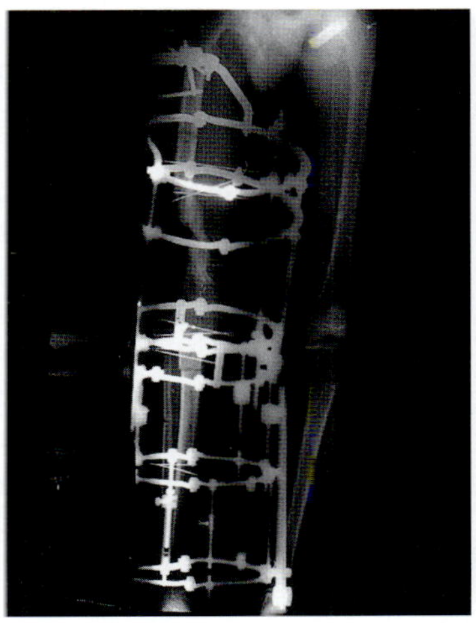

B

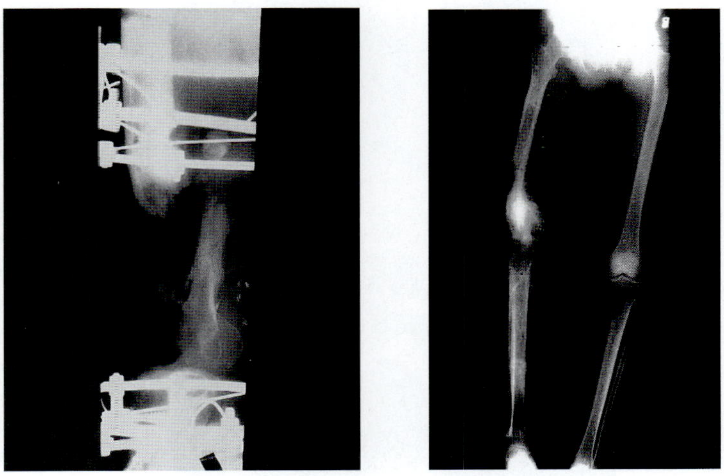

C

Figure 19.26. Distraction osteogenesis to salvage infected fracture. **A:** Severely infected supracondylar femur fracture. **B:** AP and lateral views at the onset of bifocal distraction osteogenesis. **C:** Successful knee fusion and bone regenerate. Residual leg length discrepancy managed with shoe lift. (Case courtesy of Dr. Dror Paley.)

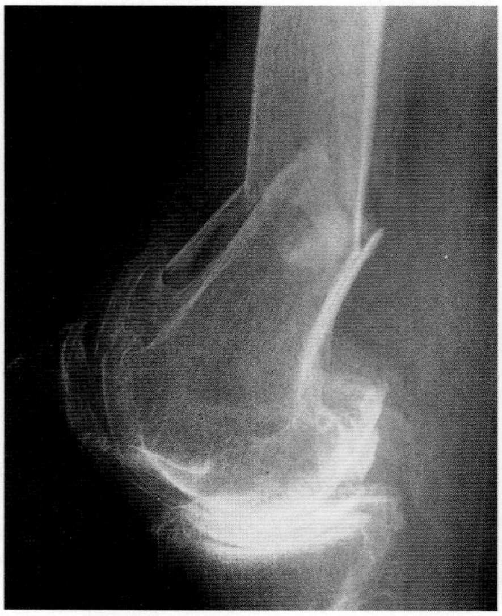

A

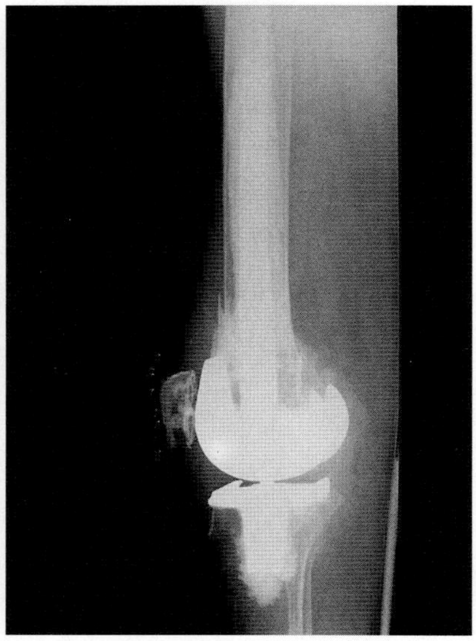

B

Figure 19.27. Infection after management of supracondylar fracture with prosthetic replacement. A: SCF fracture above arthritic knee. B: Trying to "kill two birds with one stone." Long-stem total knee arthroplasty is an excellent option in trying to provide immediate ambulation. Postoperative infection can be difficult to manage as eradication may necessitate removal of prosthesis and cemented condylar region.

graft substitutes, including bone morphogenic protein, continues.

Treatment of nonunions after previous operative intervention can be more challenging. When previous DCS/plating has been undertaken, one of three situations usually exists: (1) the lag screw has cut out distally, (2) the plate has broken, or (3) the plate has pulled off the bone proximally.

Lag screw cutout can be one of the most difficult situations to revise (Fig. 19.28). As mentioned previously, casting or bracing may be an option. Revision of the lag screw can be undertaken with the use of a larger lag screw or with a lag screw supplemented by cement fixation. In the elderly, one can consider revision to a custom distal femoral replacement prosthesis (Fig. 19.30).[89] We have not found intramedullary constructs helpful in these circumstances.

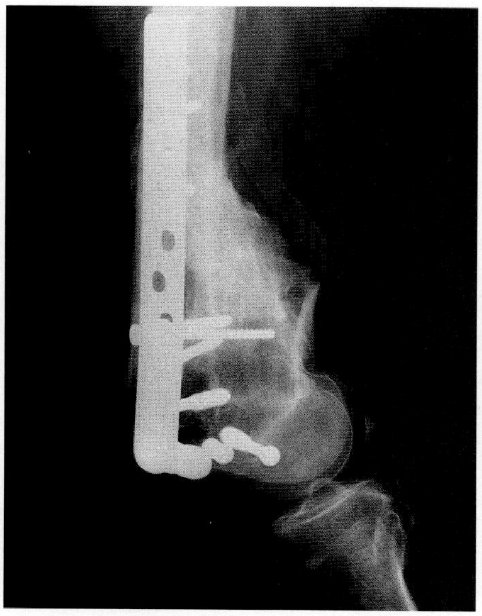

Figure 19.28. Casting a failed construct. Cast immobilization was the treatment option after hardware cutout in this elderly patient with excessive medical risks.

Plate breakage usually means that the weak link is usually the plate and not the bone quality. The usual solution is often compression of the fracture gap with repeat fixation. A second plate, at 90 degrees or medial to the previous plate, can be utilized. Segmental defects can be treated with a variety of methods discussed later.

Plate pull-off proximally can be due to the surgeon's error with insufficient proximal fixation (see Fig. 19.12). Revision surgery consists of repeat fixation with a longer plate. Cerclage wires (see Fig. 19.13) can be helpful if the nonunion is adjacent to a femoral arthroplasty component. Bone grafting and dual plating may be considered. Small gaps should be compressed. In select elderly patients with periprosthetic fractures, aggressive fixation may be considered if the potential for fracture healing is remote. Dual plating, tensioned cables, and methylmethacrylate may yield a rigid construct in these somewhat pathologic situations. Healing around the construct is occasionally observed (Fig. 19.31).

Distal femoral nonunions can occur after intramedullary nailing. Construct failure usually involves (1) breakage of the antegrade nail near one of its screw holes, (2) breakage of the retrograde nail at the level of the fracture, or (3) backout, breakage, or cutout of the locking screws in the distal femur.

Hypertrophic distal shaft nonunions can be managed

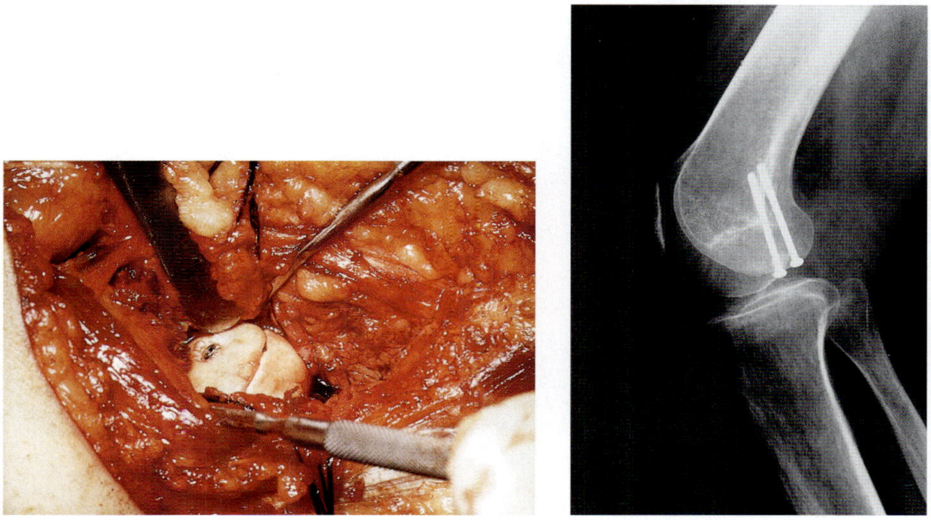

A B

Figure 19.29. Treatment of intraarticular nonunion shown in Figure 19.2. **A:** Fixation of posterior condyle nonunion with posterior approach to the knee. Posterior iliac crest bone was utilized to fill a small defect between incongruent bony surfaces. **B:** Lateral view shows union of posterior femoral condyle. Hardware was removed at later date. Knee instability was cured and the patient return to full motion and activity.

with reamed exchanged nailing. An intramedullary device that contains a dynamization slot is advantageous for revision. We often extract the broken nail fragment with a nail removal hook specially designed for this purpose, avoiding an open exposure. Bone grafting is reserved for the atrophic distal shaft nonunions, in fractures with significant bone loss, or when rod removal necessitates an open exposure of the nonunion. Screw breakage alone may cause nail dynamization and occasionally allow union. When rotational instability is present, however, eventual union is unlikely, and reamed exchange nailing is indicated.

Intramedullary nailing is less reliable for more distal or atrophic nonunions. In a study by Koval et al,[97] only four (25%) of 16 distal femoral nonunions united at an average 17 months following retrograde nailing with a statically locked nail. Therefore, the authors do not advocate retrograde nailing for atrophic or surgically treated nonunions of the distal femur, but prefer the dynamic condylar screw/plate with autogenous bone grafting (Fig. 19.32).

External fixation is also an option for distal femoral nonunions, but because of poor patient acceptance its application may be limited to patients with previous severe open fractures, free flaps, burns, extensive scarring, or unusually poor bone stock. Additionally, knee range-of-motion can be limited by the fixator's pins or wires. While external fixation is the treatment of choice for a few surgeons, the authors recommend these devices only in certain salvage situations.

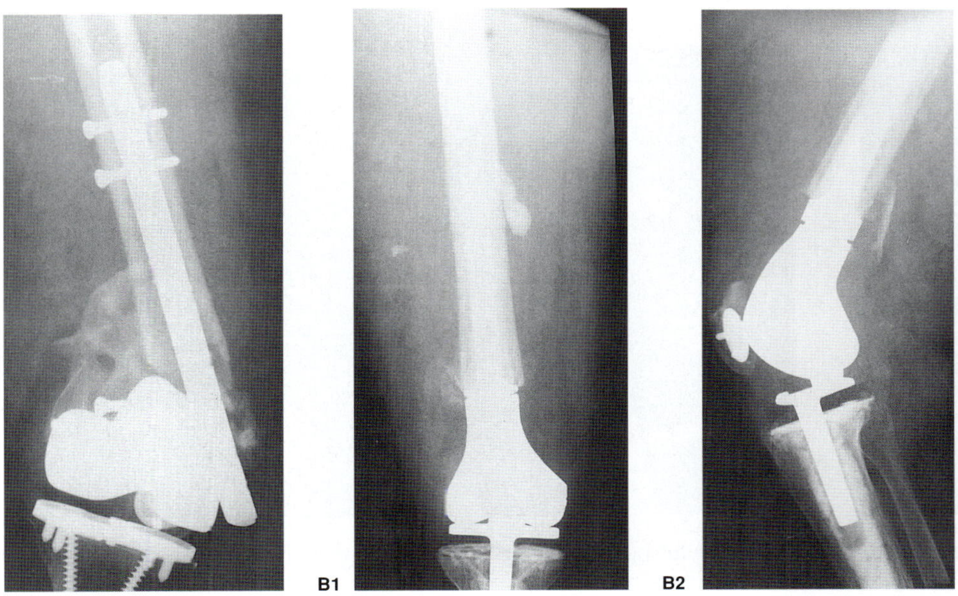

A B1 B2

Figure 19.30. Distal femoral replacement as a salvage for distal femoral nonunion in the elderly. **A:** Nonunion and flexion deformity. **B1** and **B2:** Rotating hinge distal femoral replacement as appropriate salvage. (Ref. 110)

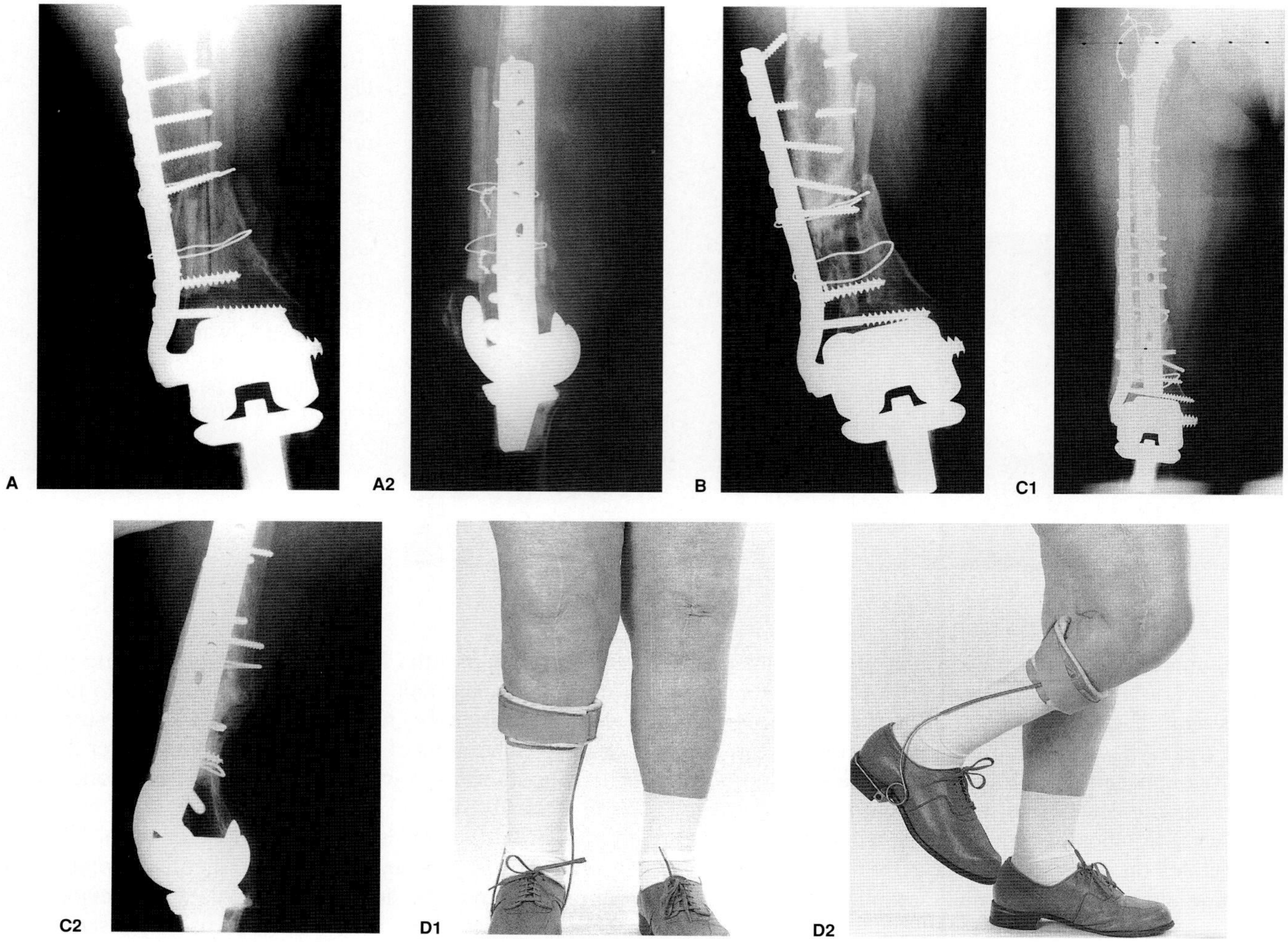

Figure 19.31. Treatment of supracondylar nonunion after proximal failure of DCS and side plate. **A:** AP and lateral views of supracondylar femur fracture above total knee and below total hip arthroplasty. Dynamic screw and plate fixation with use of medial fibular allograft. The patient suffered a tibial and peroneal nerve injury during surgery. **B:** Failure of construct with lack of incorporation of allograft. The patient suffered pain until this construct failed 1.5 years later. **C:** AP and lateral views of aggressive reconstruction with use of dual plates and multiple cerclage wires. Methylmethacrylate was used to help reinforce fixation. Healing is apparent despite massive reconstruction. **D:** Satisfactory functional result with lack of pain. The patient states that this is the first time the knee has not hurt in 2 years.

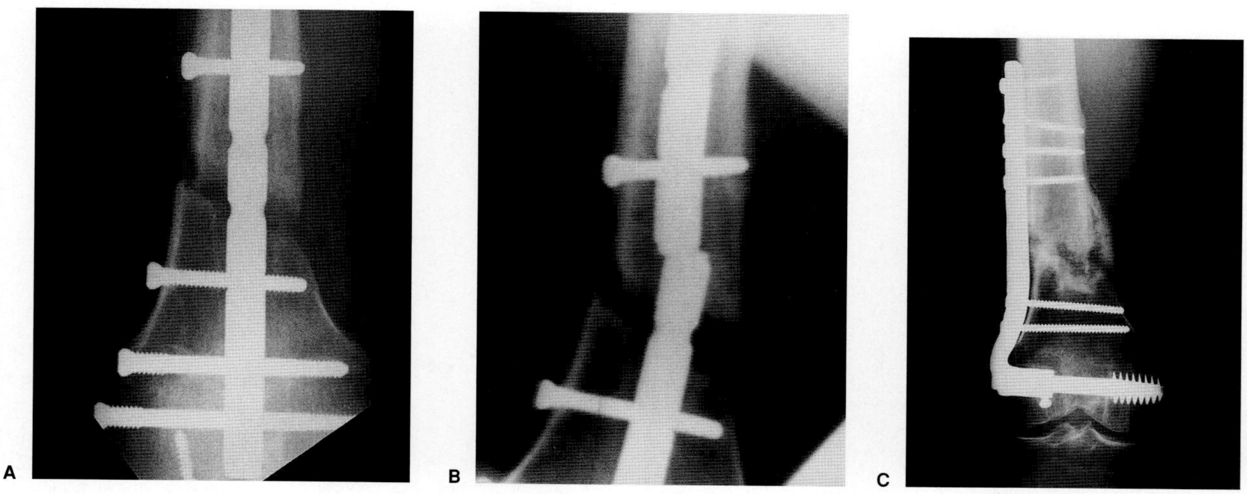

Figure 19.32. Treatment of supracondylar nonunion after retrograde nailing. **A:** Eight months after initial fixation, patient refused surgery to treat moderately painful nonunion. **B:** Increased pain is noted with nail breakage through screw hole at level of nonunion. **C:** Treatment with DCS and side plate utilizing articulating tension device and autogenous bone graft.

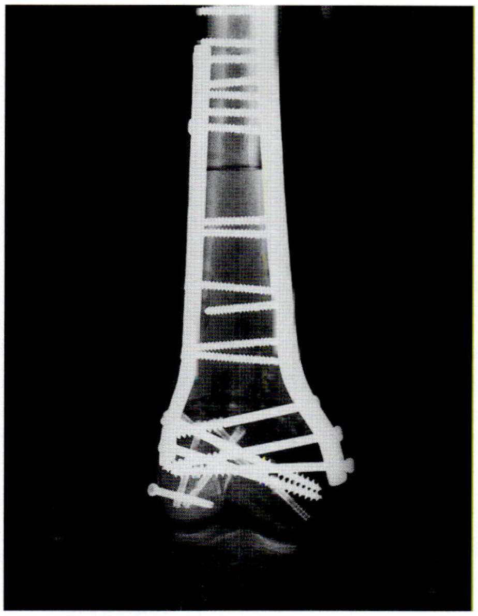

Figure 19.33. Treatment of supracondylar defect with segmental allograft and dual plates. Bone healing to an allograft may occur, but substantial replacement of a structural allograft is rarely observed. Autogenous bone grafting was planned for the junction sites. The patient was lost to long-term follow-up.

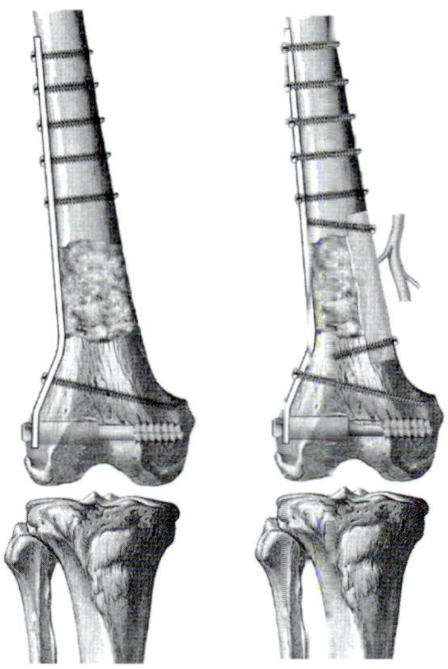

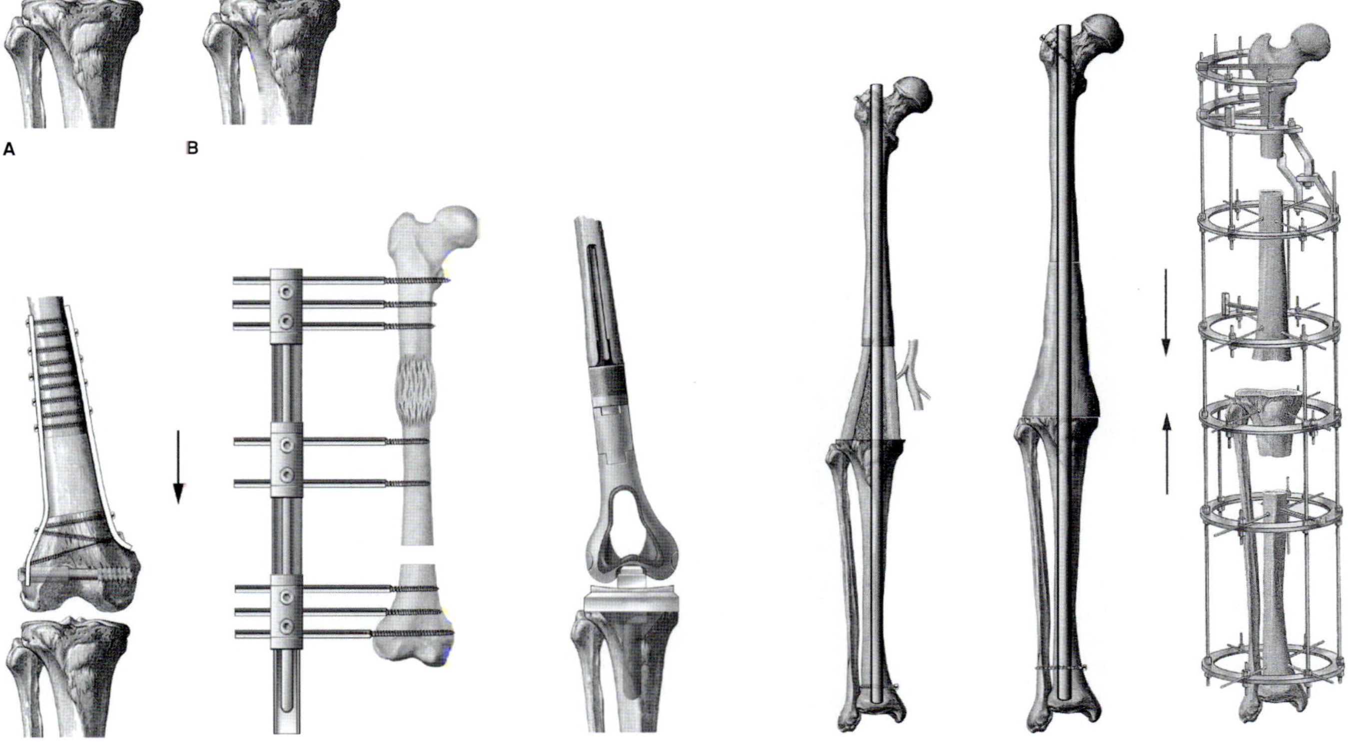

Figure 19.34. Treatment of segmental bony defects. **A:** Iliac crest bone grafting (ICBG). **B:** Vascularized fibula and ICBG. **C:** Allograft and ICGB. **D:** Distraction osteogenesis (uniplanar external fixation). **E:** Distal femoral prosthetic replacement. **F:** Vascularized fibula knee fusion. **G:** Allograft knee fusion. **H:** Distraction osteogenesis knee fusion (Ilizarov multiplane external fixator).

A particularly challenging problem is the SCF nonunion with a prominent segmental defect. Small defects can be shortened and bone grafted. A larger bone defect may require a vascularized fibular graft[84,85] in combination with iliac crest bone grafting. Segmental allograft will provide excellent early structural support, but has a poor probability of healing (Fig. 19.33). Distraction osteogenesis, although a major advance, can be cumbersome and poorly tolerated. Prosthetic distal femoral replacement is occasionally considered in the elderly patient. Significant deficiency of articular cartilage usually leads to arthrodesis or a knee arthroplasty. In the select patient, en-bloc osteochondral allografting may be indicated. The treatment options and their indications can be complex and are outlined in Fig. 19.34.

Refracture following plate or hardware removal is treated according to the principles previously cited. Bostman[98] has reported a 10% mean refracture rate at an average 26 months following plate removal. The previous use of supplemental interfragmentary screws significantly increased the risk of refracture in that series. Routine plate or rod removal is not advised.

Malunion

Intraarticular malunion usually progresses to posttraumatic arthritis (see Fig. 19.21).[50] Realignment intraarticular osteotomy is rarely indicated and reserved the younger patient. Total knee arthroplasty (TKA) can be quite useful in the elderly, especially following the development of posttraumatic arthritis.

Extraarticular malunion has decreased with the advent of modern surgical and fluoroscopic techniques. It is more common in the SCF fracture treated closed (Fig. 19.35). SCF malunion in the elderly rarely causes enough functional disability to warrant the risks of surgery.

When surgery is elected, preoperative planning is critical in the management of this complication. Deformities occur in varying degrees of angulation, translation, and rotation. Realignment osteotomies, to treat deformities either acutely or via distraction osteogenesis, are based about the CORA for most traditional methods. When there is more than one CORA, they should all be addressed or resolved. Newer, gradual, computer-assisted methods of deformity correction are beyond the scope of this chapter.

Traditionally, a closing wedge osteotomy has been the most common method of correction (Fig. 19.36). It is best applied at the closing wedge CORA to allow realignment of the mechanical axis of the limb. These corrections are usually best fixed with a plate if it can be applied on the tension side of the deformity. The articulated tensioning device or the femoral distractor can be helpful. The wedge removed is a good source of bone graft. Slight shortening is accepted.

An opening wedge osteotomy can restore length in addition to restoring normal limb alignment. It can be achieved gradually with external fixation and distraction, or acutely with bone grafting and internal fixation. These osteotomies are based on the opening wedge CORA. Bone healing with an opening wedge osteotomy is less reliable and usually limited to the pediatric population.

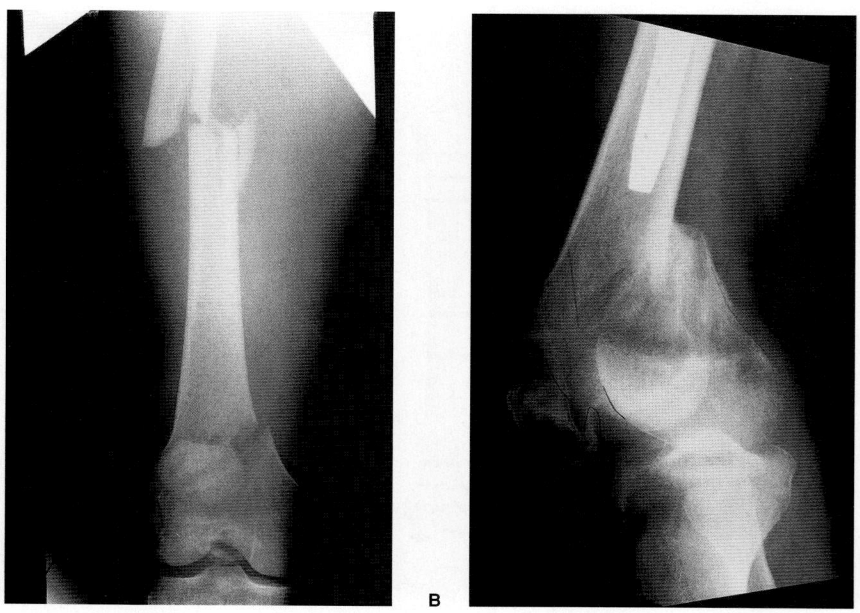

A B

Figure 19.35. Distal femoral malunion in closed treatment of supracondylar fracture. **A:** Segmental femur fracture. **B:** Diaphyseal fracture was treated with antegrade nail. Surgeon elected to do cast brace treatment of distal femoral component; malunion resulted.

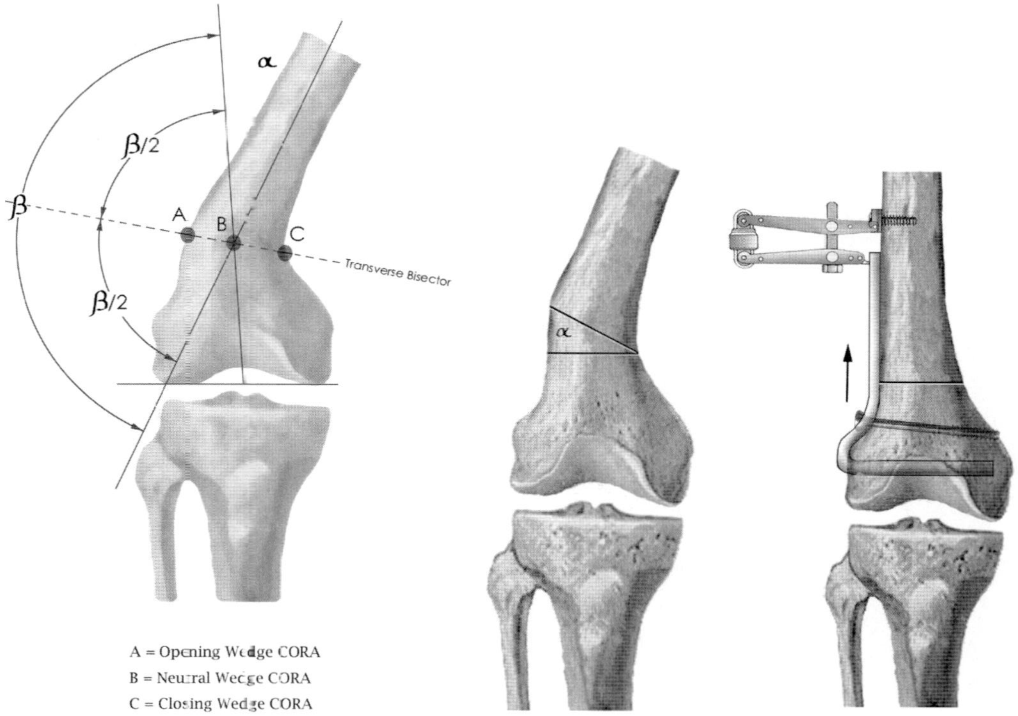

A B C

Figure 19.36. Closing wedge osteotomy. (CORA, center of rotation and angulation.)

Recently a focal dome osteotomy was described utilizing fixator-assisted nailing.[99] This technique can be performed percutaneously, but care must be taken to avoid translation during fixation (Fig. 19.37). While technically demanding, potential advantages include early union due to limited dissection.

Oblique plane osteotomy is another commonly used technique to correct SCF malunion.[100] Its advantages include excellent stability, potentially broad bone surfaces to promote union, and the potential to restore a limited amount of length (Fig. 19.38). Its disadvantages include the considerable surgical exposure and meticu-

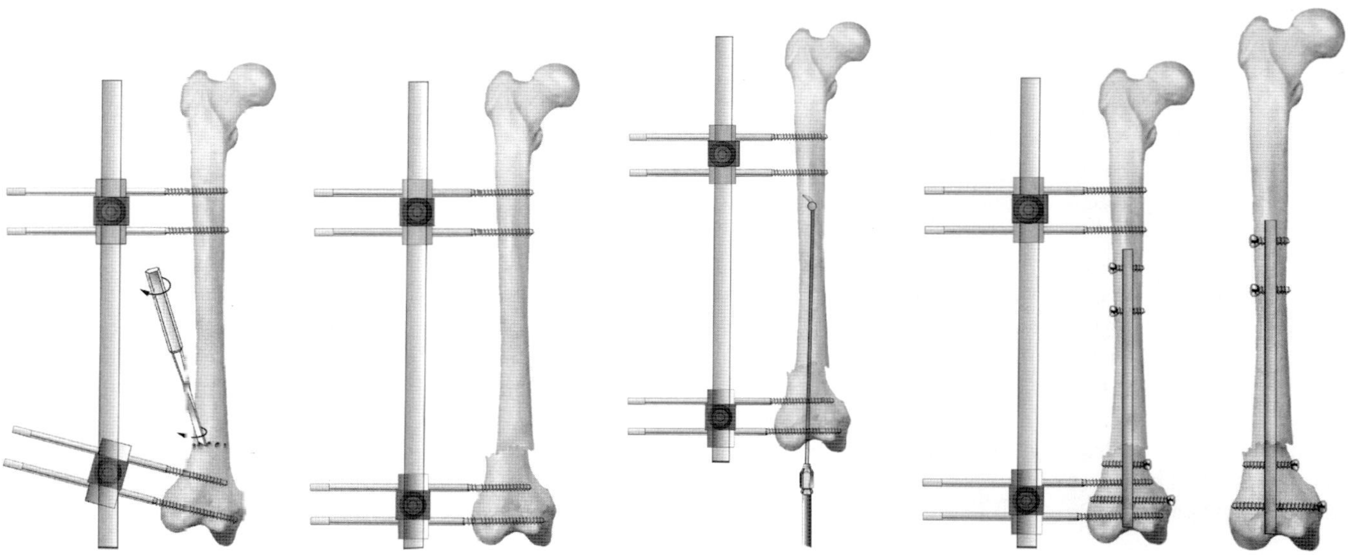

A B C D E

Figure 19.37. Fixator assisted nailing. (Adapted with permission of Dr. Dror Paley.[99])

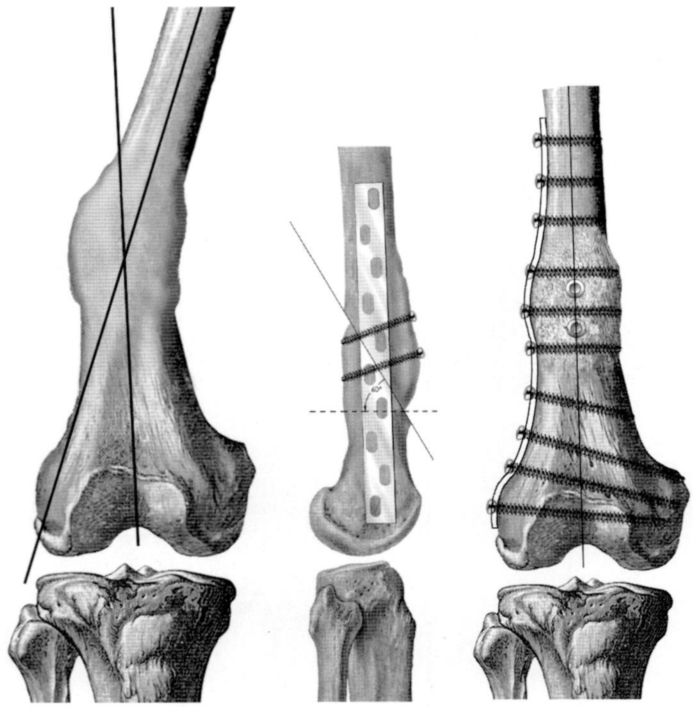

Figure 19.38. Oblique plane osteotomy.

lous preoperative planning required. Chapman[100] reported a 95% union rate with this method.

When limb length discrepancy occurs following a distal femur fracture, definitive treatment may consist of a shoe lift, limb lengthening, or contralateral limb shortening. Lengthening can be achieved acutely or with gradual distraction. Lengthening a shortened limb that has an overlapped malunion can be accomplished acutely with osteotomy, use of the femoral distractor, and internal fixation.[101] However, acute length restoration can be limited due to the risk for neurovascular compromise. Johnson[101] advocates the use of the AO/ASIF (Arbeitsgemeinschaft für Osteosynthesefragen/Association for the Study of Internal Fixation) fracture distractor applied directly to the osteotomy site, with fixation provided by either a 95-degree blade plate or an antegrade locking intramedullary nail. In his series, he was able to lengthen femora by an average of 3.2 cm, maintaining bone contact without any adverse affects. We do not recommend acute lengthening that creates a gap, even if graft is applied.

Lengthening of larger discrepancies is usually accomplished utilizing the Ilizarov technique of distraction osteogenesis. This technique relies on gradual distraction with external fixation to form new bone in the distraction gap. Preservation of the periosteal sleeve at the osteotomy site is crucial. The learning curve is steep and the regenerate is less predictable in older patients.

Femoral lengthening over an intramedullary nail (Fig. 19.39) is an option in the adult population,[45] with advantages including decreased duration of external fixation, protection against refracture, and earlier rehabilitation.[102] The technique is technically demanding as there is little room proximally for both the external fixator pins and the femoral nail. The technique is limited by retained hardware, and lengthens along the anatomic and not the mechanical axis.

Closed intramedullary shortening of the contralateral femur is a reasonable option in select patients[103] (Fig.19.40). This technique allows immediate weight bearing and functional return. Disadvantages include the shortening of stature and an operative intervention on a normal limb. The procedure can be performed closed with an intramedullary saw, and following length correction an IM nail may be inserted. Autologous bone graft may also be added to the IM canal if additional bone is needed. Dysfunction of the quadriceps and hamstrings following a femoral shaft shortening procedure has been reported. Holm and coworkers[104] demonstrated a significant decrease in muscle function up to 2 years postsurgery. They concluded that shortening the femur by 10% or more would have long-term effects.

Stiffness

When stiffness does occur, and the patient exhausts conservative measures, the surgeon may need to correct the block to range of motion. Manipulation under anes-

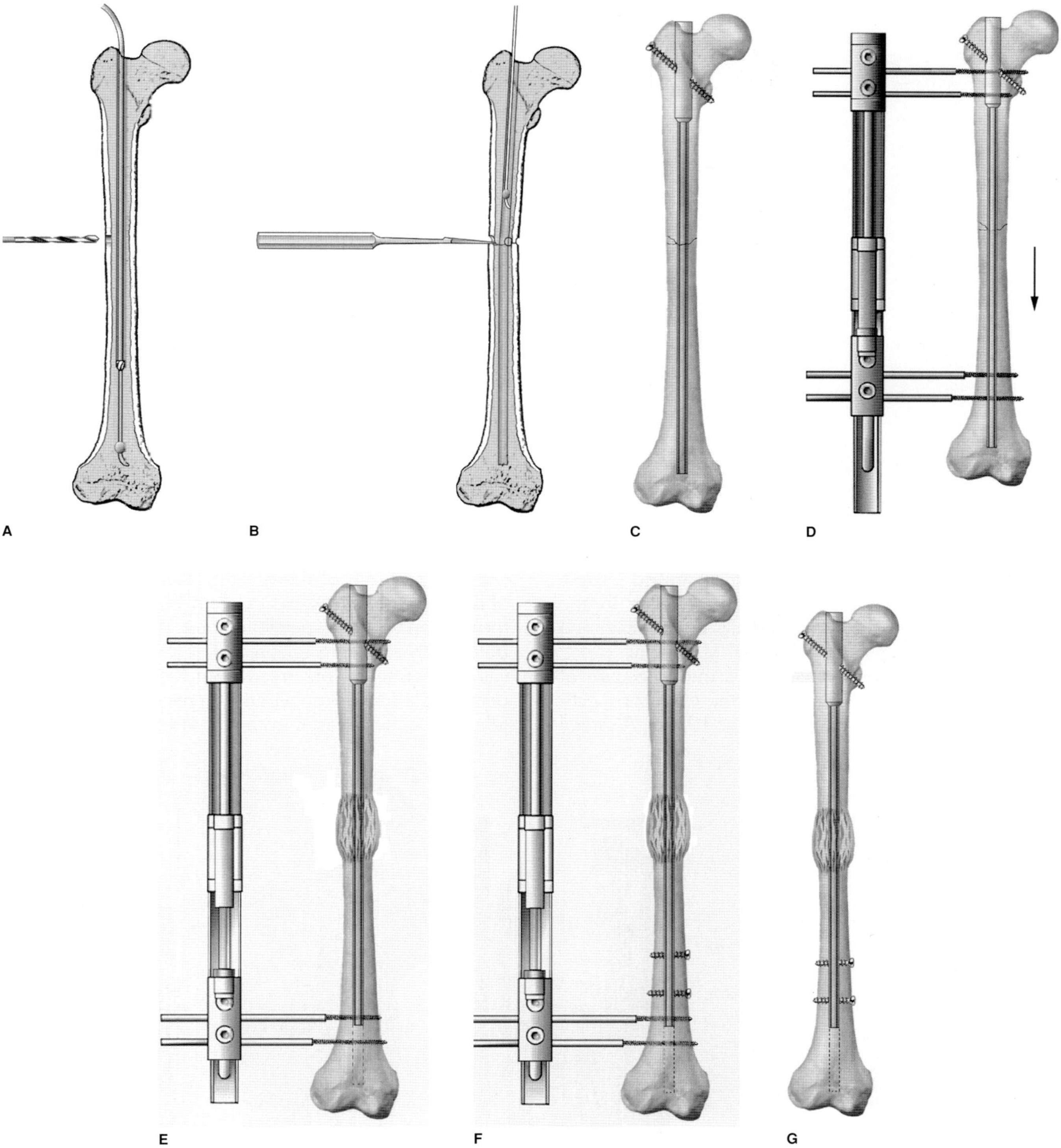

Figure 19.39. Femoral lengthening over a nail. (Adapted with permission of Dr. Dror Paley.[102])

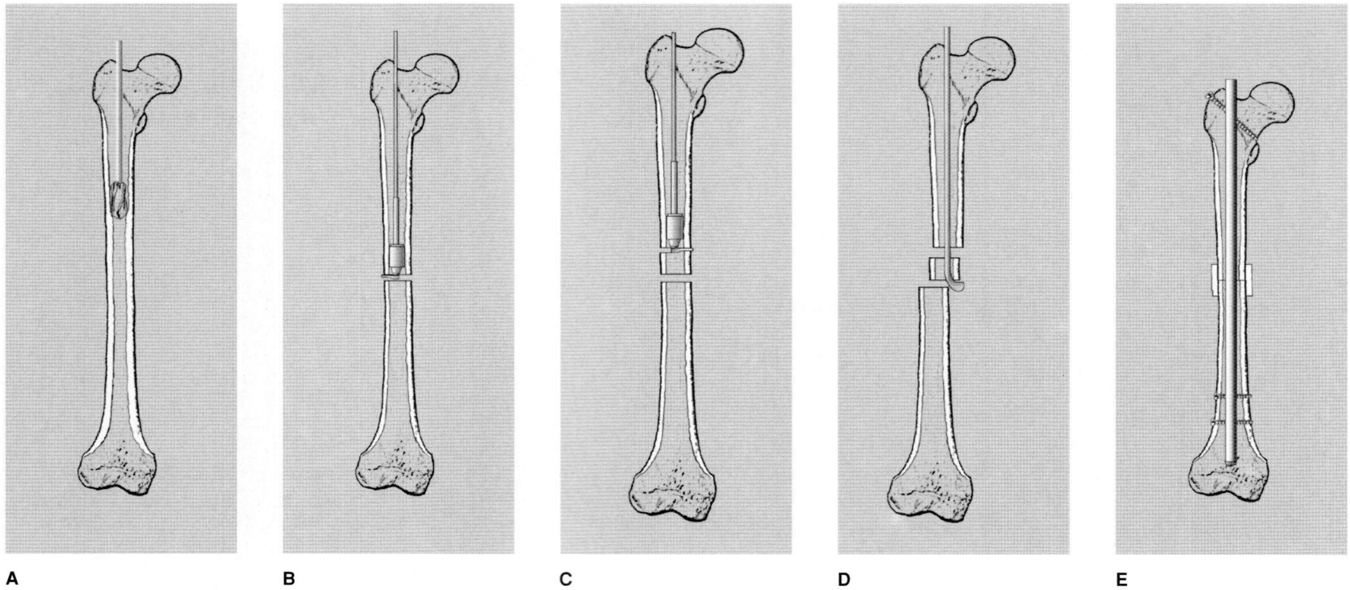

Figure 19.40. Closed intramedullary shortening of femur. (Adapted from 103, 104.)

thesia may be indicated and the risks include refracture and/or disruption of the extensor mechanism. Usually extrinsic scarring of the extensor mechanism in the supracondylar area is at least partially responsible, and therefore arthroscopy alone is rarely of benefit.

A Judet quadricepsplasty[105,106] is the procedure of choice when significant scarring of the extensor mechanism occurs to the distal femur (Fig. 19.41). A lateral approach to the knee may be extended proximally to within 4 to 5 cm of the greater trochanter depending of the exposure necessary. A lateral capsulotomy is performed and lateral patellofemoral and suprapatellar pouch adhesions are released. The vastus lateralis and vastus intermedius are freed from femur and linea aspera, and if further mobilization is necessary, the rectus femoris can be released from the pelvis. We do not rec-

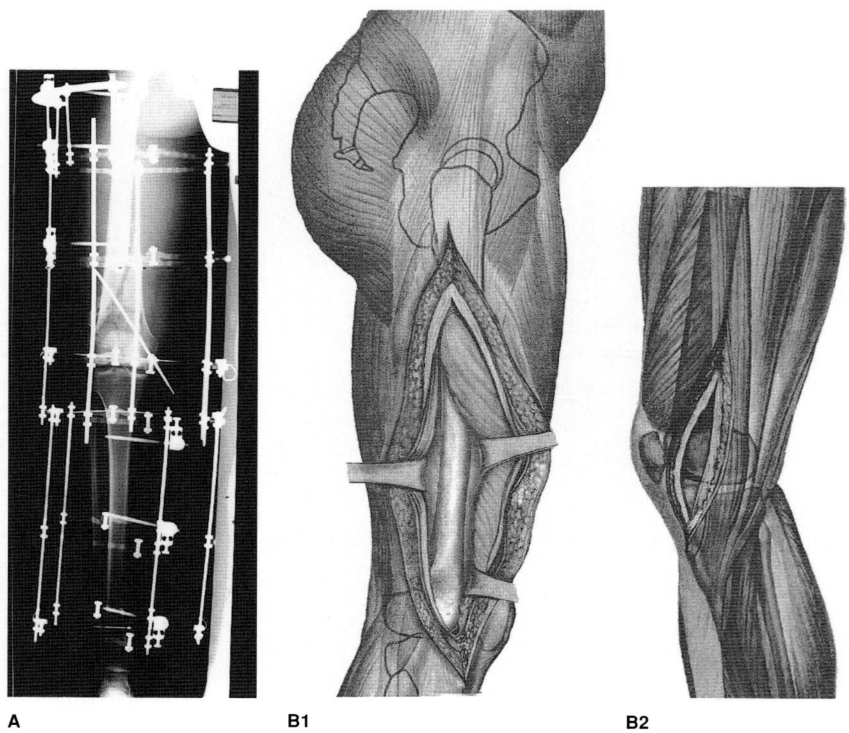

Figure 19.41. Judet quadricepsplasty. **A:** Stiffness results after long leg-knee bridging external fixation. Injury was open and comminuted. **B:** Schematic of technique of quadricepsplasty. If possible, one would like not to disrupt the continuity of the rectus femoris. Either anterior or simultaneous medial and lateral incisions can be utilized.

ommend transection of the quadriceps tendon in the supracondylar region. If necessary, an anteromedial incision may be used to free medial patellofemoral adhesions, the vastus medialis, the medial capsule, and other intrinsic contractures. Tight intrinsic and extrinsic contractures are released sequentially until the desired range of motion is obtained. Exposure must allow resection of any bony bars. Alternatively, the mentioned releases may be performed through an anterior incision that has wide medial and lateral skin flaps. The wound is closed over a drain and may be splinted in flexion. Continuous passive motion and postoperative epidural anesthesia are aids to maintaining motion.

Posterior capsular release may be considered for some flexion contractures. Hamstring lengthening or release may also be necessary. In the extreme case, gradual correction via a multiplanar external fixator with a hinge placed near the instantaneous center of rotation of knee is an option. Postoperative immobilization in extension is required following either acute or gradual correction.

Osteoarthritis

The treatment of posttraumatic arthritis is similar to that for osteoarthritis (OA). Unicompartmental OA in an active young individual may be an indication for an osteotomy.[107] The objective is usually slight overcorrection to unload the involved compartment. The osteotomy can be performed in either the femur or the proximal tibia, but preferably at the site of the major deformity.

Knee arthrodesis is a viable salvage procedure to be considered when bony injury is severe, the extensor mechanism is disrupted, the articular surface is destroyed, or fulminant infection occurs.[108,109] Fixation with a locked femoral-tibial nail is a sound technique in the absence of sepsis. The Ilizarov external fixator is useful with deformed bony anatomy or in cases involving infection (Fig. 19.42).

Joint replacement arthroplasty is an ideal solution for the elderly. Custom prostheses with long stems that are more constrained may be necessary. Contraindications for arthroplasty include sepsis or loss of the extensor mechanism. The authors have found that the posttraumatic patients are more prone to stiffness following TKA than are the typical OA patients.

Vascular Compromise

As mentioned previously, we are discussing vascular injury in this chapter so that this complication from the injury is treated appropriately. Vascular injury from the treatment of the fracture itself is extremely rare. The prevention of complication in these cases was already discussed. Figure 19.43 demonstrates the worst-case scenario of loss of limb from an inappropriately managed injury.

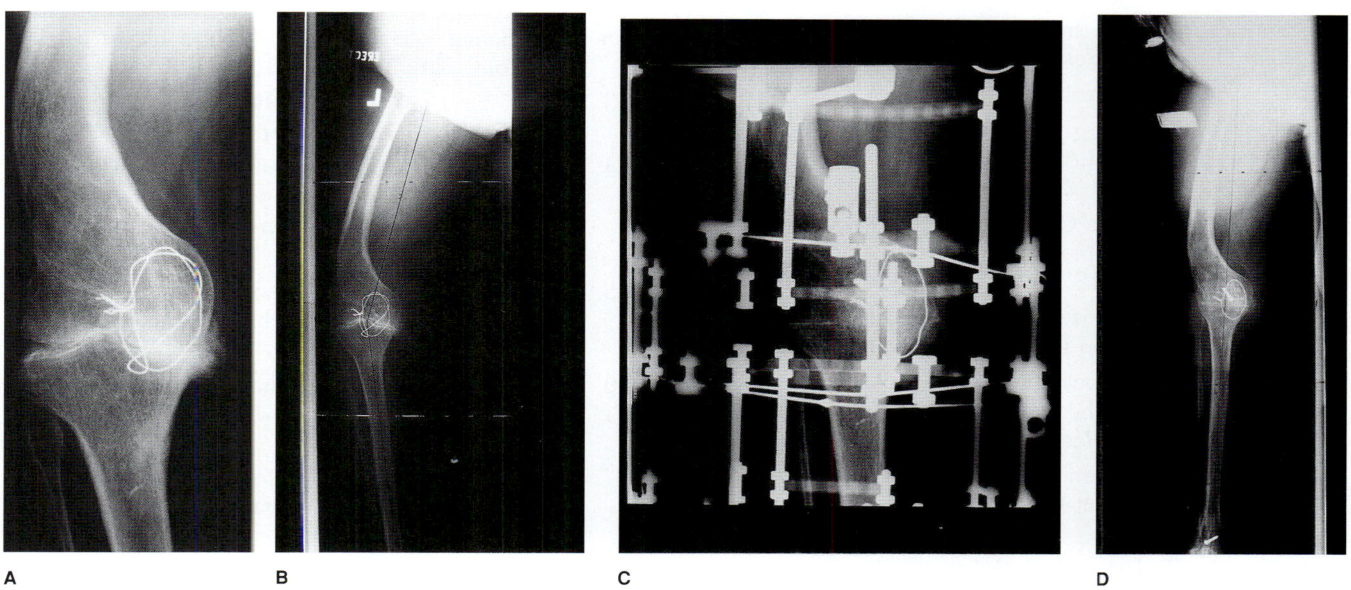

Figure 19.42. Knee arthrodesis as a salvage for osteoarthritis. **A:** Posttraumatic degenerative joint disease resulting from distal femur fracture. Knee is nearly ankylosed and painful. **B:** Longstanding view shows mechanical varus of 20 degrees. The patient has had a previous tibial-calcaneal fusion and walks on the lateral border of the foot. **C:** Surgeons opted against total arthroplasty because of prior history of infection, poor soft tissue envelope, and injury to extensor mechanism. **D:** Successful knee fusion with realignment of limb and resultant 0-degree mechanical axis. The patient's satisfaction was high not only because of the lack of knee pain, but also because of a more plantigrade foot.

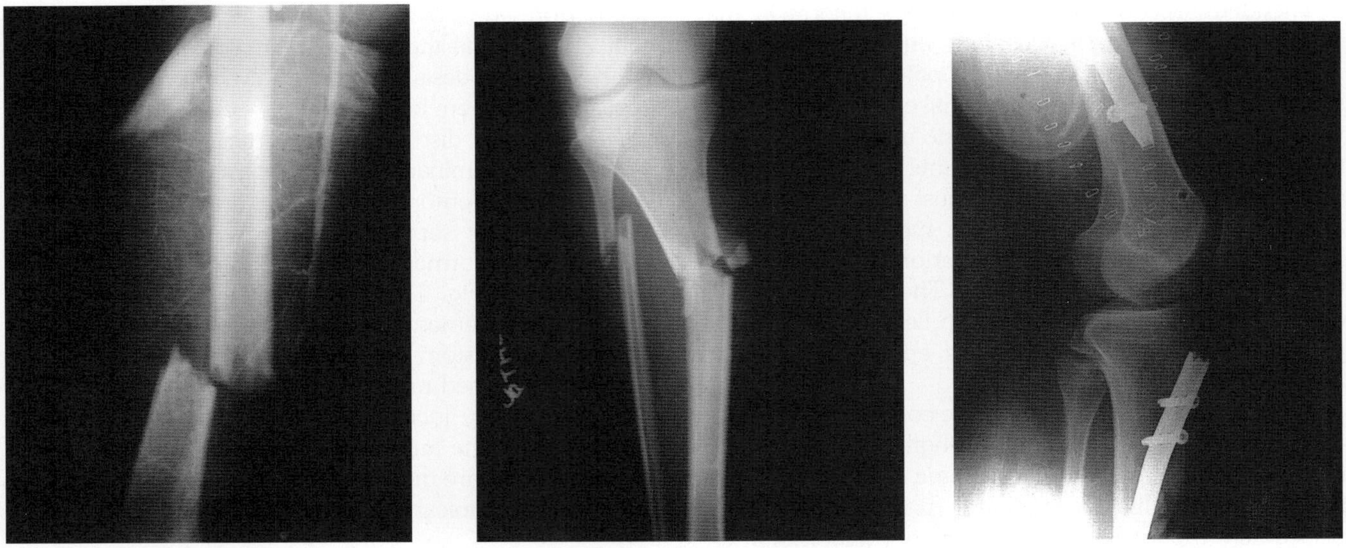

A B C

Figure 19.43. Disaster in the treatment of vascular compromise. **A** and **B:** Floating knee injury. Excessive warm ischemic time following transfer from initial facility where lack of pulse was noted in the preoperative holding area. Formal angiogram further delayed treatment. **C:** Internal fixation began after warm ischemic time of 10 hours. Fixation consisted of antegrade femoral nail, redraping for a tibial nail, followed by vascular bypass. Delayed fasciotomy did not prevent amputation days later.

References

1. Mays J, Neufeld A. Skeletal traction methods. *Clin Orthop Rel Res* 1974;102:144–151.
2. Kuntscher G. The intramedullary nailing of fractures. *Clin Orthop Rel Res* 1968;60:5–12.
3. Campbell W. *Operative Orthopedics*. St. Louis, Mosby, 1939.
4. White EH, Russin LA. Supracondylar fractures. *Kansas Med Soc* 1967;68:328–332.
5. Schatzker J, Horne G, Waddell J. The Toronto experience with the supracondylar fracture of the femur, 1966–72. *Injury* 1975;6(2):113–128.
6. Schatzker J, Lambert DC. Supracondylar fractures of the femur. *Clin Orthop Rel Res* 1979;138:77–83.
7. Chiron HS, Tremoulet J, Casey P, et al. Fractures of the distal third of the femur treated by internal fixation. *Clin Orthop Rel Res* 1974;100:160–170.
8. Neer CS, Grantham SA, Shelton ML. Supracondylar fracture of the adult femur. *J Bone Joint Surg* 1967; 49A:591–613.
9. Connolly JF, Dehne E, LaFollette B. Closed reduction and early cast-brace ambulation in the treatment of femoral fractures. *J Bone Joint Surg* 1973;55A(8): 1581–1599.
10. Mooney V, Nickel V, Harvey JP, et al. Cast-brace treatment for fractures of the distal part of the femur. *J Bone Joint Surg* 1970;52A(8):1563–1578.
11. Healy WL, Brooker AF Jr. Distal femoral fractures. Comparison of open and closed methods of treatment. *Clin Orthop Rel Res* 1983;174:166–171.
12. Olerud S. Operative treatment of supracondylar fractures of the femur: technique and result in fifteen cases. *J Bone Joint Surg* 1972;54A:1015–1032.
13. Muller ME, Allgower M, Willenegger H. *Manual of Internal Fixation.* New York: Springer-Verlag, 1979.
14. Giles JB, DeLee JC, Heckman JD, et al. Supracondylar-intracondylar fractures of the femur treated with a supracondylar plate and lag screen. *J Bone Joint Surg* 1982;64A:864–870.
15. Mize RD, Bucholz RW, Grogan DP. Surgical treatment of displaced comminuted fractures of the distal end of the femur. *J Bone Joint Surg* 1982;64A:871–879.
16. Schatzker J, Mahomed N, Schiffman K, et al. Dynamic condylar screw: a new device. *J Orthop Trauma* 1989; 3:124–132.
17. Sanders R, Swiontkowski M, Rosen H et al. Double-plating of comminuted unstable fractures of the distal part of the femur. *J Bone Joint Surg* 1991;73(3):341–346.
18. Simon JA, Hale J, Kummer F, et al. Improved fixation in osteoporotic bone: a novel locked supracondylar buttress plate. Poster presented at the Orthopaedic Trauma Association, Louisville, KT, October 1997.
19. Koval K, Hoehl JJ, Kummer FJ, et al. Distal femoral fixation: a biomechanical comparison of the standard condylar buttress plate, a locked buttress plate, and the

95-degree blade plate. *J Orthop Trauma*, 1997;11(7):521–524.

20. Rush LV. *Atlas of Rush Pin Techniques*, 2nd ed. New York: Meridian, 1976.
21. Shelbourne KD, Brueckmann FR. Rush-pin fixation of supracondylar and intercondylar fractures of the femur. *J Bone Joint Surg* 1982;64A(2):161–169.
22. Kolmert L, Egund N, Persson BD. Internal fixation of supracondylar and bicondylar fractures using a new semielastic device. *Clin Orthop Rel Res* 1983;181:204–219.
23. Zickel RE. Nonunions of fractures of the proximal and distal thirds of the shaft of the femur. *Instr Course Lect* 1988;173–179.
24. Zickel RE, Fietti VG, Lawsing JF, et al. A new intramedullary fixation device for the distal third of the femur. *Clin Orthop Rel Res* 1977;125:185–191.
25. Marks DS, Isbister ES, Porter KM. Zickel supracondylar nailing for supracondylar femoral fractures inelderly or infirm patients. *J Bone Joint Surg* 1994;76B(4):596–601.
26. Papagiannopoulos G, Clement DA. Treatment of fractures of the distal third of the femur: a prospective trial of the derby intramedullary nail. *J Bone Joint Surg* 1987;69B(1):67–70.
27. Leung KS, Shen WY, So WS, et al. Interlocking intramedullary nailing for supracondylar and intercondylar fractures of the distal part of the femur. *J Bone Joint Surg* 1991;73A:332–340.
28. Lucas SE, Seligson D, Henry S. Intramedullary supracondylar nailing of femoral fractures. *Clin Orthop Rel Res* 1993;296:200–206.
29. Sanders R, Koval KJ, Dipasquale T, et al. Retrograde reamed femoral nailing. *J Orthop Trauma* 1993;7(4):293–302.
30. Iannacone WM, Bennett FS, DeLong WG, et al. Initial experience with the treatment of supracondylar fractures using the supracondylar intramedullary nail: a preliminary report. *J Orthop Trauma* 1994;8:322–327.
31. Moed BR, Watson JT, Cramer KE, et al. Unreamed retrograde intramedullary nailing of fractures of the femoral shaft. Paper presented at the Orthopaedic Trauma Association, Louisville, KY, October 1997.
32. Ostrum RF, DiCicco J, Lakatos R, et al. Retrograde intramedullary nailing of femoral diaphyseal fractures. Paper presented at the Orthopaedic Trauma Association, Louisville, KY, October, 1997.
33. Marsh JL, Jansen H, Yoong HK, et al. Supracondylar fractures of the femur treated by external fixation. *J Orthop Trauma* 1997;11(6):405–411.
34. Sanders R, Regazzoni P, Reudi T. Treatment of supracondylar-intraarticular fractures of the femur using the dynamic condylar screw. *J Orthop Trauma* 1989;3(3):214–222.
35. Stewart MJ, Sisk TD, Wallace SL. Fractures of the distal third of the femur. *J Bone Joint Surg* 1966;48A(4):784–807.
36. Adamson GJ, Wiss DA, Lowery GL, et al. Type II floating knee: ipsilateral femoral and tibial fractures with intraarticular extension into the knee joint. *J Orthop Trauma* 1992;6(3):333–339.
37. Gustilo RB, Anderson JT. Prevention of infection in the treatment of one thousand and twenty-five open fractures of long bones: retrospective and prospective analyses. *J Bone Joint Surg* 1976;58A:453–458.
38. Gustilo RB, Mendoza RM, Williams DN. Problems in the management of type III (severe) open fractures: a new classifacation of type III open fractures. *J Trauma* 1984;24:742–746.
39. Cierny GI, Mader JT, Pennick JJ. A clinical staging system for adult osteomyelitis. *Contemp Orthop* 1985;10:17–37.
40. Tscherne H, Gotzen L. *Fractures with Soft Tissue Injuries*. Berlin: Springer-Verlag, 1984.
41. Koval K. Supracondylar and intercondylar fractures of the distal femur. In: Levine AM (ed). *OKU Trauma*. Rosemont IL: AAOS, 1996;137–144.
42. Zehntner MK, Marchesi DG, Burch H, et al. Alignment of supracondylar/intercondylar fractures of the femur after internal fixation by AO/ASIF technique. *J Orthop Trauma* 1992;6(3):318–326.
43. Mize R, Johnson E, and Hohl M. Complications of treatment of fractures and dislocations of the knee. In: Epps CH (ed). *Complications of Orthopaedic Surgery*. Philadelphia: Lippincott, 1994:475–513.
44. Green SA, Gibbs P. The relationship of angulation to translation in fracture deformities. *J Bone Joint Surg* 1994;76A(3):390–397.
45. Paley D, Herzenberg JE, Tetsworth K, et al. Deformity planning for frontal and sagittal plane corrective osteotomies. *Orthop Clin North Am* 1994;25(3):425–465.
46. DiChristina DG, Riemer BL, Butterfield SL, et al. Femur fractures with femoral or popliteal artery injuries in blunt trauma. *J Orthop Trauma* 1994;8(4):494–503.
47. Morrey BF. Post-traumatic stiffness: distraction arthroplasty. In: Morrey BF (ed). *The Elbow and Its Disorders*, vol 2. Philadelphia: WB Saunders,1993:476–491.
48. Mira A, Markley K, Greer R. A critical analysis of quadriceps function after femoral shaft fractures in adults. *J Bone Joint Surg* 1980;62A(1):61–67.
49. Salter RB, Simmonds DF, Malcolm BW, et al. The biological effect of continuous passive motion on the healing of full-thickness defects in articular cartilage. An experimental investigation in the rabbit. *J Bone Joint Surg* 1980;62A:1232–1251.
50. Llinas A, McKellop HA, Marshall GJ, et al. Healing and remodeling of articular incongruities in a rabbit fracture model. *J Bone Joint Surg* 1993;75A(10):1508–1525.

51. Lefkoe TP, Trafton PG, Ehrlich MG, et al. An experimental model of femoral condylar defect leading to osteoarthrosis. *J Orthop Trauma* 1993;7(5):458–467.
52. Egund A, Kolmert L. Deformities, gonarthrosis and function after distal femoral fractures. *Acta Orthop Scand* 1982;53:963–974.
53. Wiss D. Supracondylar and intercondylar fractures of the femur. In: Rockwood CA, Green DP, Bucholz RW, Heckman JD (eds). *Fractures in Adults*. Philadelphia: Lippincott-Raven, 1996:1972–2000.
54. Rooster B, Bengtson S, Hagglund G. Acute compartment syndrome from anterior thigh muscle contusion: a report of eight cases. *J Orthop Trauma* 1991;5(1): 57–59.
55. Bednar DA, Parikh J. Effect of time delay from injury to primary management on the incidence of deep infection after open fractures of the lower extremities caused by blunt trauma in adults. *J Orthop Trauma* 1993;7(6):532–535.
56. Norris BL, Kellam JF. Soft-tissue injuries associated with high-energy extremity trauma: principles of management. AAOS 1997;5(1):37–46.
57. Chapman JW, Olson SA. Open fractures. In: Rockwood CA, Green DP, Bucholz RW, Heckman JD, (eds). *Fractures in Adults*. Philadelphia: Lippincott-Raven, 1996: 305–352.
58. Green A, Trafton PG. Early complications in the management of open femur fractures: a retrospective study. *J Orthop Trauma* 1991;5(1):51–56.
59. Bone LB. Indirect fracture reduction: a technique for minimizing surgical trauma. *J AAOS* 1994;2(5):247–254.
60. Tornetta P III, Tiburzi D. The treatment of femoral shaft fractures using intramedullary interlocked nails with and without intramedullary reaming: a preliminary report. *J Orthop Trauma* 1997;11(2):89–92.
61. Knapp TP, Patzakis MJ, Lee J, et al. Comparison of intravenous and oral antibiotic therapy in the treatment of fractures caused by low-velocity gunshots. *J Bone Joint Surg* 1996;78A(8):1167–1171.
62. Bolhofner BR, Carmen B, Clifford P. The results of open reduction and internal fixation of distal femur fractures using a biologic (indirect) reduction technique. *J Orthop Trauma* 1996;10(6):372–377.
63. Tornkvist H, Hearn TC, Schatzker J. The strength of plate fixation in relation to the number and spacing of bone screws. *J Orthop Trauma* 1996;10(3):204–208.
64. Benum P. The use of bone cement as an adjunct to internal fixation of supracondylar fractures of osteoporotic bone. *Acta Orthop Scand* 1977;48:52–56.
65. Struhl S, Szporn MN, Cobelli NJ, et al. Cemented internal fixation for supracondylar femur fractures in osteoporotic patients. *J Orthop Trauma* 1990;4(2):151–157.
66. Rolston LR, Christ DJ, Halpern A, et al. Treatment of supracondylar fractures of the femur proximal to a total knee arthroplasty. *J Bone Joint Surg* 1995;77A(6): 924–931.
67. Healy WL, Siliski JM, Incavo SJ. Operative treatment of distal femoral fractures proximal to total knee replacements. *J Bone Joint Surg* 1993;75A(1):27–34.
68. David SM, Harrow ME, Peindl RD, et al. Comparative biomechanical analysis of supracondylar femur fracture fixation: locked intramedullary nail versus 95-degree angled plate. *J Orthop Trauma* 1997;11(5):344–349.
69. Koval KJ, Kummer FJ, Bharam S, et al. Distal femoral fixation: a laboratory comparison of the 95-degree plate, antegrade and retrograde inserted reamed intramedullary nails. *J Orthop Trauma* 1996;10(6):378–382.
70. Firoozbakhsh K, Behzadi K, DeCoster TA, et al. Mechanics of retrograde nail versus plate fixation for supracondylar femur fractures. *J Orthop Trauma* 1995;9(2): 152–157.
71. Ito K, Grass R, Zwipp H. Internal fixation of supracondylar femoral fractures: comparative biomechanical performance of the 95-degree blade plate and two retrograde nails. *J Orthop Trauma* 1998;12(4):259–266.
72. Brumback RJ, Uwegie-Ero S, Lakatos RP, et al. Intramedullary nailing of femoral shaft fractures—part II: fracture-healing with static interlocking fixation. *J Bone Joint Surg* 1988;70A:1453–1462.
73. Giannoudis PV, Furlong AJ, Macdonald DA, et al. Fractures of the femur: the osteogenic effect of reaming. Paper presented at the Orthopaedic Trauma Association, Louisville, KY, October 1997.
74. Tornetta P, Riina J, Ritter C. Risks of AP locking screws in the proximal femur. Paper presented at the Orthopaedic Trauma Association, Louisville, KY, October 1997.
75. George CJ, Lindsey RW, Noble PC, et al. Optimal location of a single distal interlocking screw in intramedullary nailing of distal third femoral shaft fractures. *J Orthop Trauma*, 1998;12(4):267–272.
76. Voor MJ, Verst DA, Mladsi SW, et al. Fatigue properties of a twelve-hole versus a five-hole intramedullary supracondylar nail. *J Orthop Trauma* 1997;11(2):98–102.
77. Fogler C, Alexander JW, Lindsey R Comparison of fracture stability in intramedullary nailing of distal femur fractures with one or two distal screws. Paper presented at the Orthopaedic Trauma Association, Boston, MA, 1996.
78. Kaysinger KK, Nicholson NC, Ramp WK, et al. Toxic effects of wound irrigation solutions on cultured tibiae and osteoblasts. *J Orthop Trauma* 1995;9(4):303–311.
79. Altman RD, Latta LL, Keer R, et al. Effect of nonsteroidal antiinflammatory drugs on fracture healing: a laboratory study in rats. *J Orthop Trauma* 1995;9(5): 392–400.

80. Finnegan MA, Guo WS, May H, et al. The effect of nicotine on the proliferation of isolated periosteal cells and bone marrow cells in culture. Paper presented at the Orthopaedic Trauma Association, Louisville, KY, October 1997.

81. DiCicco JD, Karpik K, Gregory P. Ipsilateral fractures of the femur and tibia: treatment with retrograde femoral nailing and antegrade tibial nailing. Paper presented at the Orthopaedic Trauma Association, Tampa, FL, October 1995.

82. Crag J, Spence R. Popliteal artery trauma: a high-risk injury. *Br J Surg* 1987;74:91–94.

83. Seybold EA, Buscone BD. Traumatic popliteal artery thrombosis and compartment syndrome of the leg following blunt trauma to the knee: a discussion of treatment and complications. *J Orthop Trauma* 1996;10(2): 138–141.

84. Johansen K, Bandyk D, Thiele B, et al. Temporary intraluminal shunts: resolution of a management dilemma in complex vascular injuries. *J Orthop Trauma* 1982; 22(5):395–402.

85. Rasmussen MR, Bishop AT, Wood, MB. Arthrodesis of the knee with a vascularized fibular rotatory graft. *J Bone Joint Surg* 1995;77A(5):751–759.

86. Usui M, Ishii S, Naito T, et al. Arthrodesis of knee joint by vascularized fibular graft. *Microsurgery* 1996;17:2–8.

87. Vail TP, Urbaniak JR. Donor-site morbidity with use of vascularized autogenous fibular grafts. *J Bone Joint Surg* 1996;78A(2):204–211.

88. Weiner SD, Scarborough M, Vander Griend RA. Resection arthrodesis of the knee with an intercalary allograft. *J Bone Joint Surg* 1996;78A(2):185–192.

89. Freedman EL, Hak DJ, Johnson EE, et al. Total knee replacement including a modular distal femoral component in elderly patients with acute fracture or nonunion. *J Orthop Trauma*, 1995;9(3):231–237.

90. Scheid DK, Hanel DP, Strege D. Limb salvage reconstruction in severe knee infections with associated large soft tissue and bony defects. *J Orthop Trauma* 1991; 5(1):60–65.

91. Helfet DL. Fractures of the distal femur. In: Browner BD, Jupiter JB, Levine AM et al (eds). *Skeletal Trauma.* Philadelphia: WB Saunders, 1992:1643–1683.

92. Crenshaw AH. Delayed union and nonunion of fractures. In: Crenshaw AH (ed). *Campbell's Operative Orthopaedics*, vol 3. St Louis: Mosby, 1987:20–54.

93. ZumBrunnen C, Brindley H. Nonunion of long bones (analysis of 144 cases). *JAMA* 1968;203:637.

94. Hume EL. Paper presented at the EBI Medical Systems residents conference, Parsippany NJ, February 1998.

95. Lindsey RW, Grobman J, Leggon RE et al. Effects of bone graft and electrical stimulation on the strength of healing bony defects in dogs. *Clin Orthop Rel Res* 1987;222:275–280.

96. Wu C, Shih C. Distal femoral nonunion treated with interlocking nailing. *J Orthop Trauma* 1991;31:1659–1662.

97. Koval KJ, Seligson D, Rosen H, et al. Distal femoral nonunion: treatment with a retrograde inserted locked intramedullary nail. *J Orthop Trauma*, 1995;9(4):285–291.

98. Bostman OM. Refracture after removal of a condylar plate from the distal third of the femur. *J Bone Joint Surg* 1990;72A(7):1013–1018.

99. Paley D, Herzenberg JE, Bor N. Fixator-assisted nailing of femoral and tibial deformities. *Tech Orthop* 1997; 12(4):260–275.

100. Chapman MW. Nonunions and malunions of the femoral shaft and patella. In: Chapman MW (ed). *Operative Orthopaedics*, 2nd ed. Philiadelphia: JB Lippincott, 1993.

101. Johnson EE. Acute lengthening of shortened extremities after malunion or nonunion of a fracture. *J Bone Joint Surg* 1994;76A:379–389.

102. Paley D, Hernzenber JE, Paremain G, et al. Femoral lengthening over an intramedullary nail. *J Bone Joint Surg* 1997;79A(10):1464–1480.

103. Winquist RA. Closed intramedullary osteotomies of the femur. *Clin Orthop Rel Res* 1986;212:155–164.

104. Holm I, Nordsletten L, Steen H, et al. Muscle function after mid-shaft femoral shortening. *J Bone Joint Surg* 1994;76B(1):143–146.

105. Ebraheim NA, DeTroye RJ, Saddemi SR. Results of Judet quadricepsplasty. *J Orthop Trauma* 1993;7(4): 327–330.

106. Judet R, Judet J, Lagrange J. A technique for freeing the extensor apparatus in cases of stiffness of the knee. *Mem Acad Chir* 1956;82:944–947.

107. Finkelstein JA, Gross AE, Davis A. Varus osteotomy of the distal part of the femur. *J Bone Joint Surg* 1996; 78A(9):1348–1352.

108. Hak DJ, Lieberman JR, Finerman GAM. Single plane and biplane external fixators for knee arthrodesis. *Clin Orthop Rel Res* 1995;316:134–144.

109. Rodrigo JJ. Arthrodesis of the knee. In: Chapman MW (ed.). *Operative Orthopaedics*, 2nd ed. Philiadelphia: JB Lippincott, 1993:2011–2016.

110. Morrey BF. *Joint Replacement Arthroplasty.* New York: Churchill-Livingstone, 1991.

Chapter 20

Fractures of the Patella

Robert E. Leggon, John S. Henry,
and Ronald W. Lindsey

Patella fractures account for approximately 1% of all orthopaedic fractures.[1] Injuries to the patella occur from either direct or indirect trauma. Direct injury mechanisms include blows, falls, or dashboard impacts, while indirect fractures occur due to longitudinal forces from the violent contraction of the quadriceps.

The principal goal in the treatment of patellar fractures is the surgical restoration of the extensor mechanism and anatomic reconstruction of the articular surface. Stable fixation is essential if motion is to be started early in the postoperative course. Frequently these goals can be challenging due to associated risk factors such as soft tissue injury, comminution, the subcutaneous location of the patella, poor patient compliance, and technical errors. All these factors can contribute to the development of complications.

Knee stiffness, loss of reduction (secondary to hardware failure or refracture), posttraumatic osteoarthrosis, hardware irritation, infection, nonunion, malunion, and avascular necrosis are the major complications that may arise during the treatment of patellar fractures. This chapter provides a brief historical review of the treatment of these fractures, their complications, as well as their prevention and treatment.

ANATOMY AND BIOMECHANICS

The patella, the largest sesamoid bone in the body, is a triangular bone that lies within the quadriceps tendon. The proximal portion is wide and tapers to a distal inferior pole. The articular surface is divided into medial and lateral facets separated by a vertical ridge. In the majority of patients a second vertical ridge exists near the medial border and separates the medial facet from the odd facet. The lateral facet, the largest, accounts for more than 50% of the articular surface. The proximal three-fourths of the patella is covered with thick articular cartilage (typically greater than 1 cm thick), while the distal pole is nonarticular.

The quadriceps aponeurosis inserts proximally into the superior pole of the patella. A thin layer then extends anteriorly over the patella and joins with the patellar tendon at its origin on the inferior pole. The fascia lata and iliotibial band also coalesce proximally, with the quadriceps tendon. The medial and lateral patellar retinaculi are formed by expansions from the quadriceps that pass medially and laterally to the patella as well as deep transverse fibers that originate from the epicondyles. The patellar tendon originates from the inferior pole and inserts into the tibial tubercle. The quadriceps tendon, medial and lateral retinaculi, the patella, and the patellar tendon form the extensor mechanism of the knee.

The blood supply to the patella is mainly derived from an extraosseous anastomotic ring lying over the extensor mechanism. The superior, middle, and inferior geniculate arteries supply the ring. The intraosseous blood supply is made up of the midpatella vessels that penetrate the middle third of the anterior patella, and polar vessels that enter the patella through the inferior pole. Both are derived from the anastomotic ring and this arrangement is important in understanding the mechanism of avascular necrosis and its relationship to fracture pattern.

The principal function of the patella is to increase the mechanical advantage of the quadriceps tendon. The patella transmits the force generated by the quadriceps to the patellar tendon but also serves to elevate the lever arm of the extensor mechanism from the axis of rotation of the knee. Studies have shown that the patella causes an increase in the quadriceps moment arm by almost 30% at full extension.[2] The patella also functions to protect the femoral condyles from injury and aid in nourishment of the inferior articular surface of the femur.

The loads upon the patella vary greatly with knee position. At full extension, the primary load is tension. With the knee flexed, the patella is compressed (described as the patellofemoral joint reactive force) against the distal femur, resulting in three-point bending (compression posteriorly and tension anteriorly). Anterior tension is greatest between 45 and 60 degrees of flexion.[3] Because both the posterior articular surface of the patella and the anterior articular surface of the femur are convex, only a small portion of the two articular surfaces is in contact at any given time. It has been demonstrated that through a full range of motion only 13% to 38% of the patellar surface is load bearing.[4] Therefore, due to the small patellofemoral contact and the large amount of force generated across the patellofemoral joint, the patellofemoral contact stresses exceed those of other major weight-bearing joints for virtually all activities.[5]

HISTORICAL SUMMARY

Historically the treatment of patella fractures has reflected our evolving appreciation of patellar function. Prior to the 1820s, most of these fractures were treated nonoperatively with splinting in extension. The resulting fibrous union with residual knee stiffness and decreased strength convinced some surgeons to try more invasive methods of treatment. Early stabilization consisting of external fixators with percutaneous pins connected by leather straps or metal wires to provide compression was tried.[6] A percutaneous clamp described by Malgaigne[7] soon followed.

Around 1877 Sir Hector Cameron[8] performed the first open reduction and internal fixation of a patella fracture in Scotland. His technique consisted of silver wires threaded through drill holes. By the early 1900s, open reduction and wire fixation had become the method of choice. A variety of suture materials were developed. With the development of aseptic surgery, infection, the primary objective to open reduction and internal fixation, had been overcome.

About this same time, some physicians began to question whether the patella was essential enough to preserve. Authors such as Brooke, Hey-Groves, and Watson Jones suggested the patella actually inhibited the action of the quadriceps, and patellectomy improved the strength of the extensor mechanism.[6] For a brief period, total patellectomy was thought to be reasonable for all types of patella fractures. However, as many as 50% of patellar fractures treated in this manner were complicated by poor results.[9]

Improved methods of internal fixation, research establishing the biomechanical function of the patella, and the poor results of total and subtotal patellectomy helped to disdain the view of patellectomy as the treatment of choice for all patellar fractures. Thompson,[10] who introduced partial patellectomy, helped clarify that the optimal treatment for patellar fractures consisted of reconstruction of the patella, partial patellectomy with tendon repair, or total patellectomy with extensor mechanism repair. These are the same basic options available to today's surgeons.

A major advance in the management of patellar fractures occurred in the early 1950s with Pauwel's development of the anterior tension band.[11] This biomechanically sound method was later modified by the Arbeitsgemeinschaft für Osteosynthesefragen (AO) and currently seems to offer the best results in stabilization of the majority of patellar fractures. Partial patellectomy and total patellectomy still remain options in excessively comminuted or contaminated fractures. Indications for each are dependent on the specific type of fracture to be treated. Unfortunately, early complications in the operative treatment of patella fractures can still reach 25%, even with modern techniques and the best of surgeons.[12]

COMPLICATIONS

Knee Stiffness

Decreased range of motion is the most common complication noted after treatment of patellar fractures. In fact, loss of motion after a patellar fracture has been described as the rule rather than the exception.[5] The extent of lost knee flexion is often greater than that of extension, and may be related to the tendency of many to splint in extension. Functionally, however, a small loss of extension (as little as 15 degrees) is usually more of a clinical impairment than a similar loss of flexion.

Loss of knee motion can result from both extrinsic and intrinsic causes.[13] Extrinsic contracture involves contracture of the soft tissues—the capsular, ligamentous, or muscular. Capsular and ligamentous adhesions can occur in the medial compartment, lateral compartment, or the region of the suprapatellar pouch. Ectopic calcification of ectopic bone formation can bridge these structures. Loss of elasticity and excursion of the quadriceps muscle group is usually more extensive than that of the hamstrings. Intrinsic contracture implies a cartilaginous or osseous origin. Intraarticular adhesions between the patella and femur, or between the femur and tibia, can predominate. Loss of articular cartilage, with exposed bone can accelerate this process. Rarely, union between the opposing bony surfaces can occur. Finally, intrinsic contracture can result from gross articular surface distortion due to the initial trauma, or due to inadequate or failed reduction.

Loss of Reduction and Loss of Fixation

Loss of reduction or loss of fixation prior to healing has been reported to occur in up to 20% of operatively treated patellar fractures.[14] Factors that may precipitate this complication include unrecognized comminution, inadequate or improper fixation technique, an inadequate period of postoperative joint immobilization, poor bone quality, or poor patient compliance. It is extremely uncommon following nondisplaced fractures. Proper surgical technique, with attention to the biomechanical characteristics of the construct used, is paramount, especially in the more challenging fractures. Refracture, although rare, has been reported at an incidence varying from 1% to 5%.[6]

Loss of reduction or fixation in the management of patella fractures usually culminates in functional compromise. If an articular step-off occurs and is accepted, posttraumatic arthritis may ensue. A distraction gap between fragments may lead to nonunion. Revision surgery is often indicated, but the risk of wound complications or knee stiffness may be prohibitive. Even the simplest of fractures warrant stable fixation if the joint is to be mobilized early.

Osteoarthritis

Posttraumatic patellofemoral osteoarthritis following patella fracture is not uncommon. Nummi[15] reported a long-term incidence of 56% in a study of over 700 patellar fractures. Sorensen[16] demonstrated a 70% incidence of patellofemoral arthritis in patients 10 to 30 years after fracture compared with a 31% incidence in the contralateral, uninjured knee. The development of osteoarthritis has been attributed to several factors. Damage to the articular cartilage at the time of injury can play a major role. Even a blow to the cartilage without a fracture can result in eburnation and ensuing arthritis. Continuous passive motion has been felt by some to aid in healing and remodeling of full-thickness defects in articular cartilage.[17]

The healing and remodeling of osteochondral step-offs are substantially different, however, from cartilage defects. Increased cartilage pressures are generated in the high side of the defect. While cartilage and subchondral bone can adapt to their surface incongruities by remodeling their surface, the remodeling is incomplete.[18] Continuous passive motion does not appear to improve healing or remodeling, particularly for large step-offs.

Patellar enlargement following fracture has also been shown to cause patellofemoral arthritis. Exuberant bone formation may ensue after treatment of a comminuted fracture. This bone, combined with articular cartilage injury and osteochondral step-off, can be difficult to manage (Fig. 20.1).

Comminuted patellar fractures requiring partial patellectomy are reported to account for 20% to 26% of all patellar fractures.[19] Patients treated by partial patellectomy may pose a particular problem. The patellar contact area moves proximally with increasing flexion. Loss of a comminuted fragment can signifigantly alter these forces, increase contact pressures, and subsequently become a source of patellofemoral pain and produce an increased incidence of patellofemoral arthritis. In a long-term follow-up study of 56 patients with patellar fractures treated with partial patellectomy, 55% developed radiographic arthritic changes.[19]

Patella baja or alta, or imbalance of the retinaculum causing lateral tilt, are also contributing factors. Radiologic studies including standing anteroposterior and lateral views are useful in measuring patella baja/alta and the Insall-Salvati ratio of patella ligament length/patellar length (normal less than 1.2). Axial tangential

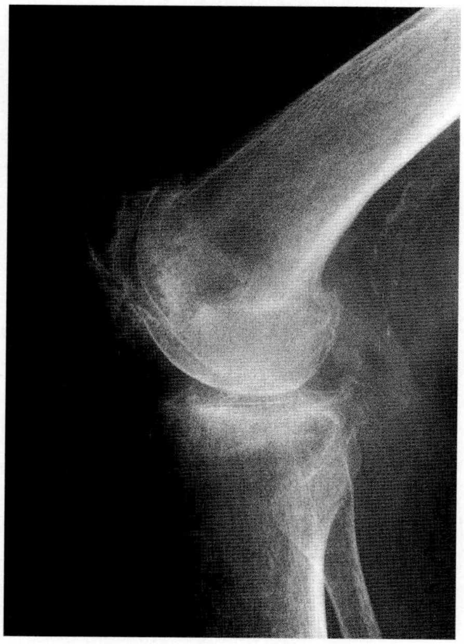

Figure 20.1. Chondral injury, osteoarticular step-off, and exuberant bone formation all contribute to patellofemoral posttraumatic arthritis.

views using knee flexion angles from 20 through 55 degrees are helpful in evaluating congruence of the patellar facets, cartilage loss, subchondral step-offs or sclerosis, and dynamic tracking.

Symptomatic Hardware

Hardware irritation of the soft tissue surrounding the patella is also very common. The subcutaneous position of the patella allows the hardware to be easily palpable. Wires and wire knots can cause irritation of the joint capsule or patellar/quadriceps tendon, while screws tend to be less irritating. Wire breakage can also be a source of pain, especially with intraarticular migration.[20]

The exact percentage of patients is unknown, but removal of the hardware secondary to irritation is necessary in at least 18%[12] of cases and in our experience even higher. Although some surgeons would not consider hardware irritation a complication, the fact that many patients require additional surgery suggests that it can have a significant influence on patient outcome. The risk of symptomatic hardware and the possible need for a second procedure should be discussed with the patient.

Infection

Infection following the surgical treatment of the patella is relatively uncommon but very significant. Reported rates range from 3% to 10%, a relatively high rate of infection in any series of open reduction and internal fixation procedures.[14] Higher infection rates have been cited following treatment of open fractures.[21]

The infection severity is dependent on the depth of the infection (superficial or deep), the adequacy of the soft tissue envelope, the extent of bony involvement, and the virulence of the infection organism(s). The subcutaneous position of the patella with its overlying skin can present a difficult problem in the treatment of patellar fractures. Interestingly, the management of the soft tissue envelope may be more challenging than the bony injury (Fig. 20.2). Unfortunately, some patients experience severe injury to the soft tissue envelope, which can lead to skin slough, the need for a muscle flap, deep infection, or spontaneous knee fusion.

The risk of an infection includes factors that are associated with the mechanism of injury, the treatment, and with the quality of the host itself.[22] Factors that are associated with the injury itself are related to the energy of the injury and the degree of contamination. Open fractures, avascular bone, comminution, soft tissue injury, loss of tissue, compartment syndrome, and vascular injury also predispose to infection. Factors associated with treatment include inappropriate antibiotic prophylaxis, extensive surgical dissection, inadequate

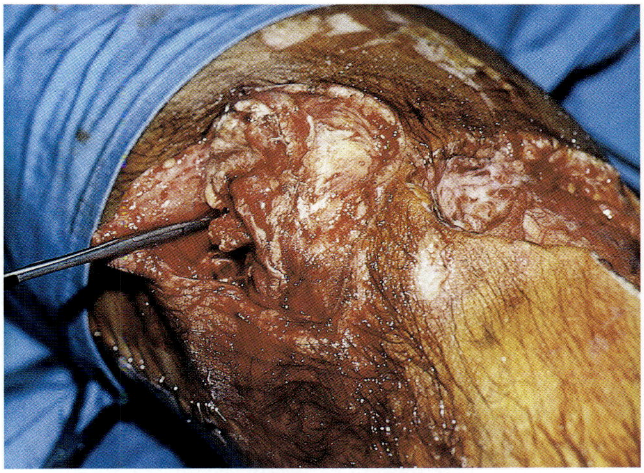

Figure 20.2. Occasionally, treatment of the soft tissue injury may be more important than that of the bony injury.

fixation, poor soft tissue management, prolonged operative time, and a delay in operative intervention. Finally, the health of the patient may significantly affect the infection potential. Conditions such as end-stage renal disease, diabetes, chronic steroid use, polytrauma, obesity, increasing age, and immunodeficiency syndromes may contribute to the type and route of infection and an increased infection rate.

Nonunion

Historically most nonunions resulted after the nonoperative treatment of widely displaced patellar fractures. Sorensen[16] reported that between 1930 to 1951, 10% to 55% of patellar fractures treated nonoperatively did not unite. Currently, nonunion is reported in less than 1% of displaced patellar fractures treated operatively,[5] an improvement principally due to modern surgical technique.

The severity of the nonunion can vary from an asymptomatic fibrous nonunion to an infected, painful nonunion, to a scarred comminuted nonunion with persistent displacement and loss of extensor capacity. A minimally displaced fibrous nonunion typically presents following an unrecognized or untreated fracture. Aseptic nonunions most often occur after failure of fixation and loss of fracture reduction. Infection may cause nonunion even without loss of fixation. Appropriate treatment is based on the etiology of the nonunion and the patient's symptoms and functional demands.

Avascular Necrosis

Displaced patellar fractures, especially transverse fractures through the middle one-third, are at increased risk for developing avascular necrosis (AVN). The proximal pole is at greater risk than the distal pole, which has a dual blood supply. The incidence of AVN has been reported to range from 3.5% to 24%.[6] Scapinelli[23] described 41 cases of AVN, 38 of which involved the proximal pole. The amount of initial separation seems to correlate with the risk of AVN. AVN occurs more frequently following circumferential stabilization techniques that occlude the peripatellar vessel blood supply.[6] The radiographic findings consistent with AVN are usually visible within 1 to 2 months following fracture.

Initially the radiographic density of the infarcted area seems normal. As the injured knee is rested the area becomes osteoporotic from disuse. The infarcted area, from having no more blood supply, cannot undergo osteoporosis and becomes relatively more dense. As creeping substitution occurs, new living bone may be deposited on the surfaces of the necrotic trabeculae, resulting in an absolute increase in the radiographic density of the repairing infarct. Occasionally, when repair stalls, calcification may also occur in the necrotic marrow.[24]

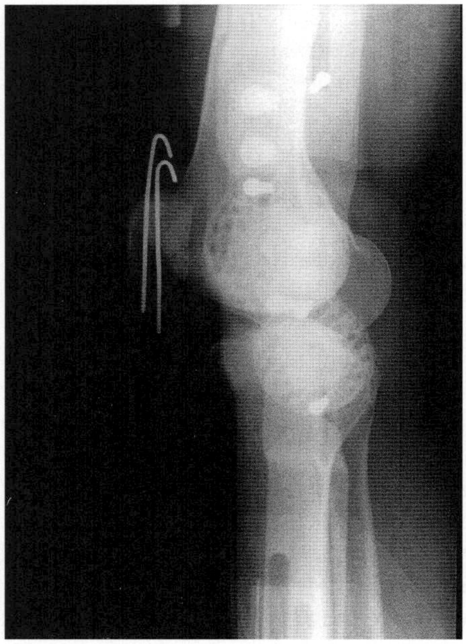

Figure 20.3. The surgeon forgot the tension band portion of the tension band wiring construct. The patient was then braced and the contracture accepted.

PREVENTION OF COMPLICATIONS

Knee Stiffness

The most important factor in preventing knee stiffness is stable fixation, which permits early active or passive motion. Modern fixation techniques generally allow knee range of motion to begin within 2 weeks postsurgery. Early motion not only is beneficial in preventing stiffness, but also may provide a beneficial effect for cartilage defect healing. According to Nummi,[15] immobilization for 4 weeks or less postoperatively provided good results in 83% of patients compared with 15% in patients immobilized 8 weeks. Once the fracture is healed, the patient should be progressed from low resistance early motion to aggressive physical therapy aimed at regaining preoperative strength as well as a functional range of motion.

Joint contracture is always the result of inactivity, and may be unavoidable due to associated complications. Frequently the complication is an unstable method of fixation, which causes the surgeon to opt for prolonged immobilization (Fig. 20.3). Pain from prominent hardware often can be especially detrimental, as the patient is reluctant to comply with physical therapy (Fig. 20.4). Other complications such as malreduction with an articular step-off, infection, and multiple surgeries can also be contributory.

Patients with closed head injuries or polytrauma who are unable to participate in appropriate postoperative physical therapy represent a particularly difficult rehabilitation challenge. A team approach coordinated with the trauma service, critical care workers, and physical and occupational therapists can affect the ultimate functional outcome. Even in the most critical patient the goal should always be early motion, either passive or active.

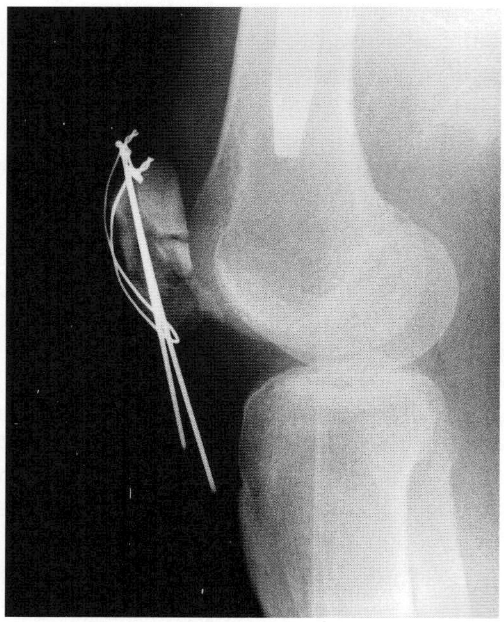

Figure 20.4. Anteropostero (AP) and lateral x-rays show unnecessarily prominent hardware inferiorly. This fixation led to pain with therapy and late stiffness.

Loss of Reduction and Loss of Fixation

Surgical error is the most common cause of loss of reduction. Recognition of the degree of comminution as well as the quality of bone available to support the chosen method of fixation are important factors in preventing loss of reduction. The type of fixation used should be influenced by the degree of comminution, fracture pattern, and surgeon expertise.

Tension band wiring is the most versatile and commonly used method for the fixation of patellar fractures (Fig. 20.5). One should include both pins and wires to prevent loss of reduction (Fig. 20.3). Additional Kirschner wires (K-wires) can be added in comminuted fracture patterns. The tension band wire can either be in a figure-of-8 or cerclage fashion. The authors prefer bending both ends of the pins to prevent migration and loss of fixation (Fig. 20.6).

Apart from the standard tension band method presented, there are many techniques available for open reduction and internal fixation of the patella, and numerous biomechanical studies have been performed test-

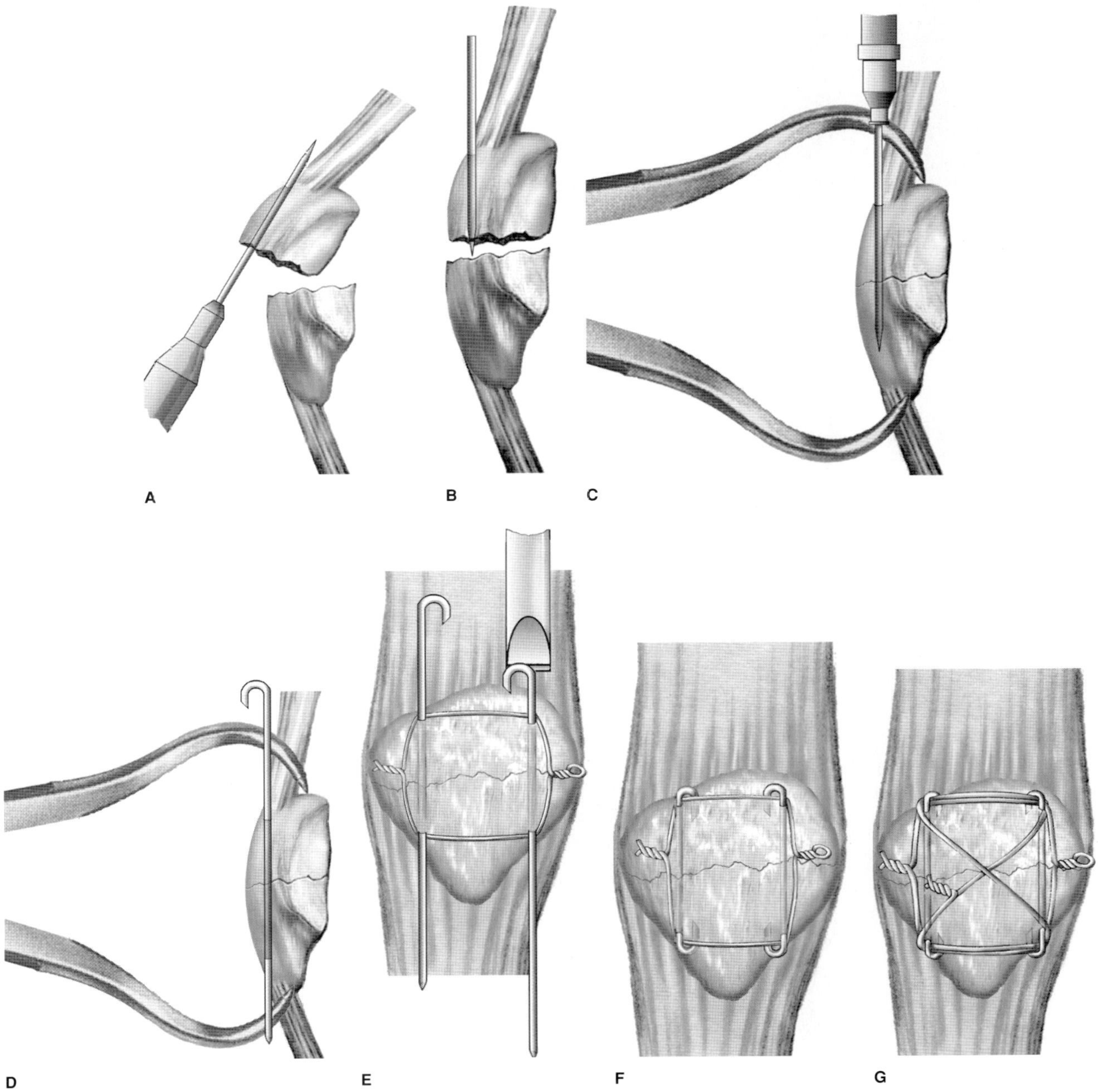

Figure 20.5. **A–G:** Modified AO technique of tension band wiring.

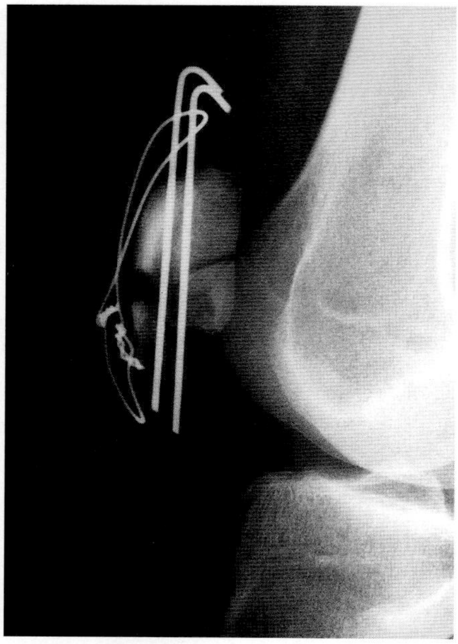

Figure 20.6. Migration of wires and loss of fixation. Bending both ends of the wire can help to prevent this complication.

ing the integrity of these various methods of fixation (Fig. 20.7). Burvant et al[25] compared the modified tension band, anterior tension band with cerclage wire (the Pyrford technique), tension band with cancellous screws, cerclage wire and cancellous screws, and cancellous screws alone in a cadaveric study of transverse patellar fractures. They found that all methods functioned adequately (no fracture gap exceeding 1 mm), but the method of tension banding supplemented with cancellous screws performed best in preventing loss of reduction. Those authors surmised that the addition of screws helped provide compression at the fracture site throughout a full range of motion.

In a similar study, the mechanical properties of the modified tension band (AO technique), two parallel 4.5-mm interfragmentary lag screws and two 4-mm cannulated screws with a tension band through the screws were compared for transverse patellar fractures. The modified tension band technique was found to be the least effective of the three in preventing fracture separation. Fractures fixed with cannulated screws and a tension band demonstrated failure at higher loads than screws alone, followed by patellae with tension band alone.[26]

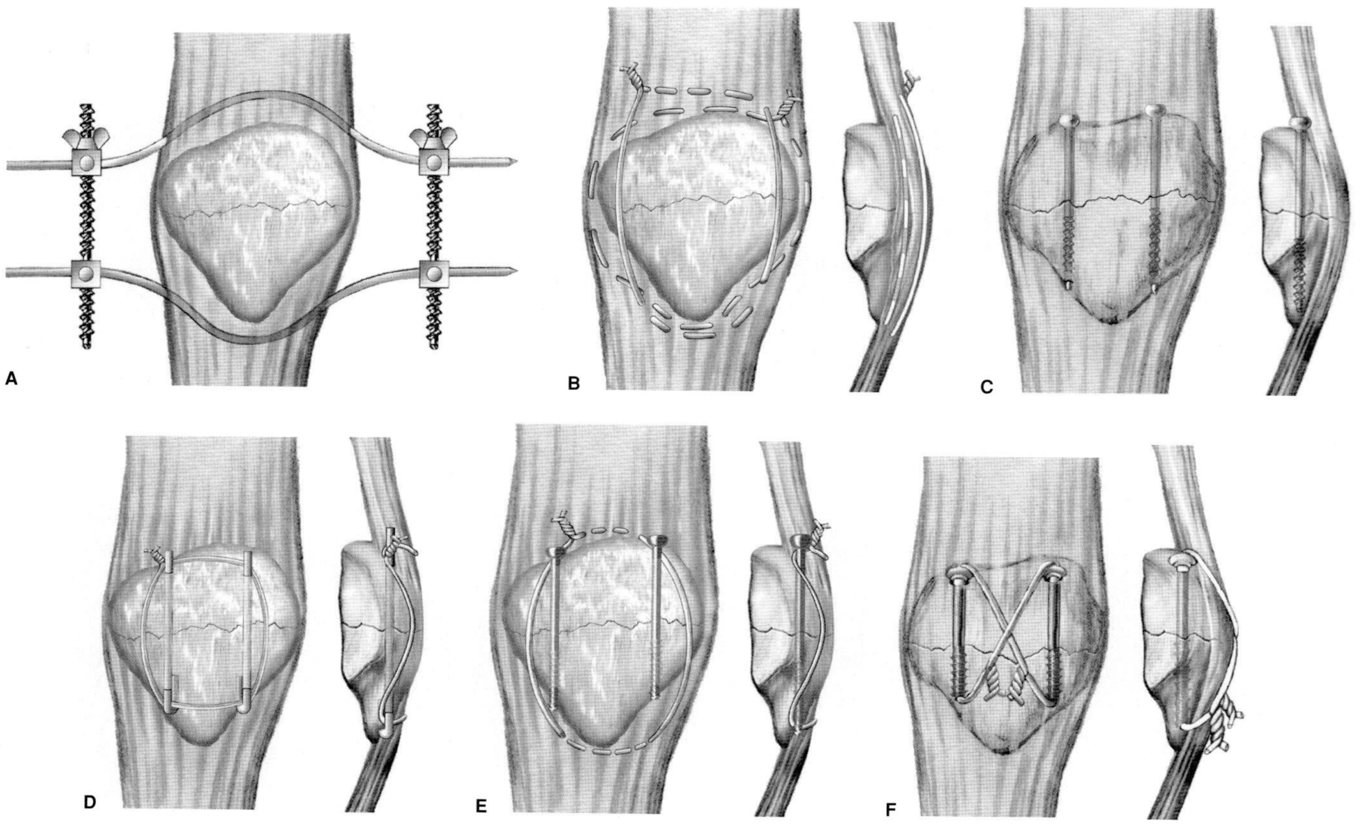

Figure 20.7. **A–F:** Six methods of fixation for transverse patellar fractures.

These studies suggest that, in transverse patellar fractures with good bone quality, interfragmentary screw fixation is superior to the modified tension band technique in preventing loss of reduction. The use of a tension band through cannulated screws provided additional strength and should be considered. One should remember, however, that these studies utilized a simple, transverse fracture pattern model. In the more comminuted fractures or complex fracture patterns, the modified tension band technique is still a very versatile and viable option. Likewise, when dealing with fractures of a petite patella, it may be difficult to use the somewhat larger screws.

Augmentation of open reduction and internal fixation (ORIF) with a load-sharing cable has been shown to be effective in preventing loss of reduction. This cable loops through a drill hole in the proximal tibia and over the superior pole of the patella. It is strongly recommended to augment the repair of an inferior pole patella fracture (Fig. 20.8). A load-sharing cable can also be used to reinforce a tenuous tension band wire repair.

A study performed by Perry[27] compared the stability of patellar fixation protected with a load-sharing cable against tension banding or interfragmentary fixation alone. For both methods the addition of a load-sharing cable resulted in a statistically lower incidence of failure. In the clinical portion of the same study, the increased stability offered by the cable allowed for earlier postoperative mobilization than with standard fixation techniques alone.

Patient compliance is an extremely important factor in preventing loss of reduction. The management of postoperative mobilization should depend on the stability of the reduction, but be modified according to the ability or willingness of the patient to comply with therapy recommendations. Frequently the surgeon must balance the potential complications of loss of reduction versus loss of motion.

Osteoarthritis

Posttraumatic osteoarthritis of the patella can be minimized by accurate fracture reduction and stable fixation. It is important to inspect the articular surface at the time of reduction, either directly via arthrotomy, or indirectly via fluoroscopy or arthroscopy (Fig. 20.9). While direct articular cartilage damage at the time of injury is unpreventable, every effort should be made to avoid additional insults to the articular cartilage during fixation.

The patella is no longer thought of as expendable due to its important role in the biomechanics of the extensor mechanism. In general every effort should be made to salvage as much of the patella as possible following fracture. At times, though, this is not possible secondary to extensive comminution or contamination, and excision of part or all of the patella is necessary.

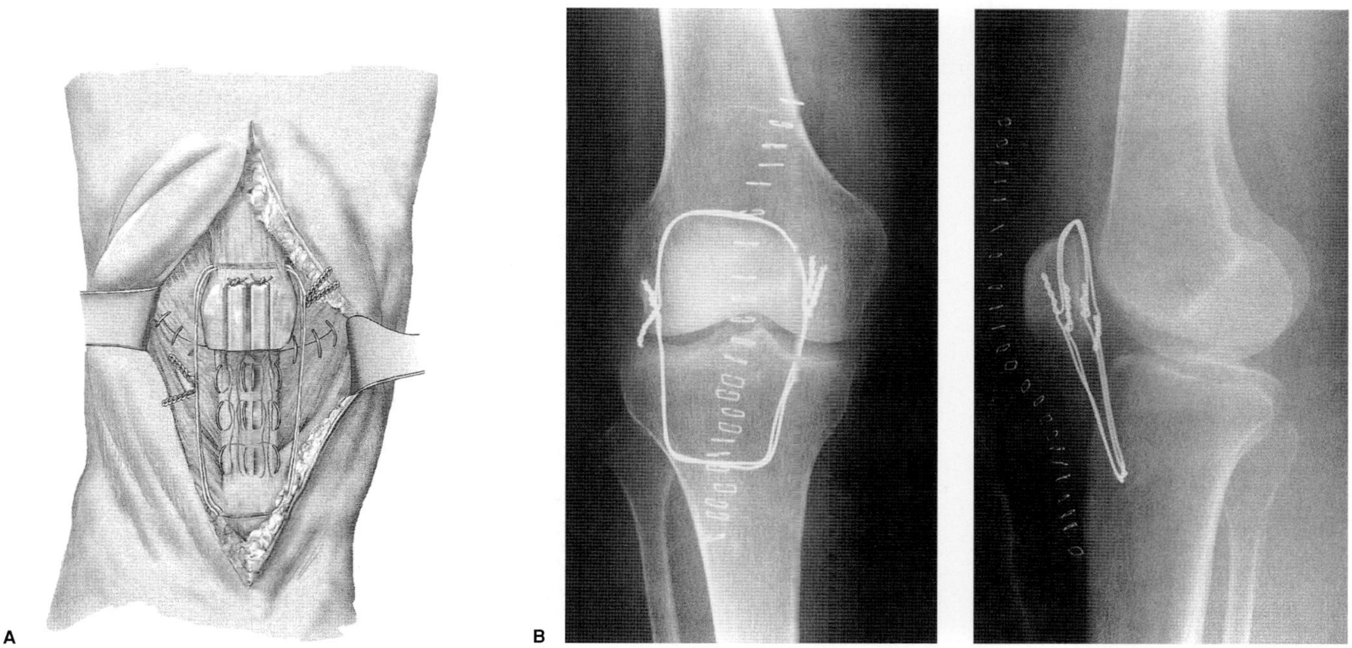

Figure 20.8. Load-sharing cable. A: Repair of an inferior pole patella fracture with debridement of comminuted inferior pole fragments; the patellar tendon is sutured to the remaining patella utilizing three drill holes. B: AP and lateral x-rays depicting doubly tensioned dual wires to protect repair.

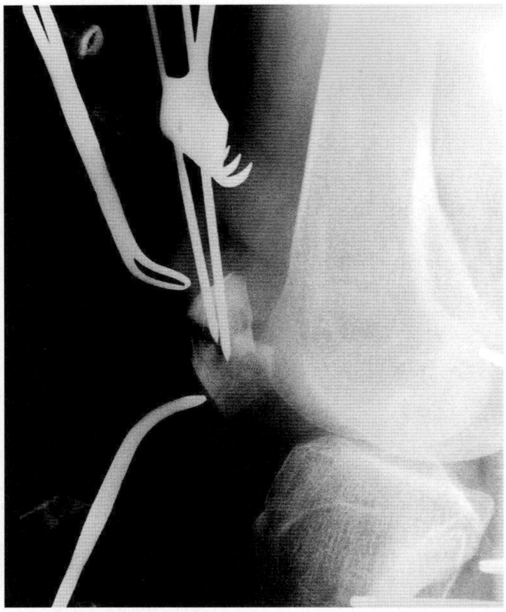

Figure 20.9. Prevention of osteoarthritis is prevention of malreduction. In surgery the dorsal surface appears congruent but the articular surface has a 5-mm step-off due to bone loss in this open fracture. The use of an accessory arthrotomy, intraoperative x-ray, intraoperative fluoroscopy, or arthroscopic assistance is the standard of care to prevent malunion.

Complete patellectomy can eliminate the rapid onset of patellofemoral arthritis, but at the expense of extensor strength (Fig. 20.10).

If the fracture is treated by partial patellectomy, the manner in which the patellar tendon is reattached is critical. Thirty years ago it was felt that if the tendon was reattached too far anteriorly, posterior rotation of the patella would occur, leading to an increased incidence of osteoarthritis, and posterior reattachment was recommended.[28] Recent studies have demonstrated that an anterior reattachment of the patellar tendon following partial patellectomy significantly decreases the contact stresses of the patellofemoral joint with excision of less than 60% of the patella. Following excision of greater than 60% of the patella, the placement of the patellar tendon had no effect on patellofemoral contact stress.[29]

Symptomatic Hardware

Hardware irritation is difficult to prevent secondary to the subcutaneous position of the patella. Obviously one must be aware that the hardware becomes more prominent with flexion (Fig. 20.11). Screws, although less irritating than wires, are more difficult to insert and remove. Wire knots and the bent ends of the K-wires should never be prominent, and attempts should be made to bury the more irritating surfaces within available soft tissue. Wires may stretch less than braided suture, but often fail months or years later (Fig. 20.12). The fragments may migrate into the surrounding soft tissues and become irritating. Heavy, braided suture is an option.

Infection

Prevention of infection following ORIF of patellar fractures begins with the basics of aseptic technique, appropriate antibiotics pre- and postoperatively, and

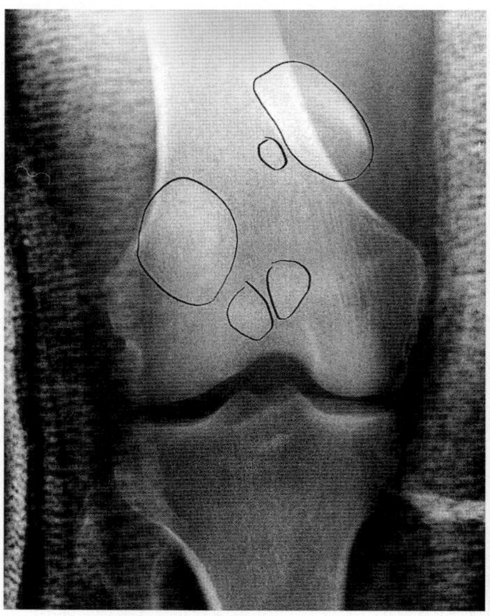

A

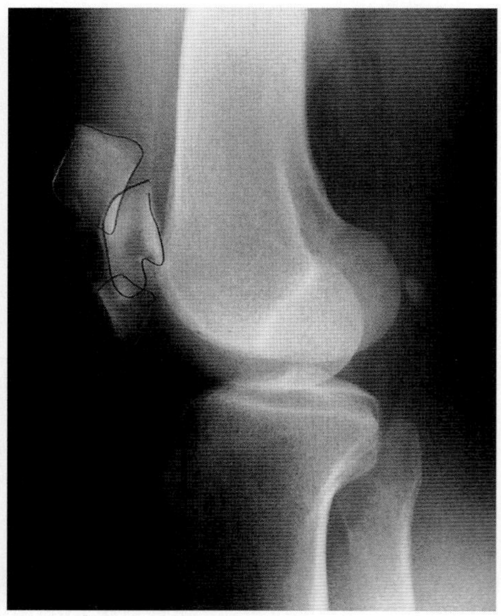

B

Figure 20.10. Patellectomy. AP and lateral x-rays show a severely comminuted patella fracture with disruption of the extensor mechanism. To avoid the likelihood of arthritis, patellectomy can be considered but at some expense of extensor strength.

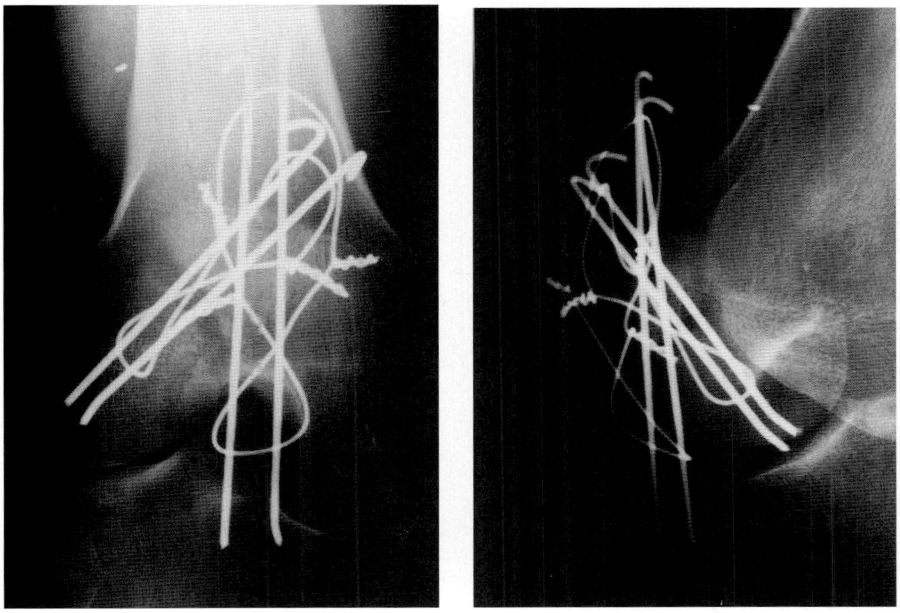

A B

Figure 20.11. AP and oblique x-rays show excessively prominent hardware.

meticulous care when handling the surrounding soft tissues. A midline, longitudinal skin incision is the preferred approach in most cases (least disvascular, most extensile, and more accommodating to revision surgery) (Fig. 20.13). A brief period of postoperative immobilization in extension may be necessary to protect injured soft tissues and prevent wound healing problems in some cases. Early detection and treatment of an infection may help prevent chondrolysis, septic arthritis, and osteomyelitis.

Open fractures are treated with immediate irrigation and debridement (repeated in 36 to 72 hours as needed), longer courses of antibiotics, and timing of fracture fixation based on wound contamination. Fracture fixation

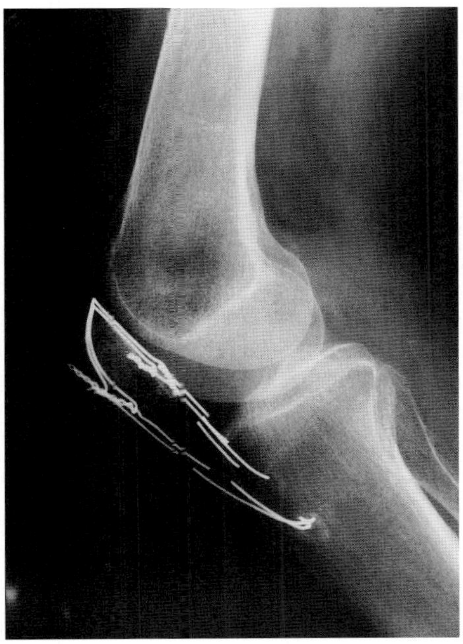

Figure 20.12. Late wire failure as a source of hardware irritation.

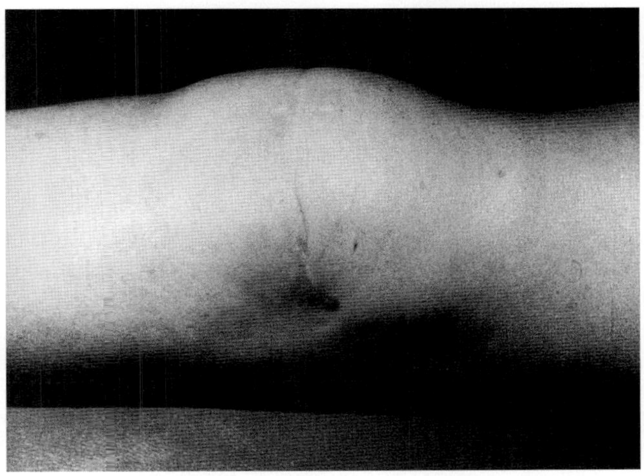

Figure 20.13. Transverse incision. Later surgery such as knee replacement is jeopardized by previous transverse incision.

should be delayed only in the most contaminated of cases. Bone grafting should be performed in a delayed fashion to minimize the risk of infection in open fractures.

Current antibiotic recommendations for grade I and II (Gustilo classification[22]) open fractures include 3 days of a first-generation cephalosporin (generally cefazolin, 1 g every 8 hours) intravenously, and for grade III open fractures, 5 days of cefazolin and gentamicin (2 mg/kg adjusted to serum levels). Addition of penicillin, 4 million units IV every 6 hours, is recommended for wounds with gross contamination (e.g., barnyard, lake, stream) to cover anareobic organisms (including *Clostridium perfringens* and *Clostridium septicum*, which can cause gas gangrene).[30] Immunization against *Colstridium tetani* also needs to be undertaken.

Open fractures of the patella represent a high-energy injury, involving not only bone but also the surrounding soft tissue.[31] Torchia and Lewallen[21] reported a postoperative deep infection rate of 10.7% with open patella fractures and noted a correlation between the incidence of postoperative infection and the magnitude of soft tissue injury. Their series included 57 open patella fractures treated with either ORIF or partial patellectomy. None of the grade I or II open fractures treated with immediate rigid internal fixation became infected, and they recommend immediate internal fixation of grade I and II open patella fractures. In the same series partial patellectomy of open, highly comminuted fractures provided results similar to those less comminuted fractures treated with internal fixation. Therefore, removal of contaminated, loose fragments may decrease the rate of infection. A 29% infection rate (two of seven patients) occurred following cerclage wiring, possibly due to circumferential damage to the surrounding blood supply.

When soft tissue coverage is necessary following an open patella fracture, usually a rotational gastrocnemius pedicle flap will suffice. If this not an option, a free flap (rectus abdominis, latissimus dorsi, etc.) is acceptable. It is important to avoid desiccation of the extensor mechanism and cartilage surfaces, as appropriate soft tissue management can aid in healing and prevent infection and chondrolysis.

When treating a fracture in a damaged soft tissue envelope, external fixation or percutaneous suture repair may seem advantageous. Unfortunately, in this anatomic region external fixation can be bulky and poorly tolerated by the patient. In addition, it carries with it the risk of secondary pin tract and late infections, and a tendency toward malreduction. Fracture displacement may be difficult to reduce percutaneously because of entrapped hematoma or soft tissue. A tendency toward anterior separation of the fracture gap with percutaneous suture repair has been noted.[32] The authors have not found this technique to be particularly reliable.

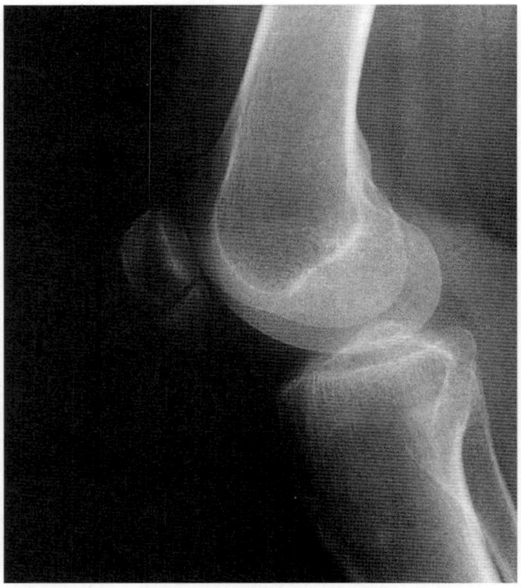

Figure 20.14. Subtle fibrous nonunion 7 months after the diagnosis of knee contusion.

Nonunion

Nondisplaced, fibrous nonunions are associated with late diagnosis. These fractures may have been inappropriately treated following the assumption of knee contusion and failure to obtain an x-ray (Fig. 20.14). Diagnosis may also be difficult in the head-injured, intubated, or polytrauma patient. The treatment of the nonunion is more difficult than that of the initial fracture, especially when the extensor mechanism becomes fixed in a shortened position (Fig. 20.15).

Attention to the basic tenets of fracture treatment cannot be overemphasized. Stable fracture fixation and attention to the blood supply and soft tissue envelope are crucial. Loss of fixation is contributory. Excessive motion at the fracture site due to unstable fixation may encourage fibrous tissue proliferation at the fracture site. Conversely, rigid stabilization with a fixed fracture gap is equally as deleterious. Incongruous bone edges can be debrided and the patellar stability and joint congruity can be improved by slightly shortening the patella. Supplemental bone grafting (autologous iliac crest) should always be considered.

Avascular Necrosis

Initial wide fragment separation and transverse fractures through the body are factors that may predispose the patella to AVN. Treatment with circumferential wiring has also been identified as a possible culprit and should be avoided.[23] Preservation of blood supply is the key to prevention.

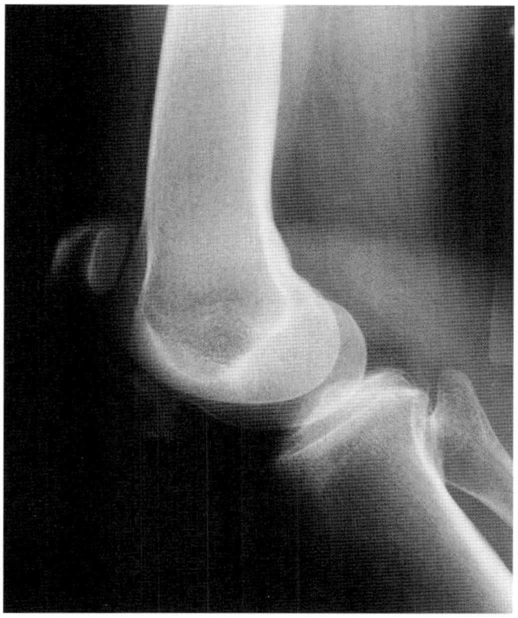

Figure 20.15. Missed patella fracture in a polytrauma patient. Treatment of the nonunion more difficult secondary to a shortened extensor mechanism.

TREATMENT OF COMPLICATIONS

Knee Stiffness

Aggressive physical therapy should begin during the process of fracture healing. If the patient fails to improve, then manipulation under anesthesia should be considered (Fig. 20.16). The surgeon should appreciate the amount of fracture healing as well as the integrity of the extensor mechanism and exercise extreme care during manipulation (especially following partial patellectomy). Noble and Hayek[33] reported a case of a boutonnière-type deformity of the knee following manipulation. Knee arthroscopy and lysis of adhesions as well as medial and/or lateral releases may also be necessary depending on the degree of patellar restriction. Hardware removal may occasionally be of benefit.

Quadricepsplasty and lysis of adhesions is reserved for the most extreme cases of arthrofibrosis (see Chapter 19, Fig. 19.41). This procedure is particularly useful when there has been concomitant injury to the distal femur and subsequent scarring and adhesion of the extensor mechanism along the distal femur. A modified Judet quadricepsplasty[34] involves the disinsertion and sliding of the quadriceps tendon. A lateral approach is used initially beginning at the level of the knee joint and may be extended proximally to within 4 to 5 cm of the greater trochanter, depending on the exposure necessary. A lateral capsulotomy is performed and lateral

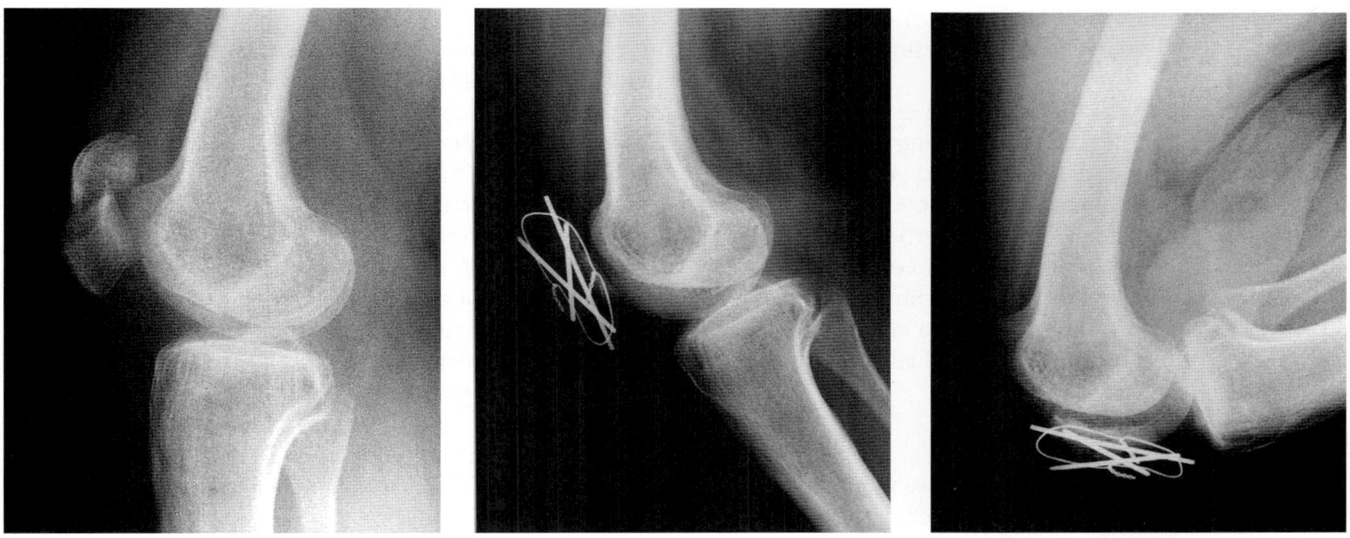

A B C

Figure 20.16. Manipulation under anesthesia to treat arthrofibrosis. **A:** Stellate fracture of the patella with limited disruption of the retinaculam but significant intraarticular stepoff. **B:** Arthroscopic-assisted open reduction and internal fixation (ORIF) resulted in union but with limitation of motion to 30 degrees of flexion. **C:** Active flexion after manipulation 3 months following initial surgery.

patellofemoral and suprapatellar pouch adhesions are released. The vastus lateralis and vastus intermedius are completely freed from the femur and the linea aspera, and if further release is necessary, the rectus femorus can be released from the pelvis. The authors do not recommend transection of the rectus femoris in the supracondylar region. If necessary an anteromedial incision may be used to free medial patellofemoral adhesions, the vastus medialis, the medial capsule, and other intrinsic contractures. Tight intrinsic and extrinsic contractures are released sequentially until the desired range of motion is obtained. Alternatively, the mentioned releases may be performed through an anterior incision that has wide medial and lateral skin flaps. The wound is closed over a drain and may be splinted in flexion. If patellar fixation allows, continuous passive range of motion is useful, and in certain cases can be supplemented postoperatively with a epidural anesthesia.

Significant losses in extension are less common. When present the common etiologies include a disrupted or redundant extensor mechanism or, conversely, a fixed flexion contracture of the posterior capsule (intrinsic) or hamstrings (extrinsic). Due to the risk of popliteal neurovascular injury, manipulation has a limited role in these situations.

Treatment of a disrupted extensor mechanism consists of repair of the involved structures. Reconstruction may be augmented by various methods (see Nonunion/Malunion, below). Imbrication may be useful for redundant tissue. Loss of the patellar lever arm following total patellectomy may result in an extensor lag and weakness.[16] The Maquet procedure moves the patella tendon forward, theoretically increasing the mechanical advantage.

Posterior capsular release may be considered for intrinsic flexion contractures. Hamstring lengthening or release is at times also necessary to address extrinsic contracture. In an extreme case, one could utilize a gradual correction via a multiplanar external fixator with a hinge placed near the instantaneous center of rotation of the knee. Slight distraction of the joint prevents chondrolysis. Postoperative immobilization in extension is required following either acute or gradual correction.

Loss of Reduction

The treatment of loss of patella fracture reduction should be individualized to the patient and fracture. X-rays should be obtained with the knee in full extension prior to revision. If reduction is achieved, a limited course of extension splinting may be successful. In patients with minimal displacement, treatment with a cylinder cast in full extension is recommended until healing is demonstrated.

Reoperation is indicated if there is greater than 3 to 4 mm of displacement or greater than 2 mm of articular step-off. As mentioned previously, conformation of an anatomic or near-anatomic reduction and attention to a sound biomechanical surgical technique can usually avoid this complication. Unfortunately, even in the best of hands, loss of reduction of the articular and nonarticular surfaces can occur with or without ultimate biomechanical failure of the construct.

Treatment requires revision of the initial construct, and is directed toward the "weak link" in the construct. If the wire tension band fails, one must add more wires, often of thicker gauge. Knot breakage can be avoided by the use of the modern crimped cable systems. Kirschner pin migration is addressed by bending each end into soft tissue of bone. Failure due to cutting out hardware should be treated with placement in more sound bone, or limitation of early motion as indicated.

Partial patellectomy can be a reasonable option if one of the bony fragments is particularly comminuted or small. This is especially common with inferior pole fractures. Total patellectomy is reserved for those situations involving the most severe degrees of comminution or osteopenia. One should remember that an augmentation loop may be added in revision surgery whether a patellectomy is performed or not (Fig. 20.17). Unfortunately, the chance of success seems inversely proportional to the number of operations performed.

Osteoarthritis

Initial treatment of posttraumatic arthritis of the patella should consist of physical therapy, injection, and nonsteroidal antiinflammatories. Debridement generally provides limited relief of pain. The authors have limited experience with arthroscopy for the treatment of posttraumatic arthritis of the patellofemoral joint. Anteriorization of the tibial tubercle has been recommended by some. Theoretically this alters the contact pressures of the patellofemoral joint and may provide pain relief. The Maquet procedure is usually indicated only for young patients with intractable knee pain.[35] Patient selection is vital, and this procedure should be considered for salvage purposes only.

Results following patellectomy for patellofemoral degenerative joint disease are still controversial. There are conflicting reports concerning the pain-reducing effects of patellectomy.[36] Despite early favorable results, others have been more skeptical. Kaufer[2] demonstrated a 15% to 30% increase in the force necessary to produce full extension after patellectomy. Smillie[37] asserted that patellectomy frequently led to the loss of the first 5 to 15 degrees of extension, and loss of protection of the exposed femoral condyles. Lind[38] concluded that the pain-reduc-

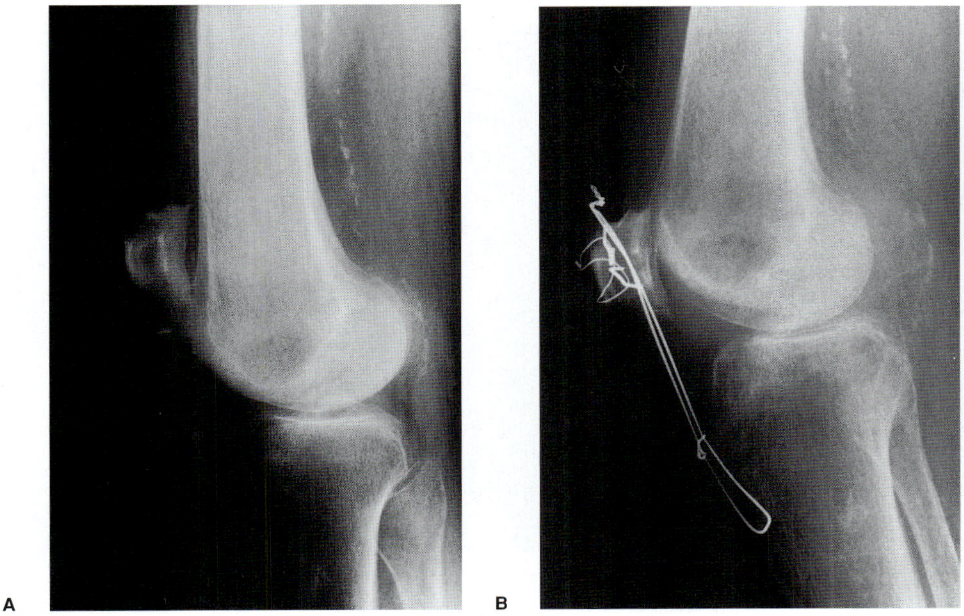

Figure 20.17. Loss of reduction of an inferior pole patella fracture. A: Disruption of the repair following simple suturing of patellar bone fragments together. B: Revision surgery including augmentation loop to protect the repair of tendon into the comminuted remaining patella.

ing effect of patellectomy is generally poor. Fewer than 50% of those who underwent patellectomy for osteoarthritis had an excellent or good result. However, Lind emphasized that the less satisfactory results were obtained when there was concomitant tibiofemoral osteoarthritis.

A more favorable experience was published by West.[39] In six of eight knees undergoing patellectomy for patellofemoral arthritis, the results were excellent or good. Patellectomy appears best indicated in cases of severe, isolated patellofemoral arthritis and pain to justify the subjective symptoms of weakness and some quadriceps atrophy that are to be expected postoperatively.[36] Patellectomy does allow for total knee replacement down the road with satisfactory results.[40]

Patellofemoral arthroplasty (prosthetic resurfacing of the patella and femoral groove) may also play a role in those patients with isolated patellofemoral osteoarthritis. In one study, the best results were obtained for patellar dislocation or fracture as compared to primary osteoarthritis or dysplasia.[41] In another study evaluating 22 patellofemoral arthroplasties, 86% of the patients had good results when the presence of tibiofemoral arthritis was excluded. No cases of mechanical failure were noted at follow-up of 5.3 years.[42] Other authors have reported varied success and note no advantage over total replacement in general.[43]

In summary, the treatment of patellofemoral arthritis can be extremely unrewarding. The authors reserve the Maquet procedure for relatively young patients with moderate, isolated patellofemoral arthritis. Total patellectomy is recommended for young and middle-aged patients with severe patellofemoral arthritis. Prosthetic replacement should be considered only in older patients, and combined with tibial-femoral replacement for multicompartment disease.

Symptomatic Hardware

The treatment of symptomatic hardware is often simple: if it hurts and it's healed, take it out. The possibility of refracture must be discussed. If it hurts and it's not healed, two options exist. First, depending on the degree of patient discomfort, the fracture should be ideally permitted to fully unite prior to removal. Second, revision of prominent hardware prior to healing is indicated to allow for patient compliance with physical therapy (Fig. 20.18). The authors do not advocate immobilization as reasonable treatment for symptomatic hardware.

Infection

Wound healing problems (or delayed healing) immediately postoperatively need to be differentiated from infection and should be managed with local wound care and immobilization until healing is complete. Occasionally patients respond best to surgical debridement and delayed primary closure. Rarely, split-thickness grafting or muscle flaps (pedicle or free) may be necessary.

Superficial wound infections should be treated with intravenous antibiotics, local wound care, and immobilization. Irrigation and debridement may be required depending on the degree of soft tissue involvement. If a deep infection is suspected, aspiration through an un-

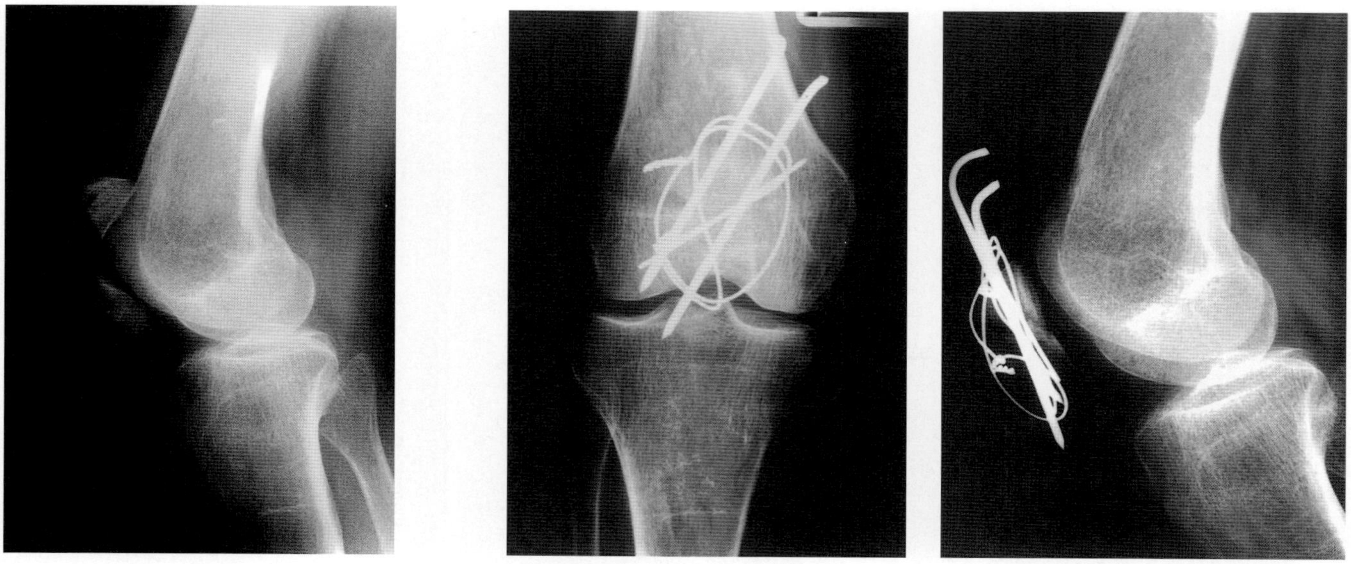

A B

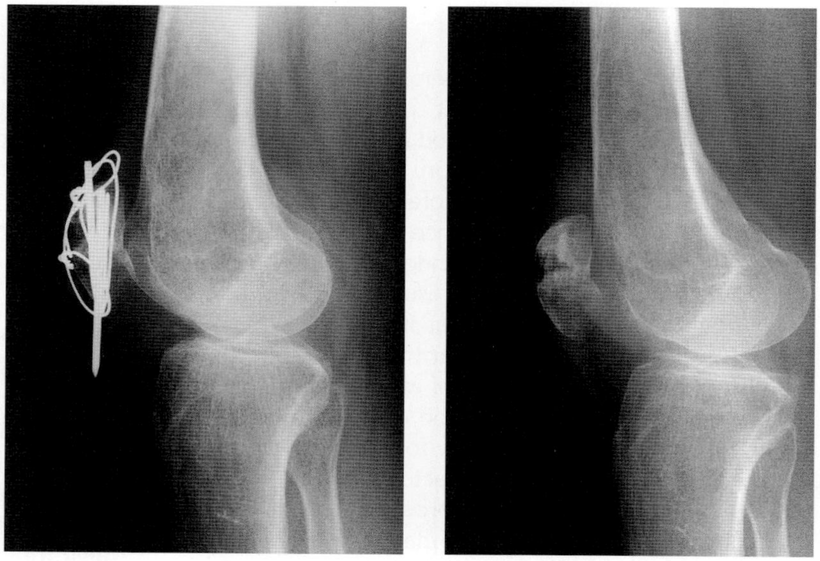

Figure 20.18. Prominent hardware and multiple surgeries. **A:** Simple transverse fracture with retinacular disruption. **B:** AP and lateral x-rays show ORIF with oversized pins prominent superiorly. **C:** Pain with flexion due to prominent pins necessitated revision prior to bony union. These pins subsequently migrated inferiorly. **D:** Union and an excellent clinical result despite some malunion. The patient had a total of three surgeries, however.

C D

involved area may be helpful in making the diagnosis. The treatment of deep infections depends on several variables: the stage of fracture healing, the stability of the fixation, and the degree of bony involvement. All should be treated with culture-specific antibiotics and formal irrigation and debridement. In wound infections prior to fracture healing with stable fixation and viable bone, the hardware may initially be left in and treated by irrigation and debridement. The wound is left to heal via secondary intention or with delayed primary closure over drains (Fig. 20.19). If infection persists, one should search for any devitalized bone and consider partial patellectomy. The timing of hardware removal is crucial. Premature removal can lead to extensor mechanism disruption with proximal retraction of the quadriceps. Delayed removal can contribute to persistent infection. In severe cases total patellectomy may be the treatment of choice. Sequential debridements are performed until it is felt the infection has cleared. Infections that develop after fracture healing are somewhat easier to manage. They should be treated with hardware removal in addition to debridement.

In the treatment of extensor mechanism infections one must be certain that the remainder of the knee joint is clear of infection. Septic arthritis, if present, may require multiple debridements in addition to antibiotics.

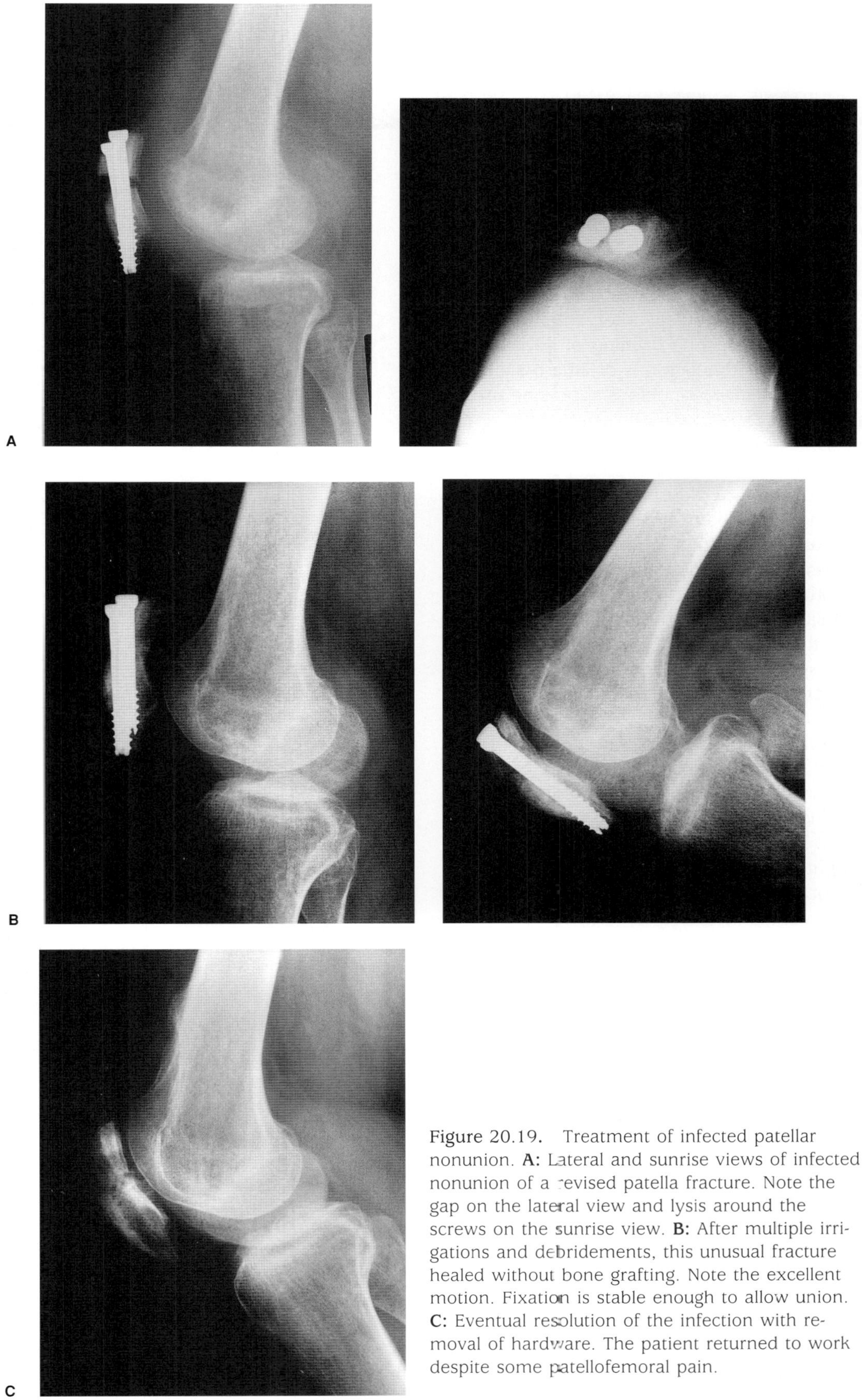

Figure 20.19. Treatment of infected patellar nonunion. **A:** Lateral and sunrise views of infected nonunion of a revised patella fracture. Note the gap on the lateral view and lysis around the screws on the sunrise view. **B:** After multiple irrigations and debridements, this unusual fracture healed without bone grafting. Note the excellent motion. Fixation is stable enough to allow union. **C:** Eventual resolution of the infection with removal of hardware. The patient returned to work despite some patellofemoral pain.

Postinfectious arthritis of the knee, if severe, is best managed by an arthrodesis achieved by external fixation. Ancient septic arthritis may be managed with a total knee arthroplasty with an acceptable infection rate as long as the infection is truly ancient.

Nonunion/Malunion

Patellar delayed unions, once identified, should be treated initially with relative rest and observation. They will usually unite without surgical intervention. Occasionally one may consider bone grafting or revision of the construct. Electrical stimulation is of little benefit.[44]

The treatment of patellar nonunions should be predicated on the patient's symptoms. Asymptomatic nonunions (painless, no extensor mechanism weakness) should be observed. This is especially so in patients with a low function demand. Extensive reconstruction of patellar nonunions should be reserved for those patients with pain and weakness. In a report of 20 patellar nonunions, Klassen and Trousdale[45] concluded that minimally symptomatic delayed unions or nonunions can be successfully treated nonoperatively, knowing that the majority of the fractures will not unite. Operative management of symptomatic patients is recommended and can be expected to achieve union and increase function of the knee.

Surgical treatment should consist of excision of intervening fibrous tissue followed by internal fixation. Tension banding with cannulated screws, compression screw fixation (Fig. 20.20), or modified tension banding is acceptable. Bone grafting may or may not be necessary. Partial patellectomy should be considered if stable fixation is not possible due to poor bone stock or if the nonunion is secondary to AVN.

Satku and Kumar[46] describe treatment of patellar nonunions with modified tension banding and achieved excellent results in their three cases. Klassen and Trousdale[45] reported union in 12 of the 13 operatively treated nonunions in their series. However, neither series dealt with infected nonunions.

Tissue loss (bone and tendon) presents a particularly challenging problem. Bone defects are best treated with autogenous graft, or with partial or complete patellectomy. Tendon defects (patellar or quadriceps) are best replaced with autogenous tendon[47–50] (semitendinousis, gracilis, fascia lata, quadriceps) or bone-tendon grafts[51–53] (fibular head-biceps femoris, patella-quadriceps, tibia-patellar tendon-patella-quadriceps tendon). Allograft,[54] or artificial materials[55–56] may also be considered. Rarely, Ilizarov external fixation[48] may be utilized in cases of late reconstruction to gradually distract the contracted extensor mechanism (and also protect the reconstruction). Massive extensor mechanism bone-tendon allografts are best avoided if possible. The clinical success of the various grafting options has not been compared. The authors have occasionally utilized both autogenous and allogenous graft materials with success. An augmentation loop should always be considered to help reinforce these constructs.

Patellar malunion treatment is uncommon. The man-

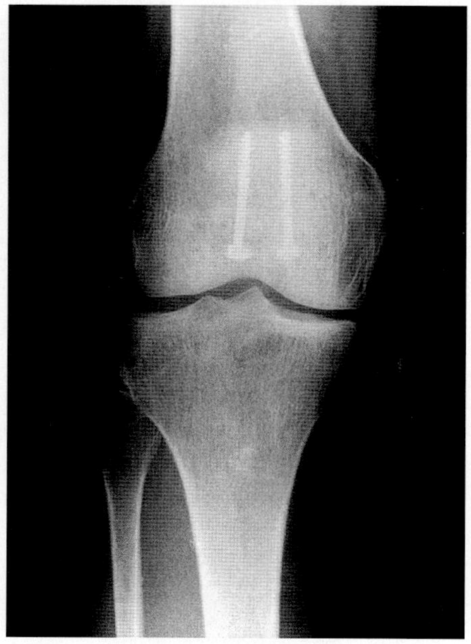

A

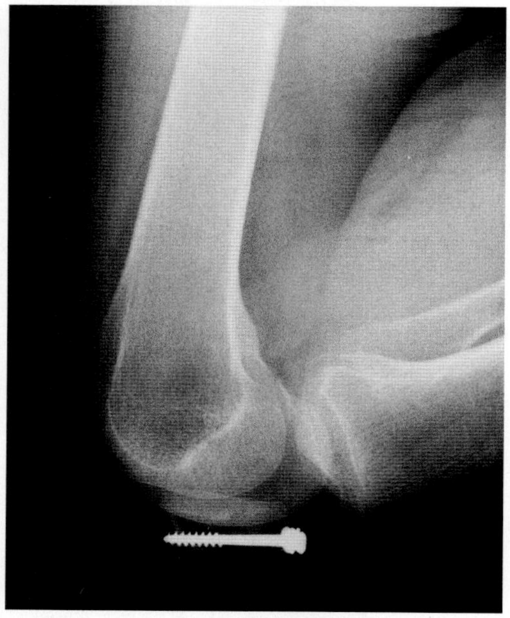

B

Figure 20.20. Treatment of fibrous nonunion (as depicted in Fig. 20.14) with compression screw fixation. AP and lateral views.

agement goals are dependent on patient symptomatology and demand. The goal is the prevention of patellofemoral arthritis. The malunion is taken down and realigned. Solid fixation is then obtained. Indications include a step-off of greater than 2 mm. The surgeon must be sensitive to the risk of trading a small malunion for a big nonunion. The rehabilitation program is then the same as with a fresh fracture, although healing may be more prolonged.

Avascular Necrosis

The natural history of patellar AVN usually entails varying degrees of patellofemoral arthritis. Treatment for avascular necrosis of the patella is generally observation. If patellofemoral arthrosis does develop and the patient is symptomatic, then treatment is as listed for osteoarthrosis.

References

1. Bostrom A. Fractures of the patella: a study of 422 patellar fractures. *Acta Orthop Scand Suppl* 1972;143:1–80.
2. Kaufer H. Mechanical function of the patella. *J Bone Joint Surg* 1971;53A:1551–1560.
3. Goldstein SA, Coate E, Weiss APC, et al. Patellar surface strain. *J Orthop Res* 1986;4:372–377.
4. Matthews LS, Sonstegerd DA, Hanke JA. Load bearing characteristics of the patellofemoral joint. *Acta Orthop Scand* 1977;48:511–516.
5. Carpenter JE, Kasman R, Matthews LS. Fractures of the patella. *J Bone Joint Surg* 1993;75A:1550–1561.
6. Johnson EE. Fractures of the patella. In: Rockwood CA, Green DP, Bucholz RW, et al (eds). *Fractures in Adults.* Philadelphia: Lippincott-Raven, 1996:1956–1972.
7. Malgaigne JF. *Dennis System of Surgery*, vol 1. Philadelphia: Lea Brothers, 1895.
8. Cameron HC. Transverse fractures of the patella. *Glasgow Med J* 1878;10:289–294.
9. Blodgett WE, Fairchild RD. Fractures of the patella. *JAMA* 1936;20:2121–2125.
10. Thompson JEM. Comminuted fractures of the patella: treatment of cases presenting with one large fragment and several smaller fragments. *J Bone Joint Surg* 1935; 17:431–434.
11. Muller ME, Allgower M, Schneider R, et al. *Manual of Internal Fixation. Techniques Recommended by the AO Group.* Berlin: Springer-Verlag, 1979:248–253.
12. Smith ST, Cramer KF, Karges F, et al. Early complications in the operative treatment of patella fractures. *J Orthop Trauma* 1997;11:183–187.
13. Morrey BF. Post-traumatic stiffness: distraction arthroplasty. In: Morrey BF (ed). *The Elbow and Its Disorders*, vol 2. Philadelphia: WB Saunders, 1993:476–491.
14. Cramer KE, Moed BR. Patellar fractures: contemporary approach to treatment. *J AAOS* 1997;5(6):323–331.
15. Nummi J. Fracture of the patella: a clinical study of 707 patellar fractures. *Ann Chir Gynaecol* 1971;60(suppl 179):1–85.
16. Sorensen KH. The late prognosis after fracture of the patella. *Acta Orthop Scand* 1964;34:198–212.
17. Salter RB, Simmonds DF, Malcolm BW, et al. The biological effect of continuous passive motion on the healing of full-thickness defects in articular cartilage. An experimental investigation in the rabbit. *J Bone Joint Surg* 1980;62A:1232–1251.
18. Llinas A, Mckellop HA, Marshall GJ, et al. Healing and remodeling of articular incongruities in a rabbit fracture model. *J Bone Joint Surg* 1993;75A:1508–1523.
19. Hung LK, Lee SY, Leung KM, et al. Partial patellectomy for patellar fracture: tension band wiring and early mobilization. *J Orthop Trauma* 1993;7(3):252–260.
20. Chen Y, Wu C, Hsu R, et al. The intra-articular migration of the broken wire: a rare complication of circumferential wiring in patellar fractures. *Chang Gung Med J* 1994;17(3):276–278.
21. Torchia ME, Lewallen DG. Open fractures of the patella. *J Orthop Trauma* 1996;10(6):403–409.
22. Gustilo RB, Gruninger RP, Davis T. Classification of type III (severe) open fractures relative to treatment and results. *Orthopedics* 1987;10:1781–1788.
23. Scapinelli R. Blood supply of the human patella: its relation to ischemic necrosis after fracture. *J Bone Joint Surg* 1967;49B:563–570.
24. Enneking WF, Berrey BH, Scarborough MT, et al. *Clinical Musculoskeletal Pathology Study Guide.* Gainesville: University of Florida, 1997:section 6, 1–6.
25. Burvant JG, Thomas KA, Alexander R, et al. Evaluation of methods of internal fixation of transverse patella fractures: a biomechanical study. *J Orthop Trauma* 1994; 8(2):147–153.
26. Carpenter JC, Kasman RA, Patel N, et al. Biomechanical evaluation of current patella fracture fixation techniques. *J Orthop Trauma* 1997;11(5):351–356.
27. Perry CR, McCarthy JA, Kain CC, Pearson R L. Patellar fixation protected with a load sharing cable: a mechanical and clinical study. *J Orthop Trauma* 1988;2: 234–240.
28. Duthie HL, Hutchinson JR. The results of partial and total excision of the patella. *J Bone Joint Surg* 1958; 40B:75–81.
29. Marder RA, Swanson TV, Sharkey A, et al. Effects of partial patellectomy and reattachment of the patellar tendon on patellofemoral contact areas and pressures. *J Bone Joint Surg* 1993;75A:35–45.
30. Chapman JW, Olson SA. Open fractures. In: Rockwood C A, Green D P, Bucholz R W, Heckman JD, (eds). *Fractures in Adults.* Philadelphia: Lippincott-Raven, 1996; 305–352.

31. Catalano JB, Iannacone WM, Marczyk S, et al. Open fractures of the patella: long-term functional outcome. *J Trauma* 1995;39:439–444.
32. Ma Y, Zhang Y, Qu K, et al. Treatment of fractures of the patella with percutaneous suture. *Clin Orthop Rel Res* 1984;191:235–241.
33. Noble HH, Hajek MR. Bountonnière-type deformity of the knee following patellectomy and manipulations. *J Bone Joint Surg* 1984;66A:137–138.
34. Ebraheim A, DeTroye RJ, Saddemi SR. Results of Judet quadricepsplasty. *J Orthop Trauma* 1993;7:327–330.
35. Maquet, PGJ. *Biomechanics of the Knee: with Application to the Pathogenesis and Surgical Treatment of Osteoarthrosis*. Berlin: Springer-Verlag, 1976.
36. Shives T C, Morrey B F. Alternative Reconstruction Procedures. In: Moorey BF (ed). *Joint Replacement Arthroplasty*. New York: Churchill Livingstone, 1991;1113–1126.
37. Smillie IS. *Injuries of the Knee Joint*. Baltimore: Williams and Wilkins, 1951.
38. Lind TH. An evaluation of patellectomy for retropatellar pain. *Acta Orthop Belg* 1986;52:831.
39. West FE. End results of patellectomy. *J Bone Joint Surg* 1962;44A:1089–1108.
40. Kang JD, Papas SN, Rubash HE, et al. Total knee arthroplasty in patellectomized patients. *J Arthroplasty* 1993; 8(5):489–501.
41. Argenson J, Guillaume J, Aubaniac J. Is there a place for patellofemoral arthroplasty? *Clin Orthop Rel Res* 1995; 321:162–167.
42. Arciero RA, Toomey HE. Patellofemoral arthroplasty. *Clin Orthop Rel Res* 1988;236:60–71.
43. Insall J, Tria AJ, Agliette P. Resurfacing of the patella. *J Bone Joint Surg* 1980;62A:933–936.
44. Lindsey RW, Grobman J, Leggon RE, et al. Effects of bone graft and electrical stimulation on the strength of healing bony defects in dogs. *Clin Orthop* 1987;222: 275–280.
45. Klassen JF, Trousdale RT. Treatment of delayed and nonunion of the patella. *J Orthop Trauma* 1997;2(3): 188–194.
46. Satku K, Kumar V. Surgical management of non-union of neglected fractures of the patella. *Injury* 1991;22: 108–110.
47. Fukui N, Cho N, Tashiro T, et al. Anatomical reconstruction of the patellar tendon: a new technique with hamstring tendons and iliotibial tract. *J Orthop Trauma* 1999;13:375–379.
48. Isiklar AU, Varner KE, Lindsey RW, et al. Late reconstruction of patellar ligament ruptures using Ilizarov external fixation. *Clin Orthop Rel Res* 1996;322:174–178.
49. Katzman BM, Silberberg S, Caligiuri DA, et al. Delayed repair of a quadriceps tendon. *Orthopedics* 1997;20: 553–554.
50. Larson RV, Simonian PT. Semitendinosus augmentation of acute patellar tendon repair with immediate mobilization. *Am J Sports Med* 1995;23:82–86.
51. Dejour J, Denjean S, Neyret P. Treatment of old or recurrent ruptures of the patellar ligament by a contralateral autograft. *Rev Chir Orthop* 1992;78:58–62.
52. Peyser AB, Makley JT. Patellar tendon reconstruction augmented by a free autograft of the biceps tendon attached to the fibular head. *Orthopedics*. 1996;19:545–549.
53. Williams RJ III, Brooks DD, Wickiewicz TL. Reconstruction of the patellar tendon using a patella-quadriceps tendon autograft. *Orthopedics* 1997;20:554–558.
54. Falconiero RP, Pallis MP. Chronic rupture of a patellar tendon: a technique for reconstruction with Achilles allograft. *Arthroscopy* 1996;12:623–626.
55. Fujikawa K, Ohtani T, Matsumoto H, et al. Reconstruction of the extensor apparatus of the knee with the Leeds-Keio ligament. *J Bone Joint Surg* 1994;76B:200–203.
56. Levin PD. Reconstruction of the patellar tendon using a dacron graft. A case report. *Clin Orthop Rel Res* 1976; 118:70–72.

Chapter 21

FRACTURES AROUND THE KNEE IN CHILDREN

Hormozan Aprin

Fractures around the knee in children include epiphyseal and metaphyseal fractures, injuries of the growth plate, fractures of the distal femur and proximal tibia, avulsion fracture of the tibial spine, fracture of the tibial tubercle, and fracture or dislocation of the patella with osteochondral fractures.

The epiphyseal injuries around the knee are rare, accounting for 1% to 6% of all epiphyseal injuries.[1–3] These injuries can occur at any age in a growing child, with the highest incidence between ages 11 and 15 years. The ligamentous injuries frequently seen in adults are rare in children.[4–7]

The clinical reviews indicate a high incidence of growth disturbances following physeal injuries.[4,5,8] Other complications may occur with a different degree of severity. These include injuries to the popliteal artery[9] and peroneal nerve,[8] stiffness of the knee, quadriceps atrophy, and osteoarthritic changes of the articular cartilage.

Treatment of these injuries requires anatomic reduction of the articular surface and growth plate. The avulsed tendons and ligaments should be repaired. The fractures heal fast in children and the period of immobilization does not exceed 4 to 6 weeks. All patients require a period of rehabilitation to regain strength and motion after a significant knee injury.

SURGICAL ANATOMY

The distal femoral epiphysis contains the medial and lateral condyle. The lateral border of the lateral condyle is in line with the lateral cortex of the diaphysis. Just proximal to the medial border of the medial condyle the metaphysis flares out to the adductor tubercle. On the posterior surface the condyles are separated by a deep intercondylar notch, which extends to the midpoint of each condyle. On the anterior surface the lateral condyle is almost vertical, while the medial condyle is more flattened and C-shaped.[10]

Most of the external surface of the distal femoral epiphysis is covered by the articular cartilage for articulation with the patella and upper tibia. The tibial surface of each femoral condyle extends to the posterior surface, and the articular cartilage reaches the posterior margin of the distal femoral growth plate. The anterior surface of the femoral epiphysis has a shallow concave midline to accommodate the vertical ridge of the undersurface of the patella.

The distal femoral growth plate is horizontal. It extends from the adductor tubercle to just above the lateral epicondyle. It is slightly tilted anteriorly.

The proximal tibial epiphysis has a slightly concave surface. The medial and lateral sides are separated by the anterior and posterior tibial eminence. The distal surface of the tibial epiphysis is concave to match the convex upper end of the proximal tibial metaphysis. The height of the epiphysis is greater on the lateral surface than on the medial side. The growth plate slopes downward and anteriorly, and extends distally under the tibial tubercle. The tibial tubercle is a downward projection of the tongue of the proximal tibial epiphysis.

The position of the growth plate in the distal femur is extraarticular. The suprapatellar pouch bulges up superiorly over the anterior surface of the distal femoral metaphysis. The synovial membrane, posterior capsule, and all the ligaments are attached to the femoral epiphysis, just distal to the growth plate. The medial and lateral collateral ligaments are also attached to the distal femoral epiphysis below the growth plate. The plantaris and two heads of the gastrocnemius muscle originate from the upper margin of the posterior surface of the distal femoral metaphysis. On the tibial side the synovial membrane and the capsule are attached to the proximal tibial epiphysis proximal to the growth plate. The cruciate ligaments are attached to the anterior and posterior tibial eminence. The lateral collateral ligament is attached to the fibula, and the medial collateral ligament is attached to the upper tibial metaphysis beyond the growth plate. The patellar ligament is attached to the tibial tubercle and superficial to the downward extension of the growth plate. The ligament then spans to either side of the tubercle and finally it is connected to the deep fascia in the upper tibial diaphysis. The patellar ligament is reinforced by the medial and lateral retinaculum. The semimembranous tendon inserts on both the epiphyseal and metaphyseal side of the growth plate in the posteromedial corner of the proximal tibia.

The patella is the largest sesamoid bone in the body. It lies deep to the quadriceps tendon, with strong attachment of the extensor mechanism to its surface.

Due to the anatomic position and bony configuration of the knee joint, the stability and strength of the knee is provided by the ligaments and tendons that surround it. A strong force puts tension on the ligaments and strain on the adjacent bone. When the amount of the force exceeds the resistant strength of the bone, the epiphysis will separate from the metaphysis.

The popliteal artery is in close proximity to the posterior surface of the distal femur. It is separated from the distal femoral metaphysis by a thin layer of fat. The superior geniculate arteries are branched just above the femoral condyle. The popliteal artery continues distally and lies on the posterior capsule of the knee joint between the femoral condyles. The middle geniculate artery originates at the level of the joint capsule. The distal portion of the popliteal artery is separated from the posterior aspect of the upper tibia by the popliteus muscle. The inferior geniculate arteries originate at this level and enter the proximal tibial epiphysis. Under the soleal arch, the popliteal artery divides into the anterior and posterior tibial arteries.

The epiphysis of the distal femur and proximal tibia have a rich blood supply from anastomosis of the geniculate arteries. Abundant blood supply in this region makes it less vulnerable to ischemic changes following injuries. The blood supplies of the patella are mainly from the superior and inferior genicular arteries, supreme genicular artery, and anterior recurrent tibial artery.[11,12] Anastomosis from branches of these arteries covers the anterior surface of the patella and enters the patella in the middle third of the patella.

The popliteal artery and its branches are prone to injury from a backward thrusting of the end of the distal femoral metaphysis at the time of the hyperextension injury, or by posterior displacement of the proximal tibial metaphysis during a physeal fracture of the proximal tibia.

Above the popliteal space, the sciatic nerve divides into the peroneal and posterior tibial nerves. The peroneal nerve travels between the biceps femoris muscle and the lateral head of the gastrocnemius muscle, to the level of the neck of the fibula. The stretching of the peroneal nerve can occur during a varus tilt and medial rotation of the distal femoral epiphysis. Moreover, the superficial location of the peroneal nerve subjects it to direct contusion from a blow on the posterolateral aspect of the knee.

CLASSIFICATION OF EPIPHYSEAL FRACTURES

The Salter-Harris classification[13] on the epiphyseal fracture is the most commonly used classification and is based on the radiographic finding of the fractures (Fig. 21.1). Ogden[14] has expanded the Salter-Harris classification by adding more subdivisions based on the different types of the epiphyseal injuries, including intraarticular injuries.

Type I: There is complete separation of the epiphysis from the metaphysis, without any fracture of the epiphysis or metaphysis.

Type II: The fracture is through the epiphyseal plate and extends through the metaphysis. A triangular segment of the metaphysis (Thurston-Holland sign) is attached to the epiphyseal plate.

Type III: The fracture is intraarticular, through the physis, and it extends to the epiphysis.

Type IV: The fracture is intraarticular. The longitudinal fracture line starts from the metaphysis, crosses the growth plate, and exits through the epiphysis.

Type V: The injury entails crushing or impacting of the growth plate with little or no displacement. This type of injury may not be visible on the initial film. In this instance, magnetic resonance imaging (MRI) demonstrates the impaction of the growth plate, marrow edema, and subperiosteal bleeding (Fig. 21.2).

Type VI: Mercer Rang[15] has added this type to the classification. This is a localized injury to the perichondral ring. A small fragment including a portion of the perichondrium and underlying bone is avulsed (Fig. 21.3). This may not be initially appreciated on the x-ray, especially if the avulsed fragment is very small. Following healing of the fracture, the bony bridge may cause angular deformity.

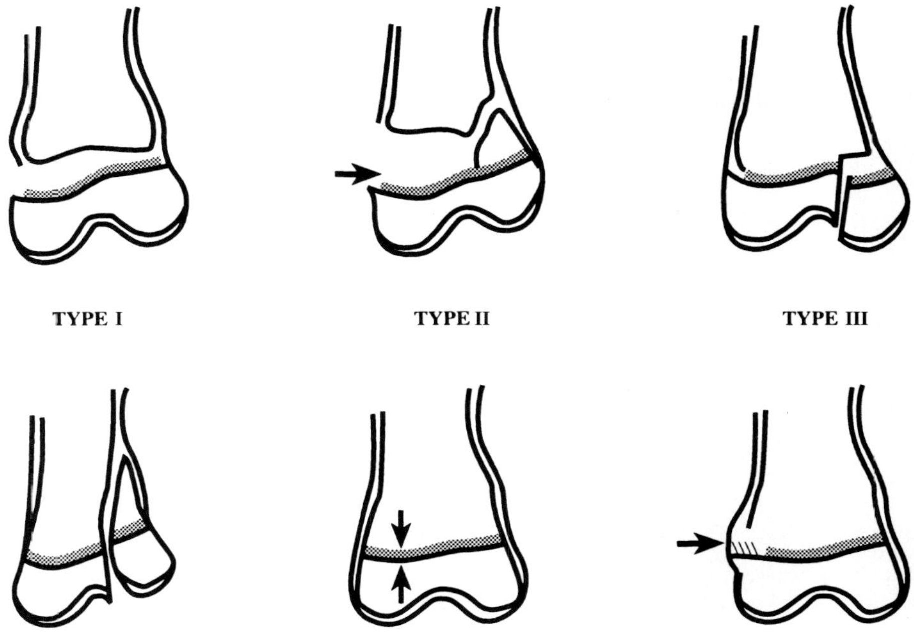

Figure 21.1. Salter-Harris classification of epiphyseal fracture separation (arrows point to epiphyseal plates). Type I fracture involves only the growth plate. The epiphysis is completely separated from the metaphysis without any fractures involving the metaphysis or epiphysis. Type II fracture is through the growth plate and exits through the metaphysis with a triangular segment of the metaphysis attached to the epiphyseal plate. Type III is an intraarticular fracture. The fracture is through the physis and exits through the epiphysis. Type IV is also an intraarticular fracture. The longitudinal fracture line starts from the metaphysis. It crosses the growth plate and exits through the epiphysis. Type V is a crushing or impacting injury of the growth plate with little or no displacement. Type VI is a localized injury to the perichondral ring. A small fragment including a portion of the perichondrium and underlying bone is avulsed. (Redrawn from ref. 15.)

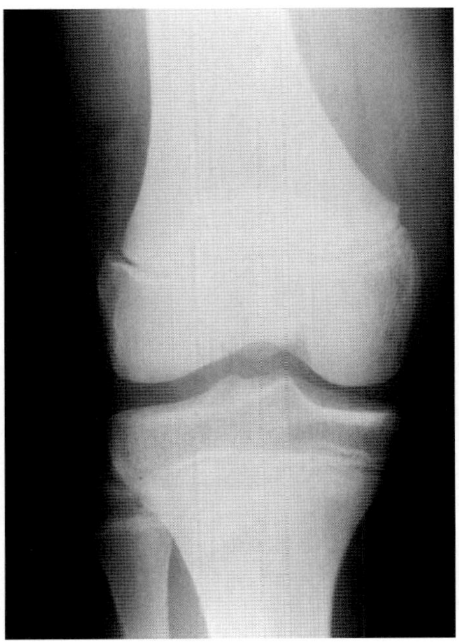

A

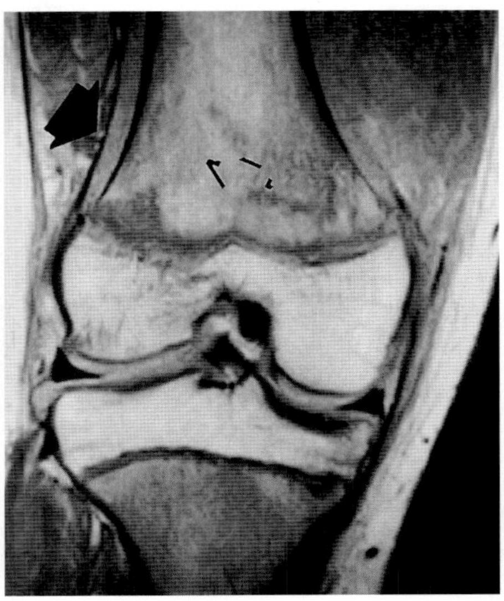

B

Figure 21.2. A Salter-Harris type V fracture may not be visible on the initial x-ray. **A:** The initial x-ray may look normal. **B:** Magnetic resonance imaging (MRI) shows periosteal elevation, subperiosteal bleeding, impaction of the growth plate, and marrow edema in the epiphysis and metaphysis of the distal femur.

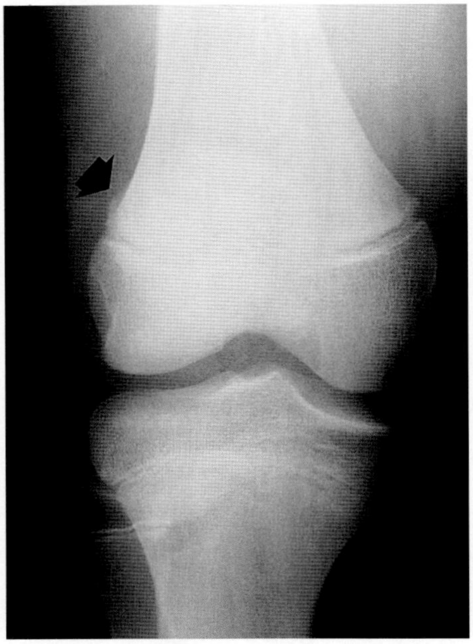

Figure 21.3. In Salter-Harris type VI fracture, the x-ray shows avulsion injury to the edge of the growth plate, with a small fragment of a portion of the perichondrium and underlying bone.

FRACTURES OF THE DISTAL FEMORAL EPIPHYSIS

The growth plate of the distal femur is the largest and most actively growing physis in the body. It covers the 70% of the length of the femur. Most of the ligaments are attached to the epiphysis of the distal femur. The growth plate and metaphysis of the distal femur have minimal ligamentus support. Thus, the distal femoral epiphysis is more prone to fracture separation than is the proximal tibial epiphysis.

Fracture separation of the distal femoral epiphysis is rare, constituting 1% of all the physeal fractures. This fracture can occur at any age in children, with the highest incidence being between ages 11 and 15 years.

Mechanism of Injury

Separation of the distal femoral epiphysis is caused by a sudden severe force applied in the region of the knee joint. The fracture is most often caused by an indirect injury.[16,17] The impact of the force causes compression of the growth plate at the site of the impact and avulsion or separation of the growth plate on the opposite side. The fracture begins with the separation of the epiphysis from the metaphysis on the tension side, and ends with an oblique fracture through the metaphysis on the compression side.

The separation of the distal femoral epiphysis in children between the ages of 6 and 12 years is mostly due to motor vehicle and pedestrian accidents. In older children and adolescents, sports-related injuries are the cause of separation of the distal femoral epiphysis.[5,8] Separation of the distal femoral physis can be detected in newborns at the time of a difficult delivery.[1,18,19] This fracture can occur in other conditions such as arthrogryposis multiplex congenita,[20] myelomeningocele,[21,22] osteomyelitis, and leukemia.

Type of Fracture

Classification of the fracture separation of the distal femoral epiphysis can be based on the anatomic pattern of the separation, or it can be based on the mechanism of injury.

Classification by Anatomic Location

The anatomic classification of Salter-Harris[13] is useful for describing the injury and treatment plan.

Salter-Harris type I is seen in newborns after birth injuries or in adolescents as a nondisplaced separation. Either one may be easily missed. Often the diagnosis is made in retrospect when the subperiosteal new bone formation is seen in the follow-up x-rays (Fig. 21.4). In obvious cases, the displacement is usually seen in the sagittal plane.

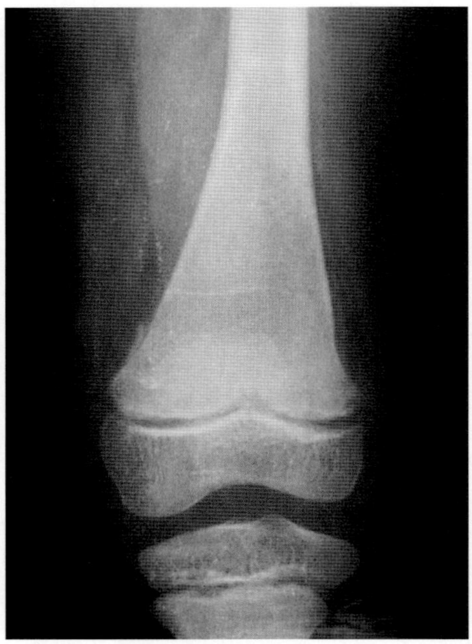

Figure 21.4. X-ray of the knee demonstrates widening of the growth plate and periosteal elevation with subperiosteal reaction, indicating a nondisplaced Salter-Harris type I fracture of the distal femur. (Courtesy of Dr. J. Richard Bowen, A.I. Dupont Institute.)

Salter-Harris type II is the most common type of separation of the distal femoral epiphysis. The displacement is usually in the coronal plane. The triangular metaphyseal fragment is on the side toward which the epiphysis is displaced (Fig. 21.5).

Type III is an intraarticular fracture. The fracture of the femoral condyle can occur in any area, but most of the time it is in line with the intercondylar notch (Fig. 21.6).

Type IV is uncommon. In this type of fracture even a slight displacement may cause premature closure of the growth plate and asymmetrical growth of the distal femur.

Type V may not be diagnosed on the initial x-rays. It is usually recognized at the time of premature growth arrest (Fig. 21.7). In this instance, MRI is very helpful for accurate diagnosis (see Fig. 21.2).

Type VI is an avulsion injury to the edge of the growth plate.[15] A small fragment including a portion of the perichondrium and underlying bone may be detached with the avulsion of the proximal attachment of the collateral ligament (see Fig. 21.3).

Classification by Type of Injury

Fractures involving the distal femoral physis can be divided into the following types according to the direction of the force causing the injury.

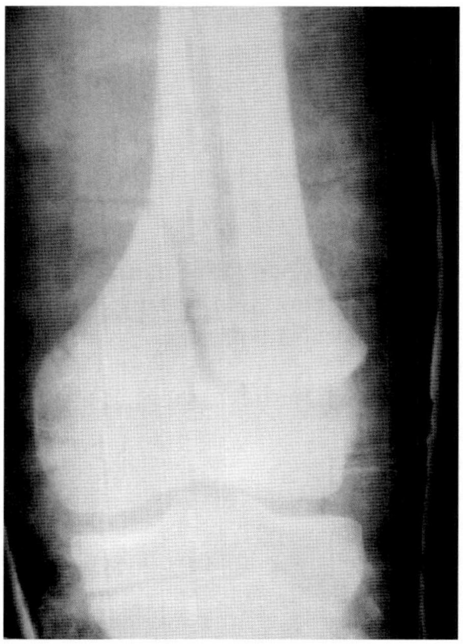

Figure 21.5. In Salter-Harris type II, the fracture line is through the epiphyseal plate and exits through the metaphysis with a triangular segment of the metaphysis attached to the epiphyseal plate. The triangular piece of the metaphysis is on the side toward which the epiphysis is displaced. (Courtesy of Dr. J. Richard Bowen, A.I. Dupont Institute.)

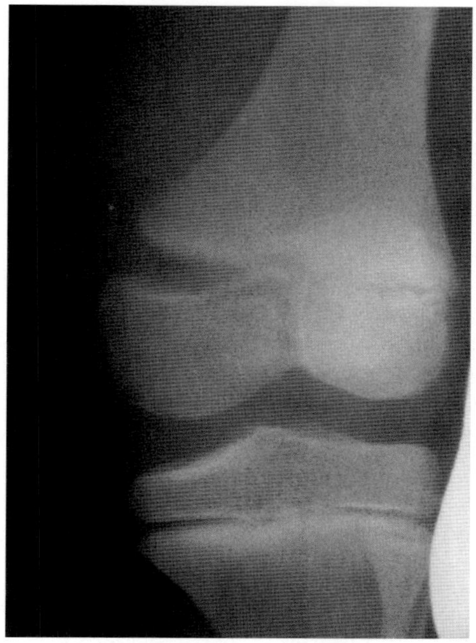

Figure 21.6. Salter-Harris type III is an intraarticular fracture. The fracture line is through the growth plate and exits through the femoral condyle. The fracture of the condyle can occur in any area, but most of the time it is in line with the intercondylar notch. (Courtesy of Dr. J. Richard Bowen, A.I. Dupont Institute.)

Abduction (valgus) type: This type of injury is caused by a blow to the lateral side of the distal femur. This usually happens in high school football games. A similar type of injury in adults causes a tear of the medial collateral ligament and cruciate ligaments. On the medial side, the periosteum is torn and the distal femoral epiphysis is displaced laterally with a trian-

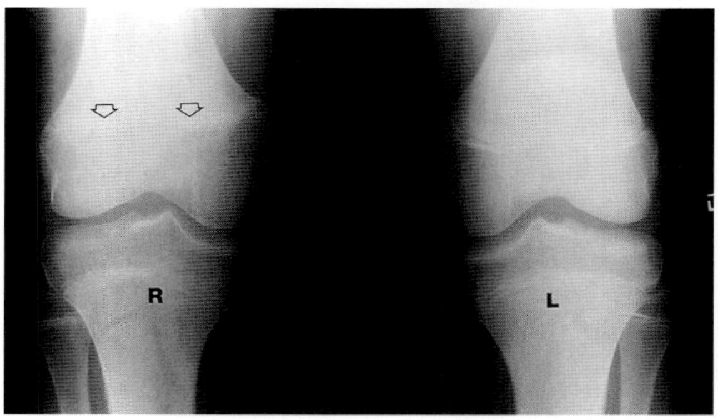

Figure 21.7. Premature closure of the growth plate of the distal right femur occurred 4 months following a Salter-Harris type V injury. The initial x-ray at the time of the injury was interpreted as normal.

gular fragment of the lateral metaphysis. This type of fracture may go into spontaneous reduction and may be missed if the triangular metaphyseal fragment is small. Abduction injuries may be interpreted as a strain or tear of the medial collateral ligament. If there is any doubt, one can obtain special abduction stress views to confirm the diagnosis.

Hyperextension type: By a hyperextension force the distal femoral epiphysis is displaced anteriorly. The displacement is exaggerated by the pull of the contraction of the quadriceps muscle. The posterior periosteum is torn and the fibers of the gastrocnemius muscle are stretched or torn. The distal femoral metaphysis is moved posteriorly into the popliteal fossa (Fig. 21.8). This injury is similar to dislocation of the knee in adults. There is a high chance of injuries to the popliteal vessels and common peroneal and posterior tibial nerves.[1]

Hyperflexion type: This is an extremely rare injury. The distal femoral epiphysis is displaced posteriorly. This fracture is due to forceful flexion injury and is usually caused by a direct blow to the distal femur.

Clinical and Radiographic Findings

There is a history of severe injury to the lower extremity. The child is in severe pain and unable to bear weight on the injured leg. The knee is swollen and is held in the position of semiflexion. The child resists any passive movement of the knee. With hyperextension injury, the femoral condyle may be palpated anterior to the distal femoral shaft. There may be fullness of the popliteal region due to the hematoma or posteriorly displaced distal femoral metaphysis. With lateral displacement there may be a valgus deformity. It is imperative to perform a complete neurovascular examination. The leg may be cold and cyanotic with absence of the posterior tibial and dorsalis pedis pulse.

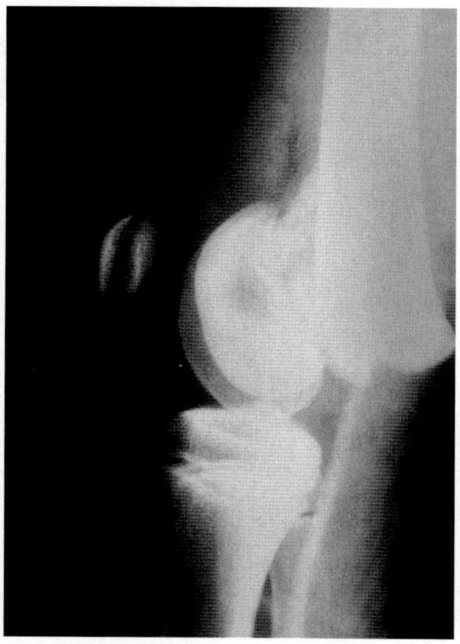

Figure 21.8. In hyperextension fracture and separation of the distal femur, the femoral metaphysis is displaced posteriorly into the popliteal fossa, which causes impingement of the neurovascular structures in the popliteal region. (From ref. 97, with permission.)

X-rays of the knee will demonstrate the type of the fracture. Sometimes the x-rays may appear normal. A careful examination of the x-rays is essential, looking for the triangular piece of the metaphyseal bone in the periphery of the growth plate. If indicated, a varus or valgus stress x-ray should be taken. If in doubt, one should obtain MRI of the knee, which will show signal changes in the region of the metaphysis and epiphysis of the distal femur (see Fig. 21.2).

Treatment

The goals of treatment of fractures of the distal femoral epiphysis are to obtain close to anatomic reduction, maintain the reduction, and avoid further damage to the growth plate. The stability of the knee joint is not affected by this type of fracture, because the ligaments and joint capsule are attached to the distal femoral epiphysis distal to the fracture line. The other objective of treatment is maintaining the functional range of motion of the knee and the strength of the muscles.

The method of reduction depends on the type of fracture. In the displaced fracture, general anesthesia is required to obtain adequate relaxation of the muscles. Prior to reduction the hemarthrosis should be aspirated to facilitate manipulation and reduction. The reduction should be performed by gentle manipulation. Prolonged and multiple forceful attempts for reduction may cause an adverse effect and further damage to the growth plate and other tissues.[13,23,24]

Closed reduction can be achieved up to 10 days after injury.[25,26] A Salter-Harris type I or type II may be spontaneously reduced before it is seen by the physician. A displaced Salter-Harris type I or type II can be easily reduced by gentle manipulation. An open reduction is usually required for the irreducible cases due to interposition of the torn periosteum, which is rolled inside the separation.

The nondisplaced Salter-Harris type I and type II fractures are immobilized in a well-padded and well-molded long leg cast. The displaced fractures are immobilized in a hip spica cast. In the anteriorly displaced fracture, the reduction is stable when the knee is held in 90 degrees of flexion. Anterior displacement usually recurs if the knee is held in less than optimal flexion.[27] After 2 weeks the cast is changed and the knee is brought to about 45-degree flexion. After 4 to 6 weeks the patient is allowed gentle active range of motion of the knee.

Unstable anteriorly displaced fractures require percutaneous pin fixation under fluoroscopy image. If the metaphyseal fragment (Thurston-Holland sign) is large enough, a threaded pin is placed transversely across the metaphyseal segments. The unstable Salter-Harris type II fracture with a large metaphyseal fragment requires internal fixation with a metaphyseal lag screw. If the metaphyseal fragment is very small, a smooth Kirschner wire (K-wire) is inserted from each condyle to the metaphysis. The direction of the pins should be through the central portion of the growth plate.

The medial and lateral displacement is reduced by gentle manipulation, and the leg is immobilized in a hip spica cast. The knee is immobilized in extension and is molded with three-point fixation. In the abduction-type injury the pressure is applied laterally at the ankle and greater trochanter, and medially at the knee joint. In the adduction or medially displaced fractures, the three-point fixation is reversed. The pressure is applied medially at the ankle and groin area, and laterally at the knee joint. The plaster immobilization is used for 4 to 6 weeks. Following removal of the cast, the patient starts gentle range-of-motion and muscle-strengthening exercises.

Hyperflexion injuries are reduced with longitudinal traction. With gentle manipulation the knee is brought into extension. The leg is immobilized in a hip spica cast with the knee in extension. In hyperflexion injuries, it is important to remember that the knee should not be immobilized in the position of semiflexion. The fracture line is distal to the attachment of the medial head of the gastrocnemius muscle. When the knee is held in extension, the medial head of the gastrocnemius muscle is stretched and acts as a dynamic splint and prevents posterior displacement of the distal femoral condyle. When the knee is placed in flexion, the medial head of the gastrocnemius muscle is relaxed, and consequently the femoral condyles will displace posteriorly.[27] If a stable reduction cannot be obtained by cast immobilization, one should consider percutaneous pinning of the fragments.

In Salter-Harris type III fracture the displacement of the fracture should be evaluated carefully. An anterior open-book–type fracture, a fracture with a gap greater than 2 mm, or any vertical step-off requires open reduction and internal fixation. During the open reduction one should take measures not to jeopardize the circulation to the distal femoral condyle. If both condyles are fractured, the articular surface should be restored by anatomic fixation of the condyles using transverse lag screws. Then the femoral condyles are attached to the femoral metaphysis by using crossed K-wires or plate fixation, depending on the age of the patient. In the comminuted fractures reconstruction of the articular surface should be done first, then alignment of the growth plate, and finally attachment to the rest of the femur.

The principles of treatment of Salter-Harris type IV fractures are the same as those for type III. Anatomic reduction is the essential part of the treatment, to restore the continuity of the articular surface and growth plate. Following open reduction, the fracture is fixed by transverse lag screws or threaded K-wires.

Type V and VI fractures are treated with a long-leg cast for 4 weeks. This is followed by early range-of-motion and strengthening exercise. Premature closure of the growth plate and bony bridge is a common complication of these type of fractures. This can be dealt with later if it becomes a problem.

Open Fractures

Classification of the open fractures in children follows the same principles used for adults.[28] The open fractures are classified based on their severity. Grade I is a fracture with a puncture wound. The wound is less than 1 cm in size. Grade II is a transitional wound. The size of the laceration is between 1 cm and 10 cm. Grade III is a big laceration. The size of the wound is greater than 10 cm. Grade III is divided into three subgroups (A, B, and C) based on the severity of soft tissue injuries.[28]

In children with grade II or III injuries, the fracture should be treated using the same guidelines that are used for adults with severe soft tissue injuries. All wounds require copious irrigation and complete debridement of all the traumatized and devitalized tissues. The fractures are reduced and stabilized by means of internal fixation or external fixation[29] and the wound is left open. Debridement of the wound is done every 2 days until the wound is clean and there is no sign of infection. Postoperatively, patients are prescribed broad-spectrum antibiotics.

Complications

Complications following fracture separation of the distal femoral epiphysis can be categorized as early or late. The early complications include injuries to the popliteal artery, neuropaxia of the peroneal nerve, and loss of reduction. The late complications include stiffness of the knee, quadriceps atrophy, leg length discrepancy, and angular deformity. Avascular necrosis of the femoral condyle has not been a problem. Because of the rapid healing of the fracture in the metaphyseal area, delayed union or nonunion has not been a problem.

Vascular Injuries

Only 18% of vascular injuries in children are caused by fractures, usually from a fall or motor vehicle accident.[30] Vascular injuries around the knee are usually seen in patients with dislocation of the knee, fractures of the distal femoral epiphysis, and fracture of the proximal tibial epiphysis[31–33] (Fig. 21.9). Epiphyseal fractures around the knee with the absence of the distal pulse is highly suggestive of vascular injury. If after manipulation and reduction the pulse does not return, the patient will need an emergency arteriogram of the involved lower extremity.[34] Disruption of the distal pulse could be due to arterial spasm, which is common in children.[35,36] An intimal tear and thrombosis may occur in the popliteal artery due to impingement.[32,37]

Even though the vascular impingement is relieved by immediate reduction of the fracture and dislocation, patients should be observed for 48 to 72 hours to rule out the subsequent thrombosis of the artery. If the patient has persistent pain with a cool and pale foot, a femoral angiogram is obtained. Vascular occlusion can happen slowly due to increasing compartment pressure of the leg. In patients with a swollen leg, pain, and paresthesia, one should consider the possibility of increased compartment pressure.[38] These patients need very close observation and measurement of the compartment pressure. All patients with increased compartment pressure of the leg require fasciotomy and decompression of the compartment pressure. The technique of fasciotomy is the same as in adults. Excision of the fibula should not be performed in children, because it may cause valgus angulation and deformity of the ankle.[31,32]

In adults the limb can be saved in 90% of cases if the circulation is restored within 6 hours of the time of injury. After 8 hours, the limb salvage rate is reduced and most patients may require amputation.[32,37] The soft tissues, especially the nerves and muscles, in children cannot withstand prolonged ischemia. A delay of more than 6 hours in repair of vascular occlusion ends in a poor result.[30]

Reduction and fixation of the fracture reduces further injury to the soft tissue and collateral circulation. Vascular repair is easier after the fracture is fixed and the limb is stable.[31] Restoration of the circulation cannot be compromised because of the delay in the reduction and fixation of the fracture. In selected cases, arterial and venus bypass can be performed for temporary restoration of the circulation to the leg. This will reduce the risk of compartment syndrome while stabilizing the fracture.[31,39,40]

Peroneal Nerve Injury

Neuropaxia of the peroneal nerve may occur because of the stretching of the nerve by the anteriorly or medially displaced distal femoral epiphysis. The nerve can also be stretched by rough manipulation of the injured leg, at the time of closed reduction.[24] It is important to document the function of the nerve prior to any manipulation and reduction. The neuropraxis usually resolves spontaneously over a period of 6 months.[4,5,8]

The peroneal nerve palsy rarely requires treatment.

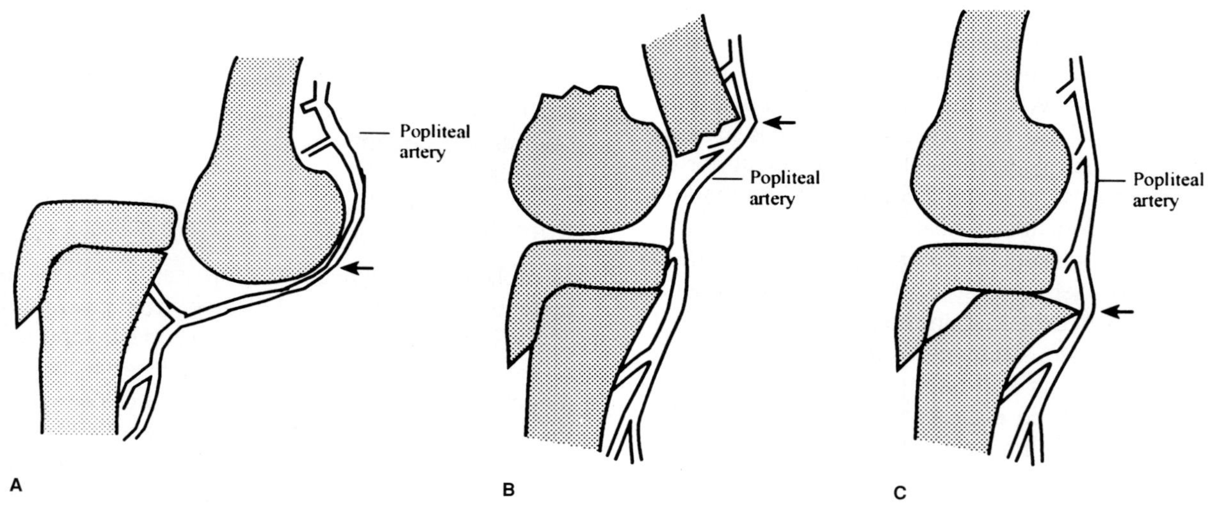

Figure 21.9. The mechanism of vascular injuries around the knee following fracture and dislocation. **A:** Vascular injury following dislocation of the knee. **B:** In hyperextension-type fracture of the distal femoral epiphysis, the mechanism of injury is the same as anterior dislocation of the knee. The popliteal artery, which is tightly attached to the proximal tibia, is stretched and pulled anterior, while the distal femoral metaphysis impinges the vessels and pushes them into the popliteal fossa. **C:** In fracture separation of the proximal tibial epiphysis, the posterior displacement of the proximal tibial metaphysis will impinge the popliteal vessels.

During recovery, the patient uses a solid ankle-foot orthosis for better ambulation and to prevent equinus deformity. Patients may also need physical therapy and electrical stimulation of the gastrocsoleus muscle to maintain its tone and excursion. If the neurologic deficit persists for 3 months, nerve conduction and electromyographic (EMG) studies are performed. These studies are repeated at 6 months postinjury. A persistent nerve conduction time delay and fibrillation of denervation are indications for exploration of the peroneal nerve.

Loss of Reduction

Separation of the distal femoral epiphysis may be quite unstable, especially if the displacement is in the sagittal plane.[9] In anterior displacement following reduction, the knee should be kept in at least 90 degrees of flexion. If the knee is placed in extension, the distal femoral epiphysis may slide and tilt forward. The position of the knee in extension will stabilize the reduction of the posterior, medial, or lateral displacement. The displacement occurs because of the instability of the fracture, inadequate casting, and a loose cast when the swelling subsides.

These patients should be followed closely. They should have x-rays every 2 or 3 days to check the reduction. If reduction is lost and a second manipulation is required, one should consider percutaneous pin fixation with smooth K-wires. Repeated manipulations increase the risk of damage to the growth plate.

Joint Stiffness

Stiffness of the knee joint can occur following separation of the distal femoral epiphysis. This can be due to intraarticular adhesions from hemarthrosis or capsular or muscular contracture. Patients will have difficulty in regaining full extension of the knee after being kept in flexion for a long time. In patients with anterior displacement, immobilization of the knee in acute flexion should not be for longer than 3 to 4 weeks. After 2 to 3 weeks, when the x-rays show signs of healing and periosteal reaction, the cast should be changed toward extension of the knee. Limitation of knee extension can be due to contractures of the posterior capsule and a stretched and atrophied quadriceps muscle.

The treatment begins after the reduction and stabilization of the fracture. If the knee is immobilized in an acute flexed position, the cast should be changed within 2 or 3 weeks of injury and changed every week. By serial casting the position of the knee can be brought to close to full extension after three to four castings.

Isometric quadriceps and hamstring exercises are begin within the first week after injury when the patient is comfortable and the acute pain has subsided. After removal of the cast, the patient will need extensive physical therapy to regain knee motion and muscular strength. The therapy should emphasize active and active-assisted range-of-motion exercise and active-resisted exercise for quadriceps, hamstrings, and hip abductors. Sometimes after extensive physical therapy the patient may not gain full range of motion and may require gentle manipulation of the knee under anesthesia.

Growth Disturbance

Progressive leg length discrepancy and angular deformity may follow a fracture separation of the distal femoral epiphysis. In older children who are within 2 years of reaching skeletal maturity, the deformity and leg length discrepancy may not be significant. In younger children there is a high chance of progressive deformity and leg length discrepancy. The leg length discrepancy secondary to growth disturbance of the distal femoral epiphysis may progress at a rate of 1 cm per year.

Progressive angular deformity following fracture of the distal femoral epiphysis is mostly due to asymmetrical retardation of growth (Fig. 21.10). Usually this happens when a portion of the growth plate is damaged by compression or shear at the time of initial injury.[2,4,41–42] It is difficult to recognize and predict the occurrence of this complication at the time of injury.

In Salter-Harris type II injury, the portion of the

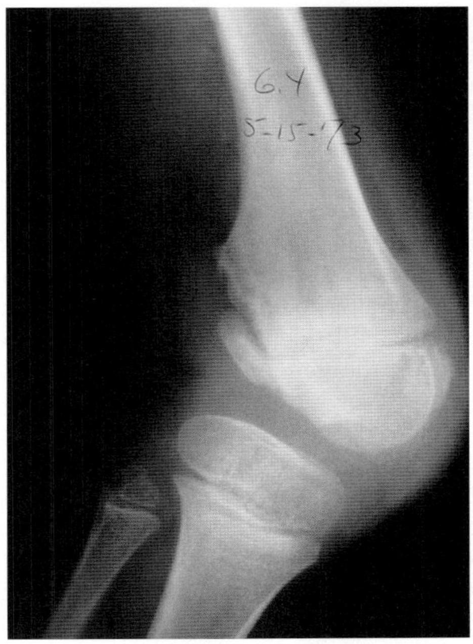

Figure 21.10. Partial growth disturbance of the distal femoral epiphysis, causing progressive angular deformity. (Courtesy of Dr. J. Richard Bowen, A.I. Dupont Institute.)

growth plate underneath the triangular metaphyseal fragment is usually spared. If the metaphyseal segment is on the medial side, a valgus deformity may be expected. If the metaphyseal fragment is on the lateral side, a varus deformity may result. In Salter-Harris type III and type IV there will be bony bridge between the epiphysis and metaphysis across the fracture line. Salter-Harris type V may cause symmetrical premature growth arrest (see Fig. 21.7). This will generally cause leg length discrepancy rather than angular deformity. Avulsion injury to the edge of the growth plate or Salter-Harris type VI may lead to localized premature closure of the growth plate and angular deformity.[15]

Patients who demonstrate progressive angular deformity following separation of the distal femoral epiphysis need further evaluation. This include a tomogram of the distal femur, MRI, and three-dimensional reconstructed computed tomography (CT) scan to map the location and size of the bony bridge. If the area of the bony bridge is found to be less than one-third of the total area of the physis, one should consider excising the bony bridge and filling the defect with autogenous fat, Silastic, or methylmethacrylate.[27,43–45] Tethering of the growth plate in a patient who is close to maturity should be treated by partial epiphysiodesis of the remaining open growth plate to prevent further angular deformity. The partial epiphysiodesis is performed if the predicted leg length discrepancy will not be more than 2 cm. Patients with angular deformity who have reached skeletal maturity will require a corrective osteotomy.[46,47] An open wedge osteotomy is preferred if there is associated leg length discrepancy.

If epiphyseal fracture separation of the distal femur is complicated by premature closure of the growth plate, a progressive leg length discrepancy should be expected. Patients who develop leg length discrepancy should be followed closely. Every 6 months a clinical and radiographic evaluation should be done. Scanograms and x-ray of the hand are obtained every 6 months for 2 years. Following the gathering of all the information, the amount of the leg length discrepancy can be calculated based on the Green-Anderson[48] chart of the remaining growth, or Moseley's[49] straight line graph.

If the predicted leg length discrepancy at skeletal maturity is less than 2.5 cm, no surgical treatment is indicated. If discrepancy is expected to be between 2.5 and 5 cm, consideration should be given to shortening of the opposite lower extremity. This can be done by epiphysiodesis of the distal femur, proximal tibia, and fibula, or a combination of femur and tibia based on the age of the patient and the amount of remaining growth. Femoral lengthening should be considered (Fig. 21.11), if the predicted leg length discrepancy is more than 5 cm.[47,50–54]

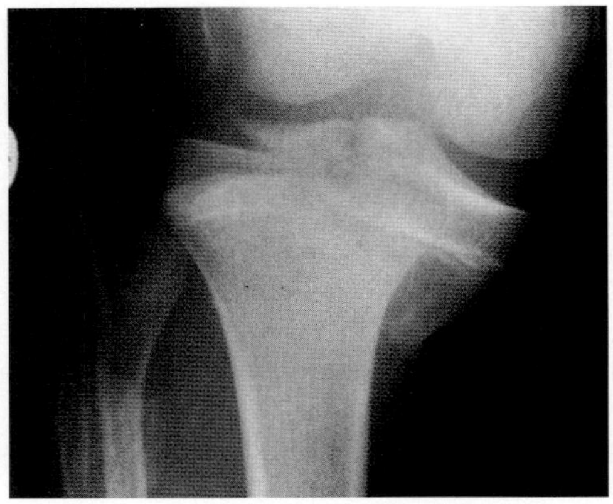

Figure 21.11. Femoral lengthening by callus distraction and cortical apposition (Z-osteotomy). Six weeks after lengthening the x-ray demonstrates healing of the osteotomy with ossification of the distracted callus.

Degenerative Articular Changes

Degenerative articular changes may occur following intraarticular injuries of the distal femoral epiphysis. The changes are usually due to the irregular articular surface resulting from Salter-Harris type III and IV injuries. The changes can occur at the tibiofemoral articulation or patellofemoral articulation, depending on the location of the epiphyseal fracture. All patients with Salter-Harris type III and type IV require open anatomic reduction and internal fixation.

Knee Joint Instability

Laxity or instability of the knee joint may occur following separation of the distal femoral epiphysis.[4,41] This could be due to the tear of the collateral or cruciate ligaments, which can happen simultaneously with a separation of the distal femoral epiphysis.[41] Ligament injuries are the main cause of knee joint instability after healing of the fractures of the distal femoral epiphysis. It would be difficult to recognize an associated ligamentous injury at the time of initial examination. With any signs and symptoms of instability of the knee, patients should have a complete evaluation for possible ligamentous injury. This includes a complete examination, MRI, and arthroscopy of the knee. Ligamentous injury should be treated properly to prevent problems in the future.

FRACTURE SEPARATION OF THE PROXIMAL TIBIAL EPIPHYSIS

Fracture separation of the proximal tibial epiphysis is a relatively rare injury, constituting 0.8% to 2% of all epiphyseal separations.[2,3,25,55,56] The proximal tibial epiphysis is less prone to fracture than the distal femoral epiphysis, due to the relative lack of ligamentous attachments to the proximal tibial epiphysis. In the posteromedial corner of the proximal tibia, the superficial fibers of the medial collateral ligament are attached to the metaphysis beyond the growth plate, and the semimembranous muscle is inserted into both the epiphysis and metaphysis on either side of the growth plate. The anterior portion of the physis is protected by the beak-shaped tibial tubercle, which is advanced distally and overhangs the metaphysis. The lateral collateral ligament is attached to the head of the fibula. The proximal end of the fibula is tightly attached to the tibia. These anatomic structures around the proximal tibia protect the tibial epiphysis from injury.

Mechanism of Injury

Fractures of the proximal tibial epiphysis can be due to either a direct or indirect trauma. A direct trauma can happen when a child's leg is caught between the bumpers of two cars or is run over by the wheels of a car. In indirect trauma the leg is forced into hyperextension or abduction against the fixed knee. This type of fracture can happen in adolescents due to sports-related injuries, motor vehicle accidents, or a fall from a height. Less commonly this type of fracture can occur during a difficult delivery. It can also happen with passive manipulation of the knee in children, with arthrogryposis multiplex congenita, and with myelomeningocele. Pathologic fractures can occur secondary to bone tumors and osteomyelitis.

Type of Fracture

The fracture separation of the proximal tibial epiphysis, like physeal separation of the other long bones, is classified based on the Salter-Harris[13] classification (Fig. 21.12).

Salter-Harris type I fractures are usually difficult to detect if they are nondisplaced. In displaced type I fractures the separation takes place across the growth plate and tibial tubercle near the posterior border of the attachment of the patellar tendon. The distal metaphyseal

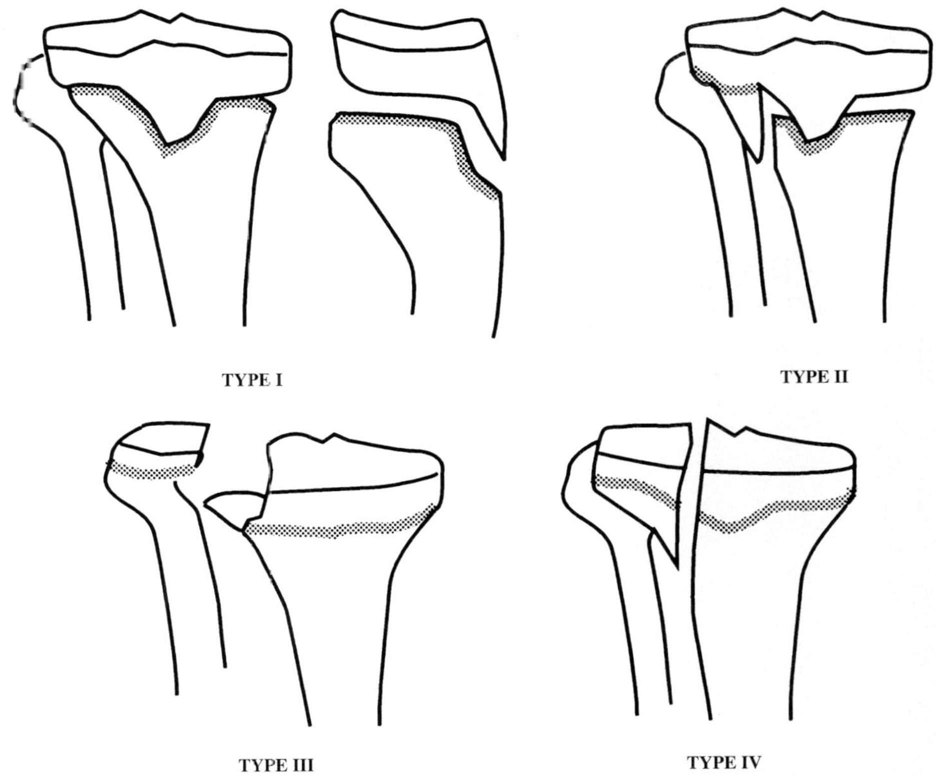

Figure 21.12. Salter-Harris classification of the proximal tibial epiphyseal fracture separation. In type I the fracture separation takes place across the growth plate and tibial tubercle near the posterior border of the attachment of the patellar tendon. The type II is the most common type. The separation occurs in the line between the proximal tibial epiphysis and the tibial tubercle. In type III fracture there is a vertical fracture line through the proximal tibial epiphysis. In type IV the fracture involves either medial or lateral condyle. The fracture line is through the epiphysis and metaphysis of the proximal tibia. (Redrawn from ref. 97, with permission.)

fragment can be displaced medially or posteriorly. Anterior displacement of the metaphysis is prevented by overhanging of the tibial tubercle. The lateral displacement is prevented by a tightly attached proximal fibula to the lateral side of the proximal tibia. This fracture is usually associated with fracture of the diaphysis of the upper end of the fibula or separation of the upper fibular epiphysis (Fig. 21.13). A medially displaced fracture of the proximal tibial epiphysis without fracture of the proximal fibula can be associated with diastasis of the interosseous ligament between the upper tibia and fibula.

Salter-Harris type II separation is the most common type of fracture of the proximal tibial epiphysis. The separation occurs in the line between the proximal tibial epiphysis and tibial tubercle. The displacement is usually in a posteromedial or posterolateral direction. When the metaphysis is displaced medially, the triangular metaphyseal fragment is attached to the lateral side of the epiphysis. This causes a valgus deformity. There is usually an associated fracture of the upper fibula.

In Salter-Harris type III fracture there is a vertical fracture through the proximal tibial epiphysis. The fracture line starts from the articular surface, extends through the epiphysis, and exits in the line of the growth plate. Fracture of the lateral condyle is more common, but either the medial or lateral condyle can break depending on the type and direction of the forces. The fracture may be quite unstable. In some Salter-Harris type III fractures, there is a partial closure of the growth plate in the posterior part of the proximal tibia. This type of fracture is similar to the Tillaux fracture at the ankle.[2]

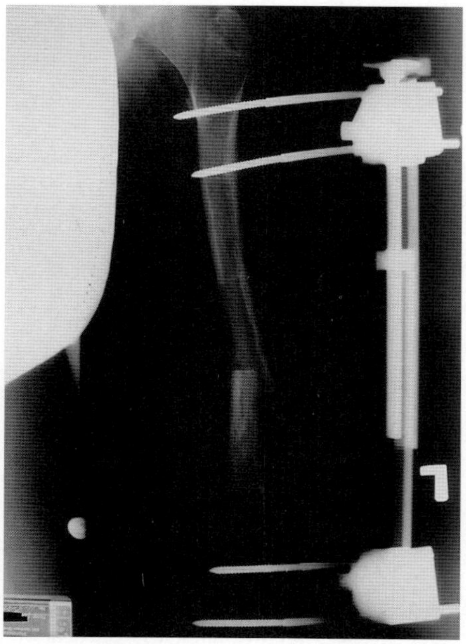

Figure 21.13. X-ray shows a type I fracture separation of the proximal tibial epiphysis. There is associated fracture of the diaphysis of the proximal fibula. (From ref. 97, with permission.)

In Salter-Harris type IV the fracture involves either the medial or lateral condyle. The vertical fracture line starts from the upper surface of the tibial epiphysis and extends downward and crosses the growth plate and exits through the metaphyseal cortex. The fracture line can be in the intercondylar area or through either condyle. Fracture of the lateral condyle is associated with a valgus deformity. With fracture of the medial condyle there may be a varus deformity.

Salter-Harris type V fracture is rare. It may be in conjunction with a fracture of the proximal tibial metaphysis or the tibial diaphysis. Salter-Harris type V injury may not be diagnosed on the initial evaluation. Assumption of the original injury is usually made when the patient develops a progressive angular deformity or leg length discrepancy.

Clinical and Radiographic Findings

The child who has sustained a fracture separation of the proximal tibial epiphysis complains of constant severe pain and swelling of the knee. Passive extension and flexion of the knee is limited because of muscle spasm and splinting. There is tenderness over the proximal tibial growth plate. With posterior displacement of the distal segment there will be a step-off or concavity at the level of the tibial tubercle. The knee joint may feel unstable.[57] If apparent instability of the knee is present during the initial examination, stress radiographs are needed to differentiate the physeal separation from ligamentous injuries. The initial evaluation should focus on a detailed neurovascular examination.

X-rays will show a significant hemarthrosis and expansion of the knee joint. In a nondisplaced fracture the x-rays may look normal. Stress x-rays will demonstrate a partial separation of the proximal tibial epiphysis. The stress views may also show a medial, lateral, or posterior opening of the physis depending on the type of the injury. The x-rays should be examined for a fracture line through the epiphysis or metaphysis of the proximal tibia. In nondisplaced fractures, the fracture line may be visible only on oblique views. A tilt of the epiphysis in relation to the metaphysis may indicate an epiphyseal separation. A valgus tilt represents medial displacement and a forward tilt of the epiphysis is a sign of posterior displacement. If in doubt, one should obtain tomograms and MRI of the knee.

Treatment

Before starting treatment, all patients should have a thorough neurovascular evaluation. Patients with absent dorsalis pedis and posterior tibialis pulse require immediate reduction of the fracture. If after reduction the pulse does not return, patients should have an emergency arteriogram and vascular consultation to repair the vascular injury. If after reduction the distal pulse is restored, patients should be kept under close observation for the possibility of a thrombosis of the popliteal artery.

Nondisplaced Salter-Harris type I and type II fractures are treated with a long leg cast with 30-degree flexion at the knee. The cast and underlying padding are split. X-rays are taken to confirm the reduction. The anterior part of the cast can be removed for neurovascular examination. If after 1 week there is no displacement or loss of reduction, the cast is reinforced by further casting material. The cast is removed at 4 to 6 weeks after injury, and patients are started on physical therapy. Patients will continue active range-of-motion and strengthening exercises until a full recovery is attained.

A displaced Salter-Harris type II and some type I fractures may be unstable. The unstable fractures require percutaneous pin fixation using smooth K-wires across the physis to maintain the reduction. In Salter-Harris type II fractures with a large metaphyseal fragment, internal fixation is achieved by using a cancellous screw across the metaphysis. The screw is placed parallel to the growth plate to avoid damaging it.

The displaced type III fractures require anatomic reduction to realign the articular surface and the growth plate. Following open reduction the fragments are transfixed by two K-wires or a transphyseal lag screw. The same principles should be used for Salter-Harris type IV fractures. Fragments should be fixed internally even if they are minimally displaced, to maintain congruity of the joint surface and prevent the formation of a bony bridge across the growth plate. All patients with vascular injury require internal fixation to avoid further damage to the arterial repair, which can happen if further manipulation of the leg is required.

Open injuries to the upper tibia carry a much worse prognosis than closed fractures. All open fractures require copious irrigation and complete debridement of devitalized and necrotic tissues. The fractures are reduced and stabilized by internal or external fixation. The closure of the wound is delayed until there is clean granulation tissue and no sign of infection. Postoperatively patients should be kept on an intravenous broad-spectrum antibiotic.

Complications

Possible complications of a fracture of the proximal tibial epiphysis are the same as those reported earlier for fractures of the distal femoral epiphysis. The principles of management of complications of fractures around the knee are also the same, including fractures involving the distal femoral epiphysis and proximal tibial epiphysis.

Loss of Reduction

Displaced Salter-Harris type II, III, and IV fractures and some type I fractures are unstable. This is particularly true if the initial displacement is posterior. If, after closed reduction of the fracture, the reduction cannot be maintained, patients need percutaneous pin fixation using smooth K-wires, or they may need open reduction and internal fixation. If after closed reduction the fracture appears to be stable, a long leg cast is applied. Patients need periodic x-rays during the first week following treatment to check the alignment. With any sign of loss of reduction, patients require remanipulation and pin fixation or open reduction and internal fixation.

Vascular Injuries

Vascular compromise is the worst complication that can occur with the fractures of the proximal tibia. It is due to the anatomic location of the popliteal artery and its two major branches. The popliteal artery is tightly attached to the posterior surface of the proximal tibial epiphysis. A hyperextension injury with posterior displacement of the upper end of the metaphysis may cause stretching and tearing of the popliteal artery (see Fig. 21.9).

Arterial injuries may be due to a complete tear of the popliteal artery.[58] It may also be due to arterial occlusion, which can occur as a result of the arterial thrombosis. Vascular compromise can also be due to progressive compression of the vessels in the swollen compartments of the leg due to increased compartment pressure.[56]

All patients with fracture of the proximal tibial epiphysis require close observation for vascular problems and the presence of the compartment syndrome. The guidelines for assessment of compartment pressure are given by Mubarak et al.[38] Delay in recognition of vascular insufficiency and its treatment will cause catastrophic results.

Growth Disturbance

The growth plate of the upper end of the tibia grows at a rate of approximately 6 mm per year. Premature closure of the growth plate can occur following all types of Salter-Harris fracture, which may lead to leg length discrepancy and angular deformity. The final amount of the angular deformity and leg length discrepancy depends on the age of the patient at the time of the injury. Patients with predicted leg length discrepancies of less than 2.5 cm do not require treatment. Patients with discrepancies of more than 2.5 cm require treatment to correct the leg length discrepancy. This can be done either by epiphysiodesis of the opposite leg at the appropriate time, or by a lengthening procedure, depending on the age of the patient and the amount of the remaining growth.

Angular deformities occur with partial closure of the growth plate. The degree of progressive angulation depends on the proximity of the growth arrest to the periphery of the growth plate and on the age of the patient. In young children, resection of the bony bridge is indicated if the area of the growth arrest is less than one-third of the total area of the physis.[27,43–45] If patients are close to maturity, a partial epiphysiodesis or stapling of the remaining open growth plate should be considered to prevent the angular deformity. Patients with established angular deformity require corrective osteotomy of the proximal tibia.

Other Complications

Stiffness of the knee joint can occur following fracture of the proximal tibial epiphysis. To minimize the occurrence of this complication, cast immobilization should be minimized to 4 to 6 weeks, and following that, patients should be placed on vigorous and extensive physical therapy.

Ligamentous injury, especially tear of the medial collateral ligament, may occur with fracture separation of the proximal tibial epiphysis. Following fixation of the fracture any ligamentous injuries should be repaired to prevent future instability of the knee.

Degenerative articular changes may develop if the fracture involves the condyles of the tibia. This is more common in Salter-Harris type III and IV fractures. All patients with type III and IV fractures require open anatomic reduction and fixation.

AVULSION FRACTURE OF THE TIBIAL TUBERCLE

Avulsion fracture of the tibial tubercle is a rare injury. It entails a traumatic separation of the physis deep to the ossific nucleus of the tubercle. It should be differentiated from the Osgood-Schlatter lesion, in which there is separation of the anterior surface of the apophysis without displacement from the tibial metaphysis.[59,60] In the avulsion fracture of the tibial tubercle the level of the separation is deep to the ossific nucleus of the tubercle.

The tibial tubercle is a bony prominence on the anterior surface of the proximal tibia. The development of the tibial tubercle can be divided in four stages based on Ehrenborg's[61] classification. In the beginning the tubercle has the histologic appearance of fibrocartilage. This is called the cartilaginous stage. The second stage is the apophyseal stage, in which the ossification center appears in the tongue of the cartilage. The third stage is the epiphyseal stage, in which the formation of bone, or a secondary ossification center, is completed and it is separated from the tibial metaphysis by the epiphyseal line. The fourth stage is completion of the ossification of the tibial tubercle and fusion of the tubercle to the tibial metaphysis.

The tibial tubercle has a rich blood supply. It receives its main supply from multiple small branches that originate behind the quadriceps tendon. The tibial tubercle also receives some of its blood supply from adjacent periosteal and metaphyseal vessels.[59,62]

Mechanisms of Injury

A complete avulsion of the tibial tubercle is due to a strong pulling force that is applied by the patellar ligament. It usually happens during the forceful flexion of the knee against the resistance to the contraction of the quadriceps muscle. The injury can also happen during a severe contraction of the quadriceps muscle against the fixed tibia.

Avulsion of the tibial tubercle is common in adolescent boys between 14 and 16 years of age. It is also common in children who have preexisting Osgood-Schlatter disease. These patients usually have a strong quadriceps muscle and tight hamstrings.[59] Traumatic avulsion of the tibial tubercle occurs during sports activities such as gymnastics, football, and basketball.[25,41,63–65] It can also happen after a fall from a height.[59,65]

Type of Fracture

Watson-Jones[16] has classified these fractures into three types. This classification was modified by Ogden et al[59] based on the degree and severity of displacement (Fig. 21.14).

In type I avulsion fracture of the tibial tubercle the separation occurs between the secondary center of ossification and the portion of the physis under the tibial tubercle. In type II the separation line is through the area bridging the tibial tubercle and the proximal tibial epiphysis. In type III the separation involves the anterior portion of the tibial epiphysis. Separation starts from underneath the tibial tubercle and extends proximally into the proximal tibial epiphysis and ends in the joint under the meniscus or anterior fat pad. The amount of displacement depends on the amount of the force exerted at the time of injury.

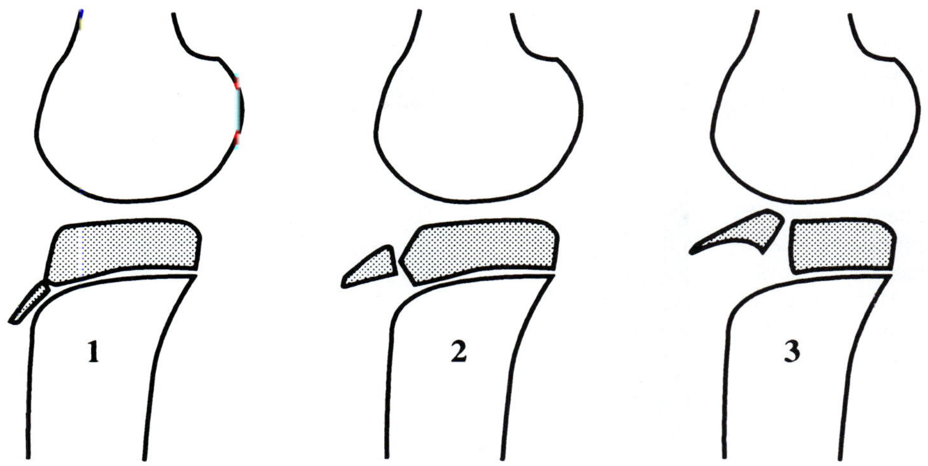

Figure 21.14. Classification of avulsion fracture of the tibial tubercle. In type I there is minimal displacement. The separation is between the secondary center of ossification and part of the physis under the tibial tubercle. In type II the separation line is through the area bridging the tibial tubercle and the proximal tibial epiphysis. In type III the separation is through the anterior portion of the tibial epiphysis and involves the articular surface of the proximal tibia.

Clinical and Radiographic Findings

There is swelling and tenderness in the area of the tibial tubercle. In type III, with an intraarticular fracture there is joint effusion and hemarthrosis. In a completely separated tibial tubercle, a movable fragment of bone can be palpable between the upper tibia and femoral condyle. The position of the tubercle depends on the amount of displacement and on the superior migration of the extensor mechanism of the knee. A defect in the area of the tibial tubercle may or may not be palpable. This depends on the amount of soft tissue swelling and hematoma. The knee joint is held in slight flexion and the patient resists passive extension of the knee due to hamstring spasm. In type I avulsion, the patient may be able to partially extend the knee because of attachment of the medial and lateral retinaculum. In type II and III avulsion, the patient is unable to actively extend the knee.

The lesion is best seen on the lateral projection radiographs of the knee. In type I fracture there is anterior and slightly superior displacement of the distal end of the tibial tubercle. It may look like an Osgood-Schlatter lesion. In type II the avulsed tubercle is larger. It is separated from its bed and hinged near the proximal tibial physis. In type III the fracture line extends through the proximal tibial epiphysis into the joint. The degree of separation and patella alta can be well seen on the lateral x-rays of the knee in different degrees of flexion.

In type I and II separations, the x-rays may not show the extent of the injury. MRI shows the separation of the tubercle, the hematoma between the tibial tubercle and proximal tibial metaphysis, and marrow changes in the tibial epiphysis, indicating a trauma and fracture through the proximal tibial epiphysis (Fig. 21.15).

Treatment

The minimally displaced type I avulsion in patients who have active extension of the knee is treated by closed reduction. The fragments can be pushed together by direct finger pressure. Following the reduction, the patients are treated in an above-knee cast with the knee in extension. The type II avulsion fractures are treated by closed reduction. The presence of a gap between the tibial tubercle and tibial metaphysis on the postreduction x-rays indicates an incomplete reduction. This could be due to interposition of the periosteal flap at the fracture site. These patients require open reduction and fixation either by K-wires or by suturing of the fibrocartilaginous portion of the tubercle to the adjacent periosteum. All type III fractures require open reduction and internal fixation with a cancellous screw or multiple threaded Steinmann pins. Following reduction, the knee is immobilized in a long leg or a cylinder cast for 4 to 6 weeks. Following removal of the cast, the knee is protected in a posterior splint or a knee immobilizer for an additional 3 weeks. During this time patients are allowed active range of motion of the knee, isometric exercise, and gentle quadriceps strengthening exercise. After 6 weeks patients receive vigorous active range-of-motion and quadriceps-strengthening exercise.

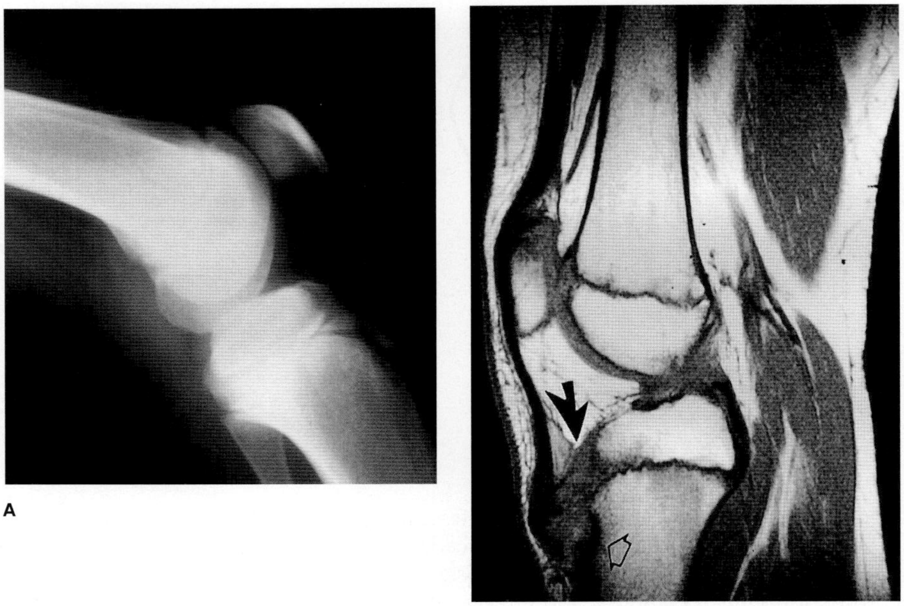

A

B

Figure 21.15. Avulsion of the tibial tubercle. **A:** The lateral x-ray of the knee demonstrates elevation of the ossific nucleus of the tibial tubercle, which may be mistaken for an Osgood-Schlatter lesion. **B:** MRI shows separation of the tibial tubercle, hematoma between the tubercle and proximal tibial metaphysis (hollow arrow), and marrow changes in the tibial epiphysis, indicating a trauma and fracture through the proximal tibial epiphysis (solid arrow).

Complications

The healing of the avulsion fracture of the tibial tubercle occurs by epiphysiodesis of the tibial tubercle to the anterior tibial physis. In spite of anterior epiphysiodesis, genurecurvatum does not develop, because most of the injuries occur in children close to the age of skeletal maturity, with little growth remaining from the proximal tibial physis. Other minor complications can be expected, such as loss of full flexion of the knee, atrophy of the quadriceps muscle, and enlargement and prominence of the tibial tubercle.[63–65]

FRACTURE OF THE INTERCONDYLAR EMINENCE OF THE TIBIA (TIBIAL SPINE)

The intercondylar eminence of the tibia is located between the two articular surfaces of the proximal tibia. It has a triangular shape with its base over the anterior border of the proximal tibia. In young children, the structure of the proximal surface of the eminence is mostly cartilage. Therefore, the actual size of the avulsed fragment is always larger than its x-ray images. The intercondylar eminence is located directly beneath the intercondylar notch of the femur. The cruciate ligaments and menisci are directly attached to the intercondylar eminence.

Fracture of the intercondylar eminence occurs most frequently in children between 8 and 13 years of age. The fracture can occur through the anterior or posterior intercondylar eminence. Avulsion fracture of the posterior intercondylar eminence is a rare injury in children. The ratio of the fracture of the anterior intercondylar eminence to the fracture of the posterior intercondylar eminence is 10 to 1.[66] In Torisu's[67] report, the youngest patient who had fracture of the posterior tibial spine was 15 years of age. Due to the rarity of the avulsion fracture of the posterior tibial spine in children, this injury is not discussed here.

Mechanisms of Injury

Fractures of the intercondylar eminence are due to avulsion of the anterior or posterior cruciate ligament with its bony attachment. The anterior cruciate ligament is tight when the knee is in the position of flexion or hyperextension. A direct blow to the femoral condyle in a flexed knee displaces the femur posteriorly and results in avulsion of the anterior tibial spine. A forceful medial rotation of the tibia in relation to the femur increases tension on the cruciate ligament and leads to avulsion of the anterior tibial spine.[66,68] Bicycle injuries are the most common type. The child falls from the bicycle and lands on the front of the flexed knee. This can also happen during a fall from a bicycle when the child extends the knee to break the fall. Avulsion of the posterior tibial spine is caused by a direct force to the proximal part of the tibia when the knee is flexed. This pushes the proximal tibia in the posterior direction against the femur. It can also be the result of a hyperextension injury to the knee. In this condition there is always an associated tear of the posterior capsule.

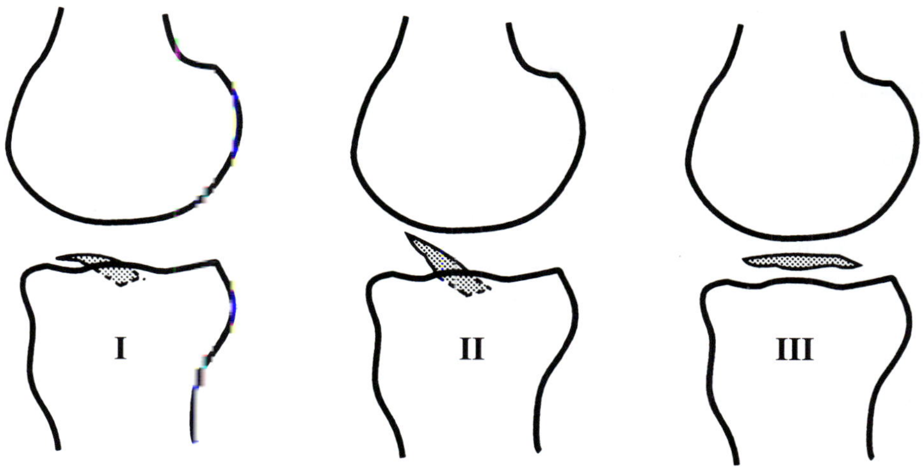

Figure 21.16. Classification of the fracture of the intercondylar eminence of the proximal tibia in children (according to Meyers and McKeever[68]). In type I there is little displacement of the avulsed fragment with only slight elevation of its anterior margin. In type II there is more displacement. The anterior rim of the avulsed fragment is lifted from its bed. The fragment hinges on its posterior margin, which is attached to the proximal surface of the tibia. In type III the entire fragment is detached and elevated. Often the avulsed fragment is rotated and the fracture surface is faced anterior. (Redrawn from ref. 68, with permission.)

Type of Injury

Meyers and McKeever[68] classified the fractures of the intercondylar eminence of the proximal tibia into three types based on the degree of the displacement of the avulsed fragment (Fig. 21.16). In type I there is relatively little displacement of the avulsed fragment, with only slight elevation of its anterior margin. In type II there is greater displacement. The anterior rim of the avulsed fragment is lifted from its bed. The fragment hinges on its posterior margin, which is still attached to the proximal surface of the tibia. In type III the entire fragment is detached from the proximal tibia and is completely elevated and often rotated so that the fracture surface is facing anteriorly.

Clinical and Radiographic Findings

There is a history of injury to the knee, commonly a fall from a bicycle. There is hemarthrosis and swelling of the knee. The knee is held in flexion due to muscle spasm, and any passive extension of the knee is extremely painful. Restriction of motion is due to muscle spasm, not to the displacement of the avulsed fragment. If the medial collateral ligament is intact, the anterior drawer sign will be negative. If there is an associated tear of the medial collateral ligament, patients will have signs of knee joint instability with a positive anterior drawer sign, and medial opening of the joint on valgus stress.

The avulsion fracture of the anterior tibial spine is best seen on the lateral x-ray of the knee (Fig. 21.17). The bony portion of the avulsed fragment can be very thin and small, especially in younger children, because most of the avulsed fragment is cartilage and may not be appreciated on x-ray. There can be a variable degree of displacement. On the anteroposterior x-ray one should outline the margins of the fracture. If the width of the fragment is narrow and is located in the central portion of the intercondylar eminence, closed reduction will be easy. In a fracture with a wide base, which is extended underneath the articular surface, the anterior horn of the menisci, especially the lateral meniscus, can be displaced and entrapped between the displaced fragment and its base. It is extremely important to obtain adequate x-rays to determine the type of fracture. If in doubt, one should obtain a CT scan or MRI of the knee.

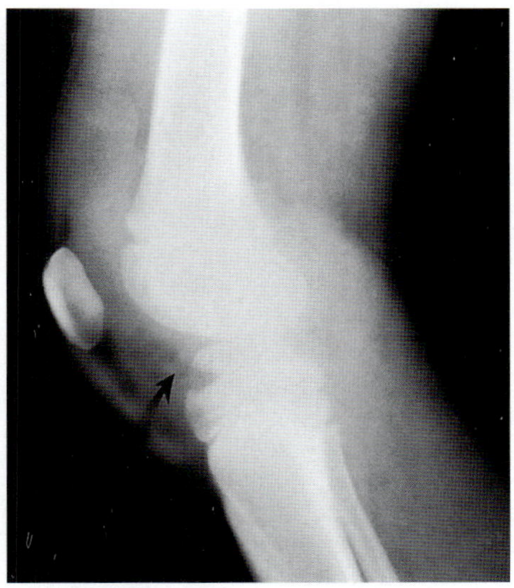

Figure 21.17. Displaced avulsion fracture of the anterior tibial spine, which is best seen on lateral x-ray of the knee. There can be a variable amount of displacement.

Treatment

Nondisplaced or minimally displaced type I and type II fractures require closed reduction and immobilization of the knee in a cylinder cast with the knee in 15 to 20 degrees of flexion. Excessive manipulation and hyperextension of the knee are not indicated because they may further displace the avulsed fragment as a result of tightening of the anterior cruciate ligament when the knee is placed into hyperextension. Prior to reduction patients require aspiration of the knee to reduce the amount of pain. Immobilization is continued for 6 to 8 weeks or until there are radiographic signs of the healing of the fracture. After removal of the cast, patients start physical therapy with active-resistive quadriceps exercise and range of motion of the knee.

Displaced type III fracture of the anterior tibial spine requires open reduction and internal fixation.[67,69,70] At open reduction the joint is irrigated for better visualization, and the small, loose fragments of bone are removed. The interposition of the anterior horn of the lateral meniscus under the avulsed fragment is corrected and the meniscus is moved out with a small hook or forceps. Following repositioning of the meniscus, the reduction can be easily obtained by pushing the tibial spine toward its base or by extending the knee. Internal fixation can be obtained by a variety of methods, such as using a wire loop, pins, small screws, or heavy absorbable sutures through the avulsed fragment into the adjacent epiphysis (Fig. 21.18). Crossing the growth plate should be avoided during internal fixation. Meyers and McKeever[69] have suggested suturing the fragment to the adjacent meniscus to hold the fragment in reduced position. Reduction can then be maintained by holding the knee in extension.

Older children can be treated by arthroscopy. Following irrigation the detached fragment is visualized through the arthroscope. The interposed anterior horn of the meniscus is freed by a hook. The avulsed fragment is reduced by direct pressure. Following reduction the knee joint is extended and is checked for stability of the reduction. If the reduction is stable, the knee is immobilized in a cylinder cast with the knee in neutral extension. Hyperextension of the knee should be avoided to prevent displacement of the fragment.

Following healing of the fracture, patients require extensive physical therapy to improve range of motion of the knee and strength of the quadriceps muscle.

Complications

Limitation of extension of the knee can occur if the displaced fragment is not adequate reduced. This can be avoided by making sure the patient has full extension of the knee before applying the cast. A displaced and malunited fracture that is causing limitation of extension of the knee requires operative treatment. This can be done either by excision of the fragment without damaging the cruciate ligaments or by lifting the tibial spine and removing the bone from the intercondylar eminence and placing the tibial spine in a deeper position.[71]

The instability of the knee joint following avulsion

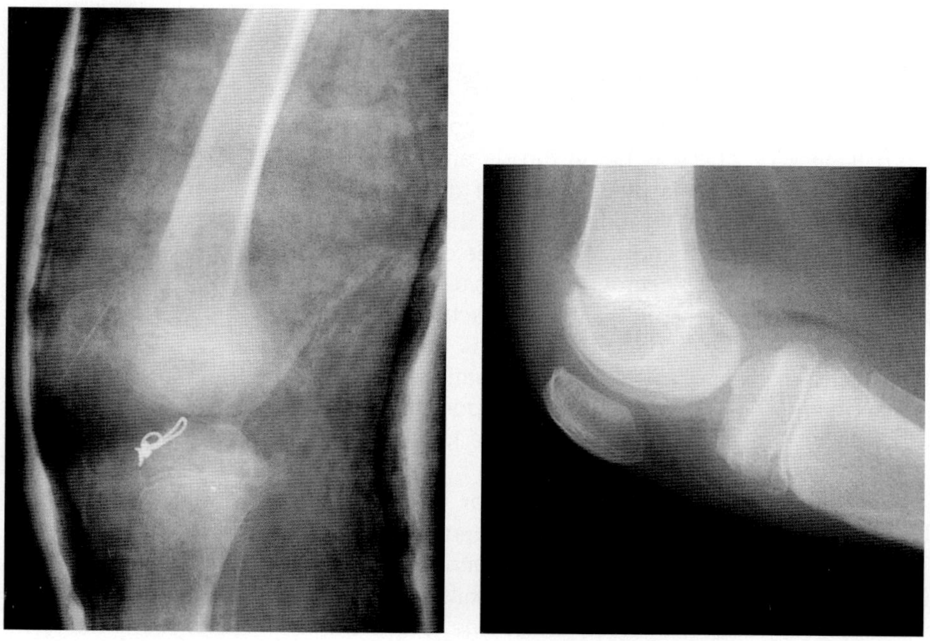

A B

Figure 21.18. Lateral x-ray of the knee shows the method of internal fixation of the fracture of the anterior tibial spine by the wire-loop technique. **A:** The placement of the wire through the anterior tibial spine into the upper margin of the tibial epiphysis. The growth plate of the proximal tibia should not be crossed during the internal fixation. **B:** Healing of the fracture 4 months after the injury.

fracture of the anterior tibial spine is usually due to an undetected tear of the medial collateral ligament. The instability can also happen following menisectomy for an associated torn meniscus.

Other complications, including postoperative infection, stiffness of the knee, and quadriceps atrophy, can be avoided by appropriate postreduction treatment, such as postoperative antibiotic therapy and extensive physical therapy following healing of the fracture.

FRACTURES OF THE PATELLA

Fractures of the patella are rare in children, accounting for fewer than 1% of fractures of the patella,[72,73] because the osseous part of the patella is small and is surrounded by large cartilage tissue that protects the patella from direct trauma.[74] Because of the cartilaginous nature of the patella in children, the actual size of the fragment may not be the size seen on x-rays.

At birth the structure of the patella is mostly cartilage. The ossification center appears at 2 or 3 years of age but may be delayed until the sixth year. The patella usually has one center of ossification. It may begin with more than one center, and gradually these separate ossific nuclei will unite and ossification will continue until the entire patella is ossified.

About 2% to 3% of patellae have a secondary center of ossification. The secondary ossification center usually appears at age 12 but may be seen as young as 8 years and may persist until adult life. The secondary ossification center gives a bipartite shape to the patella. The bipartite patella is located in the upper lateral corner of the patella where it may look separated or partially fused to the main body of the patella. Other types of bipartite patella with a different location of the secondary ossific center have been reported in the literature.[75,76] The bipartite patella is more common in boys than girls, and about 50% of cases are bilateral.[75]

Most of the blood supply to the patella is from its anterior surface and lower pole. There are minimal blood vessels entering the patella from the proximal pole, medial margin, or lateral margin. Scapinelli[12] found a high incidence of delayed union or nonunion of the marginal fractures due to poor circulation in the margin of the patella. He also found that disruption of the circulation through the anterior surface of the patella may cause avascular necrosis of the superior pole of the patella.

Mechanisms of Injury

Fracture of the patella can be due to a direct blow to the patella, sudden contraction of the quadriceps muscle against a fixed flexed knee, or a combination of both. A direct blow to the patella will crush the patella against the femoral condyle and result in a transverse or comminuted fracture.[17,72] Lateral or medial marginal fracture can occur when the direct blow is applied to the periphery rather than the central portion of the patella. Avulsion fracture of the inferior pole of the patella can be a result of an indirect force, usually during jumping or after a fall.[77,78] The sleeve fracture of the patella is usually seen in children between 8 and 12 years of age. This is an avulsion fracture of a small bony fragment of the inferior pole of the patella, along with a large sleeve of the articular cartilage and retinaculum.[78]

Clinical and Radiographic Findings

Clinically, there is local pain, swelling, effusion, and tense hemarthrosis. Palpation of the knee reveals a gap between the separated fragments of the patella. With complete separation, patients are not able to actively extend the knee. If the medial and lateral retinaculum are intact, patients are able to extend the knee when gravity is eliminated. In marginal fractures, there is tenderness over the medial or lateral margin of the patella. In marginal fractures, since the continuity of the quadriceps mechanism is intact, patients are able to perform straight leg raising but with some extensor lag.

Transverse fractures are best seen on lateral x-rays with the knee in 30 degrees of flexion to fully appreciate the displacement. Presence of the wide anterior opening and minimal posterior opening may indicate that the articular cartilage is intact.[72]

In sleeve fracture, the avulsed fragment has minimal bone and is difficult to see on x-rays. It may be completely separated from the patella.[78,79] A combination of a small avulsed fracture of the inferior pole of the patella with a high-riding patella is highly suggestive of a sleeve fracture. The sleeve fracture should be differentiated from accessory ossification,[80] overuse syndrome, apophysitis of the inferior pole of the patella, or Sinding-Larsen–Johansson lesion.[81] If in doubt, one should obtain an MRI of the knee to visualize the small bony fragment and separation of the articular cartilage from the undersurface of the patella.

A bipartite patella is seen as a crescent radiolucent line in the superior and lateral corner of the patella. This is best seen on anteroposterior x-rays of the knee. The marginal fractures are best seen on skyline views. The fracture lines are vertically oriented and involve the entire thickness of the patella.

Treatment

Treatment of the fractured patella in children follows the same principles that are used in adults. Nondisplaced fractures with an intact extensor mechanism of the knee are treated by closed reduction and immobilization of the knee in a cylinder cast. Prior to application of the cast, the knee joint is aspirated to relieve the pain from extensive hemarthrosis.

Transverse patella fractures, with displacement of less than 2 mm and no vertical step-off in the articular cartilage, are treated by cast immobilization in a cylinder cast. Fractures with displacement of more than 2 mm and step-off in the articular cartilage are treated by open reduction and internal fixation. Many methods of fixation have been described in the past, including fixation with nonabsorbable sutures through longitudinal drill holes, circumferential wiring through the adjacent soft tissue around the patella, and tension-band wiring.[17,72,77,82] The cerclage wiring or tension band wiring with a wire loop over two longitudinal K-wires remains the treatment of choice (Fig. 21.19). Following internal fixation, repair of the extensor mechanism of the knee is an essential part of the treatment.[25,63,83]

Controversy remains about the treatment of the comminuted fractures of the patella in children. One should try to preserve the patella by fixing the fragments and repairing the extensor mechanism of the knee. Medial marginal fractures require open reduction and fixation with transverse K-wires if they contain a large portion of the articular cartilage.[84–86] The lateral marginal fractures and some small medial marginal fractures of the patella are best treated by surgical excision and repair of the extensor mechanism because of a high incidence of nonunion or fibrous union, which can cause persistent pain.[86]

The sleeve fractures of the patella are seen only in children. The avulsed fragment from the inferior pole of the patella has minimal bone and is often difficult to see on x-rays. If in doubt, one should obtain an MRI of

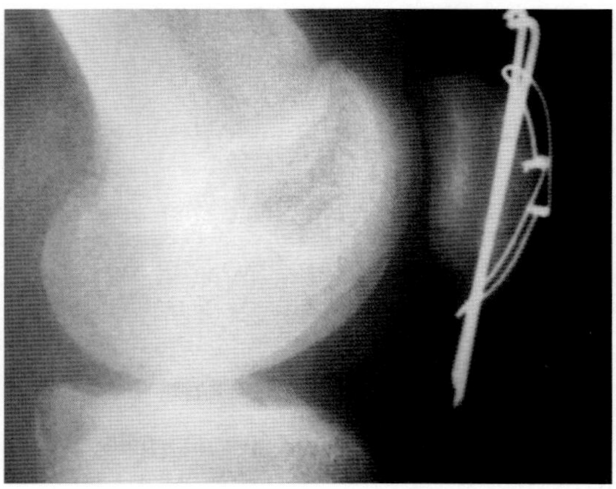

Figure 21.19. Lateral x-ray of the knee demonstrates the technique of internal fixation of the transverse fracture of the patella by tension band wiring. The wire loop is tightened over two longitudinal K-wires. (From ref. 97, with permission.)

the knee and even a diagnostic arthroscopy to evaluate the articular cartilage and the amount of separation of the articular cartilage. The nondisplaced sleeve fracture is treated with a cylinder cast. A displaced sleeve fracture of the patella with disruption of the extensor mechanism of the knee requires open reduction and internal fixation.[78]

Following either closed or open reduction, the knee is immobilized in a cylinder cast. Isometric exercise is started as soon as possible. Patients are instructed to do straight leg raising, and they should be able to perform this exercise within the first week following the treatment. The cast is removed in 6 weeks, and then patients start active-resistive exercise for the quadriceps muscle, hip abductors, and hip extensors. The range of motion of the knee should begin slowly. Patients start with active-assisted range-of-motion exercise and gradually advance to more vigorous and passive range-of-motion exercise.

Complications

All displaced fractures of the patella require anatomic reduction and restoration of the articular cartilage and extensor mechanism of the knee. An unreduced displaced fracture results in high-riding patella and patella alta. The change in the position and length of the extensor apparatus ultimately affects the extensor mechanism of the knee.[87,88] These changes cause disuse atrophy of the quadriceps muscle and extensor leg. The defect in the articular cartilage and irregularity of the articular cartilage cause degenerative changes and chondromalacia of the patella. Osteonecrosis of the patella can occur following circular wire fixation.[12] This may cause retardation of the growth of the patella, especially in younger children. Stiffness of the knee joint can be due to prolonged immobilization. Patients will require extensive physical therapy to correct this problem.

DISLOCATION OF THE PATELLA AND OSTEOCHONDRAL FRACTURES OF THE KNEE

Acute dislocation of the patella, in a normal knee, is a rare injury in children. The injury is caused by a direct blow to the medial side of the patella. A sudden contraction of the quadriceps muscle results in lateral dislocation of the patella, when the knee is fixed in flexion and varus position. The patella is usually dislocated laterally. On rare occasions the patella can be displaced medially, due to a direct blow to the lateral margin of the patella. Other conditions that predispose chronic subluxation or recurrent dislocation of the patella include internal torsion of the femur, hypoplasia of the lateral femoral condyle, external torsion of the tibia, genu valgum, patella alta, and quadriceps insufficiency.[82,89]

In a complete lateral dislocation, the patella is pushed over the lateral femoral condyle and lies on the lateral surface of the condyle. The incomplete dislocation occurs when the patella is displaced laterally and rests on the lateral edge of the femoral condyle. With complete dislocation of the patella, there is always a soft tissue injury to the medial side of the knee, such as a tear of the medial retinaculum, joint capsule, synovial membrane, or part of the vastus medialis. The degree of soft tissue injury is less with incomplete dislocation of the patella.

A sudden lateral dislocation and spontaneous reduction of the patella may cause osteochondral fracture of the lateral femoral condyle or patella.[84,90–92] Osteochondral fractures of the femoral condyle can also occur after direct trauma to the medial or lateral femoral condyle. A fall on a flexed knee can cause osteochondral fracture of the medial femoral condyle. Osteochondral fractures of the lateral condyle can be due to a direct blow to the lateral condyle. The osteochondral fractures can also be due to the rotation and compression of the articular surface of the tibia against the distal femur.[93,94]

Clinical and Radiographic Findings

Most dislocated patellae are spontaneously reduced or are reduced by another person—coach, trainer, or emergency personnel—at the time of injury. Diagnosis of a recently reduced dislocation of the patella is based on the history and clinical findings of hemarthrosis, tenderness on the medial side of the patella, and lateral subluxation of the patella. In an unreduced dislocated patella, the patient has pain and swelling in the knee and the knee is kept in flexed position. The patient is unable to actively flex or extend the knee. The patella can be palpated on the lateral side of the knee, and femoral condyles can be easily palpated under the skin in the anterior surface of the knee.

The patient with osteochondral fracture of the knee may give a history of a direct blow to the front of the knee, or may describe a severe twisting injury in the flexed knee or a history of dislocation of the patella. There is extensive effusion of the knee joint. There is localized tenderness over the femoral condyle or medial margin of the patella. There may be subluxation and instability of the patella when it is pushed laterally. Aspiration of the knee shows bloody fluid containing fatty droplets.

It is difficult to visualize an osteochondral fracture on plain x-rays. The loose osteochondral fragment may be obscured by overlapping femoral condyles. A lateral view may show a loose fragment in the suprapatellar pouch. The anteroposterior view may show entrapment of the loose fragment beneath the medial or lateral collateral ligament or adjacent to the patella. The tunnel view may show the fragment when it is in the intercondylar notch. The skyline view may show the loose osteochondral fragment in the medial or lateral parapatellar region, or adjacent to the femoral condyle (Fig. 21.20). A double-contrast arthrogram of the knee may show the loose fragment. Routine radiographs will fail to show the fracture bed on either the femoral condyle or the undersurface of the patella. MRI of the knee may

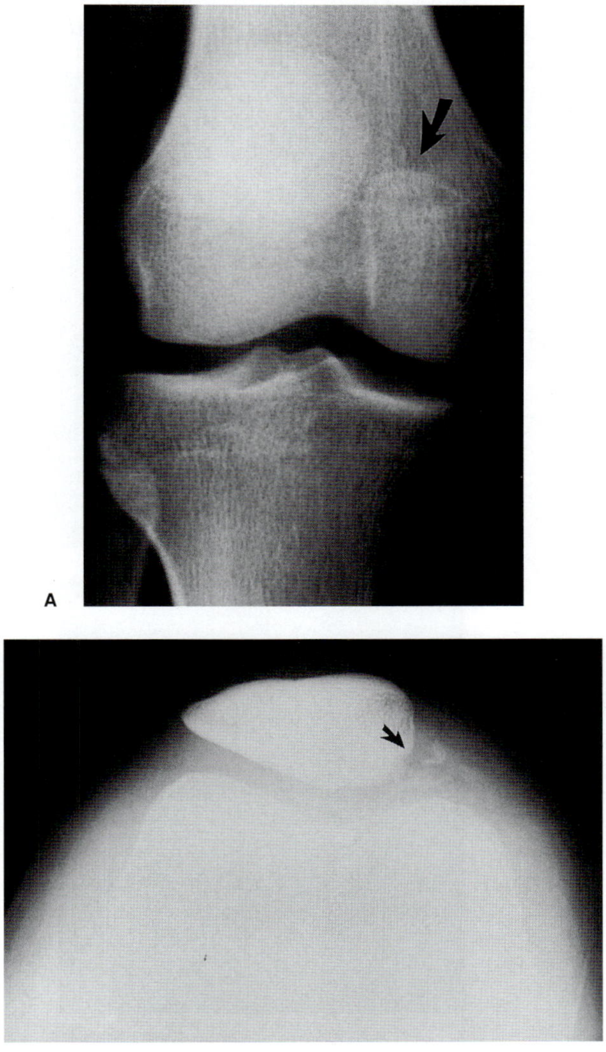

Figure 21.20. The x-rays of the knee shows the osteochondral fracture following dislocation of the patella. **A:** The anteroposterior view of the knee shows the osteochondral fragment (arrow), which is overlapped by the medial femoral condyle. **B:** The skyline view shows the osteochondral fragment (arrow) near the medial facet of the patella.

localize the osteochondral fragment and its bed, and will show a defect in the articular cartilage and marrow edema in the subchondral region of the patella or the femoral condyle. With dislocation of the patella, MRI will show subluxation of the patella and edema of the medial retinaculum (Fig. 21.21).

Treatment

A dislocated patella is easily reduced. The hip is flexed to relax the rectus femoris. The knee is slowly brought into extension and the patella is gently pushed anteriorly and medially into the intercondylar area. The procedure does not require general anesthesia. Some patients may require intravenous sedation for relaxation.

A

B

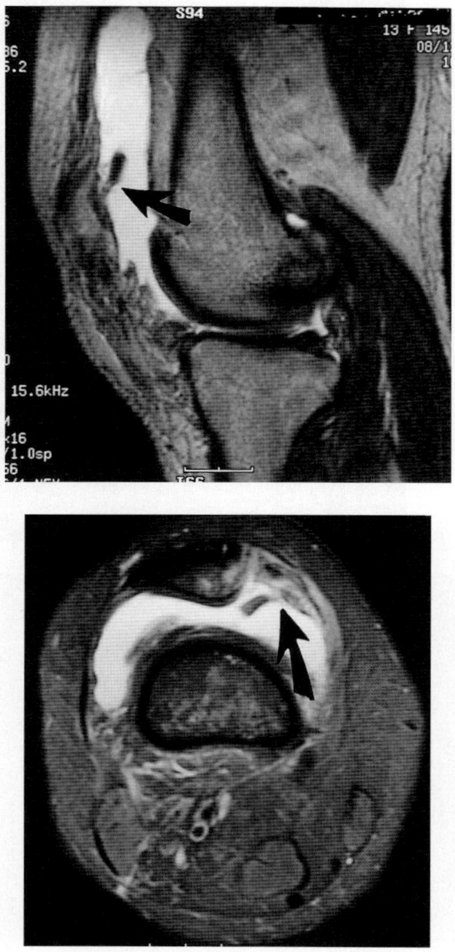

Figure 21.21. MRI of the knee following dislocation of the patella. **A:** On the lateral view MRI shows joint effusion and a loose osteochondral fragment (arrow) in the suprapatellar area. **B:** On the cross-section view MRI demonstrates edema and partial disruption of the medial retinaculum, and the loose osteochondral fragment (arrow). It also shows an osteochondral defect and subchondral edema of the medial facet of the patella.

After reduction, the hemarthrosis should be aspirated. The fluid is checked for droplets of fat, and if positive, one should consider the possibility of an osteochondral fracture. Following reduction, the knee is immobilized in a cylinder cast holding the knee in full extension. The cast is used for a period of 4 weeks. After removal of the cast, patients receive physical therapy for strengthening of the quadriceps muscle, especially the vastus medialis.

Patients with first-time dislocation of the patella require surgical repair if there is a wide, palpable gap in the medial retinaculum and capsule. All patients with chronic subluxation or recurrent dislocation of the patella require realignment of the patella, which is performed by lateral release and imbrication of the medial capsule and retinaculum. For more stability, the vastus medialis muscle can be advanced distally and anteriorly.

For accurate diagnosis and localization of the osteochondral fracture, patients require further diagnostic studies, including MRI of the knee and arthroscopy. Operative treatment should be considered as the treatment of choice for acute osteochondral fractures.[91,95,96] Small, loose osteochondral fragments from the margin of the femoral condyle or patella are removed. The defects involving the articular surface are smoothed and drilled down to the bleeding bone. The small defects will fill with fibrocartilage tissue. Reduction of the loose osteochondral fragments is indicated if the fragments are large and the defects are in the weight-bearing area.[86,89] Following reduction, the fragment is internally fixed by drilling a threaded pin or a compression screw through the osteochondral segment into the femoral condyle or patella. The fixating wire or screw should be countersunk in the articular surface.[86,89] The operative repair of the medial retinaculum and joint capsule is recommended at the time of the replacement of the large osteochondral fragment.[84,91,95]

Complications

An unrepaired or stretched medial retinaculum results in persistent instability of the patella, chronic subluxation, and recurrent dislocation. Patients with instability of the patella have limited athletic activities. They complain of tiring easily and weakness of the quadriceps muscle, and they hesitate to squat. All patients with chronic instability of the patella require realignment of the patella.

The defect and irregularity of the articular cartilage may cause chondromalaclia and osteoarthritic changes of the joint, with persistent recurrent pain. Other complications include quadriceps atrophy, stiffness, and reactive synovitis of the knee due to the penetration of the fixating pin into the joint.

References

1. Tachdjan MO. *Pediatric Orthopaedics*. Philadelphia: WB Saunders, 1972.
2. Neer CS II, Horwitz BS. Fractures of the proximal humoral epiphyseal plate. *Clin Orthop* 1965;41:24–31.
3. Peterson CA, Peterson HA. Analysis of the incidence of the injuries to the epiphyseal growth plate. *J Trauma* 1972;12:275–281.
4. Lombardo SJ, Harvey JP Jr. Fractures of the distal femoral epiphysis. Factors influencing prognosis: a review of thirty-four cases. *J Bone Joint Surg* 1977;59A:742–751.
5. Roberts JM. Fracture separation of the distal femoral epiphysis. In: Proceedings of the American Academy of Orthopaedics Surgeons. *J Bone Joint Surg* 1973;55A: 1324.
6. Ogden S. *Skeletal Injury in the Child*. Philadelphia: WB Saunders, 1990:787–790.
7. Clanton TO, Delee JC, Sanders B, et al. Knee ligament injuries in children. *J Bone Joint Surg* 1979;61A:1195–1201.
8. Stephens DC, Louis DS, Louis E. Traumatic separation of the distal femoral epiphyseal cartilage plate. *J Bone Joint Surg* 1974;56A:1383–1390.
9. Basset FH III, Goldner JL. Fracture involving the distal femoral epiphyseal growth line. *South Med J* 1962;55: 545–557.
10. Goss CM (ed). *Gray's Anatomy of the Human Body*, 29th ed. Philadelphia: Lea & Febiger, 1973:664.
11. Crock HV. The arterial supply and venous drainage of the bones of the human knee joint. *Anat Rec* 1962; 144:199–217.
12. Scapinelli R. Blood supply of the human patella: its relation to ischemic necrosis after fracture. *J Bone Joint Surg* 1967;49B:563–570.
13. Salter RB, Harris WR. Injuries involving the epiphyseal plate. *J Bone Joint Surg* 1963;45A:587–622.
14. Ogden JA. Skeletal growth mechanism. Injury pattern. *J Pediatr Orthop* 1982;12:371–377.
15. Rang ML. *The Growth Plate and Its Disorders*. Edinburgh: E&S Livingstone, 1969:139.
16. Watson-Jones R. *Fractures and Joint Injuries*, 4th ed. Edinburgh: E&S Livingstone, 1955–56.
17. Weber BG, Brunner C, Freuler F. *Treatment of Fracture in Children and Adolescents*. New York: Springer-Verlag, 1980.
18. Snedecor ST, Wilson HB. Some obstetrical injuries to the long bones. *J Bone Joint Surg* 1949;31A:378–384.
19. Burman MS, Langsam MJ. Posterior dislocation of lower femoral epiphysis in breech delivery. *Arch Surg* 1939; 38:250–260.
20. Diamond LS, Alegado R. Perinatal fractures in arthrogryposis multiplex congenita. *J Pediatr Orthop* 1981; 189–192.
21. Edwardsen P. Physeo-epiphyseal injuries of lower extremities in myelomeningocele. *Acta Orthop Scand* 1972;43(6):550–557.
22. Wenger DR, Jeffcoat BT, Heering JA. The guarded prognosis of physeal injury in paraplegic children. *J Bone Joint Surg* 1980;62A:241–246.
23. Hutchinson J Jr. Lectures on injuries to the epiphysis and their results. *Br Med J* 1894;1:669–673.
24. Kurlander JJ. Slipping of the lower femoral epiphysis. *JAMA* 1931;96:513–517.
25. Bohler L. *The Treatment of Fractures*, vol 2, 5th ed. New York: Grune and Stratton, 1957.
26. Peterson WJ. Separation of lower femoral epiphysis. *Can Med Assoc J* 1929;21:301–303.
27. Aitken AP, Magill HK. Fractures involving the distal femoral epiphyseal cartilage. *J Bone Joint Surg* 1952; 34A:96–108.
28. Buckley SL, Smith G, Sponseller PD, et al. Open fractures of the tibia in children. *J Bone Joint Surg* 1990; 72A:1462–1469.
29. Tolo VT. External skeletal fixation in children's fracture. *J Pediatr Orthop* 1983;3:435–442.
30. Stamford JR, Evans WE, Morse TS. Pediatric arterial injuries. *J Vasc Dis* 1976;27:1–7.
31. Friedman RJ, Jupiter JB. Vascular injuries and closed extremity fractures in children. *Clin Orthop* 1984;188: 112–119.
32. Greene NE, Allen BL. Vascular injuries associated with dislocation of the knee. *J Bone Joint Surg* 1977;59A: 236–239.
33. Navarre JR, Cardillo PJ, et al. Vascular trauma in children and adolescents. *Am J Surg* 1982;143:229–231.
34. Smith PL, Lim WN, Ferris EJ, et al. Emergency arteriography in extremity trauma: assessment of indications. *AJR* 1981;137:803–807.
35. Russo VJ. Case report: traumatic arterial spasm resulting in gangrene. *J Pediatr Orthop* 1985;5:486–488.
36. Samson R, Pasternak BM. Traumatic arterial spasm—rarity or nonentity. *J Trauma* 1980;20:607–609.
37. Fabian TC, Turkleson ML, Connelly TL, et al. Injury to the popliteal artery. *Am J Surg* 1982;143:225–228.
38. Mubarak SJ, Hargens AR, Owen CA, Garetto LP, Akenson WM. The Wick catheter technique for measurement of intermuscular pressure. *J Bone Joint Surg* 1976; 58A:1016–1020.
39. Lange RH, Bach AW, Hansen ST Jr, et al. Open tibial fractures with associated vascular injuries: prognosis for limb salvage. *J Trauma* 1985;25:203–208.
40. Bach A, Johansen K. Limb salvage using temporary arterial shunt following traumatic near amputation of the thigh. *J Pediatr Orthop* 1982;2:187–190.

41. Poland J. *Traumatic Separation of the Epiphysis*. London: Smith, Elder, 1898.

42. Salter RB, Czitrom A, Willis RB. Fractures involving the distal femoral epiphyseal plate. In: Kennedy JC (ed). *Injury to the Adolescent Knee*. Baltimore: Williams & Wilkins, 1979.

43. Bright RW. Operative correction of partial epiphyseal plate closure by osseous-bridge resection and silicone rubber implant. *J Bone Joint Surg* 1974;56A:655–664.

44. Bright RW, Burstein AH, Elmore SM. Epiphyseal plate cartilage. A biomechanical and histological analysis of failure modes. *J Bone Joint Surg* 1974;56A:688–703.

45. Langenshiold A. An operation for partial closure of an epiphyseal plate in children and its experimental basis. *J Bone Joint Surg* 1975;57B:325–330.

46. Abbott LC, Gill GG. Valgus deformity of the knee resulting from injury to the femoral epiphysis. *J Bone Joint Surg* 1942;24:97–113.

47. Wagner H. Surgical lengthening or shortening of femur and tibia: technique and indications. *Prog Orthop Surg* 1977;1:71–94.

48. Anderson M, Green WT, Messner MB. Growth and predictions of growth in the lower extremities. *J Bone Joint Surg* 1963;45A:1–14.

49. Moseley CF. A straight line graph for leg-length discrepancies. *J Bone Joint Surg* 1977;59A:174–179.

50. Aprin H. Femoral lengthening by callus distraction and cortical apposition (Z-osteotomy). *Clin Orthop* 1994; 309:222–229.

51. DeBastiani G, Aldegheri R, Renzi-Brivio L. Limb lengthening by callus distraction (callotasis). *J Pediatr Orthop* 1987;7:129–134.

52. Kojimoto H, Yasui N, Goto T, Matsude S, Shimomura Y. Bone lengthening in rabbits by callus distraction. *J Bone Joint Surg* 1988;70B:543–546.

53. Ilizarov GA, Deviatov AA, Torkhova VG. Surgical lengthening of the shortened lower extremities. *Vestn Khir* 1972;107:100–106.

54. Monticelli G, Spinelli R. Limb lengthening by closed metaphyseal corticotomy. *Ital J Orthop Traumatol* 1982;4: 139–145.

55. Shelton WR, Canale ST. Fractures of the tibia through the proximal tibial epiphyseal cartilage. *J Bone Joint Surg* 1979;61A:167–173.

56. Barkhart SS, Peterson HA. Fractures of the proximal tibial epiphysis. *J Bone Joint Surg* 1979;61A:996–1002.

57. Welch PH, Wynne GF Jr. Proximal tibial epiphyseal fracture separation: case report. *J Bone Joint Surg* 1963; 45A:782–784.

58. Nicholson JT. Epiphyseal fractures about the knee. *Instr Course Lect* 1967;18:74–83.

59. Ogden JA, Tross RB, Murphy MJ. Fractures of the tibial tuberosity in adolescents. *J Bone Joint Surg* 1980; 62A:205–215.

60. Smillie IS. *Injuries to the knee joint*, 4th ed. Baltimore: Williams & Wilkins, 1970.

61. Ehrenborg G. The Osgood-Schlatter lesion: a clinical and experimental study. *Acta Chir Scand* Suppl 1962;288: 1–36.

62. Truenta J. *Studies of the Development and Decay of the Human Frame*. London: Heinemann, 1968.

63. Hand WL, Hand CR, Dunn AW. Avulsion fractures of the tibial tubercle. *J Bone Joint Surg* 1971;53A:1579–1583.

64. Christie MJ, Dvouvh VM. Tibial tuberosity avulsion fracture in adolescents. *J Pediatr Orthop* 1981;1:391–394.

65. Levi JH, Coleman CR. Fracture of the tibial tubercle. *Am J Sports Med* 1976;4:254–263.

66. Roberts JM, Lovell WW. Fractures of the intercondylar eminence of the tibia. In: Proceedings of the American Academy of Orthopaedic Surgeons. *J Bone Joint Surg* 1970;52A:827.

67. Torisu T. Isolated avulsion fracture of the tibial attachment of the posterior cruciate ligament. *J Bone Joint Surg* 1977;59A:68–72.

68. Meyers MH, McKeever FM. Fracture of the intercondylar eminence of the tibia. *J Bone Joint Surg* 1959; 41A:209–222.

69. Meyers MH, McKeever FM. Follow-up notes: fractures of the intercondylar eminence of the tibia. *J Bone Joint Surg* 1970;52A:1677–1684.

70. Zaricznyj B. Avulsion fracture of the tibial eminence: treatment by open reduction and pinning. *J Bone Joint Surg* 1977;59A:1111–1114.

71. Garcia A, Neer CS II. Isolated fractures of the intercondylar eminence of the tibia. *Am J Surg* 1958;95: 593–598.

72. Belman DAJ, Neviaser RJ. Transverse fracture of the patella in a child. *J Trauma* 1973;13:917–918.

73. Bostrom A. Fracture of the patella. *Acta Orthop Scand* Suppl 1972;43:1–80.

74. Crawford AH. Fractures about the knee in children. *Orthop Clin North Am* 1976;7:639–656.

75. Green WT Jr. Painful bipartite patellae: a report of three cases. *Clin Orthop* 1975;110:197–200.

76. Kohler A, Zimmer EA. *Borderlands of the Normal and Early Pathologic in Skeletal Roentgenology*, 3rd ed. New York: Grune and Stratton, 1968.

77. Blount WP. Fractures of the patella. In: Blount WP. *Fractures in Children*. Baltimore: Williams & Wilkins, 1955.

78. Houghton GR, Ackroyd CE. Sleeve fractures of the patella in children. A report of three cases. *J Bone Joint Surg* 1979;61B:165–168.

79. Devas MB. Stress fractures of the patella. *J Bone Joint Surg* 1960;42B:71–74.

80. Beddow FH, Corkery PM, Shatwell GL. Avulsion of the ligamentum patellae from the lower pole of the patella. *J R Coll Surg* Edinb 1963;64–65:66–69.

81. Sinding-Larsen MF. A hitherto unknown affection of the patella in children. *Acta Radiol* 1922;1:171–173.

82. Ogden JA. *Skeletal Injury of the Child*. Philadelphia: Lea & Fibiger, 1982.

83. Griswood AS. Fractures of the patella. *Clin Orthop* 1954;4:44–56.

84. Rorabeck CH, Bobechko WP. Acute dislocation of the patella with osteochondral fracture: review of eighteen cases. *J Bone Joint Surg* 1976;58B:237–240.

85. Peterson L, Stener B. Distal disinsertion of the patellar ligament combined with avulsion fracture at the medial and lateral margins of the patella. *Acta Orthop Scand* 1976;47:680–685.

86. Smillie IS. *Injuries of the Knee Joint*, 5th ed. Edinburgh: Churchill-Livingstone, 1978.

87. Lieb FJ, Perry J. Quadriceps function: an anatomical and mechanical study using amputated limbs. *J Bone Joint Surg* 1968;50A:1535–1548.

88. Lieb FJ, Perry J. Quadriceps function. An electromyographic study under isometric conditions. *J Bone Joint Surg* 1971;53A:749–758.

89. Kennedy JC. *The Injured Adolescent Knee*. Baltimore: Williams & Wilkins, 1979.

90. Rosenberg NJ. Osteochondral Fracture of the Lateral Femoral Condyle. *J Bone Joint Surg* 1964;64A: 1013–1026.

91. Ahstrom JP. Osteochondral fracture in the knee joint associated with hypermobility and dislocation of the patella. Report of eighteen cases. *J Bone Joint Surg* 1965; 47A:1491.

92. Coleman HM. Recurrent osteochondral fracture of the patella. *J Bone Joint Surg* 1948;30B:153–157.

93. Cofield RH, Bryan RS. Acute dislocation of the patella: results of conservative treatment. *J Trauma* 1977;17: 526–531.

94. McManus F, Rang M, Heslin DJ. Acute dislocation of the patella in children. The natural history. *Clin Orthop* 1979;139:88–91.

95. Bassett FH III. Acute dislocation of the patella, osteochondral fractures, and injuries to the extensor mechanism of the knee. *Instr Course Lect* 1976;25:40–49.

96. Johnson EW, Mcleod TL. Osteochondral fragments of the distal end of the femur fixed with bone pegs. Report of two cases. *J Bone Joint Surg* 1977;59A;677–679.

97. Hensinger RN. Operative Management of Lower Extremity Fractures in Children. *AAOS Monograph Series*, 1992:34.

Chapter 22

HIGH TIBIAL OSTEOTOMY

Martin W. Korn

Painful knees with varus or valgus angular deformity and mainly unicompartmental noninflammatory arthritis can be symptomatically improved by corrective osteotomy about the knee. This is believed to be due to transferring the excessive weight-bearing forces from the diseased compartment to the less involved one. As larger and more intact articular surfaces share the weight-bearing forces, pressure decreases, degeneration of the overloaded compartment may slow or reverse, and pain diminishes or ceases. Coventry,[1] Maquet,[2,3] Fujisawa et al,[4] and Oldenbring et al[5] reported that correction of angular deformity can lead to regrowth of an articular surface, which is thought to mature to a fibrocartilage. Analysis of the biomechanical forces involved in arthritic deformity has been published by Maquet,[6] Chao,[7] and Harding.[8]

This chapter addresses valgus high tibial osteotomy (HTO) for the varus knee, which is a more common and successful procedure for a more common problem than is distal femoral osteotomy for the valgus knee. A brief discussion of distal femoral osteotomy will follow the section on HTO. In discussions of HTO, it is often described as a difficult procedure with a high risk of complications. As with all surgery, meticulous attention to detail, careful preoperative planning and preparation, and experience combine to improve outcomes and limit problems.

HISTORY

Osteotomy of the tibia to correct deformity has been used since Richard Volkmann's report in 1885. Lange treated deformity produced by ricketts, poliomyelitis, and trauma. Tibial osteotomy for degenerative joint disease of the knee was first reported by Jackson and Waugh[9] in 1958. In 1961 they reported the use of a "ball and socket" osteotomy at the level of the tibial tubercle to treat varus and valgus deformity in patients with a "useful" range of motion.[10] Coventry's[1] preliminary report of 30 knees further stimulated interest in HTO. He and others have continued to report their postsurgical and long-term results.

Early total knee replacement research and practice emphasized the use of long, standing x-rays for accurate mechanical axis and femoral-tibial angle measurement, and the intraoperative use of guides to establish correct lower limb alignment. Arthroscopic knee joint inspection, debridement, and abrasion arthroplasty had all been introduced by 1981 and improved the planning and performance of HTO.

Prior practice most often depended on short x-rays without determining magnification, paper tracings and cutouts of the short x-rays for preoperative planning, and intraoperative standard x-rays, since portable fluoroscopy was not generally available. In addition, osteotomes alone were used to cut bones since saws were not available, and osteotomy fixation was often with only a cast, or with internal staple(s) and a cast. The fact that so many patients did so well is a tribute to the surgeons and to the soundness of the rationale for HTO.

COMPLICATIONS, PITFALLS, AND SALVAGE

General complications that may be associated with any type of knee surgery are not discussed in this chapter. Prevention and treatment are discussed under the following major categories of HTO complications and pitfalls:

- poor patient selection
- undercorrection
- overcorrection
- delayed union or nonunion
- nerve or vascular injury
- metal protruding into the medial joint space and fracture of the proximal tibial fragment
- fixation placement problems
- conversion to total knee replacement
- ligament laxity

Poor Patient Selection

Inappropriate patient selection decreases the likelihood of a satisfactory result, but many factors influence this decision.

The Ideal Candidate
The ideal candidate is younger than 65 years of age, active, not obese, and has isolated medial unicompartmental osteoarthritis. The genu varum is less than 10 degrees (femoral-tibial angle). There is at least 100-degree range of motion without extension lag. If there is a flexion contracture, it is less than 20 degrees. There is no major ligament instability and muscle strength is adequate. Pain is mostly medial, severe, and due to osteoarthritis. The patient can use crutches or a walker and can participate in a postoperative rehabilitation program. Unfortunately, the ideal candidate is rarely seen.

Specific Criteria

Age and Activity Level. Total knee replacement (TKR) is most often considered for patients older than 65 years, but older patients who are "physiologically young," are in relatively good health, and have an active lifestyle can be strong candidates for HTO. For a sedentary patient over 65 years of age with similar disease a TKR would usually be more appropriate. Similarly, patients younger than 65 years of age, who are active, working, and in good health, but whose joint deformity and degenerative disease are more severe than ideal for HTO may be offered arthroscopy and osteotomy, because the alternative is prosthetic knee replacement. Whereas HTO results can improve over time as new fibrocartilage develops and knee range of motion increases, the result from a TKR is rarely better than after the initial 6 to 12 months postoperative.

I have done valgus HTO on a few younger patients (35 to 50 years of age) whose deformity and/or degenerative joint disease was sufficiently severe that they were better candidates anatomically for TKR. Their postoperative results were quite gratifying, which confirms Maquet's advice to do HTO first, even with advanced osteoarthritis, since it often suffices, and a TKR can be done later if needed. However, except for young patients, I believe our TKR technique and equipment have now improved to the point that TKR would be preferable in those cases with more advanced degenerative joint disease or deformity.

Type and Location of Arthritis. Tibial osteotomy has been more successful in unicompartmental osteoarthritis in the medial joint space than in other profiles of the disease. The results of tibial osteotomy in patients with rheumatoid or other inflammatory arthritis have been less favorable, and they are usually better managed with TKR. I consider inflammatory arthritis a specific contraindication for HTO.

Degree of Varus Deformity and Range of Motion. The genu varum should ideally be less than 10 degrees (femoral-tibial angle). Varus of more than 15 degrees on weight-bearing preoperative radiographs is a relative contraindication to osteotomy. Severe limitation of range of motion (less than 70 to 80 degrees), a flexion contracture of more than 20 degrees, or a limitation of flexion beyond 80 degrees is a contraindication for this type of surgery.

Bone Loss and Instability. Instability of a collateral ligament may confuse the preoperative osteotomy planning. Although some advise varus and valgus stress radiographs, I concur with most surgeons in my preference for a single-leg, standing, anteroposterior, weight-bearing radiograph on 91- or 130-cm films (36- or 51-inch), which minimizes the effect of collateral ligament laxity. A weight-bearing anteroposterior film (of any length) helps to differentiate between ligamentous instability and instability due to cartilage or bone loss. A severe bone loss (greater than 10 mm) of the medial tibial plateau may contribute significantly to instability after osteotomy and to a "teeter-totter" effect on the tibial eminence.

There is controversy over the correction of ligament instability. Maquet[2,3] reported that sufficient correction by osteotomy produces ligamentous tightening by the end of the first postoperative year, regardless of the preoperative laxity. I have not tightened collateral ligaments, and have not observed subsequent symptomatic ligament laxity, though it required 2 years for one knee with a lax lateral collateral ligament to tighten up.

Subluxation of the Tibia. Lateral subluxation of the tibia has been reported in about 50% of knees with 10 to 15 degrees of varus deformity, and in almost 100% with more than 15 degrees of varus deformity. Some surgeons consider more than 1 cm of lateral subluxation of the tibia a contraindication to osteotomy. I agree with Keene and Dyreby[12] and associates, however, who did not find a correlation between the degree of tibial subluxation and the final clinical scores.

Obesity. Obesity, by adding major weight-bearing stress to the knee joint, aggravates the deleterious biomechanical effects of angular deformity. However, clinical judgment should prevail when faced with the option of unicompartmental or total knee replacement in a very painful knee with mainly unicompartmental osteoarthritis. In my practice, obese patients have been vigorously counseled to lose weight before surgery, which has been delayed for this purpose, but no one has been denied HTO solely because of obesity. Osteotomy is more likely to be selected in less than ideal circumstances for younger patients and patients with strenuous occupational stress. Obesity may be an even greater threat to the long-term stability and success of TKR.

In summary, a young, active patient involved in strenuous activities but with relative contraindications of severe osteoarthritis and/or deformity, obesity, or tibial subluxation may still be considered for HTO,[13] whereas the same findings in a patient over 60 years of age would lead to a TKR. Surprisingly good results can be achieved by correcting the angular deformity in these challenging cases, as originally advised by Maquet.[2,3]

As always, surgical decision making is done one case at a time, and not rigidly "by the book."

Undercorrection

Undercorrection is the most common cause of poor results with valgus HTO. Two main reasons for undercorrection are failure to initially obtain the desired valgus angle ("didn't get it"), and failure to maintain the initial correction ("didn't keep it").

Failure to Initially Obtain the Desired Valgus Angle

This failure can be due to either preoperative x-ray technical problems or problems with preoperative planning, or intraoperative technical problems.

Radiographic Protocol. Consistent technical accuracy in taking the x-rays must be achieved to determine the precise degree of initial preoperative varus or valgus, to plan the surgery accurately, and to follow the postoperative changes over time with accuracy and consistency for outcome determinations in each patient and in a series of patients.

Positioning when obtaining these films is the essential factor; it must be consistent. In particular, the radiographic technologist must take special care to avoid limb rotation from true anteroposterior, posteroanterior, or lateral projections. Failure to do so introduces considerable error into the measurement of angles. Flexion contractures also make accurate angular measurement difficult.

For the preoperative initial x-ray protocol, the following four views are recommended:

1. A 91-cm (36-inch) or 130-cm (51-inch) single leg standing anteroposterior view of the involved leg.[7] The mechanical axis and femoral tibial angle are accurately measured on this view, as well as the height of the medial and lateral joint spaces and a relatively anterior tibiofemoral contact area. The hip and ankle joint should also be adequately visible for evaluation, even though the x-rays are diverging proximally and distally.
2. A 45-degree flexion posteroanterior view of both knees.[14] The height of the medial and lateral joint spaces at a relatively posterior tibiofemoral contact area can be accurately measured. The degenerative joint changes are usually more severe in this more posterior region, and therefore these measurements add sensitivity by recording the narrowest joint spaces.
3. A 20-degree standing lateral view. The patellar index is measured on this view. The quadriceps contraction keeps the patellar tendon taut and thus helps to avoid positioning artifact of patellar position or patellar tendon length. The patellar index is normal if the patellar tendon is within 20% of the length of the patella. This is particularly useful for diagnosing patella infera. Patellar degenerative joint disease may be seen as well.
4. A 45-degree Merchant patellar axial view. Patellar degenerative joint disease is well seen on this view as well as patellofemoral congruity, or lack thereof, at this physiologically functional angle. At more than 45 degrees of knee flexion, the patella is almost always congruous, and therefore the traditional sunrise view with greater knee flexion is not as useful.

Additional x-ray views may be obtained if needed, but these four provide the essentials for accurate preoperative determination of the severity of the arthritis and the precise amount of varus or valgus, for preoperative planning, and for postoperative follow-up.

Based on anteroposterior long, standing x-rays and standing 45-degree flexion posteroanterior weight-bearing films, overall assessment of the severity of the osteoarthritic degenerative changes of the medial compartment is made according to the classifications of Ahlback[15]:

Grade I:	Joint space narrowing.
Grade II:	Joint space obliteration.
Grade III:	Mild bone destruction (less than 5 mm).
Grade IV:	Moderate bone destruction (5 to 10 mm).

Grade V: Lateral subluxation (more than 5 mm) of the tibial plateau, which may include lateral arthrosis and more than 10 mm of bone destruction.

For preoperative x-ray planning, it is important to obtain accurately positioned x-ray views, which include at a minimum the first three views listed above for preoperative initial x-ray protocol. Mechanical axis and femoral-tibial angle measurements define the severity of the deformity.

The magnification of these images must be determined so that surgical decisions are based on the actual dimensions of the proximal tibia. Magnification markers (either a radiopaque 10-mm ball or two radiopaque marks 10 cm apart on a bar) can be taped to the skin halfway between the anterior and posterior proximal tibial borders when taking the long anteroposterior standing film. Alternatively, a long radiopaque ruler can be taped to the skin in the same manner for the long anteroposterior standing x-ray. This allows direct measurement of the tibia, since the ruler is magnified to the same degree as the bone.

For the closing wedge HTO, the ruler technique is more accurate and easier than making tracings and cutouts. For the dome or wedge HTO, the divergence angle of proximal and distal pins can be calculated (see below) from the long anteroposterior single leg standing view.

In summary, undercorrection is often a technical problem starting with the preoperative x-rays. Preoperative radiographs may not have been weight bearing (leading to failure to account for cartilage or bone loss or ligamentous laxity), may have been too short for accurate determination of the deformity, or may have been rotated (leading to underestimation of the angular deformity). Failure to compensate accurately for x-ray magnification can also produce intraoperative error.

Recommended Terminology for Lower Limb Radiographs and Their Measurement. The literature contains varying and not always clearly defined references to x-ray views and techniques. The inconsistent terminology for measurement of these x-ray views makes it difficult to evaluate the published results. We need a standard nomenclature. I propose the following:

A *short film* may be taken on any standard cassette normally used for knee x-ray films.

A *long film* is taken on cassettes with dimensions of 35 by 91 cm (14 by 36 inches) or 35 by 130 cm (14 by 51 inches). The goal is to visualize the entire limb from the femoral head to the ankle joint. This is the more accurate format, and its use is strongly recommended. It should be obtained as an anteroposterior, single-leg standing film.

The *anatomic axis of the femur* (Fig. 22.1) is a line down the "center" of the diaphysis (shaft) of the femur. This is most accurately located by connecting two points. One method is to measure the center of the femoral condyle at the intercondylar notch as point 1 and to use a point at the measured center of the upper femoral shaft diameter (as high as the film length allows) or the point of convergence of the lateral portion of the superior femoral neck and the greater trochanter as point 2. A second method establishes point 1 at the measured

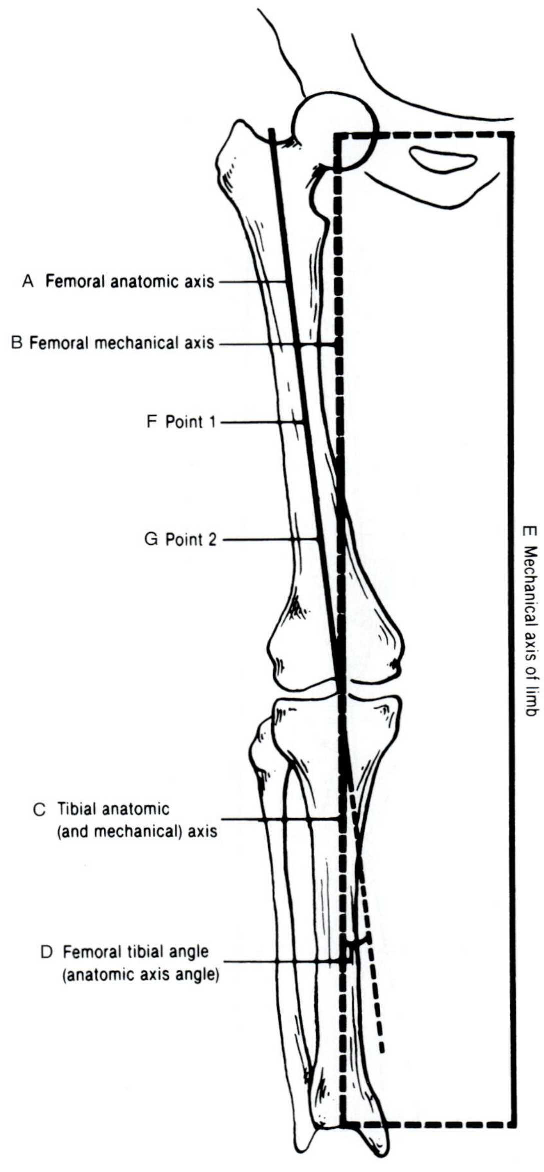

Figure 22.1. Normal lower extremity alignment. The femoral-tibial angle is made by crossing the femoral and tibial anatomic axes. **A:** Femoral anatomic axis. **B:** Femoral mechanical axis. **C:** Tibial anatomic (and mechanical) axis. **D:** Femoral-tibial angle (anatomic axis angle). **E:** Mechanical axis of limb. **F:** Point 1. **G:** Point 2.

center of the femoral shaft diameter halfway between the proximal and distal ends of the femur. Point 2 is 10 cm above the knee joint at the measured center of the femoral shaft. These two methods may yield slightly different results.

The *anatomic axis of the tibia* (Fig. 22.1) is a line from the measured center of the ankle joint (i.e., the center of the articular portion of the distal tibia at the ankle joint) to the measured center of the proximal tibial plateau. Because in taller patients a 1-m cassette may exclude the ankle joint, it is acceptable (and occasionally necessary) to mark the distal tibial point in the measured center of the tibial shaft as far distal as possible.

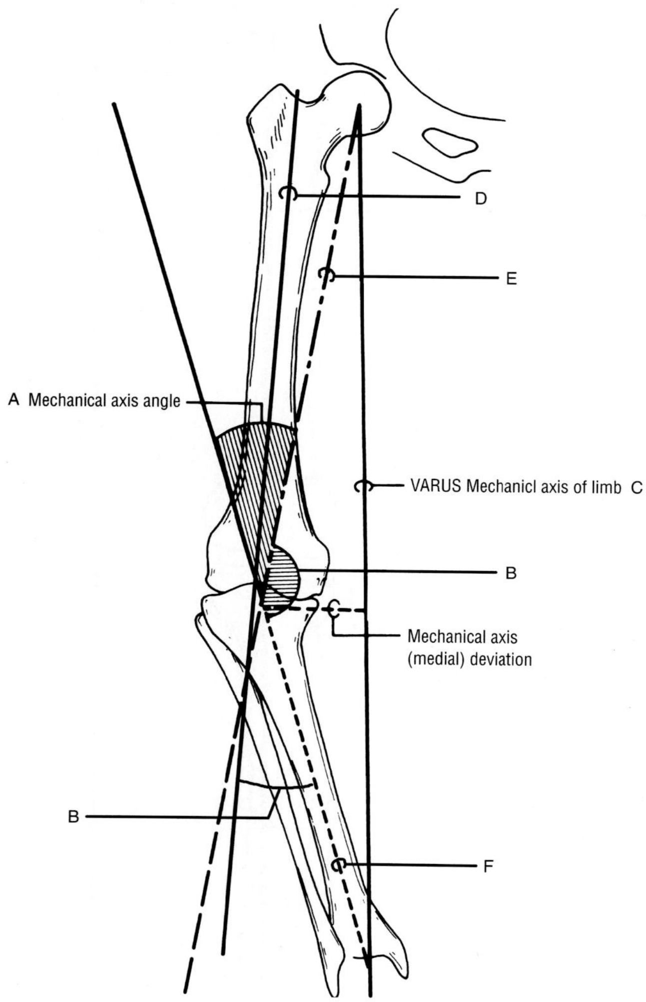

Figure 22.2. Severe varus deformity. The mechanical axis angle is made by crossing the femoral and tibial mechanical axes. **A:** Mechanical axis angle. **B:** Femoral-tibial angle (anatomic axis angle). **C:** Mechanical axis of limb in varus. **D:** Femoral anatomic axis. **E:** Femoral mechanical axis. **F:** Tibial mechanical (and anatomic) axis.

The *mechanical axis of the tibia* (Fig. 22.2) is the same as the anatomic axis of the tibia.

The *femoral-tibial angle* (Fig. 22.2) is the angle in the coronal plane formed by the intersection of the *anatomic axes* of the femur and tibia. It is often called the "anatomic axis" but perhaps should be called the "anatomic axis angle." It should be obtained with the patient standing, ideally on one leg only, with no more than balance support from the opposite limb. It is best taken on anteroposterior long films. The shape of the tibia or femur will influence the angle obtained.

The *mechanical axis of the femur* (Fig. 22.2) is a line between the center of the femoral head (established by eye estimation) and the measured center of the femoral condyles at the intercondylar notch or one of several almost contiguous points.

The *mechanical axis of the lower limb* (Fig. 22.2) is a line from the center of the femoral head (established by eye estimation) to the center of the ankle joint, as in the tibial anatomic axis. In a normal knee, this line passes within 3 to 4 mm of the center of the joint, which can be established at the measured midpoint of the tibial plateau. This axis defines the weight-bearing line of the limb for practical purposes. It should be obtained from a long single-leg weight-bearing film.

The *mechanical axis angle of the lower limb* (Fig. 22.2) is formed in the coronal plane by the intersection of the mechanical axis of the femur with the mechanical axis of the tibia. The term *mechanical axis* is often used to denote either of these measurements and may be a source of confusion. As with the femoral-tibial angle and mechanical axis, it is best obtained from a single-leg weight-bearing film, although patient inability may require it to be obtained from a two-leg weight-bearing view on a long film. In a normal knee, this angle is very close to 0 degrees and the mechanical axis of the femur overlies that drawn for the mechanical axis of the lower limb. If there is any angular deformity, the mechanical axis angle is different from the mechanical axis. "Mechanical axes are more reliable than anatomic axes in defining knee joint deformity."[7]

The *mechanical axis deviation* (Figs. 22.3 and 22.4) is the distance in millimeters or centimeters that the mechanical axis of the limb is displaced from the measured midpoint of the tibial plateau (subchondral plate). It is a simple and consistent measure of deformity and of its correction, which permits a percentage of deviation to be derived that is a consistent comparison between x-ray exams over time, and between patients. For example, "The mechanical axis is medially deviated 2.0 cm over a 4.0-cm hemitibia." This describes a mechanical axis medial deviation of 50% of the medial hemitibia.

The *deviation angle of the mechanical axis* is the angle between the mechanical axis of the limb and the

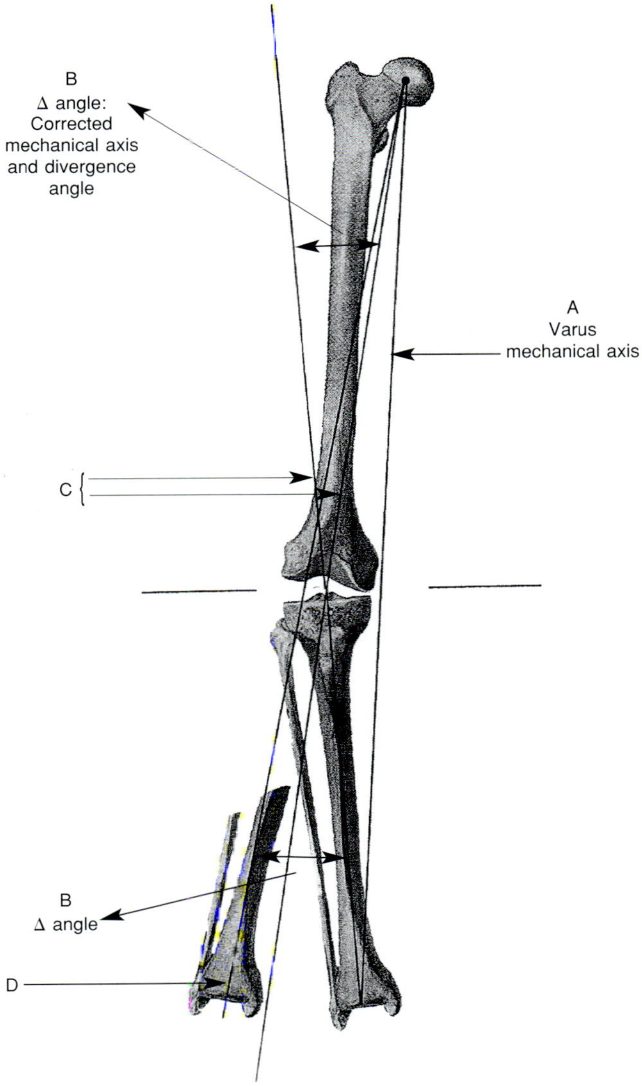

Figure 22.3. Varus knee with preoperative x-ray measurement. **A:** Mechanical axis in varus. **B:** Medial deviation of mechanical axis. **C:** Delta angle or angle of change after osteotomy. This is the corrected mechanical axis angle (CMA) and the divergence angle of two pins or screws in the tibia, which, when brought parallel, provide the desired valgus. **D:** The two intersection lines that made the delta angle (corrected mechanical axis angle). They are drawn from the center of the femoral head and the center of the ankle, intersecting in the lateral compartment at 30–50% lateral deviation to produce the desired postoperative mechanical axis. **E:** New leg position after valgus high tibial osteotomy correction.

tibial mechanical axis when the patient is standing. It is normally 0 degrees. This measurement is seldom used, but it can sometimes be informative.

The *tangential tilt angle* is the angle between the femoral condyle and the tibial plateaus, measured from

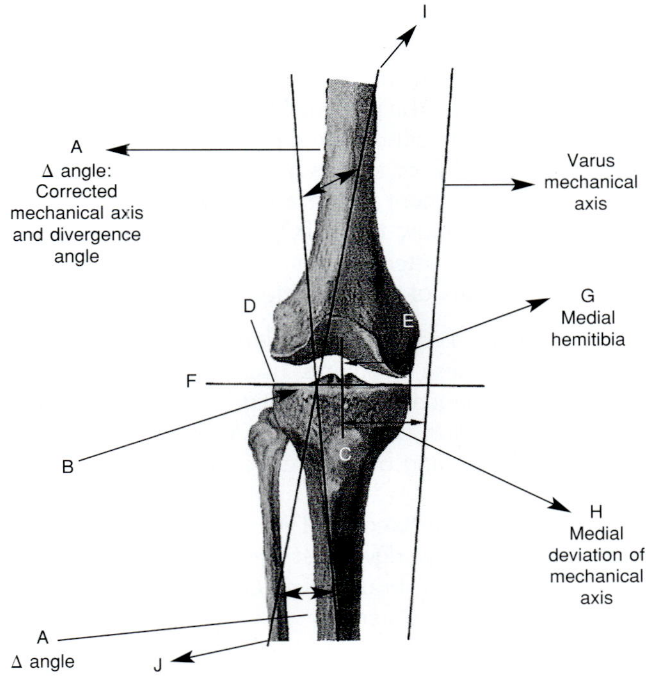

Figure 22.4. Expanded view of varus knee with all of the routinely used preoperative measurements. **A:** Delta angle (corrected mechanical axis and divergence angle). **B:** 30–50% lateral deviation of mechanical axis is desired postoperative result. **C:** Measured midpoint of tibia. Considered the midpoint of the knee for x-ray measurements. **D:** Lateral tibial bony border. **E:** Medial tibial bony border. **F:** Subchondral plate of tibia. **G:** Hemitibia. **H:** Medial deviation of mechanical axis. **I:** To center of femoral head. **J:** To center of ankle.

a coronal x-ray projection with the patient standing. This is no longer considered useful or clinically relevant.

A *45-degree posteroanterior flexion weight-bearing x-ray view*[14] assesses the relative narrowing of the tibiofemoral joint space and is useful for comparing the compromised joint space in a varus or valgus knee with that in the opposite knee. It is also more accurate and sensitive than the standard weight-bearing anteroposterior x-ray film taken with the knee in full extension. The femoral-tibial contact area on this projection is more posterior than the anteroposterior standing view with the knee(s) extended to 0 degrees. Osteoarthritic changes are usually more severe in the posterior tibial and femoral articular surfaces and therefore this view usually reveals the most compromised area(s) of the joint.

The *corrected mechanical axis* (angle) or the *mechanical axis correction angle* (Figs. 22.1–22.4) is formed by the intersection of one line drawn from the center of the femoral head (established by eye estimation) through the lateral tibia subchondral plate (tibial plateau) at a point 25% to 30% laterally deviated from the measured center of the tibial plateau, and a second line drawn from the center of the tibial articular surface at the ankle through the same point on the lateral tibial subchondral plate. The proximal and distal angles formed are the same, and either one equals the *divergence angle* of the two pins or screws in the lateral tibial (one in the proximal fragment above an HTO, and one in the distal fragment below the HTO), which, when brought parallel after the osteotomy is completed, will achieve the desired valgus of the corrected mechanical axis.

Intraoperative Technical Problems Causing Undercorrection. These problems usually begin preoperatively with inadequate x-rays, failure to determine the bone magnification on x-ray, and imprecise preoperative surgical planning of the wedge or dome procedure to be performed.

With the closing wedge HTO, all of the preoperatively determined wedge must be removed. Failure to plan well may result in undercorrection due to excision of a wedge that is too small.

The expectation that 1 mm of bone at the base of the lateral based wedge is equivalent to approximately 1 degree of angular correction is true only for a tibial width of 56 mm. Most tibias have a greater width, and will therefore require more than 1 mm to achieve 1 degree of angular correction.

Medial soft tissue release is sometimes needed to gain all of the desired valgus correction, especially if there is severe varus of more than 10 degrees. This is true for most HTO techniques.

The stabilizing lateral strut function of the fibula must be released in most cases, or all of the desired valgus correction will not be achieved or retained. Different ways to release the fibular strut are discussed under below (see Nerve Injury). This is true for most HTO techniques.

In the closing wedge technique, it is common to leave too much posterior cortical bone (usually because of concern for the adjacent major neurovascular structures). If not removed, this can prevent adequate closure of the wedge, even if it was correctly planned.

In the dome technique there is occasionally impaction of the proximal and distal fragment lateral tibial cortices, which limits the amount of valgus that can be obtained. A periosteal elevator in the lateral osteotomy can disimpact the cortices.

Intraoperative mechanical axis measurement, use of divergence angle (Figs. 22.3 and 22.4), and composite long x-rays can improve the accuracy of valgus correction.

Failure to Maintain the Initial Correction and Loss of Correction Producing Undercorrection

The usual causes of loss of the surgically obtained valgus correction can best be categorized by the interval after surgery when the loss occurs.

In the first few weeks postoperatively, loss of bony fixation at the osteotomy is the most common cause. For example, if external fixator pins become infected and require early removal prior to bony union at the osteotomy, there is increased risk of a loss of valgus correction. In this situation, it would be best to consider application of a well-molded long-leg cast in extension with full three-point valgus pressure applied while the cast material sets. This can be later converted to a cylinder cast, if there is x-ray evidence of early bony union and if the leg is sufficiently thin that a well-molded cylinder cast will stay up. Alternatively, a valgus orthotic can be applied and kept locked in extension for at least the first 4 to 6 weeks, depending on x-ray evidence of bony union. Touchdown weight bearing with two crutches or a walker is required until good bony union is evident.

Staple fixation can fail as well in the early weeks before bony stability at the osteotomy has occurred. Treatment would be the same as for early external fixator removal.

After the second or third month postoperative, loss of correction is commonly due to delayed union or nonunion at the osteotomy. Diagnosis is usually made with plain x-rays, but computed tomography (CT) scan and bone scan can assist when the diagnosis is uncertain (see below).

Some loss of correction can occur years after HTO and is probably due to progression of the medial compartment degenerative joint disease. This is a consistent observation of all long follow-up studies. There is no prevention, and the treatment is conversion to TKR if significant pain and disability have recurred.

Overcorrection

Overcorrection is not common. However, the causes of overcorrection usually start preoperatively, as with undercorrection, with inadequate x-rays (too short, rotated, not weight-bearing), failure to determine the bone magnification on x-ray, and imprecise planning of the wedge or dome procedure to be performed. During surgery, it is important to try to confirm how much valgus correction has been achieved before committing to the final fixation of the osteotomy. The same methods can be used that were discussed for undercorrection. If there appears to be excessive valgus, correction, if possible, should be done then. If a closed-wedge HTO has been done, it is worth trying to replace some of the wedge laterally, and morcellizing the rest to fill the space between the proximal and distal fragments as needed. Since solid contact between two flat surfaces (the ideal) has been lost, longer postoperative touchdown weight bearing may be necessary, depending on x-ray evidence of bony union. More secure fixation than staples, or staples and cast, may also be beneficial. Blade plates, plates and screws, or external fixators are all generally available and may be advisable depending on the surgeon's assessment of the osteotomy stability.

If a barrel vault (dome) HTO has been done, it is relatively easy to decrease the valgus at surgery. Even in the first 1 to 2 weeks postoperatively, the valgus can be reduced, especially if an external fixator has been used. It requires only releasing the external fixator, repositioning the alignment, and then resecuring and compressing the external fixator. If internal fixation has been used, it is still possible to reduce the valgus in the first 1 to 2 weeks postoperatively, but only with major open surgery. This may not be the better decision unless the postoperative femoral tibial angle is 15 to 20 degrees or more. However, the specific situation will have to be individually assessed.

For most patients, a mild to moderate amount of increased valgus in the range of 12 to 15 degrees (femoral tibial angle) is well tolerated. In the early postoperative period, the main patient concern is usually cosmetic. This concern can often be minimized by reminding the patient that the goal of the operation was to convert their "bowlegged" knee to a "knock-knee." Having reviewed their x-rays with them preoperatively and having explained the rationale of the procedure, they usually remain content, even with a bit more valgus than needed to accomplish symptom relief. It is also consistently true that relief of medial pain allays most patients' concern regarding some increased valgus. In fact, for some, the valgus is visible evidence of the reason their knee feels better.

However, over the years, excessive valgus may predispose some knees to earlier increasing lateral degenerative joint disease and lateral knee pain than might otherwise have resulted. There is no objective or consistent measure regarding this issue, which is why whether to do major open surgery to reduce valgus must remain an individual decision between surgeon and patient in each instance. If nothing is done to correct excessive valgus in the immediate postoperative period, it is probably best to continue the usual postoperative care. Should significant lateral pain later develop, there is always the option of joint replacement, if needed. This too should always be discussed preoperatively with the patient.

Foot pain may develop in the presence of significant genu valgum, due to compensatory subtalar and midfoot varus. A shoe orthotic will often help relieve the symptoms.

Delayed Union or Nonunion

Delayed union and nonunion are not common problems with HTO due to the large cancellous surfaces of the osteotomy. Each occurrence, however, is a very individual problem that may defy specific diagnosis despite an extensive evaluation. Some specific possible causes and some management options follow.

Clinically evident infection can cause a delayed or nonunion, though bone healing may continue even with infection, especially if adequate osteotomy immobilization can be maintained. In this era of "high tech" solutions, it is important to use the time-tested basic treatment methods for wound infection, including appropriate antibiotics and route of administration per culture and sensitivity, incision and drainage as the wound requires, and lower limb immobilization at least for a few weeks. In addition, limb elevation and rest are needed as are minimal and protected touchdown-only ambulation with two crutches or a walker, and good nutrition. Removal of the fixation device may be required to control the infection. In this situation, a valgus knee orthosis should be considered until bony union is achieved.

After the infection is controlled, a persistent failure of bone healing may require bone grafting. My strong preference remains fresh, posterior iliac crest, autogenous bone, which provides a large graft volume and a long successful history of producing bone union. Bone banks and non–human-derived grafting materials can be used when an autogenous source is not available or is contraindicated, but I would not consider them as the first choice until they can be shown to be as successful in the long term as fresh autogenous bone.

Subclinical "suspected" infection can be difficult, and sometimes impossible, to diagnose and may only be suspected. A patient can present with some, but rarely all of the following:

Early postoperative observations (first 2 to 3 weeks) can include wound erythema, induration, or edema; a small hematoma or seroma that is not drained or cultured; low-grade temperature elevations; borderline elevated white blood count with neutrophils shifted minimally to the left; negative fever of unknown origin workup including blood cultures; and difficulty regaining knee range of motion.

Later postoperative observations (after 6 to 8 weeks) can include persistence of any of the earlier problems except hematoma or seroma, which would have either resolved or become a more obvious problem needing drainage with culture and sensitivity, and treatment as indicated. In addition, continued or increasing proximal tibial pain may now be present, whereas pain should be mostly absent by this interval, with knee range of motion close to the preoperative values.

After 3 to 4 months postoperatively there may be failure to achieve solid bony union combined with some of the earlier postoperative observations which were suspicious of, but were not diagnosed as, infection. Attention at this point focuses on whether the delayed union is due to infection. I have found it helpful to involve consultants in infectious disease and nuclear medicine at this stage, and often earlier as well when a "suspicion" of infection existed.

Some of the techniques that have been helpful include computed axial tomography scan, magnetic resonance imaging (MRI), and bone scan with isotopes that can help differentiate bone from soft tissue infection (if present at all). Needle biopsy of bone can be used, but by this time if there is no clear diagnosis of infection, surgery is probably indicated and the biopsy can be done at that time. The procedure I have used in four cases involved open inspection of the osteotomy area anteriorly with tissue biopsy of the osteotomy site for stat Gram stain, culture and sensitivity, and histology. None had infection. Only one osteotomy had a nonunion (although it was expected in all four), and this was curetted and packed with fresh autogenous posterior iliac cancellous bone and healed. No instability was evident, so only a protective postoperative orthotic was used. The fact that the other three cases clearly had some peripheral bony bridging anteriorly at the time of direct surgical visualization and therefore no nonunion, demonstrates that even a CT scan can miss a thin rim of healing bone. All four went on to heal.

The value of ultrasound or electrical bone stimulation in these or other delayed unions needs further clarification, but seems promising at this time. I have had four or five cases in which I think bony union was accelerated with either electrical or ultrasound stimulation, but without adequate controls these results are only anecdotal.

Once active infection has been controlled, or shown not to be present, additional issues may arise, such as whether to attempt to regain lost valgus correction if the initially obtained valgus has indeed drifted back into varus, and whether to alter or reinsert fixation. Bone grafting may need to be part of this additional intervention. Use of a valgus orthosis may help maintain valgus correction until bone union is secure. I have found these orthotics helpful and well tolerated, especially when it is understood that their use is temporary.

Inadequate bone contact at the osteotomy may delay, but rarely prevents, bone union. If the osteotomy surfaces are irregular due to technical problems, these may touch only at the "peaks," producing inadequate bone surface contact. Separation of the proximal and distal tibial fragments will produce inadequate bone contact as well.

Though a medial gap may remain after good bone union has occurred in the lateral one-half to two-thirds of the osteotomy, it will reliably close by 12 to 24 months postoperatively and should therefore not be a cause for concern.

Too little compression may favor inadequate bone contact as well as allowing some motion at the osteotomy, either of which can delay union.

There is a subtle problem involving the fixation device that I believe I have seen twice, resulting in one delayed union and one nonunion. This problem can occur with either an external fixator or an internal blade plate. The interference with bony union appears to be caused by distal migration of the proximal tibial fragment fixation (either 5.0 mm external fixator screws or the blade of the blade plate) into the lateral part of the osteotomy itself. I believe the compression applied through the fixation device near the end of the procedure produces this distal migration through the relatively soft cancellous bone of the proximal fragment. Further compression only compresses the proximal fragment metal against the distal tibial fragment, and this is primarily against the dense lateral tibial cortical bone of the distal fragment. If this occurs, there may be no effective compression remaining in the lateral contact area of the osteotomy, and in fact there may even be some distraction, especially if excessive compression is applied, which can bend the distal screws and can produce a proximally directed force on the medial portion of the proximal fixation device (screw or blade of blade plate). This problem can be avoided by being careful to place the proximal fragment fixation screw or blade at least 1 cm above the osteotomy, particularly laterally, and by not compressing the osteotomy excessively. Although I think most of this problem starts intraoperatively, it is possible that it progresses somewhat in the early postoperative period as the knee is moved, stressing the proximal fixation.

Nerve or Vascular Injury

Nerve Injury

There is a consistent risk of peroneal nerve injury associated with HTO. Most larger studies report some cases, though the incidence varies widely. Peroneal nerve injury is associated with division of the fibular shaft. The incidence of peroneal nerve palsy (partial or complete) is most often reported with fibular neck osteotomy, followed by osteotomy in the middle and distal thirds of the fibular shaft. The junction of the middle and distal thirds is the safest region of the fibular shaft for osteotomy or short ostectomy. Safer still is a proximal tibiofibular joint capsulotomy, a medial fibular head minimal ostectomy, and "springing" the fibular head away from the tibia (with a $3/4$-inch curved osteotome) to ensure adequate fibular mobility when valgus tibial correction is achieved. This last technique is fully described and illustrated in the description of the HTO technique I have been using for the past 11 years.

The best prevention of peroneal nerve injury (often just some weakness of the extensor hallucis longus) is to avoid any surgery on the fibular shaft. Between January 1987 and now, I have done 116 HTOs. However, in the prior years (1983 to 1986), I had three peroneal nerve palsies. All three were associated with fibular osteotomy 10 to 15 cm below the fibular head, which is a common location for fibular osteotomy. Two were initially a drop-foot and the third a great toe weakness and numbness. They have all resolved to the point that only a small amount of residual great toe weakness remains.

Vascular Injury and Posterior Tibial Neurovascular Bundle Injury

The incidence of this rare complication of HTO can be even further decreased by attention to some anatomic details. Although the neurovascular bundle lies in close proximity to the posterior tibia, it is somewhat mobile. Therefore, careful dissection next to the bone is not likely to cause injury. However, the neurovascular bundle does not "fall away" from the tibia when the knee is flexed, even to 90 degrees. Knee flexion does, however, relax the musculotendinous structures adjacent to the neurovascular bundle, thus enhancing the normal mobility of the bundle, and knee extension accomplishes the opposite. Anteriorly directed pressure behind the knee can "trap" the neurovascular bundle against the posterior tibia. For this reason, it is essential to avoid bolsters or hands behind the knee during HTO. I have found it helpful to use a leg holder (Fig. 22.5) to maintain the desired flexion during surgery. This frees an assistant from having to control knee position and hip rotation, and helps to avoid a hand from inadvertently straying behind the knee.

The placement of most internal fixation devices on the lateral tibial surface can endanger the anterior tibial artery or its branches. This occurs because dissection and retraction to the posterior portion of the lateral tibial shaft, near the interosseous membrane, is often necessary to gain exposure and secure fixation of the osteotomy with the usual blade plates or plates and screws. The anterior tibial artery and its branches penetrate into this same space anterior to the interosseous membrane at the proximal tibia, and are thus at risk. Bleeding from one of the branches of the anterior tibial artery can be difficult to control because they are deep in the wound, which at that location is bounded by the rigid fibula, tibia, and interosseous membrane. This makes retraction and dissection for better visualization quite challenging.

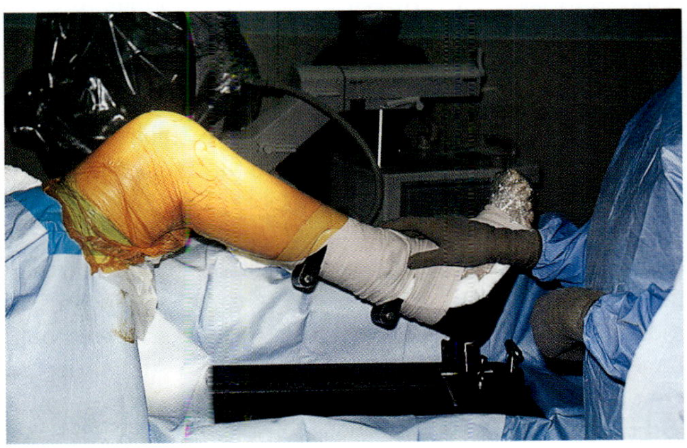

Figure 22.5. Leg holder (Innomed, Mentone, IN).

Completing the anterior compartment fasciotomy started proximally by the anterior exposure will help avoid anterior compartment syndrome, which is always a risk with tibial fracture, even when surgically produced.

Pin or screw insertion from lateral to medial for external or internal fixation of the tibia can produce vascular injury if the device penetrates too far posteriorly. If there is any question regarding the location of the hardware, obtain additional projections with the portable fluoroscope, especially lateral and external rotation views.

Metal Protruding into the Medial Joint Space and Fracture of the Proximal Tibial Fragment

These are intraoperative technical problems that can usually be avoided by generous use of portable fluoroscopy. If a screw, pin, or blade is introduced from anterolateral to posteromedial, the x-ray external rotation view can bring the metal to 90 degrees from the central x-ray beam, thus showing the true length and tip position of the metal. This view can be used beneficially, therefore, in addition to the usual anteroposterior and lateral views if needed.

There is a risk of fracture of the proximal fragment in the closing wedge HTO if the medial cortex is left intact and a strong valgus force is applied. It is therefore important to at least weaken the medial cortex with drill holes or a partial osteotomy so that the valgus force passes through the proximal tibia in the plane of the osteotomy.

Fixation Placement Problems

For high tibial valgus osteotomy, internal or external fixation is usually inserted from the lateral tibial surface. It is highly desirable to direct the fixation from anterolateral to posteromedial. There are several reasons for this:

1. As discussed above (see Nerve or Vascular Injury), it is important to stay anterior on the lateral tibial surface in order to avoid the anterior tibial artery and

its branches, which lie posteriorly at the proximal tibia.

2. It is technically easier for visualization and instrumentation, and gentler to soft tissues and periosteum, to stay more anterior in the anterior compartment.
3. Good bone purchase and control can be achieved without needing to go more posterior.
4. Only the anterior 1.5 to 2.0 cm of the lateral tibial shaft needs to be exposed where the fixation is to be inserted. The anterior tibial muscle that is released from the tibia in this area is gently retracted. The fixation is inserted through the exposed bone and not through the muscle. This minimizes muscle injury, bleeding, and pain, as well as decreases the risk of peroneal nerve injury.

If an external fixator is used, the skin edges should be held temporarily approximated (with a suture, towel clip, etc.) when the external fixator pins or screws are inserted through the skin. This prevents the pin or screw from holding the skin edges apart, which necessitates replacing the external fixator when attempting to close the wound at the end of the operation. However, after passing the pin or screw through the skin, I advise exposing the wound as needed for each pin or screw so as to retract the anterior compartment muscle out of the way. If directed from anterolateral to posteromedial, the external fixator pin or screw thus passes essentially from skin to bone and minimally or not at all through muscle.

These comments regarding anterior compartment muscle apply only to the fixation device at the *distal* fragment, since there is so little soft tissue over the *proximal* tibial fragment's lateral and anterolateral surface.

Conversion to Total Knee Replacement

Some authors state that doing a TKR after a closing wedge HTO is more like a revision TKR than a primary one. This has not been the case in my experience after dome HTO.

With wedge HTO, I believe the difficulty when present stems from the more common occurrence of patella infera and the loss of metaphyseal bone with resulting "step-off" laterally, inherent in the closing wedge technique. If a significant tibial bone segment must be removed for the TKR, the surgeon risks looking at the "bottom of the ice cream cone" and at a major decrease in medial-lateral tibial diameter. This can result in a significant mismatch between the medial-lateral femoral and tibial diameters, or less than adequate bone support for the lateral part of the tibial component. A thinner tibial cut can be planned if a lateral prosthetic wedge or block is used as a lateral filler. A V-Y quadriceps tenoplasty can help adjust for patella infera, but this displaces the patella distally, which changes its contact area on the femoral trochlea.

Ligament Laxity

Preoperative exam will detect significant ligament laxity. Single-leg, standing, anteroposterior x-ray will usually clarify functional ligament balance and laxity issues. It is rarely necessary to consider varus-valgus stress x-rays.

Lateral ligament laxity is of special concern, and if severe is probably a contraindication to vagus HTO since retention of the valgus correction may not be possible, resulting in a teeter-totter effect.

Anterior cruciate ligament (ACL) laxity is rarely a practical problem in these patients, since they usually have low-demand knees. It is preferable to do the HTO, correct the bony alignment, and then observe whether the ACL laxity is symptomatic. With this approach an ACL reconstruction may not be necessary.

Significant medial or posterior laxity in this patient group is very rare. If encountered, it is best approached like ACL laxity. I have no experience with collateral ligament tightening as part of an HTO, and have not found it necessary.

DISTAL FEMORAL OSTEOTOMY

This procedure is reserved for lateral compartment osteoarthritis with genu valgum. Correction should be to 0 degrees, or to 3 to 4 degrees of valgus, but should not be overcorrected into varus (in contrast to the varus knee, which is beneficially slightly overcorrected into valgus). Preservation of the joint line parallel to the ground is the reason for correcting the excessive genu valgum above the knee joint. Joint obliquity can result when a significant valgus deformity is corrected by an HTO. Either a medial or lateral approach to the supracondylar femur can be used. The same three techniques as used for HTO for intraoperatively checking the amount of angular correction can be used for distal femoral osteotomy. Fixation must be rigid due to the anatomic requirements of the femur, which has a thick cortex, a relatively small bone contact surface, and much less cancellous bone than the proximal tibia. Due to the large circumference of the thigh, because of the thigh muscles, cast immobilization is not adequate. External fixation is also not a good choice due to the large muscle mass through which the external fixator screws would have to penetrate. Staples do not provide sufficient mechanical strength. Therefore, a blade plate or plate and screws are the fixation of choice for a distal femoral osteotomy. The supracondylar location of the osteotomy rules out current techniques of intramedullarly fixation.

Results of distal femoral osteotomy for valgus knees

Figure 22.6. Saw bones: plate of instrumentation unit secured to tibia with one uni- or bicortical screw.

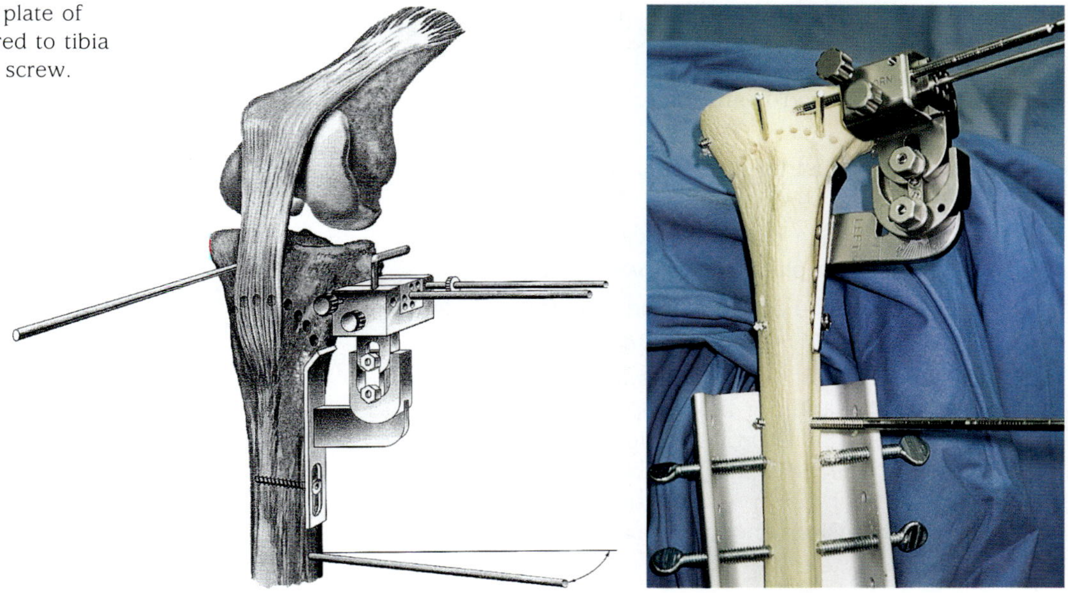

A B

are not as good as HTO for varus knees. Because there are far more knees with varus deformity, distal femoral osteotomy is a less common procedure than HTO. As a result, most orthopedic surgeons have relatively little experience with distal femoral osteotomy. The patient group tends to be older, and there may be a hereditary influence. Due to the poorer results of distal femoral osteotomy (compared to HTO), patients over 50 years old with significantly painful lateral knee osteoarthritis with genu valgum may be advised to have a unicompartmental or a total knee replacement. Therefore, patients with moderate genu valgum and mild to moderate pain that can be reasonably controlled by nonoperative means can be treated conservatively until pain and disability progress to the level that joint replacement can be appropriately recommended.

I believe that some of the previously discussed potential complications of HTO can be prevented by using a high tibial dome (vault) osteotomy. I have developed appropriate instrumentation for this technique (Figs. 22.6 and 22.7) that is not commercially available at present. This blade plate instrumentation helps to re-

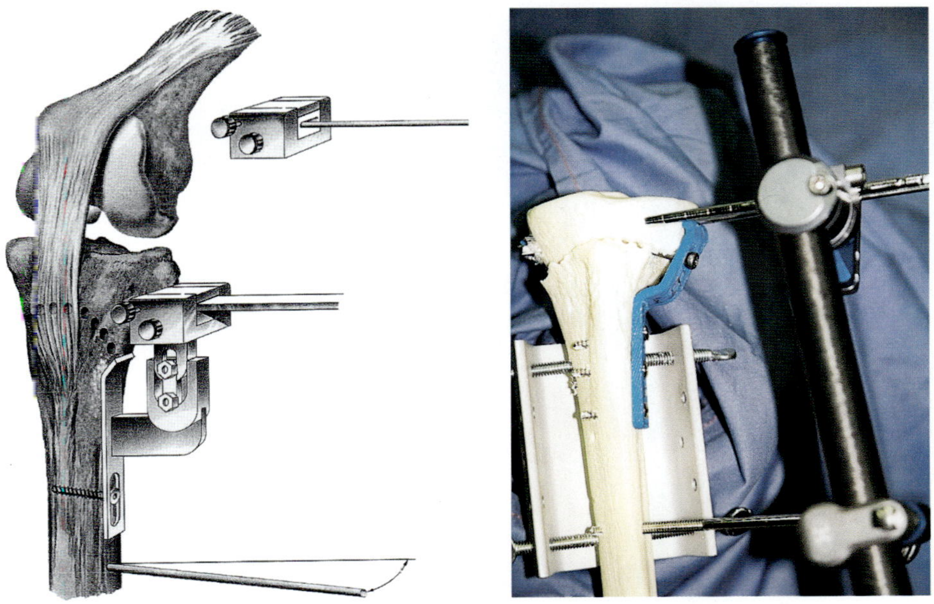

Figure 22.7. Saw bones: temporary intraoperative external fixator securing and gently compressing the proximal and distal 5-mm screws and osteotomy. The screws are now parallel.

A B

solve many of the internal fixation problems encountered with a valgus HTO:

The blade is directed from anterolateral to posteromedial.

The plate is applied far anteriorly on the lateral tibial shaft.

Since this is a blade plate, it provides more stability and rigidity than a plate and screws, or staples.

Compression can be applied to the osteotomy as desired before placing screws in the plate.

The instrumentation unit and this technique confine dissection to the anterior tibia, improve the accuracy of angular correction, provide a template for the final blade-plate angle if the final blade-plate implant needs to be bent, and provides three intraoperative checks of the desired angular correction.

References

1. Coventry MB. Osteotomy of the upper portion of the tibia for degenerative arthritis of the knee. *J Bone Joint Surg* 1965;47A:984.
2. Maquet P. Biomechanics of the knee and surgical possibilities of healing ostioarthritic knees. *Clin Orthop* 1980; 146:102.
3. Maquet P. The treatment of choice in osteoarthritis of the knee. *Clin Orthop* 1985;192:108.
4. Fujisawa Y, Masuhara K, Shiomi S. The effect of high tibial osteotomy on osteoarthritis of the knee. *Orthop Clin North Am* 1979;10:585.
5. Oldenbring S, Egund N, Lindstrand A, et al. Cartilage regeneration after proximal tibial osteotomy for medial gonarthrosis. *Clin Orthop* 1992;277:210–216.
6. Maquet P. *Biomechanics of the Knee.* New York: Springer-Verlag, 1984.
7. Chao E. Biomechanics of high tibial osteotomy. In: *American Academy of Orthopaedic Surgeons Symposium on Reconstructive Surgery of the Knee.* St. Louis: CV Mosby, 1978.
8. Harding ML. A fresh appraisal of tibial osteotomy for osteoarthritis of the knee. *Clin Orthop* 1976;114:223.
9. Jackson JP, Waugh W. First high tibial osteotomy report for knee degenerative joint disease. *J Bone Joint Surg* 1958;40B:826.
10. Jackson JP, Waugh W. Tibial osteotomy for osteoarthritis of the knee. *J Bone Joint Surg* 1961;43B:746.
11. Johnson LL. Arthroscopic abrasion arthroplasty, historical and pathological perspective: present status. *Arthroscopy* 1986;2:54–69.
12. Keene J, Dyreby J. High tibial osteotomy in the treatment of osteoarthritis of the knee. *J Bone Joint Surg* 1983;65A:36–42.
13. Korn MW. Combined arthroscopy and high tibial osteotomy. In: Shahriaree H (ed). *Textbook of Arthroscopic Surgery.* Philadelphia: JB Lippincott, 1992:437–548.
14. Rosenberg T, Paulos L, Parker R, et al. The 45 degree posterior-anterior flexion and weight-bearing radiograph of the knee. *J Bone Joint Surg* 1988;70A:1479.
15. Ahlback S. Osteoarthrosis of the knee: a radiographic investigation. *Acta Radiol Suppl* 1968;277:1–7.

Section VI

Complications, Pitfalls, and Salvage in Prosthetic Knee Arthroplasty

Chapter 23

Overview of Complications of Total Knee Arthroplasty

Felicia M. Ollivierre and M. Mike Malek

Over the past two decades, total knee arthroplasty has evolved into a procedure with reliable and predictable results. The reported 10- to 15-year survivorship of a total knee replacement is as high as 95% to 98%.[1–3] Refinements in prosthetic designs, recognition of the importance of ligamentous balancing, and modifications in instrumentation to achieve appropriate alignment contribute to the improved success rate. Despite the improvement in surgical outcome, however, complications continue to occur.

An understanding of the potential complications and pitfalls of primary and revision total knee reconstruction is essential for prevention. The common complications of total knee arthroplasty include infection, loosening, thromboembolism, arthrofibrosis, periprosthetic fracture, extensor mechanism dysfunction, and bone loss. There are also neurovascular and wound-related complications.

This chapter reviews the common complications and pitfalls of total knee replacement procedures. For each complication, the incidence, etiology, predisposing risk factors, and management options are discussed.

SOFT TISSUE COMPLICATIONS

The incidence of wound-related complications following primary and revision total knee arthroplasty is reported to be as high as 10% to 22%.[4] Types of wound problems include delayed wound healing, prolonged or persistent drainage, hematoma, superficial infection, and necrosis. The significance of wound healing problems is that they lead to an increased risk of developing deep infection; 17% to 50% of prosthetic infections are associated with a history of prolonged wound drainage.[5]

Compared to the hip, the knee is a superficial joint with a relatively thin soft tissue envelope. The superficial nature of the joint can complicate an otherwise minor wound problem. In addition, the knee has a unique vascular anatomy. The blood supply to the soft tissues of the anterior knee is random and arises from the contributions of multiple vessels. An anastomosis of arteries forms a ring around the patella.[6] Arising from the popliteal artery, the inferior and superior genicular arteries supply terminal branches to the anastomotic ring. Additional arteries contributing branches to the ring include the lateral circumflex femoral, a branch of the profunda femoris artery; the supreme genicular, from the superficial femoral artery; and the anterior tibial recurrent, from the tibial artery.[7]

The blood supply to the skin of the lower extremity typically arises from direct cutaneous vessels, musculocutaneous perforators, and fasciocutaneous perforators.[8] However, the anterior knee does not have intermuscular septa or muscles to provide arterial perforators to the skin. In addition, except for the medial saphenous region of the knee, there are no direct cutaneous vessels.[9] The arterial blood supply is not located superficially near the dermis.[10] Anteriorly, the circulation of the skin is dependent on the dermal plexus. This plexus originates from arterioles traveling with the subcutaneous fascia.[5] Undermining the subcutaneous layer and raising skin flaps superficial to this fascia can disrupt skin circulation and potentially lead to wound compromise.[4] To preserve skin circulation, it is recommended to leave the fascia attached to the subcutaneous layer.

Choosing the appropriate skin incision is important to reduce the risk of developing a wound complication. Midline skin incisions are generally the least disruptive to the blood supply.[4,5] The appropriate incision for primary and revision arthroplasty is one that allows sufficient exposure but avoids the creation of hypovascular flaps. Patients at greatest risk for developing severe wound complications following total knee arthroplasty have a history of prior knee skin incisions[5,7,10,11] (Figs. 23.1–23.6).

Unfortunately, many patients in need of primary and revision total knee replacements have had prior operative interventions and may have numerous scars of varying orientations and locations. Performing a new surgical approach in the presence of preexisting incisions can potentially compromise the circulation. For the previously operated knee, it is recommended to place the incision at or near the midline.[10] When possible, preexisting scars should be utilized.[5,11] In addition, old incisions can be incorporated, if they lie near the midline.

Previous straight medial and lateral incisions, such as those used for collateral ligament repairs, cannot be easily incorporated with a standard midline approach and most often can be ignored.[7] Also, prior short parapatellar incisions can generally be ignored.[5] If necessary, previous incisions can be crossed at 90-degree angles without significant risk of soft tissue complications.[7]

Although midline incisions are preferred, an exception is made when there are prior longitudinal incisions, such as an old medial or lateral parapatellar incision. In this setting, use of the previous approach is preferred

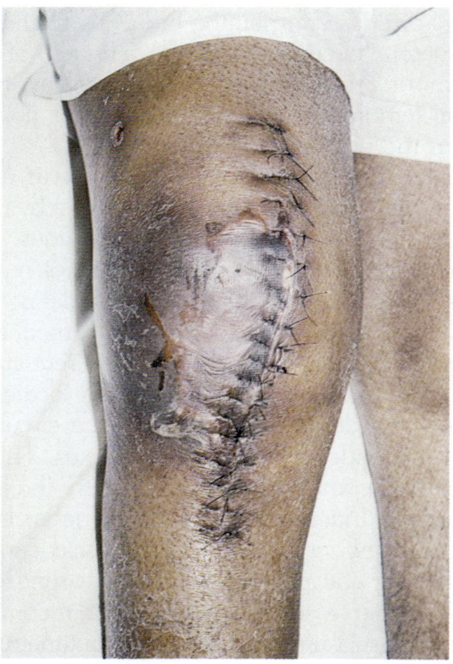

Figure 23.1. An avascular flap 5 days post–total knee arthroplasty in a patient with multiple prior surgeries and incisions on the knee.

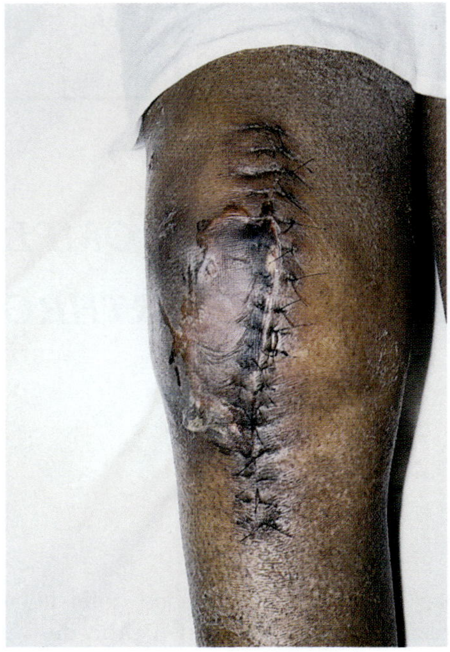

Figure 23.2. Gradual process of necrotic flap development, which appeared to be superficial. No generalized signs of infection and no joint involvement 9 days postoperatively.

over the creation of a new midline incision. The skin between scars has an increased potential for inadequate vascularity. Also, when there are multiple longitudinal scars about the anterior knee, it is generally recommended to choose the most lateral scar.[5,7] The rationale for use of the lateral incision is based on the vascular pattern, which is richer on the medial side of the knee compared to the lateral side. In addition, transcutaneous oxygen measurements show reduced oxygen tension in the lateral skin region.[4,5,12]

Associated with a high incidence of wound complications are curved medial incisions with large laterally based flap.[10–12] Typically, the more medial the incision, the larger the lateral skin flap is required for adequate exposure. However, the blood supply of these flaps is random and may be poorly vascularized. In addition, the base to width ratio may not be sufficient to support the flap, resulting in ischemia.[13] Moreover, wide scars with underlying atrophic soft tissue may suggest prior subdermal circulatory compromise and should be approached with caution.

In addition to previous scars, other significant risk factors for the development of soft tissue complications are skin compromised by burns, irradiation, or prior wound healing problems. Irradiated tissue is associated with atrophy, fibrosis, and poor tissue repair secondary to residual endothelial cell injury and endarteritis.[14]

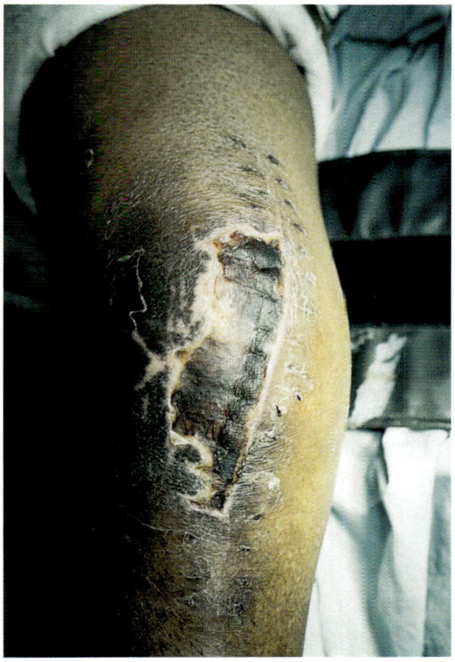

Figure 23.3. At 2 weeks postoperation, the skin lesion has completely demarcated. No drainage and no sign of joint involvement are present.

Another factor that can adversely affect wound healing is cigarette smoking.[15] Substances contained in cigarettes such as nicotine and its breakdown product cotinine cause systemic vasoconstriction.[7,15] Systemic vasoconstriction potentially decreases microcirculation to the skin. Smoking can also affect cellular healing by inhibiting factors involved in wound epithelialization.[7,15]

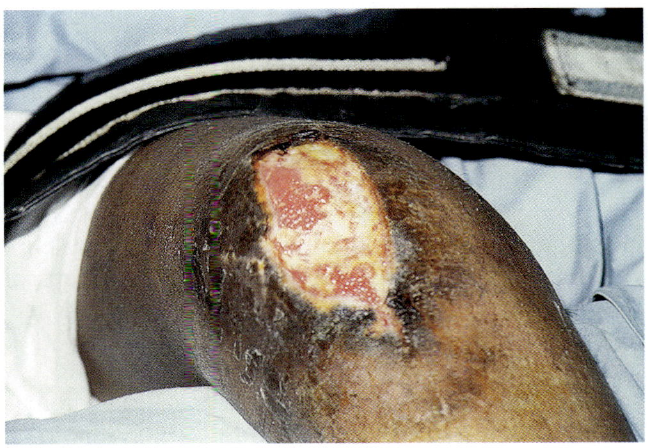

Figure 23.4. At 15 days postoperation, the skin lesion and surrounding necrotic tissues are debrided. Split-thickness skin graft will be applied.

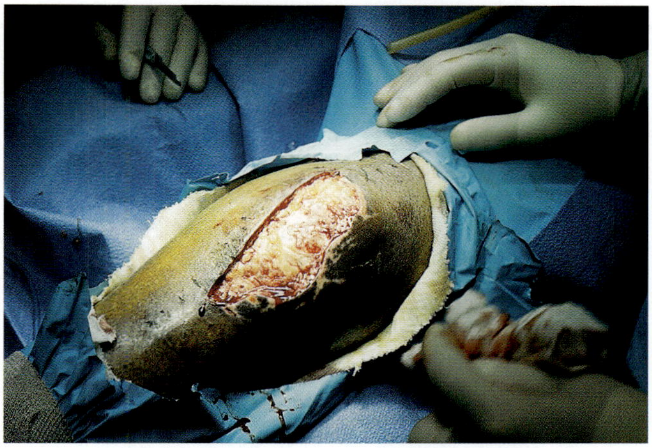

Figure 23.5. Debridement completed prior to application of split-thickness skin graft.

Other less significant risks for wound-related problems include chronic steroid use.[16] Steroid use can be associated with poor tissue turgor and poor skin vascularity.[4] Wound inflammation, epithelialization, and collagen synthesis are reduced.[14] Cortisone causes an in-

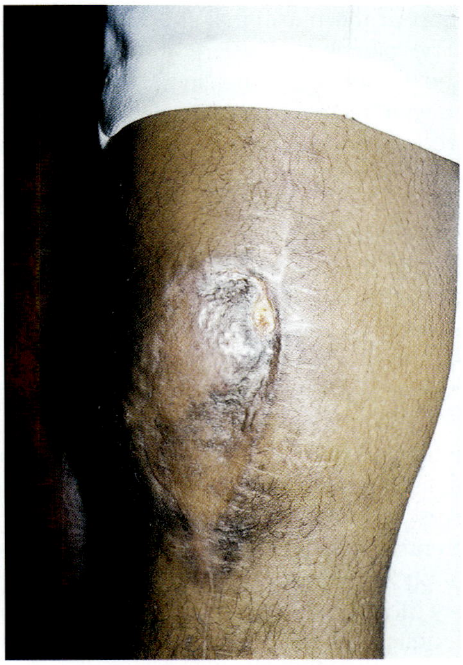

Figure 23.6. At 3 months postoperation, the skin graft has healed. No further skin problems or joint problems encountered. At the time of this writing, the patient is 12 years postoperation and continues to be asymptomatic and has not required revision.

crease in collagenase activity, causing collagen destruction.[11] Inhibited fibroblast proliferation and collagen accumulation may result in decreased tensile wound strength.[11] Steroid use in the early postoperative period may potentially impair healing.[14] However, at this time, there is not an established need to eliminate steroids prior to surgery when they are required for disease control and prevention of addisonian crises. Chronic steroid users are theoretically at greater risk for developing wound complications.[4]

It has been reported that wound-related complications are more common in rheumatoid arthritis than osteoarthritis. It has been observed that there is some reduction in skin thickness in patients with rheumatoid arthritis, which may occur as a result of altered collagen metabolism.[16] However, the predilection for soft tissue complications is likely to be related to steroid use for patients with rheumatoid arthritis.

Another potential deleterious effect on wound healing is malnutrition.[17] A total lymphocyte count of less than 1,500 cells per cubic millimeter and serum albumin less than 8.5 g per deciliter are associated with a greater frequency of developing a major wound complication following total joint arthroplasty.[18] Preoperative screening of nutritional parameters may identify patients at risk for developing major wound problems. To avoid potential wound-related problems, preoperative optimization of the nutritional status is recommended.

The hypovolemia and severe anemia have also been found to be detrimental to healing. These conditions are associated with decreased oxygen delivery to the wound. Wounds require adequate oxygenation for healing.[19] Inadequate hydration may reduce tissue perfusion and oxygen delivery to the soft tissues, resulting in wound necrosis.[7] Severe anemia with concomitant hypovolemia potentially reduces tissue oxygenation. However, for normovolemic patients, mild to moderate anemia is not a factor causing poor wound healing because blood oxygen does not adversely affect collagen activity.[14]

Impaired wound healing has been found in diabetes mellitus.[5,7,14] Decreased collagen synthesis, delayed tensile strength, and delayed capillary ingrowth have been proposed as possible contributing factors.[7] Also, peripheral vascular disease is common in diabetics. To avoid potential wound problems, blood sugar control should be optimized preoperatively in diabetic patients and closely monitored in the postoperative period.[4,7] In addition, meticulous wound closure is recommended to optimize wound healing.[20]

Morbid obesity can also contribute to delayed wound healing and an increased incidence of wound drainage following total knee arthroplasty.[21] In substantially obese patients, the skin is less adherent to the underlying soft tissues and can become separated during retraction. Adipose tissue also lacks good circulation, which makes it particularly vulnerable to devascularization. The use of longer incisions and multiple layer closure may be helpful in reducing the risk of wound healing problems postoperatively.

The effect of immunosuppressive medication such as methotrexate has not been reliably demonstrated in the literature to contribute adversely to wound healing.[22] Chemotherapeutic agents, however, may slow wound healing because of their affect on dividing cells.[14] Also, use of continuous passive motion (CPM) machines has not shown a major difference in wound healing. However, there is controversial support for not allowing CPM knee flexion greater than 40 degrees during the early postoperative period.[4,5,23]

Vigilance is required postoperatively to detect early signs of soft tissue complications, particularly for patients with known risk factors. Early treatment of wound problems reduces the risks for developing deep infection. In addition, prompt treatment can prevent loss of soft tissue envelope and subsequent exposure of the prosthesis. There are three categories of wound problems: prolonged drainage or delayed healing, superficial necrosis, and full-thickness necrosis.[4,5] The need for surgical intervention is dependent on the extent of skin compromise.

Early superficial drainage can be observed when it is associated with a benign-appearing wound and no other findings typical of infection such as tenderness, erythema, or purulence. A temporary period of immobilization and local wound care may be sufficient for treatment. Cultures of superficial drainage should be interpreted with caution. The drainage fluid is often contaminated by skin flora and may not correlate with deep infecting organisms. Antibiotics, however, should be avoided without first obtaining culture and sensitivity of the joint fluid.

The incidence of culture-proven deep prosthetic infection for patients with prolonged drainage ranges from 17% to 50%.[5] Prompt surgical intervention for chronic drainage may prevent deep infection. It is advocated that patients with serous drainage persisting longer than 5 to 7 days for infection should be taken to the operating room for exploration and debridement.[5] The need for surgical exploration is dependent on the overall appearance of the wound, the notation of other signs of infection, and the existence preoperatively of risk factors for wound-related problems.

Hemarthrosis and hematoma formation can be associated with persistent wound drainage.[4] Hematomas can adversely affect wounds from local pressure. The release of toxic breakdown products of hemoglobin also potentially threatens skin viability. In addition, hematomas are a good culture medium for organisms and are not well penetrated by antibiotics. Large hematomas with signs of impending skin necrosis or drainage should be surgically drained and the patient placed on prophylactic antibiotics.

Early signs of skin blood flow compromise include ecchymosis and bullous formation (Fig. 23.1). Removal of the blister should be considered to better assess underlying skin viability. Superficial necrotic areas measuring less than 3–4 cm in diameter and marginal necrosis may be treated conservatively with local wound care. However, the dermal layer must be intact. Caution must be exhibited with nonoperative management, as a small tract may lead from the skin directly to the prosthesis. Surgical excision of the necrotic area can be considered. However, a tension-free secondary closure may not be achievable following debridement, and soft tissue reconstruction may be required. Following surgical debridement, superficial lesions greater than 3 cm may require skin grafting or fasciocutaneous flap coverage (Figs. 23.5 and 23.6). Skin graft coverage, however, requires a period of immobilization to promote vascular ingrowth. Skin grafts provide coverage when wound healing by secondary intention is not suitable.[7]

Full-thickness necrosis requires aggressive surgical management. Debridement of full-thickness lesions can leave the prosthesis exposed. Loss of the protective soft tissues over implants leads to catastrophic results including infection and prosthetic failure.[24,25] Muscle flap reconstruction and split-thickness skin grafting can be used to provide soft tissue coverage.[13,26] Available muscles for flap reconstruction are local rotational flaps, such as the medial or lateral heads of the gastrocnemius muscle, or free vascular flaps from a distant site, such as the latissimus dorsi or rectus abdominis.[27] The most commonly preferred muscle used for flap coverage of the knee is the medial gastrocnemius.[7,24] The medial gastrocnemius muscle is versatile and has a large arc of rotation for coverage of soft tissue defects about the knee and proximal leg.[25,28] Also, it can provide coverage for the patella and proximal tibia where the incidence of skin necrosis is the greatest. The lateral gastrocnemius muscle has a shorter rotational arc and is best for coverage of soft tissue defects of the lateral aspect of the knee.[25] Free flaps are best suited for massive soft tissue defects.[7,25] Muscle flaps can also be done prophylactically for patients with adherent skin and scarring secondary to prior surgery. Muscle flaps following total knee arthroplasty have a greater chance for success when performed for wound dehiscence and necrosis in the early postoperative period or for prophylaxis.[27] The disadvantages of gastrocnemius muscle flap reconstruction are largely cosmetic, including the bulk of the flap and donor-site defect.[7] In addition, typically a period of restricted knee motion is required for flap viability.

Muscle flaps and skin grafts that show signs of compromise can be treated with hyperbaric oxygen. Hyperbaric oxygen therapy (HBOT) involves intermittent breathing of 100% oxygen in a pressure chamber of elevated atmospheric pressure.[29] Oxygen is a necessary requirement for wound healing.[19] Hyperbaric oxygen raises the tissue tension of oxygen. It promotes phases of wound healing including collagen synthesis, matrix deposition, angiogenesis, and epithelialization.[19,29,30] Hyperbaric oxygen has additional bactericidal effects for wounds such as direct killing of certain anaerobes and restoring of neutrophil-mediated bacterial killing in previously hypoxic tissues.[30,31] The Hyperbaric Oxygen Therapy Committee of the Undersea and Hyperbaric Medical Society regulates the guidelines for hyperbaric oxygen treatment.[30,32] The approved indications for HBOT include the enhancement of healing in selected wound problems and compromised skin grafts and flaps.[29,30] Hyperbaric oxygen therapy is beneficial when there is a known decrease in the microcirculation or hypoxia. It will not heal normal wounds more rapidly.[32] Disadvantages of hyperbaric oxygen use include the limited number of pressure chambers available and cost. Common pitfalls of its use include temporary ocular side effects, barotrauma of the middle ear, and oxygen toxicity.[29–31]

Another option for the prevention of wound complications following total knee arthroplasty is tissue expansion.[33–35] Scarring from prior trauma or surgery can interrupt the cutaneous vasculature and predispose to ischemia. In addition to being poorly vascularized, the skin and underlying soft tissues may become thin, contracted, or adherent to underlying bone. Knees with severe angular deformity in combination with scarred immobile skin may also be at risk for insufficient skin coverage following correction of the deformity.[33] To prevent wound dehiscence or necrosis, prophylactic use of tissue expanders can increase the volume of skin for subsequent closure.[34] Tissue expansion devices are inserted subcutaneously and are placed in an area of good-quality skin that is adjacent to the scar.[35] The balloon-like expansion device is gradually inflated in an outpatient setting with serial injections of sterile saline until the desired amount of expansion is achieved.[33] As the device expands, the skin stretches and increases its volume. In addition to the wound closure, sufficient expansion may allow excision of the scarred area during the second-stage knee reconstruction procedure. Tissue expansion can also be used in preparation for flap coverage. Tissue expanders have been used successfully prior to primary and revision total knee arthroplasty.[33] However, the potential complications of tissue expansion are numerous, but appear to be related to the anatomic site expanded. To reduce complications associated with the use of the devices, it is recommended that expanders be placed underneath areas of healthy-appearing tissue and that the expansion process occur slowly and gradually.[33–35]

Avoiding the pitfalls of wound-related complications after total knee arthroplasty begins with a careful preoperative history to identify risk factors. Where possible, the condition of underlying medical problems should be optimized. In addition, the physical examination should include an evaluation of the peripheral circulation and an assessment of any preexisting scars. Intraoperatively, optimal choice of the skin incision preserves the blood supply to the skin and subcutaneous tissues. Gentle soft tissue handling, meticulous hemostasis, and tension-free wound closure can protect the vascularity and integrity of the soft tissue envelope. Lastly, prompt management of persistent drainage or soft tissue necrosis postoperatively will reduce the incidence of infection, exposure of the prosthesis, and subsequent failure of the knee reconstructive procedure.

THROMBOEMBOLISM

Without prophylaxis, the reported incidence of deep venous thrombosis (DVT) following total knee replacement is 40% to 88%.[36–38] Most thrombi occur in the calf veins, with 85% to 90% found distal to the trifurcation of the popliteal vein.[38] The majority of calf thrombi are small, measuring less than 3 cm in length.[39] Small clots in the calf may resolve without symptoms.[40,41] However, up to 30% of calf thrombi may propagate to proximal veins, leading to symptomatic DVT and pulmonary emboli.[42] In addition, patients who have bilateral total knee replacement procedures under one operative setting are at high risk for developing DVT.[41,43] Also, DVT can occur solely in nonoperated legs in 10% to 15% of patients.[38] The development of DVT in both the operated and nonoperated lower extremities reportedly occurs in 3% to 15% of patients.[11,44]

In contrast to total hip arthroplasty, the incidence of proximal vein thrombosis following total knee replacement procedures occurs less frequently.[11] Thrombus located proximally in the popliteal, femoral, and pelvic veins is at higher risk of embolism compared to thrombus located distally in calf veins.[37,40,43] Femoropopliteal thrombosis is noted in 10% to 15% of patients after total knee reconstruction.[11,38] Proximal thromboses in the total knee patients are typically continuous extensions of preexisting calf thrombi.[11,38] Segmental thrombi are not commonly seen following total knee arthroplasty. Calf thrombi, measuring greater than 5 to 6 cm in length, are at risk for proximal extension and embolization.[40]

Deep venous thrombi can resolve without clinical sequelae.[41] However, the significance of DVT is the subsequent development of pulmonary embolism, which is potentially life threatening. As with proximal DVT, patients with calf thrombi are also at risk for symptomatic and asymptomatic pulmonary embolism.[41,45] Asymptomatic pulmonary embolism occurs in 7% to 17% of patients as detected by abnormal ventilation-perfusion scans.[40,41,44] The incidence is likely underestimated, as the diagnosis is frequently missed due to the lack of symptoms or attribution of symptoms to other cardiac and pulmonary problems. Symptomatic pulmonary embolism is seen less frequently, with an incidence of 0.5% to 3%.[41,46] Fatal pulmonary embolism, one of the most dreaded complications of total knee arthroplasty, reportedly occurs in less than 1% to 2% of patients without the use of pharmaceutical prophylaxis.[39,47,48] Fatal pulmonary emboli can occur weeks to months following total knee replacement.[41] The late occurrence of pulmonary embolism may be related to proximal migration of calf thrombi.[11]

The etiology of DVT is multifactorial. Virchow's triad, consisting of stasis, hypercoagulability, and endothelial injury, is the basis for understanding the development of deep venous thromboses.[40,49] All three elements of Virchow's triad can occur following total knee arthroplasty. Hypercoagulability likely occurs as a result of intramedullary canal instrumentation.[38] It is believed that embolized fat and other marrow contents can activate the endogenous clotting cascade.[38]

Another factor contributing to the development of thrombi is venous stasis. Stasis and congestion may occur as a result of kinking of blood vessels during knee hyperflexion while performing the arthroplasty procedure.[41] Venous stasis can occur due to the application of a tourniquet.[41] However, there are conflicting reports regarding the detrimental effects of the tourniquet.[38] Tourniquet release is associated with the stimulation of fibrinolytic factors that may offset the effects created by stasis.[11,38] Also, relative immobility due to limited ambulation in the postoperative period can lead to the occurrence of DVT in both the operated and nonoperated legs.[41] Endothelial cell damage leads clot formation by causing platelet aggregation and activation.[40] The blood coagulation cascade is also initiated by damage to the endothelial lining of blood vessel walls.[38] Use of the tourniquet and knee manipulation can cause endothelial cell damage, leading to the formation of deep thromboses.[38]

In addition to Virchow's triad, there are intrinsic and extrinsic risk factors for the development of thrombi. Intrinsic factors include prior history of deep venous thrombosis or pulmonary embolism, malignancy, cardiovascular disease, major medical illness, and age greater than 40.[47,50] Extrinsic factors involve prolonged immobility, paralysis, major trauma, and major surgery.[47,50] Major knee surgery is a risk factor for the development of DVT.

The administration of regional anesthesia, specifically continuous epidural anesthesia, reportedly reduces the occurrence of DVT.[51] Epidural anesthesia has a sympathetic effect, which increases venous blood flow and returns blood to the central circulation system. The anesthetic may also have a direct effect on the vascular endothelium, causing an increase in fibinolysis and a decrease in platelet adhesion.[40] Regional anesthesia appears to selectively reduce thrombus formation in calf veins.[40]

The clinical presentation of DVT varies.[40] Many times there are no signs or symptoms. Symptoms, when present, can included calf pain, swelling, febrile illness, and skin discoloration.[40] Swelling and calf pain, however, can be seen following knee surgery and these findings are not specific for making the diagnosis of DVT. The accuracy of clinical diagnosis for DVT in hospitalized patients varies from 14% to 50%.[40] Certain tests can aid in the diagnosis of DVT when they are correlated with the clinical presentation. Diagnostic tests for DVT include duplex ultrasound and venography. Doppler ultrasound has excellent sensitivity in the detection of DVT.[52] Ultrasound has the additional advantage of being noninvasive. Venography is considered the gold standard for diagnosis DVT.[40] However, this study is invasive and is associated with numerous complications.[40,52]

Postphlebitic syndrome is a potential complication of DVT.[38,41] High intravenous pressure in the superficial venous system occurs secondary to outflow obstruction, narrow recanalization of thrombosed veins, or valve destruction.[38] The consequences of this increased pressure can include lower swelling, edema, induration, pigmentation, and possible skin ulceration.[38,42] This syndrome can occur even months to years after the development of DVT.[38]

The majority of DVTs attributed to performing total knee replacement procedures form during the intraoperative or immediate postoperative period.[46] Prevention is the best solution for the problem of thromboembolic disease. The goal of treatment is to prevent clot embolization, which can lead to fatal pulmonary embolism. In addition, prophylaxis reduces the risks of developing complications of DVT or pulmonary emboli such as postphlebitic syndrome and pulmonary hypertension, respectively. Anticoagulants and mechanical devices, used in combination, are popularly employed for DVT prophylaxis. The prophylactic regimen can be adjusted to meet the individual needs of patients.

For pharmacologic prophylaxis of DVT following total knee replacement, the most commonly used anticoagulants are warfarin, aspirin, and low molecular weight heparin.[37] Warfarin or Coumadin is taken orally. It inhibits the synthesis of active vitamin K–dependent coagulation factors and anticoagulation proteins.[53] Warfarin may limit clot propagation and embolization, but it does not appear to consistently decrease the incidence of DVT in total knee patients.[41,54] Therapeutic anticoagulation typically occurs 24 to 72 hours after administration.[41] There is a need to monitor the prothrombin (PT) time. The dose is adjusted to maintain the PT between 1.3 and 1.5 times control and the international normalized ratio (INR) between 2.0 and 2.5.[11,41] Coumadin can be started on the night of surgery or the night before. The major pitfalls of warfarin use are the risks of bleeding complications and skin necrosis.[53]

Aspirin can also be used for pharmacologic DVT prophylaxis.[37] It inhibits the enzyme cyclooxygenase in platelets, which leads to the inhibition of the synthesis of thromboxane-2. The overall result is decreased platelet adhesiveness. Aspirin is usually taken, 325 to 650 mg twice daily by mouth.[40] Aspirin gained popularity following early reports of the low incidence of DVT in total hip replacement patients.[41] Subsequently, however, the efficacy of aspirin for total joint replacement was questioned.[41] In a large European study of 9,000 randomized patients, it was found that antiplatelet agents including aspirin reduced both DVT and fatal pulmonary embolism.[55] The study advocates use of antiplatelet medication for elective orthopedic cases. Aspirin may also be efficacious when used in combination with mechanical devices.[56] The advantages of aspirin for prophylaxis include low cost and ease of administration. Pitfalls of its use include dose-related gastric complications, including gastritis and ulcer formation.[41]

Low molecular weight heparin (LMWH) is an anticoagulant that can be used for DVT prophylaxis after total knee reconstruction.[37,54,57] LMWH is fractionated heparin that effectively binds antithrombin III, inactivating factor Xa.[37] A fixed dose is initially administered subcutaneously 12 to 24 hours following the total knee arthroplasty procedure, and then every 12 hours.[37] LMWH is typically continued for 2 weeks postoperatively. Unlike heparin, routine monitoring with laboratory tests is not required. Lovenox (enoxaparin) is the most popular brand name available. With enoxaparin, the incidence of DVT has been reported to range from 17% to 25% when administered twice daily.[41,57] There are several pitfalls of LMWH including high cost compared to other anticoagulants and the need for self-injection following hospital discharge. In addition, major bleeding complications occur in 0% to 2.8% of patients.[41] Postoperative wound drainage may be slightly prolonged with LMWH use.

Intermittent pneumatic compression appears to be the best modality for prophylaxis to prevent DVT following total knee arthroplasty. When used alone, sequential compression boots or stockings reduced the incidence of DVT to 22%.[58] In addition, a metanalysis, conducted on 25 studies found in an English literature search, compared several prophylactic regimens.[41] Pneumatic devices had the lowest DVT rate of 18%, followed by LMWH, warfarin, and aspirin. Intermittent compression devices are available in calf or thigh lengths. Pneumatic devices are believed to reduce venous stasis by periodically raising venous pressure, accelerating the emptying of the venous system, and increasing fibrinolytic activity. Pulsatile pneumatic plantar devices or foot pumps are also available.[59,60] Foot pumps reduce venous stasis similar to sequential leg devices. In addition, the devices cause the forceful ejection of blood from the plantar venous plexus into the femoropopliteal veins.[59,60]

Pneumatic compression devices can be applied to the contralateral nonoperated leg, which is also at risk for developing DVT. For the operated limb, use of calf length boots or foot pumps avoids coverage of the knee. The mechanical devices are typically removed once the patient is independently ambulatory.[41] The advantages of mechanical devices use include relatively low cost and complication risk. However, a potential disadvantage is lack of compliance with wearing the device.[59] Sequential compression devices should be avoided when significant peripheral vascular disease is present.[41]

Graduated compression stockings, CPM machines, and early mobilization can be used in the prevention of DVT. However, they are not highly effective when used alone for prophylaxis in patients undergoing total knee arthroplasty.[40] Also, routine screening for DVT with duplex ultrasound or venography can be done prior to hospital discharge. However, this may be cost prohibitive for routine use.

Treatment of DVT is dependent on the location of the lesion. Distal calf thrombi are typically treated with Coumadin for anticoagulation to prevent the clot from propagating to proximal veins. If anticoagulation is not used, follow-up duplex ultrasonography should be performed to detect possible proximal migration.[52]

The presence of large proximal thrombi or symptomatic pulmonary embolism in the early postoperative period requires aggressive intervention. The management team may include vascular surgery or pulmonology, depending on the institution. Intravenous heparin is begun until a therapeutic level of warfarin is achieved. Warfarin is typically recommended for 6 weeks to 3 months for proximal thrombi and for 3 to 6 months for pulmonary emboli.[38] Intravenous fluid hydration, oxygen, and possible ventilation support may also be required in managing symptomatic pulmonary embolism. The major complication of heparin and warfarin use is bleeding.[53] Bleeding most commonly occurs at the operative site or gastrointestinal tract. For intravenous heparin, bleeding occurs at the operative site in 50% of patients when started within 6 days of surgery.[61]

Vena caval interruption devices, such as the Greenfield filter, can prevent catastrophic embolism of a DVT in total joint patients.[62] Inferior vena cava filters prevent the migration of emboli to the lungs without interrupting blood flow. Vena cava filters can be inserted prophylactically in patients at high risk for thromboembolism.[62] In addition, the filters are indicated for patients with a history of recurrent DVT or pulmonary embolism despite anticoagulation.[40,43,62] Patients with a contraindication or prior complication related to anticoagulation are also suitable candidates for vena caval interuption.[40,43,62] The filters do not have a direct effect on thrombi and will not reduce the risk of developing postphlebitic syndrome.[40] Complications can occur with insertion and use of vena cava filters, but not commonly.[62]

Pulmonary Embolism

The signs and symptoms of pulmonary embolism are varied and can be nonspecific. Symptoms of pulmonary embolism can include dyspnea, pleuritic pain, tachypnea, tachycardia, and fever.[40] Symptoms of DVT may be present. Patients in whom pulmonary embolism is suspected should be examined for the concomitant presence of DVT. The diagnostic workup includes arterial blood gas analysis, which typically shows a low Po_2 with an increased A-a gradient.[40] In addition, an electrocardiogram can show classic lead changes, T-wave inversion, or new-onset atrial fibrillation. Possible chest radiograph findings include wedge-shaped infarct shadows, atelectasis, reduced lung volumes, or small pleural effusions.[40] Ventilation perfusion scintigraphy (V/Q scan) is noninvasive and can assist in detecting pulmonary embolism. However, VQ scans are sensitive but not specific for the presence of pulmonary emboli. Lastly, pulmonary arteriography is the most accurate for in detecting pulmonary emboli. Arteriography is invasive and associated with potential complications. Fatal pulmonary embolism is associated with more than 75% occlusion of the pulmonary arterial circulation.[42]

PERIPROSTHETIC FRACTURES

Femur Fractures

The most common periprosthetic fracture is the supracondylar femur fracture. A periprosthetic supracondylar fracture occurs within 15 cm of the joint line or within 5 cm of the proximal extent of the intramedullary femoral component.[63] The incidence of supracondylar fracture after total knee replacement ranges from 0.3% to 2.5%.[64] Fractures can occur intraoperatively or postoperatively.

Trauma is the most common cause of supracondylar fractures following total knee arthroplasty.[65] Fractures can occur with low-energy trauma such as a simple fall, particularly in those patients with predisposing risk factors. Most patients who sustain these fractures are elderly, with a female to male predominance of 4:1.[66] Less commonly, periprosthetic fractures of the femur occur as a result of major trauma such as motor vehicle accidents.[64]

Multiple predisposing risk factors for periprosthetic supracondylar femur fractures are identified. Predisposing risk factors include conditions that result in osteopenia such as senility, disuse, or medication-induced osteoporosis.[67] Patients with rheumatoid arthritis may be at risk for periprosthetic fractures because of osteopenia secondary to the use of chronic steroid medication. However, rheumatoid arthritis itself may be a predisposing risk factor and is associated with periprosthetic fractures.[64,67–69] Additional predisposing factors include arthrofibrosis, bone defects, certain neurologic conditions, notching of the anterior femoral cortex, and revision arthroplasty in conjunction with distal femoral bone loss or constrained implants.[65,68–72]

Several neurologic conditions are associated with periprosthetic fractures such as seizure disorder, Parkinson's disease, myasthenia gravis, polio, and cerebral palsy.[71] Fractures in these neurologic patients may be attributed to gait disturbance or medication-induced osteoporosis.[70]

Arthrofibrosis after total knee replacement is identified as a predisposing factor to periprosthetic fracture. The mechanism associated with occurrence of fractures in these patients is increased stress in the distal femur metaphysis.[69,70] Fractures can occur in patients with stiff knees most commonly as an intraoperative complication of manipulation.

The association between notching of the anterior aspect of the distal femur during total knee replacement and subsequent supracondylar fracture is debated in the literature (Figs. 23.7 and 23.8). Several reports associate breeches of the anterior femoral cortex with periprosthetic fractures. It is postulated that notching the anterior femoral cortex interrupts the smooth transition of forces from cancellous to cortical bone at the diaphyseal-metaphyseal junction during weight bearing.[68] In addition, it is postulated that significant loss of the anterior cortex of the distal femur due to notching decreases the torsional strength of the bone.[71] Other potential contributing factors include stress shielding of bone, inadequate bone remodeling, and differing elastic modulus between the implant and the distal femoral cortical bone.[72]

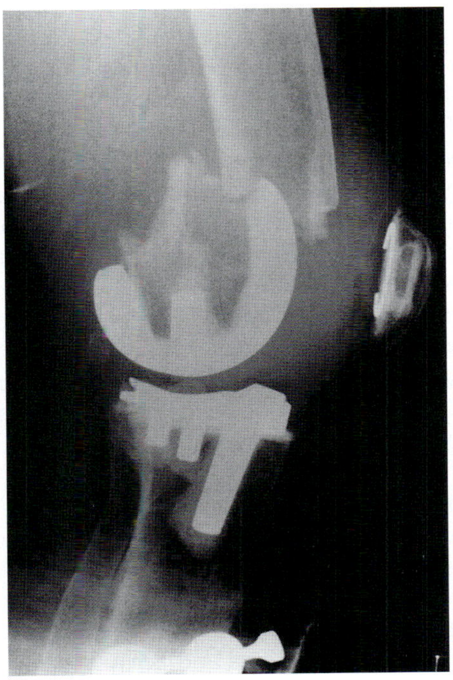

Figure 23.7. Supracondylar fracture occurred 4 years postoperation in a 72-year-old woman following a fall.

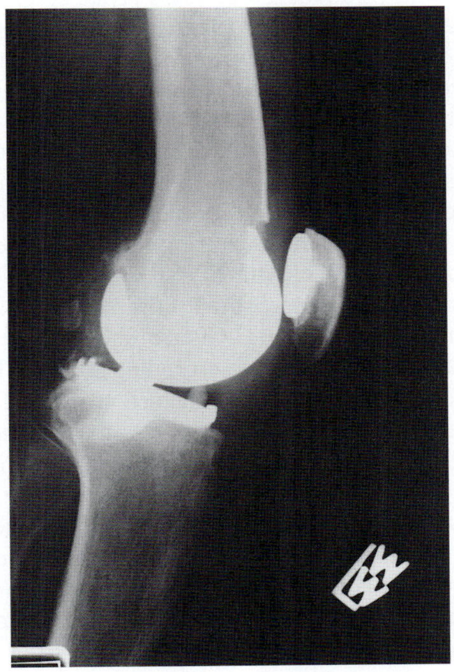

Figure 23.8. Notching of the femur usually occurs in association with excessive flexion of the femoral prosthesis or retroversion of the component.

In fracture series, the incidence of notching of the anterior femoral cortex is 0% to 50%, with an average of 35%, but the fracture rate for severely notched femurs is 0% to 42%.[73] The discrepancy in the incidence of anterior femoral cortical notching and supracondylar femur fractures suggest that the etiology of periprosthetic fractures is likely multifactorial. While fracture may not occur in every instance, notching of the anterior femur cortex during total knee replacement is best avoided, particularly in osteopenic bone.[69,71,73,74]

Bone cysts associated with rheumatoid or degenerative arthritis located near the proximal aspect of the femoral flange may serve as stress risers and increase the risk for fracture.[70,75] For fracture prevention, these lesions may require bone grafting and protection with a stemmed femoral component. Also, polyethylene wear can lead to osteolysis adjacent to the femoral component. Osteolytic defects in the distal femur can create stress risers that may lead to late supracondylar femur fracture.[76]

Treatment goals for managing a supracondylar fracture proximal to total knee arthroplasty include returning the patient to prefracture functional status.[70] Functional goals can be best achieved with restoration of alignment, retention of prosthetic fixation, union of the fracture, and maintenance of adequate extensor function and range of motion.

Good-quality radiographs are obtained in the evaluation of fractures about a total knee replacement and are compared to prefracture films. Comminution, bone quality, displacement, alignment, and prosthetic loosening are all factors that are taken into consideration in the treatment decision.[63]

There is not an universally accepted classification system for periprosthetic supracondylar femur fractures. The Neer classification of supracondylar fractures can be used to describe the fracture pattern, but it does not take into account the status of the prosthesis.[77] A treatment protocol for periprosthetic supracondylar fractures of the femur proposed by DiGioia and Rubash[63] is based on a modification of the Neer grading system. The proposed acceptable results of fracture treatment include less than 5 mm of displacement, less than 5 degrees of angulation in the varus-valgus plane, less than 10 degrees of angulation in the anteroposterior plane, and no more than 1 to 2 cm of shortening.[63] Additional acceptable results include pain-free fracture union in less than 6 months and, depending on the prefracture range of motion, greater than 90 to 100 degrees of knee range of motion is maintained.[73]

Conservative management is proposed for secure implants associated with nondisplaced or minimally displaced fractures with less than 5 mm of displacement or 5 degrees of angulation. If intervention is indicated, alignment of the fracture and mechanical axis of the limb should be easily restored and maintained by closed reduction. Options for nonsurgical management include functional bracing or cast immobilization. In addition, a period of skeletal traction may be required prior to functional bracing. Close monitoring is required to assess progressive loss of alignment during fracture healing. Comminuted fractures that are treated nonoperatively are at risk for collapse and subsequent varus malalignment. Even for stable, nondisplaced fractures, the existence of prefracture malalignment, osteolysis, and polyethylene wear may necessitate revision or partial revision as part of the fracture management to prevent subsequent failure.

An advantage of nonoperative management appears to be the ability to achieve good results with stable nondisplaced fractures. Statistical analysis of published studies of ipsilateral supracondylar femur fractures reveals that 83% of nondisplaced fractures treated nonoperatively have satisfactory outcomes.[75] However, the pitfalls of traction include the development of decubitus ulcerations, DVTs, and other complications linked with recumbency, especially in elderly patients. Other complications of nonoperative management including immobilization are limited knee motion, malunion, and nonunion. Malunion may result in late prosthetic loosening. For patients who have poor arthroplasty outcomes as a result of nonoperative periprosthetic fracture management, revision arthroplasty often yields satisfactory results.[67] However, the advantages of immediate surgical treatment of the fracture must be weighed against delayed surgery to manage the complications of nonoperative fracture treatment. Delayed surgical treatment is an option for patients who are not medically stable.

Surgical intervention is recommended when satisfactory alignment cannot be achieved or maintained by closed reduction or if there is radiographic evidence of prosthetic loosening. Proponents of internal fixation believe that surgical treatment provides the best restoration of mechanical alignment of the limb, permits early mobilization, and may maximize healing potential in a region where blood supply is already compromised. When rigid fixation is achieved, internal fixation can optimize the patient's return to prefracture functional status.[70]

In most cases, surgical intervention is elective and the timing of the procedure should allow for thorough preoperative medical evaluation of the patient. Underlying medical conditions that may have contributed to the patient's fall such as cardiac arrhythmia or electrolyte imbalance should be identified and addressed. In addition, the failure to recognize remote sites of infection and nutritional deficiencies may adversely affect surgical outcome.

Surgery can be challenging in the treatment of periprosthetic supracondylar femur fractures, especially in the presence of osteopenia, comminution, and intercondylar extension of the fracture. Operative management typically includes open reduction and internal fixation, revision arthroplasty, or a combination of both. Bone grafting may also be required. Surgical planning includes having the instruments available as well as the implants for both standard fracture management and long-stem revision total knee replacement. Revision knee replacement may become necessary if stable internal fixation of the fracture cannot be obtained or if previously unrecognized loosening of the implant is discovered intraoperatively. Bone grafting may also be required to optimize the change for healing.

The choices of internal fixation devices are numerous. Condylar buttress plates, supracondylar blade plates, supracondylar compression screws and side plates, and intramedullary nails have been used in the management of periprosthetic supracondylar femur fractures.[69] Screw and side plate fixation works best when there is minimal comminution of the distal fragment and for more proximal fractures. The technique for using the lateral plate and screws is exacting.

The condylar buttress plate is preferable when there is comminution of the distal fragment, because it allows the use of multiple screws to fix the distal fragment. It is more versatile than the blade plate/condylar compression screw, which provides a single point of fixation in the distal fragment. The buttress plate may be beneficial for patients who have osteopenia of the distal femur and comminution of the fracture extending into the intercondylar region.

With surgical management, care must be taken to avoid excessive soft tissue dissection, especially medially, which may disrupt the blood supply. Indirect reduction techniques minimize soft tissue stripping. A femoral distractor or external fixator applied temporarily may be useful to apply distraction to achieve an indirect reduction.

Using the anterior midline approach that incorporates the previous total knee scar is recommended.[69] Extending the midline incision laterally and proximally and continuing in the midline off the tibial crest distally can provide additional exposure. If indicated, the anterior incision also allows for dual plating and for revision arthroplasty. A midline approach also provides visualization of the distal femur in the medial-lateral plane, which is helpful in correcting varus malalignment of the supracondylar fracture.

Another option in the treatment of supracondylar femur fractures is a lateral incision. The straight lateral approach exposes the lateral cortex of the femur for hardware placement. This approach avoids violation of the knee joint.[65,70] However, for those knees with preexisting anterior scars, a lateral approach can potentially cause skin bridge necrosis. The soft tissue blood supply is at risk, especially in the region of the tibial tubercle.[69]

Internal fixation with an intramedullary rod inserted in a retrograde manner through the knee joint has been used successfully to treat supracondylar fractures above knee replacements.[78–80] The rods are designed to allow the placement of locking transverse screws proximal and distal to the fracture site. The intramedullary canal is accessed through the intercondylar notch of the femoral prosthesis.

The potential advantages of supracondylar intramedullary rods are numerous. Intramedullary nails have relative simplicity of instrumentation and surgical technique compared to lateral plate and screw fixation. Intramedullary fixation is also biomechanically stronger and less prone to failure than is lateral plate fixation, which has higher bending moments. In addition, intramedullary rods are load-sharing devices that may have an advantage, particularly in treating these patients who typically have osteopenia of the distal femoral metaphysis with poor cortical bone quality. With intramedullary nails, fixation can be achieved without directly exposing the fracture site, disrupting the fracture hematoma, or stripping the soft tissues.[70] The exposure for rod placement allows for assessment and revision of the prosthetic implants.[81] With rigid fixation, early range of motion of the knee can be allowed. Postoperatively, functional bracing and partial weight bearing supplement the treatment protocol. Good short-term clinical results are reported with the use of supracondylar intramedullary rods; however, these results are based on a small series of patients.[78,79,81] Long-term results have not been reported.

A potential pitfall of retrograde nailing is lack of access to the intramedullary canal due to the design of the femoral component. A minimum intercondylar distance of 12 mm is required for retrograde insertion of an intramedullary rod. In addition to published intercondylar distances for commonly used prostheses, the distance can also be obtained from the manufacturer of the implant.[78] High-speed burrs can be used to make minor adjustments such as widening the intercondylar opening or shortening rods. However, femoral components with closed housings or long stems are not amenable to retrograde intramedullary nailing. In addition, exposure of the prosthesis during placement of the rod potentially risks the development of an infection.[73] Other possible complications include rod migration into the knee joint, femoral shortening, arthrofibrosis, and nonunion.[81]

Additional fracture fixation options include the use of antegrade intramedullary nails. However, adequate bone stock distal to the fracture is required to allow for two screws to be placed in the distal fragment.[70] Antegrade intramedullary nails are best suited for more proximal fractures. Also, rush rods are available for fracture fixation in certain situations.[82] Rush condylar rods can be inserted through the medial and lateral epicondyles of the distal femoral. The treatment protocol typically includes the use of a knee immobilizer and protected weight bearing until fracture healing occurs.

Also, external fixators have been described in the treatment of periprosthetic femur fractures, with successful results.[83] However, the use of external fixation is precluded for supracondylar femur fractures because of the need to cross the knee joint and to place pins near the prosthetic implant. Furthermore, the prosthesis is potentially exposed to infection secondary to pin-site infection.[81]

Revision total knee replacement using a long-stem femoral component is recommended for patients who have loosening of the femoral component associated with supracondylar femur fracture or extension of the fracture to the prosthetic interface. In addition, revision arthroplasty may be required in cases where acceptable alignment and joint motion cannot be obtained by other methods. A success rate of 93% has been reported with revision arthroplasty.[75]

During revision total knee replacement for the management of supracondylar fractures, it is recommended that the collateral ligaments be retained and cement extrusion into the fracture site be avoided. Most revisions are amenable to the use of press-fit implants. Distal femoral allograft and a revision femoral component with intramedullary stems may be required for the management of difficult fractures associated with intercondylar extension, severe comminution, or bone deficiency. Reconstruction with large-segment allografts and long-stem femoral components may also be useful for salvage when previous attempts at fracture stabilization with conventional methods fail.[84]

Overall, the pitfalls of treatment of periprosthetic supracondylar femur fractures are malalignment, malunion, arthrofibrosis, nonunion, and infection. Hardware failure and infection may also complicate surgical management. The treatment decision is based on numerous local and systemic factors including the presence of displacement, comminution, osteopenia, bone deficiency, and prosthetic loosening. The prefracture status of the implant and surgical candidacy of the patient are also important. A satisfactory outcome can be accomplished when care is taken to select the appropriate method of treatment for the individual patient.

In addition to supracondylar fractures, fractures of the proximal femur and femoral shaft can also occur as a result of total knee replacement procedures. Fractures of the femoral neck may be caused by forceful femoral component compaction.[64,81] Femoral neck fractures are typically seen in osteopenic bone and are likely to be discovered postoperatively when weight bearing is attempted.[64] Fractures of the femoral shaft are seen in association with intramedullary instrumentation and stemmed femoral component use.[64,81] Osteopenia, deformity of the femoral shaft, and narrow canal width canal may be contributing factors.[64,81] Fracture treatment may include internal fixation techniques, and bone grafting, if necessary. Also, in the distal femure, condylar fractures can occur. However, these fractures are typically seen in association with the preparation of a box-shaped cut in the distal femur intercondylar region, to accommodate certain posterior stabilized femoral designs. Internal fixation with a lag screw may be sufficient for fracture stabilization.

Tibia Fractures

Periprosthetic fractures of the tibia occur infrequently. In contrast with periprosthetic supracondylar femur fractures, there are relatively few reports of tibia fractures in the literature. The majority of tibia fractures occur in the tibial plateau and adjacent to the prosthetic tibial stem in the proximal metaphysis or diaphysis. Less frequently, fractures occur in the tibia shaft distal to the prosthetic stem or involve the tibia tubercle.[85] Predisposing risk factors for tibia fractures include osteoporosis and component malposition. Fractures can also occur following the use of hinged prostheses and tibial tubercle osteotomies.[72]

Important variables for the management of periprosthetic tibia fractures include fracture displacement, anatomic location, prosthetic fixation, and bone quality.[85] The goal of treatment is the maintenance of appropriate limb alignment and knee motion. An important factor in determining appropriate treatment is the status of the prosthetic fixation. Generally, fractures associated with a loose prosthesis will require revision arthroplasty as part of fracture management. Also, the basic principles of fracture management are applicable. Methods of internal fixation include cancellous screws, plate with screws, or intramedullary fixation with long-stem revision components. In some cases, bypassing the fracture site with a long-stem tibial component can provide fracture stabilization.

Fractures of the tibia can occur intraoperatively or postoperatively. Intraoperative fractures can occur at all stages of a primary or revision arthroplasty procedure. Fractures of the tibial metaphysis are typically vertical and can occur during impaction of the tibial component.[81] Fractures can also occur secondary to impingement of prosthetic stems. Treatment options include cancellous screw fixation. Cement fixation of the implant can also be done to protect the fracture.[81] Diaphyseal fractures cause by stem impingement may not disrupt the periosteum. However, these fractures are subject to displacement and angulation with weight bearing. Patellar tendon–bearing functional braces may be useful for management and permit early weight bearing.

Postoperative tibia fractures can occur as a result of trauma, including minor trauma such as a simple fall. Fractures of the tibia plateau, however, may not be associated with trauma. Stress fractures of the medial tibia plateau occur most frequently in knees with varus malalignment and tilting of the anterior tibial component.

Tibia plateau fractures are typically of the depression or split type.[85] Nondisplaced fractures with acceptable alignment and stable implant fixation are amenable to closed treatment. Functional bracing, cast immobilization, and protective weight bearing are among the treatment options. In the presence of a stable implant, displaced fractures may be treated with standard internal fixation techniques. Tibial plateau fractures associated with a loose prosthesis require revision arthroplasty in addition to the possible need for fracture fixation.

Tibia fractures of the metaphysis or proximal diaphysis adjacent to prosthetic stems can also occur.[85] The presence of a constrained or long-stem prosthesis may affect the fracture location. For loose prostheses, open reduction and internal fixation as well as revision arthroplasty with long-stem tibial components may be indicated. Patients with medial stress fractures associated with varus alignment are also candidates for revision arthroplasty. Depressed areas of the plateau can be addressed with bone grafting and wedge augmentation of the tibial component. Reconstruction with allograft prosthetic composites may be useful when there is extensive tibial osteolysis.

Fractures of the tibia shaft, occurring distal to the prostheses, rarely involve loosening and have the best prognosis for long-term survival of the knee prosthesis.[85] Also, avulsion fractures of the tibia tubercle can occur secondary to trauma. Nondisplaced fractures can be treated nonoperatively. Avulsion fractures are rarely seen in conjunction with prosthetic loosening. Displaced fractures are best treated with open reduction and internal fixation. Following tibia tubercle osteotomy, avulsions of the osteotomized fragment can occur due to fixation failure, especially when there is poor bone.[86] In addition to avulsions, the extended tibia tubercle osteotomy can weaken the upper tibia, predisposing it to fracture.[87]

The general principles for the management of periprosthetic tibia fractures are similar to those described for periprosthetic supracondylar femur fractures. Fractures occurring in association with secure implants may be treated with standard fracture care. However, those fractures associated with prosthetic loosening require revision arthroplasty in addition to fracture treatment.

ARTHROFIBROSIS

The development of a flexion or extension contracture after total knee arthroplasty is a potentially debilitating complication. In addition to problems with range of motion, there is usually pain. A stiff knee after total knee replacement is defined as having a total range of motion of less than 50 degrees or a contracture of more than 20 degrees.[88] Severe arthrofibrosis is associated with the formation of excessive scar tissue and intraarticular adhesions with obliteration of the suprapatellar pouch and contracture of the extensor mechanism.

The incidence of stiffness following total knee arthroplasty is unknown. Fibrous ankylosis, a severe form of arthrofibrosis, is defined as 0 degree of motion. The incidence of this rare complication after total knee replacement is reported to be 0.1% to 0.3%.[89]

Range of motion and functional status are interdependent. A minimum of 90 degrees of flexion is required for daily activities.[89] Ninety degrees of motion or greater is necessary to descend stairs and 105 degrees are needed to easily get out of a chair.[90] For patients with bilateral knee involvement, flexion of more than 90 degrees is needed in at least one knee.[89] In addition, a fixed flexion contracture can lead to gait disturbance, with early fatigue occurring as a result of increased energy expenditure.[91]

Knee stiffness in the immediate postoperative period is not considered pathologic. Not uncommonly, stiffness subsides 6 to 8 weeks following total knee reconstruction.[92] Knee range of motion then steadily improves during the first 3 months. Progressive gains in motion can continue during the 12 months following surgery.

The reported average range of motion following total knee arthroplasty is 107 degrees, with a range of 95 to 123 degrees.[92] Balancing the soft tissues in flexion and extension intraoperatively improves postoperative range of motion. With the appropriate alignment, tissue balancing and prosthetic design flexion greater than 120 degrees can be achieved.[93,94,95]

The etiology of stiffness and loss of motion following total knee arthroplasty is multifactorial. Postoperative range of motion is dependent on preoperative, intraoperative, and postoperative factors. Surgical technique, prosthetic design, patient compliance, psychological status, and rehabilitation play a significant role in range of motion achieved postoperatively. Deterioration of range of motion after total knee arthroplasty is associated with infection, mechanical considerations secondary to component malposition, impending arthrofibrosis, and reflex sympathetic dystrophy. Late onset of stiffness following total knee arthroplasty may represent infection, synovitis in patients with a history of inflammatory arthritis, synovitis or tendinitis secondary to overuse, and prosthetic loosening or breakage.

Preoperative risk factors that may affect postoperative range of motion include the preoperative range of motion. Poor preoperative motion appears to predispose to problems with motion postoperatively.[96] Body habitus can also play a role. An obese lower extremity may lead to decreased flexion because of the bulk of posterior soft tissues. Preoperative adhesions involving the extensor mechanism and quadriceps contracture, if not adequately corrected, may also limit postoperative range of motion. Patients with rheumatoid arthritis have a greater incidence of postoperative flexion contracture than osteoarthritis. Motion problems are more likely to occur in primary compared to revision total knee reconstruction.

There are numerous intraoperative factors that can result in the limitation of knee motion postoperatively. Prosthetic technique and surgical technique are significant in that they are under the control of the surgeon. For instance, overfilling the flexion gap secondary to inadequate bone resection or an oversized femoral component can tighten the collateral ligaments, leading to limited flexion and postoperative pain.[97] Also, inadequate resection of the patella and anterior placement of the femur can overfill the patellofemoral joint. This tightens the extensor mechanism and results in loss of knee flexion.[92]

Failure to restore the joint line can alter joint mechanics. Lowering the joint line leads to relative tightening of the extensor mechanism and limited knee flexion. Raising the joint line potentially alters ligament tension, causing tightness during knee flexion greater than 90 degrees.[92] Also, patella baja can occur as a result of raising the joint line, leading to flexion restraint.

An important cause of stiffness is inadequate release of capsular and ligamentous structures. In addition, a tight retained posterior cruciate ligament may contribute to the development of poor flexion and extension. In addition, removal of posterior osteophytes from the distal femur improves knee flexion. Postoperative flexion contractures most commonly occur as a result of insufficient posterior capsular release and bone resection.

Achieving appropriate knee alignment is also important. Residual varus or valgus malalignment due to failure to adequately release the soft tissues or improper placement of cutting guides may affect the range of motion achievable postoperatively. Tilting of the components in the sagittal plane can adversely affect motion. Posterior tilting of the femoral component should be avoided. Additionally, anterior tilting of the tibial component may cause impingement of the extensor mechanism or contribute to tightness of the posterior cruciate ligament in flexion.

There are also numerous postoperative risk factors. The lack of preoperative education leads to unrealistic patient expectations. In addition, poor motivation and unrecognized psychiatric or psychological issues can adversely affect patient compliance with the postoperative rehabilitation protocol.

The development of patellofemoral dysfunction postoperatively may cause pain and contribute to the development of stiffness secondary to disuse. Patellofemoral conditions may include insufficient lateral release, patella maltracking, asymmetric patella resection, joint line elevation, internal rotation of the femoral prosthesis, patella fracture, and patella component loosening.[11]

Postoperative preventive measures, including the use of a CPM machine, may help to achieve early flexion. For optimal effectiveness, CPM should be used early in the postoperative period, prior to the development of adhesions or fibrosis. During the first 3 postoperative days, decreased transcutaneous oxygen tension of the wound edges can occur with CPM flexion beyond 40 degrees.[5,23] However, impaired wound healing and infection as a direct result of early CPM use have not been demonstrated.[26] Also, excessive postoperative pain can lead to limitation of motion. Adequate pain control is recommended. In addition, to analgesic medication, cryotherapy can also be utilized.

Supervised physical therapy is also essential for preventing soft tissue contracture and intraarticular adhesions. Excessive scar formation and intraarticular adhesions can lead to obliteration of the suprapatellar pouch causing stiffness. Overzealous and forceful passive range of motion by the therapist should be avoided.

An uncommon complication following total knee arthroplasty with a reported incidence of 0.8% is reflex sympathetic dystrophy (RSD). Patients with RSD may complain of disproportionate pain, skin hypersensitivity, and marked limitation of motion. Skin discoloration may also occur. However, RSD has varying presentations and may exist despite lacking the full complement of physical findings classic of RSD.[98] Despite potential diagnostic challenges, it is important to recognize this condition. RSD may worsen with aggressive physical therapy, manipulation, or surgical intervention.

Heterotopic ossification is also a rare cause of knee stiffness. Heterotopic ossification can be seen in 1% to 42% of stiff knees.[99] Few cases, however, require excision of the heterotopic bone for management and this is typically done at the time of revision arthroplasty.

In the evaluation of the stiff total knee replacement,

serial physical examinations to establish range of motion and functional status are important. Radiographs are obtained within the first 6 weeks after knee replacement and are repeated for persistent or progressive pain and stiffness.[92] Plain films may reveal patellofemoral subluxation, inadequate bone resection, and oversized femoral components. Technetium-99 MDP bone scans are useful in late presentations of infection. A triple-phase bone scan may demonstrate increased uptake of one or more of the prosthetic components in all three phases. Bone scans, however, are typically not useful during the first year after total knee replacement when bone activity is considered normal. Arthrocentesis to obtain joint fluid for culture and sensitivity is indicated for patients with a history of progressive stiffness, pain, and swelling. If the knee culture is negative but the clinical suspicion for infection remains high, arthroscopy or arthrotomy may be required to obtain tissue for culture.

The treatment of knee stiffness can be challenging. Physical therapy alone is not typically effective for range of motion less than 50 degrees. The use of dynamic splints, such as Dynasplints (Dynasplint Systems, Severna Park, MD), or static splints, such as JAS splints (Joint Active Systems, Effingham, IL) may have a role in the early treatment.[100]

Manipulation in the early postoperative period is controversial and may not improve final knee flexion. Manipulation may result in complications such as supracondylar fracture of the femur, patella ligament avulsion, wound dehiscence, and hemarthrosis.[98]

Arthroscopic lysis of adhesions and lateral release may improve range of motion. It may also reveal retained cement, loose bodies, subclinical infection, and prosthetic wear and loosening. Gentle closed manipulation under anesthesia can also be done in conjunction with arthroscopic surgery.

For more severe stiffness or arthrofibrosis, however, arthroscopic management is inadequate. An arthrotomy and extensive soft tissue release may be required to address extraarticular adhesions or contracture. Fibrosis of the vastus intermedius, shortening of rectus femoris, adhesions of the suprapatellar pouch, fibrosis, and shortening of the lateral and medial vastus expansion are associated with severe stiffness. The surgical exposure can be technically challenging. Care must be taken to prevent patellar tendon avulsion from occurring during exposure of the knee. A tibial tubercle osteotomy or quadriceps release may be required to facilitate exposure and to protect the extensor mechanism.[101–105] There are numerous proximal releases available including the quadriceps or rectus snip, modified rectus snip, patella turndown, V-Y quadricepsplasty, and femoral peel.[103–106] Complications of the procedures that transect the quadriceps include potential extensor lag and weakness. Potential complications of tibial tubercle osteotomy such as nonunion, tibia tubercle avulsion, tibia fracture, and fixation failure can occur, particularly in cases of deficient tibial bone stock.[87,88]

An important issue in correcting or improving an arthrofibrotic knee is the re-creation of the suprapatellar pouch. This is done through an arthrotomy and requires the excision of all fibrotic scar tissue in the suprapatellar pouch as well as the lateral and medial gutters. There may be a need to release and separate the extensor mechanism and quadriceps from the femur, especially in cases where calcification has occurred in those areas. One method of preventing this condition from recurring is temporary usage of silicone sheath interposition arthroplasty. A 0.2-mm sheath of silicone is wrapped around the femur from the joint line up to 8 inches above the joint line. The area from 8 o'clock to 4 o'clock is sutured to soft tissues with absorbable sutures. After the procedure is completed, the knee is gently manipulated and wound closure is performed in routine fashion. The postoperative course includes physiotherapy and usage of CPM. Generally 12 to 16 weeks postoperatively, the silicone sheath is removed through a small 2- to 3-cm incision in the supralateral aspect of the knee. Care should be exercised to remove the sheath in all one piece. In cases of sheath fragmentation, the knee should be irrigated and all pieces are suctioned out. In our hands, this has been an excellent alternative in dealing with severe cases of arthrofibrosis following total knee arthroplasty (Fig. 23.9–23.11).

In addition, malpositioned prosthetic components require revision in conjunction with soft tissue release and lysis of adhesions. The classic technique of ligamentous balance with matching flexion and extension gaps should be followed. Additional bony resection of the distal fe-

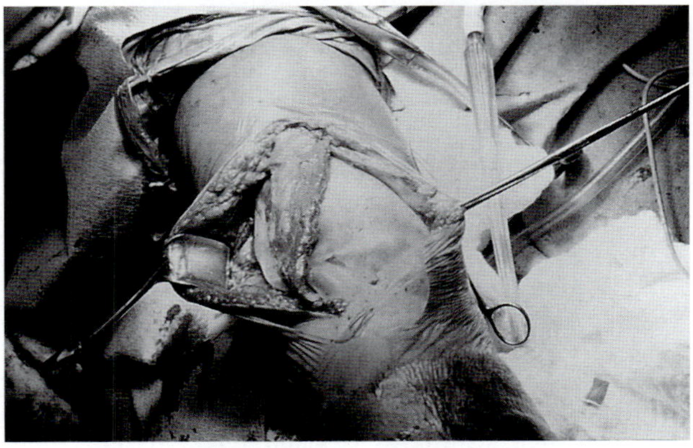

Figure 23.9. Silastic sheet implanted after extensive debridement and controlled manipulation. The tibial tubercle was detached for better exposure and complete release.

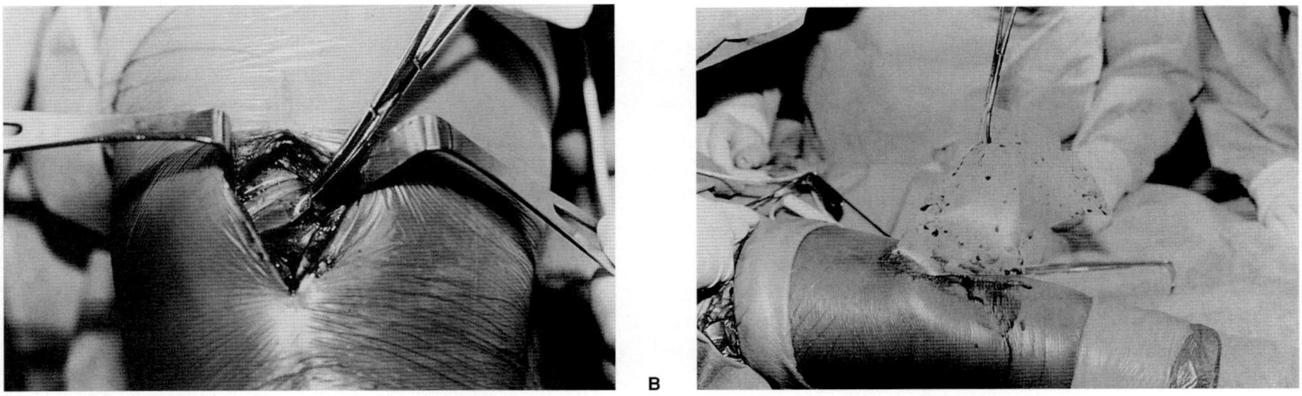

Figure 23.10. **A** and **B**: Twelve weeks postimplantation, the Silastic sheet was removed through a small incision all in one piece.

mur may be needed. Also, posterior osteophytes, if present, require removal for optimal range of motion. The posterior cruciate ligament (PCL), posterior capsule, and gastrocnemius may require elevation to establish the posterior recess. The PCL can be proximally released from its insertion on the medial femoral condyle. It can also be lengthened with sequential sectioning or multiple perforations. Posterior instability occurring as a result of sacrificing the ligament is addressed with the use of a cruciate substituting design. For severe contractures, posterior capsule transection may also be required.

An important pitfall of treating knee stiffness after total knee arthroplasty is the failure to correctly establish the identifying cause such as referred pain from primary hip or spine disease, emotional or psychological disturbance, RSD, or infection.

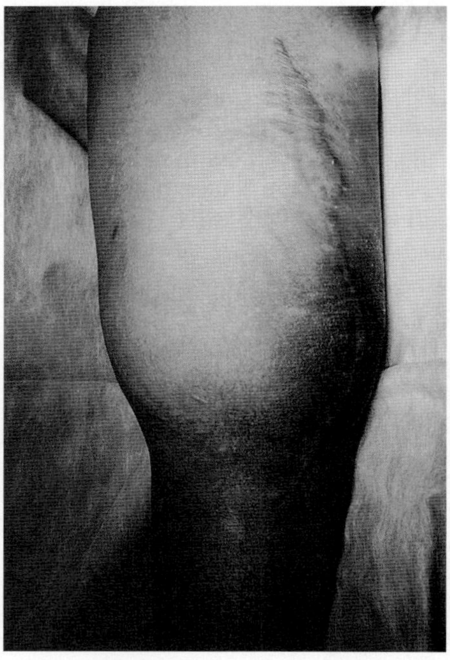

Figure 23.11. A 59-year-old woman, a known rheumatoid arthritis patient, with gross swelling, pain, and limitation of motion was not diagnosed as having a prosthetic infection for 14 months. She was treated by her primary orthopedic surgeon with physical therapy, analgesics, and antiinflammatory medication.

NEUROLOGIC COMPLICATIONS

The most common major nerve complication associated with total knee arthroplasty is peroneal nerve palsy. Complete peroneal palsy results in weakness of foot extensors and evertors, causing a foot drop.[106] This is typically accompanied by sensory impairment of the anterolateral leg and dorsum of the foot. The cumulative prevalence of peroneal nerve palsy following total knee reconstruction is 0.6% as reported the literature.[107] However, the incidence may vary depending on the severity of the case mix for a given surgeon or institution.[11] The incidence is likely higher than reported if partial palsies with mild motor involvement or sensory impairment are considered.

The etiology of peroneal nerve palsy after total knee arthroplasy is multifactorial. Risk factors associated with peroneal nerve palsy include a preoperative valgus deformity and/or flexion contracture of more than 20 degrees.[107] In addition, possible mechanisms of injury to the peroneal nerve include traction during surgical correction of a severe deformity and restoration joint alignment; ischemia secondary to stretching of the surrounding soft tissue, which causes small vessel occlusion; and direct pressure caused by a tight dressing, splint, or hematoma.[11] For some patients, no identifiable cause can be determined.

It is not uncommon to have a delayed presentation

of peroneal nerve injury following total knee reconstruction. Peroneal nerve palsy is most commonly diagnosed within 2 days of surgery.[11] A delay in diagnosis may be related to the postoperative use of epidural anesthesia, which may cause prolonged sensory and motor blockade.[108] Late nerve compromise can also occur during the postoperative period with improper positioning of the operated limb in CPM machines. In addition, external pressure from bed rails, knee immobilizers/splints, and excessively tight dressings have been implicated in causing peroneal nerve palsy, especially for patients who continue to receive epidural anesthesia postoperatively.

Early treatment of peroneal nerve palsy is directed primarily at preventing additional injury. It is recommended to remove constrictive dressings and place the knee in 20 to 30 degrees of flexion.[11,109] These measures may result in partial sensory or motor recovery when nerve injury is recognized early.[11,109] Passive range of motion of the ankle should be performed to maintain ankle mobility. The use of a foot-drop splint or ankle-foot orthosis can prevent equinus contracture and assist in ambulation.

Observation may reveal spontaneous complete or partial nerve recovery. Early surgical management is limited to the drainage of compressive hematomas.[11] Electrodiagnostic tests should be performed for at least 3 weeks postoperatively and can document the extent of the nerve lesion. At 2 to 3 months, significant neurologic deficits may benefit from surgical exploration.[107,110] Following operative decompression, Krackow et al[110] reported subjective improvement in five of five patients with peroneal palsy complicating total knee replacement. The decompression procedure was performed 5 to 45 months after their index total knee arthroplasty procedures. The time to improvement for the total knee replacement patients included in that series ranged from 3 weeks to 3 months. Also, in a follow-up series of these patients as well as those with other causes of peroneal palsy, 97% of 31 patients had subjective and functional improvement following operative decompression.[107] Surgery was performed after at least 2 months of conservative management.

Prophylactic exploration of the peroneal nerve is proposed for patients with severe fixed valgus with angulation greater than 15 degrees.[106] Through a separate incision, the peroneal nerve is dissected and released of its soft tissue constraints prior to performing the total knee replacement procedure. However, previously it was reported that prophylactic nerve release did not consistently preventing palsy from occurring following total knee arthroplasty.[106,109]

The prognosis is good for partial peroneal nerve palsy.[111] Patients with initial partial palsy had better function compared to patients with complete palsies.[111] With complete palsy, a variable amount of recovery is expected and full recovery is rare. Bilateral nerve palsy is unusual and likely occurs secondary to an occult generalized peripheral neuropathy or underlying neurologic disorder.

Preventive strategies in patients at high risk for developing nerve injury include resection of adequate amounts of bone during the correction of flexion or valgus deformities, to prevent excessive bowstringing of the peroneal nerve. In addition, tight dressings are avoided and knee flexion is allowed in the recovery room to prevent stretch on the peroneal nerve. There has been no demonstrated advantage to exploring and prophylactically releasing the peroneal nerve at the time of total knee arthroplasty in high-risk patients.

VASCULAR COMPLICATIONS

Vascular complications following total knee arthroplasty are rare. Types of vascular complications associated with total knee replacement include arterial occlusion, arterial laceration, arterial aneurysm, and arteriovenous fistula formation.[112] The incidence of vascular injury has been reported as 0.05% in primary total knee arthroplasty.[113] The incidence of vascular trauma for revision arthroplasty is not reported in the literature. However, the occurrence of vessel injury is likely higher than in knees that require extensive dissection in the presence of scar formation, contracture, and anatomic distortion.[106] Careful surgical technique and knowledge of vascular anatomy can avoid the pitfall of vascular injury during total knee reconstruction.

The popliteal artery is the most common vessel at risk for injury during total knee reconstruction procedures.[106] Popliteal artery injuries can occur due to penetration of the posterior capsule during meniscal excision and PCL resection.[114] This vessel is also at risk during posterior capsular release procedures. In addition, the use of saw blades, penetrating instruments, and excessively long screws for the fixation of allografts or cementless tibia components can potentially traumatize the neurovascular structures in the posterior knee.

In addition to the popliteal artery, other arterial vascular structures at risk for direct trauma during total knee replacement procedures include the inferior medial and lateral geniculate arteries. Partial lacerations of arteries and their adjacent veins can lead to the formation of a false aneurysms and arteriovenous (AV) fistulas. Rare reports exist of inferior medial geniculate artery AV fistula associated with false aneurysm following total knee replacement.[115,116] This is a potential complication of subperiosteal release of the medial soft tissue for ligamentous balancing.[116] AV fistulas can be prevented by attention to hemostasis.[118] False aneurysms typically present with a palpable mass.[117]

During tibial screw preparation and insertion, the popliteal artery, and vein, anterior tibial artery, and common peroneal nerve are potentially vulnerable to injury.[116] These neurovascular structures may be located only 3 to 8 mm from the proximal tibia plateau.[118] To illustrate the relationships, key neurovascular structures about the proximal tibia have been compared to the face of a clock.[114,118] Rubash et al[118] propose a clock orientation such that the lateral aspect of the knee corresponds to the 3 o'clock position and the tibial tubercle to the 6 o'clock position. The center of the clock is the center of the tibial plateau. The popliteal artery and vein are typically found directly posterior, between the 12 and 1 o'clock positions.[114,118] For the right knee, the tibial nerve lies medial to the vein, at 1 o'clock.[118] For the left knee, the nerve lies at the 11 o'clock position.[114] For both knees, neurovascular structures at risk are located from the 11 to 1 o'clock positions.[115,119]

Additionally, more distally along the proximal tibia, the popliteal artery bifurcates, forming anterior and posterior tibial arteries. The bifurcation occurs in the 2 o'clock position for left knees and 10 o'clock for right knees. The common peroneal nerve wraps around the fibular head near the 3 o'clock position for the left and 9 o'clock for the right knee. Neurovascular structures from 11 to 3 o'clock in left knees and 1 to 9 o'clock in right knees can be injured, particularly with penetration of the tibial cortex during screw placement.

Tourniquet release prior to wound closure depends on the preference of the surgeon. However, if a vascular injury is suspected, tourniquet deflation is recommended, ideally prior to insertion of the prosthetic components. Popliteal artery laceration is typically readily recognized when the tourniquet is deflated prior to wound closure. When the tourniquet is deflated after wound closure and application of postsurgical dressings, monitoring blood loss and circulation can help assess the vascular status. An expanding popliteal mass, lack of return of distal pulses, and voluminous bleeding are indications for intraoperative arteriography and a vascular surgery consult.[114] With prompt identification of vascular compromise and restoration of circulation, a good outcome can be expected.[112]

Vascular compromise is treated by the vascular surgeon with direct anastomosis or grafting depending on the extent of vessel damage and the ability to achieve full knee extension. Following a vascular insult and revascularization procedure, compartment syndrome can occur. The pitfall of direct vascular injury during total knee replacement is under the control of the surgeon. Vessel injury is avoided with attention to surgical technique. Using the scalpel blade parallel to the posterior tibia while pulling forward the meniscus during meniscal resection can avoid penetration of the posterior structures. Also, care is taken during resection of the PCL, which lies in front of the popliteal vessels. To prevent accidental vessel injury, a portion of the PCL can be retained. In addition, using a periosteal elevator to lift the posterior capsule directly from the tibia and distal femur is generally safer than transection of the capsule at the joint line.

In addition to direct penetration, indirect vascular compromise occurs due to partial or complete vessel popliteal artery occlusion.[106] Patients with peripheral vascular disease and severe flexion contractures are at risk for developing arterial insufficency following total knee arthroplasty.[117] For patients with flexion contractures, the popliteal artery can become entrapped in scar tissue. Correction of flexion contractures can result in arterial intimal tears, fascial obstruction, spasm, and thrombosis.[119] Arterial damage may result from traction on the vessel that occurs as the knee is fully extended.[120]

The risk of arterial insufficiency following total knee arthroplasty is also associated with severe peripheral vascular disease. Subtle ischemia may manifest as skin necrosis and delayed wound healing Acute arterial insufficiency typically occurs due to trauma or thrombosis of atherosclerotic blood vessels. Arterial thrombosis is also associated with knee manipulation and tourniquet use.[120,121] Mechanical tourniquet pressure can cause compression of diseased arteries, resulting in the fracture or embolization of atheromatous plaques.[117,119–121] In addition, lack of blood flow in atheromatous vessels is also a possible causative factor.[120] Use of the tourniquet is not recommended for patients with poor distal pulses, and preoperative radiographs that show severe vessel calcification.[117] Vascular contraindications to total knee arthroplasty include a history of severe vascular claudication and the presence of skin ulceration due to venous stasis disease or arterial insufficiency or limb necrosis. Preoperative evaluation should include skin inspection and palpation of the dorsalis pedis and posterior tibial pulses.

Preoperative consultation with a vascular surgeon is highly recommended for patients with a history of severe peripheral vascular disease, poor distal pulses, or extensive vessel calcification as seen on radiographs. The vascular assessment may include the measurement of the ankle/brachial pressure index. An index less than 0.5 is associated with increase risk of vascular compromise.[114] Arteriography may be required for patients in need of vascular bypass prior to total knee arthroplasty. Bypass surgery is not a contraindication to performing total knee replacement, but a tourniquet should not be used and the operative time is kept to a minimum. Total knee replacement can be performed without the use of a tourniquet. Dry bone surfaces can be achieved for cement techniques.[122] In addition, operating time and blood loss can be comparable to those cases in which a tourniquet is utilized.[122]

Acute arterial occlusion is a rare but serious complication with the potential for poor outcome, including amputation.[116] This complication can be avoided by careful preoperative screening. Patients with vessel calcification on radiographs should have inspection of the entire lower limb for signs of severe peripheral vascular disease and documentation of the presence and strength of distal arterial pulses. For those patients with poor or absent pedal pulses or other risk factors, the vascular surgery consultation is recommended. If necessary, total knee arthroplasty procedures can be done without the use of the tourniquet. Following correction of severe flexion contractures, the circulation should be monitored postoperatively. After tourniquet deflation, an assessment of pedal pulses and distal capillary refill may result in early detection and treatment of acute arterial insufficiency, improving the ultimate outcome.

INFECTION

Infection is a potentially devastating complication of total knee arthroplasty procedures. Deep infection is associated with patient morbidity and high treatment costs.[123,124] It can adversely affect joint function and threaten limb preservation. Over the years, numerous advances have lowered the rate of infection including the routine use of prophylactic perioperative antibiotics.[125] The infection rate following primary total knee arthroplasty currently ranges from 1% to 2%.[126–128] The reported rate of infection after revision arthroplasty is as high as 5.6%.[126]

Many variables influence the development of deep infection including operating room environment, surgical technique, operative time, implant selection, patient factors, and wound status.[125,127–131] Predisposing wound factors include dehiscence, prolonged drainage, skin necrosis, skin infection, and hematoma formation.[128,131] Important patient risk factors include altered immune status, prior surgery, prior knee infection, concurrent sepsis, psoriasis, medical illness such as rheumatoid arthritis and diabetes mellitus, malnutrition, and morbid obesity.[125,127–129,131]

Bacterial organisms gain access to the operative site by endogenous or exogenous sources.[127,128] The operating room is the chief source of exogenous bacteria.[127] The skin harbors microorganisms, which shed continuously into the environment. Some operating room personnel shed bacteria at a rate of 1 to 10,000 bacteria per minute.[127,128,132] Bacteria reach the operative site from direct contact with contaminated equipment or by an airborne route.[128]

Endogenous bacteria are found within the patient.[128] The bacterial source may be located at a site distant from the knee such as a dental abscess or genitourinary tract infection. Bacteria gain access to the operative wound by direct invasion due to skin compromise or by a hematogenous route. Types of skin compromise that predispose to infection include skin necrosis or wound dehiscence.[128] Wound drainage is associated with 25% of prosthetic infections.[131]

Patient factors associated with increased infection rates include a prior history of deep sepsis such as septic arthritis or osteomyelitis.[127–129] In addition, prior surgery on the affected knee increases the risk of deep infection. Previous surgical intervention is associated with scarring and adverse changes in blood supply about the knee. Revision total knee arthroplasty has a higher risk of sepsis than primary knee replacement for the reasons indicated for prior surgery. Additional contributing factors to the infection rate for revision procedures are the presence of knee stiffness, soft tissue contracture, and poor bone quality.[128]

Rheumatoid arthritis may predispose to a higher risk of deep sepsis, particularly those patients with multiple system involvement. The infection rate is reported to be 2.5 times greater in rheumatoid compared to osteoarthritic knees.[133] Rheumatoid patients are at high risk for developing late hematogenous sepsis. The risk of late infection is as high as 50% during the patient's lifetime.[125,133] For patients with American Rheumatism Association class III and IV function, the most common mode of late prosthetic failure is delayed infection.[134] It is proposed that rheumatoid patients with multiple-system involvement may be more immunocompromised than those with rheumatoid arthritis of less severity.[127,135] Rheumatoid patients are at higher risk for single and multiple prosthetic infections compared to osteoarthritic patients.[135] Previous total joint arthroplasties are at risk for developing infection from hematogenous spread in rheumatoid patients, particularly those with advanced functional involvement.[135]

Moreover, diabetes mellitus, morbid obesity, and malnutrition are considered factors for deep sepsis.[125,127,129] These conditions likely pose a risk of infection due to the increased incidence of wound-related problems. Recurrent urinary tract infections, pneumonia, dental bacteremia, skin ulcerations, and invasive procedures may predispose to infection from a distant site.[129] Organ transplantation, coexisting renal or hepatic disease, neoplasm, and other conditions may predispose to infection from altered or diminished host immune function.[127,128]

Sepsis after total knee arthroplasty may involve a variety of microorganisms. The most common pathogens are aerobic gram-positive bacteria, usually *Staphylococcus aureus* or *Staphylococcus epidermidis*.[127,128,136] Less commonly, streptococcal, enterococcal, gram-negative, or mixed polymicrobial infections occur.[128,130] Infections caused by gram-negative bacilli and mixed polymicrobial organisms can be encountered when there is prolonged wound drainage.[127,131,136] Furthermore, antibiotic-resistant bacterial strains can develop as a result of chronic antibiotic suppression.[127] Resistant bacterial infections are associated with the production of a glycocalyx film that adheres to the implant, impairing antibiotic penetration and macrophage attack.[128,129] In addition to the bacteria that produce a glycocalyx, other virulent organisms include methicillin-resistant staphylococci, gram-negative bacteria, enterococci, and group D streptococci.[129] Other pathogens that have been isolated from infected total knee arthroplasties include mycobacteria and fungi. These organisms may be responsible for infections in patients with immunocompromised immune systems.[128,136]

Numerous preventive measures reduce the incidence of infection following total knee arthroplasty. Perioperative intravenous antibiotics are important in the prevention of infection. The selection of the correct antibiotic for prophylaxis depends on the microorganisms responsible for infection in each hospital environment.[136]

Since staphylococcal organisms are responsible for causing most total joint infections, antibiotic selection is typically directed at these organisms.[136] A first-generation cephalosporin such as cefazolin is relatively inexpensive and penetrates bone; 1 g of cefazolin is administered intravenously 30 minutes prior to surgery and is continued after surgery every 8 hours for three to six doses.[130] The minimum time necessary to achieve significant antibiotic concentration in the tissues is 5 or 10 minutes before tourniquet inflation.[137] Antibiotic concentration in bone was negligible when administered after inflation of the tourniquet.

If the patient is allergic to cephalosporins, vancomycin is an alternative and is active against methicillin-resistant *S. aureus*[130]; 1 g of vancomycin is administered over 30 minutes prior to surgery. It is continued after surgery every 12 hours for two to four doses. The vancomyacin dose may need to be adjusted, depending on the patient's renal function.

In addition to prophylactic antibiotics, numerous preventive measures are available to reduce infection. The length of the hospitalization preoperatively is minimized to prevent colonization of the skin with potential antibiotic-resistant organisms.[127] Also, cleansing the skin with hexachlorophene daily for 2 to 4 days prior to the total knee arthroplasty can reduce the bacterial population and protects the skin for a limited period of time.[138]

Intraoperative measures that reduce the risk of infection include the preparation of the operative site with a germicidal agent to kill transient endogenous bacteria.[127,128] In addition, iodophor-impregnated drapes that adhere to the skin help to lower the number of bacteria in the wound.[127,128,138] Minimizing the number of personnel and amount of traffic in the operating room potentially decreases bacterial contamination.[125,128] In addition, the use of hoods and masks provides a temporary reduction in bacterial shedding.[127] Other intraoperative measures include the use of double gloves and impermeable surgical gowns and drapes, which protect both the patient and the surgeon.[127,128] Helmet aspirator or body exhaust suits, typically used by surgeons and assistants, can prevent bacterial shedding.[125,127–129] Also important for the operating room is appropriate air filtration and circulation.[127,139] Vertical laminar flow and ultraviolet lights have been used with success to reduce environmental contamination in the operating room.[125,127]

Surgical technique is also important in preventing infection. Preventive measures include utilizing previous incisions, careful handling of the wound tissues, and avoiding the formation of flaps. Copious lavage of the wound prior to wound closure removes debris that can provide an ideal environment for bacterial growth.[128] Efficient use of operative time reduces the risk for wound contamination.[128] The potential risk of deep infection increases with the length of time in the operating room.[128]

Deep infections may present in the early or late postoperative period. An intermediate category of infection is also described. There are varying classifications describing the time frame for infections. Acute infections occur within the first 2 to 3 weeks of surgery.[125,127] Acute infections may be associated with local wound complications such as delayed healing, skin slough, or hematoma formation.[139] Intermediate or delayed infections can also occur. Intermediate infections may result from contamination that occurred during the perioperative period or from hematogenous spread.[127,128,140] Late infections are more common than early infections.[127,128] Late infections are usually due to hematogenous spread of microorganisms from a distant site. An early time of onset of the infection and the virulent nature of the organism are important when formulating a treatment strategy that will result in a functional knee that is free of pain and ongoing infection.

Prompt diagnosis and treatment of prosthetic infection potentially reduces morbidity. If infections are treated in a timely and aggressive fashion, the potential for salvage without implant removal exists. However, if treatment is neglected, the septic process will extend to involve the bone-cement interface, necessitating implant removal. In addition, the infectious process may migrate proximally, especially in cases where the diagnosis is delayed and appropriate treatment and intervention has not been carried out (Figs. 23.11–23.15).

Presenting symptoms of infection range from persistent pain to life-threatening systemic sepsis.[128] Fulminant infection is readily diagnosed when the clinical presentation includes systemic fever and a knee with warmth, erythema, swelling, and limitation of motion.[125,127] Pain and swelling can be seen in 95% of acute prosthetic infections.[128] In contrast to acute infections, chronic low-grade infections can be a diagnostic challenge.[127,128] The presenting symptom in intermediate or late infection may be pain.[128,129] Pain at rest may be a sign of infection in late presentations.[127] The symptoms may additionally include increased knee warmth or limited range of motion. The development of acute pain and swelling or limited range of motion following a total knee replacement that had been asymptomatic should raise the suspicion of infection. Other issues that should increase the clinical suspicion for infection include a history of known risk factors for contamination such as prolonged wound drainage, problems with wound healing following the initial arthroplasty, and reoperation for any reason.

Routine hematologic testing is done but may not be helpful in establishing the diagnosis of an infected total knee arthroplasty. The blood leukocyte count may be elevated or normal. The C-reactive protein, however, is

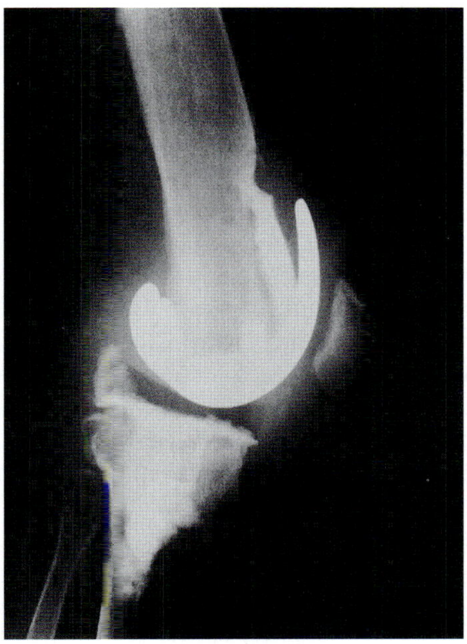

Figure 23.12. Gross loosening of the femoral component.

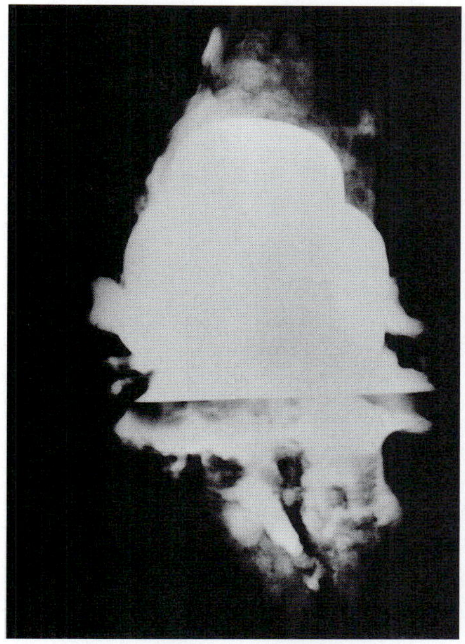

Figure 23.13. Arthrographic appearance of the knee in the anteroposterior (AP) plane.

typically increased. A baseline erythrocyte sedimentation rate (ESR) is obtained.[128] The ESR is not consistently elevated with deep prosthetic infection. A normal ESR may exist in the patient with an infected total knee arthroplasty. Also, the ESR can be elevated following

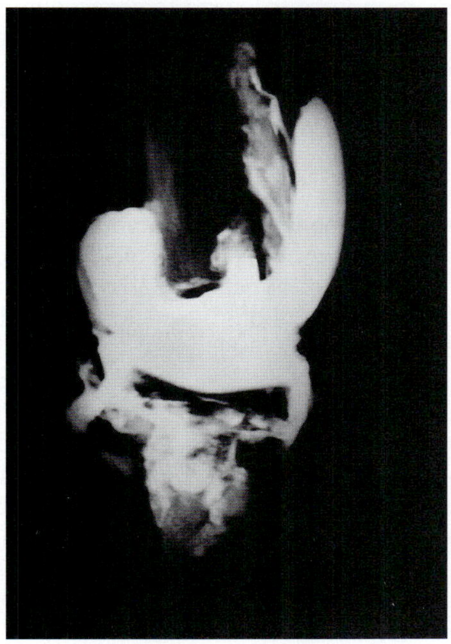

Figure 23.14. Arthrographic appearance of the knee in the lateral plane.

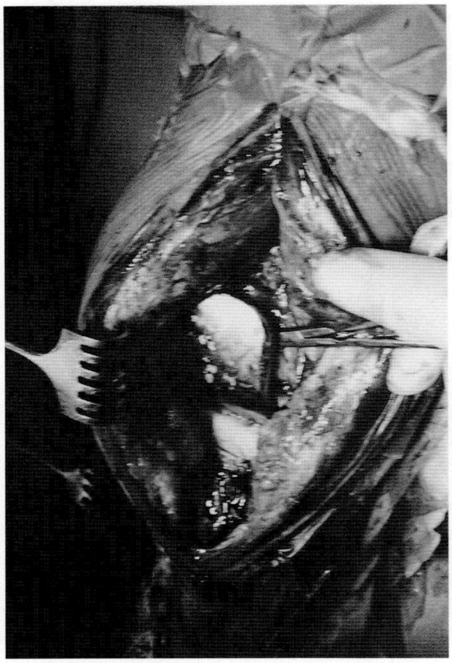

Figure 23.15. At exploration, gross loosening identified. Note the thickening of the soft tissue envelope around the knee due to chronicity of infection. Unfortunately, this knee was not salvageable and the patient ended up with an above-knee amputation.

routine total knee reconstruction and remain elevated for 3 or more months following the procedure.[129] The ESR can be helpful when used to monitor the response to treatment.

Periprosthetic osteolysis is the most frequency radiographic finding of an infected total knee arthroplasty. Radiographic technique is important in detecting early osteolysis. The radiographic beam must be tangential to the bone-cement–bone-implant interface. Progressive osteolysis in the absence of a mechanical etiology should raise the suspicion of infection. Radiographic findings such as periosteal new bone formation are highly suggestive of infection, but rarely present.[125]

Nuclear medicine studies are available to assist in the diagnosis of infection. However, these studies may not conclusively detect the presence of infection following total knee replacement.[129,140] Technetium-99m methylene disphonphonate (Tc-99m MDP) or technetium bone scan is the standard for bone scintigraphy.[127] Technetium bone scans detect bone metabolic activity, which is present with infection. However, accelerated bone turnover due to remodeling is also present following routine total knee arthroplasty. The specificity of a bone scan or the triple-phase bone scans, which can enhance the detection of bone infection, can be poor in the presence of a recent total knee replacement. Bone scan may be positive during the first postoperative year, limiting its usefulness in detecting prosthetic infections during that time.[141] In addition, gallium 67 citrate scans are often done in conjunction with bone scans to enhance the detection of infection. However, like bone scans, gallium scans can be positive in the presence of bone remodeling.[127] Indium 111–labeled white cell scans can also detect prosthetic infection, but are technique dependent.[142] In addition, indium scans are less accurate for evaluating total knee replacement compared with total hip arthroplasty.[142] Because of false-positive and -negative studies, correlation of the indium-labeled scan with the clinical evaluation is recommended.[142]

Aspiration of the joint is recommended for the diagnosis of a prosthetic infection.[143] Arthrocentesis is performed under sterile conditions to minimize risk of contamination of the specimen with skin flora.[143] Synovial fluid analysis includes a cell count, specifically a white cell count. A white cell count greater than 25,000 per millimeter with more than 75% polymorphonuclear cells is suggestive of infection.[140] Furthermore, the fluid should be sent for glucose and protein levels.[140] Low glucose and elevated protein level compared to plasma levels are also compatible with infection. A Gram stain of the synovial fluid will show microorganisms in 25% of cases.[128]

Synovial fluid cultures with antibiotic sensitivities are the gold standard for determining the existence of deep infection. In addition to standard cultures for aerobic and anaerobic bacteria, additional cultures for fungi and acid-fast bacilli may be indicated.[131] The cultures of draining fluid and superficial wounds are often contaminated by skin flora and may not reflect the infecting microorganism found deep in the knee.

In some knees that appear clinically infected, synovial fluid cultures will be negative.[128] Patients who have received antibiotics within a month of the culture may have false-negative results due to suppression.[127,140] In addition, intraoperative wound cultures, obtained at the time of initial arthroplasty, may not correlate with the postoperative infecting organism.[128]

If an infected total knee arthroplasty is suspected, but efforts fail in identifying an infecting organism, an open biopsy for pathologic evaluation may be indicated.[129] Tissue specimens can be obtained by arthroscopy or arthrotomy. In the setting of a painful, loose prosthesis, culture of the implants or cement fragments may result in identification of the organism. Histopathology of the periprosthetic tissue often reveals an acute inflammatory response with polymorphonuclear leukocytes (PMNs). However, acute inflammatory may be present without sepsis in other conditions such as rheumatoid arthritis.[128] Sometimes only chronic inflammatory changes are present, which can be difficult to differentiate from changes associated with prosthetic material. The finding of five PMNs per high power field in five sections is suggestive of infection.[127]

The primary goal of treatment for infected total knee arthroplasty is the eradication of infection.[128] There are numerous treatment options including antibiotic suppression, irrigation and debridement with component retention, one-stage or two-stage reimplantation, resection arthroplasty, arthrodesis, and amputation.[125,127–129,139–140] The management team includes the orthopedic surgeon and infectious disease consultant.[128]

Factors taken into consideration in deciding the ideal treatment option include chronicity of the infection, presence of an immunosuppressive conditions, age and functional demand of the patient, virulence of the infecting organism, quality of bone stock, type of prosthesis, and integrity of the soft tissues

Surgical debridement with implant retention is useful in the management of acute infections diagnosed within 3 to 4 weeks of the index arthroplasty procedure.[139] Debridement is indicated for acute infections that occur in association with a securely fixed implant and low virulent infecting organism.[125,128,129,139,144] The procedure includes a synovectomy. Following debridement, the wound is closed over suction drains. Debridement is followed by a 4- to 6-week course of intravenous antibiotics.[145] A pitfall of implant retention is unrecognized extension of the septic process extension to the bone-cement or bone-implant interface.[125,128,129,139]

Prosthetic exchange can be performed immediately following debridement or in a delayed fashion after a course of intravenous antibiotics.[125,128,129,139,145–148] Delayed exchange is the gold standard.[131] It allows for the eradication of infection and preservation of knee function. Two-stage reimplantation is associated with the highest success rates for the treatment of infection.[125,128,129,139,146,147] Most reported success rates with delayed exchange are 90% or greater.[126,140,145–148] Candidates for exchange have susceptible organisms, adequate bone stock, competent immune systems, intact extensor mechanisms, and adequate soft tissues including the skin and collateral ligaments.[125] The long-term functional results, reinfection rate, and survivorship for two-stage reimplantation is reportedly comparable to the results of reconstruction for aseptic failure.[82]

For success of delayed exchange, debridement includes removal of the implant and all foreign material.[146] An antibiotic impregnated polymethylmethacrylate spacer is commonly inserted. The insertion of a hand-molded cement spacer into the joint space following implant removal has several potential advantages. It can provide high-dose local antibiotic delivery, allow better patient mobility, and reduce soft tissue contracture following implant removal.[149] To fabricate the spacer, the antibiotics commonly mixed during the preparation of the cement are tobramycin or vancomycin.[125] The tobramycin dose is 1.2 g per 40 g of polymethylmethacrylate used.[125] The dose of vancomycin is 500 mg per 40 g of cement.[125] The potential pitfalls of cement spacers include the presence of foreign material within the infected joint. In addition, on removal of the spacer, further bone loss can occur if the cement becomes fixed to bone at the time of insertion. With some cement block designs, range of motion and weight bearing is limited.

Following surgery, intravenous antibiotics are continued for 4 to 6 weeks. Some surgeons prefer an additional period of oral antibiotics. A minimum serum bactericidal level of 1:8 is maintained.[128,140,146] The white blood count (WBC), ESR, and C-reactive protein are monitored. After the antibiotic course is completed, repeat arthrocentesis is performed.[128] A positive culture is a contraindication to reimplantation.[125] During revision implantation, antibiotic-impregnated cement is routinely utilized.[125,140]

An alternative to the antibiotic impregnated spacer is the insertion of a temporary implant as described by Hofmann et al.[126] Following debridement, the femoral component is sterilized by autoclave. The femoral prosthesis and a new polyethylene tibial implant are inserted using tobramycin-impregnated cement. The cement is inserted in a doughy stage to prevent significant interdigitation with bone and facilitate removal. Range of motion and partial weight bearing are allowed as tolerated.

Another temporary functional spacer that can be used for delayed exchange is Prostalac (*pros*thesis of *a*ntibiotic-*l*oaded *ac*rylic cement).[149] Prostalac is a prosthetic implant coated with antibiotic-impregnated acrylic cement.[150] The goal of the temporary implant is to deliver local antibiotics while maintaining limb length and anatomic relationships.[150] The design of the second-generation system allows for improved joint stability and patient mobility.[150] The use of antibiotic-loaded cement, typically in higher doses than that for cement spacer blocks, appears to offset any adverse effects of the presence of foreign material in the Prostalac implant.[150]

Unlike two-stage exchange arthroplasty, immediate prosthetic exchange has limited indications. It is reserved with caution for immunocompetent patients who meet other criteria for prosthetic exchange and have a highly susceptible infecting organism. In addition, antibiotic suppression can be used for the elderly or severely medically compromised patients. Best suited for suppression are infections with a low-virulence organism that are sensitive to oral antibiotics in the presence of a stable implant. Eradication of infection with suppression is not likely. As a routine, the prolonged use of antibiotics should be avoided without confirmation of infection. Pitfalls of chronic antibiotic suppression are the potential development of infection by antibiotic-resistant bacterial strains, antibiotic toxicity, and eventual painful prosthetic loosening.

Resection arthroplasty is a useful salvage procedure and is an alternative to arthrodesis. Severely disabled patients, such as those with rheumatoid arthritis who have polyarticular involvement and limited functional goals, are best suited for the procedure. Also, arthrodesis is indicated for immunocompromised hosts. Some range of motion can be expected after surgery, and a brace is usually needed for support during ambulation. The pitfalls of this procedure include persistent pain and instability.

For single-joint involvement, arthrodesis is the option of choice for infections likely to fail reimplantation.[128,140,145] Staged arthrodesis, following debridement and component removal, is recommended. Suitable candidates for fusion have infections with highly virulent organisms, inadequate extensor mechanism or soft tissue envelope, insufficient bone stock to support a prosthetic replacement, or failed implant exchange. Surgical techniques for arthrodesis include external fixation, intramedullary nailing, and compression plating with supplemental cast immobilization. Compression plating and intramedullary nails have higher fusion rates than external fixation. The patient's ability to ambulate independently following arthrodesis is dependent on the function of adjacent joints. The pitfalls of arthrodesis include lack of knee motion, shortening, gait disturbance, persistent infection, fracture, and nonunion. A potential complication of external fixation is pin-tract infection. A pitfall of knee fusion obtained by intramedullary rodding is the spread of infection to previously unaffected bone.

Amputation is a final salvage procedure, reserved for patients with life-threatening infection such as that caused gas-forming microorganisms.[128,131,140] Other candidates for amputation have failed other treatment options, and have extensive bone loss and significant soft tissue destruction.

Lastly, somewhat controversial in the prevention of late prosthetic infections is the use of antibiotic prophylaxis prior to dental, invasive diagnostic, or therapeutic procedures. Most patients undergoing routine cleaning and other dental manipulation experience transient bacteremia. However, there appears to be a low risk for bacterial seeding of the prosthesis, and antibiotic prophylaxis is of questionable value when given after the first 2 years of surgery. The recommended antibiotic regimen is in accordance with the guidelines developed by the American Heart Association for prophylaxis of bacterial endocarditis in the presence of prosthetic heart valves.[151]

EXTENSOR DYSFUNCTION

Patellofemoral Instability

Complications related to the extensor mechanism are a common reason for reoperation following total knee replacement.[152–156] Despite improvements in prosthetic design, alignment guide systems, and surgical technique, the incidence of extensor mechanism complications remains high. Problems related to component position and soft tissue balance can contribute to a variety of patellofemoral complications following total knee arthroplasty.[155] Common patellofemoral complications include instability, failure of the patella component, rupture of the extensor mechanism, and soft tissue impingement.

Patella instability is the most common complication of the extensor mechanism.[152] The incidence of patella tracking problems is been reported as high as 29% following total knee replacement procedures.[157,158] Patella instability includes subluxation and dislocation. Subluxation occurs more frequently than frank dislocation (Fig. 23.16).[154,159]

There are multiple causes of patellofemoral instability: extensor mechanism imbalance, component malposition, inferior component design, asymmetric patellar resection, capsular repair disruption, patella alta, trauma, and soft tissue impingement.[154,156,159]

A common cause of patellofemoral instability is soft tissue imbalance of the extensor mechanism.[152] A typical physical finding is excessive tightness of the lateral retinaculum. The imbalance may also be accompanied by weakness of the vastus medialis muscle. Patients with preoperatively valgus knee deformity, chronic lateral patella subluxation, or a history of instability are particularly at risk for developing patella tilt or instability following total knee replacement.[155] Valgus malalignment creates an abnormal Q angle, altering the resultant force of the quadriceps muscle on the patella.[154,159]

Malpositioning of the prosthetic components also predisposes to patellofemoral instability.[152,154,159] Internal rotation of the femoral component can result in lateral displacement of the patella relative to the trochlear groove. Similarly, excessive medial translocation of the femoral component on the femur adversely affects tracking of the patella in the femoral groove. Also, placement of the femoral component in excessive valgus can alter the resultant muscle pull on the patella.[154]

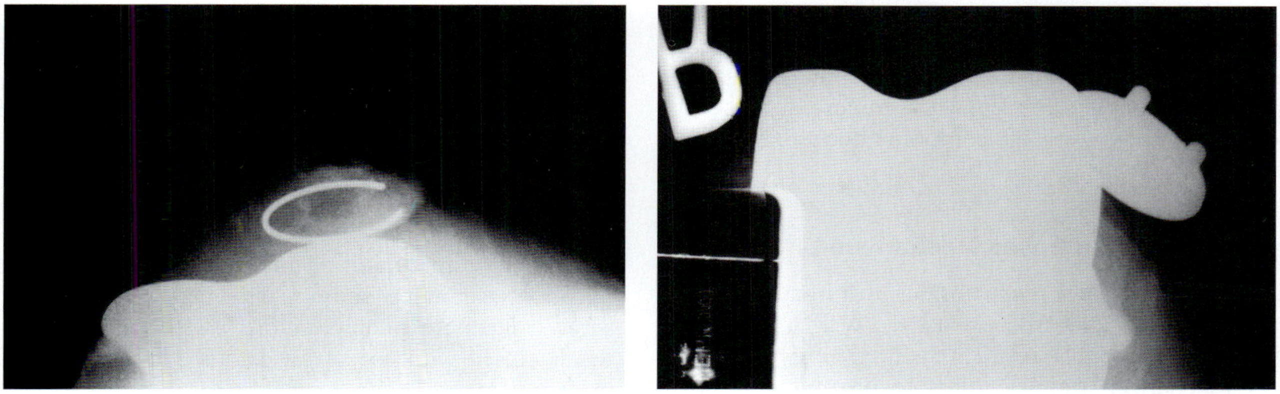

A B

Figure 23.16. A: Patellar subluxation post–total knee arthroplasty without frank dislocation. B: Recurrent dislocation following total knee arthroplasty. Situations like this may require bony procedures in addition to soft tissue realignment.

Another cause of patella maltracking is excessive internal rotation of the tibial component.[152,154,159] Tibial component malalignment can cause external rotation of the tibia relative to the femur and lateralization of the tibia tubercle. The Q angle also increases, which can predispose to patella subluxation. In addition, lateral placement of the patellar component on the patella can cause maltracking.

Asymmetrical resection of the patella can also lead to patellofemoral instability. An asymmetric cut with excessive resection of the lateral patella facet can result in laterally tilting of the patella.[152,154,159] In addition, the overall patellar height should be preserved. Excessive patella-patella composite thickness increases quadriceps tension and the load across the patellofemoral joint, resulting in patellar dysfunction.[152,154,160,161] Caliper measurement of the patella following resection and component placement can assist in maintaining appropriate patella height.[155]

Certain prosthetic designs predispose to problems with patellar tracking.[152,159] Kinematic rotating-hinge prostheses and rigid hinge designs are associated with relatively high rates of patellofemoral instability.[152] Also, patients with imbalance of the extensor mechanism reconstructed with rotationally unconstrained prostheses are at risk for patellofemoral instability, if excessive external rotation of the tibia and lateralization of the tibia tubercle are allowed to occur.[152] Similarly, patients with collateral and posterior cruciate ligament insufficiency who undergo total knee arthroplasty may be at increased risk for patella instability.[152]

Disruption of the capsular repair following total knee arthroplasty also can cause patellar maltracking or instability.[152,154,155] Capsular disruption can occur due to failed closure of the medial arthrotomy, hemarthrosis, aggressive physical therapy, and trauma. Physical findings on examination include a palpable capsular defect. Revision of the capsular repair may be indicated for cases of acute disruption.

Many causes of patella instability can be prevented with good surgical technique. The intraoperative assessment of patella tracking is critical. The tourniquet can have a binding effect on the extensor mechanism and can be released, if necessary, during the assessment of patella tracking. The evaluation of patella during flexion and extension should occur without medially directed stabilization such as that provided by the surgeon's thumb.[152,155] Achieving soft tissue balance is essential for normal patella tracking. Patella component medialization may also enhance patella tracking.[161–163] Medialization is achieved by centering the component over the median ridge, which corresponds to the high point of the patella prior to resection.

Patellofemoral instability is treated on the basis of its etiology. Nonoperative measures include intensive quadriceps rehabilitation; external patellofemoral bracing; and avoidance of activities, such as squatting or stair climbing, which involve heavy loading of the patellofemoral joint.[155]

When the extensor mechanism does not respond to nonoperative measures, proximal realignment may be indicated.[152,154,155,164,165] A lateral retinacular release alone may not sufficiently correct the malalignment.[152,154] The lateral release is often combined with advancement or imbrication of the vastus medialis.[154]

Medial transfer of the tibia tubercle in conjunction with osteotomy of the tibial tubercle is an option for instances of severe malalignment that cannot be corrected with soft tissue procedures alone. However, nonunion is a potential complication of the procedure.[152]

Prosthetic revision can be performed for patients who have significant malpositioning of the components that is not amenable to simpler realignment procedures.

The pitfalls of patella instability are increased risk of patella fracture as well as component loosening and wear.

Rupture of the Extensor Mechanism

Rupture of the extensor mechanism is an infrequent complication of total knee reconstruction, with a reported prevalence ranging from 0.17% to 2.5%.[152,158,166] Extensor mechanism rupture refers to disruption of the soft tissue component of the extensor mechanism, specifically the patella and quadriceps tendons. The patella tendon ruptures occur more often than those of the quadriceps tendon.[167,168] Ruptures may occur as a result of trauma. However, patella tendon ruptures are most often atraumatic. The etiology may be related to underlying vascular, mechanical, and surgical technique factors.

Quadriceps tendon rupture following total knee arthroplasty is rare. When it does occur, it is usually in patients who have had a lateral retinacular release.[152] Surgical disruption of the tendon's blood supply may contribute to subsequent rupture.[165,166] Additionally, extension of a lateral release too far anteriorly with disruption of the tendinous fibers of the quadriceps is a possible contributing factor.[152] Malpositioning of the femoral component in flexion causes impingement and attritional wear of the quadriceps tendon. Other suspected risk factors for rupture of the quadriceps are inflammatory arthritides, chronic steroid use, and previous surgery.[155]

Repair or reconstruction of a quadriceps tendon rupture can be challenging. Often there is insufficient tissue for end-to-end anastomosis. The results of operative repairs are often unsatisfactory due to extensor lag, weakness, or limited range of motion.[152] Reinforcement or reconstruction with autograft such as the semitendinosus tendon may be required. With appropriate surgical technique, the outcome should not be altered.

The risk of patellar tendon ruptures after total knee arthroplasty is increased in patients who have had previous operations involving the knee, such as distal extensor alignment.[167] In addition, partial detachment of the patellar tendon, done to enhance exposure at the time of arthroplasty, increases the risk of acute rupture.[167] At particular risk of avulsion of the tendon from the tibia tubercle is stiff knees with limited preoperative flexion. Acute tendon ruptures can also occur as a complication of forceful closed manipulation of the knee following total knee reconstruction. The most common type of patellar tendon rupture is the distal avulsion from the tibial tubercle.[167] Proximal and midsubtance tears occur less often.[167]

Late attritional patellar tendon ruptures may be associated with devascularization from the surgical exposure or impingement of the tendon on the prosthesis. Late traumatic ruptures are associated with falls or significant contraction of the quadriceps with a slightly flexed knee (Figs. 23.17–23.21).

Numerous treatment options exist including cast application, ligament suture, wire fixation, staples or screws, ligament augmentation, and reconstruction of the ligament with use of an extensor mechanism allograft.[167]

Generally, acute repairs of extensor tendon ruptures do better than late repairs. Long-standing ruptures are associated with soft tissue contracture, joint stiffness, and extensor lag. Following patellar tendon rupture, the patella migrates proximally. Late presentations of patellar tendon ruptures are associated with concomitant quadriceps tendon contracture. Mobilization of the extensor mechanism may be required as part of the reconstruction. When the tendon is of poor quality or cannot be mobilized sufficiently, several options exist for management. An allograft comprising the quadriceps tendon, patella, patellar ligament, and tibia tubercle can be used reconstruction.[169] Despite functional improvement following reconstruction, moderate extensor lag can occur.[170] Alternatively, reconstruction with autogenous semitendinosus tendon has been described.[170] The

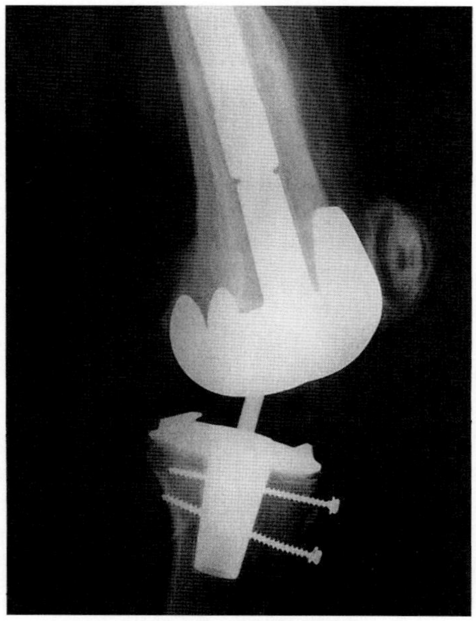

Figure 23.17. Traumatic rupture of the patellar tendon status post–revision arthroplasty of the knee. At exposure, there is significant shortening of the remaining patellar tendon, which was not suitable for repair or reattachment.

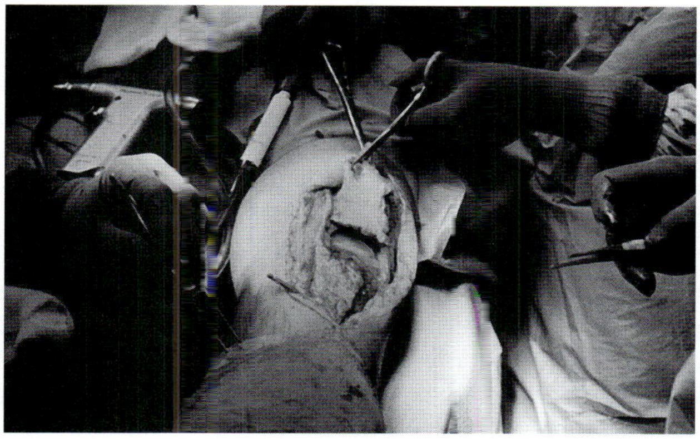

Figure 23.18. Traumatic rupture patellar tendon one year after revision total knee arthroplasty.

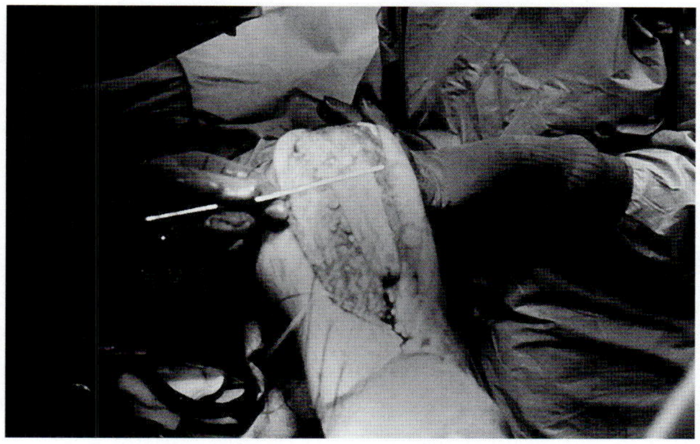

Figure 23.19. Reconstruction of patellar tendon rupture with Achilles tendon allograft.

semitendinosus tendon is detached proximally, passed through a channel made in the distal pole of the patella, and then sutured to itself at its insertion on the tibia or to adjacent periosteum.[170] For a short or small-caliber semitendinosus tendon, augmentation of the reconstruction can be done using the gracilis tendon.[170] Also, the semitendinosus tendon can be woven into the quadriceps tendon combined with a turndown of a tongue of the quadriceps inferiorly for reinforcement. Use of autogenous hamstring tendon appears to be superior to staple or suture fixation alone. It may also be advantageous over allograft tissue for patients with soft tissue devascularization from previous surgical procedures or compromised connective tissue from systemic disease.[170]

For patients who do not have adequate bone stock for use of the semitendinosus reconstruction, a medial gastrocnemius or extended gastrocnemius flap is an alternative.[171] Gastrocnemius flap reconstruction can also be considered for patients with patellar ligament rupture, failed quadriceps tendon repair, poor soft tissue coverage, or an exposed prosthesis associated with loss of the extensor mechanism.[170] This flap provides a blood supply to enhance healing of the reconstruction and does not require good bone quality of the patella or proximal tibia.

Low-demand, medically compromised patients not considered suitable candidates for surgery can be treated with bracing.[167] Knee arthrodesis is a salvage procedure. Knee fusion is an option when other treatment methods fail and stability is preferred.

Preventive strategies for acute patellar tendon rupture include protecting the patellar tendon during surgery, using a longer capsulotomy and extensile exposure for tight knees or revision arthroplasty, and avoiding partial patellar tendon release. When necessary, the tibial tubercle can be osteomized for better exposure and reattached at the completion of the proce-

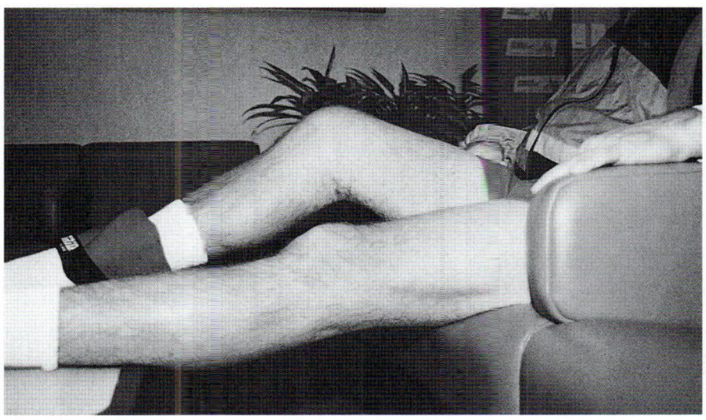

Figure 23.20. At 6 months postoperation, range of motion from −5 degrees (shown here) to 120 degrees with independent ambulation

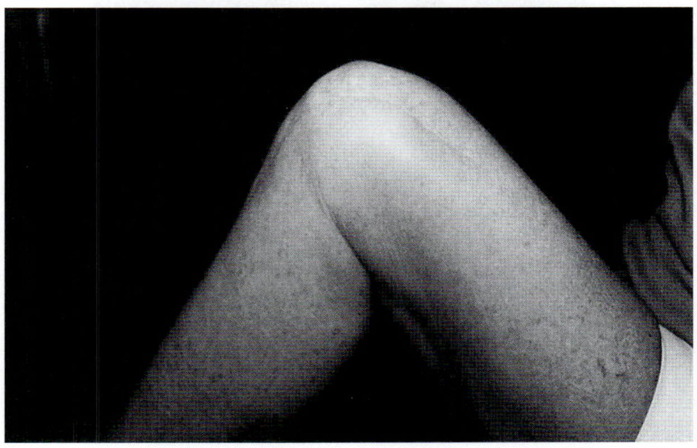

Figure 23.21. At 6 months postoperation, range of motion of the knee is −5 degrees to 120 degrees (shown here) with independent ambulation.

dure.[101] Extensile exposures can be accomplished with a proximal release of the quadriceps such the rectus snip or modified V-Y quadricepsplasty or an extended tibial tubercle osteotomy.[86,102,103,105]

Patella Fracture

Patella fracture is an uncommon complication of total knee reconstruction. However, the reported incidence is as high as 21%.[152] The fracture rate is higher for revision total knee replacement compared to primary arthroplasty. Patella fractures may not be associated with any specific traumatic event and can be asymptomatic.[172] Fatigue fractures are more common following total knee arthroplasty than traumatic fractures.[172]

Numerous causes of patella fracture have been proposed. Fractures are associated with patellar subluxation, improper patellar resection, avascular necrosis, component design, component malpositioning, increased knee flexion, and revision arthroplasty. Conditions that weaken bone such as osteopenia and thermal necrosis from cement use are also contributing factors (Fig. 23.22).[152]

An important cause of patella fracture is patella malalignment. Contact forces substantially increase with patellofemoral malalignment.[152,172] Both the eccentricity and the magnitude of patellofemoral loads on the patella increase the risk of fracture.

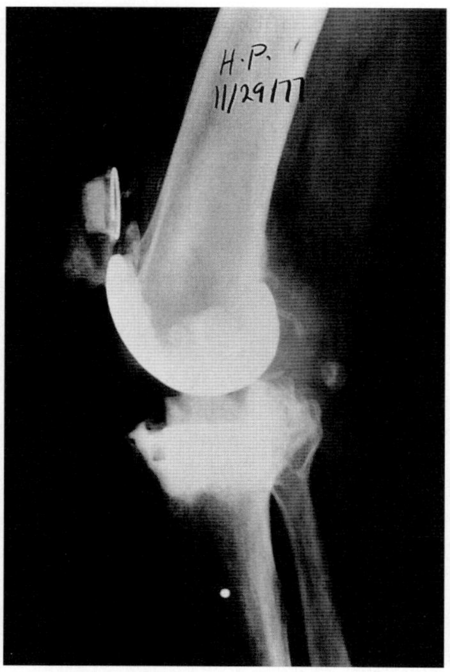

Figure 23.22. Patella fracture with dislocation of the patellar component secondary to malpositioning of the femoral component.

Also, excessive patellar resection predisposes the patella to fracture. Removal of subchondral bone causes weakness of the patella.[167] Following resection, a residual patellar thickness of less than 15 mm substantially increases anterior patellar strain.[160] Conversely, too little patellar resection creates a thick patella–patella component composite. Increased patellar height increases patellofemoral joint reaction forces and quadriceps tendon tension. Use of an oversized femoral component with an excessive anteroposterior diameter or placement of the femoral component in a flexed position also alters joint reaction forces and can lead to patella fracture.[167]

Patella component design has been linked to patella fractures.[152,172] Components with large central pegs are at higher risk for fractures than those designed with multiple smaller pegs.[152] Fractures may be related to penetration of the anterior cortex with a drill during preparation for resurfacing.

Disruption of the blood supply of the patella can result in osteonecrosis and subsequent fracture.[152,155,173] The patella vascular supply can be disrupted in performing routine total knee arthroplasty. During the medial peripatellar arthrotomy, the medial superior, medial inferior, and supreme genicular arteries may be divided. In addition, the lateral inferior genicular artery can be damaged during lateral menisectomy or fat pad excision. The lateral superior genicular artery is at risk when a lateral retinaculum release is performed.[164,165] Another factor linked to avascular necrosis is cement technique. Heat generated from the use of polymethylmethacrylate may exceed the coagulation temperature of tissue proteins, resulting in thermal necrosis of bone.[152]

A variety of fracture patterns can occur. Nonoperative management of patella fractures is suitable for fractures associated with an intact extensor mechanism and a well-fixed patella component.[152,155,172] These fractures usually have less than 5 mm of displacement and little to no comminution. Treatment options include cast immobilization or bracing for 4 to 6 weeks, followed by progressive knee range of motion and rehabilitation.

Integrity of the extensor mechanism and fixation of the patella component are important factors in determining the need for operative management. In addition, the extent of fracture displacement and comminution are also considered. Treatment options include open reduction and internal fixation. If the fracture is associated with a large single fragment, partial patellectomy and repair of the extensor mechanism is indicated. If there is not sufficient bone stock to permit patella component reimplantation, partial patellar resection or patellectomy is performed. For fractures associated with implant loosening, a temporary period of immobilization may allow sufficient bone consolidation to permit resurfacing with a new patella component.

Soft Tissue Impingement

Soft tissue impingement following total knee arthroplasty involves a spectrum of problems related to soft tissue formation about the patella.[155] Some fibrous tissue formation around the patella component is expected after total knee replacement.[154,174] However, more aggressive fibrous tissue formation leads to symptoms related to impingement including pain, limitation of motion, crepitus, and catching.[175] Two types soft tissue fibrosis amenable to surgical treatment are patella clunk syndrome and intraarticular band formation.

In patella clunk syndrome, a prominent fibrous nodule develops at the junction of the posterior aspect of the quadriceps tendon and the proximal pole of the patella.[176] Associated symptoms include anterior knee pain. In addition, a catch or clunk of the patella is typically noted with knee extension.

During knee flexion, the nodule enters the intercondylar notch of the femoral prosthesis.[176] As the knee extends, the quadriceps tendon and the patella migrate proximally and the nodule catches on or becomes entrapped within the notch. With further extension, tension placed on the fibrous nodule by the extensor mechanism causes it to dislodge from intercondylar notch. The latter stage is associated with an audible or palpable clunk.

Prosthetic design and surgical technique are believed contribute to the etiology of patella clunk syndrome.[152,176] The syndrome has been linked to the use of a type of posterior stabilized prosthesis in which the femoral component has sharp edges in the region of the intercondylar notch.[153,176] The sharp outline of the notch may cause local irritation of the extensor mechanism, resulting in nodule formation.

Technical errors associated with the development of the syndrome include malposition of the patella component in which the component proximally overhangs the patella. Also, excessive thickness of the patella and patella baja resulting from the failure to restore the normal joint line may be contributing factors.[155]

Nonoperative measures are not likely to be successful in eradicating symptoms. Recommended surgical treatment includes open or arthroscopic debridement.[152,155,174–177] Arthrotomy is usually reserved for patients requiring component revision to address malpositioning or loosening.[155]

The formation of intraarticular adhesions following total knee arthroplasty is not unusual. However, the formation of thick intraarticular fibrous bands that can result in tethering of the patella is pathologic. The etiology of the intraarticular band syndrome is unknown. There are three types of hypertrophic fibrous bands[175]: Type 1 bands are located superiorly and transversely and can prevent the patella from seating properly. Type 2 bands tether the patella laterally during knee range of motion. Type 3 bands tether the patella inferiorly. The bands can be removed successfully with arthroscopic debridement.

Failure of the Patella Component

Loosening of the patella component occurs more frequently with cementless design.[167] Risk factors for patella implant failure are multifold. Patient-related risks include trauma, morbid obesity, knee flexion above 115 degrees, and high activity level.[155,178–183] Technical errors associated with increased patellofemoral loading and subsequent component failure include malalignment, excessive patella–patella component composite thickness and patella component malposition.[152] Additional errors are the placement of an oversized femoral component or the femoral component in flexion, and failure to restore the prosthetic joint line to an anatomic level.[152] Prosthetic design is also an important factor contributing to patella implant failure.[161]

Metal-backed patella components were designed to allow fixation of the implant without use of cement and to reduce patella strain.[184] However, failure rates for metal-backed patella components are relatively high, with failure usually occurring early within a few years following arthroplasty.[180] Because of high failure rates, the use of metal-backed patella has largely fallen out of favor.[179] However, not well known is that failure of metal-backed patella appears to be limited with proper component design, surgical technique, and patella alignment.[161,185] Using the Natural Knee system (Intermedics Orthopedics, Austin, TX) over the last 10 years, our experience with metal-backed patellae has been favorable compared to cemented patellae.

Many metal-backed designs failed due to wear and fracture of the polyethylene, dissociation of the polyethylene from the metal plate, dissociation of the pegs from the metal plate, and fracture of the metal plate. With entire component thickness limited, the thickness of polyethylene is reduced to accommodate the metal base. Also associated with premature failure were components with thin layers at their outer margin or no polyethylene at the periphery to cover the metal plate.[166,182] The use of a thin layer of polyethylene predisposes to increased wear rates.[166]

For metal-backed patella designs, failure may occur at the peg attachment sites to the metal plate. Bone ingrowth around fixation pegs but not the component itself leads to failure. Shear loads are resisted at the peg-plate junction. Over time, fatigue fractures occur at the junction with the plate and can cause the metal plate to break free from the patella and the embedded ingrown lugs.

Cementless systems with reportedly favorable results have design features that minimize patellofemoral forces. Design factors include a modified dome-shaped patella, a deep-dished trochlea groove of the femoral component, a 3-mm-minimum polyethylene button, a partially countersunk patella component, and smooth press-fit patella pegs cast to the metal-backed disk.[161] The patellofemoral design in combination with soft tissue balancing and proper component sizing may contribute to successful bone ingrowth.[185]

Clinical signs of failure of the patella component include effusion and crepitus. Clinical symptoms often appear suddenly following activities associated with increased patellofemoral loading, such as climbing stairs, squatting, or rising from a seated position.

Intraoperative findings include wear and fragmentation of the polyethylene with exposure of the metal plate and black staining of the synovial membrane with metal debris. Damage can occur to the femoral component from metal-to-metal contact (Figs. 23.23 and 23.24). Depending on the design, loose, porous, coated beds or titanium fiber mesh fragment may be found embedded in the polyethylene of the patella as well as the tibia component. Additionally, complete dislodgment of the component inferiorly may be association with patellar tendon rupture.

A major factor in decision making is adequacy of the remaining patella bone stock following removal of the failed component. If sufficient bone, revision can be performed. If bone is insufficient to allow resurfacing, the options include patellar resection arthroplasty or patellectomy. Extensor weakness following patellectomy is not unexpected.

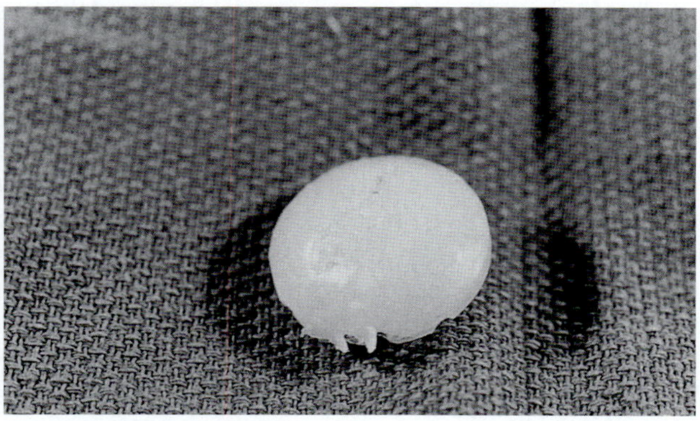

Figure 23.23. Polyethylene wear on a patella component, which produces particles in the joint with secondary swelling and pain.

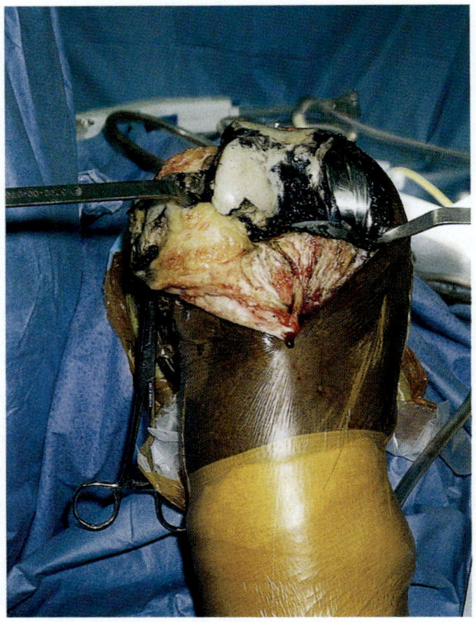

Figure 23.24. Black staining of the joint from metal-to-metal contact.

Overall, patella component failure rates have improved with advancements in prosthetic design, proper patella resection, and bone preparation and centralized patellar tracking.

PROSTHETIC FAILURE

Failure of a total knee arthroplasty may occur for a variety of reasons.[186–192] Excluding infection, types of failure include aseptic loosening, polyethylene wear, pain, and inadequate motion. Soft tissue imbalance and malalignment are significant factors in the development of failure following total knee replacement.[186–189] Prosthetic designs allow some rotational motion, which must controlled by appropriate soft tissue tension for proper kinetic function. Malalignment and soft tissue imbalance lead to ligament instability, bone and soft tissue overload, and polyethylene overload.

The most frequent cause of revision following total knee reconstruction is aseptic loosening.[186] The incidence of aseptic component loosening is difficult to quantify because of many variations of prosthetic design and modes of fixation. The most common cause of loosening is mechanical failure of the prosthesis-bone interface (Fig. 23.25 and 23.26). Failure of fixation typically occurs because of osteolysis due to wear debris or

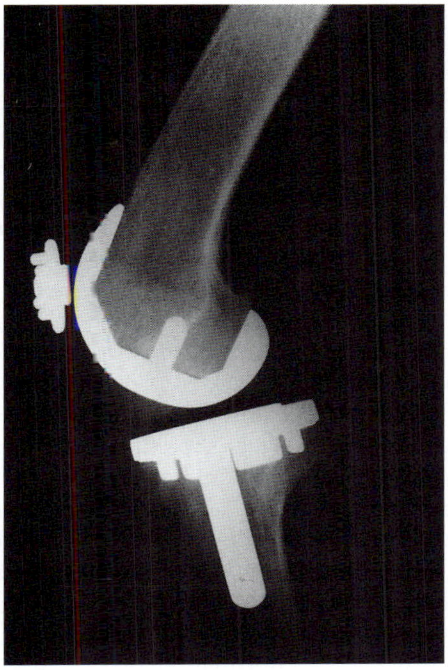

Figure 23.25. Well-positioned total knee arthroplasty with noncemented components.

failure of cancellous bone support of the tibial component secondary to overload. Patient selection, surgical technique, and prosthetic implant design all influence survivorship after total knee arthroplasty.

Several patient characteristics affect implant survival. Age, body weight, and activity level are important factors. Younger patients have poorer survival rates than older patients. Poorer survival rates are also seen with excessive weight or morbid obesity. In addition, patients

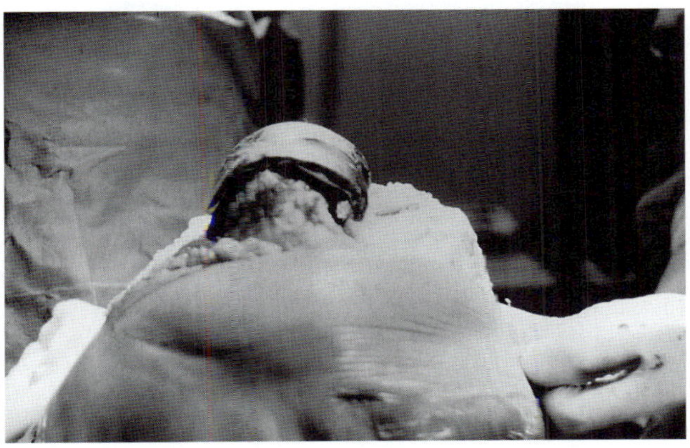

Figure 23.26. The patient in Fig. 23.25 10 years postoperation with complete resorption of femoral condyles behind the posterior flares of the femoral component and overall loosening of the prosthesis.

with a prior total knee arthroplasty and those with posttraumatic or osteoarthritis generally have implant survival rates lower than do those with rheumatoid arthritis.

Surgical technique is also an important factor affecting prosthetic survivorship. Increased attention to limb alignment and ligament balance are attributed to the improved survival rate associated with modern condylar implant designs.[187,189] Failure to correct limb alignment causes eccentric loading of the prosthetic components and ultimately contributes to loosening. The assessment of alignment for total knee arthroplasty, however, involves more than the anteroposterior and coronal planes. Rotation and translocation of the components in other planes are also important. For the femur and tibia, there are 6 degrees of freedom with regard to malalignment: valgus-varus, flexion-extension, proximal-distal, internal-external rotation, anterior-posterior, and medial-lateral.

Varus malalignment contributes to early failure (Fig. 23.27). The mechanical axis of the limb passes from the hip to the ankle through the center of the knee. Components are generally oriented at a right angle to the mechanical axis to allow transmission of compressive forces to the fixation interface. For the average patient, the knee is placed in 5 to 7 degrees of valgus alignment in the anteroposterior (AP) plane. Mild varus alignment of the femoral prosthesis alone may not contribute to failure. It is the overall alignment of the limb, particularly

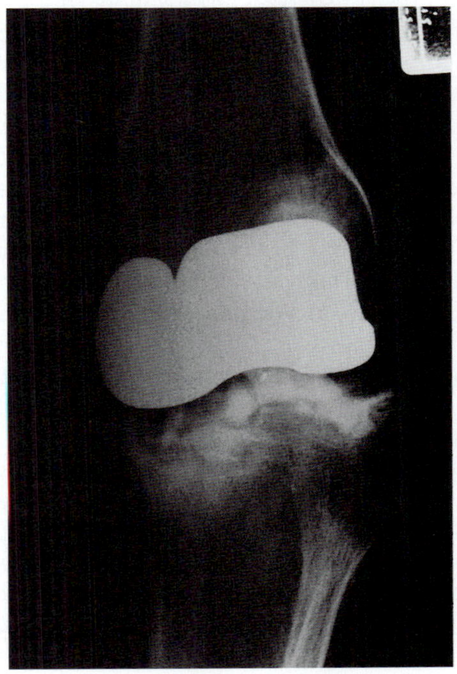

Figure 23.27. Varus malalignment, which led to failure of the total knee arthroplasty in 9 months.

in neutral or varus alignment, which can lead to premature failure. Typically there is a contribution to overall alignment by the tibial component. Varus alignment of the tibial component is associated with premature failure of fixation and accelerated polyethylene wear.

The restoration of axial alignment solely for the bony structures is insufficient. Soft tissue balance is also linked to mechanical alignment. Failure to adequately release contracted ligaments, especially medially and laterally, leads to malalignment. If a ligamentous balance is not achieved, compressive forces can occur on the contracted side and tensile forces can be seen on the noncontracted side, leading to uneven distribution of forces across the knee. Ligamentous release is anticipated for knees with significant preoperative varus or valgus deformity. Similar to the results of component malalignment, residual ligament imbalance postoperatively leads to early fixation failure or accelerated polyethylene wear. Postoperatively, excessive valgus alignment is generally better tolerated than neutral or varus alignment. However, valgus malalignment, especially in an obese individual, may lead to a cosmetically unsatisfactory result.

Medial placement or internal rotation of the femoral component can alter patellofemoral tracking. A lateral retinacular release may compensate for minor translocation or rotation. However, medial placement or internal rotation of the femoral prosthesis can lead to premature failure of the polyethylene of the patella component. In addition, other patellofemoral complications can result, such as subluxation, dislocation, or patella fracture. Surgical management may also require revision arthroplasty to address the femoral component malalignment as well as the patellofemoral issues. Malrotation can occur, particularly in knees with posterior femoral condyle deficiency. Distortion of anatomy and loss of landmarks can make it difficult for accurate prosthetic placement. Proper assessment of femoral component rotation may not be achievable with the use of routine intramedullary guides. The epicondylar axis is an acceptable adjunct to standard alignment systems. In addition, the AP axis is an alternative guide used to evaluate external rotation for femoral component placement. As with femoral rotation, rotational alignment of the tibial component is important. External rotation reduces the Q angle and improves patella femoral tracking.

Knee replacements have a tendency to fail with subsidence medially and anteriorly. Placement of the tibial component to cover the anterior cortical bone is preferred to more posterior placement where the bone is of inferior quality. More posterior placement increases the risk of the component subsiding anteriorly. In addition, the highest quality of cancellous bone in the proximal tibia is located beneath the subchondral plate. Excessive depth of the tibial bone resection is generally avoided to prevent subsidence into weaker cancellous bone.

An advantage to the use of cement for fixation is that it provides strength to support the tibial component. In cemented designs, stress at the interface of the bone is similar to that for the cement. However, cement is generally stronger than cancellous bone in compression, tension, and shear. Cement interdigitation to bone is essential to resist stresses at the interface. In addition, stemmed prostheses also reduce stress at interface. The use of a long-stem implant in conjunction with cement is advocated for fixation in poor quality bone.

Long-term success with press-fit fixation is dependent on the design of implant system. In addition, bone should be of adequate quality to provide stable fixation. If tight fixation cannot be obtained with press-fit components, then the implants should be cemented.

Ultra-high molecular weight polyethylene (UHMWPE) is the bearing material of choice in total knee reconstruction.[1] However, its use in well-aligned, balanced knees is attributed to long-term survival of total knee arthroplasty. However, the lifetime of UHMWPE is not indefinite. Polyethylene particles at the bone implant interface are a major contributing factor to aseptic loosening. The biologic response to wear debris leads to bone resorption and loosening of the implant at the bone interface. Polyethylene wear in total knee arthroplasty typically occurs secondary to high contact stresses, with resulting polyethylene damage and debris formation (Figs. 23.28–23.30). Among the findings

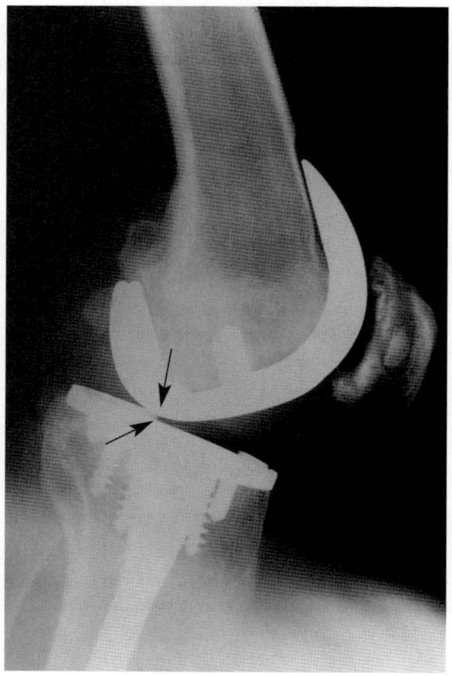

Figure 23.28. Loss of polyethylene space and failure of total knee arthroplasty 8 years postoperation. Arrows point to metal-to-metal contact.

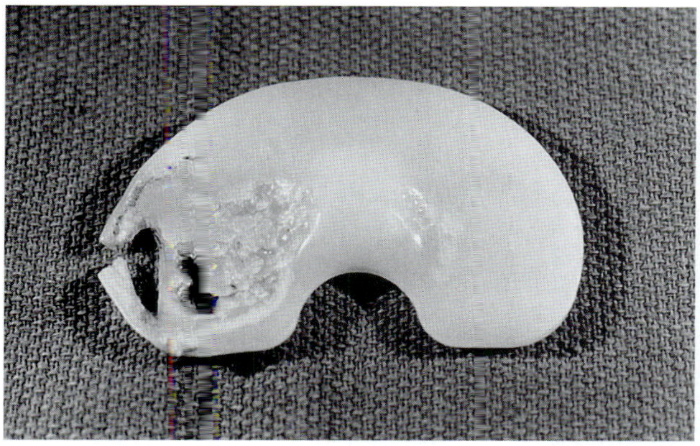

Figure 23.29. Destruction and fragmentation of the polyethylene component.

consistent with damage in retrieved polyethylene implants are pitting, delamination, abrasion, burnishing, scratching, deformation, and fracture. The size of polyethylene particles found around total knee replacements is larger than that typically found associated with total hip replacements. However, the wear particle patterns are attributed to differences in the kinematics, loading, and geometry of the knee. Higher stresses are generated in the knee with relatively lower conformity of the implants. In addition, the femoral component has additional motions of rolling and sliding during gait that contribute to differing wear compared to hip prostheses. The prior use of thin polyethylene implants is a risk factor for catastrophic wear and early failure. It is now recognized that polyethylene has a minimum acceptable thickness for optimal durability and longevity.

Also important for the longevity of polyethylene is its sterilization and oxidation. Gamma irradiation, which had been used until the 1990s, is associated with the generation of polyethylene debris and osteolysis.[1] Also, with exposure to oxygen, degradation of polyethylene occurs. Specifically, oxidation of polyethylene causes changes in its quality, physical properties, and wear resistance. Currently, ethylene oxide gas or gas plasma are used for sterilization. Modifications in sterilization and cross-linking are among the advances intended to improve wear properties of polyethylene, with further advances anticipated in the future.

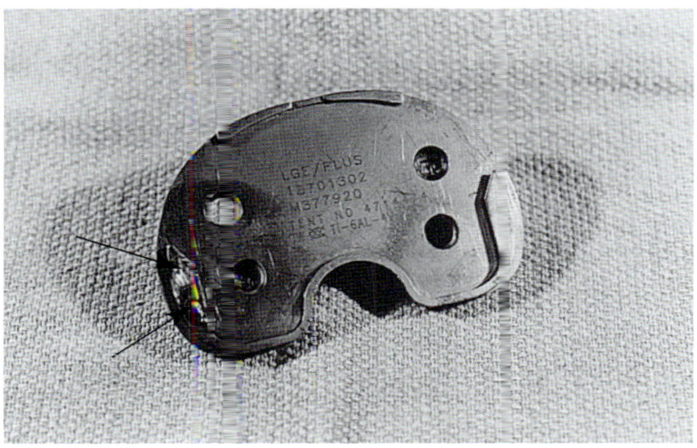

Figure 23.30. Arrows point to secondary deformation of the tibial metal tray.

BONE LOSS

Osseous deficiency can be seen in primary and revision total knee arthroplasty. In primary knees, proximal tibial bone deficiency is seen more often than distal femoral deficiency. Proximal tibial bone defects typically result from varus or valgus knee deformity.[193–195] The most common lesion encountered in primary total knee arthroplasty is located in the posterior medial tibia and is associated with a varus knee deformity. Central defects of the proximal tibia usually occur with valgus knees. In primary knees, bone defects can result from a sliding motion that replaces the normal rolling action of knee flexion or from overload of the subchondral bone, which causes collapse.

There are several options available for the management of bone defects that typically occur with primary knees. Alteration of the surgical procedure and bone preparation can be used for managing small defects. Additional options include the use of polymethylmethacrylate, metal wedges or spacers, custom prostheses, or bone graft.

In revision knees, bone loss can have a range of severity. Early failed total knee arthroplasties are typically associated with smaller bone defects. Most small to intermediate-sized defects found in revision knees can be managed similarly to defects commonly found in primary knees. However, in cases of late prosthetic failure with aseptic loosening, more extensive bone loss can occur.[196] Particulate debris leads to enzymatic destruction of bone that can cause bone loss as well as implant migration. The management of massive bone loss in revision total knee arthroplasty can be particularly challenging. Inadequate bone stock may be only one of several problems encountered during revision total knee arthroplasty. Multiple surgical options include arthrodesis, amputation, custom total knee arthroplasty, autograft, or allograft.[193,194,196,197]

Selecting the most appropriate option for the treatment of bone deficiency depends on a number of variables including the severity of the disease process, the anatomic location of the deformity, the existence of previous surgical reconstruction, and the need for sufficient support for the prosthetic components.

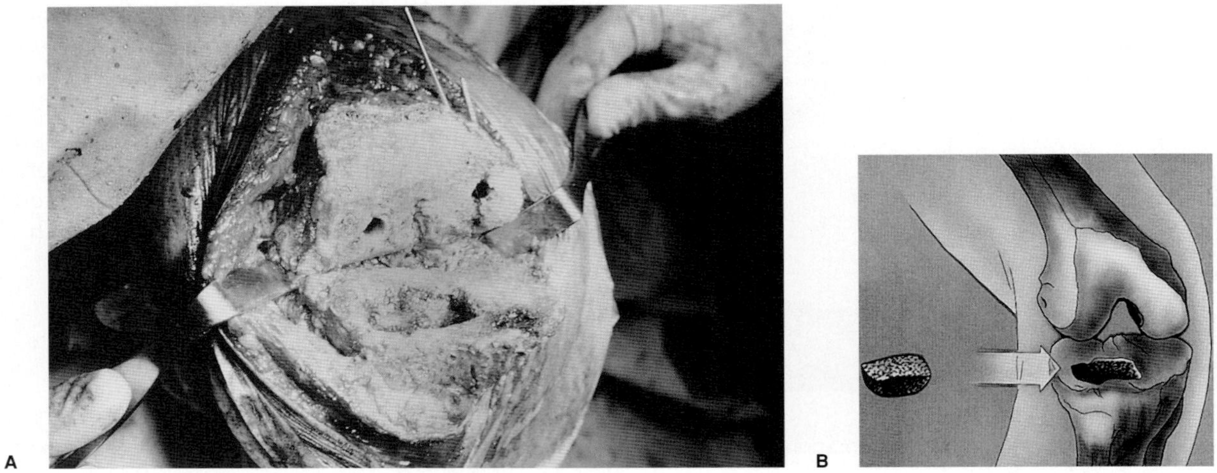

Figure 23.31. **A** and **B**: Type I (Rand) lesion associated with focal bone loss with some metaphysical and cortical bone remaining intact.

Classification

Several classification schemes exist for the evaluation of bone loss in revision total knee arthroplasty. These schemes can also be applied to bone loss found in primary knees. Plain AP and lateral radiographs are inspected for the presence of bone defects and/or the reduction in the profile and dimension of the metaphyseal segment of the femoral condyles or tibia plateau. Bone defects, particularly those found in primary total knee arthroplasty, tend to be peripheral or central in location.[193,198] Contained defects have an intact cortical rim. Defects lacking a cortical shell are considered noncontained.

Mow and Wiedel[199,200] described bone deficiency as segmental, cavitary, or a combination of the two. Segmental defects imply a significant amount of cortical bone loss. Cavitary bone defects involve loss of metaphyseal bone with an intact cortical shell. In combination lesions, there is loss of both metaphyseal and cortical bone.

In the classification scheme proposed by Rand, a type 1 lesion is associated with the focal loss of bone, with some metaphyseal and cortical bone remaining intact (Fig. 23.31).[193] In type 2 defects, there is loss of metaphyseal bone and a cortical rim of bone remains intact (Fig. 23.32).[193] In type 3 lesions, there is gross or global loss of both metaphyseal and cortical bone.[193]

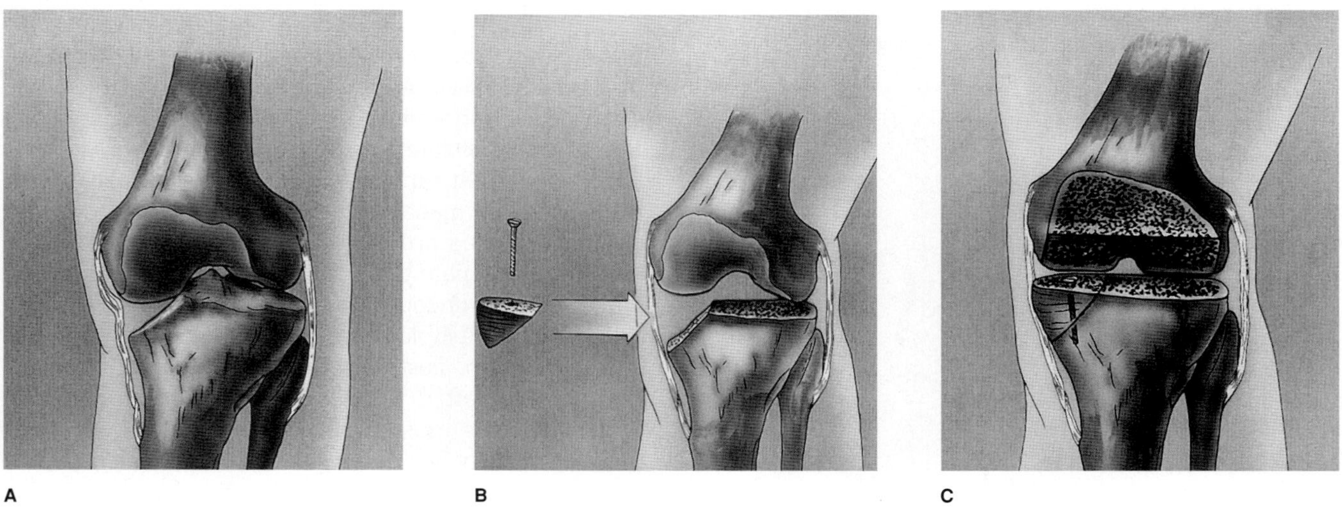

Figure 23.32. **A–C**: Type 3 lesion when global loss of both metaphysical and cortical bone exists.

Alternatively, the Anderson Orthopaedic Research Institute (AORI) classification also addresses bone loss patterns in revision surgery.[196] This classification not only addresses bone loss patterns but also proposes treatment options based on the pattern. The AORI classification is applied separately to the femur (F) and tibia (T). In a type 1 defect, the metaphyseal bone is intact. Typically, there are minor bone defects that do not compromise the stability of the prosthesis. For type 2 defects, there is loss of cancellous bone in the metaphysis. Type 2A bone defects involve one femoral or tibial plateau. In type 2B lesions, both condyles or plateaus are involved. In a type 3 defect, the metaphyseal bone is deficient and compromises a major portion of either condyle or plateau. These severe defects are occasionally associated with patellar or collateral ligament detachment.

In general, the F1-T1 classification is applied when cancellous bone is present at a normal joint line level that permits use of standard nonstemmed implants. The F2-T2 categories included cases with damaged cancellous bone that require augmentation or repair to restore joint line and knee stability. The F3-T3 category should be reserved primarily for severe cases in which the damaged metaphyseal segment of bone must be repaired with major bone grafts, custom components, or hinges in order to reconstruct the damaged bone.[196]

Femoral Bone Deficiency

Distal femoral defects are rare in primary knee surgery. Tibial deficiency is more common.[193] However, bone deficiency can occur following trauma. In addition, distal femur fractures may result in condylar malunion or angular deformity, which can complicate treatment with total knee arthroplasty. Also, loss of viable bone occurs in avascular necrosis.[193] Removal of avascular bone may result in a significant bone defect.

There are several options available for the management of femoral deficiency. Cancellous bone graft easily manages the majority of lesion found in the distal femur. In addition, cement can also be used for smaller contained osseous lesions, but is not the preferred option. Modular wedges can be attached to augment the femoral component.

Autogenous graft can be obtained from resected femoral or tibial bone that is harvested in performing the primary total knee arthroplasty procedure. If there is not sufficient bone available, allogeneic graft bone can be used. For larger defects, structural graft may be necessary. Fresh frozen allograft from femoral heads is commonly used as a source of allogeneic bone. As with autograft, allograft bone can be morselized and impacted into areas of loss.[201] Alternatively, allograft bone can

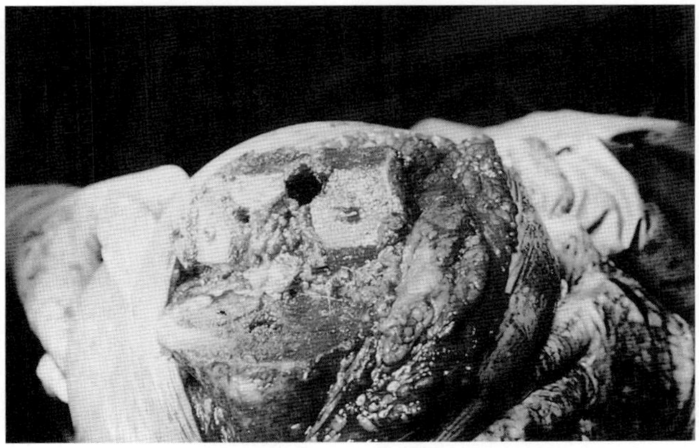

Figure 23.33. In femoral condylar insufficiency allograft or autograft can be utilized to re-create the anatomic integrity and a base so that the prosthesis can be applied. Any minor deficiency then can be packed with additional cancellous material.

be shaped into bony blocks matching the pattern of loss (Fig. 23.33). When stability of the component is not compromised, bone graft is necessary only to fill the defect and not to support the component.

Despite involvement of the weight-bearing area, there is usually adequate distal femoral bone stock in a typical failed total knee arthroplasty. For smaller bone defects, treatment options in revision surgery are similar to those of primary total knee reconstruction. As with primary knees, bone graft is commonly used to treat deficiencies.[202,203] Morselized cancellous autograft or allograft can be successfully used for the management of smaller cavitary lesions in revision total knee arthroplasty. Cement also can be used to fill contained defects.[193] The augmentation of the femoral prosthesis with metal wedges is another available option with many revision knee systems.[198] Structural bone grafts are often required for the management of noncontained bone lesions.[204–206]

In revision total knee arthroplasty, severe femoral bone loss may be present due to osteolysis.[193,196] The femur often has a funnel-shaped appearance, with absent cancellous bone in the distal femur (Fig. 23.34). The available surgical options include the use of structural allograft to restore bone stock. The restoration of bone stock is important in the event of future revision surgery. Bone graft offers numerous advantages including biocompatibility, availability, and versatility in its ability to be shaped to fit the pattern of the patient's deficient bone. It also can be used to restore bone stock. If necessary, ligaments can be reattached to large bulk allografts. Other options included fixed or modular wedges that can be applied to the distal femoral component or custom prosthetic components.[198]

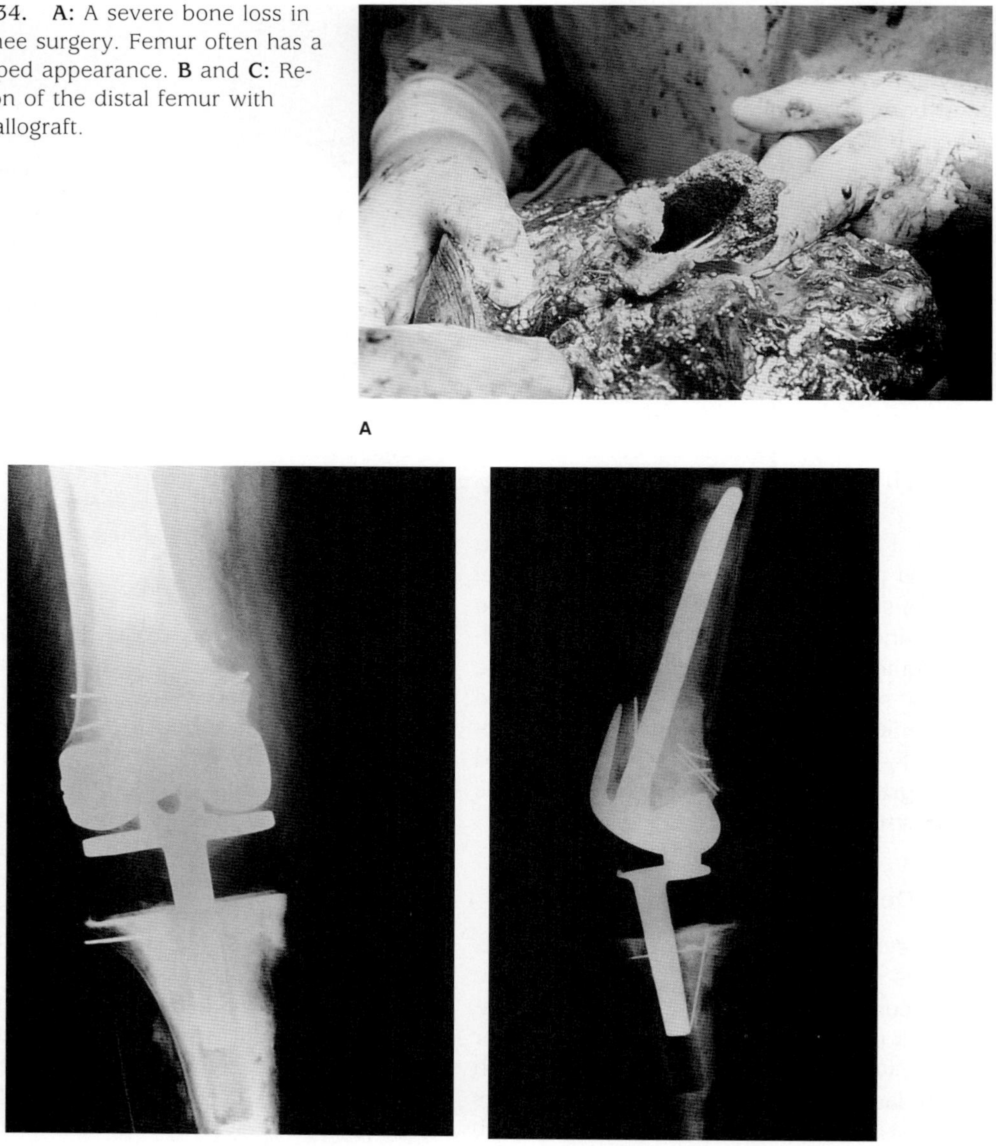

A

B

C

Figure 23.34. **A:** A severe bone loss in revision knee surgery. Femur often has a funnel-shaped appearance. **B** and **C:** Reconstruction of the distal femur with structural allograft.

Tibial Bone Deficiency

In primary and revision total knee arthroplasty, bone deficiency most commonly occurs in the proximal tibia. Bone loss is often associated with varus or valgus angular deformity.[193,194,198] Even mild to moderate bone loss can be seen in primary knees in the presence of angular malignment. The most common bone defect is located in the posteromedial third of the proximal medial tibial condyle. This metaphyseal bone lesion is located in the peripheral aspect of the proximal tibia.[193] These peripheral lesions may or may not preserve the cortical rim of the tibial condyle.[193] In addition, peripheral deficits are often associated with varus deformity. The typical depth of most bone defects does not exceed 5 to 6 mm.[193] The majority of lesions are usually removed with proximal tibia resection during the routine arthroplasty procedure. In contrast, central tibia lesions are usually found in the metaphyseal region and are associated with valgus knees. More commonly, the cortical rim is preserved in central defects. However, the rim may be involved in extensive lesions.

The treatment of the bone deficiency is dependent on the extent of the lesion following routine tibial resection and whether the cortical rim is preserved. Defects are described as central or peripheral depending on their location in the tibial metaphysis. For contained defects, the cortical margins are preserved. Cortical ero-

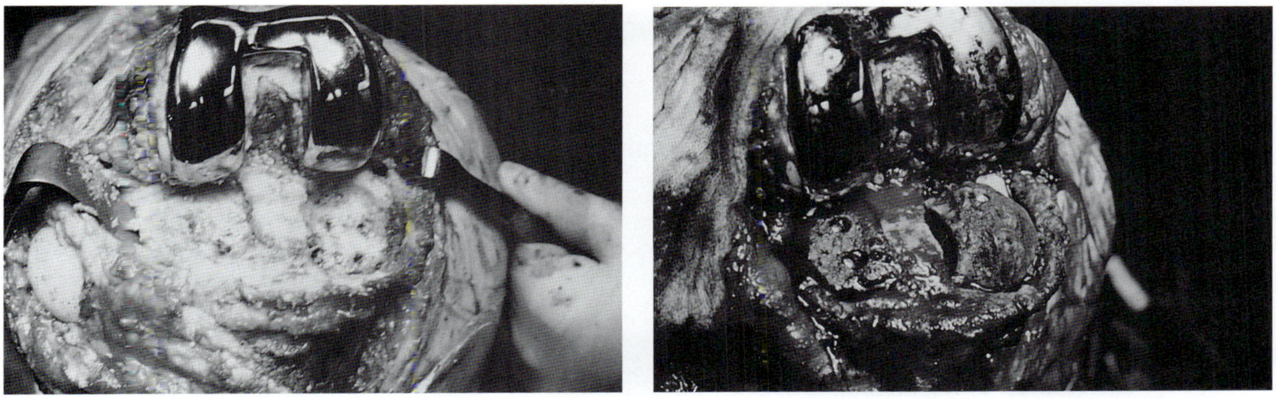

A B

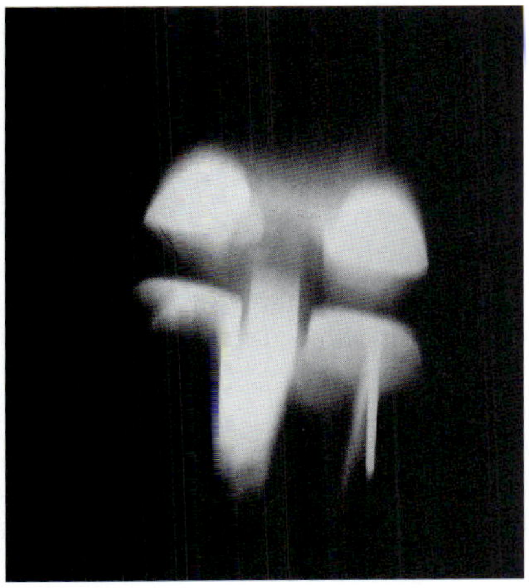

C

Figure 23.35. **A:** Tibial defect involving over 50% of a tibial condyle prior to debridement. (depth 12 and 14 mm). **B:** Defects after preparation and grafting with femoral head allografts, prior to insertion of tibial component. **C:** Tomogram 24 months postoperation shows complete incorporation of grafted area.

sion is associated with noncontained defects. Defects associated with implant instability exceed 5 mm in depth following tibial resection and encompass over 50% of a tibial condyle (Fig. 23.35).[193] Advantages and disadvantages of the options for management of these defects are addressed.

Lowering the tibial resection line is mechanically unsound and may cause result in less than optimal support for the prosthesis (Fig. 23.36).[207–209] This option is feasible only for small areas of bone loss. The strength of the tibial bone decreases below the subchondral margin. A bone resection 12 mm below the joint line typically results in removal of more than 80% of the cancellous bone and may place the implant on cortical, rather than metaphyseal, bone.[197] With more distal cuts, there is danger of compromise of important ligament attachments. Therefore, it is not recommended to routinely resect tibial defects to their bases.

Strategic positioning of the tibial tray can be used to avoid a bone deficit.[195,210] However, this may require the use of a smaller than ideal implant with the potential for long-term consequences.

The most common management of central and peripheral bone defects is with the use of bone graft.[198] However, for small to medium-sized defects, there are numerous options available to the surgeon including cement fill, metal wedges, augmentation of the tibial prosthesis with metal wedges or spacers, and modular stems.[198]

Cement

The indications for use of polymethylmethacrylate (PMMA) or cement to fill bone defects is limited. PMMA can be used for contained bone defects measuring less than 5 to 10 mm in height.[193,195] Advantages of PMMA include availability and simplicity. It achieves full strength shortly after curing. The techniques for preparation and insertion of cement are not technically demanding.

The disadvantages of cement, however, are numerous. The modulus for elasticity for cement is less than that of bone. The addition of screws and mesh to cement for reinforcement do not provide sufficient structural support. Also, adequate penetration of cement into bone may not be adequate, and there are not good

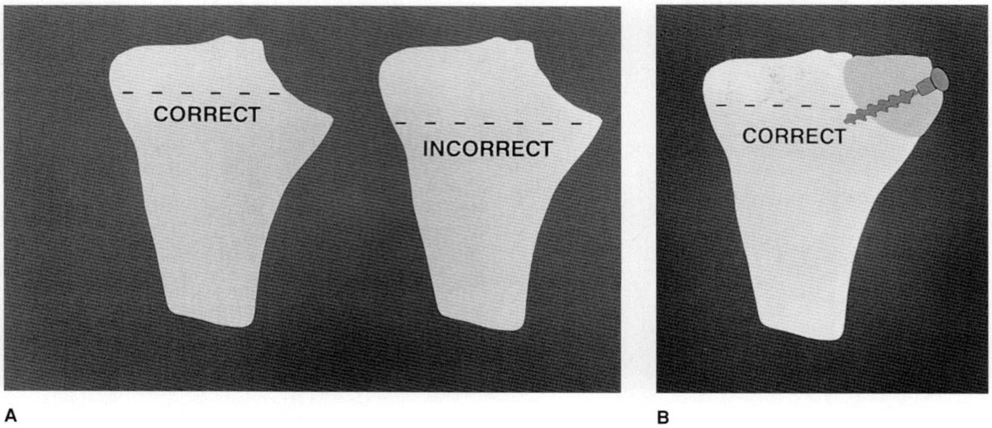

Figure 23.36. **A:** Lowering the tibial resection line is mechanically not sound. **B:** Resection should be minimal combined with grafting of the defect, which is a more mechanically sound procedure.

methods to secure cement. Cement is inferior in its ability to resist fixation failure. Furthermore, laminations within PMMA are associated with subsequent fragmentation and loss of component fixation.[195,210]

Cement is also not acceptable for use in large bone defects. Problems associated with large amounts cement include the generation of excessive heat, shrinkage in volume during curing, susceptibility to infection, and unacceptable strain at the bone-prosthesis interface under axial and varus loading.

In addition, PMMA is not a viable option for the managing peripheral bone defects with the loss of the cortical shell. Cement placed in oblique areas of bone loss does not achieve adequate purchase and is subject to loosening.[197]

Metal Wedges
Metal wedges or spacers are most commonly attached to tibial prosthetic components.[195–198] They are readily available with most primary and revision total knee arthroplasty systems.[197] In addition to convenience and simplicity, they can be applied relatively quickly to the prosthesis. The modular design of the wedge allows it to be placed in multiple positions and it comes in a variety of sizes.

Wedges have been used in the treatment of peripheral bone lesions such as a deficient condyle. For tibial deficiency, wedges have been used to manage defects involving up to 50% of the medial or lateral plateau.[195] Wedges can be used in addition to bone graft. In revision knees, wedges are useful in instances where it is desirable to avoid the use bone graft. Biomechanically, they provide sufficient resistance to applied loads and optimize stress distribution.

However, the long-term durability of metal wedges and spacers has not been established. Short-term studies are encouraging. However, there has not been sufficient follow-up documenting lasting clinical effectiveness. Therefore, wedges are most suitable for small to intermediate-sized bone defects in low-demand patients. They are not advocated in the management of large defects.

Modular Knee Designs
Modular knee designs are available for use in managing bone loss. Modular systems, however, can be expensive. In this era of managed care and cost containment, the expense of a design system is noteworthy. In revision cases, the use of modular stems and wedges can cost several times more than reconstruction with bone allograft and certain total knee replacement systems.[193,195]

Custom Implants

Custom implants are an option for the management of severe bone deficiency. Because they are designed to the pathology of the individual patient, they theoretically offer optimal fit and restoration of biomechanical force transmission. However, despite careful preoperative planning, the custom prosthesis may not fit as planned or not at all.[200,211]

Another potential disadvantage of custom designs is an unacceptable time delay during the fabrication of the design.[211] Furthermore, additional bone sacrifice may be required during the insertion of the implants, which may be problematic in cases of future revision surgery. Also, in cases of custom prosthetic failure, further bone loss may occur.[197]

Compared to off-the-shelf designs, however, custom implants are expensive. Custom prostheses are not cost-effective for widespread use. In addition, long-term studies using custom systems are lacking. The indications for custom design are limited to problems that cannot be addressed by other options.

Bone Graft

Techniques for Tibial Deficiency

Central defects of the tibia are not problematic if the remaining rim can support the tibia component. If the defect is large and involves a considerable proportion of the cancellous bone of the tibia plateau, bone grafting is a preferable treatment option.[193] Bone grafting provides support for the component that is physiologic and offers the opportunity for durability in the long term. The strength of tibial cancellous bone decreased with the distance from the subchondral plate.[197] In larger lesions, it is recommended to build up the deficient bone rather than resect the tibia to the base of the defect.[193,197]

Sculco's group[210] describes a technique for management of peripheral lesions. This technique may be used for peripheral defects involving only metaphyseal bone as well as those in which the cortical bone of the tibial plateau is also eroded. The eroded tibia is osteotomized, leaving a flat surface of cancellous bone. The cancellous surface of bone graft from the resected distal femur condyles is placed over the osteotomized defect. The graft is temporarily attached with Kirschner wires (K-wires) or Steinmann pins. Excess bone is cut flush with the tibia plateau. The plateau is prepared for insertion of tibia trial prosthesis. The pins are then replaced with bone screws.

In addition, for peripheral or central tibial bone defects, Insall[212] describes a technique for management. Following removal of sclerotic bone from its base, the defect is also sculpted into a rectangular or trapezoidal shape. A block graft, typically from the resected distal femur, is fashioned to a matching rectangular or trapezoidal shape. The graft is then inserted and tapped into place. Excess bone is removed with a saw and the tibia plateau is prepared for the trial prosthesis.

Altchek et al[207] reported on 14 patients who had undergone autogenous bone grafts using the Sculco technique. The average follow-up was 4.3 years, with a range of 2 to 7.5 years. For all patients, there was graft union by clinical and radiographic means. The Insall technique is a viable option for small to medium-sized defects. The bone graft creates a physiologic support for the prosthesis and adds to the bone stock.

General Principles

Autogenous or allogeneic bone graft has long been accepted in the management of tibial and/or femoral bone deficiency.[193,195,197] Autogenous metaphyseal bone graft is an ideal material in the treatment of bone defects because of its cancellous structure, strength, and osteoconductive properties. Osteoblasts in the graft material have osteogenic potential, which promote bone healing. Healed bone graft offers durable support for prosthetic components.

The key to success in bone grafting is preparation of the host bone. The preparation includes removal of all sclerotic and nonviable bone from the bone defects. An effort is made to preserve the cortical rim and viable cancellous host bone. In revision knees, any cement, membranous tissue, or other debris is thoroughly removed. Such debris can interfere with graft incorporation. Multiple drill holes are placed into the defect to promote vascularization.

There are many advantages of bone graft for the management of bone deficiency. Among the advantages are availability and economy.[193,213] Bone resected from femoral of tibial condyles can be a ready source of autogenous bone graft for managing focal deficiencies in primary and revision total knee arthroplasty procedures. At this time, however, the autogenous iliac crest bone is not routinely utilized. Iliac crest bone harvest unnecessarily increases the morbidity of the total knee arthroplasty procedure.

Bone graft is versatile and can also be obtained in a wide variety of sizes and shapes. Size ranges from morcellized cancellous chips that are more commonly used to fill contained defects to bulk proximal tibia or distal femoral allografts for massive bone deficits.[195,213] With the use of saw, burrs, and other instruments, bone can be fashioned to match shape of the bone deficit.

Other advantages of bone graft include its biocompatibility. In addition, the mode of elasticity of bone graft is comparable to the host.[193,195,197,213] Load transfer is more physiologic with bone grafting than with cement fill or custom components. Bone graft offers the additional advantage of restoring bone stock. This is especially important if revision surgery is later required. Healing of the graft to host bone occurs with autogenous and allogeneic bone. Autogenous bone graft is particularly advantageous because of its ability to incorporate rapidly.

Indications for bone grafting includes tibial or femoral defects exceeding 10 mm, a defect involving greater than 25% to 50% of the tibial surface, large contained defects of the femur or tibia, and absence of the distal femur or tibia (Fig. 23.37).[195]

The appropriate type of bone graft depends on the nature of the bone deficit. The goal is to provide a firm foundation for the components. Localized bone grafts are indicated for use in deficits involving less than 50% of the compartment surfaces. Local graft can be best obtained from resected distal femoral condyles. While autograft is the material of choice, it is not available in

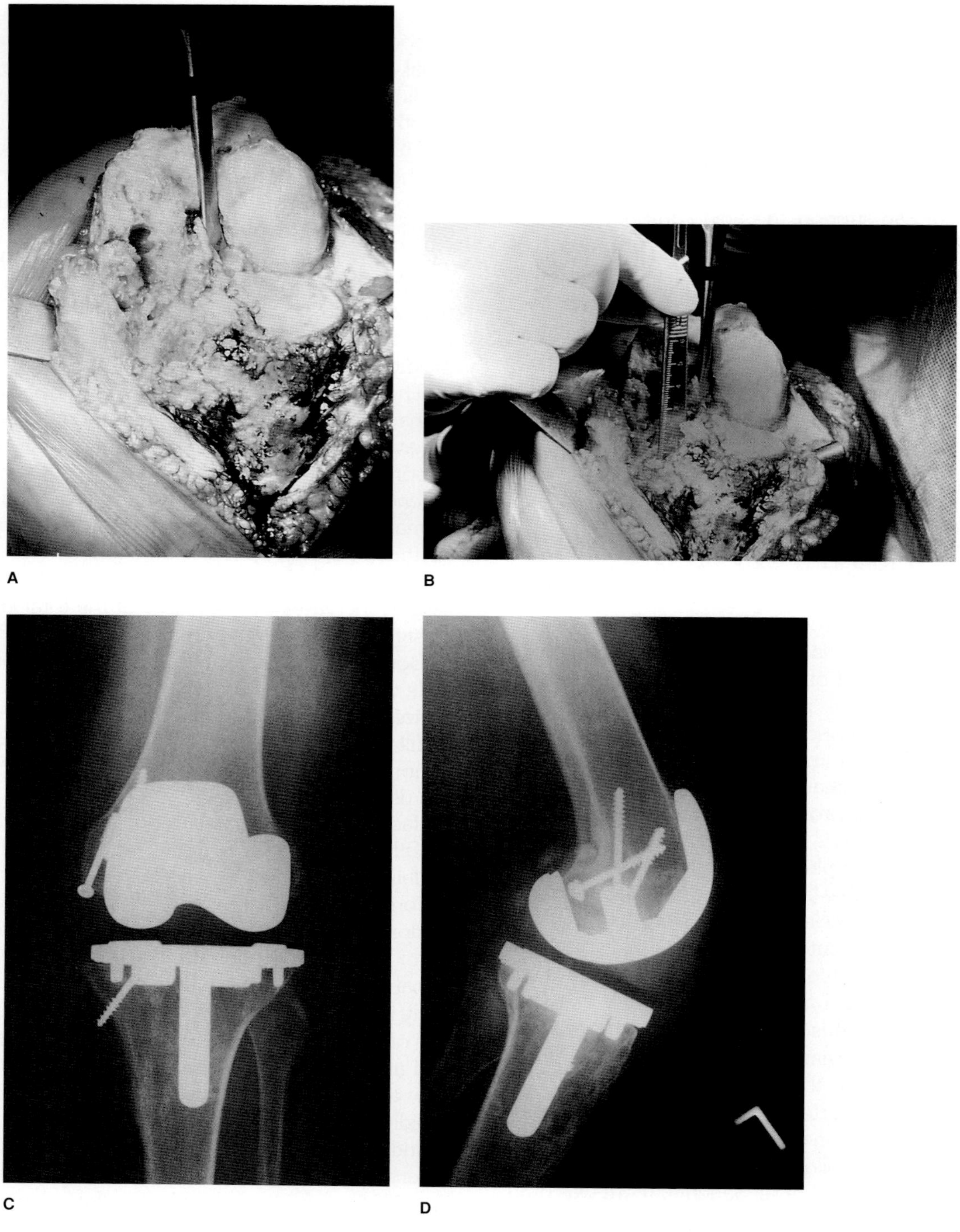

Figure 23.37. **A:** Femoral defect exceeding 10 mm in depth. **B:** Tibial defect approximately 25 mm in depth involving the entire medial condyle. **C** and **D:** After bone grafting of both condyles, a noncemented total knee arthroplasty is performed. Postoperative films at 6 months.

sufficient quantity to reconstruct larger defects. If the deficit is greater than 10 mm or more than 50% of the tibial condyle, then the use of allograft is indicated.[193] Morcellized allograft can be for defects that do not compromise support for the prosthetic component. For larger lesions structural allograft is more commonly used. Bulk allografts consisting of entire proximal tibia or distal femoral segments may be necessary in cases of global bone loss.[206] For larger lesions, long-stem prosthetic components are used to decrease load.[206]

Mechanisms of bone graft failure include varus angular malalignment, poorly prepared or avascular host bone bed, incomplete coverage of the graft by the prosthetic component, inadequate press fit of the graft to host bone, and cement extravasation into the host-bone interface.

Hill and Phillips[208] presented the results of 42 total knee arthroplasty procedures using autologous bone graft. The defects averaged 7.3 mm laterally and 10 mm medially in extent. The average follow-up was 3.9 years. Ninety-eight percent of grafts incorporated to the host bone.

Allograft

The quantity of autograft may not be sufficient, particularly during revision total knee arthroplasty where there may have been previous bone resection from prior surgery or more extensive bone loss. Allograft is advantageous in that it can restore bone stock with a material that is structurally similar to host bone.[213] It also has the ability to heal to host bone. Allogeneic bone is also available in a variety of shapes and sizes. Femoral heads obtained during total hip arthroplasty are a ready source of bone graft. Allograft bone can be morcellized and impacted into defects. Alternatively, it can be used as a structural graft in block form.

For larger bone defects, metal wedges or spacers attached to augment the prosthetic component may not be sufficient for adequate reconstruction. The insertion of a structural allograft, such as a femoral head graft, along with a stemmed prosthetic component is an excellent option for treatment of large bony deficits in both primary and revision total knee arthroplasty.

Bulk allograft can be used to replace bone absent from the distal femur and/or tibia.[213–216] If necessary, ligaments can be reattached to large structural allografts. Reconstruction can also include the management of extensor mechanism loss by replacement with an allograft containing an attached patellar tendon–patella–quadriceps extensor complex. When a proximal tibia or distal femur allograft is used as a whole segment, it is attached to host bone as a composite with the implant.

Allograft is a viable alternative that when applied properly can yield successful results. Important principles for graft success must be applied such as preparation of the host bone. Avascular sclerotic host bone, cement, and soft tissue must be debrided from the defect until healthy bleeding bone appears. Also important is an excellent fit of the graft to the host, even without necessary adjunctive fixation.

The bone graft is contoured to allow for maximal surface contact with host bone. Interference fit of the graft into host bone is ideal. At cortical junctions, step cuts at the graft-host bone interface can provide some additional rotational stability. Fixation can be achieved with cancellous or cortical screws. If necessary, plates may also be utilized. In addition, fixation of the prosthesis has a guarded prognosis if it relies on the allograft bone for support.

The use of a long-stem tibial prosthesis that engages the diaphysis enhances the success of larger grafts by reducing loads by 30%.[213] Stemmed prostheses help protect the grafts during the incorporation process by reducing stress at the bone-implant–host-bone interface.[213,216] By reducing stress, long-stem components may extend the fatigue life of the graft. Cement may be used to fix the implants. Press-fit components have been used. However, allograft is avascular. Bony ingrowth of allograft bone to the porous implant may not occur.

The disadvantages of bone allografts include slow incorporation, weakening during the revascularization phase with resultant collapse or fracture, nonunion, resorption, and infection.[193,213] There is also a risk of disease transmission.[213] However, living donors provide the opportunity for extensive testing and screening. For structural allografts, protected weight bearing is required until incorporation is seen. It may take months for radiologic signs of incorporation to be seen. In addition, an extended period of rehabilitation is required. There is also a potential for the risk of immunogenicity. However, this risk is minimized if the marrow elements are not removed.

An allograft technique described by Engh and Parks[195] is effective for large tibial or femoral bone loss. Structural allograft is provided with the use of a fresh frozen femoral head. Acetabular reamers are used to precisely contour the graft and host and maximize surface contact. Male acetabular reamers are used to prepare the host bone. After a vascular bed of cancellous bone is created. A female acetabular reamer is utilized to contour the femoral head allograft. Interference fit is accomplished by sizing the graft 2 mm larger than the host site. The graft is provisionally fixed with K-wires. The tibia or femoral plateau is prepared to receive the trial prosthesis. Later the wires are removed and cortical or cancellous screws are used to secure the graft to the host bone.

Engh et al[216] reported the Anderson clinic experience using femoral head allograft in revision total knee reconstruction. There were 21 grafts used in 21 patients. The average follow-up was 51 months. Modular or custom prosthetic components were used. Cemented revisions averaged 87 on the Knee Society Score. Four custom prostheses were used without cement. Clinical results with cementless fixation were not as encouraging. Three of the four press-fit components subsided within the first 2 years and patients reported mild pain with walking. There were no revisions or reoperations.

Other authors reviewed the results of bone grafting for treating bone defects in primary and revision total knee arthroplasty and allograft. Overall, the results are encouraging. Complications in some cases were high. However, this does not diminish the overall effectiveness of bone grafting. In spite of complications and failure, numerous authors continue to advocate the use of bone graft in the management of osseous deficiency. Many complications reviewed in retrospect could have been avoided.

Overall, authors emphasize the need for meticulous preoperative planning and operative technique. To reduce failures, basic principles must be followed. For example, a vascular host bed is required for graft healing. In addition, a stable graft-host prosthesis construct is essential. A precisely contoured graft with interference fit to the host bone also is ideal. Structural allografts must be attached to the host bone with sound internal fixation techniques including screw fixation and, if necessary, plates. Long-stem components are also recommended to reduce stress on the underlying bone. Finally, protected weight bearing is required until the graft incorporates.

The use of cement for implant fixation is a matter of debate in the literature. However, if cement is used, most favor applying it to the tibial plate, not the stem or the intramedullary canal in its path.

In addition, Samuelson[215] presented the results of 22 patients with allograft and press-fit implants of the tibia. At an average of 15 months, 16 of 22 grafts showed radiographic signs of incorporation.

Revision Total Knee Arthroplasty. Bone deficiency commonly accompanies failed cemented total knee arthroplasty. Early failure associated with stable components usually results in minor bone loss. However, tibial bone loss can be particularly extensive following cemented total knee arthroplasty. Cancellous tibial metaphyseal bone as well as the peripheral cortical rim may become eroded. In revision surgery, the proximal tibia or distal femoral bone may appear to have a funnel shape due to the loss of metaphyseal bone. There may be complete erosion of the distal femur or proximal tibia. A biologic response to particulate wear debris ultimately weakens the mechanical bone between the implant and the host bone, causing aseptic component loosening and osteolysis. Component migration and collapse may further compromise underlying bone.

Also, bone remodeling under cemented or noncemented total knee replacement components is associated with a reduction in bone strength. Following implant removal, the underlying cancellous bone may be soft and easily compressed with digital pressure. In addition to bone deficiency, there may be fibrosis and contracture of the extensor mechanism. Extensile surgical approaches are required for adequate exposure. Thus, reconstruction of large bone defects in revision total knee arthroplasty can be challenging.

In massive tibial femoral bone loss, the options for management includes arthrodesis, amputation, custom prostheses, and bone allograft.

Contemporary revision knee arthroplasty components offer canal-filling stems to enhance component stability and reduce stress on the metaphysis. The implants can be augmented fixed or modular wedges to compensate for the bone loss and restore the joint line. However, with large or massive bone loss augmented components may not be sufficient. Bulk structural allografts consisting of entire proximal tibia or distal femur segments may be required for management.

Mnaymneh et al[217] evaluated 14 allograft-prosthesis constructs for severe bone loss. Extensive loss of an entire bone end was treated with distal femoral or proximal tibial segmental allograft. The average follow-up was 40 months. There was an 86% host-graft union rate.

Stockley et al[218] reported a 100% graft union rate in their series of 32 allografts used to reconstruct large bone deficits. There were 18 revision and two primary total knee arthroplasties performed in 20 knees. The bulk allografts replaced the distal femur in 12 of 16 femoral reconstructions and 11 of 16 tibial defects. While three infections occurred, they were not believed to have originated from the allograft. The average follow-up was 4.2 years.

Mow and Wiedel[199,200] reported the results the University of Colorado's experience with structural allografts for managing large bone defects in cementless revision total knee arthroplasty. There was an average follow-up of 5.6 years with a range of 2.4 to 10 years. There were 17 revisions in 16 patients. Only one tibial component loosened. In an earlier report, 13 of 15 allografts in patients with revision total knee arthroplasty showed radiographic signs of incorporation of the graft.

In addition, Tsahakis et al[219] reviewed 36 allografts in 21 revision total knee arthroplasties. There was an average follow-up of 3.5 years. All allografts incorporated or healed to host bone. No complications were reported.

Also, Whiteside[220,221] presented the results of 56 bone grafts with cementless revision total knee arthroplasty. The short-term results showed only one incident of tibial component loosening.

Furthermore, Malefijt et al[222] studied 36 patients with bone grafting and cemented total knee arthroplasty. Twenty-three patients had morcellized grafts; 22 had solid structural grafts. There was a mean follow-up of 3 years. The mean IKS clinical score was 90. In 11 of 14 cases in which morcellized graft was used, graft incorporation was seen.

A small study by Ullmark and Hovelins[201] reported the results of three cases of intramedullary impaction with morcellized bone graft for tibial deficiency. Despite these encouraging preliminary results with morcellized graft for large bone defects, Engh and others advocate that morcellized graft offers minimal support for the anticipated axial loads during weight bearing. The stability of the component is less dependent on the prosthetic stem when a structural graft is used for mechanical support.

Elia and Lotke[223] presented the results of a series of 40 revision total knee arthroplasties in 38 patients. Patients were followed for an average of 41 months with a range of 2 to 9 years; 75% of knees were considered excellent or good results. However, in this study there was a 30% complication rate, the majority of which were wound complications.

CONCLUSION

Bone loss is seen in both primary and revision total knee arthroplasty. Bone loss is associated with angular deformity in primary knees and osteolysis in revision knees. Multiple options exist for management depending on the location, severity, and extent of the bone deficiency. Selecting the most appropriate treatment option depends on numerous variables including quality of the patient's bone stock, availability of materials, and surgeon experience. With good surgical technique and adherence to basic principles, good results can be obtained.

References

1. Li S. Ultra-high-molecular-molecular weight polyethylene: the weak link. In: Lotke P, Garino J (eds). *Revision Total Knee Arthroplasty*. Philadelphia: Lippincott-Raven, 1999 43–88.
2. Ranawat C, Flynn W, Saddler S, et al. Long-term results of the total condylar knee arthroplasty. *Clin Orthop* 1993;286:94–101.
3. Ritter M, Herbst S, Keating E, et al. Long-term survival analysis of a posterior cruciate-retaining total condylar total knee arthroplasty. *Clin Orthop* 1994;309:136–145.
4. Klein N, Cox C. Wound problems in total knee arthroplasty. In: Fu F, Harner C, Vince K (eds). *Knee Surgery*. Baltimore: Williams & Wilkins, 1994:1539–1552.
5. Dennis D. Wound complications in total knee arthroplasty. *Instr Course Lect* 1997;46:165–169.
6. Scapinelli R. Studies on the vasculature of the human knee joint. *Acta Anat* 1968;70:305–331.
7. Craig S. Soft tissue considerations in the failed total knee arthroplasty. In: Scott W (ed). *The Knee*. Orlando: Mosby, 1994:1279–1295.
8. Ackland R, Shusterman M, Godine M, et al. The saphenous neurovascular free flap. *Plast Reconstr Surg* 1981;67:763–774.
9. Hallock G. Salvage of total knee arthroplasty with local fasciocutaneous flaps. *J Bone Joint Surg* 1990;72A:1236–1239.
10. Peters P. Surgical exposures for revision total knee arthroplasty. In: Engh G, Rorabeck C (eds). *Revision Total Knee Arthroplasty*. Baltimore: Williams & Wilkins, 1997:195–204.
11. Ayers D, Dennis D, Johanson N, et al. Common complications of total knee arthroplasty. *J Bone Joint Surg* 1997;79A:278–311.
12. Johnson D. Midline or parapatellar incision for knee arthroplasty. *J Bone Joint Surg* 1988;70B:656–658.
13. Rothaus K. Plastic and reconstructive surgery. In: Rand J (ed). *Total Knee Arthroplasty*. New York: Raven Press, 1993:1193–1202.
14. Adzick N. Wound healing. In: Sabiston D, Lyerly H (eds). *Textbook of Surgery*, 15th ed. Philadelphia: WB Saunders, 1997:207–220.
15. Kwiatkowski T, Hanley E, Ramp W. Cigarette smoking and its orthopaedic consequences. *Am J Orthop* 1996;25:590–597.
16. Garner R, Mowat A, Hazelman B. Wound healing after operations on patients with rheumatoid arthritis. *J Bone Joint Surg* 1973;55B:134–144.
17. Barbul A, Purtill W. Nutrition in wound healing. *Clin Dermatol* 1994;12:133–140.
18. Greene K, Wilde A, Stulberg B. Preoperative nutritional status of total joint patients. *J Arthroplasty* 1991;6:321–325.
19. LaVan F, Hunt T. Oxygen and wound healing. *Clin Plast Surg* 1990;17:463–472.
20. England S, Stern S, Insall J, et al. Total knee arthroplasty in diabetes mellitus. *Clin Orthop* 1990;260:130–134.
21. Winiarsky R, Barth P, Lotke P. Total knee arthroplasty in morbidly obese patients. *J Bone Joint Surg* 1998;80A:1770–1774.

22. Perhala R, Wilke W, Clough J, et al. Local infectious complications following large joint replacement in rheumatoid arthritis patients treated with methotrexate versus those not treated with methotrexate. *Arthritis Rheum* 1991;34:146–152.

23. Johnson D. The effect of continuous passive motion on wound healing and joint mobility after knee arthroplasty. *J Bone Joint Surg* 1990;72A:421–426.

24. Gerwin M, Rothaus K, Windsor R, et al. Gastrocnemius muscle flap coverage of exposed or infected knee prostheses. *Clin Orthop* 1993;286:64–69.

25. LaRossa D, Low D. Postoperative complications of wounds and skin necrosis. In: Lotke P, Garino J (eds). *Revision Total Knee Arthroplasty*. Philadelphia: Lippincott-Raven, 1999:447–459.

26. Nahabedian M, Orlando J, Delanois R, et al. Salvage procedures for complex soft tissue defects of the knee. *Clin Orthop* 1998;356:119–124.

27. Markovich G, Dorr L, Klein N, et al. Muscle flaps in total knee arthroplasty. *Clin Orthop* 1995;321:122–130.

28. Hemphill E, Ebert F, Muench A. The medial gastrocnemius muscle flap in the treatment of wound complications following total knee arthroplasty. *Orthopedics* 1992;15:477–480.

29. Boykin J. Hyperbaric oxygen therapy: a physiologic approach to selected problem wound healing. *Wounds* 1996;8:183–198.

30. Roth R, Weiss L. Hyperbaric oxygen and wound healing. *Clin Dermatol* 1994;12:141–156.

31. Leach R, Rees P, Wilmshurst P. Hyperbaric oxygen therapy. *Br Med J* 1998;317:1140–1143.

32. Kindwall E, Gottlieb L, Larson D. Hyperbaric oxygen therapy in plastic surgery: a review article. *Plast Reconst Surg* 1991;88:898–906.

33. Gold D, Scott S, Scott W. Soft tissue expansion prior to arthroplasty in the multiply-operated knee. *J Arthroplasty* 1996;11:512–521.

34. Santore R, Kaufman D, Robbins A, et al. Tissue expansion prior to revision total knee arthroplasty. *J Arthroplasty* 1997;12:475–478.

35. Namba R, Diao E. Tissue expansion for staged reimplantation of infected total knee arthroplasty. *J Arthroplasty* 1997;12:471–474.

36. McKenna R, Galante J, Bachmann F, et al. Prevention of venous thromboembolism after total knee replacement by high-dose aspirin or intermittent calf and thigh compression. *Br Med J* 1980;280:514–517.

37. Zimlich R, Fulbright B, Friedman R. Current status of anticoagulation therapy after total hip and total knee arthroplasty. *J Am Acad Orthop Surg* 1996;4:54–62.

38. Pellegrini V. Thromboembolic disease. *Instr Course Lect* 1997;46:185–189.

39. Lotke P, Ecker M. Deep venous thrombosis after total knee surgery. In: Rand J (ed). *Total Knee Arthroplasty*. New York: Raven Press, 1993:409–416.

40. Mosca P, Haas S. Thromboembolic disease. In: Fu F, Harner C, Vince K (eds). *Knee Surgery*. Baltimore: Williams & Wilkins, 1994:1493–1506.

41. Haas S. Postoperative complications of deep venous thrombosis. In: Lotke P, Garino J (eds). *Revision Total Knee Arthroplasty*. Philadelphia: Lippincott-Raven, 1999:437–446.

42. Leclerc J. Natural history of venous thromboembolism. In: Leclerc J (ed). *Venous Thromboembolic Disorders*. Philadelphia: Lea & Febiger, 1991:166–175.

43. Insall J, Haas S. Complications of total knee arthroplasty. In: Insall J, Windsor R, Scott W, et al (eds). *Surgery of the Knee*, 2nd ed. New York: Churchill-Livingstone, 1993:891–934.

44. Stulberg B, Insall J, Williams G, et al. Deep-vein thrombosis following total knee replacement. *J Bone Joint Surg* 1984;66A:194–201.

45. Haas S, Tribus C, Insall J, et al. The significance of calf thrombi after total knee arthroplasty. *J Bone Joint Surg* 1992;74A:799–802.

46. Maynard M, Sculco T, Ghelman B. Progression and regression of deep venous thrombosis after total knee arthroplasty. *Clin Orthop* 1991;273:125–130.

47. Cladgett G, Anderson F, Heit J, et al. Prevention of venous thromboembolism. *Chest* 1995;108(suppl):S312–S334.

48. Ansari S, Warwick D, Ackroyd C, et al. Incidence of fatal pulmonary embolism after 1,390 knee arthroplasties without routine prophylactic anticoagulation, except in high risk cases. *J Arthroplasty* 1997;12:599–602.

49. Virchow R. Nuer fall von todlicher emboli der kungerarteries. *Arch Pathol Anat* 1856;10:225.

50. Paltiel O. Epidemiology of venous thromboembolism. In: Leclerc J (ed). *Venous Thromboembolic Disorders*. Philadelphia: Lea & Febiger, 1991:166–175.

51. Neilsen P, Jorgensen L, Albrecht-Beste E, et al. Lower thrombosis risk with epidural blockade in total knee arthroplasty. *Acta Orthop Scand* 1990;61:29–31.

52. Grady-Benson J, Oishi C, Hanson P, et al. Postoperative surveillance for deep venous thrombosis with duplex ultrasonography after total knee arthroplasty. *J Bone Joint Surg* 1994;76A:1640–1657.

53. Hirsh J. Oral anticoagulant drugs. *N Engl J Med* 1991; 324:1865–1875.

54. RD Heparin Arthroplasty Group. RD heparin compared with warfarin for prevention of venous thromboembolic disease following total hip or total knee arthroplasty. *J Bone Joint Surg* 1994;76A:1174–1185.

55. Antiplatelet Trialists' Collaboration, Collaborative overview of randomised trials of antiplatelet therapy—III: reduction in venous thrombosis and pulmonary embolism by antiplatelet prophylaxis among surgical and medical patients. *Br Med J* 1994;308:235–246.

56. Clayton M, Thompson T. Activity, air boots, and aspirin as thromboembolism prophylaxis in knee arthroplasty:

a multiple regimen approach. *Orthopedics* 1987;10: 1525–1527.

57. Leclerc J, Geerts W, Desjardins L, et al. Prevention of deep vein thrombosis after major knee surgery—a randomized double blind trial comparing a low molecular weight heparin fragment (enoxaprin) to placebo. *Thromb Haemost* 1992;67:417–423.
58. Haas S, Insall J, Scuderi G, et al. Pneumatic sequential-compression boots compared with asprin prophylaxis of deep-vein thrombosis after total knee arthroplasty. *J Bone Joint Surg* 1990;72A:27–31.
59. Westrich G, Sculco T. Prophylaxis against deep venous thrombosis after total knee arthroplasty. *J Bone Joint Surg* 1996;78A:826–834.
60. Wilson N, Das S, Kakkar V, et al. Thrombo-embolic prophylaxis in total knee replacement. *J Bone Joint Surg* 1992;74B:50–54.
61. Patterson B, Marchand R, Ranawat C. Complications of heparin therapy after total joint arthroplasty. *J Bone Joint Surg* 1989;71A:1130–1134.
62. Emerson R, Cross R, Head W. Prophylactic and early therapeutic use of the Greenfield filter in hip and knee joint arthroplasty. *J Arthroplasty* 1991;6:129–135.
63. DiGioia A, Rubash H. Periprosthetic fractures of the femur after total knee arthroplasty. *Clin Orthop* 1991; 271:135–142.
64. Lewis P, Rorabeck C. Periprosthetic fractures. In: Engh G, Rorabeck C (eds). *Revision Total Knee Arthroplasty*. Baltimore: Williams & Wilkins, 1997:275–295.
65. Healy W, Schmitz M, & Siliski J. Femoral fractures above total knee arthroplasty. In: Siliski J (ed). *Traumatic Disorders of the Knee*. New York: Springer-Verlag, 1994: 409–415.
66. Sochart D, Hardinge K. Nonsurgical management of supracondylar fracture above total knee arthroplasty. *J Arthroplasty* 1997;12:830–834.
67. Merkel K, Johnson E. Supracondylar fracture of the femur after total knee arthroplasty. *J Bone Joint Surg* 1986;68A:29–43.
68. Aaron R, Scott R. Supracondylar fracture of the femur after total knee arthroplasty. *Clin Orthop* 1987;219: 136–139.
69. Ayers D. Supracondylar fracture of the distal femur proximal to a total knee replacement. *Instr Course Lect* 1997;46:197–203.
70. Chmell M, Moran M, Scott R. Periarticular fractures after total knee arthroplasty: principles of management. *J Am Acad Orthop Surg* 1996;4:109–116.
71. Culp R, Schmidt R, Hanks G, et al. Supracondylar fracture of the femur following prosthetic knee arthroplasty. *Clin Orthop* 1987;222:212–222.
72. Ritter M, Faris P, Keating M. Anterior femoral notching and ipsilateral supracondylar femur fracture in total knee arthroplasty. *J Arthroplasty* 1988;3:185–187.
73. Booth R. Supracondylar fractures: all or nothing. *Orthopedics* 1995;18:921–922.
74. Figgie M, Goldberg V, Figgie H, et al. The results of treatment of supracondylar fracture above total knee arthroplasty. *J Arthroplasty* 1990;5:267–276.
75. Chen F, Mont M, Bachner R. Management of ipsilateral supracondylar femur fractures following total knee arthroplasty. *J Arthroplasty* 1994;9:521–526.
76. Rand J. Supracondylar fracture of the femur associated with polyethylene wear after total knee arthroplasty. *J Bone Joint Surg* 1994;76A:1389–1393.
77. Neer C, Grantham S, Shelton M. Supracondylar fracture of the adult femur. *J Bone Joint Surg* 1967;49A: 591–613.
78. Jabczenski F, Crawford M. Retrograde intramedullary nailing of supracondylar femur fractures above total knee arthroplasty. *J Arthroplasty* 1995;10:95–101.
79. Murrell G, Nunley J. Interlocked supracondylar intramedullary nails for supracondylar fractures after total knee arthroplasty. *J Arthroplasty* 1995;10:37–42.
80. Rolston L, Christ D, Halpern A, et al. Treatment of supracondylar fractures of the femur proximal to a total knee arthroplasty. *J Bone Joint Surg* 1995;77A: 924–931.
81. Engh G, Ammeen D. Periprosthetic fractures adjacent to total knee implants. *J Bone Joint Surg* 1997;79A: 1100–1113.
82. Ritter M, Keating M, Faris P, et al. Rush rod fixation of supracondylar fractures above total knee arthroplasties. *J Arthroplasty* 1995;10:213–216.
83. Biswas S, Kurer M, Mackenney R. External fixation for femoral shaft fracture after Stanmore total knee replacement. *J Bone Joint Surg* 1992;74B:313–314.
84. Kraay M, Goldberg V, Figgie M, et al. Distal femoral replacement with allograft/prosthetic reconstruction for treatment of supracondylar fractures in patients with total knee arthroplasty. *J Arthroplasty* 1992;7:7–16.
85. Felix N, Stuart M, Hanssen A. Periprosthetic fractures of the tibia associated with total knee arthroplasty. *Clin Orthop* 1997;345:113–124.
86. Reis M, Richman J. Extended tibial tubercle osteotomy in total knee arthroplasty. *J Arthroplasty* 1996;11: 964–967.
87. Ritter M, Carr K, Keating M, et al. Tibial shaft fracture following tibial tubercle osteotomy. *J Arthroplasty* 1996;11:117–119.
88. Aglietti P, Windsor R, Buzzi R, et al. Arthroplasty for the stiff or anklylosed knee. *J Arthroplasty* 1989;4:1–5.
89. Papagelopoulos P, Brodersen M. Knee stiffness after reconstruction. In: Morrey B (ed). *Reconstructive Surgery of the Joints*, 2nd ed. New York: Churchill-Livingstone, 1996:1701–1710.
90. Kettlekamp D, Johs R, Schmidt G, et al. An electrogoniometric study of knee motion in normal joints. *J Bone Joint Surg* 1970;58A:754–765.

91. Lombardi A Jr, Mallory T. Dealing with flexion contractures in total knee arthroplasty. In: Insall J, Scott W, Scuderi G (eds). *Current Concepts in Primary and Revision Total Knee Arthroplasty*. Philadelphia: Lippincott-Raven, 1996:191–202.
92. Johanson N. The stiff total knee replacement: causes, treatment, and prevention. *Instr Course Lect* 1997; 46:191–195.
93. Jordan L, Olivio J. Stiffness and limitation of motion: prevention and management. In: Lotke P, Garino J (eds). *Revision Total Knee Arthroplasty*. Philadelphia: Lippincott-Raven, 1999:461–467.
94. Hofmann A, Tkach T, Evanisch C, et al. Patella component medialization in total knee arthroplasty. *J Arthroplasty* 1997;122:155–160.
95. Montgomery W, Insall J, Haas S, et al. Primary total knee arthroplasty in stiff and anklylosed knees. *Am J Knee Surg* 1998;11:20–23.
96. Anouchi Y, McShane M, Kelly F. Range of motion in total knee replacement. *Clin Orthop* 1996;331:87–92.
97. Moreland J. Mechanisms of failure in total knee arthroplasty. *Clin Orthop* 1988;226:49–64.
98. Vince K, Eissmann E. Stiff total knee arthroplasty. In: Fu F, Harner C, Vince K (eds). *Knee Surgery*. Baltimore: Williams & Wilkins, 1994:1529–1538.
99. Harwin S, Stein A, Stern R, et al. Heterotopic ossification following primary total knee arthroplasty. *J Arthroplasty* 1993;8:113–116.
100. Hepburn G. Case studies: contracture and stiff joint management with Dynasplint. *J Orthop Sports Phys Ther* 1987;8:498–504.
101. Whiteside L. Exposure in difficult total knee arthroplasty using tibial tubercle osteotomy. *Clin Orthop* 1995; 321:32–35.
102. Insall J. Surgical approaches. In: Insall J, Windsor R, Scott W, et al (eds). *Surgery of the Knee*, 2nd ed. New York: Churchill-Livingstone, 1993:135–148.
103. Barrack R. Specialized exposure for revision total knee arthroplasty: quadriceps snip and patellar turndown. *J Bone Joint Surg* 1999;881A:138–141.
104. Windsor R, Insall J. Exposure in revision total knee arthroplasty: the femoral peel. *Tech Orthop* 1988;3: 1–4.
105. Trousdale R, Hanssen A, Rand J, et al. V-Y quadricepsplasty in total knee arthroplasty. *Clin Orthop* 1993; 286:48–55.
106. Zimmerman G, Crossett L, Rubash H. Intraoperative complications of revision total knee arthroplasty. In: Lotke P, Garino J (eds). *Revision Total Knee Arthroplasty*. Philadelphia: Lippincott-Raven, 1999:411–436.
107. Mont M, Dellon L, Chen F, et al. The operative treatment of peroneal nerve palsy. *J Bone Joint Surg* 1996;78A:863–869.
108. Idusuyi O, Morrey B. Peroneal nerve palsy after total knee arthroplasty. *J Bone Joint Surg* 1996;78A: 177–184.
109. Rose H, Hood R, Otis J, et al. Peroneal-nerve palsy following total knee arthroplasty. A review of the Hospital for Special Surgery experience. *J Bone Joint Surg* 1982;64A:347–351.
110. Krackow K, Maar D, Mont M. Surgical decompression for peroneal palsy after total knee arthroplasty. *Clin Orthop* 1993;292:223–228.
111. Asp J, Rand J. Peroneal nerve palsy after total knee arthroplasty. *Clin Orthop* 1990;261:233–237.
112. Hozack W, Cole P, Gardner R, et al. Popliteal aneurysm after total knee arthroplasty: case reports and review of the literature. *J Arthroplasty* 1990;5:301–305.
113. Heck D, Blaha J, Windsor R. Knee reconstruction. In: Kasser J (ed). *Orthopaedic Knowledge Update V*. Rosemont: American Academy of Orthopaedic Surgeons, 1996:481–498.
114. Johanson N. Neurovascular complications following total knee replacement: causes, treatment, and prevention. *Instr Course Lect* 1997;46:181–184.
115. Dennis D, Neumann R, Toma P, et al. Arteriovenous fistula with false aneurysm of the inferior medial geniculate artery. *Clin Orthop* 1987;222:255–260.
116. Kumar S, Chapman J, Rawlins I. Vascular injuries in total knee arthroplasty. *J Arthroplasty* 1998;13:211–216.
117. Rand J. Neurovascular complications of total knee arthroplasty. In: Rand J (ed). *Total Knee Arthroplasty*. New York: Raven Press, 1993:417–422.
118. Rubash H, Berger R, Britton C, et al. Avoiding neurologic and vascular injuries with screw fixation of the tibial component in total knee arthroplasty. *Clin Orthop* 1993;286:56–63.
119. Hagan P, Kaufman E. Vascular complication of knee arthroplasty under tourniquet: a case report. *Clin Orthop* 1990;257:159–161.
120. Rush J, Vidovich J, Johnson M. Arterial complications of total knee replacement. *J Bone Joint Surg* 1987; 69B:400–402.
121. McAuley C, Steed D, Webster M. Arterial complications of total knee replacement. *Arch Surg* 1984;119: 960–962.
122. Abdel-Salam A, Eyres K. Effects of tourniquet during total knee arthroplasty. *J Bone Joint Surg* 1995;77B: 250–253.
123. Sculco T. Economic issues: the economic impact of infected joint arthroplasty. *Orthopedics* 1995;18:871–873.
124. Herbert C, Williams R, Levy R, et al. Cost of treating an infected total knee replacement. *Clin Orthop* 1996; 331:140–145.

125. Pellegrini V. Management of the patient with an infected knee arthroplasty. *Instr Course Lect* 1997;46:215–219.

126. Hofmann A, Kane K, Tkach T, et al. Treatment of infected total knee arthroplasty using an articulating spacer. *Clin Orthop* 1995;321:45–54.

127. Barrack R, Wolfe M. Diagnosis of the infected total knee replacement. In: Engh G, Rorabeck C (eds). *Revision Total Knee Arthroplasty*. Baltimore: Williams & Wilkins, 1997:355–370.

128. Rand J. Sepsis following total knee arthroplasty. In: Rand J (ed). *Total Knee Arthroplasty*. New York: Raven Press. 1993:349–375.

129. Hanssen A, Rand J. Evaluation and treatment of infection at the site of a total hip or knee arthroplasty. *J Bone Joint Surg* 1998;80A:910–922.

130. Osmon D, Stuckelberg J, Wilhelm M, et al. Medical management of total knee arthroplasty infection. In: Rand J (ed). *Total Knee Arthroplasty*. New York: Raven Press, 1993:377–390.

131. Windsor R, Insall J. Management of the infected total knee arthroplasty. In: Insall J, Windsor R, Scott W, et al. (eds). *Surgery of the Knee*, 2nd ed. New York: Churchill-Livingstone, 1993:959–974.

132. Ritter M. Intraoperative controls for bacterial contamination during total knee replacement. *Orthop Clin North Am* 1989;20:49–53.

133. Wilson M, Kelley K, Thornhill T. Infection as a complication of total knee arthroplasty. *J Bone Joint Surg* 1990;72A:878–883.

134. Luessenhop C, Higgins L, Brause B, et al. Multiple prosthetic infections after total joint arthroplasty: risk factor anaylsis. *J Arthroplasty* 1996;11:862–868.

135. Rodriguez J, Saddler S, Edelman S, et al. Long-term results of total knee arthroplasty in class 3 and 4 rheumatoid arthritis. *J Arthroplasty* 1996;11:141–145.

136. Fitzgerald R. Medical and surgical management of the patient with an infected total knee arthroplasty. In: Lotke P, Garino J (eds). *Revision Total Knee Arthroplasty*. Philadelphia: Lippincott-Raven, 1999:371–386.

137. Friedman R, Freidrich L, White R, et al. Antibiotic prophylaxis and tourniquet inflation in total knee arthroplasty. *Clin Orthop* 1990;260:17–23.

138. Tanzer M, Miller J, Richards G. Preoperative assessment of skin colonization and antibiotic effectiveness in total knee arthroplasty. *Clin Orthop* 1994;299:163–168.

139. Mont M, Waldman B, Banerjee C. Multiple irrigation, debridement and retention of components in infected total knee arthroplasty. *J Arthroplasty* 1997;12:426–433.

140. Windsor R, Bono J. Infected total knee replacements. *J Am Acad Orthop Surg* 1994;2:44–53.

141. Sacchetti G, Ghisellini F, Brambilla M, et al. Quantitative scintigraphic evaluation of total knee arthoplasties. *Clin Orthop* 1996;325:181–189.

142. Rand J, Brown M. The value of indium leukocyte scanning in the evaluation of painful or infected total knee arthroplasties. *Clin Orthop* 1990;259:179–182.

143. Duff G, Lachiewicz P, Kelley S. Aspiration of the knee joint before revision arthroplasty. *Clin Orthop* 1996; 331:132–139.

144. McLaren A, Spooner C. Salvage of infected total knee components. *Clin Orthop* 1996;331:146–150.

145. Petty W. Operative management of the infected knee. *Orthopedics* 1995;18:927–929.

146. Insall J, Thompson F, Brause B. Two-stage reimplantation for the salvage of infected total knee arthroplasty, *J Bone Joint Surg* 1983;65A:1087–1098.

147. Goldman R, Scuderi G, Insall J. 2-stage reimplantation for infected total knee replacement. *Clin Orthop* 1996;331:118–124.

148. Wasielewski R, Barden R, Rosenberg A. Results of different surgical procedures on total knee arthroplasty infections. *J Arthroplasty* 1996;11:931–938.

149. Booth R, Lotke P. The results of pacer block technique in revision of infected total knee arthroplasty. *Clin Orthop* 1989;248:57–60.

150. Masri B, Duncan C, Beauchamp C. The modified two stage exchange arthroplasty in the treatment of the infected total knee replacement: the Prostalac system and other articulated spacers. In: Engh G, Rorabeck C, (eds). *Revision Total Knee Arthroplasty*. Baltimore: Williams & Wilkins, 1997:394–424.

151. Dajani A, Bisno A, Chung K, et al. Prevention of bacterial endocarditis: recommendations by the American Heart Association. *JAMA* 1990;264:219–222.

152. Dennis D. Extensor mechanism problems in total knee arthroplasty. *Instr Course Lect* 1997;49:171–180.

153. Rand J. The patellofemoral joint in total knee arthroplasty. *J Bone Joint Surg* 1994;76:612–620.

154. Hozack W. Patellar complications related to tracking. In: Fu F, Harner C, Vince K (eds). *Knee Surgery*. Baltimore: Williams & Wilkins, 1994:1459–1472.

155. Kolessar D, Rand J. Extensor mechanism problems following total knee arthroplasty. In: Morrey B (ed). *Reconstructive Surgery of the Joints*, 2nd ed. New York: Churchill-Livingstone, 1996:1533–1547.

156. Rand J. The patellofemoral joint in total knee arthroplasty. *J Bone Joint Surg* 1994;76A:612–620.

157. Cameron H, Fedorkow D. The patella in total knee arthroplasty. *Clin Orthop* 1982;165:197–199.

158. Lynch A, Rorabeck C, Bourne R. Extensor mechanism complications following total knee arthroplasty. *J Arthroplasty* 1987;2:135–140.

159. Cadambi A, Schmidt R. The extensor mechanism in revision total knee arthroplasty. In: Engh G, Rorabeck C (eds). *Revision Total Knee Arthroplasty*. Baltimore: Williams & Wilkins, 1997:205–223.

160. Reuben J, McDonald C, Woodard P, et al. Effect of

patella thickness on patella strain following total knee arthroplasty. *J Arthroplasty* 1991;6:251–258.

161. Evanich C, Tkach T, Von Glinski S, et al. 6- to 10-year experience using countersunk metal-backed patellas. *J Arthroplasty* 1997;12:149–154.

162. Yoshii I, Whiteside I, Anouchi Y. The effect of patella button placement and femoral component design on patella tracking in total knee arthroplasty. *Clin Orthop* 1992;275:214–219.

163. Kewonowski K, Dorr L, McPherson E, et al. Medialization of the patella in total knee arthroplasty. *J Arthroplasty* 1997;12:161–167.

164. Johnson D, Eastwood D. Lateral patellar release in knee arthroplasty. *J Arthroplasty* 1992;7(suppl):427–431.

165. Scuderi G, Scharf S, Meltzer L, et al. The relationship of lateral releases to patella viability in total knee arthroplasty. *J Arthroplasty* 1987;2:209–214.

166. Rand J, Morrey B, Bryan R. Patella tendon rupture after total knee arthroplasty. *Clin Orthop* 1989;244: 233–237.

167. James D, Scott R. Extensor mechanism complications. In: Rand J (ed). *Total Knee Arthroplasty*. New York: Raven Press, 1993:393–401.

168. Emerson R. Extensor mechanism rupture. In: Fu F, Harner C, Vince K (eds). *Knee Surgery*. Baltimore: Williams & Wilkins, 1994:1483–1490.

169. Emerson R, Head W, Malinin T. Reconstruction of patella tendon rupture after total knee arthroplasty with an extensor mechanism allograft. *Clin Orthop* 1990; 260:154–161.

170. Cadambi A, Engh G. Use of a semitendinosis tendon autogenous graft for rupture of the patellar ligament after total knee arthroplasty. *J Bone Joint Surg* 1992; 74:974–979.

171. Jaureguito J, Dubois C, Smith S, et al. Medial gastrocnemius transposition flap for the treatment of disruption of the extensor mechanism after total knee arthroplasty. *J Bone Joint Surg* 1977;79:866–873.

172. Kraay M, Goldberg V. Patellar fracture and breakage. In: Fu F, Harner C, Vince K (eds). *Knee Surgery*. Baltimore: Williams & Wilkins, 1994:1473–1482.

173. Tria A, Harwood D, Alicea J, et al. Patella fractures in posterior stabilized knee arthroplasties. *Clin Orthop* 1994;299:131–138.

174. Markel D, Luessenhop C, Windsor R, et al. Arthroscopic treatment of peripatellar fibrosis after total knee arthroplasty. *J Arthroplasty* 1996;11:293–297.

175. Thorpe C, Bocell J, Tullos H. Intra-articular fibrous bands. *J Bone Joint Surg* 1990;72A:811–814.

176. Beight J, Yao B, Hozack W, et al. The patella "clunk" syndrome after posterior stabilized total knee arthroplasty. *Clin Orthop* 1994;299:139–142.

177. Bocell J, Thorpe C, Tullos H. Arthroscopic treatment of symptomatic total knee arthroplasty. *Clin Orthop* 1991;271:125–134.

178. Rosenberg A, Andriacchi T, Barden R, et al. Patella component failure in cementless total knee arthroplasty. *Clin Orthop* 1988;226:106–114.

179. Rosenberg A. Management of the failed metal-backed patella. *Orthopedics* 1996;19:813–815.

180. Bayley J, Scott R. Further observations on metal-backed patella component failure. *Clin Orthop* 1986;236:88–105.

181. Bayley J, Scott R. Further observations on metal-backed patellar component failure. *Clin Orthop* 1988;286: 82–87.

182. Stulberg S, Stulberg B, Hamati Y, et al. Failure mechanisms of metal-backed patella components. *Clin Orthop* 1988;236:88–105.

183. Berry D, Rand J. Isolated patella component revision of total knee arthroplasty. *Clin Orthop* 1988;236:82–87.

184. Goldstein S, Coale E, Weiss A, et al. Patella surface strain. *J Orthop Results* 1986;4:372–377.

185. Bloebaum R, Bachus K, Jenson J, et al. Porous-coated metal-backed patella components in total knee replacement. *J Bone Joint Surg* 1998;80A:518–528.

186. Engh G, Dwyer K. Mechanical failure: implant breakage and loosening. In: Fu F, Harner C, Vince K (eds). *Knee Surgery*. Baltimore: Williams & Wilkins, 1994:1507–1527.

187. Faris P. Soft tissue balancing and total knee arthroplasty. In: Fu F, Harner C, Vince K (eds). *Knee Surgery*. Baltimore: Williams & Wilkins, 1994:1385–1389.

188. Ayers D. Polyethylene wear and osteolysis following total knee replacement. *Instr Course Lect* 1997;46:205–213.

189. Hungerford D. Alignment in total knee replacement. *Instr Course Lect* 1996;45:455–468.

190. Hungerford D, Mont M. The issue of ligament balance in revision total knee replacement. In: Lotke P, Garino J (eds). *Revision Total Knee Arthroplasty*. Philadelphia: Lippincott-Raven, 1999:77–87.

191. Bartel D. The effect of design on long term survivorship. In: Lotke P, Garino J (eds). *Revision Total Knee Arthroplasty*. Philadelphia: Lippincott-Raven, 1999: 17–29.

192. Garino J. Successes and failures. In: Lotke P, Garino J (eds). *Revision Total Knee Arthroplasty*. Philadelphia: Lippincott-Raven, 1999:3–14.

193. Dorr L. Management of bone defects. In: Rand J (ed). *Total Knee Arthroplasty*. New York: Raven Press, 1993:309–317.

194. Dorr L, Ranawat C, Sculco T, et al. Bone graft for tibial defects in total knee arthroplasty. *J Bone Joint Surg* 1977;79A:1030–1039.

195. Morrey B. Bone deficiency. In: Morrey B (ed). *Reconstructive Surgery of the Joints*, 2nd ed. New York: Churchill-Livingstone, 1996:1569–1585.

196. Engh G, Parks N. The management of bone defects in

revision total knee arthroplasty. *Instr Course Lect* 1997;46:227–236.

197. Laskin R, Saddler S. Bone defects in total knee arthroplasty. In: Fu F, Harner C, Vince K (eds). *Knee Surgery*. Baltimore: Williams & Wilkins, 1994:1399–1405.

198. Rand J. Bone deficiency in total knee arthroplasty: use of metal wedge augmentation. *Clin Orthop* 1991:271; 63–71.

199. Mow C, Wiedel J. Structural allografting in revision total knee arthroplasty. *J Arthroplasty* 1996;11:236–241.

200. Mow C, Wiedel J. Noncemented revision total knee arthroplasty. *Clin Orthop* 1994;309:110–115.

201. Ullmark G, Hovelius L. Impacted morsellized allografts and cement for revision total knee arthroplasty. *Acta Orthop Scand* 1996;67:10–12.

202. Cameron H, Turner D, Cameron G. Results of bone grafting in tibial defects in uncemented total knee replacements. *Can J Surg* 1988;31:30–32.

203. Aglietti P, Buzzi R, Srobe F. Autologous bone grafting for medial tibial defects in total knee arthroplasty. *J Arthroplasty* 1991;6:287–294.

204. Ghazavi M, Stockley I, Yee G, et al. Reconstruction of massive bone defects with allografts in revision total knee arthroplasty. *J Bone Joint Surg* 1977;79A:17–25.

205. Harris A, Poddar S, Gitelis S, et al. Arthroplasty with a composite of an allograft and a prosthesis with severe deficiency of bone. *J Bone Joint Surg* 1995;77A: 373–386.

206. Kraay M, Goldberg V, Figgie M, et al. Distal femoral replacement with allograft/prosthetic reconstruction for treatment of supracondylar fractures in patients with total knee arthroplasty. *J Arthroplasty* 1992;7:7–16.

207. Altchek D, Sculco T, Rawlins B. Autogenous bone grafting for severe angular deformity in total knee arthroplasty. *J Arthroplasty* 1989;4:151–155.

208. Hill R, Phillips H. Bone grafting in primary total knee arthroplasty. *J Arthroplasty* 1992;7:81–86.

209. Laskin R. Total knee arthroplasty in the presence of large bone defects of the tibia and modified knee instability. *Clin Orthop* 1989;248:66–70.

210. Windsor R, Insall J, Sculco T. Bone grafting of tibial defects in primary and revision total knee arthroplasty. *Clin Orthop* 1986;205:132–137.

211. Wilde A, Schickendantz M, Stulberg B, et al. The incorporation of tibial allografts in total knee arthroplasty. *J Bone Joint Arthroplasty* 1990;72:815–824.

212. Insall JN. Total knee replacement. In: Insall J (ed). *Surgery of the Knee*. New York: Churchill-Livingstone, 1984:587.

213. Dennis D. Structural allografting in revision total knee arthroplasty. *Orthopedics* 1994;17:849–851.

214. Rosenberg A. The use of bone graft for managing bone defects in complex total knee arthroplasty. *Am J Knee Surg* 1977;10:42–48.

215. Samuelson K. Bone grafting and noncemented revision arthroplasty of the knee. *Clin Orthop* 1988;226:93–101.

216. Engh G, Herzwurn P, Parks N. Treatment of major defects of bone with bulk allografts and stemmed components during total knee arthroplasty. *J Bone Joint Surg* 1977;79A:1030–1039.

217. Mnaymneh W, Emerson R, Borja F, et al. Massive allografts in salvage revisions of failed total knee arthroplasties. *Clin Orthop* 1990;260:144–153.

218. Stockley I, McAuley J, Gross. Allograft reconstruction in total knee arthroplasty. *J Bone Joint Surg* 1992; 74B:393–397.

219. Tsahakis P, Beaver W, Brick G. Technique and results of allograft reconstruction in revision total knee arthroplasty. *Clin Orthop* 1994;303:86–94.

220. Whiteside L. Cementless reconstution of massive tibial bone loss in revision total knee replacement. *Clin Orthop* 1989;248:80–86.

221. Whiteside L. Cementless revision total knee arthroplasty. *Clin Orthop* 1993;286:160–167.

222. Malefijt M, Van Kampen A, Slooff T. Bone grafting in cemented knee replacement. *Acta Orthop Scand* 1995;66:325–328.

223. Elia E, Lotke P. Results of revision total knee arthroplasty associated with significant bone loss. *Clin Orthop* 1991;271:114–121.

Chapter 24

HETEROTOPIC OSSIFICATION FOLLOWING TOTAL KNEE ARTHROPLASTY

Vincent D. Pellegrini, Jr.

In contrast to the well-known association with total hip arthroplasty, heterotopic ossification (HO) following total knee replacement has largely been regarded as a coincidental radiographic curiosity of little clinical importance. While rarely impuned as responsible for any compromise in the functional result of prosthetic knee arthroplasty, there have been isolated case reports of such dramatic magnitude as to attract the attention of the knee surgeon. In its most florid form bony ankylosis may result; inflammation and ossification within the suprapatellar extensor mechanism is a more frequent sequela of lesser degrees of involvement. Notwithstanding these noteworthy reports, the true clinical significance of ectopic bone formation about the knee following prosthetic arthroplasty remains to be defined.

THE CLINICAL PROBLEM

Unlike after total hip arthroplasty, heterotopic bone formation following total knee arthroplasty (TKA) is an infrequent and poorly defined event. Case reports of questionable clinical significance populated the early literature on the subject. In 1973 Freeman[1] noted a case of ectopic calcification following cemented primary TKA in a patient with a previously ankylosed knee. Engelbrecht et al[2] in 1976 and Booth and King[3] in 1979 then each reported two cases of myositis ossificans that occurred following constrained and tricompartmental primary TKA, respectively. McClelland and Rudolf[4] in 1986 added a case of myositis ossificans that occurred following porous ingrowth primary TKA. Two years later Scott et al[5] noted HO in a patient with severe osteoarthritis and a preoperative range of motion of only 30 degrees. More recently, symptoms related to snapping of the extensor mechanism over a prominent mass of ectopic bone on the anterior femur and painful stiffness associated with a defined mass of HO within the quadriceps tendon have been reported to be amenable to surgical resection of the offending bone.

Notwithstanding these sporadic examples of clinically meaningful HO following TKA, radiographic surveys provide the best approximation of the magnitude of the problem. In a purely radiographic study, Lovelock and colleagues[6] in 1984 reviewed roentgenograms from 224 TKAs performed over a 6-year period in a population with a diagnosis of osteoarthritis in 66% and with Spherocentric (Howmedica, Rutherford, NJ) components implanted in 60% of knees. They noted some degree of HO in 22 knees (10%); in 18 only a few bony fragments were observed in the soft tissues as an incidental radiographic finding. Of the four knees with moderate HO, two involved the quadriceps mechanism and were felt to be associated with painful limitation of motion, although no surgical treatment was undertaken. They noted an additional 5 patients (2%) with aseptic periostitis about the distal femur of uncertain clinical significance and concluded that severe HO does not occur following TKA.

Subsequently HO after TKA has been the subject of five clinical series in which radiographic appearance was correlated with functional outcome.[7–11] A total of 1,058 TKA were reviewed in these studies with a 14% (149 of 1,058 knees) overall radiographic prevalence of HO, ranging from 3.8% to 42% in the individual series. Each report proposed a different classification scheme, precluding aggregate analysis of radiographic severity of HO, but a total of only 5 (0.5%) patients offered symptomatic complaints that were attributed to the HO by the respective authors. If the radiographic series of Lovelock is included, an overall prevalence for HO of 13.3% (171 of 1,282 knees) has been observed following TKA, with less than 0.5% (7 of 1,282 knees) producing symptoms of pain, snapping of the extensor mechanism, or stiffness. Of these seven symptomatic knees, two (0.2%) underwent reoperation for removal of a bothersome mass of heterotopic bone.

As a more sensitive measure of the effect of HO on the functional performance of TKA, objective assessment of the postoperative range of motion has been correlated with the radiographic appearance of HO.[9,11] A statistically significant reduction of 14 degrees, compared with a loss of 3 degrees in control knees, from preoperative to postoperative flexion range was observed in association with HO measuring greater than 5 cm in length within the extensor mechanism.[9] This resulted in mean maximum flexion of 92 degrees in the 8% of knees with grade B HO compared with maximum flexion of 104 degrees in knees without such extensive HO. Furthermore, such a loss of postoperative flexion of 12 degrees was felt to represent a clinically meaningful compromise in knee function. Unlike the *extent* or *grade* of HO, whether the HO was attached to the anterior femur or free-floating in the soft tissues of the extensor mechanism (*class*) had no influence on final knee flexion. Therefore, the extent of HO, as assessed by radiographic grade, was a better predictor of follow-up range of motion than the location of HO, as assessed by radiographic class. In another series, Anapolle and Stuchin[11] observed a 5.9-degree improvement in postoperative range of motion in patients without HO compared with a 4.3-degree loss in patients with any radiographic evidence of HO following TKA.

The most significant implication is that HO may act as a marker for an abnormality of soft tissue maturation. Limitation of knee flexion in the more severely involved knees may possibly result from direct interference with the extensor mechanism by the bulk of the HO. Alternatively, it is more likely that HO is only a local manifestation of a systemic predisposition for fibrosis and joint stiffness following surgical insult. Biochemical and histologic studies have highlighted differences in osteoblasts derived from heterotopic bone. In culture, HO-derived osteoblasts produced three times as much osteoid as similar cells from age-matched controls; this observation may reflect a generalized metabolic hyperactivity of the cell populations associated with this tissue.[12] Similarly, it is plausible that HO is mechanistically related to the condition of arthrofibrosis as observed most commonly following acute knee injury or reconstruction of the anterior cruciate ligament. As such, the appearance of HO following TKA may herald a compromised range of motion based on a pathologically aggressive healing response of the pericapsular tissues to operative trauma about the knee. Better identification of the population at risk may allow preoperative pharmacologic intervention directed at modifying the healing response in these patients.

CLINICAL PRESENTATION

Prior to the appearance of radiographic signs of bone formation needed to establish the diagnosis of HO, the patient with this condition following TKA is indistinguishable from a much larger group of patients who struggle through a stormy early postoperative course. Most unfortunately, these radiographic hallmarks of the condition are not apparent on plain x-rays for 6 to 8 weeks following operation. Once mechanical causes of restricted range of motion are ruled out, such as flexion-extension gap imbalance or an overstuffed patellofemoral joint, the challenge to the surgeon is to distinguish the largely benign condition of HO from others with a much poorer prognosis that require prompt therapeutic intervention.

The clinical presentation is one of a painful, warm, swollen, and often visibly inflamed and erythematous knee. Physical therapy progresses slowly and the early gains in range of motion quickly disappear to leave an unsatisfactory arc during the first few months. The differential diagnosis at this time includes an ominous list of dreaded complications, most noteworthy of which are deep infection and reflex sympathetic dystrophy (RSD). A painfree arc usually exists, albeit less than expected by both patient and surgeon, which helps to differentiate this condition from the septic prosthetic joint. The sedimentation rate is usually normal in the setting of HO but may be elevated in its acute inflammatory phase. Should concerns over the diagnosis remain, the joint must be aspirated to rule out deep sepsis. RSD is less readily distinguished from the patient with HO in the early inflammatory phase. Both conditions are marked by pain out of proportion to the physical examination and signs of sympathetic overflow and inflammation may appear indistinguishable. A diagnostic and therapeutic trial of a lumbar sympathetic blockade may be helpful but is infrequently pursued at this early stage postoperatively. Tricyclic antidepressants and related agents with efficacy in the setting of neurogenic pain assist the RSD patient, while nonsteroidal antiinflammatory agents ameliorate the symptoms of HO. However, neither class of drugs has therapeutic specificity to allow a definitive diagnosis to be made until the surgeon and patient have both suffered through a seeming eternity of 6 to 8 weeks until the radiographic appearance of the typical ossification pattern on the routine postoperative films (Fig. 24.1).

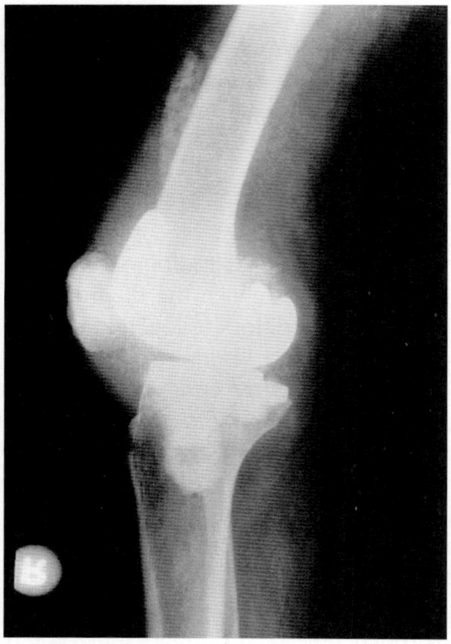

Figure 24.1. Two-month postoperative radiograph of a patient following total knee arthroplasty who manifests pain, swelling, erythema, and stiffness in her early postoperative course. Aspiration of the knee to rule out infection produced clear sterile fluid. At 1 year postoperatively she had a range of 10 to 90 degrees and was pain free and independent of assistive devices for ambulation.

After the radiographic diagnosis of HO is made, empirical continuation of nonsteroidal antiinflammatory agents is appropriate and assists in controlling symptoms. The impact of such a regimen on the ultimate radiographic or functional outcome, however, has not been determined in any clinical trial and remains a matter of conjecture. Symptoms usually abate over the first 3 months and range of motion will again improve, provided the regimen of physical therapy is followed for 6 to 12 months. The final range of motion is less than that observed after otherwise uncomplicated TKA and takes longer to obtain, but most patients will enjoy a 90-degree arc with modest functional limitation. As already mentioned, the rare patient will experience persistent symptoms of pain, tenderness, or snapping of the extensor mechanism referable to a mass of ectopic bone inconveniently located on the anterior surface of the distal femur. Even fewer will require resection of the mass to control symptoms.

RADIOGRAPHIC ASSESSMENT

The radiographic diagnosis of HO is one with little ambiguity after the appearance of progressive calcifications within the soft tissues or sessile bony outgrowths from the femur or tibia on the postoperative x-rays. While bony excrescences have been noted on all surfaces of the femur and tibia, the location most closely associated with symptomatic ossification or restriction of motion is the anterior surface of the distal femur. Several authors have proposed radiographic classification systems for assessment of the severity of HO following knee arthroplasty. If the value of any classification schema lies in its ability to predict clinical outcome and direct subsequent intervention, that of Furia and Pellegrini[9] is of greatest utility. Based on the relationship of the ossified mass to the surface of the distal femur (class) and the extent of ossification (grade), this system has been shown to correlate closely with both postoperative range of motion and subjective patient complaints.

Heterotopic ossification is first sought on the 6-week postoperative and all subsequent anteroposterior and lateral radiographs. HO is identified as bone islands or spurs most readily seen on the lateral radiograph. Findings consistent with HO must progress in size and/or mineralization on postoperative radiographs to be considered ectopic bone formation, as distinguished from static postsurgical changes or ossification residual from a previous operation. Class I consists of islands of bone localized to the extensor mechanism and suprapatellar soft tissue areas of the distal femur (Fig. 24.2). Class II bone is organized into sessile areas of ossification contiguous with the anterior surface of the distal femur (Fig. 24.3). The two grades of HO are defined based on the size of the largest segment of bone: grade A <5 cm and grade B ≥5 cm (Figs. 24.4 and 24.5). Five centimeters was empirically chosen as the transition point

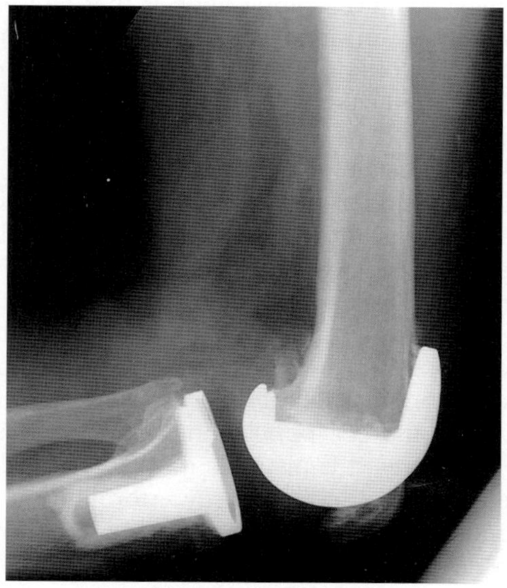

Figure 24.2. Lateral radiograph of class I grade A heterotopic ossification in the suprapatellar soft tissues anterior to the distal femur.

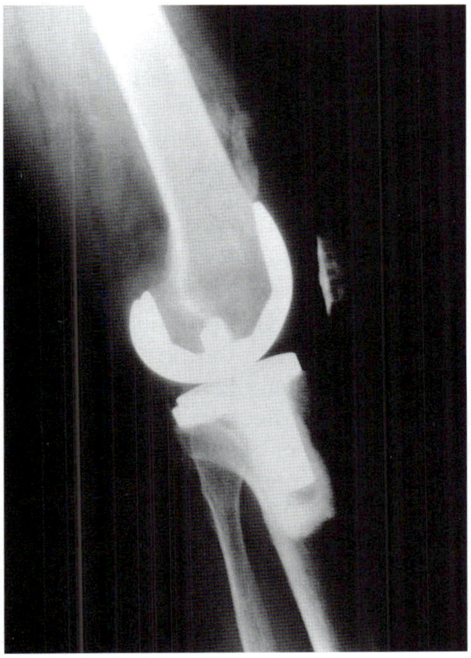

Figure 24.3. Lateral radiograph of class II grade A heterotopic ossification contiguous with the anterior surface of the distal femur.

between grades because of a naturally occuring split at this value separating knees with normal from those with restricted range of motion. The extent of ossification, or grade, was most closely associated with decreased functional outcome of the knee arthroplasty.[9]

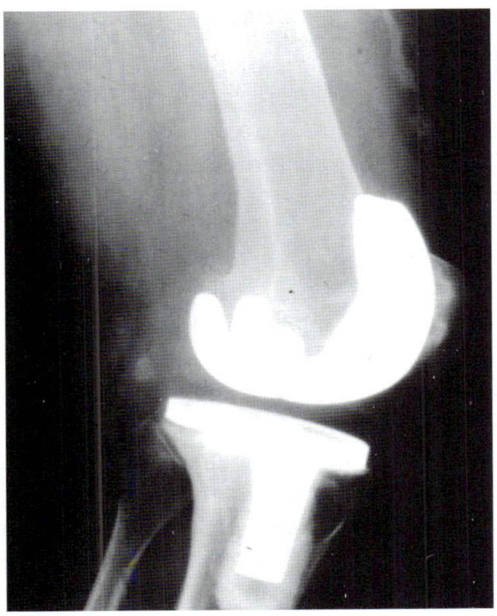

Figure 24.4. Lateral radiograph of class I grade B heterotopic ossification in the suprapatellar soft tissues measuring 5 cm in length.

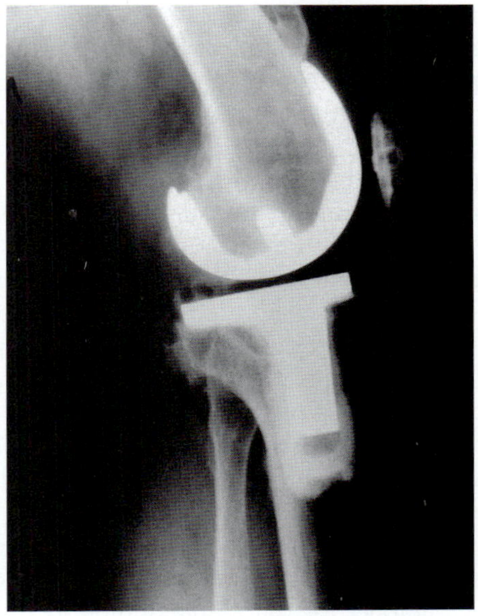

Figure 24.5. Lateral radiograph of class II grade B heterotopic ossification with a segment of ectopic bone attached to the anterior femur greater than 5 cm in length

PATHOPHYSIOLOGY

Owing to the greater prevalence of HO complicating surgery about the hip, much of the basic science investigation on this subject has utilized either a hip surgery or long-bone fracture model. Nonetheless, with the notable difference that the knee is endowed with a less abundant muscle envelope than the hip, the biologic mechanisms operative about the hip are equally applicable to the knee.[13]

The cellular mechanisms of HO remain unclear. Essential to this issue is the question of anatomic origin of the pluripotential mesenchymal cells participating in the process of bone formation within the soft tissues. Transformation of local cells into bone-producing elements has been proposed by many investigators.[14–19] Geschickter and Maseritz[15] hypothesized that trauma to muscle leads to hemorrhage, muscle degeneration, and proliferation of perivascular connective tissue, and finally culminates in the production of heterotopic bone. Studies in an animal model using ^{3}H-labeled thymidine and uridine demonstrated that local soft tissue fibroblasts adjacent to an implanted demineralized bone fragment were induced to transform into pluripotential mesenchymal cells that differentiated into osteoblasts.[20] Pluripotential mesenchymal cells are ubiquitous in the soft tissues and periosteum, and it is postulated that these cell lines may be induced to undergo atypical differentiation into osteogenic stem cells capable of participating in the process of HO. Maturation of these cells down either osteoblastic or chondroblastic stem cell lines could then lead to the formation of detectable heterotopic bone. However, to date a specific initiating agent and local tissue factors have not been identified in the local regional milieu following operative trauma.

Alternatively, other authors have postulated that distant migratory hematopoietic stem cells may be essential to inducing local connective tissue elements to form heterotopic bone.[14,15,21] Pluripotential mesenchymal cells and osteocytes are liberated from the marrow space of neighboring bones during arthroplasty surgery and are likely present in the local hematoma. They may contribute to the process of HO either by direct bone formation or indirectly via stimulation of local cells to express osteogenic phenotypes. Distant hematopoietic stem cells transported to the wound by virtue of the normal inflammatory response to surgical injury also possess the capability to mature along osteogenic cell lines under the influence of mitogenic stimuli in the wound environment.

In 1975 Chalmers and associates[14] postulated that three requisite conditions must be met to allow heterotopic bone formation: (1) the presence of an inducing agent, (2) an osteogenic precursor cell, and (3) an environment conducive to osteogenesis. Relative to the stimulatory agent, Urist and colleagues[22–24] have isolated a bone-inducing factor that they have used to reproduce the process of HO in a laboratory animal model. Puzas and associates[12,25] have reported that "bone dust" recovered from patients who formed heterotopic bone stimulated the proliferation of isolated bone progenitor cells in culture sixfold that of similar material extracted from patients who did not form heterotopic bone. The exact mechanism of this stimulation appears to be related to an exceptionally high level of detectable growth factors in the heterotopic bone matrix and remains under investigation.[26] Similarly attesting to the metabolic hyperactivity of this tissue, histomorphometric and biochemical data have demonstrated heterotopic bone to contain more than twice the number of active osteoclasts and to have a rate of appositional new bone formation nearly three times that of normal age-matched bone.[25] A stimulatory protein, isolated in greater amounts from heterotopic bone than normal control bone, has been shown to induce both osteoprogenitor cell proliferation and collagen synthesis.

Regardless of the site of origin of these pluripotential mesenchymal cells, HO would seem to be clearly dependent on cellular differentiation down osteoprogenitor cell lines. Likewise, ionizing radiation is known to exert its greatest influence on rapidly dividing cells by interfering with the normal production of nuclear deoxyribonucleic acid (DNA).[21,27,28] Tonna and Cronkite[19] have demonstrated in mice that differentiation of pluripotential mesenchymal cells into osteoblasts began 16 hours following fracture of the femur and peaked at approximately 32 hours postinjury. In their model the critical events of cellular differentiation occurred in the immediate postoperative period. A similar chronology may be extrapolated to the sequence of HO, even though the actual heterotopic bone is not detectable radiographically for several weeks following operation. Therefore, to be most effective, it would seem essential that irradiation or other intended prophylactic agents be administered early enough in the postoperative period to prevent osteoblastic differentiation of pluripotential mesenchymal stem cells, effectively arresting osteoid and subsequent heterotopic bone formation in the initial phases of cellular reorganization.

Further analysis of the clinical data concerning radiation prophylaxis is instructive. Both limited field portals and radiation administered preoperatively have been shown to be as effective as conventional postoperative expanded field irradiation in preventing heterotopic bone formation about the hip. These clinical results imply that the source of the osteoprogenitor cells is the local operative environment rather than a distant source providing cells via a chemotactic attraction to the surgical wound. The responsible cells would then logically be present in the immediate operative field at the time of operation in order to be modified by a restricted field radiation beam applied prior to the time of surgical trauma. This hypothesis would seem to lend itself nicely to the situation of HO about the knee. In this setting there is a sparse muscle envelope and the preponderance of heterotopic bone forms in close association with the anterior cortex of the distal femur or the immediately adjacent soft tissues of the extensor mechanism. A rational, yet scientifically unproven, assumption would be that the responsible osteoprogenitor cells reside in the periosteal tissues of the distal femur and are liberated during operative exposure and preparation of this region during TKA.

RISK FACTORS AND PROPHYLAXIS

Heterotopic ossification has been associated with numerous conditions including hip surgery,[29–50] spinal cord trauma,[51,52] burns,[53] head injury,[54] and fractures.[55,56] Most common after total hip arthroplasty (THA), HO is now also recognized to occur after knee,[1,3–5,57] shoulder,[58] and elbow arthroplasty. In comparison to the figures presented for knee replacement, the radiographic prevalence of HO following primary THA has been reported to be between 8% and 90%, and is clinically significant in 5% to 10% of cases where extensive heterotopic bone formation will cause pain and result in a diminished range of motion, which may negate the anticipated functional benefits of the operation.[17,29–50,59–63] Risk factors following surgery about the hip have included male gender,[42,46,64] previous HO,[34,45,46,64] diffuse idiopathic skeletal hyperostosis,[35,65] ankylosing spondylitis,[31,49] and hypertrophic osteoarthritis. The combination of such an overwhelming frequency of HO after hip surgery, well-established risk factors, and the severe functional compromise that may ensue have resulted in well-defined guidelines for the application of either external beam irradiation or nonsteroidal antiinflammatory agents as methods of prophylaxis following THA in high-risk patients.

In contrast, neither risk factors nor recommendations for prophylaxis are clearly defined as they relate to HO following TKA, owing largely to the less severe consequences of HO after knee replacement compared with hip arthroplasty and the relatively recent appreciation of the condition after TKA. Clearly defined risk factors include hypertrophic osteoarthritis with tricompartmental disease and prominent osteophytes, especially on the lateral view of the patella, measuring 2 cm or more in length.[9] Posttraumatic arthritis and a fixed combined biplanar deformity of the knee greater than 15 degrees are significantly associated with development of HO, albeit without compromise in clinical function.[7] Notably, the same authors observed no increase in risk of HO with soft tissue release for even a severe single-plane fixed deformity about the knee. Previous HO, of either the contralateral knee or about another joint, is associated with greater risk of HO after TKA, attesting to the systemic nature of the diathesis for this process. In one series, eight of 11 patients (73%) with preexisting heterotopic bone at other sites developed HO in the index knee following primary TKA.[9] Finally, in the rare instance of takedown of a knee arthrodesis with conversion to TKA, analagous to the similar situation about the hip, prophylactic irradiation has been useful in discouraging recurrent ossification and ankylosis across the new prosthetic knee joint.

A systemic diathesis for this condition is further supported by the finding that elevated mean lumbar spine bone mineral density (BMD) predicted formation of HO in patients undergoing TKA.[9] One-way analysis of variance (ANOVA) demonstrated a significant elevation of the lumbar BMD in the region of vertebrae two through four in patients with HO after TKA compared to age-, gender-, weight-, and height-matched controls ($p < .01$). For all patients with HO, mean BMD at each individual level from the first to the fourth lumbar vertebrae was also significantly elevated compared to the control group. Furthermore, for all patients with HO mean lumbar spine BMD was significantly elevated compared with a matched control group of patients undergoing TKA but not forming HO ($p < .05$). HO following primary TKA correlates with limitation of postoperative knee flexion and was predicted by increased lumbar BMD. Preoperative assessment of spinal BMD may identify those patients at risk for HO and provide a quantitative measure for institution of preoperative prophylaxis and modification of postoperative rehabilitation to optimize functional outcome following TKA in these patients.

At-risk situations for HO peculiar to the knee include extensive dissection and injury to the periosteum and soft tissues anterior to the knee as well as anterior cortical notching of the femur. While both cementless application of the femoral component and use of methylmethacrylate have been implicated as factors, there is no convincing evidence to reliably support either claim as a risk factor for HO.[11,66,67] On the other hand, manipulation of the knee for poor recovery of range of motion following prosthetic replacement has been strongly associated with not only occurrence of HO but also with functional compromise attributable to stiffness and a mass effect from the ectopic ossification. Daluga et al[68] specifically investigated the outcome of manipulation following TKA and noted HO in 17 of 60 patients (28%) whose knees were manipulated. Despite this association, in their series HO affected neither the final range of motion nor the Hospital for Special Surgery (HSS) knee score, and was regarded as an incidental radiographic finding. However, numerous other anecdotal reports of HO following manipulation of the prosthetic knee provide strong circumstantial evidence for the association of clinically significant HO in this setting.[7,8,66,69]

CONCLUSION

Numerous factors influence postoperative function and range of motion following TKA, including preoperative range of motion, component alignment, change in position of the joint line, posterior cruciate retention or sacrifice, knee laxity, the type of prosthesis, surgical technique, and the systemic predisposition of the patient.[57,70–77] Given the variability of pathologic anatomy about the knee and operative approaches to its treatment, it is impossible to control all of these clinical variables for a rigid scientific analysis. Nonetheless, there is considerable evidence to establish a relationship between the occurrence of heterotopic ossification and compromise in function of the knee following total joint replacement.

As is true following total hip arthroplasty, HO following TKA is manifest by restricted joint motion, as well as pain in the early inflammatory phase, compromising an otherwise technically successful operation. Clinically, this presentation in the early postoperative period must be distinguished from a similar constellation of signs and symptoms associated with RSD as well as deep infection. The diagnosis is easily made after the radiographic appearance of ossification in the soft tissues anterior to, or contiguous with, the distal femur on the lateral radiograph. The Brooker classification of HO following total hip arthroplasty is well accepted, and is based on the location and severity of the ectopic ossification.[32] A comparable scheme for HO following TKA has noted that the extent or size of the focus of HO (grade) is more predictive of final knee flexion than is the location (class) of the ectopic ossification.[9] Despite more profound stiffness in the first few months following operation, continued diligence in physical therapy most often results in a range of motion 10 to 15 degrees less than observed in unaffected knees after a more protracted period of 6 to 12 months postoperatively.

Identification of the at-risk population holds the potential for preemptive intervention in mitigating the effects of HO after knee arthroplasty.[78,79] While routine screening for elevated BMD may not be cost-effective, in patients with preexisting HO, hypertrophic osteoarthritis, or severe fixed biplanar deformity about the knee, preoperative measurement of BMD may be an effective method for quantitatively assessing this at-risk population. In this subset of patients, some form of HO prophylaxis may be indicated and a more prolonged course of postoperative rehabilitation, aided by pharmacologic or radiation-induced modification of the healing response, may ultimately prove to be beneficial in achieving maximum range of motion and optimizing functional outcome following TKA. The practical benefit of these theoretically rational interventions remains to be proven in controlled clinical trials.

References

1. Freeman PA. Walldius arthroplasty. A review of 80 cases. *Clin Orthop Rel Res* 1973;94:85–91.
2. Engelbrecht E, Siegel A, Rottger J, Buchholz HW. Statistics of total knee replacement: partial and total knee replacement, design St. Georg: a review of a 4-year observation. *Clin Orthop Rel Res* 1976;00(120):54–64.
3. Booth CM, King JB. Myositis ossificans following porous-ingrowth total knee replacement. *Orthop Rev* 1979;25: 223–227.
4. McClelland SJ, Rudolf LM. Myositis ossificans following porous-ingrowth TK replacement. *Orthop Rev* 1986;15: 223–227.
5. Scott WN, Rubinstein M, Scuderi G. Results after knee replacement with a posterior cruciate-substituting prosthesis. *J Bone Joint Surg* 1988;70A:1163–1173.
6. Lovelock JE, Griffiths HJ, Silverstein AM, Anson PS. Complications of total knee replacement. *AJR* 1984; 142:985–992.
7. Figgie HE III, Goldberg VM, Heiple KG, Moller HS III. The incidence and significance of heterotopic ossification following total knee arthroplasty. *Adv Orthop Surg* 1986;10:12–17.
8. Harwin SF, Stein AJ, Stern RE, Kulick RG. Heterotopic ossification following primary total knee arthroplasty. *J Arthroplasty* 1993;8:113–116.
9. Furia JP, Pellegrini VD Jr. Heterotopic ossification following primary total knee arthroplasty [see comments]. *J Arthroplasty* 1995;10:413–419.
10. Rader CP, Barthel T, Haase M, Scheidler M, Eulert J. Heterotopic ossification after total knee arthroplasty: 54/615 cases after 1–6 years' follow-up. *Acta Orthop Scand* 1997;68:46–50.
11. Anapolle DM, Stuchin SA. Heterotopic ossification following total knee arthroplasty. *Am J Knee Surg* 1994; 7:82–86.
12. Puzas JE, Brand JS, Evarts CM. Endogenous factors regulate bone formation: a possible cause of heterotopic bone growth after surgery. *Surg Forum* 1981;32: 529–531.
13. Pellegrini VD Jr, Evarts CM. Radiation prophylaxis of heterotopic bone formation following total hip arthroplasty: current status. Semin *Arthroplasty* 1992;3:156–166.
14. Chalmers J, Gray DH, Rush J. Observations on the induction of bone in soft tissues. *J Bone Joint Surg* 1975;57B:36–45.
15. Geshickter CF, Maseritz IH. Myositis ossificans progressiva. *J Bone Joint Surg* 1929;11A:157.
16. Hall BK. Histogenesis and morphogenesis of bone. *Clin Orthop Rel Res* 1971;74:249–268.
17. Jowsey J, Coventry MB, Robins PR. Heterotopic ossification: theoretical considerations, possible etiologic factors, and a clinical review of total hip arthroplasty patients exhibiting this phenomenon. In: Murray WR (ed). *The Hip: Proceedings of the Fifth Open Scientific Meeting of the Hip Society*. St. Louis: CV Mosby, 1977: 210–221.
18. Ostrowski K, Wlodarski K. Induction of heterotopic bone formation. In: Bourne GH (ed). *The Biochemistry and Physiology of Bone*, vol 3. New York: Academic Press, 1971:299.
19. Tonna EA, Cronkite EP. Autoradiographic studies of cell proliferation in the periosteum of intact and fractured femora of mice utilizing DNA labelling with 3H thymidine. *Proc Soc Exp Biol Med* 1961;107:719.
20. Tornkvist H, Nilsson OS, Bauer FC, Lindholm TS. Experimentally induced heterotopic ossification in rats influenced by anti-inflammatory drugs. *Scand J Rheumatol* 1983;12:177–180.
21. Craven PL, Urist MR. Osteogenesis by radioisotope labelled cell populations in implants of bone matrix under

the influence of ionizing radiation. *Clin Orthop Rel Res* 1971;76:231–233.

22. Urist MR, Silverman BF, Buring K, Dubuc FL, Rosenberg JM. The bone induction principle. *Clin Orthop Rel Res* 1967;53:243–283.
23. Urist MR, Hay PH, Dubuc F, Buring K. Osteogenetic competence. *Clin Orthop Rel Res* 1969;64:194–220.
24. Urist MR, Strates BS. Bone formation in implants of partially and wholly demineralized bone matrix, including observations on acetone-fixed intra- and extracellular proteins. *Clin Orthop Rel Res* 1970;71:271–278.
25. Puzas JE, Brand JS, Howard GA, Liu CC, Evarts CM. Heterotopic bone formation after operation: a quantitative histologic and biochemical study. *Surg Forum* 1984; 35:521–523.
26. Puzas JE, Evarts CM, Brand JS. The stimulus for bone formation. In: Brand RA (ed). *The Hip: Proceedings of the 14th Open Scientific Meeting of the Hip Society.* St. Louis: CV Mosby, 1986:25–38.
27. Bonarigo BC, Rubin P. Nonunion of pathologic fracture after radiation therapy. *Radiology* 1967;88:889–898.
28. Friedlander GE. The influence of various physical modalities and drugs on bone regeneration and ingrowth. In: Fitzgerald R (ed). *Noncemented Total Hip Arthroplasty.* New York: Raven Press, 1988:135–141.
29. Ahrengart L, Lindgren U. Functional significance of heterotopic bone formation after total hip arthroplasty. *J Arthroplasty* 1989;4:125–131.
30. Bergstrom B, Lindberg L, Persson BM, Onnerfalt R. Complications after total hip arthroplasty according to Charnley in a Swedish series of cases. *Clin Orthop Rel Res* 1973;95:91–95.
31. Bisla RS, Ranawat CS, Inglis AE. Total hip replacement in patients with ankylosing spondylitis with involvement of the hip. *J Bone Joint Surg* 1976;58A:233–238.
32. Brooker AF, Bowerman JW, Robinson RA, Riley LH Jr. Ectopic ossification following total hip replacement. Incidence and a method of classification. *J Bone Joint Surg* 1973;55A:1629–1632.
33. Charnley J. The long-term results of low-friction arthroplasty of the hip performed as a primary intervention. *J Bone Joint Surg* 1972;54B:61–76.
34. DeLee J, Ferrari A, Charnley J. Ectopic bone formation following low friction arthroplasty of the hip. *Clin Orthop Rel Res* 1976;121:53–59.
35. Fahrer H, Koch P, Ballmer P, Enzler P, Gerber N. Ectopic ossification following total hip arthroplasty: is diffuse idiopathic skeletal hyperostosis a risk factor? *Br J Rheumatol* 1988;27:187–190.
36. Foster DE, Hunter JR. The direct lateral approach to the hip for arthroplasty. Advantages and complications. *Orthopedics* 1987;10:274–280.
37. Hierton C, Blomgren G, Lindgren U. Factors associated with heterotopic bone formation in cemented total hip prostheses. *Acta Orthop Scand* 1983;54:698–702.
38. Johnston RC. Clinical follow-up of total hip replacement. *Clin Orthop Rel Res* 1973;95:118–126.
39. Kromann-Andersen C, Sorensen TS, Hougaard K, Zdravkovic D, Frigaard E. Ectopic bone formation following Charnley hip arthroplasty. *Acta Orthop Scand* 1980;51:633–638.
40. Lazansky MG. Complications revisited. The debit side of total hip replacement. *Clin Orthop Rel Res* 1973;95:96–103.
41. Nolan DR, Fitzgerald RH Jr, Beckenbaugh RD, Coventry MB. Complications of total hip arthroplasty treated by reoperation. *J Bone Joint Surg* 1975;57A:977–981.
42. Pedersen NW, Kristensen SS, Schmidt SA, Pedersen P, Kjaersgaard-Andersen P. Factors associated with heterotopic bone formation following total hip replacement. *Arch Orthop Trauma Surg* 1989;108:92–95.
43. Pellegrini VD Jr, Konski AA, Gastel JA, Rubin P, Evarts CM. Prevention of heterotopic ossification with irradiation after total hip arthroplasty. Radiation therapy with a single dose of eight hundred centigray administered to a limited field. *J Bone Joint Surg* 1992;74A:186–200.
44. Riegler HF, Harris CM. Heterotopic bone formation after total hip arthroplasty. *Clin Orthop Rel Res* 1976; 117:209–216.
45. Ritter MA, Vaughan RB. Ectopic ossification after total hip arthroplasty. Predisposing factors, frequency, and effect on results. *J Bone Joint Surg* 1977;59A:345–351.
46. Shaffer B. A critical review. Heterotopic ossification in total hip replacement. *Bull Hosp Joint Dis Orthop Inst* 1989;49:55–74.
47. Soballe K, Christensen F, Kristensen SS. Ectopic bone formation after total hip arthroplasty. *Clin Orthop Rel Res* 1988;228:57–62.
48. Sundaram NA, Murphy JC. Heterotopic bone formation following total hip arthroplasty in ankylosing spondylitis. *Clin Orthop Rel Res* 1986;207:223–226.
49. Williams E, Taylor AR, Arden GP, Edwards DH. Arthroplasty of the hip in ankylosing spondylitis. *J Bone Joint Surg* 1977;59B:393–397.
50. Wilson PD Jr, Amstutz HC, Czerniecki A, Salvati EA, Mendes DG. Total hip replacement with fixation by acrylic cement. A preliminary study of 100 consecutive McKee-Farrar prosthetic replacements. *J Bone Joint Surg* 1972;54A:207–236.
51. Garland DE. Clinical observations on fractures and heterotopic ossification in the spinal cord and traumatic brain injured populations. *Clin Orthop Rel Res* 1988;233: 86–101.
52. Lal S, Hamilton BB, Heinemann A, Betts HB. Risk factors for heterotopic ossification in spinal cord injury. *Arch Phys Med Rehabil* 1989;70:387–390.
53. Peterson SL, Mani MM, Crawford CM, Neff JR, Hiebert JM. Postburn heterotopic ossification: insights for management decision making. *J Trauma* 1989;29:365–369.

54. Garland DE, Blum CE, Waters RL. Periarticular heterotopic ossification in head-injured adults. Incidence and location. *J Bone Joint Surg* 1980;62A:1143–1146.

55. Bosse MJ, Poka A, Reinert CM, Ellwanger F, Slawson R, McDevitt ER. Heterotopic ossification as a complication of acetabular fracture. Prophylaxis with low-dose irradiation. *J Bone Joint Surg* 1988;70A:1231–1237.

56. Brumback RJ, Wells JD, Lakatos R, Poka A, Bathon GH, Burgess AR. Heterotopic ossification about the hip after intramedullary nailing for fractures of the femur [see comments]. *J Bone Joint Surg* 1990;72A:1067–1073.

57. Edwards E, Miller J, Chan KH. The effect of postoperative collateral ligament laxity in total knee arthroplasty. *Clin Orthop Rel Res* 1988;236:44–51.

58. Kjaersgaard-Andersen P, Frich LH, Sojbjerg JO, Sneppen O. Heterotopic bone formation following total shoulder arthroplasty. *J Arthroplasty* 1989;4:99–104.

59. Evarts CM, Ayers DC, Puzas JE. Prevention of heterotopic bone formation in high-risk patients by postoperative irradiation. In: Brand R (ed). *The Hip: Proceedings of the 14th Open Scientific Meeting of the Hip Society*. St. Louis: CV Mosby, 1986:70–83.

60. Ilstrup DM, Nolan DR, Beckenbaugh RD, Coventry MB. Factors influencing the results in 2,012 total hip arthroplasties. *Clin Orthop Rel Res* 1973;95:250–262.

61. Kjaersgaard-Andersen P, Hougaard K, Linde F, Christiansen SE, Jensen J. Heterotopic bone formation after total hip arthroplasty in patients with primary or secondary coxarthrosis. *Orthopedics* 1990;13:1211–1217.

62. Nollen AJ, Slooff TJ. Para-articular ossifications after total hip replacement. *Acta Orthop Scand* 1973;44:230–241.

63. Parkinson JR, Evarts CM, Hubbard LF. Radiation therapy in the prevention of heterotopic ossification after total hip arthroplasty. In: Nelson JP, ed. *The Hip: Proceedings of the 10th Open Scientific Meeting of the Hip Society*. St. Louis: CV Mosby, 1982:211–227.

64. Sawyer JR, Myers MA, Rosier RN, Puzas JE. Heterotopic ossification: clinical and cellular aspects. *Calcif Tissue Int* 1991;49:208–215.

65. Resnick D, Linovitz RJ, Feingold ML. Postoperative heterotopic ossification in patients with ankylosing hyperostosis on the spine (Forestier's disease). *J Rheumatol* 1976;3:313–320.

66. Freedman EL, Freedman DM. Heterotopic ossification following total knee arthroplasty requiring surgical excision. *Am J Orthop* 1996;25:559–561.

67. Austin KS, Siliski JM. Symptomatic heterotopic ossification following total knee arthroplasty. *J Arthroplasty* 1995;10:695–698.

68. Daluga D, Lombardi AV Jr, Mallory TH, Vaughn BK. Knee manipulation following total knee arthroplasty. Analysis of prognostic variables. *J Arthroplasty* 1991; 6:119–128.

69. Pham J, Kumar R. Heterotopic ossification after total knee arthroplasty. *Am J Orthop* 1997;26:141–143.

70. Maloney WJ, Schurman DJ. The effects of implant design on range of motion after total knee arthroplasty. Total condylar versus posterior stabilized total condylar designs. *Clin Orthop Rel Res* 1992;278:147–152.

71. Ritter MA, Stringer EA. Predictive range of motion after total knee replacement. *Clin Orthop Rel Res* 1979;143: 115–119.

72. Schurman DJ, Parker JN, Ornstein D. Total condylar knee replacement. A study of factors influencing range of motion as late as two years after arthroplasty. *J Bone Joint Surg* 1985;67A:1006–1014.

73. Walker PS, Garg A. Range of motion in total knee arthroplasty. A computer analysis. *Clin Orthop Rel Res* 1991; 262:227–235.

74. Ryu J, Saito S, Yamamoto K, Sano S. Factors influencing the postoperative range of motion in total knee arthroplasty. *Bull Hosp J Dis* 1993;53:35–40.

75. Chiarello CM, Gundersen L, O'Halloran T. The effect of continuous passive motion duration and increment on range of motion in total knee arthroplasty patients. *J Orthop Sports Phys Ther* 1997;25:119–127.

76. Gotlin RS, Hershkowitz S, Juris PM, Gonzalez EG, Scott WN, Insall JN. Electrical stimulation effect on extensor lag and length of hospital stay after total knee arthroplasty. *Arch Phys Med Rehabil* 1994;75:957–959.

77. Stulberg SD. Extensor mechanism complications after total knee arthroplasty. *Orthopedics* 1995;18:919–920.

78. Pellegrini VD Jr. Radiation prophylaxis of heterotopic ossification [editorial] [see comments] [published erratum appears in Int J Radiat Oncol Biol Phys 1995; 32(1):283]. *Int J Radiat Oncol Biol Phys* 1994;30: 743–744.

79. Pellegrini VD Jr, Gregoritch SJ. Preoperative irradiation for prevention of heterotopic ossification following total hip arthroplasty. *J Bone Joint Surg* 1996;78A:870–881.

Chapter 25

Recurrent Hemarthrosis After Total Knee Arthroplasty

Kirk A. Kindsfater

Spontaneous recurrent hemarthrosis after total knee arthroplasty (TKA) is an uncommon but well-recognized clinical entity. It occurs in less than 1% of TKAs and is seen primarily by surgeons who perform a large number of total joint arthroplasties.

Although spontaneous hemarthrosis after TKA is rare, when it does occur it is often recurrent and can be disabling to the patient. In addition, this entity often presents a diagnostic and treatment challenge to the orthopedic surgeon, as there is a paucity of literature on this subject, which is limited to a few case reports and a moderately sized study of 30 patients [1–4]

DEMOGRAPHICS

Patients with hemarthrosis after TKA most often present with spontaneous development of knee swelling, warmth, pain, and a grossly bloody effusion upon aspiration. Antecedent trauma is occasionally present, but most cases occur de novo.[1,2]

The underlying diagnosis present prior to TKA does not appear to influence the risk of recurrent hemarthrosis, as this entity has occurred in total knees performed for osteoarthritis, inflammatory arthropathies, and avascular necrosis. Most knees in which recurrent hemarthroses have presented have been cemented knees, but they have also occurred in press-fit arthroplasties.[1] There does not appear to be any relationship between recurrent bleeds and whether the prosthesis is cruciate sparing or cruciate substituting or sacrificing.[1]

Intrinsic disorders of coagulation increase the risk of recurrent hemarthrosis, but most patients who develop this entity do not have a known coagulation disorder. Approximately one-third of patients reported in the literature may have been predisposed to bleeding secondary to the administration of medication with anticoagulant properties, e.g., warfarin, aspirin, or nonsteroidal antiinflammatories.

The average interval from implantation of the prosthesis until the first hemarthrosis averages approximately 2 years, but has ranged from 2 weeks to 12 years.[1] Most patients have multiple recurrences. In the study by Kindsfater and Scott,[1] the average number of recurrences was 5.5 with a range of 1 to 20. The interval between bleeds can range from a few days to 1 year.[1]

PATHOGENESIS

Recurrent hemarthrosis of the native knee is a common clinical entity, and multiple causes have been described, including hemophilia, pigmented villonodular synovitis, intraarticular and juxtaarticular vascular tumors, chondrocalcinosis, gout, and degenerative tears of the posterior portion of the lateral meniscus.[5–11]

In contradistinction, recurrent hemarthrosis after TKA is uncommon and its causes are less well defined. The most common identifiable cause of recurrent hemarthrosis after prosthetic arthroplasty appears to be entrapment of synovial tissue or the fat pad between prosthetic surfaces (Fig. 25.1). However, over 50% of all recurrent bleeds do not have an identifiable etiology and are therefore felt to be idiopathic. If tissue entrapment is not elucidated as the cause of recurrent bleeding, a juxtaarticular tumor or intraarticular vascular malformation can be identified with angiography, but this is extremely rare.

Pigmented villonodular synovitis has been described

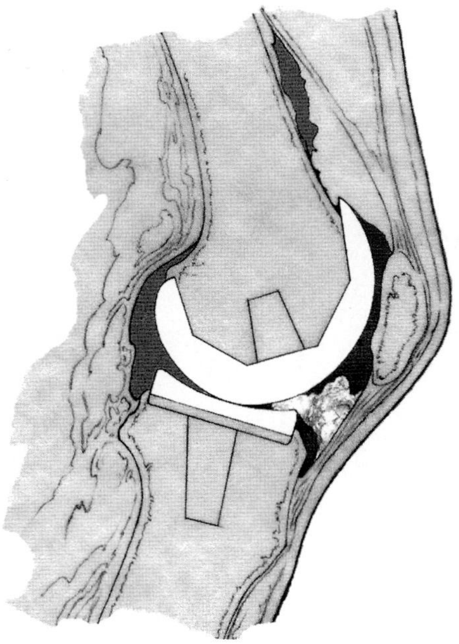

Figure 25.1. Schematic demonstrating entrapment of hypertrophic fat pad between the tibial and femoral components.

as a cause of recurrent hemarthrosis after TKA, but this has been identified in only one patient.[6]

I believe that synovial entrapment may be more likely in patients who develop a proliferative synovitis after TKA. This proliferative synovitis has been noted at the time of both primary and revision arthroplasties of the knee.[12–14] This proliferative synovium may become traumatized easily by the repetitive motion of the joint, leading to recurrent bleeds and the development of a pigmented/hypertrophic synovium.

The wide variation in the interval between implantation and the onset of hemarthrosis may be related to these factors. Patients who bleed early in the postoperative course may have a loose tag of synovial tissue or fat pad remaining from surgery that becomes entrapped early in the postoperative course, whereas others may slowly develop a proliferative synovium that over time eventually becomes entrapped and may lead to late hemarthrosis.

HISTOLOGY

A study of the synovium from prosthetic knees with recurrent hemarthrosis has delineated consistent features, including focal synovial hyperplasia, increased histiocytic infiltration, and significant hemosiderin deposition. Foreign-body giant cells and dense fibrosis are less common. Gross fibrous nodules have not been noted. Although these findings are similar to those of pigmented villonodular synovitis (PVNS), certain features appear to be missing. Grossly no fibrous nodules have been noted and often the synovium is only focally reactive, whereas pigmented villonodular synovitis usually affects the entire synovial lining and contains fibrous nodules. Histologically, PVNS demonstrates osteoclast-type giant cells, a polyhedral stroma, and, though not pathognomonic, foam cells—findings that have not been seen in most knees with recurrent hemarthrosis after TKA.[15–18] Therefore, patients with recurrent hemarthrosis after TKA who have a pigmented synovium should not blindly be labeled as having PVNS unless the appropriate histologic features are present.

PREVENTION

Over half of all recurrent bleeds after TKA do not have an identifiable cause; thus, complete prevention of this complication is not possible. However, the risk of this entity can be decreased by paying meticulous attention to the soft tissues during the arthroplasty. Hypertrophic synovium at the time of primary arthroplasty should be considered for excision, preferably with total synovectomy. If total synovectomy is not performed, then excision of the hypertrophic synovium from areas susceptible to entrapment by the prosthesis should be considered. These areas include the medial and lateral gutters at the level of the joint line and any tissue that may become entrapped in the patellofemoral articulation.

A hypertrophic fat pad should be trimmed if any evidence of potential impingement in the patellofemoral or tibiofemoral articulation is noted. If the fat pad is abundant, closure of this layer separately from the capsular closure may help to decrease the mobility of the fat pad and hence decrease the likelihood of its entrapment within the joint.

Finally, adherence to the basic principles of knee arthroplasty with respect to alignment and soft tissue balancing helps to prevent excessive polyethylene wear that results from a poorly aligned or balanced prosthetic knee. This may help to decrease the risk of developing a proliferative synovitis secondary to polyethylene debris.

MANAGEMENT OF RECURRENT HEMARTHROSIS AFTER TOTAL KNEE ARTHROPLASTY

When recurrent hemarthrosis develops after TKA, the diagnosis should be confirmed by aspiration of the joint. Gross bloody fluid will be obtained if the aspiration is performed acutely. Conservative care is initiated including rest, ice, compression, and elevation. If the patient is taking any medication that may affect platelet function or the coagulation cascade, then this medication should be stopped. In some cases, medical concerns prevent the discontinuation of the anticoagulant medication.

A gradual return to activities should be allowed as the knee becomes less symptomatic.

If the hemarthrosis recurs more than once, a medical workup for potential disorders of coagulation should be instituted. This workup should include investigations into drug-induced thrombocytopenias, von Willebrand's disease, and defective platelet function. In addition, factor deficiencies, fibrinolytic defects, and circulating anticoagulants or inhibitors should be ruled out. If an intrinsic disorder of the coagulation system is not found, and all extrinsic factors have been managed appropriately, then surgical intervention should be considered.

Although arthroscopic investigation and synovectomy can be considered, this mode of treatment has been shown to be less effective than open synovectomy with a higher recurrence rate of hemarthrosis.[1] Therefore, open synovectomy and exploration of the joint is preferred.

A thorough investigation of the soft tissues of the joint at the time of arthrotomy should be undertaken to rule out an entrapped or traumatized piece of soft tissue or a vascularized leash of soft tissue. If such a piece of tissue is found, this should be excised. In addition, a complete synovectomy should be performed and the polyethylene insert should be removed to allow access to the posterior aspect of the joint. The surgeon should, as always, be prepared to revise any portion of the joint that may incidentally be found to be loose or have failed otherwise. This technique has proven successful in 93% (14 out of 15) of knees reported on previously by this author.[1] If recurrent hemarthrosis continues after open synovectomy, then angiography may be necessary to rule out an occult juxtaarticular vascular malformation or tumor.

References

1. Kindsfater K, Scott RD. Recurrent hemarthrosis after total knee arthroplasty. *J Arthroplasty Suppl* 1995;10: S52–S55.
2. Oishi S, Elliot M, Colwell C. Recurrent hemarthrosis following a total knee arthroplasty. *J Arthroplasty Suppl* 1995;10:S56–S58.
3. Kitridiou RC, Shumacher HR, Sbarbaro TL, Hollander JL. Recurrent hemarthrosis after prosthetic knee arthroplasty: identification of metal particles in synovial fluid. *Arthritis Rheum* 1969;12:530–537.
4. Worland R, Jessup D. Recurrent hemarthrosis after total knee arthroplasty. *J Arthroplasty* 1996;11:977–978.
5. Gilbert M. Musculoskeletal manifestations of hemophilia. *Mt Sinai J Med* 1977;44:339–351.
6. Ballard N, Clark K, Callaghan JJ. Recurrent spontaneous hemarthrosis nine years after a total knee arthroplasty: a presentation with pigmented villonodular synovitis. *J Bone Joint Surg* 1993;75A:764–767.
7. Meyers B, Masi A, Feigenbaum S. Pigmented villonodular synovitis and tenosynovitis: a clinical epidemiological study of 166 cases and literature review. *Medicine* 1980; 59:223–238.
8. Visuri T. Recurrent spontaneous hemarthrosis of the knee associated with a synovial and juxta-articular hemangiohamartoma. *Ann Rheum Dis* 1987;49:554–556.
9. Menkes D, Rondier J. Idiopathic hemarthrosis with chondrocalcinosis. *Ann Rheum Dis* 1987;46:85.
10. Martin D, Merenda G, McDonald D, Sundaram M. Recurrent hemarthrosis associated with gout. *Clin Orthop* 1992;277:262–265.
11. Kawamura H, Ogata K, Miura H, et al. Spontaneous hemarthrosis of the knee in the elderly patient: etiology and treatment. *Arthroscopy* 1994;10:171–175.
12. Ewald FC, Sledge CB, Carson J, et al. Giant cell synovitis associated with failed polyethylene patellar replacements. *Orthopedics* 1976;115:213–219.
13. Tong I, Beardmore T, Kaufman R. Prosthetic synovitis: a consideration in painful prosthetic joints. *Arthritis Rheum* 1981;24:62–69.
14. Weissman B, Scott RD, Brick G, Corson J. Radiographic detection of metal induced synovitis as a complication of arthroplasty of the knee. *J Bone Joint Surg* 1991;73A: 1003–1007.
15. Ghadially F. Ultrastructure of pigmented villonodular synovitis. *J Pathol* 1979;127:19–27.
16. Mirra J. *Bone Tumors: Clinical, Radiological and Pathologic Correlations*. Philadelphia: Lea and Feibiger, 1989.
17. Robbins SL, Cotran RC, Kumar V. The musculoskeletal system. In: Robbins SL, Cotran RC, Kumar V (eds). *Pathologic Basis of Disease*, 3rd ed. Philadelphia: WB Saunders, 1984:1304–1369.
18. Wylie JC. The stromal cell reaction of pigmented villonodular synovitis: an electron microscopic study. *Arthritis Rheum* 1969;12:205–211.

Chapter 26

UNICONDYLAR ARTHROPLASTY

Gérard P. Deschamps and Philippe Cartier

Unicompartmental knee arthroplasty (UKA) is a very special form of knee replacement. It constitutes a viable and useful, though not indispensable, alternative to total knee replacement, which remains the technique of choice of a number of authors.[1] It is, however, of indisputable value in the management of unicompartmental osteoarthrosis (OA) in the elderly, since it has very little morbidity, leads to rapid recovery, and, in all cases, gives a good range of motion (ROM). In spite of these advantages, it has not yet been universally accepted because of the particular demands made in terms of patient selection, surgical technique, and hardware selection. Ignorance or violation of the stringent rules that govern UKA have, until quite recently, been responsible for failures that have cast doubt on the viability of the concept of unicompartmental replacement.

The concept of unicompartmental replacement was defined by MacIntosh[2] as early as 1958: "To correct deformity, restore stability, and relieve pain." These principles have not changed; however, as we shall demonstrate in the light of our experience and of a search of the recent literature, some qualifications of MacIntosh's statement are now required.

The first qualification, and one that is of paramount importance, is that the only possible purpose for which UKA should be employed is the correction of the wear element of the deformity—to correct wear and nothing else. The limit as far as axial correction is concerned is the restoration of the natural axis that the limb had prior to the arthrotic process. The reference for the choice of thickness of the implant is the retensioning, without overtightening, of the ligaments on the concave side of the deformity. Techniques that will not meticulously produce this result, or which leave the knee with excessively taut ligaments, have been responsible for most of the failures that are discussed in the first part of this chapter. We shall be concentrating mainly on wear and loosening in the short, medium, and long term, which are now the main issues.

Our own experience, and that of all those who have written about UKA (be they proponents or opponents), is that, of all the knee arthroplasties, UKA has the lowest intra- and postoperative morbidity. In particular, the rate of thromboembolic complications is twice as low as that of total knee arthroplasty (TKA) and of osteotomies. There are no reports in the literature of intraoperative fatalities, and the rate of infection is less than 1%, even in the earliest studies and in the multicenter studies.[3,4] Also, many authors have stressed the fact that blood loss during this procedure is very slight.[5–8] More often than not, there is no need for transfusions, with all their attendant risks.

These advantages, plus the rapid rehabilitation of the patients, and the fact that the eventual ROM is as good as, or better than, that before surgery,[5,9–12] are the main arguments in favor of using UKA rather than TKA or osteotomies. It is because of these benefits that surgeons, to this day, remain interested in UKA. The study of what has gone wrong and why, which is presented in this chapter, is vital, since it allows us to define the role of UKA in the management of OA of the knee joint, to define the rules of how UKA should be employed, and to describe in greater detail the current hardware options.

UNICOMPARTMENTAL FAILURES

At the 1995 SOFCOT (Société française de chirurgie orthopedique et traumatologie) symposium in Paris,[13] we presented the results of 680 unicompartmental prostheses; this exercise, together with a search of the literature, allows us to analyze the failures of unicompartmental knee replacements and to attempt to establish whether these failures are attributable to an inherently faulty concept, or whether they have occurred because of mistakes made in the application of what is, in itself, a sound and sensible concept. If the latter were to be true, then an analysis of this kind could be used to prevent the recurrence of the mistakes and failures of the past.

Analysis of Failures

Our study involved 680 unicompartmental prostheses (483 medial, 197 lateral).[13] The main design used was the Lotus I (Howmedica). The mean follow-up was 5.5 years (range: 1 to 20 years). There were 90 failures (13%) necessitating revision. Leaving aside five cases of infection (0.7%), failure was chiefly due to mechanical causes. Among these, loosening was the most frequent (33 cases), followed by instability (22 cases); progression of the arthrotic process to the other compartments only came third, together with other causes such as polyethylene (PE) wear.

While all authors, including ourselves, have reported the same failure causes, the percentage distribution of the different causes varies in the literature, due to a number of factors such as patient selection, implant patterns (of which some are no longer in use, while others have been modified), and the UKA experience of the individual surgeon. These aspects will also be analyzed.

Loosening

In Our Series. In 595 cases available for review, the tibial component loosening rate (56 cases = 9.4%) was slightly higher than that of femoral component loosening (50 cases = 3.4%). There was a significant difference between medial and lateral UKAs; medial UKAs (483 cases) had more instances of tibial component loosening (10% of cases), while femoral component loosening was less frequently seen (3.7%). Conversely, lateral UKAs (197 cases) had more femoral component loosening (4.7%), and less tibial component loosening (3.6%). As will be shown below, the failure of lateral UKAs is more frequently associated with instability than with loosening. The statistical analysis also allowed us to establish a correlation between certain technical errors or inappropriate patient selection on the one hand, and loosening on the other hand.

Tibial component loosening was significantly correlated with a preoperative deformity >20 degrees, especially in varus knees; postoperative overcorrection of the deformity (transformation of a preoperative varus into a valgus, or vice versa); and a residual instability after surgery, either in the sagittal plane (anterior instability) or gaping on the opposite side in the coronal plane (medial gaping with a lateral UKA). There was also a significant correlation with femoral component malposition in the coronal plane, and with an increase in the anteroposterior (AP) diameter of the femoral condyle, creating excessive thickness of the femoral component at the back.

Femoral component loosening was correlated with mediolateral instability, either in the form of a persistent lateral subluxation of the tibia on the femur with medial UKAs, or of medial gaping with lateral UKAs, and, as in tibial component loosening, with an increase in the AP diameter of the femoral condyle, resulting from an excessively thick posterior portion of the femoral component. It should be noted that, in our series, the main pattern used was the Lotus (Howmedica), with an all-PE tibial plateau.

In the Literature. Our results were borne out by the data in the literature; however, in our search, we came across some interesting information regarding failure causes. Barrett and Scott,[14] in 29 revisions, found loosening to be the main cause of failure of the first procedure (55% of cases). Swank et al,[15] in a series of 82 UKAs followed up for up to 8 years, found a loosening rate of 3.5%, while Callahan et al,[16] in a metaanalysis of 2,391 UKAs and 884 TKAs, found a UKA loosening rate of 3.6% as against a TKA rate of 2.4%. Conversely, Rougraff et al,[5] in a comparison between 120 UKAs and 81 TKAs over the same period of 5 to 6 years, found 4% UKA loosening as against 11% for the TKAs.

As for the causes of loosening, Takai et al,[17] using a finite element method, showed that the increased stress levels resulting from undercorrection promote tibial component loosening. Scott,[18] in a review of 20 years of UKA at the Brigham and Women's and New England Hospitals, attributed femoral component loosening to the narrow femoral runners of the original design, and, as in our study, found that the lack of secure posterior prosthetic fixation promotes component loosening.

The crucial study to show the increased risk of femoral component loosening inherent in the design of porous coated anatomic (PCA) UKAs was performed by Lindstrand et al,[19] who compared 772 PCA, 1,564 Marmor, and 1,441 St. Georg sledge devices. The authors found a cumulative revision rate that differed significantly at 2 years, and eventually increased to 15% for the PCA, as against 5% and 7%, respectively, for the two other designs. This study was borne out by the findings of Harilainen et al[20] and Gacon and Ferreira.[21] These studies show how nefarious the effects of certain implant designs can be. However, that does not mean that UKA as a concept should be condemned.

It is also interesting to note that while most authors feel that obese patients should be selected for UKA only upon careful reflection, only one study, that by Heck et al,[7] has shown a correlation between loosening and excess body weight. Voss et al[22] reported that 62% of the partial radiolucencies in their series were found in patients weighing 90 kg or more. In our own series, there was no statistical correlation between these factors. However, all the participants in the SOFCOT symposium were in favor of not selecting patients weighing over 85 kg for UKA,[13] especially where the deformity is pronounced or when there is osteoporosis.

Wear

In Our Series. We found that wear eventually occurs, and is seen in virtually all cases at more than 10 years, regardless of the thickness of the PE. In our patients, who had mainly received a non–metal-back plateau, mean wear was found to be 1.83 (±0.094) mm on the medial side, and 1.45 (±0.151) mm on the lateral side. The mean value found beyond 10 years was 3.26 (±0.23) mm. In two-thirds of the cases, lateral films showed the wear to be central.

Wear was seen to correlate with a preoperative deformity >20 degrees and postoperative varus/valgus overcorrection of the deformity ($p = .05$), which may be related to overstress from excessive tightening of the ligaments in the concavity. It also correlated with instability, either in the coronal plane (lateral tibial translation in medial UKAs, medial gaping with lateral UKAs, $p = .0001$), or in the sagittal plane (anterior instability, $p = .0009$)—in the latter case, with posterior wear. There was also a very important correlation of wear with insufficient plateau thickness (6 mm, $p = .001$) and with length of follow-up ($p = .001$).

In the Literature. The data in the literature confirm our findings. In particular, Engh et al,[23] in their analysis of 86 PE inserts removed at 39.5 months from TKAs or UKAs, found major wear with delamination and/or associated deformation in 51% of cases. This wear correlated with the length of follow-up (time in situ), the lack of congruency of the implant surfaces, and insufficient PE thickness. Engh et al emphasize the deleterious effect of metal backing if the metal-backed PE is too thin, especially around the rim of the implant and above the screw holes in cementless implants. They recommend a minimum thickness of 6 mm above the metal backing, and as much as 8 mm of PE above the screw holes. This view is borne out by a number of articles that emphasize that the heightened wear risk in implants associating metal backing and insufficiently thick PE.[18,24]

There are, however, other factors that may play a role, such as changes in the PE subsequent to sterilization, especially with gamma radiation. Langlais[25] recommends either gamma sterilization in a vacuum, or ethylene oxide sterilization, while Cartier[26] prefers ethylene oxide. In a prospective study of 120 PCA units, Lindstrand and Stenström[27] stressed the risks inherent in the heat-pressing of PE, which makes the component more prone to wear, with a very distinctive delamination pattern.

The main problem of UKA is the undercorrection of the deformity, which, as we shall see, is one of the planks of this arthroplasty concept. The study by Berger et al[28] showed a correlation between adduction moment and alignment. Residual malalignment subjects the implant to abnormally high loads and may increase the prospect of device failure, as compared with a TKA, where the object of surgery is to produce a neutral axis. Thus, wear is thought to be inevitable. However, this somewhat gloomy statement should be considered in the light of Bensadoun's[29] findings that, with a slight (5-degree) undercorrection, the stress pattern is 54% on the implanted side, as against 46% in the opposite compartment, because of the gradient of elasticity between the two compartments.

Wear is, however, frequently seen at revision. While some designs and some manufacturing techniques[27] may give rise to delamination, we must consider wear in connection with undercorrection, especially when determining the age range of patients who may benefit from UKA. It should also be noted that conforming designs, such as Goodfellow's Oxford Knee,[30] have good wear function; unfortunately, this pattern is fraught with major stability problems.

Instability

In our series, instability was to blame for a quarter of the failures encountered.[13] As a failure cause, it came second after loosening. Instability is a serious problem, because it may lead to early implant failure, which may be difficult to revise. A distinction should be made between instability in the coronal and in the sagittal plane, since the effects and the causes of the two patterns are different, although they may occur in association with each other.

In the Coronal Plane. Lateral instability associated with medial tibiofemoral OA is rare. Failures have been mainly attributable to medial instability in conjunction with lateral tibiofemoral compartment OA; in these cases, clinically demonstrable instability was associated with wear of the tibial or loosening of the femoral component. The problem may be caused by dysplasia of the ipsilateral hip. In such patients, it would have been preferable to perform a TKA, after treating the hip condition. Instability of this kind may also be found in post-traumatic lateral compartment OA.

In our series of 197 lateral UKAs, there were 17 revisions in the first 5 years; of these, two-thirds were for instability. These cases are distressingly difficult to revise. In some cases, very constrained implants have had to be, or ought to have been, used (Fig. 26.1). Scott[18] and Bonutti and Kester[31] also consider medial instability in lateral compartment OA as a contraindication to UKA. Interestingly, the pattern on the medial side was the inverse of that seen in the lateral compartment, with two-thirds of the revisions required for loosening or wear.[32]

In the Sagittal Plane. We were among the first to emphasize that UKA failure may be associated with anterior cruciate ligament (ACL) deficiency.[33] In our series, anterior instability was a particular factor with medial UKAs, causing tibial component loosening (p = .04) and PE wear, with a characteristic pattern of posterior plateau wear (p = .001).

We found two distinct patterns: The first—and the more dangerous—is one where the ACL deficiency can be seen at the preoperative workup, which requires a weight-bearing lateral view. If the anterior drawer measured under these conditions is ≥10 mm, with a posterior wear defect (Fig. 26.2), we have invariably found on the postoperative lateral films (also taken as weight-bearing views) an anterior drawer >10 mm, which would progress and, after a very short time of less than 3 years, lead to complete posterior wear of the plateau and the need for implant revision. In our opinion, this is the typical pattern of OA secondary to anterior instability, as described by Dejour et al.[34] Associated posteromedial ligament deficiency means that the UKA does not stand a chance, since its flat plateau cannot control the instability. Patients with this pattern should not be managed with UKA.

The second pattern is one in which the ACL deficiency is noted at surgery, but where the preoperative lateral weight-bearing films showed an anterior drawer <10 mm. In our patients, this pattern was observed in 54% of the cases that were ACL deficient. In these cases, the UKA will fail much more gradually (some-

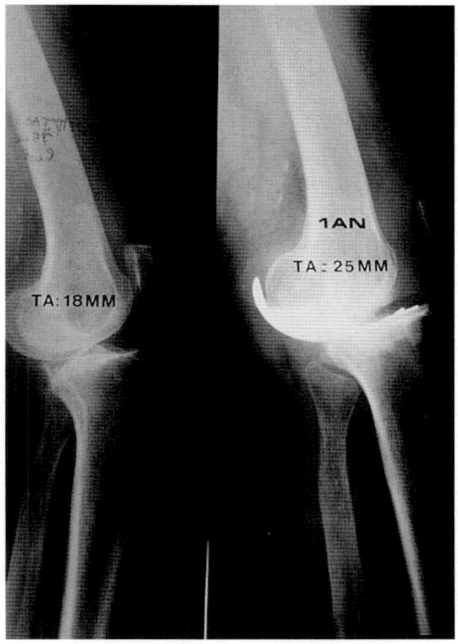

Figure 26.2. Weight-bearing lateral radiograph; preoperative anterior tibial translation >10 mm. The postoperative film shows immediate recurrence of the anterior subluxation, which led to early failure.

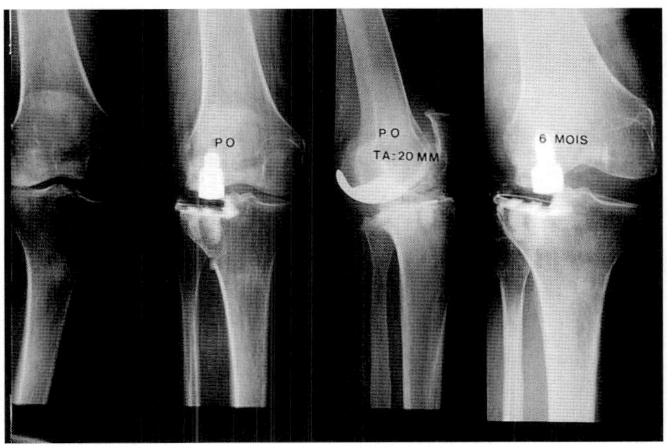

Figure 26.1. Lateral compartment osteoarthritis (OA) with medial instability, in a patient with ipsilateral developmental dysplasia of the hip. Failure from stretching of the medial ligaments required revision to a constrained prosthesis at 6 months.

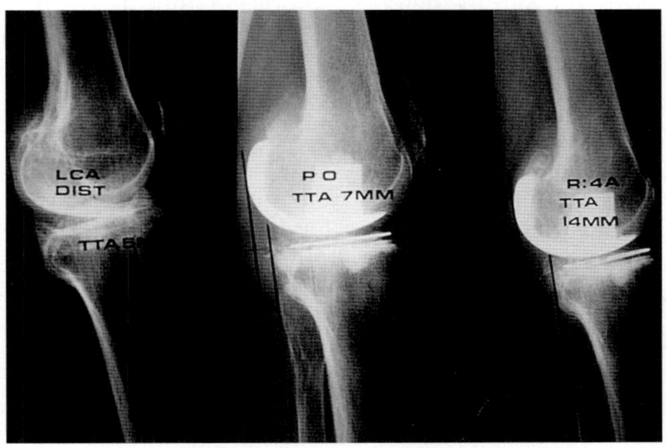

Figure 26.3. Stretching of the anterior cruciate ligament (ACL) found at surgery; no anterior tibial translation had been seen on the preoperative weight-bearing film. Slow but inexorable progression to anterior subluxation with posterior plateau wear occurred within 4 years.

times only after 7 years) (Fig. 26.3); however, the implant will eventually fail. Also, compared with patients with an intact ACL, the International Knee Society (IKS) score will always be significantly poorer, from the outset, even if there is no obvious dislocation. Undoubtedly, this poorer score is largely accounted for by the patients' adoption of a quadriceps avoidance gait, which is not normally seen in patients managed with (ACL-sparing) UKAs. The role of the quadriceps has been emphasized by Chassin et al[35] and by Berger et al.[28]

Although with this second pattern, deterioration may be slow, ACL deficiency should still be considered a contraindication to UKA. On this, there is now agreement in the literature.[31,36,37] The effects of this deficiency are particularly severe in the Oxford Knee, where it causes the bearing dislocations reported by Goodfellow et al[37,38] and by other authors using that design.[3]

As for the origin of the rupture of the ACL, the question arises as to whether the ACL tear precedes the insertion of the UKA, or whether it is secondary to the arthroplasty and linked to the flat design of the plateau. Bartley et al[39] studied 147 UKAs, of which 18 failed; 11 of the failures were in PCA devices, with progressive anterior subluxation of the tibia and posterior PE wear. In all these cases, the ACL had been intact at surgery. The authors concluded that the fate of the ACL after UKA cannot be predicted, since the causes of ACL attrition are unknown. Without being able to give a definitive answer, we may state that in our series of 680 UKAs, there were only eight cases of secondary rupture; however, no precipitating factor could be found.[40]

On the other hand, the statistical analysis performed failed to show any correlation between, for example, the slope of the plateau and the presence of anterior subluxation on the postoperative films. The only factor that correlated with the deterioration of the implant was preoperative damage to or loss of the ACL. Goodfellow et al[38] emphasized the pattern of ACL degeneration seen in some OA patients: the ligament has lost its synovial covering and is split into numerous bundles; when probed, it will readily tear. Such a ligament is functionally useless. ACL damage of this kind may account for a certain number of failures that have been wrongly considered to be secondary ACL tears of unknown origin.

Progression of OA to the Other Knee Compartments

In our series, this was the least frequently encountered cause of UKA failure.[13] A distinction must be made between patellofemoral compartment and opposite compartment involvement, since the consequences of the two patterns are different.

Patellofemoral Compartment Involvement. This compartment was seen to remain stable over time. In 74% of the cases, no changes were seen during the follow-up period; 18% showed mild degenerative changes, while 8% developed patellofemoral OA. Also, of the knees that had mild changes, only 10% went on to patellofemoral OA in the longer term. The presence of patellofemoral OA did not affect the knee score; it did, however, slightly lower the function score, since reciprocating stairs was not as good. It should also be noted that no patients had to be revised because of patellofemoral problems. We feel that Stern et al[1] are being unduly restrictive, and would agree with Kozinn and Scott[41] that the patellofemoral compartment must be examined clinically. The mere presence of radiographic abnormalities should not rule out UKA.

Opposite Compartment Involvement. In the study presented to the SOFCOT symposium, 19% of the initially healthy opposite compartments went on to osteophyte formation, and 9% to loss of joint space from full-blown OA.[42] There was a significant difference between medial and lateral UKAs, since there was a 14% rate of opposite compartment OA after lateral, and only a 7% rate after medial compartment replacement.

Opposite compartment OA had a significant adverse effect on the knee score; however, the effect was less pronounced with lateral UKA. The main cause of opposite compartment deterioration is overcorrection of the deformity. In our study, overcorrection led to loss of opposite compartment joint space in 29% of the cases, both after medial and after lateral compartment replacement. Many other authors have found the same.[18,43–45]

In patients who were not overcorrected, however, there was a 3% rate of opposite compartment space loss after medial, and a 9% rate after lateral compartment replacement. We have, in fact, seen a natural tendency for the opposite compartment to deteriorate over time. This phenomenon may be related to PE debris. However, unless there is malalignment, the condition will remain comparatively asymptomatic. Swank et al[15] also found progression of OA in 2.4%, in nonovercorrected knees. One possible explanation of the phenomenon is afforded by the experimental study of compartment stresses after UKA by Bensadoun.[29] This study showed that overcorrection by as little as 5 degrees results in 88% of the stresses being transferred into the opposite compartment, and that even with correction to normal alignment, 65% of the stresses will still be concentrated in the nonimplanted compartment.

In the light of our study, there is another way in which the phenomenon may be explained: Even in the absence of overcorrection, we found that merely raising the implant joint line in relation to the healthy tibial plateau could cause opposite compartment deterioration and space loss. We will be emphasizing later in this chapter how dangerous it is to try to correct the deformity at all costs, by increasing the thickness of the implant beyond the amount required to make up for wear. UKA can only compensate for wear; it cannot correct bony malalignment such as a tibial varus. It is also interesting to see that the phenomenon was observed mainly with medial UKA. However, overcorrection remains the chief cause of opposite compartment compromise, which will give rise to pain, often of early onset, and will ultimately require revision to a TKA.

Origin of the Failures

Going beyond a review of failures, we must ask ourselves what makes UKAs fail. If it can be shown that most failures are due to inappropriate patient selection, technical errors, or poor and/or badly designed hardware, then preventive action may be taken, and the concept of UKA need not be abandoned. If, however, no definite cause can be found, or if it is seen that the root cause of the problem is the very concept of unicompartmental replacement, then UKA is doomed.

In the literature, there is virtual unanimity on this subject. Only Bartley et al.[39] have reported failure from unpredictable causes; however, these related to 11 PCA devices out of a total of 18 failures. Other studies, such as those by Lindstrand et al,[19] Gacon and Ferreira,[21] and Harilainen et al,[20] stress the high failure rate of this device, and discuss reasons for its failure. In the series reported by Insall and Aglietti[46] and Laskin,[47] the failures observed were related to inappropriate use of the UKA, since attempts had been made—especially with medial UKA—to overcorrect as for an osteotomy, or because a concomitant patellectomy had been performed. As pointed out by Bonutti and Kester,[31] these studies belong to an earlier period, and are not representative of present-day UKA practice. However, as we have seen with the PCA[19,27] and the Oxford knee,[3] even the more recent models may lead to design-related failures. In particular, the survival rate of the PCA UKA appears to match that of the PCA TKA, which, in turn, is worse than that of the Insall TKA. What we see, in fact, is that failure is much more a consequence of the design of the implants used than of the concept of UKA or TKA as such. UKA is an alternative to TKA, rather than an indispensable management principle, while the value of total knee replacement has been established beyond any doubt. This being so, some authors feel—wrongly, to our way of thinking—that there is no need for UKA.

Recent studies using properly designed implants have produced much more encouraging results, which also reflect more accurately what can be achieved with contemporary UKAs. Ten-year implant survivorship has been seen to be in the 81% to 93% range,[5,7,48,49] which comes very close to what can be achieved with TKA.

Two Swedish studies are of interest, because they involved a UKA vs. TKA comparison. Stenström et al[50] compared the failure rate of Marmor UKAs with that of Insall's total condylar device implanted between 1975 and 1989; these devices had not undergone any major design modifications during that period. The study showed an improvement in the implant survival rates, by a drop in the failure rate from 11% in 1975–1977 to 5% in 1984–1986, in the Marmor group, and from 10% in 1978–1980 to 2% in 1984–1986, in the total condylar group. The UKA failure rate remained higher since, as the authors point out, the UKA was used almost exclusively by two-thirds of the participating centers, which meant that some of the patients managed with the device were not, in fact, suitable candidates for UKA. Knutson et al[51] analyzed 30,003 arthroplasties performed between 1976 and 1992. The TKA survival rate gradually improved over this period, to a final failure rate of 4%, while the UKA survival rate remained stable, at 8% of failures, because of the disappointing results of some of the more recent designs (PCA, Oxford knee). Stenström et al[50] reported the results of an unpublished study by Lewold, which excluded the newer UKA designs; this comparison of 15,749 TKAs, 8,425 medial UKAs, and 788 lateral UKAs showed a cumulative failure rate of 7% for the TKAs, of 9% for the medial, and of 11% for the lateral UKAs. This study appears to give an accurate picture of what is happening nowadays, when UKAs are used on a large scale by skilled but not hyperspecialized teams. While there is a slight difference in the failure rates, we would agree with Stenström et al that a failed UKA is much easier to revise than a failed total knee replacement. Also, the postoperative course is much more straightforward following UKA than TKA, and the ROM achieved is better. To us, this means that it is right and proper to continue our policy of recommending UKA.

FAILURE PREVENTION

Since, as we have seen, UKA failure is the result of the faulty use of a sound principle, failure prevention is of paramount importance. The analysis presented above suggests how UKA failure may be prevented. The aspects to be considered are patient selection, surgical technique, and proper hardware selection.

Patient Selection

In 1989, Kozinn and Scott[41] laid down the clinical criteria governing patient selection. In 1991, Chesnut[6] added radiologic criteria. The analysis of the study presented at the SOFCOT symposium[13] allowed us to produce an updated version of the selection criteria for UKA.[52] Broadly speaking, patient selection must comply with the nature of unicompartmental knee replacement: A UKA is a "spacer" designed to correct the intraarticular component of wear in a deformed knee, involving only one tibiofemoral compartment. It may be used in primary as well as in posttraumatic OA, and in osteonecrosis; however, it is unsuitable for the management of inflammatory (rheumatoid) conditions.

In the light of our failure analysis, we have refined our clinical and radiologic criteria. Progress in imaging techniques has been such as to provide reliable preoperative information to guide the decision-making process. This is important, since changing tactics mid-procedure is fraught with many problems and should be avoided at all costs.

Clinical Criteria

The criteria drawn up by Kozinn and Scott[41] remain a benchmark: age over 60 years, body weight <82 kg, low level of activity, minimal knee pain at rest, preoperative flexion ≥90 degrees, flexion contracture <5 degrees; angular deformity <15 degrees, intact ACL, and no cartilage damage in the weight-bearing areas of the opposite compartment. Three of these items need to be considered in more detail:

> Angular deformity, as we shall see, must be looked at on radiographs, and in particular on stress views. To our way of thinking, a global angle is meaningless in patients considered for UKA. What is required is a distinction between the wear element, which may be fully compensated for, and the bony element, which neither can nor should be corrected by the unicompartmental spacer inserted into the joint.
>
> For the fixed flexion deformity, a global figure of 5 degrees appears to us to be unduly restrictive, especially if the deformity is due to impingement on osteophytes. The study by Voss et al[22] showed that 18% of the flexion contracture cases in the series had ≥10 degrees before arthroplasty, which was readily corrected to a mean of 1.6 degrees. These results are borne out by our own experience.
>
> As an additional item, the condition of the ipsilateral hip should be included in the clinical decision-making process before surgery, since, on the one hand, the hip must be dealt with before the knee is tackled, and, on the other hand, a dysplastic hip associated with a valgus deformity of the knee is, to us, an absolute contraindication to a lateral UKA, because of the medial instability that is invariably encountered under these circumstances.

Radiographic Criteria

In every patient, weight-bearing AP and lateral views must be obtained, as well as a skyline view in 30 or 45 degrees of flexion, and stress views. If necessary, posteroanterior (PA) radiographs in 45 degrees flexion should also be taken.[6] If the patient appears to be a suitable candidate for UKA, a stress hip-knee-ankle (HKA) film is important, to guide both patient selection and the performance of the arthroplasty.

Weight-Bearing and Stress Views. The weight-bearing AP view in extension is the basic radiograph. It shows the unicompartmental loss of joint space and the stage to which the condition has progressed. Above all, it allows two contraindications to be detected:

> In medial compartment OA, the existence of a lateral subluxation of the tibia in the coronal plane, with impingement of the medial aspect of the lateral condyle and the tibial spine, especially if uncorrected by a valgus stress maneuver (Fig. 26.4), is a contraindication to UKA, since the impingement would persist after the replacement of the compartment. This pattern has also been described by Capra and Fehring.[48] Where it is seen, a search should be made for ACL compromise, which was seen in 60% of our patients whose weight-bearing AP films showed this pattern.[40]
>
> In lateral compartment OA, medial gaping on weight bearing is an absolute contraindication. Of our lateral UKAs that had to be revised before 5 years, 62% required revision for instability.

The weight-bearing PA view in 45-degree flexion, also known as the Rosenberg or (in France) as the schuss

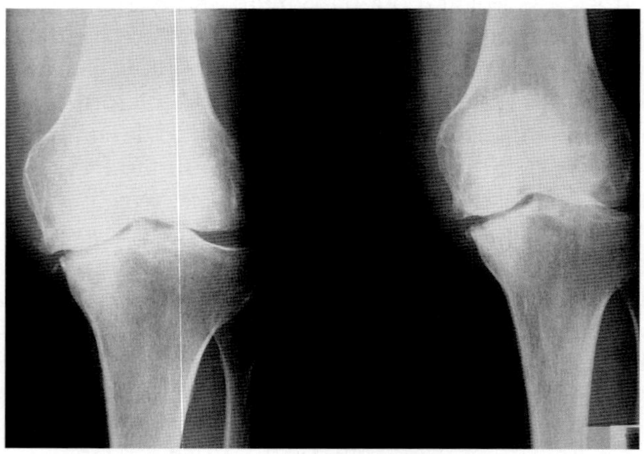

Figure 26.4. Medial compartment OA with lateral tibial translation and impingement of the lateral femoral condyle on the tibial spine, uncorrected by valgus stress. Unsuitable for unicompartmental knee arthroplasty (UKA).

view, is required if the weight-bearing AP film in extension does not show loss of joint space, whereas the weight-bearing lateral view shows such a loss and the clinical examination of the unlocked knee joint demonstrates instability on the concave side of the deformity, suggestive of wear. This wear may sometimes be further toward the back of the condyle—hence the need for a Rosenberg view. As stated also by Chesnut,[6] patients with this pattern are excellent candidates for UKA.

AP stress views must be taken in full extension. They show the extent to which the deformity may be reduced, rule out loss of opposite compartment joint space, and show whether the worn compartment tends to be overcorrected, in which case extreme caution should be exercised, since UKA may lead to the knee being overcorrected. However, these views are useless if there is an associated fixed flexion deformity, or if the films are not taken strictly AP and in full extension, since, under those conditions, they may wrongly suggest that there is overcorrection.

Weight-bearing lateral views are useful in that they show the wear defect. The existence of a posterior defect with anterior subluxation of the tibia >10 mm, which shows up only on the weight-bearing view (Fig. 26.5), is evidence of ACL deficiency, and absolutely rules out UKA. Unfortunately, this pattern is not always seen. In our series, 54% of the knees with a torn ACL failed to show it. Since, in our view, it is crucial to detect ACL deficiency, we would recommend that, in case of doubt, magnetic resonance imaging (MRI) be resorted to.

Skyline Views of the Patella. The radiographic pattern of the patella is often cited by the opponents of UKA as an argument against unicompartmental replacement. However, in our series,[13] no patient had to be revised for patellofemoral problems. This does not, however, mean that the condition of the patellofemoral compartment should be ignored. While simple osteophytes do not constitute a contraindication, the well-known rule that anything that is seen on an x-ray should be compared with the results of the clinical examination applies particularly to the patellofemoral joint.

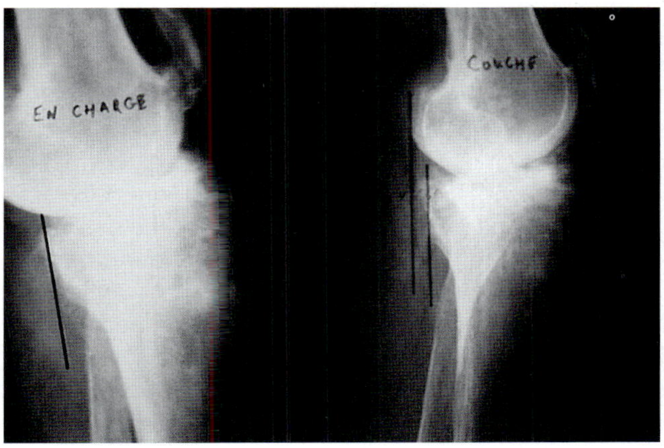

Figure 26.5. Lateral radiographs of the same patient as in Fig. 26.4. The supine view does not reveal the ACL deficiency, which is seen only on the weight-bearing lateral view, where the anterior tibial translation exceeds 10 mm.

Thus, symptomatic patellofemoral OA, with anterior knee pain on maximum flexion, or interference with knee flexion, would, to us, constitute a contraindication to UKA, especially in patients with lateral compartment OA. Equally, the presence of linear opacities, as evidence of true chondrocalcinosis, would make the patient unsuitable for UKA.

The mere presence of osteophytes, however, which can also often be detected on the lateral view, in a patient over 80 years with passive painless flexion >100 degrees, would not be as much of a contraindication as it would in a patient under 70 who is still active. In the latter subject, UKA may give rise to mild patellar pain, which frequently abates over time, but is nonetheless a problem to be taken into account.

Stress HKA Film. If, in the light of the clinical and radiographic workup described, the patient appears to be an appropriate candidate for UKA, a stress HKA film should be obtained. We have been using this technique for some time, and have found it to be a valuable source of information to guide both patient selection and the actual surgical procedure. Unfortunately, this view is not easy to obtain. The film must be taken with the patient supine, the knee in full extension, and with a 7-kg load applied to the knee on the convex side of the deformity in order to reduce the varus or valgus (valgus stress in medial compartment OA; varus stress in lateral compartment OA). The necessary distance between the x-ray source and the patient means that a height-adjustable table that can be lowered right down to floor level will need to be used.

The stress HKA film is superior to the standard weight-bearing HKA film in that it gives an accurate idea of the axis that will be obtained following UKA (Fig. 26.6; also see Fig. 26.8A). The standard HKA film allows a measurement of the overall mechanical axis only. It does not permit a separate assessment of the three components of the deformity—the bony component, the wear component, and a possible instability on the convex side. It should be borne in mind that UKA can only correct wear, while leaving the two other components unaffected.

Thus, a knee with a 15-degree varus deformity may have wear as the chief problem: Once the wear has been compensated for, the residual deformity will be 4 degrees. Under these conditions, UKA is safe. However,

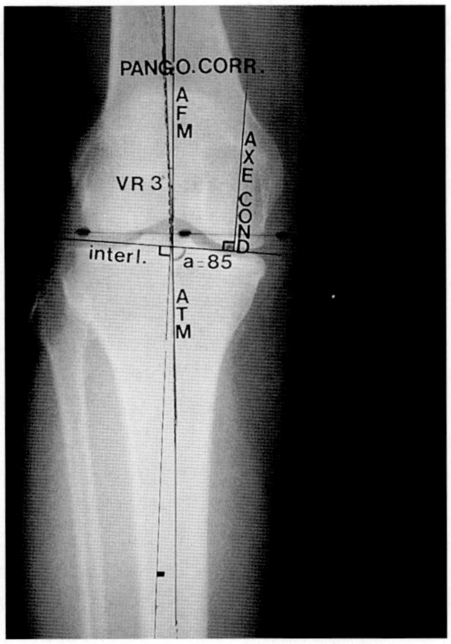

Figure 26.6. Stress hip-knee-ankle (HKA) film. This view allows measurement of the residual lower limb mechanical axis angle (varus = 3 degrees) and of the angle between the joint line and the mechanical axis of the tibia, which provides the tibial resection angle in the coronal plane (85 degrees).

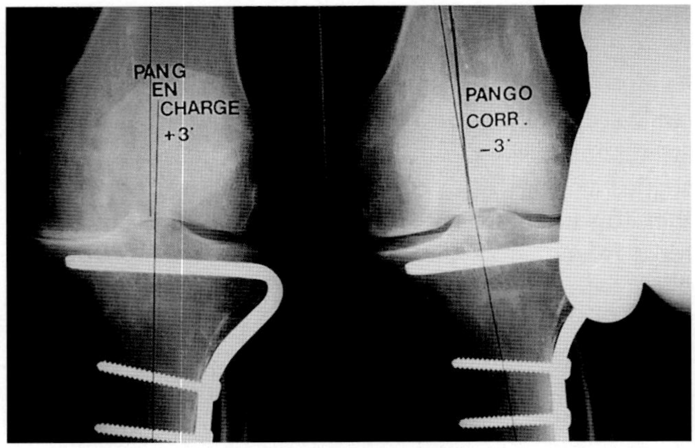

Figure 26.7. Failed high tibial valgus osteotomy. The standard weight-bearing HKA film shows 3 degrees of varus, responsible for the failure. The stress HKA film shows that the axis goes into 3 degrees of valgus, which means that UKA may result in overcorrection.

if the deformity is mainly bony in origin, and if after the application of a valgus stress the residual deformity is 10 degrees despite good correction of the wear, then a UKA would be very likely to deteriorate in the long term. In that case, the failure would not be attributable to undercorrection (a technical error on the part of the surgeon) but to an excessive residual varus deformity (inappropriate patient selection).

In our series,[13] the most durable results were seen in patients who had not been overcorrected, and whose postoperative mechanical axis did not exceed 5 degrees of residual varus in medial UKA, or 5 degrees residual valgus in lateral UKA. The residual deformity after compensation for wear by the implant can be derived only from the stress HKA film. In common with Capra and Fehring,[48] we have found that when UKA is performed to revise a failed valgus osteotomy, the results are excellent if the axis remains in varus; however, if it goes into valgus, the opposite compartment rapidly fails. Once again, the stress HKA film shows in advance whether, after correction of the wear, the overall axis will remain in varus or—as may happen—go into valgus, with all the attendant risks of curtailed implant survival (Fig. 26.7). The stress HKA film is also useful in that it provides information to guide the planning of the bone cuts.

Prevention of Technique-Related Failures

Without going into all the details of surgical technique, here are some vital points to be observed.

Preoperative Planning

Two questions are of crucial importance: (1) What is the target axial correction? and (2) Which are the principles to be observed in order to achieve this target?

Target Axial Correction. In the literature, there is no agreement on this subject. While everybody recommends "slight" undercorrection or correction to normal alignment, and condemns overcorrection, the values accepted by the different authors vary widely: 3 to 7 degrees valgus alignment (Kozinn et al[9]), 3 degrees valgus for medial and 8 degrees valgus for lateral replacements (Scott et al[49]), and correction to within 5 degrees of neutral (Voss et al[22]).

The one fundamental point that needs to be understood in unicondylar knee replacement is that, unlike osteotomies and TKA, which are used to correct an overall deformity including the bony element, UKA can correct only the wear element underlying the deformity. Any attempts to use UKA beyond its inherent capabilities would be inappropriate. The implant would have to be thicker than the spacer required to compensate for wear, which, in turn, would raise the joint line of the implanted compartment, creating wear stress not only in the implant but in the opposite compartment as well, even if the overall axis has not been overcorrected.[42,53] Providing that the joint line level is correct, some degree of implant malposition may be surprisingly well tolerated.[15] However, this tolerance is predicated upon an implant thickness that does not exceed the height required to make up for wear.

There is no ideal correction angle that could be specified; all that can be given are limits that must not be exceeded (see above). The residual angle will be a function of the wear component in the knee, as measured on the stress HKA film, which shows what the residual angle after UKA will be, and whether that angle will meet the patient selection criteria mentioned above.

How to Achieve the Target. *In the coronal plane:* Once again, much can be learned from the stress HKA film, which will, in particular, allow the level of the joint line to be drawn (line joining the midpoints of the medial and the lateral compartment joint lines), and to measure the angle between the joint line and the mechanical axis of the tibia (Fig. 26.7). These measurements show that the cut in the coronal plane will very rarely be at 90 degrees to the mechanical axis of the tibia, especially on the medial side (case of a straight tibia). More often than not, there will be a tibial varus, and the joint line will slope slightly downward and inward. In this situation, a 90-degree cut will unavoidably lead to poor seating of the femoral implant on the tibial plateau (Fig. 26.8C), and any attempt to remedy this situation by increasing the thickness of the plateau beyond what is needed to compensate for wear (Fig. 26.8D) will raise the compartment joint line, and overcorrect the deformity, placing excessive stress on the PE.[42,53] The only thing that can be done is to use a tibial cut that slopes in the coronal plane, to reproduce the natural slope of the joint line (Figs. 26.8B and 26.9). To this end, we have developed tibial cutting guides that can be adjusted in the coronal plane (HLS UNI, Tornier, Saint-Ismier, France; and Cartier Mod. III, Richards, Orthez, France).

In the sagittal plane: To prevent excessive posterior pressure during flexion, it is necessary to restore the ideal level of the joint line also in the AP direction (sagittal plane). Ideally, the cut should be made in such a way as to match the preoperative articular slope. Once again, no ideal mean value can be specified: The surgeon will need to be guided by the individual patient's pattern. Since we are dealing with centered OA (cases with posterior defects and anterior subluxation having been ruled out at the selection stage), and since there must be an intact ACL, restoring the slope of the plateau should be safe, up to 10 degrees posterior slope as measured from the axis of the tibia on the lateral view. This is in line with what has been recommended by Kozinn et al[9] and Voss et al.[22] Møller et al[54] go so far as to state that horizontal placement of the tibial component in the sagittal plane will lead to severe stress being placed on the ACL during flexion. If, when flexing the patient's knee during surgery, lifting off of the anterior part of the tibial plateau, extrusion of the plateau, or extrusion

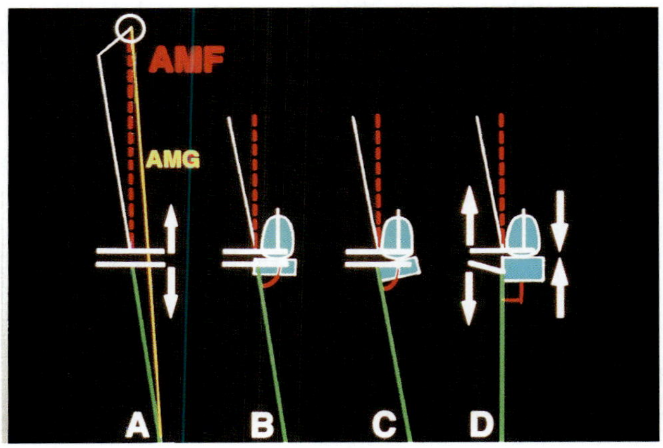

Figure 26.8. **A:** Mechanical axes plotted on stress HKA films. **B:** Ideal orientation of the plateau in the coronal plane, paralleling the joint line of the healthy compartment. **C:** Plateau positioned at 90 degrees to the mechanical axis of the tibia, but below the joint line, which prevents overcorrection. This is a disturbed femoral-on-tibial component pattern. **D:** Misguided attempt to correct this pattern by inserting a thicker plateau. This causes overcorrection of the deformity, with the risk of PE and of opposite compartment wear.

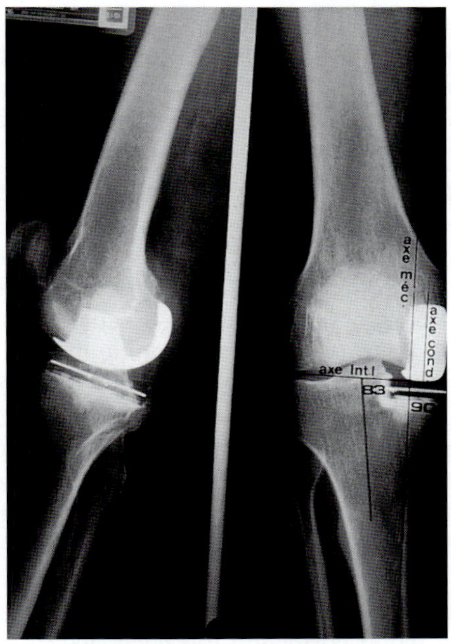

Figure 26.9. Radiograph of a well-inserted implant. Note the tibial resection angle in the coronal plane paralleling the healthy compartment joint line; this allows proper seating of the femoral component on the plateau, and places the joint line at the correct level.

of the femoral component are noted, the slope should be immediately checked and, if need be, adjusted. These technical rules must be obeyed in order to make the UKA the resurfacing prosthesis it is designed to be. As stressed by Swienckowski and Page[55] and Cartier and Cheaib,[56] the immediate success and the long-term results of the arthroplasty will depend on the surgeon's observance of these principles.

General Points Concerning Technique

Four points are of crucial importance:

1. The approach chosen must satisfy two requirements. First, it must be in keeping with the less invasive nature of unicompartmental replacement, so as to allow rapid recovery after surgery. To use Cartier's well-known phrase, a UKA is not "half a TKA." Large incisions, and eversion of the patella, should be avoided wherever possible. Second, the approach should allow for future revision, should the need arise. For a medial replacement, it should be anteromedial; for a lateral replacement, it should be strictly anterolateral, without crossing the tibial tubercle.
2. *Ligament release* should not be performed on any patient.[57] Since (with proper patient selection) the deformities will be inherently reducible, the ligaments on the concave side are the only possible guide to the thickness of the unicompartmental spacer needed to make up for wear. In fact, a minor residual laxity of 2 to 3 mm in slight flexion, on the implanted side, is desirable,[55] since it is the best guarantee of undercorrection.
3. Specific lateral UKA problems, which have been studied in depth by Cartier and Landreau,[58] mainly concern the seating of the femoral component. Centering the component in rotation may be difficult because of dysplasia, which may lead to excessive internal rotation in the positioning of the femoral component. This will cause impingement of the anterior part of the component on the lateral tibial spine during extension, and with the patella during flexion. Therefore, the preparation of the implant bed differs from what is required for a medial compartment replacement. Any lateral marginal osteophyte will need to be left in place, since this is often the only support zone for the anterior part of the femoral component when correcting the excessive internal rotation of the lateral femoral condyle. However, osteophytes in the notch should be dealt with exactly as in medial compartment replacement: they should be removed, to protect the ACL.
4. Stability check before cementing is vital. The trial components must remain stable during the ROM trial with the patella in situ. Any instability noted must be remedied before the definitive implant is cemented in place. The cement should be applied in a thin layer, without any invasive plugs that would cause problems should revision be required at a future date.

Selection of Hardware

Since this is a somewhat sensitive subject, we will outline the broad principles that have emerged from our analysis of past UKA failures.

Instrumentation

The instruments must enable the surgeon to perform a limited approach. Extramedullary alignment is preferable to the use of intramedullary rods, which are more invasive, may give rise to postoperative haemorrhage, and, with lateral UKAs, may cause problems since the rod entry point is very close to the articular surface of the medial femoral condyle.

Implants

Femoral Component. In his description of the history of the Brigham device, Scott[18] showed the way in which the femoral component evolved, through a number of design modifications, to become wider. We feel that this increased width is a welcome feature. Lindstrand et al[19,27] as well as Gacon and Ferreira[21] and Harilainen et al[20] have stressed the specific risks inherent in the PCA UKA, which has suffered from a high rate of femoral component loosening. This experience has confirmed us in our preference for resurfacing implants over those requiring bone resection, even though the latter give better control of the level of the joint line and permit cementless fixation (a controversial subject in its own right). We also feel that the radius of the posterior curvature must be degressive, to allow the component to self-stabilize in maximum flexion, without any risk of extrusion or of excessive pressure on the posterior part of the plateau.

Tibial Component. The top of the component should be flat, to allow physiologic rolling-sliding, made possible by the preservation of the cruciates. Unfortunately, this design is prone to wear in the long term. This is why a different concept has been evolved, which is represented by the Oxford meniscal-bearing UKA, in which conforming components are used to prevent wear. This attractive concept, however, is fraught with two problems: First, several authors[3,50] and the designers themselves[37] have reported bearing dislocation. Second, the procedure involves complex balancing of the ligaments, and the search for perfect stability may result in the insertion of an excessively thick plateau, and, hence, overcorrection.[3]

All-Polyethylene vs. Metal Backing

As early as 1979, Marmor[59] had stressed the wear risk inherent in 6-mm plateaus. A study by Ryd et al[60] showed that cold flow may occur even in 12-mm PE components. The study by Walker et al[61] showed the importance of metal backing in the reduction of cold flow. This technique, widely used in TKAs, was then applied to UKAs. Unfortunately, as pointed out above, UKA-specific problems related to the thickness of the PE above the metal backing were encountered, and some models were found to be extremely prone to wear.[18–20,27] To control this problem, Engh et al[23] recommend a minimum thickness of 6 mm of actual PE above the metal backing, and of as much as 8 mm over any screw holes in implants for cementless fixation. Bartley et al[39] found wear to be sometimes more pronounced peripherally, where the PE is thinner.

As for the loosening risk, a finite element analysis by Takai et al[17] suggests that metal backing improves the stress distribution; conversely, in a similar study, Blankevoort et al[62] found that the rigidity of the metal backing combined with the loading pattern in flexion and extension may increase the stresses at the implant-bone interface. This latter idea seems to be borne out by an in-vivo study by Witvoët et al,[36] which showed a larger number of radiolucencies in the group of 180 (metal-backed) Lotus II devices than in 135 (non–metal-backed) Lotus I. These considerations also prompted Heck et al[7] as well as Lindstrand and Stenström[27] to question the utility of metal backing.

Our experience is somewhat different, since Cartier uses either all-PE or metal backing with at least 7 to 8 mm of PE, depending on the patient's body weight, while the senior author, after having used all-PE for a long time, now has an original design that features a PE component set in a metal ring. This provides the best of both worlds, in that it allows full PE thickness in the weight-bearing zone and prevents cold flow thanks to the encircling metal ring. However, a longer follow-up will be required to see whether this innovative design is as beneficial as it is thought to be.

The problems of PE as such, and of the sterilization of the material, have been discussed above.

Cemented vs. Cementless

On this question, the jury is still out. We feel that the disadvantages of cementing are minimal, providing that the cement is used sparingly, and that no attempt is made to use cement to remedy a lack of stability of the trial components. The trials must be perfectly stable without any cement, before the definitive components are cemented in place.

Apart from some rare cases in which a cement fragment missed at surgery has had to be removed subsequently,[8] we find cementing to be superior in a number of ways to cementless fixation, which requires femoral resection and a metal-backed tibial component. Also, with cementless implants, the patients may have to be kept off weight bearing in the early postoperative period. This would negate one of the benefits of UKA that is much appreciated by our elderly patients—the ability to walk and bear weight very early on. Moreover, the possible defects caused in the event of a revision for conditions other than loosening would militate against cementless fixation.

One interesting possibility at present being explored is the use of hydroxyapatite-coated implants.[63]

REVISION OF FAILED IMPLANTS

Even with good patient selection, meticulous surgery, and judicious hardware selection, UKAs may have to be revised. Three questions need to be answered: (1) Are UKAs inherently difficult to revise? In other words, does UKA mean that the patient will have a less good result next time around? Or, to put it differently, is UKA a conservative arthroplasty, as claimed by Scott[18]? (2) How can we prevent difficult revision surgery? and (3) How should revision be performed?

Are UKAs Difficult to Revise?

On the question of the ease or difficulty of revision, opinions are divided. Much would seem to depend on what failures had been encountered by the different authors, and what had led to the failures in the first instance. Thus, two studies—by Padgett et al[45] and Barrett and Scott[14]—showed major difficulties, especially with loss of bone stock, which was found in 76% of Padgett's 21 revisions. However, Barrett and Scott felt that the results have improved with the advent of newer and better models.

These studies contrast with the much larger number of studies[4,9,18,44,51,64] reporting no major problems being encountered at revision, and stating that the patients were not worse off concerning the final result than they would have been if they had been given a TKA first time around. Also, Jackson et al,[65] in a comparison of 23 revisions following high tibial valgus osteotomy and 20 revisions following UKA, found a 30% complication rate in postosteotomy, and no complications in post-UKA revisions. Levine et al[44] stated that the results of UKA-TKA conversion were comparable to the results for primary TKA, and superior to those for TKA-TKA conversion, with a much lower primary revision rate, which was also seen by Knutson et al.[51] Our experience has been along the same lines. We may, therefore, conclude that, when correctly used, UKA does not in itself make for more difficult revision surgery, neither does it put the patient at a disadvantage in the event of a revision.

How to Prevent Difficulties at Revision

This issue is important, since inappropriate patient selection, poor primary surgery, and certain UKA designs can set the stage for problems at revision. Patient selection raises difficulties when there is medial instability associated with, or complicating, a lateral compartment replacement. This is the only case in which we have had major problems, and where we have had to resort to very constrained patterns (Fig. 26.1).

There are also technique and hardware factors to consider. Excessive tibial resection and invasive cement plugs cause loss of bone stock, which makes revision less straightforward. Devices requiring major resection and/or very large pegs may cause damage, either immediately or in difficult removal cases (cementless implants). This damage would be worse than that caused by the insertion of a "lightly" cemented implant.

Patient monitoring is rarely mentioned; however, the analysis of our series[13] has shown how vital this follow-up can be. Some of our patients appeared to tolerate their failed implants, and especially femoral component loosening, surprisingly well. This may have been due to their age or to the fact that they were not very active. In our study presented at the SOFCOT symposium,[13] of the 67 radiologically overt loosenings, only 30 were revised. In these cases, we found deep subsidence of the implants into the bone, and had to use a much more aggressive technique for revision, thereby negating a potential benefit of UKA. Because of the surprising tolerance seen in some of our patients, we have now set up a system to ensure that all patients are routinely examined once a year.

How to Revise a Failed UKA

UKA or TKA?

In common with Knutson et al,[51] we recommend that a failed UKA should be revised to a TKA: In our study,[13] 71% of the 14 patients with failed UKAs (isolated wear) who were revised to another UKA had a repeat failure early on.

Which TKA?

The choice will need to be made in light of the cause of failure and of the extent of bone loss following the removal of the failed UKA. In our series, more than half (52%) of the 50 revisions to a TKA were done using a standard implant. Similarly, Levine et al,[44] in 31 UKA-to-TKA conversions (21 for tibial PE wear; 10 for progression of OA), used primary posterior cruciate ligament (PCL)-sparing TKAs in 30 cases and one PCL-sacrificing TKA.

The filling of bone defects depends on the depth of the defect(s). The tibial cut must not be more than 10 mm compared with the unaffected side. The existing damage should not be made worse by overzealous immediate curetting of the bed for the new implant. A minimal resection should be performed, as soon as the UKA has been removed; after that, the extent of the defect may be assessed. More often than not, no filling will be required. For contained defects, simple filling with cement or a bone autograft will suffice. For noncontained defects, with a loss of bone stock of more than two-thirds of the surface, we prefer the use of metal augments to that of bone grafts. Whenever tibial or femoral bone defects have had to be filled, a stemmed component will need to be used.

In summary, difficulties at revision basically stem from two causes:

The index UKA may have been done in the wrong kind of patient, or using a faulty technique (major bone resection; overuse of cement). These errors will produce an unduly large number of difficult-to-revise cases.[45]

The revision hardware may be unsuitable, or insufficient provision may have been made for unforeseen situations at surgery. These deficiencies will result in improvisation, which may lead to the need for a second revision. That eventuality is all the more worrying in that the patients concerned are elderly.

In light of these considerations, we have produced a specification for the ideal revision device, which should have a stemmed tibial component and come in modular form, with stem extensions and metal augments for the femoral and tibial components.

Whether the revision implant should be cruciate-retaining or posterior-stabilized is left to the individual surgeon's preference. The only exception to this rule concerns the revisions of UKAs for ACL deficiency with major anterior subluxation of the tibia on the weight-bearing lateral views. In such cases, we would prefer a posterior-stabilized device, which is more constrained, to prevent the recurrence of the AP instability that a TKA retaining only the PCL would produce.[66] Where the failure is due to mediolateral instability, especially in medial instability after lateral compartment replacement, a very constrained implant (in some cases, a hinge prosthesis) should be used, unless the ligaments can be perfectly retuned by the use of a posterior-stabilized device.

These recommendations are the result of our experience, which has shown that preoperative planning—vital though it is—may not allow the surgeon to foresee every eventuality. A modular revision device should make it possible to handle unforeseen circumstances and would be better than "customized" implants, which, even nowadays, cannot be relied upon to produce satisfactory results in each and every patient. Where these recommendations have been followed, the second revision rate after initial UKA-to-TKA revision has been seen to be much lower than that after TKA-to-TKA revisions.[51,67]

The revision operation itself has fewer complications.[44,64] Also, many authors feel that the result of a properly performed revision from a UKA is identical to that of a primary TKA.[18,44,51] In our series of 50 UKAs revised to TKAs,[64] the only difference observed was a lower rate of excellent results, and a slightly poorer mean ROM as compared with primary TKAs.

CONCLUSION

Our study clearly shows that unicompartmental arthroplasty is a valid concept that should be an integral part of the range of treatment options offered to the elderly patient with unicompartmental OA. Compared with osteotomy, UKA has the advantages of early weight bearing, greater and more lasting pain relief,[10,43] and of easier revision in case of failure.[65] UKA is superior to TKA because it has low morbidity, does not require transfusion, allows rapid recovery, and has a superior ROM outcome.[5,10,16,68] Also, revision is easier.[67]

The only drawback is that UKA is demanding in terms of surgical technique, choice of hardware, and, above all, patient selection. However, the proportion of patients suitable for UKA is probably nearer the 10% to 20% mark[9,21] than the 6% suggested by Stern et al.[1] The reluctance on the part of surgeons in some countries to practice this form of arthroplasty stems from a shortage of centers teaching the technique, or from purely financial considerations,[31,69] which should be reviewed and revised before long, to take account of the fact that UKA has much to offer to the elderly, who make up an ever-increasing proportion of our demographic pattern.

References

1. Stern S, Becker M, Insall J. Unicondylar knee arthroplasty. An evaluation of selection criteria. *Clin Orthop* 1993;286:143–148.
2. MacIntosh D. Hemiarthroplasty of the knee using a space occupying prosthesis for painful varus and valgus deformities. *J Bone Joint Surg* 1958;40A:1431.
3. Lewold S, Goodman S, Knutson K, et al. Oxford meniscal bearing knee versus the Marmor knee in unicompartmental arthroplasty for arthrosis. A Swedish multicenter survival study. *J Arthroplasty* 1995;10:722–731.
4. Marmor L. Unicompartmental knee arthroplasty. Ten- to 13-year follow-up study. *Clin Orthop* 1988;226:14–20.
5. Rougraff B, Heck D, Gibson A. A comparison of tricompartmental and unicompartmental arthroplasty for the treatment of gonarthrosis. *Clin Orthop* 1991; 273:157–164.
6. Chesnut W. Preoperative diagnostic protocol to predict candidates for unicompartmental arthroplasty. *Clin Orthop* 1991;273:146–150.
7. Heck D, Marmor L, Gibson A, et al. Unicompartmental knee arthroplasty. A multicenter investigation with long-term follow-up evaluation. *Clin Orthop* 1993;286:154–159.
8. Rosenberg A, Galante J, Voss F, et al. Miller-Galante unicompartmental knee arthroplasty at two to five year follow-up. In: Cartier P, Epinette J, Deschamps G, Hernigou P, (eds). *Unicompartmental Knee Arthroplasty*, vol 61. Paris: Expansion Scientifique Française, 1997:220–222.
9. Kozinn S, Marx C, Scott R. Unicompartmental knee arthroplasty. A 4.5–6-year follow-up study with a metal-backed tibial component. *J Arthroplasty* 1989;4(suppl): S1–S10.
10. Jefferson R, Whittle M. Functional biomechanical results of unicompartmental knee arthroplasty compared with total condylar arthroplasty and tibial osteotomy. *J Bone Joint Surg* 1990;72B:161–162.
11. Hernigou P, de Ladoucette A, Raou D, et al. L'arthroplastie unicompartimentale interne dans la gonarthrose. Résultat de 483 prothèses avec un recul maximum de 20 ans. *Rev Chir Orthop* 1996;82(suppl 1):27–30.
12. Broughton N, Newman J, Baily R. Unicompartmental replacement and high tibial osteotomy for osteoarthritis of the knee. A comparative study after 5–10 years' follow-up. *J Bone Joint Surg* 1986;68B:447–452.
13. Hernigou P, Deschamps G. Prothèses unicompartimentales du genou. Symposium. *Rev Chir Orthop* 1996; 82(suppl 1):25–60.
14. Barrett W, Scott R. Revision of failed unicondylar unicompartmental knee arthroplasty. *J Bone Joint Surg* 1987;69A:1328–1335.
15. Swank M, Stulberg S, Jiganti J, et al. The natural history of unicompartmental arthroplasty. An eight-year follow-up study with survivorship analysis. *Clin Orthop* 1993; 286:130–142.
16. Callahan C, Drake B, Heck D, et al. Patient outcomes following unicompartmental or bicompartmental knee arthroplasty. A meta-analysis. *J Arthroplasty* 1995;10: 141–150.
17. Takai S, Yoshino N, Hirasawa Y, et al. Stress analysis of the proximal tibia after unicompartmental knee arthroplasty with finite element method. In: Cartier P, Epinette J, Deschamps G, Hernigou P (eds). *Unicompartmental Knee Arthroplasty*, vol 61. Paris: Expansion Scientifique Française, 1997:61–67.

18. Scott R. Mistakes made and lessons learned after 2 decades of unicompartmental knee replacement. In: Cartier P, Epinette J, Deschamps G, Hernigou P (eds). *Unicompartmental Knee Arthroplasty*, vol 61. Paris: Expansion Scientifique Française, 1997:163–166.

19. Lindstrand A, Stenström A, Lewold S. Multicenter study of unicompartmental knee revision. PCA, Marmor and St. Georg compared in 3,777 cases of arthrosis. *Acta Orthop Scand* 1992;63:256–259.

20. Harilainen A, Sanselin J, Ylinen P, et al. Revision of the PCA unicompartmental knee: 52 arthrosis knees followed for 2–5 years. *Acta Orthop Scand* 1993;64:428–430.

21. Gacon G, Ferreira A. Results of PCA cementless unicompartmental knee replacement. An analysis of 110 cases at a mean follow-up of five years. In: Cartier P, Epinette J, Deschamps G, Hernigou P (eds). *Unicompartmental Knee Arthroplasty*, vol 61. Paris: Expansion Scientifique Française, 1997:223–229.

22. Voss F, Sheinkop M, Galante J, et al. Miller-Galante unicompartmental knee arthroplasty at 2- to 5-year follow-up evaluations. *J Arthroplasty* 1995;10:764–771.

23. Engh G, Dwyer K, Hanes C. Polyethylene wear of metal-backed tibial components in total and unicompartmental knee prostheses. *J Bone Joint Surg* 1992;74B:9–17.

24. Neyret P, Chatain F, Deschamps G. Unicompartmental knee replacement: biomaterials and design. In: Cartier P, Epinette J, Deschamps G, Hernigou P (eds). *Unicompartmental Knee Arthroplasty*, vol 61. Paris: Expansion Scientifique Française, 1997:56–60.

25. Langlais F. Le polyéthylène en 1997. Cahiers d'Enseignement de la SOFCOT. *Conférences d'Enseignement* 1997; no. 5:53–69.

26. Cartier P. Unicompartmental knee arthroplasty: Where do we stand? Where do we go? In: Cartier P, Epinette J, Deschamps G, Hernigou P (eds). *Unicompartmental Knee Arthroplasty*, vol 61. Paris: Expansion Scientifique Française, 1997:287–294.

27. Lindstrand A, Stenström A. Polyethylene wear of the PCA unicompartmental knee. Prospective 5 (4–8) year study of 120 arthrosis knees. *Acta Orthop Scand* 1992; 63:260–262.

28. Berger R, Andriacchi T, Galante J. Biomechanics of unicompartmental knee arthroplasty. Gait analysis for the study of knee replacement. In: Cartier P, Epinette J, Deschamps G, Hernigou P (eds). *Unicompartmental Knee Arthroplasty*, vol 61. Paris: Expansion Scientifique Française, 1997:32–39.

29. Bensadoun J. Biomechanical aspects of unicompartmental arthroplasty. In: Cartier P, Epinette J, Deschamps G, Hernigou P (eds). *Unicompartmental Knee Arthroplasty*, vol 61. Paris: Expansion Scientifique Française, 1997:3–11.

30. Goodfellow J, O'Connor J. The mechanics of the knee and prosthesis design. *J Bone Joint Surg* 1978;60B: 358–369.

31. Bonutti P, Kester M. Unicompartmental knee arthroplasty: a US experience. In: Cartier P, Epinette J, Deschamps G, Hernigou P (eds). *Unicompartmental Knee Arthroplasty*, vol 61. Paris: Expansion Scientifique Française, 1997:260–266.

32. Landreau P, Cartier P. Résultats des prothèses unicompartimentales externes. *Rev Chir Orthop* 1996;82(suppl 1):30–32.

33. Deschamps G, Lapeyre B. La rupture du ligament croisé antérieur: une cause d'échec souvent méconnue des prothèses unicompartimentales du genou. A propos d'une série de 79 prothèses Lotus revues au delà de 5 ans. *Rev Chir Orthop* 1987;73:544–551.

34. Dejour H, Deschamps G, Walch G, et al. Arthrose du genou sur laxité chronique antérieure. *Rev Chir Orthop* 1987;73:157–170.

35. Chassin E, Mikosz R, Andriacchi T, et al. Functional analysis of cemented medial unicompartmental knee arthroplasty. *J Arthroplasty* 1996;11:553–559.

36. Witvoët J, Aubriot J, Pidhorz L, et al. The Lotus knee prosthesis in unicompartmental osteoarthrosis of the knee. In: Cartier P, Epinette J, Deschamps G, Hernigou P (eds). *Unicompartmental Knee Arthroplasty*, vol 61. Paris: Expansion Scientifique Française, 1997:202–209.

37. Goodfellow J, O'Connor J. Retention of the anterior cruciate ligament in arthroplasty of the knee. *J Bone Joint Surg* 1988;70B:333.

38. Goodfellow J, O'Connor J, Murray D. Principles of meniscal bearing arthroplasty for unicompartmental knee replacement. In: Cartier P, Epinette J, Deschamps G, Hernigou P (eds). *Unicompartmental Knee Arthroplasty*, vol 61. Paris: Expansion Scientifique Française, 1997:174–180.

39. Bartley R, Stulberg D, Robb W, et al. Polyethylene wear in unicompartmental knee arthroplasty. *Clin Orthop* 1994;299:18–24.

40. Deschamps G. Prothèses unicompartimentales: Causes d'échec ligamentaires. *Rev Chir Orthop* 1996;82(suppl 1):34–36.

41. Kozinn S, Scott R. Unicondylar knee arthroplasty. *J Bone Joint Surg* 1989;71A:145–150.

42. Dejour D, Chatain F, Habi S. Rôle de l'articulation fémoro-patellaire et du compartiment opposé dans la dégradation du résultat fonctionnel des prothèses unicompartimentales. *Rev Chir Orthop* 1996;82(suppl 1): 37–39.

43. Weale A, Newman J. Unicompartmental arthroplasty and high tibial osteotomy for osteoarthrosis of the knee. A comparative study with a 12- to 17-year follow-up period. *Clin Orthop* 1994;302:134–137.

44. Levine W, Ozuna R, Scott R, et al. Conversion of failed modern unicompartmental arthroplasty to total knee arthroplasty. *J Arthroplasty* 1996;11:797–801.

45. Padgett D, Stern S, Insall J. Revision total knee arthroplasty for failed unicompartmental replacement. *J Bone Joint Surg* 1991;73A:186–190.

46. Insall J, Aglietti P A five- to seven-year follow-up of unicondylar arthroplasty. *J Bone Joint Surg* 1980;62A: 1329–1337.

47. Laskin R. Unicompartmental tibiofemoral resurfacing arthroplasty. *J Bone Joint Surg* 1978;60A:182–185.

48. Capra S, Fehring T. Unicondylar arthroplasty. A survivorship analysis. *J Arthroplasty* 1992;7:247–251.

49. Scott R, Cobb A, McQueary F, et al. Unicompartmental knee arthroplasty. Eight- to 12-year follow-up evaluation with survivorship analysis. *Clin Orthop* 1991;271: 96–100.

50. Stenström A, Lindstrand A, Lewold S. Unicompartmental knee arthroplasty with special reference to the Swedish knee arthroplasty register. In: Cartier P, Epinette J, Deschamps G, Hernigou P (eds). *Unicompartmental Knee Arthroplasty*, vol 61. Paris: Expansion Scientifique Française, 1997:159–162.

51. Knutson K, Lewold S, Robertson O, et al. The Swedish knee arthroplasty register. A nation-wide study of 30,003 knees 1976–1992. *Acta Orthop Scand* 1994;65:375–386.

52. Deschamps G. Prothèses unicompartimentales—l'indication idéale. *Rev Chir Orthop* 1996;82(suppl 1):53–54.

53. Dejour H, Dejour D, Habi S. Fate of the patellofemoral and of the opposite tibiofemoral compartment, following unicompartmental knee replacement. In: Cartier P, Epinette J, Deschamps G, Hernigou P (eds). *Unicompartmental Knee Arthroplasty*, vol 61. Paris: Expansion Scientifique Française, 1997:147–150.

54. Møller J, Weeth R, Keller J. Unicompartmental arthroplasty of the knee. Cadaver study of tibial component placement. *Acta Orthop Scand* 1985;56:115–119.

55. Swienckowski J, Page B. Medial unicompartmental arthroplasty of the knee. Use of the L-cut and comparison with the tibial inset method. *Clin Orthop* 1989; 239:161–167.

56. Cartier P, Cheaib S. Unicondylar knee arthroplasty: 2–10 years of follow-up evaluation. *J Arthroplasty* 1987;2: 157–162.

57. Emerson R, Head W, Peters P. Soft tissue balance and alignment in medial unicompartmental knee arthroplasty. *J Bone Joint Surg* 1992;74B:807–810.

58. Cartier P, Landreau P. Technique de la prothèse unicompartimentale externe. *Rev Chir Orthop* 1996; 82(suppl 1):25–60.

59. Marmor L. Marmor modular knee in unicondylar disease. Minimum four-year follow-up. *J Bone Joint Surg* 1979; 61A:347–353.

60. Ryd L, Lindstrand A, Stenström A, et al. Cold flow reduced by metal-backing. An in vivo roentgen stereophotogrammetric analysis of unicompartmental tibial components. *Acta Orthop Scand* 1990;61:21–25.

61. Walker P, Greene D, Reilly D, et al. Fixation of tibial components of knee prostheses. *J Bone Joint Surg* 1981;63A:258–267.

62. Blankevoort L, Van As R, Huiskes R. Finite element analysis of the Guépar Lotus I and II unicompartmental knee prostheses. In: Cartier P, Epinette J, Deschamps G, Hernigou P (eds). *Unicompartmental Knee Arthroplasty*, vol 61. Paris: Expansion Scientifique Française, 1997:68–73.

63. Epinette J, Edidin A. Hydroxyapatite-coated unicompartmental knee replacement. A report of five to six years' follow-up of the HA Unix tibial component. In: Cartier P, Epinette J, Deschamps G, Hernigou P (eds). *Unicompartmental Knee Arthroplasty*, vol 61. Paris: Expansion Scientifique Française, 1997:243–259.

64. Deschamps G, Cartier P. Revision of unicompartmental prostheses. In: Cartier P, Epinette J, Deschamps G, Hernigou P (eds). *Unicompartmental Knee Arthroplasty*, vol 61. Paris: Expansion Scientifique Française, 1997:152–155.

65. Jackson M, Sarangi P, Newman J. Revision total knee arthroplasty: comparison of outcome following primary proximal tibial osteotomy or unicompartmental arthroplasty. *J Arthroplasty* 1994;9:539–542.

66. Julliard R. Communications particulières. 65ème réunion annuelle de la SOFCOT—Paris 1991. *Rev Chir Orthop* 1991;77(suppl 1):161.

67. Stuart M, Larson J, Morrey B. Reoperation after condylar revision total knee arthroplasty. *Clin Orthop* 1993; 286:168–173.

68. Laurencin C, Zelicof S, Scott R, et al. Unicompartmental versus total knee arthroplasty in the same patient. A comparative study. *Clin Orthop* 1991;273:151–156.

69. Grelsamer R. Unicompartmental osteoarthrosis of the knee. *J Bone Joint Surg* 1995;77A:278–292.

Chapter 27

PATELLOFEMORAL COMPLICATIONS FOLLOWING TOTAL KNEE ARTHROPLASTY

Phillip J. Lewandowski and Gerard A. Engh

Total knee arthroplasty (TKA) is a predictable and durable means of alleviating pain associated with knee arthrosis. The evolution of component design and surgical techniques has resulted in excellent functional results and increased range of motion. This success has been due in part to the addition of patellofemoral joint resurfacing. However, because of the potential for complications, including patellofemoral instability, soft tissue impingement, component failure, and loosening,[1–3] the role of patellar resurfacing in TKA remains controversial. To understand the nature of these complications, knowledge of the pertinent extensor mechanism biomechanics and current literature on patellar resurfacing is necessary. Hence, a review of patellofemoral complications and their prevention and management is presented first.

EXTENSOR MECHANISM BIOMECHANICS

The patellofemoral articulation and the extensor mechanism are crucial to the biomechanical function of the knee. The patella creates a mechanical advantage for the quadriceps by centralizing its forces and increasing its moment arm, while providing an articulating surface with a low coefficient of friction. The patella also protects the anterior knee joint from trauma, prevents attritional wear of the quadriceps tendon, and improves the cosmetic appearance of the knee.

The contact force at the patellofemoral joint is equal to the resultant force generated by tension of the quadriceps muscle and the patellar tendon. At full extension the patellofemoral joint reaction force is zero and increases with increasing knee flexion angle up to 90 degrees.[4,5] Beyond 90 degrees of flexion, the quadriceps tendon contacts the femoral articular surface and at 120 degrees of flexion supports as much as one-third of the total contact force on the extensor mechanism.[5,6] Studies have demonstrated the high contact forces at this articulation. The patellofemoral joint reaction force is one-half to one times body weight with level walking, three to four times body weight with stair climbing, and as high as seven to eight times body weight with deep knee bending.[1–7]

EXTENSOR MECHANISM BIOMECHANICS AND TOTAL KNEE ARTHROPLASTY

Total knee arthroplasty alters knee kinematics by changing patellar motion relative to the femur and decreasing the patellofemoral contact area. Patellar components must be able to withstand high-contact forces and provide a stable articulation throughout a wide range of motion. The success of the resurfacing also depends on the patellar component's ability to withstand the eccentric forces generated during rotational, translational, and tilting movements of the patella without unacceptable loosening.[6] The most extreme examples of altered kinematics following knee arthroplasty occur with constrained, hinged devices that reduce the complex multiaxis motion of the knee to a single axis of rotation, thereby increasing patellofemoral complications, especially patellar instability.[8]

Patellofemoral joint function after TKA is dependent on several factors: (1) total thickness of the resurfaced patella; (2) alignment of the femoral, tibial, and patellar components in all three planes; (3) changes in joint line position; and (4) functional patellar ligament length. A neutral alignment of the prosthetic components has been shown to establish excellent patellofemoral joint function and range of motion with fewer component failures. To achieve optimal alignment, the surgeon should reestablish the prosthetic joint line to within 8 mm of the natural joint line. Ideally the tibial component should be placed at or posterior to the midcoronal line of the tibia to optimize the extensor mechanism moment arm. The inferior pole of the prosthetic patella should be placed 1 to 3 cm above the joint line.[9]

PATELLAR RESURFACING: PROS AND CONS

Before the advent of patellofemoral resurfacing, anterior knee pain was reported in up to 50% of patients undergoing TKA with such designs.[7,10] As a result, prostheses were modified to include a trochlear flange on the femoral component and an optional polyethylene patellar implant. Many authors believe that patellar resurfacing has contributed to improved function and the alleviation of anterior knee pain.[1] Unfortunately, with the addition of patellar resurfacing, new complications have emerged, including those that are discussed in this chapter.

Some surgeons recommend routinely resurfacing the patella,[10–12] some resurface selectively,[7,13,14] and others not at all.[15–17] After reviewing the literature, Rand[8] developed guidelines recommending patellar resurfacing for all patients who have rheumatoid or other inflammatory arthritis, eburnated bone in the patellofemoral joint, cystic changes in the patella, a lack of congruency between the patella and the trochlear groove of the prosthesis, or maltracking of the patella. His only contraindication to resurfacing the patella is insufficient bone stock.

One way to evaluate resurfacing of the patella is to study patients with bilateral TKA, with one side resurfaced and the other side not resurfaced. In 25 patients with advanced patellofemoral disease, Enis et al[11] compared the clinical results in 22 patients with resurfacing of the right patella but not the left. Of these patients, 10 initially preferred the knee with the resurfaced patella and 12 were undecided. However, later follow-up showed a trend toward preference of the resurfaced knee. After considering subjective and objective data, the authors of this study concluded that (1) patellar resurfacing offers a stronger and more pain-free knee; (2) lateral retinacular release is needed more frequently to achieve proper soft tissue balance with patellar resurfacing; and (3) patellar resurfacing should not be carried out in younger, heavier patients if a congruous, well-aligned patella can be attained.[11]

A preferable way to study patellofemoral resurfacing is by a randomized, prospective study evaluating resurfacing versus not resurfacing the patella. In one such study of 118 knees (86 patients) followed for an average of 30 months, 58 knees underwent patellar resurfacing while 60 knees retained the patellar surface. No significant difference was detected with respect to clinical score or patient satisfaction. Thirty-two of these patients had a bilateral TKA with patellar resurfacing in one knee and retention of the patella in the other. None of these patients expressed a clear preference for either knee. However, 10% of the unresurfaced patellae required subsequent resurfacing for unremitting anterior knee pain. Unfortunately, the development of postoperative anterior knee pain or the need for subsequent patellar resurfacing could not be predicted by the presence of preoperative anterior knee pain, obesity, or a high grade of intraoperatively observed chondromalacia.[18]

Ultimately, long-term results of randomized, prospective studies will determine the better choice between resurfacing and not resurfacing the patella. The articular cartilage of a nonresurfaced patella articulating with a metal prosthesis may gradually deteriorate, develop painful arthrosis, and require patellar resurfacing. Many surgeons believe the current standard in TKA is to resurface the patella. Careful attention to technique with patellar resurfacing has provided very predictable, long-term success and low complication rates.[10,13,19]

SOFT TISSUE COMPLICATIONS

Patellofemoral Instability

Whether it is resurfaced or not, the patella may subluxate after TKA, but it is more likely with patellar resurfacing.[8,20] Patellar instability may cause patellofemoral pain, crepitus, component wear, failure, loosening, and fracture of the bony remnant.[1] The incidence of subluxation following TKA has been reported to be as high as 29%.[21] However, large series have reported the prevalence of symptomatic patellar instability requiring reoperation to be only 0.5% to 0.8%.[20,22] Though patellar dislocation is rare, it obviously manifests itself more dramatically than subluxation (Fig. 27.1). However, both subluxation and dislocation are usually caused by a similar combination of underlying problems, including (1) limb malalignment, (2) component malalignment, (3) improper component design, (4) improper patellar preparation, (5) surgical approach, and (6) trauma leading to disruption of the medial capsular repair.[2,10,20,23–25]

Prevention of Instability: Component Positioning

Patellar instability can occur with excessive valgus of the anatomic femorotibial axis or with malposition of any

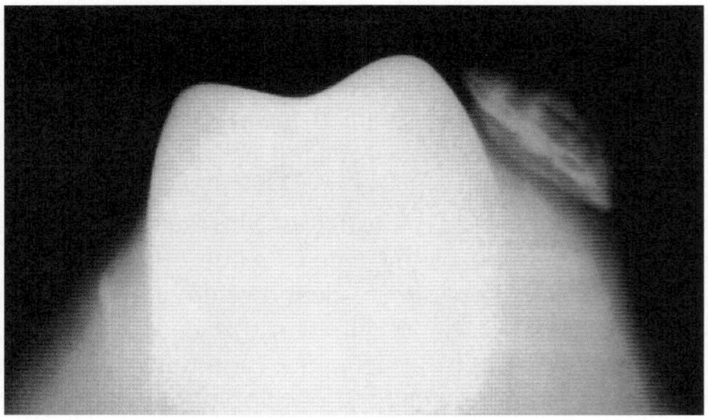

Figure 27.1. Sunrise radiograph demonstrating the dramatic presentation of a dislocated patella following total knee arthroplasty (TKA).

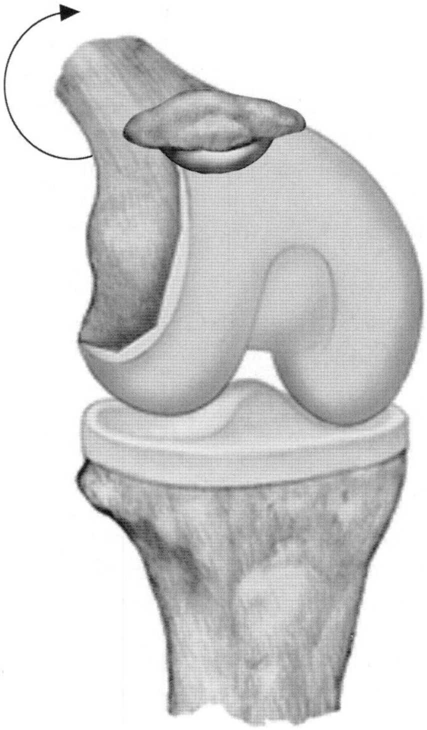

Figure 27.2. The result of internally rotating the femoral component is medialization of the trochlear groove and lateral subluxation of the resurfaced patella.

of the three prosthetic components. For instance, medial translation or internal rotation of the femoral component will result in lateral tracking of the patella relative to the femoral component. This problem can be avoided by placing the center of the femoral component just lateral to the central portion of the intercondylar notch. However, excessive lateral translation of the femoral component must be avoided, as the implant may impinge on the posterior cruciate ligament (PCL), popliteus tendon, or lateral retinaculum.

The relative thickness of bone removed from each of the posterior femoral condyles establishes the rotational alignment of the femoral component. Although external rotation of the femoral component improves patellar stability, it will affect posterior condylar bone resections. Symmetrical knee stability in flexion must be preserved by maintaining the rectangular flexion space (Fig. 27.2). Several referencing methods have been used to attain this goal.

Referencing Methods for Femoral Component Positioning

Insall's original referencing technique was to rotate the femoral cutting block to create a posterior femoral cut parallel to the transverse cut of the tibia. With this method, ligament releases are performed before bone cuts. Currently, Insall advocates the transepicondylar axis reference, which assumes that the plane of knee flexion parallels a line through the epicondyles. Posterior bone resections are made parallel to the transepicondylar line to maintain ligament balance in flexion.[26]

Anteroposterior (AP) axis referencing is another way to establish rotational alignment of the femoral component. A line is drawn from the base of the trochlear groove to the center of the intercondylar notch, and posterior condylar resections are made perpendicular to this line.[26]

Arima et al[26] compared the AP axis, transepicondylar axis, and the posterior condylar axis as landmarks for rotational alignment of the femoral component in cadavaric femora. They found the AP axis to be the most reproducible. However, an in vivo study by Poilvache et al[27] of 100 knees undergoing TKA found the transepicondylar axis to be a more reliable landmark for orientation of the femoral component. These authors felt that trochlear dysplasia, wear, or intercondylar osteophytes may distort the true AP axis for rotational alignment.

The balanced resection technique is another method of establishing femoral component rotation while accounting for the anatomic variation seen from case to case. This technique removes from each posterior condyle an amount of bone equal in thickness to the bone removed from the respective distal femoral condyle, with a 6-degree valgus distal resection. Ligament stability is preserved since the flexion gap matches the extension gap medially, independent of the flexion-extension gap balance in the lateral compartment.

Tibial Component Positioning

The central portion of the tibial tray should be placed over the medial one-third of the tibial tubercle. A cautery or methylene blue can be used to mark the position of the appropriately placed trial component to ensure proper placement of the final components. Relative external rotation or lateral translation of the tibial component improves extensor mechanism stability by internally rotating the tibial tubercle, which decreases the Q-angle.

Femoral Component Geometry

Patellofemoral stability is also influenced by femoral component geometry (Fig. 27.3). Deepening of the trochlear groove increases the resistance to patellar dislocation, but also increases stress on the fixation interface of the patella. Yoshii et al[28] demonstrated an increase in patellofemoral stability by deepening the femoral groove from 3 to 4 mm and raising the height of the lateral flange. Although the raised lateral flange effectively prevents patellar subluxation, it can be a potential source of soft tissue irritation, increased patellar polyethylene stress and wear, and increased patellar fracture.[29] Anatomic femoral component designs with right and left components are probably the most favorable for enhancing patellofemoral tracking. Although universal femurs that can be used for either a right or left TKA reduce component inventory, centrally directed patellofemoral grooves provide less predictable patellofemoral stability.

Patellar Component Design

Patellar components generally come in two basic designs: an anatomic implant with medial and lateral facets, and a dome-shaped implant. For most designs, an anatomic component conforms more with the femoral groove and is more stable than the dome-shaped design. Malalignment of an anatomic patella, however, can lead to accelerated component wear or patellofemoral instability. Most surgeons choose a dome-shaped component because it is easier to position the implant.[10,30,31]

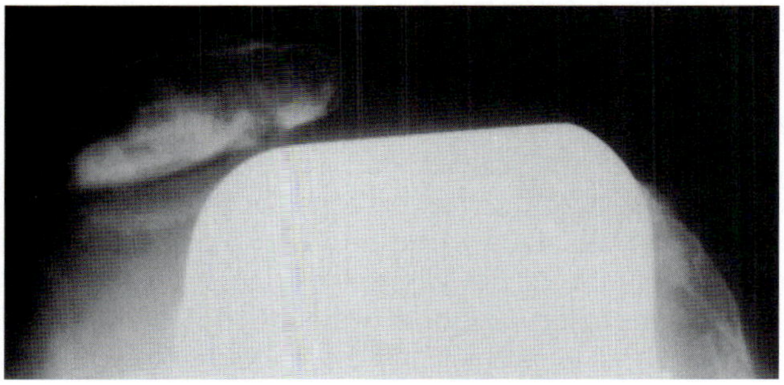

Figure 27.3. Femoral components without a trochlear groove contribute to patellofemoral instability, as seen on the sunrise radiograph.

Preparing the Patella

The asymmetric shape of the patella may lead to errors in its preparation that can result in maltracking.[1,32] Proper patellar bone exposure required for optimal patellar cuts is accomplished when enough peripatellar fat and synovium are removed to visualize the quadriceps and patellar tendon. The patellar bone should be resected parallel to its anterior surface to create a uniformly thick remnant for attachment of the patellar component. This resection is frequently performed without instrumentation, but requires frequent inspection, palpation, and often secondary cuts to eliminate any asymmetry. Measuring with calipers before and after patellar cuts increases the accuracy of resection.[33]

Prevention of Instability: Soft Tissue Techniques

Surgical Approach

The surgical approach has not traditionally been considered a factor contributing to patellofemoral joint instability. However, Engh et al[34] compared the incidence of lateral retinacular releases in TKA with a midvastus muscle-splitting approach versus a standard medial parapatellar arthrotomy. The patient groups were similar in gender, age, weight, and diagnosis; the surgical approach was the only variable. Fifty percent of the 88 knees that underwent a medial parapatellar approach required lateral retinacular release, a rate similar to other reports in the literature[35]; only 3% of cases in the group of 88 knees that had a midvastus approach required lateral releases. The authors concluded that any surgical approach that avoids incisions into the quadriceps tendon significantly reduces the chance of creating patellar instability.

Intraoperative Assessment of Patellar Tracking

Proper extensor mechanism balance without excessively tight lateral structures and a strong vastus medialis muscle help prevent patellar instability. Patellar tracking must be thoroughly assessed before wound closure to avoid extensor mechanism imbalance. To evaluate patellofemoral tracking properly, some surgeons advocate tourniquet release to eliminate its binding effect on the quadriceps mechanism.[1,36] Before retinacular repair, the knee should be flexed and stability checked without using the thumb to stabilize the patella. Patellar subluxation or tilting on this "no-thumb" test have been described as indicating the need for a lateral retinacular release.[1,37]

However, the "one-stitch" test described by Rae et al[19] may be more indicative of true patellofemoral joint stability. This test involves placing a single suture to approximate the medial repair. If the suture cuts out during flexion, then the lateral retinaculum is overly tight. Ogata et al[38] measured the tension of a suture placed in the medial retinaculum following TKA. They concluded that lateral release is not always needed if retinacular tension shows no significant increase with flexion, even if the patella dislocates when the no-thumb test is used.

Lateral Retinacular Release

A lateral retinacular release can be performed either external to the synovial cavity ("outside-in") or from within the joint capsule ("inside-out"). The first step is the release of any thickened synovial bands extending from the femur to the patella (patellofemoral ligaments). If patellofemoral joint instability persists, then a formal lateral retinacular release is appropriate. An effective and commonly used technique is an intracapsular approach, which releases the retinaculum 1.5 to 2 cm lateral to the patellar border. With care, this technique can preserve the superolateral genicular vessels that help maintain skin viability and patellar vascularity.[23,39,40]

DIAGNOSIS AND MANAGEMENT OF PATELLAR SUBLUXATION

In TKA patients with patellofemoral joint instability, diffuse anterior knee discomfort is occasionally present and is often aggravated when the patient climbs hills or stairs. However, the most common patient complaint is an insecure feeling or "giving-way" of the knee. In this situation, patellofemoral crepitation and knee swelling may be present.

Factors that may predispose the patient to patellofemoral instability are (1) excessive preoperative valgus with extensor mechanism malalignment, (2) medial retinacular attenuation, (3) a weak vastus medialis or overly strong vastus lateralis, and (4) a contracted iliotibial band.[22] When the knee is flexed from a fully extended position, the patella may also tilt laterally as it moves medially. This lateral tilt is caused by the patellar component's engaging with the trochlea of the femoral component.

Radiographic Evaluation of Instability

To assess axial alignment of the knee and the prosthetic components, radiographic examination should include a full lower extremity AP view. Sunrise views of the patellofemoral articulation taken with the knee in 45 degrees of flexion help determine patellar position with respect to the trochlear groove of the femur. Though rotational alignment of the femoral and tibial components cannot be determined by plain radiography, computed tomography (CT) has been described as effective in measuring femoral and tibial component rotation. Berger et al[41] compared 30 patients with normal axial alignment and isolated patellofemoral complications to 20 patients with well-functioning total knees. When the epicondylar axis and tibial tubercle were used as references, CT evaluation demonstrated a direct correlation between the combined femoral and tibial component internal rotation and the severity of the patellofemoral complication. The authors concluded that CT rotational evaluation can be helpful in determining femoral and/or tibial component rotational malalignment and in evaluating the need for revising one or both of the components to correct patellofemoral instability.

Management of Instability

The nonsurgical management of patellofemoral joint instability includes aggressive quadriceps rehabilitation, external patellofemoral bracing, and avoidance of activities such as squatting or stair climbing that heavily load the patellofemoral joint.[1] Nonsurgical treatment should not be considered if a component is grossly malpositioned or malaligned.[8] If conservative measures fail and an underlying cause of patellar instability is apparent, surgical intervention is directed at the cause of the patellofemoral instability. The revision of an internally rotated tibial component is preferable to a transfer of the tibial tubercle. Bone is preserved as much as possible when the tibia is revised by retaining stable cement and applying new bone cement to old cement and correctly positioning the tibial component.

Revision of the femoral component, however, is more complex because changing femoral component rotation affects ligament balance in flexion. At the time of arthrotomy, the surgeon can use the transepicondylar axis to assess the degree of femoral component malrotation directly. If the femur is rotated internally by tight medial structures, a medial collateral ligament release may correct the internally rotated femur and relieve the patellofemoral instability. If the soft tissues are balanced appropriately and the femoral component rotated internally relative to the transepicondylar axis, the femoral component will need to be revised. Correction of the internal rotation of the femoral component will require selective resection of bone from the posterior medial femoral condyle and/or use of a posterolateral augmentation block to rotate the femoral component externally (Fig. 27.4A and B). An oversized femoral component may be needed with a posterolateral augment to avoid anterolateral notching of the femoral cortex.

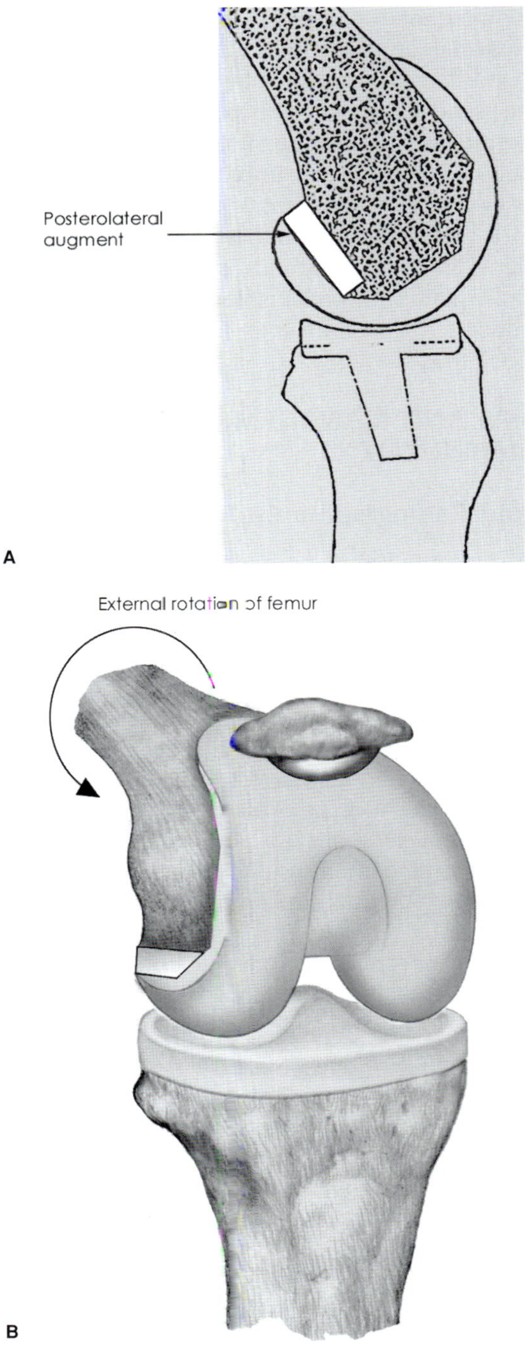

Figure 27.4. A and B: To correct an internally rotated femoral component, the surgeon revises the anterior, posterior, and chamfer cuts and uses a posterolateral augment.

Extensor mechanism realignment procedures can be used to improve patellar stability when the components are well aligned. Lateral retinacular release alone, either open or arthroscopic, is rarely successful in eliminating patellofemoral instability.[42] Proximal soft tissue realignment, combining a lateral retinacular release with vastus medialis advancement, has been successful in addressing a poorly aligned extensor mechanism. Merkow et al,[23] who treated 10 patients with proximal realignment for patellofemoral joint instability, reported improved knee scores and no redislocation. Grace and Rand[22] had limited success with proximal realignment with four recurrent subluxations in their series of 14 patients.

Distal realignment procedures change the Q-angle and avoid the medial patellar tilt associated with isolated proximal realignment procedures. A modification of the Trillat procedure has been successful when a lateral retinacular release along with a medial displacement osteotomy of the tibial tubercle is used.[42,43] However, patellar tendon rupture has been cited as a potential complication. Grace and Rand[22] reported two patellar tendon disruptions in nine patients who underwent proximal and distal realignment. Careful dissection with preservation of soft tissue flaps and use of an extended osteotomy may minimize such complications. A concomitant lateral retinacular release, avoidance of anterior translation of the osteotomized segment, and secure fixation with screws, staples, or wires are also recommended.[42,43]

On rare occasions, disruption of the medial capsular repair may occur. Excessive hematoma, aggressive physical therapy, or trauma may cause this problem and may lead to patellofemoral instability. Unlike most other forms of patellofemoral instability, this disruption is managed best by early surgical intervention.[1]

SOFT TISSUE IMPINGEMENT

Patellar Clunk

Insall et al[44,45] first described peripatellar synovial hypertrophy as a cause of symptomatic anterior femoral clicking and catching in the posterior stabilized TKA. The most recognized presentation of this soft tissue impingement is called the patellar clunk syndrome. Hozack et al[46] first described this entity in three patients who experienced a painful catching sensation when they extended the knee. The cause of this syndrome was found to be a prominent fibrous nodule at the junction of the proximal pole of the patella and the quadriceps tendon. Beight et al[47] reviewed 484 posterior stabilized total knee replacements and found 20 cases with patellar clunk syndrome in 19 patients. The average time to presentation in these patients was 10.6 months following their initial procedure. Pettine and Bryan[48] reported on five patients who developed enlarged painful infrapatellar masses that reduced their knee motion. The authors were unable to identify a cause for these masses.

Intraarticular Fibrous Bands

Thorpe et al[49] described another variation of peripatellar synovial hypertrophy. Over a 5-year period, 11 of 635 TKA patients experienced patellofemoral dysfunction, consisting of painful popping, catching, grinding, or maltracking of the patella. Arthroscopically these symptoms were found to be caused by intraarticular fibrous bands. On the basis of their observations, these authors described three anatomic varieties of fibrous bands. Type I bands course superiorly and transversely, type II bands extend laterally, and type III bands run from the distal pole of the patella to the intercondylar notch.

Prevention of Soft Tissue Impingement

Since the cause of synovial hypertrophy and entrapment is unknown, it is difficult to develop preventive measures for this problem.[48,49] Hozack et al[46] conceded that the pathogenesis of the proximal fibrous nodule is not clear, but they presented two possible explanations. The first involved impingement of the anterior edge of the intercondylar box of posterior stabilized femoral components on the quadriceps tendon in flexion. This impingement is made worse when an undersized patellar component fails to lift the quadriceps tendon away from the femoral component. The second mechanism involves impingement of the patellar component on the quadriceps tendon. If the patellar component overhangs the patella proximally, the component may contact the quadriceps tendon and cause irritation when the knee is flexed. On the basis of these proposed causes for patellar clunk syndrome, Hozack et al recommended the following steps to avoid synovial entrapment: (1) using the largest patellar component that covers the patellar remnant without overhang, (2) placing the center hole of the patellar button 1 to 2 mm distal to the patellar center to avoid impingement on the quadriceps tendon, and (3) maintaining an anatomic prosthetic joint line.

Hozack et al's[46] third recommendation was based on findings that patellar clunk occurred mostly in cases where the patellar height, relative to the joint line, was less than 10 mm or greater than 30 mm.[9] Beight et al[47] reported that posterior-stabilized femoral components with a sharp anterior border of the intercondylar box were more likely to experience patellar clunk syndrome. However, the same authors suggested that the disorder was multifactorial and could not be solely attributed to component design. In their study, only one of six patients with bilateral posterior stabilized knee arthroplasties of identical design developed bilateral patellar clunk syndrome.

Excising synovial tissue at the superior pole of the patella at the time of posterior stabilized TKA is frequently recommended to avoid tissue hypertrophy and potential synovial entrapment. However, Pettine and Bryan[48] found that excising the infrapatellar fat pad and surrounding synovial tissue did not prevent patellar clunk. In describing intraarticular fibrous bands, Thorpe et al[49] could not specifically implicate trauma, faulty prosthetic design, error in operative technique, previous operation, or abnormal patellar height. However, nine of 11 patients in their study did have posterior stabilized prostheses and four patients had undergone a previous operation.

DIAGNOSIS AND MANAGEMENT OF SOFT TISSUE IMPINGEMENT

Clinical and Radiographic Evaluation

The clinical presentation of peripatellar synovial hypertrophy may vary, depending on the location and extent of the impinging tissue. Patients often complain of anterior knee pain exacerbated by activities such as rising from a chair or climbing stairs. Audible popping, catching, or cracking usually accompany these activities. Palpable crepitus, and sometimes visible movement of the patella are evident when active, resisted knee extension from deep-knee flexion is performed. Most patients are able to reproduce a clunk or crepitation with active knee extension. The impingement usually occurs at about 90 degrees of flexion. Although radiographs usually appear normal, they should be taken to rule out component malalignment or loosening. In their radiographic evaluation of 20 patients with patellar clunk syndrome, Beight et al[47] found one loose and one proximally placed patellar component.

Management

The initial treatment of peripatellar synovial hypertrophy includes wearing a patellar knee sleeve, strengthening the quadriceps and hamstring muscles, a trial of oral antiinflammatory medication, and possibly a cortisone injection. Conservative measures are unlikely to eliminate the symptoms, but may be successful in reducing their severity. Nonoperative treatment proved successful in 4 of the 20 cases reported by Beight et al.[47]

Arthrotomy and excision of the hypertrophied tissues have been highly successful in eliminating symptoms of synovial entrapment (Fig. 27.5).[44–48] Insall et al[44,45] described open peripatellar synovectomy as the successful treatment for anterior knee clicking and catching. Hozack et al,[46] in their initial description of patellar clunk syndrome, were able to relieve the symptoms in three patients by surgically removing the fibrous nodule.

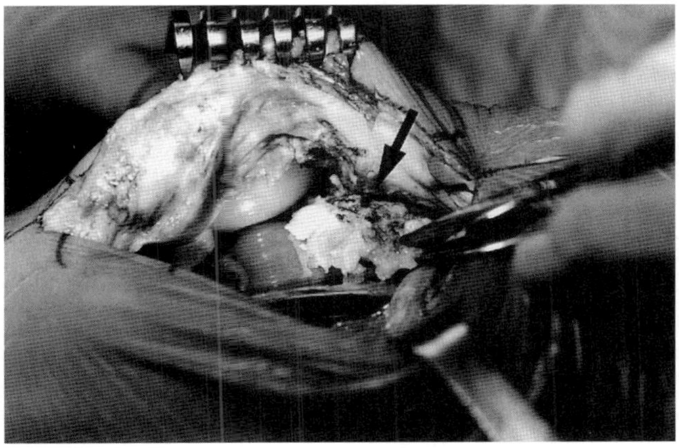

Figure 27.5. Excision of hypertrophied synovial tissue (arrow) has been successful in eliminating symptoms of synovial entrapment. (From ref. 65, with permission.)

They also advised the surgeon to be prepared for patellar component revision at the time of the arthrotomy.

Arthroscopic treatment of peripatellar synovial hypertrophy has been an equally effective technique.[47,49–51] Vernace et al[50] first reported their experience in successfully treating five cases of patellar clunk syndrome with arthroscopy. They stated that the ability to evaluate the patellofemoral joint effectively without disruption of the joint capsule was a distinct advantage of arthroscopy over arthrotomy. A superolateral portal along with inferomedial and superomedial portals is needed to aid in complete excision of the fibrous nodule. Thorpe et al[49,51] also advocate arthroscopy as an effective tool for diagnosis and treatment of the intraarticular fibrous bands.

An effective approach to the treatment of peripatellar synovial hypertrophy appears to be the algorithm described by Beight et al,[47] who state that a brief period of nonoperative management, as described above, is appropriate. If conservative management is unsuccessful, arthroscopic debridement should be attempted in cases without radiographic evidence of component abnormality. Arthrotomy and excision of the hypertrophied or fibrous synovium are indicated if symptoms recur. Obviously malpositioned or loose components should be revised and patients should be advised of the limitations of arthroscopy and the possibility of recurrence of their symptoms despite adequate operative debridement.

PATELLAR COMPONENT COMPLICATIONS

All-polyethylene patellar component failure is extremely uncommon and is described only in case reports in the literature.[52,53] Excellent clinical results have been achieved with these components although the polyethylene often exhibits deformation at the time of retrieval.[3,10,54] Loosening of cemented, all-polyethylene patellar components has been relatively rare, with the reported incidence in large series ranging from 0.6% to 1.3%.[13,20] A thin, central fixation peg on the implant, component malpositioning, and trauma have been cited as factors associated with loosening of cemented patellar components.[20] In reporting on the use of three-pegged patellar components in 577 total knee replacements, Mason et al[55] found no component loose at an average follow-up of 3 years.

Despite the clinical success of cemented, all-polyethylene patellar components, metal-backed patellar implants were introduced in the mid-1980s.[56] This design modification was influenced by the introduction of cementless, metal-backed acetabular and tibial components, which exhibited decreased polyethylene deformation and improved load transfer with mechanical testing.[30] Concerns about the longevity and biocompatibility of polymethyl methacrylate added to the enthusiasm for biologic fixation and led to an increased use of porous-coated patellar components.

The disadvantages of adding metal backing to patellar components have far outweighed the proposed advantages. In contrast to the effectiveness of all-polyethylene designs, catastrophic failure and biologically accelerated generation of wear debris have been frequent complications with metal-backed patellar implants.[8,37] The two modes of metal-backed patella failure are polyethylene dissociation from the metal backing and fracture of fixation pegs at the point where they attach to the metal plate.[37,56,57]

To avoid "overstuffing" the patellofemoral joint while trying to maintain reasonable thickness of the patella–patellar component composite, designers have reduced the polyethylene thickness considerably with metal backing. As predicted by Wright and Bartel[58] on the basis of their study of polyethylene thickness in metal-backed tibial components, a significant amount of wear has been seen with metal-backed patellar components.[37,56–60] As a result most of the literature on patellar component failure deals with the metal-backed designs. Bayley et al[59] described 25 patients with failed, metal-backed patellar components. Several manufacturers and designs were involved in these cases in which failure resulted from wear or fracture of the polyethylene, dissociation of the polyethylene, or fracture of the anchoring pegs from the base plate. Rosenberg et al[56] reported a 10% failure rate in 122 patients with metal-backed patellar components at an average follow-up of 24 months. At 6-year follow-up, Rader et al[60] found a failure rate of 33% in 30 patients. Obviously, these authors urge caution to those considering the use of metal-backed patellar components in TKA. However, a more recent study by Evanich et al,[61] which included 212 knees with metal-backed patellae, reported a 96% survivorship at 7½-year follow-up. They credited their success to the design of the component, with a modified dome-shaped patella articulating with a deep-dish trochlear groove. They also report that they optimized patellar tracking by medializing the patellar component and minimized stress on the implant by countersinking the metal-backed patella.

Prevention

Patellar component success can be optimized by appropriate (1) bone preparation, (2) component placement, (3) patellar thickness after resurfacing, and (4) patellofemoral joint tracking.[61] Josefchak et al[62] set out to determine the optimum level of a patellar osteotomy and to define the ideal fixation peg location. Their study of nine cadaver patellae found that the subchondral bone gave the best support and that peg placement was not critical to fixation strength. They cautioned that metal-backed patellar components, which require increased bone resection and removal of subchondral bone, may increase the incidence of patellar fracture significantly. Some authors recommend countersinking the patellar component 2 to 3 mm to avoid overthickening of the patella–patellar component complex, a condition that leads to excessive loading across the patellofemoral joint.[61]

One of the most important factors in the success of the patellar component is establishing a balanced extensor mechanism. This procedure requires meticulous attention to component alignment, patellar bone preparation, and soft tissue balancing (Fig. 27.6). To prevent excessive patellofemoral joint loading and rapid component failure, the surgeon should avoid using oversized femoral components. The femoral component should be placed in slight flexion, and the prosthetic joint line should be reestablished at anatomic levels.[1,56–57,59] Other methods for minimizing component loosening and failure include avoiding use of this prosthesis with deficient bone, positioning the components properly, and resecting the patella symmetrically. The risk factors associated with patellar loosening include subluxation or fracture, osteonecrosis, osteoporosis, loosening of other prosthetic components, and failure of bone ingrowth into porous-coated implants.[1,20] Patient variables associated with patellar component failure include excessive body weight, postoperative knee flexion beyond 115 degrees, high activity levels, and male gender.[1,56–57,59]

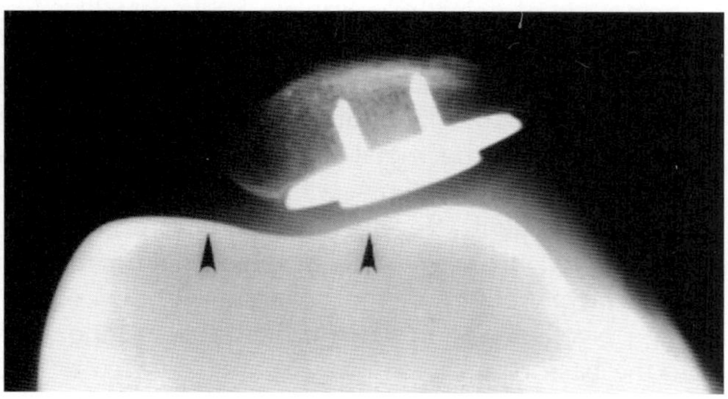

Figure 27.6. This case demonstrates several technical errors in patellar component implantation. Asymmetric patellar bone cuts, lateralization of the component, and poor soft tissue balancing lead to predictable failure in metal-backed patellar components.

DIAGNOSIS AND MANAGEMENT OF PATELLAR COMPONENT FAILURE

Clinical Evaluation

The clinical presentations of patients with a loose patellar component vary. For example, a loose patellar component may be relatively asymptomatic if stabilized by its surrounding patellar meniscus. However, some patients describe a sudden onset of pain and audible grating associated with significant knee flexion and loading of the patellofemoral joint. This acute presentation, representing catastrophic failure of a metal-backed patellar component, was present in 15 of 25 patients described by Bayley et al.[59] Only 5 of those 15 patients experienced sudden onset of symptoms with heavy loading activities such as rising from a chair or climbing stairs. However, the onset of symptoms for the remaining 10 patients occurred while they were walking on level ground.

A high index of suspicion should be associated with metal-backed patellar components with known failure mechanisms.[37,57,59] Recognizing metal-backed patellar component failure early avoids damage to the femoral component and potential catastrophe. Therefore, patients with this type of component require annual follow-up with meticulous evaluation and a high index of suspicion regardless of the absence of symptoms. Alignment and patellar tracking should be assessed with clinical examination. It is also necessary that the surgeon palpate the anterior knee to check for crepitus or grating during patellofemoral loading activities, such as rising from a chair or resisting knee extension. A dislodged component on occasion is palpable in the suprapatellar pouch.

This diagnostic process is aided by plain radiography, which is useful in diagnosing implant loosening or failure at the junction of the pegs and metal backing (Fig. 27.7). Complete radiolucency along the patellar com-

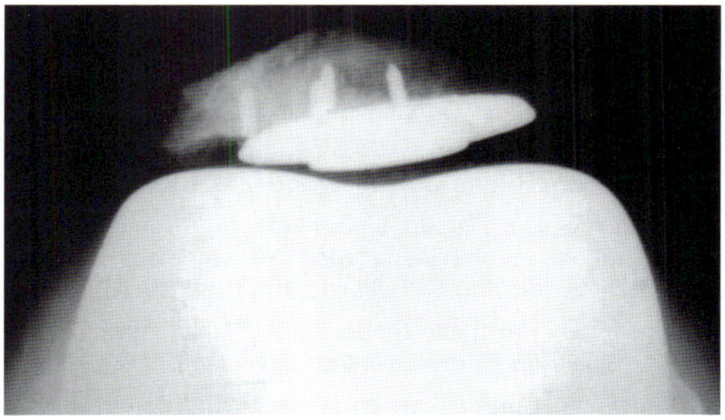

Figure 27.7. Radiograph demonstrating metal-backed patellar component failure at the junction of the pegs and metal backing.

ponent indicates implant loosening. Occasionally a dissociated polyethylene component will be visible as a radiolucency in the peripatellar region (Fig. 27.8). Merchant and other tangential views should be studied to assess decreasing space between the patellar metal backing and the femoral component.

Regardless of the type of implant, polyethylene wear alone may provoke synovitis and effusion, along with varying degrees of peripatellar pain. When a significant effusion is present, sterile aspiration may reveal darkened synovial fluid with metallic and polyethylene particles.[59] Weissman et al[63] described the "metal-line" sign, a radiodense line formed by metal debris that defines a portion of the capsule or articular surface of a knee joint. This line was found retrospectively in 11 of 18 patients with known metal-induced synovitis following failed TKA. Histologic examination of available synovial specimens showed a correlation between dense deposits of metallic particles and the metal-line sign. Titanium was the offending metal in 10 of the 11 cases, reflecting its increased vulnerability to wear and to the production of metal particles.

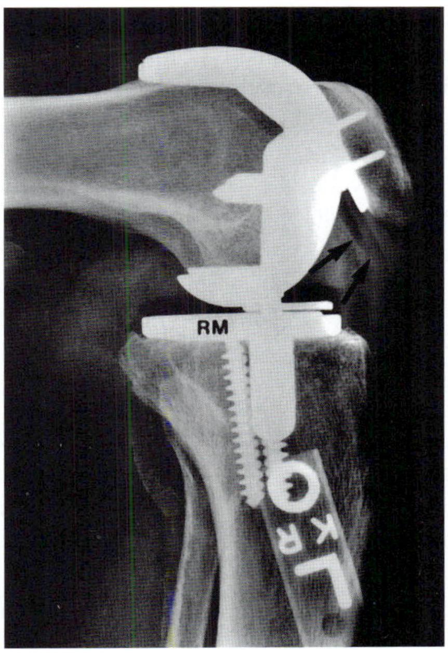

Figure 27.8. Lateral radiograph showing a dissociated polyethylene portion of a metal-backed patellar implant.

Intraoperative Evaluation

Intraoperative findings vary, depending on the type of implant and mode of failure. The most dramatic findings occur with failed titanium, metal-backed designs that result in the patellar metal backing articulating with the femoral component (Fig. 27.9). Stulberg et al[57] described their intraoperative findings in 16 knees in which the patellar polyethylene had dissociated from the metal backing. These authors encountered thin black joint fluid, and striking black synovium with minimal proliferation. They also found embedded in the polyethylene of the patellar and tibial components metallic beads that added to the abrasive wear on the femoral component. These findings were confirmed by Bayley et al,[59] who reported metal-induced synovitis in 23 of 25 failed metal-backed patellar components with considerable femoral component wear in 11 patients. In cases such as these with advanced metallosis and polyethylene wear, a thorough synovectomy is required at the time of revision.

Implant Revision

Removal of a bone-ingrown component can significantly challenge the preservation of bone stock. One effective

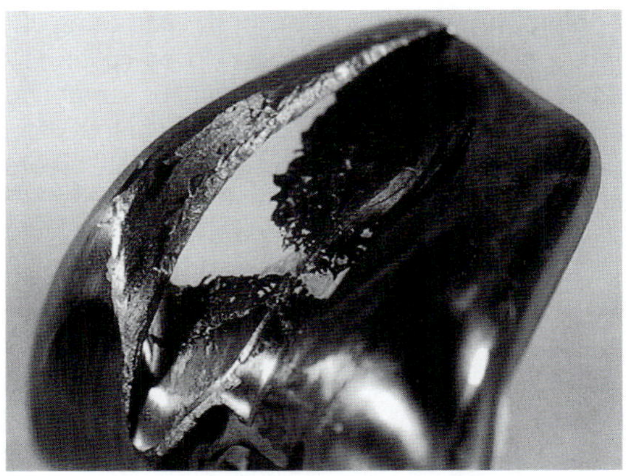

Figure 27.9. The dramatic results seen when the metal backing of a patellar component articulate with the femoral component. (From ref. 57, with permission.)

method of implant removal is to use a flat, wheel-shaped, high-speed burr to cut the pegs from the component. A pencil-tipped, high-speed burr is used to remove the pegs from the bone. Another method uses thin, flexible osteotomes to release the bone-implant interface. Overaggressive levering of the osteotome may cause fracture of the relatively avascular patellar remnant. However, risk of fracture can be diminished by stacking the osteotomes and levering of the metal implant against a metal base. After implant removal, fibrous tissue and sclerotic bone should be debrided.

Once a failed component has been removed, the patellar bone must be assessed to determine if sufficient bone is present for stable patellar resurfacing. The patellar remnant must be at least 10-mm thick for patellar replacement. In cases where inadequate bone is present, either a patelloplasty or a partial patellectomy is performed. Patelloplasty is accomplished by smoothing the undersurface of the remaining patellar bone. Following patellectomy, some surgeons use a lateral release and "tubulation" of the extensor mechanism, allowing for improved tracking and mechanical function of the remaining soft tissues. In one study an autogenous iliac crest bone graft sutured into the extensor mechanism has led to satisfactory restoration of patellar function in six of seven knees with an average 6-year follow-up.[64] The graft restores the moment arm of the extensor mechanism and improves the appearance of the anterior knee.

CONCLUSION

The most common patellofemoral complications following TKA are instability, soft tissue impingement, and component loosening. Taking steps to prevent these complications by balancing the extensor mechanism, positioning the components properly, and using all-polyethylene patellar components should be routine. When a patient presents with patellar pain or instability, the options described in this chapter should help to pinpoint the problem and determine the appropriate treatment.

References

1. Dennis DA. Extensor mechanism problems in total knee arthroplasty. *Instr Course Lect* 1997;46:171–180.
2. Doolittle KH II, Turner RH. Patellofemoral problems following total knee arthroplasty. *Orthop Rev* 1988;17: 696–702.
3. Insall J, Tria AJ, Scott WN. The total condylar knee prosthesis. The first five years. *Clin Orthop* 1979;145: 68–77.
4. Matthews LS, Sonstegard DA, Henke JA. Load bearing characteristics of the patello-femoral joint. *Acta Orthop Scand* 1977;48:511–516.
5. Huberti HH, Hayes WC. Patellofemoral contact pressures. The influence of Q-angle and tendofemoral contact. *J Bone Joint Surg* 1984;66A:715–724.
6. Goldberg VM, Figgie HE III, Figgie MP. Technical considerations in total knee surgery. Management of patella problems. *Orthop Clin North Am* 1989;20:189–199.
7. Scott RD. Prosthetic replacement of the patellofemoral joint. *Orthop Clin North Am* 1979;10:129–137.
8. Rand JA. Current concepts review: the patellofemoral joint in total knee arthroplasty. *J Bone Joint Surg* 1994; 76A:612–619.
9. Figgie HE III, Goldberg VM, Heiple KG, et al. The influence of tibia-patella femoral mechanical axis on patella femoral function in the posterior stabilized condylar knee prosthesis. *J Bone Joint Surg* 1986;68A:1035–1040.
10. Ranawat CS. The patellofemoral joint in total condylar knee arthroplasty. *Clin Orthop* 1986;205:93–99.
11. Enis JE, Gardner R, Robledo MA, et al. Comparison of patellar surfacing versus nonresurfacing in bilateral total knee arthroplasty. *Clin Orthop* 1991;260:38–42.
12. Levai JP, McLeod HC, Freeman MA. Why not resurface the patella? *J Bone Joint Surg* 1983;65B:448–451.
13. Boyd AD, Ewald FR, Thomas WH, et al. Long-term complications after total knee arthroplasty with or without resurfacing of the patella. *J Bone Joint Surg* 1993;75A: 674–681.
14. Picetti GD III, McGann WA, Welch RB. The patellofemoral joint after total knee arthroplasty without patella resurfacing. *J Bone Joint Surg* 1986;72A:1379–1382.
15. Abraham W, Buchanan JR, Daubent H, et al. Should the patella be resurfaced in total knee arthroplasty? Efficacy of patellar resurfacing. *Clin Orthop* 1988;236:128–134.
16. Levitsky KA, Harris WJ, McManus J, et al. Total knee arthroplasty without patellar resurfacing. Clinical outcomes and long-term follow-up evaluation. *Clin Orthop* 1993;286:116–121.
17. Smith SR, Stuart P, Pinder IM. Nonresurfaced patellar in total knee arthroplasty. *J Arthroplasty* 1989;4(suppl): 81–86.
18. Barrack RL, Wolfe MW, Waldman DA, et al. Resurfacing of the patella in total knee arthroplasty. A prospective randomized double-blinded study. *J Bone Joint Surg* 1997;79A:1121–1131.
19. Rae RJ, Noble J, Hodgkimsen JP. Patellar resurfacing in total condylar knee arthroplasty. Techniques and results. *J Arthroplasty* 1990;5:259–265.
20. Brick GW, Scott RD. The patellofemoral component of total knee arthroplasty. *Clin Orthop* 1988;231:163–178.
21. Cameron HU, Fedockow DM. The patella in total knee arthroplasty. *Clin Orthop* 1982;165:197–199.

22. Grace JN, Rand JA. Patellar instability after total knee arthroplasty. *Clin Orthop* 1988;237:184–189.

23. Merkow RL, Soudry M, Insall JN. Patellar dislocations following total knee replacement. *J Bone Joint Surg* 1985; 67A:1321–1327.

24. Clayton ML, Thirupathi R. Patellar complications after total condylar arthroplasty. *Clin Orthop* 1982;170:131–140.

25. Mochizuki RM, Schurman DJ. Patellar complications following total arthroplasty. *J Bone Joint Surg* 1979;61A: 879–883.

26. Arima J, Whiteside LA, McCarthy DS, et al. Femoral rotational alignment based on the anteroposterior axis in total knee arthroplasty in a valgus knee. A technical note. *J Bone Joint Surg* 1995;77A:1331–1334.

27. Poilvache PL, Insall JN, Scuderi GR, et al. Rotational landmarks and sizing of the distal femur in total knee arthroplasty. *Clin Orthop* 1996;331:35–46.

28. Yoshii I, Whiteside LA, Anoudin YS. The effect of patellar button placement and femoral component design on patellar tracking in total knee arthroplasty. *Clin Orthop* 1992;275 211–219.

29. Rhoads DD, Noble PC, Reuben JD, et al. The effect of femoral component position on patellar component trading after total knee arthroplasty. *Clin Orthop* 1990;260: 43–51.

30. Hungerford DS, Kenna RV. Preliminary experience with a total knee prosthesis with porous coating used without cement. *Clin Orthop* 1983;176:95–107.

31. Cepulo AJ, Stabruski TM, Mocau JM, et al. Mechanical characteristics of patellofemoral replacements. *Trans Orthop Res Soc* 1983;8:41.

32. Lynch AF, Rorabeck CH, Bourne RB. Extensor mechanism complications following total knee arthroplasty. *J Arthroplasty* 1987;2:135–140.

33. Rand JA. Patellar resurfacing in total knee arthroplasty. *Clin Orthop* 1990;260:110–117.

34. Engh GA, Parks NL, Ammeen DJ. Influence of surgical approach on lateral retinacular releases in total knee arthroplasty. *Clin Orthop* 1996;331:56–63.

35. Ritter MA, Keating EM, Faris PM. Clinical, roentgenographic and scientrographic results after interruption of the superior lateral genicular artery during total knee arthroplasty. *Clin Orthop* 1989;248:145–151.

36. Dennis DA, Clayton ML, O'Donnell S, et al. Posterior cruciate condylar total knee arthroplasty. Average 11-year follow-up evaluation. *Clin Orthop* 1992;281:168–176.

37. Lombardi AV, Engh GA, Volz RG, et al. Fracture/dissociation of the polyethylene in metal-backed patellar components in total knee arthroplasty. *J Bone Joint Surg* 1988;70A:675–679.

38. Ogata K, Ishinishi T, Hara M. Evaluation of patella retinacular tension during total knee arthroplasty. Special emphasis on lateral retinacular release. *J Arthroplasty* 1997;12:651–656.

39. Johnson DP, Eastwood DM. Lateral patellar release in knee arthroplasty. Effect on wound healing. *J Arthroplasty* 1992;7:427.

40. Kaylor DE, Lyttle D. Surgical interruption of patellar blood supply by total knee arthroplasty. *Clin Orthop* 1988; 229:221–227.

41. Berger RA, Crosset LS, Jacobs JJ, et al. Patellofemoral complications following total knee arthroplasty. The consequences of malrotation with normal axial alignment. Abstracts from the American Association of Hip and Knee Surgeons seventh annual Meeting, November, 1997. *J Arthroplasty* 1998;13(2):234.

42. Briard JL, Hungerford DS. Patellofemoral instability in total knee arthroplasty. *J Arthroplasty* 1989;4(suppl):87–97.

43. Kirk P, Rorabeck CH, Bourne RB, et al. Management of recurrent dislocation of the patella following total knee arthroplasty. *J Arthroplasty* 1992;7:229–233.

44. Insall JN, Binazzi R, Soudry M, et al. Total knee arthroplasty. *Clin Orthop* 1985;192:13–22.

45. Insall JN, Lachiewicz PF, Burstein AH. The posterior stabilized condylar prosthesis. A modification of the total condylar design. Two- to four-year clinical experience. *J Bone Joint Surg* 1982;64A:1317–1323.

46. Hozack WJ, Rothman RJ, Booth RE, et al. The patellar clunk syndrome. A complication of posterior stabilized total knee arthroplasty. *Clin Orthop* 1989;241:203–208.

47. Beight JL, Binnan Y, Hozack WJ, et al. The patellar "clunk" syndrome after posterior stabilized total knee arthroplasty. *Clin Orthop* 1994;299:139–142.

48. Pettine KA, Bryan RS. A previously unreported cause of pain after total knee arthroplasty. *J Arthroplasty* 1986; 1:29–33.

49. Thorpe CD, Bocell JR, Tullos HS, et al. Intra-articular fibrous bands. Patellar complications after total knee replacement. *J Bone Joint Surg* 1990;72A:811–814.

50. Vernace JV, Rothman RH, Booth RE, et al. Arthroscopic management of the patellar clunk syndrome following posterior stabilized total knee arthroplasty. *J Arthroplasty* 1989;4:179–182.

51. Bocell JR, Thorpe CD, Tullos HS. Arthroscopic treatment of the symptomatic total knee arthroplasty. *Clin Orthop* 1991;271:125–134.

52. Conway WF, Gilula LA, Serot DI. Breakage of the patellar component of a kinematic total knee arthroplasty. A case report. *Orthopedics* 1986;9:532–534.

53. Wasilewski SA, Frankel U. Fracture of polyethylene of patellar component in total knee arthroplasty, diagnosed by arthroscopy. *J Arthroplasty* 1989;4:519–522.

54. Figgie MP, Wright TM, Santner T, et al. Performance of dome shaped patellar components in total knee arthroplasty. *Trans Orthop Res Soc* 1989;14:531.

55. Mason MD, Brick GW, Scott RD, et al. Three pegged all polyethylene patellar: 2- to 6-year results. *Orthop Trans* 1994;17:991.

56. Rosenberg AG, Andriacchi TP, Barden R, et al. Patellar component failure in cementless total knee arthroplasty. *Clin Orthop* 1988;236:106–114.
57. Stulberg SD, Stulberg BN, Hamati Y, et al. Failure mechanisms of metal-backed patellar components. *Clin Orthop* 1988;236:88–104.
58. Wright TM, Bartel DL. The problem of surface damage in polyethylene total knee components. *Clin Orthop* 1986;205:67–74.
59. Bayley JC, Scott RD, Ewald FC, et al. Failure of the metal-backed patellar component after total knee replacement. *J Bone Joint Surg* 1988;70A:668–674.
60. Rader CP, Lohr JO, Wittman R, et al. Results of total knee arthroplasty with a metal-backed patellar component. A 6-year follow-up study. *J Arthroplasty* 1996;11:923–930.
61. Evanich CJ, Tkach TK, Von Glinski S, et al. 6- to 10-year experience using countersunk metal-backed patellas. *J Arthroplasty* 1997;12:149–154.
62. Josefchak RG, Finlay JB, Bourne RB, et al. Cancellous bone support for patellar resurfacing. *Clin Orthop* 1987;220:192–199.
63. Weissman BN, Scott RD, Brick GW, et al. Radiographic detection of metal-induced synovitis as a complication of arthroplasty of the knee. *J Bone Joint Surg* 1991;73A:1002–1007.
64. Buechel FF. Patellar tendon bone grafting for patellectomized patients having total knee arthroplasty. *Clin Orthop* 1991;271:72–78.
65. Engh GA, Rorabeck CH (eds). *Revision Total Knee Arthroplasty*. Baltimore: Williams & Wilkins, 1997:221.

Chapter 28

Extensor Mechanism Complications Following Total Knee Arthroplasty

Michael R. Woolfrey and Robert B. Bourne

The extensor mechanism is very important for optimal functioning of a total knee arthroplasty. There tends to be more focus on the tibiofemoral joint rather than on the patellofemoral articulation. In fact, extensor mechanism problems following total knee arthroplasty account for complication rates ranging from 1.5% to 55%.[1–6]

Our group has been involved with several studies concentrating on extensor mechanism complications. In 1987, we published the data of 281 kinematic (dome patellar component) and porous coated anatomic (PCA, anatomic patellar component) knee arthroplasties.[7] The incidence of complications was 10%. There were three quadriceps tendon ruptures, five patellar fractures, four patellar tendon ruptures, 11 recurring patellar subluxations, four cases of patellar pain, and one malrotated patella. Of these, 3% required further surgery. We noted that these complications often occurred early after arthroplasty, often less than 1 year from surgery. In addition, there was a higher proportion of complications in rheumatoid versus osteoarthritic patients.

More recent contemporary total knee arthroplasty designs have attempted to address extensor mechanism problems by incorporating femoral external rotation and deepening of the femoral groove, which has resulted in a lower incidence of lateral retinacular releases. Recently, we critically reviewed patients with greater than 4-year follow-up with SAL I (self-aligning knee [Sulzer-Medica-Intermedics, Austin, TX]) and Genesis 1 (Smith Nephew Richards, Memphis, TN) contemporary knee arthroplasties performed by our two senior surgeons (Rorabeck and Bourne). Eighty-three SAL knees with 4- to 7-year follow-up had a 12% incidence of extensor mechanism problems (excluding asymptomatic tilted patellas) (Table 28.1). Also reviewed were 156 Genesis 1 knees with a follow-up of 4 to 8 years. With this prosthesis the patellofemoral problem rate was 8%.

It is clear that there is a high percentage of problems related to the extensor mechanism that can lead to significant morbidity following surgery. Some of the complications are due to patient and component design factors. However, many are preventable if the surgeon pays attention to surgical detail and patellar tracking during each operation. The best treatment is prevention.

This chapter focuses on the various extensor mechanism complications following total knee arthroplasty, associated factors, and how to prevent these problems or treat them when they do occur.

ANATOMY

The extensor mechanism includes the quadriceps muscle and tendon, patella, medial and lateral patellar retinacula, and patellar tendon. The blood supply to the area is very important. Damage to the arterial blood supply of the extensor mechanism may increase the risk of tendon rupture or avascularity of the patella. The blood supply consists of extraosseous and intraosseous components. Figure 28.1 illustrates the extraosseous supply, while the intraosseous components are extensions of blood vessels from the quadriceps tendon, fat pad, and midpatellar regions. The figure also demonstrates how the surgeon's method of exposure may cause compromise. As well, excision of the fat pad for exposure is associated with a degree of avascularity and this should be considered routinely by those who excise it.

Table 28.1. Extensor mechanism problems with two contemporary total knee arthroplasty systems

	SAL (n = *83)*	*Genesis I* (n = *156)*
Asymptomatic tilting	6	3
Symptomatic tilting	2	4
Anterior knee pain	2	4
Undisplaced fractures	4	2
Aseptic loosening	2	3
Subluxed/dislocated	2	1
Revisions of patellar component	1	2

SAL, self-aligning knee.

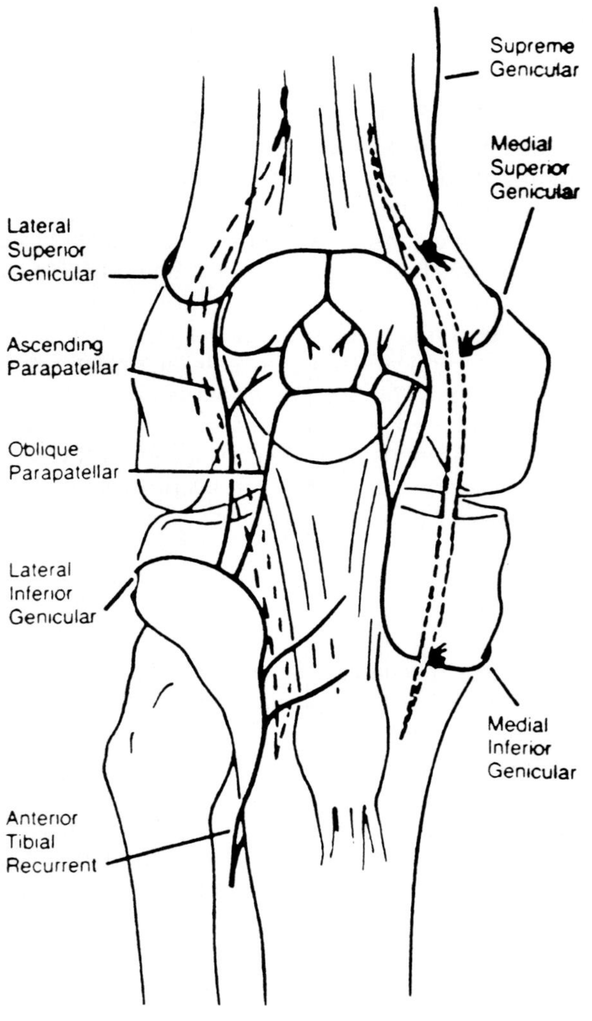

Figure 28.1. Extraosseous blood supply of the patella. A medial parapatellar incision or a lateral incision done for a lateral release, quadriceps turndown, or a lateral parapatellar approach can damage various aspects of the patellar blood supply as indicated.

BIOMECHANICS

The primary function of the extensor mechanism is to extend the knee. The patella increases the moment arm to improve quadriceps power to help with this function. This is illustrated by the fact that patients who have had their patellas removed require at least a 30% increase in quadriceps force to obtain knee extension. These patients have more difficulty with stair climbing and experience more posterior knee pain as a result of increased stresses on the posterior soft tissue structures. Secondary functions of the extensor mechanism include anterior knee protection and dynamic knee stabilization.

Forces across the patellofemoral joint can be quite considerable. Often, we think of the tibiofemoral joint as the area of the knee exposed to the greatest forces. In fact, the patellofemoral joint may exceed the forces generated across the tibiofemoral joint during certain functions.[8] Compressive loads of 0.5 to 1 times body weight occur during walking. This increases to three to four times body weight with stair climbing, and seven to eight times body weight with squatting. These features correlate with the fact that most patients with patellofemoral joint degeneration are most symptomatic on stairs or on rising from a chair.

ANTERIOR KNEE PAIN

Anterior knee pain following the arthroplasty has been noted in several patients at our center. The reported incidence in the literature is 5% to 15%.[9] It can be quite a difficult problem because the exact cause is often unknown and investigations may be negative. There have been many proposed etiologies (Table 28.2). The treatment depends on the exact cause, but if the cause is unknown, treatment may be difficult. The surgeon may have to follow the patient in hope that the pain will resolve or diminish with time.

Table 28.2. Etiologies of anterior knee pain

Tendinopathy
Arthritic exposed lateral facet of patella
Prominent lateral femoral component
Patellar component loosening
Fracture of patella
Patellar component impingement (patella baja)
Maltracking
Posterior cruciate laxity
Unresurfaced patella

PATELLAR CLUNK

Often, soft tissue problems related to the extensor mechanism resolve with time, and reassurance is often all that is needed. To help in the recovery of these problems, quadriceps rehabilitation and the use of mild pain medications or antiinflammatory agents may be helpful.

One soft tissue complication that may require surgery is patellar clunk. It is a phenomenon originally described by Hozack.[10] Patellar clunk is due to a nodule of fibrous tissue at the junction of the posterior distal aspect of the quadriceps tendon and the proximal pole of the patella in cruciate-sacrificing total knee replacements (Fig. 28.2). The problem arises in knee flexion when the nodule enters the intracondylar notch, and then with knee extension to 30 to 45 degrees the nodule becomes trapped, causing a "clunk" as the nodule snaps out of the notch.

The cause appears to be the result of implant design. Posterior stabilized components with a central box and a sharp edge at the superior aspect of the notch may cause development of the nodule in patients who have achieved greater degrees of flexion postoperatively. Several patients with an anatomic medullary knee (AMK) (DePuy, Warsaw, IN) arthroplasty at our center have experienced this problem. Symptoms have resolved with surgery and excision of the nodule. In addition changes have been made to the component in recognition of this complication. Other possible causes may be malpositioning of the patellar component beyond the proximal border of the patella, generalized postoperative scarring, and alterations of patellar height and thickness. Another factor may be elevation of the joint line resulting in patella baja, which could cause impingement of the patellar component in the notch.[11]

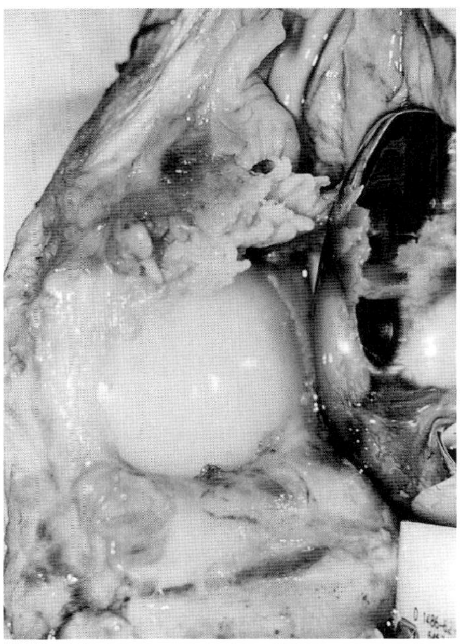

Figure 28.2. Hypertrophied tissue above the superior pole of the patella, causing patellar clunk.

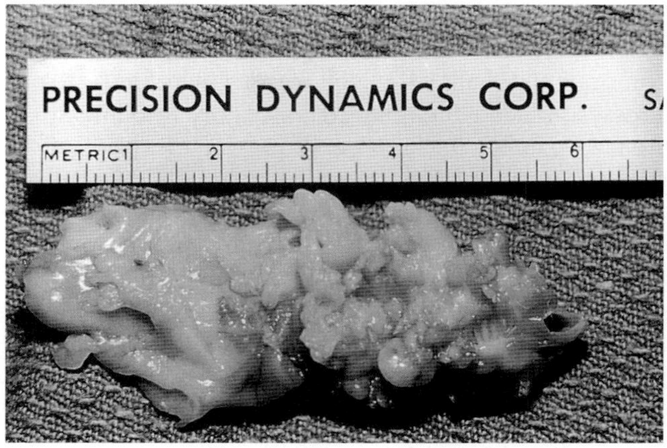

Figure 28.3. Excised tissue responsible for patellar clunk.

Clinically, patellar clunk usually occurs within the first 1 to 2 years postoperatively.[12] It can be associated with audible clicks, snapping, or crepitus. Some patients may experience pain or the sensation that the knee is unstable.

The treatment can be divided into nonoperative and operative measures. Nonoperative treatment includes similar methods for other soft tissue problems as described above. In addition, some patients may feel better simply with a knee sleeve. However, often nonoperative measures are not completely effective in relieving symptoms, and the treating surgeon has to resort to operative measures, including open or arthroscopic surgery. The operation involves addressing one of the above possible causes and resecting the nodule (Fig. 28.3). Arthroscopic treatment appears to be less successful with four recurrences out of 11 surgeries in one published study.[12]

PATELLAR FRACTURES

The incidence of patellar fractures in total knee arthroplasty varies from as high as 21%[13] to about 0.2%[14] with modern primary knee arthroplasty. There is a greater incidence in patients who have rheumatoid arthritis,[7] possibly due to weaker bone and altered circulation. Revision arthroplasty also has a high rate of patellar fractures, with an incidence of 0.61%.[13]

There are many proposed etiologies, including patellar malalignment, knees with 120 degrees or more flexion, selecting too large a femoral component in the anterior/posterior dimension, and flexion of the femoral component,[15] all of which cause increased patellar stresses. Inadequate patellar resection resulting in increased patellar thickness and, conversely, overzealous patellar resection with a final thickness less than 14 mm can also lead to fracture.[16,17] Proper intraoperative attention to patellar tracking, femoral sizing, and pre- and postresection measurements of the patella could help prevent these problems. Other patellar factors include asymmetric cuts, which may decrease bone strength, especially if occurring laterally. A patellar component with a single central peg appears to cause more fractures than those with three peripheral pegs.[18,19] Peg hole problems can also occur if the patellar component is placed too medially, which may result in the pegs being situated in sclerotic peripheral bone, predisposing the patella to avulsion fractures. Even the surgical dissection can be implicated in causing fractures by disrupting the patellar blood supply and causing avascular necrosis of the patella.[20,21] Weakening of the bone can be seen with long-term wear and osteolysis of the patella, again predisposing it to fracture. However, in the postoperative period, many fractures simply occur as the result of trauma.

The classification of periprosthetic patellar fractures varies. They can be thought of simply as undisplaced versus displaced, traumatic versus atraumatic, and by orientation—vertical, transverse, comminuted, or avulsion. Goldberg[22] describes a four-category classification: type 1, avulsion fractures without involvement of the implant/cement composite or quadriceps mechanism; type 2, compromise of the implant/cement composite or quadriceps mechanism, often with an extension lag greater than 30 degrees (Fig. 28.4); type 3, fracture of the inferior pole of the patella with subclassification into types A, in which there is associated patellar ligament disruption, and type B, without ligament involvement; and type 4, more severe, and involving a fracture dislocation of the patella.

Treatment depends most importantly on whether the extensor mechanism is intact, which is influenced by displacement, location, and orientation of the fracture. Fragment size, comminution, and patellar component stability also affect treatment options.

If the patient can do a straight leg raise with a fracture displaced less than 5 mm and has a stable patellar component, the fracture can usually be treated without an operation. A cylinder cast or knee immobilizer can be used. With displaced transverse fractures, the extensor mechanism is dysfunctional and the patellar component is often loose. Treatment options include open reduction and internal fixation, removal of the patellar component if it is loose, with excision of fracture fragments and salvage of the largest fragment. The patella can be left unresurfaced or can be resurfaced if the remaining fragment is large enough. If severely comminuted, patellectomy may have to be performed. It is important to obtain a stable repair of the extensor mechanism. A lateral release may be done at the time of surgery if patellar tracking is an issue.

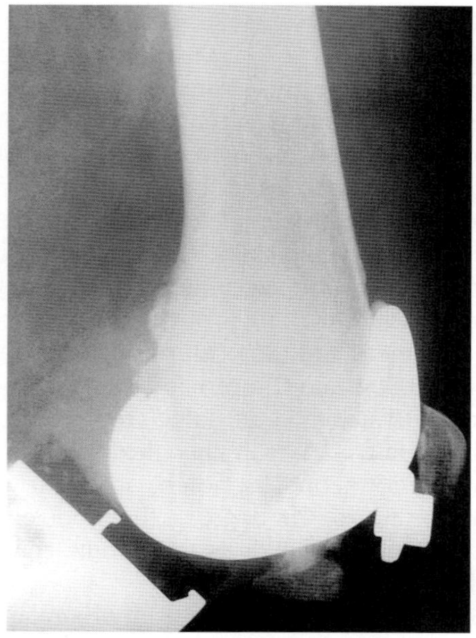

Figure 28.4. Displaced horizontal periprosthetic patellar fracture.

When considering the Goldberg classification, type 1 fractures are treated the same as undisplaced fractures, described above. Type 2 fractures are associated with an extensor lag, and are treated with tension band wiring or Bunnell suturing if there is an avulsion of the superior pole. Type 3 fractures are treated with Bunnell suturing through the tendon and then through vertical drill holes. Type 4 treatment depends on the exact fracture pattern.

PATELLOFEMORAL INSTABILITY

Patellofemoral instability is the most common extensor mechanism problem in total knee arthroplasty, with an incidence as high as 29%[13] (Fig. 28.5). It can result in clicking or catching in the knee, especially with stair climbing and rising from a seated position. Associated anterior knee pain and crepitus are common complaints. The final result may be component wear, loosening, or fracture.

The key to dealing with this problem is identifying the cause. Several etiologies may result in instability. An

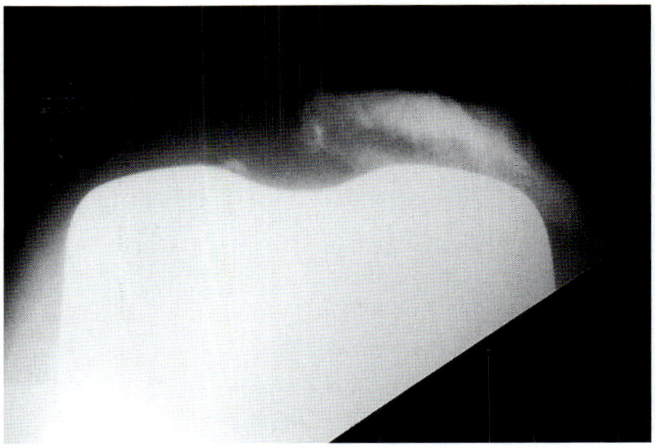

Figure 28.5. Lateral subluxed patella.

imbalance of the extensor mechanism occurs when there is a tight retinaculum, or a weak vastus medialis resulting in lateral tilting, subluxation, or dislocation. Similar findings may result if there is a disruption of the medial retinacular repair postoperatively or if there is excessive valgus of the lower limb. Imbalance of soft tissue tension may be a cause if there is a difference in patellar bone resection from medial and lateral sides. Simmons[23] reported on 12 patients treated for patellar dislocation because of patella alta. They were all treated by transposing the patellar tendon distally with medialization. Another factor to consider is component positioning. Instability is seen if the tibial or femoral components are internally rotated or medially shifted, or if there is lateral placement of the patellar component. When considering placement of the tibial component, the center of the tray should be placed over the medial one-third of the tibial tubercle. The femoral component should be about 3 degrees of external rotation (which is now built into most instrumentation). The surgeon can also consider one or all three of the following references to ensure accurate femoral positioning: Insall[24] lines up the component with the transepicondylar line; Whiteside[25] places the femoral component perpendicular to a line drawing in the center of the patellofemoral notch of the femur; the third option is to make the tibial cut first, then if there is a rectangular space between the tibia and femur in flexion, the femoral component will be accurately positioned. Finally, certain component designs predispose to instability of the extensor mechanism. For example, Campbell[26] reported a 5% incidence of patellar maltracking with the MG1. Poor design features include a shallow patellofemoral groove and a poor entrapment zone.[27]

Another bad design is seen with rigid hinges, which do not allow internal rotation in early flexion. In contrast, some prosthesis rotating platform designs allow some rotation of the tibial prosthesis on the femur in both flexion and extension, making exact positioning unnecessary.

Assessment of possible instability should occur intraoperatively. Placement of the patella in the trochlear groove and flexing and extending the knee with the tibia slightly internally rotated while assessing tracking (no-thumb technique) should be carried out and any cause of instability should be addressed. Also, direct observation of the patella in the trochlear groove with flexion of the knee should be done to ensure central tracking with no tilting.

Treatment can be divided into nonoperative and operative. The nonoperative methods include vastus medialis obliquus strengthening, bracing the patellofemoral joint, and having the patient avoid provocative activities such as squatting or stair climbing. Operative measures are aimed at correcting one of the possible causes. In general, the surgeon may consider a lateral retinacular release or realignment procedure. Proximal realignment can be done with a vastus medialis advancement. Distal procedures include tibial tubercle osteotomy with medialization such as the Emslie-Trillat procedure.[28]

PATELLAR RESURFACING

Most early knee prosthesis designs had no provision for patellar replacement; therefore, the patellofemoral joint was neglected when considering the arthroplasty (Fig. 28.6). Contemporary knee arthroplasty systems have a capacity for patellar resurfacing, and more attention is now paid to this area. There is support for resurfacing in rheumatoid arthritis patients,[21,29,30,31] but for osteoarthritic patients opinions vary on whether to resurface

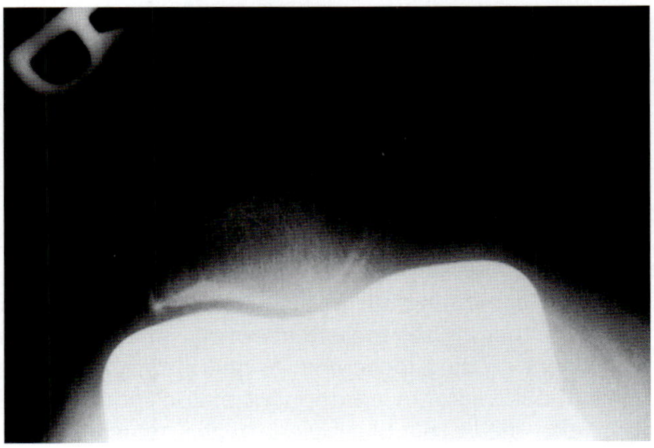

Figure 28.6. Total knee arthroplasty with an unresurfaced patella.

or not. Proponents say that it gives predictable results,[6,32–34] while others argue that the reoperation rate is similar if the patella is resurfaced or not.[13,35] The prevalence of patellar pain when the patella is not resurfaced ranges from 5% to 45%.[36,37] However, these studies are retrospective and the implants used were poorly designed to deal with the patellofemoral joint. Sledge[38] reviewed 891 knee arthroplasties and found a higher rate of revision and peripatellar pain in the nonresurfaced group, whereas Greenwald reviewed 52 patients with bilateral knee arthroplasties and found no difference in pain when the patella was resurfaced or not. Our group studied 100 patients with osteoarthritis; patients were randomized into resurfaced or nonresurfaced groups.[39] Four patients (8%) in the nonresurfaced group have required reoperation within the first 5 years because of anterior knee pain with resolution of their pain after resurfacing. However, the nonresurfaced group had significantly less anterior pain, and better knee flexion torques. This study did not take into account intraoperative findings, but as Scott[40] has stated, it was not possible from preoperative and interoperative findings to predict which patients might have patellofemoral symptoms following surgery.

This leaves the surgeon with one of three possible strategies: always resurface the patella, never resurface the patella, or resurface the patella depending on clinical and intraoperative guidelines.

We think absolute indications for resurfacing the patella would be rheumatoid arthritis, or when the operation is done for patellofemoral arthrosis. Relative indications include moderate to severe patellofemoral arthritis and when the knee implant used has a nonanatomic patellofemoral joint.

PATELLAR COMPONENT LOOSENING

The incidence of patellar component loosening is less than 2% in the cemented versus 0.6% to 13.5% in cementless components[2,6,41] (Fig. 28.7). Component loosening can be subdivided into aseptic and septic etiologies. Aseptic loosening has many causes, including loosening as a result of poor bone quality as seen in patients with osteonecrosis or osteoporosis. Loosening can also occur if the surgeon utilizes poor cementing technique or if cementing into deficient bone results in poor fixation. Other causes include abnormal stresses on the component causing loosening, as seen in patients with patellar subluxation or component malposition. Malposition also leads to polyethylene wear, which in turn can cause debris-induced osteolysis disrupting the bone/cement interface. The yield strength of ultra-high molecular weight polyethylene is less than the patellofemoral joint reaction forces, which can result in cold flow, deformation, and particulate debris formation if proper component positioning, conformity, and constraint are not achieved. Finally, some component designs have been implicated as the cause of loosening.

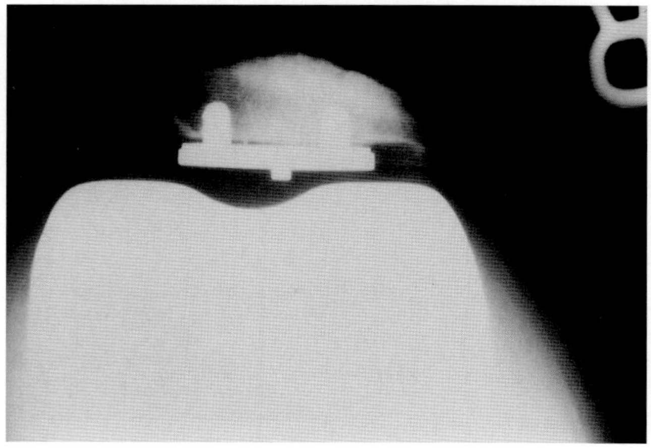

Figure 28.7. Probably loose patellar component with radiolucency between the component and bone.

The diagnosis is confirmed by correlating the patient's symptoms and signs with radiographic findings. On radiographs one may see a progressive radiolucency between the bone and component/cement interface or even a displaced component. A diagnosis of displacement of the polyethylene is made easier if it contains a radiolucent marker. However, a loose patellar component may be relatively asymptomatic if it is stabilized by the surrounding soft tissue. Often during revision surgery, this can be seen as a meniscus-like structure around the edges of the polyethylene. But, with advanced wear, peripatellar pain and an effusion will develop.

Treatment depends on the mode of failure. If a cause of the loosening is found, it should be corrected and then the component revised. Patellar revision alone can be achieved with good results if the etiology is found to be isolated to the patella, but complication rates between 24% and 33%[42] have been reported with single component revision of the patella. A new patellar component can be inserted if adequate bone stock remains (greater than 10–14 mm thick). If bone stock is not adequate, then retaining the remaining patella after smoothing of prominent edges results in good function. However, some surgeons prefer not to resurface at all in revision knee arthroplasty cases. (Lotke[27] also thinks this is the best method of salvage with a loose patellar component associated with osteonecrosis.) If adequate patella is not available during the revision, a technique described by Buechel[43] can prove useful. He reports use of bone graft sutured into the extensor mechanism to help restore patellar function.

METAL-BACKED PATELLA

Metal-backed patellar components were introduced in an attempt to reduce forces in the implants, cement, and bone; however, polyethylene wear has become a significant problem with this design[44–47] (Figs. 28.8 and 28.9). Problems arise because the metal occupies space, leaving a decreased thickness of polyethylene, which in turn leads to increased wear. The polyethylene is especially thin at the periphery, which predisposes to wear. Exposed metal is the result and causes scratching of the femoral component, leading to more wear, debris, and osteolysis. These changes are often seen in the first 2 years postoperatively.[44–47] Other modes of failure include the metal not extending all the way out to the periphery of the polyethylene, leading to deformation and possible breakage.[47] In addition, fatigue fractures may occur at the peg-plate interface if the pegs are securely ingrown but the plate is not. Finally, as wear occurs, the polyethylene may dislodge from the metal if the locking mechanism is affected.

The clinical signs of this occurrence include crepitus (audible and palpable) and an effusion. Confirmation with a radiograph is useful. A Merchant view is best and may show metal-on-metal, displaced polyethylene or metal synovitis (metal line sign).

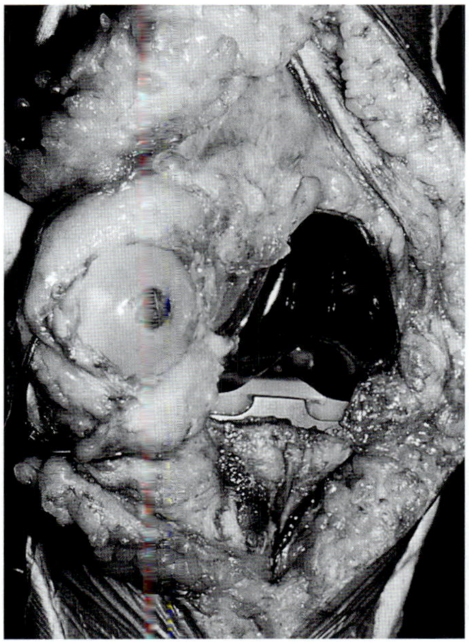

Figure 28.8. Metal-backed patella with polyethylene wear.

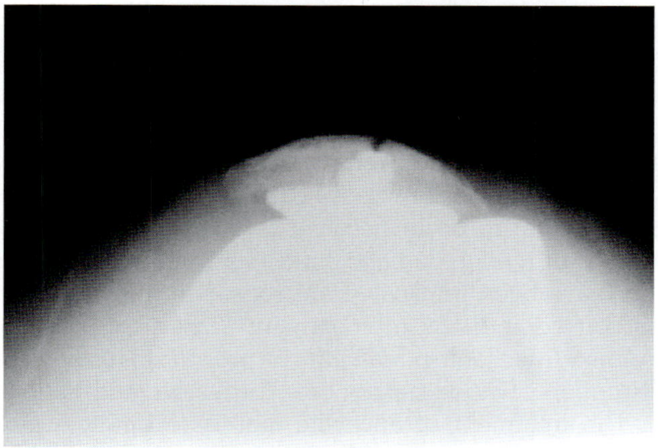

Figure 28.9. Radiograph of a metal-backed patella with polyethylene wear.

Treatment is to revise the knee arthroplasty. The extent of the revision depends on the degree of damage. Intraoperatively, the surgeon may encounter extensive debris and black staining of the synovium. A synovectomy should be part of the procedure. These metal particles may be found ground into the tibial polyethylene as well. Also noted is patellar polyethylene wear and scoring of the femoral component. This situation requires a complete revision to be performed. At time of revision, the metal may be solidly ingrown and require burrs or osteotomes to remove the component.

REPAIR OF PATELLAR POUCH

Most surgeons pay attention to proper repair of the patellar pouch while closing a knee arthroplasty, realizing that inadvertent obliteration of the pouch leads to reduced knee flexion. Often while repairing the superior aspect of a medial parapatellar incision, the pouch may be included with wide bites of the suture. This could lead to a decreased volume of the pouch, which may lead to decreased knee flexion. Some failures attributed to poor knee flexion in the postoperative period may be related to this problem, which in turn may leave the patient with significant disability.

LOSS OF EXTENSOR MECHANISM

Loss of the extensor mechanism results in a poorly functioning knee arthroplasty, which usually ends in failure. Weakness or a nonfunctioning extensor mechanism and a loss of anterior/posterior stability occurs. Loss of the extensor mechanism is seen in various conditions including acute or chronic ruptures of the patellar or quadriceps tendon or paralysis of the quadriceps muscle.

Quadriceps Tendon Rupture

Quadriceps tendon rupture is less common than patellar tendon disruption[7,48] (Fig. 28.10). There are various situations in which a patient may be more likely to sustain a rupture of the tendon. It occurs more frequently if a lateral retinacular release has been performed.[7] It is also thought to occur because of possible vascular disruption or tendon damage during surgery. Other factors that have been implicated are repeat steroid injection, patellar component impingement, a previous proximal extensor mechanism realignment procedure resulting in disruption of blood supply, scar formation, and trauma.

The treatment of an acute tear is repair by suture techniques. The tear usually occurs near or at the patellar attachment. A good method is to use Merseline no. 5 suture and perform a grasping stitch (i.e., Bunnell) in the tendon, and then bring the two ends out through the distal aspect of the torn tendon. Next, drill holes are placed longitudinally from the superior pole to the inferior pole of the patella. The superior pole surface is prepared by roughening the bone surface to the point of bleeding to help in the healing of the tendon to the patella. Next, each of the suture ends are passed through one of the tunnels. This can be achieved by straightening out the needle with two large needle drivers, or by using a suture passer. The ends are then tied together after the tendon has been secured tightly to the patella. The remainder of the torn soft tissue cuff can be oversewn. This usually results in a good repair, which allows early range of motion and prevents stiffness of the knee. Occasionally, a bone fragment will be avulsed with the quadriceps tendon, and in this situation the stability of the patellar component (if present) should be assessed.

Patellar Tendon Rupture

Patellar tendon rupture is a complication feared by all orthopedic surgeons who perform total knee arthroplasty, as the result can be devastating (Fig. 28.11). Prevention is the key, and great care is taken intraoperatively to prevent any damage to the tendon. Our group often places a ⅛-inch pin through the patellar tendon at the level of the tibial tubercle to stress relieve the tendon insertion in these situations. For very tight exposures, the options include a quadriceps snip, quadriceps turndown, or tibial tubercle osteotomy. Care should be taken when carrying out a tibial tubercle osteotomy, or the surgeon may create the same problem he was trying to prevent. A butt joint implemented proximally can help prevent migration, and if the osteotomy is done properly, the nonunion rates are low.[49] Other intraoperative factors that could result in patellar tendon disruption include blood supply disruption with removal of

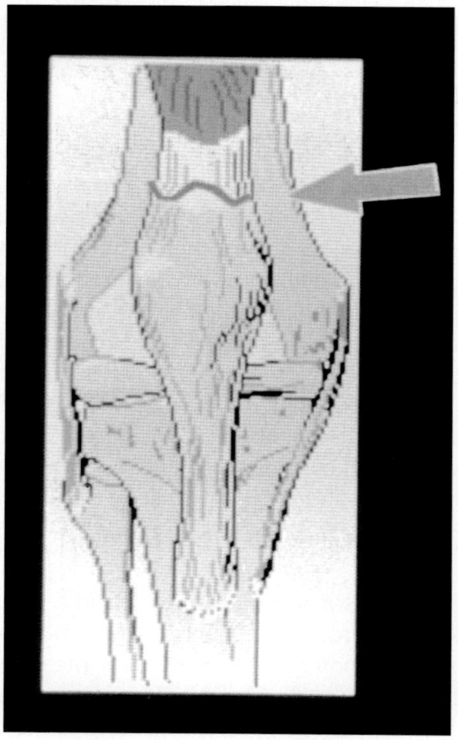

Figure 28.10. Quadriceps tendon rupture (arrow).

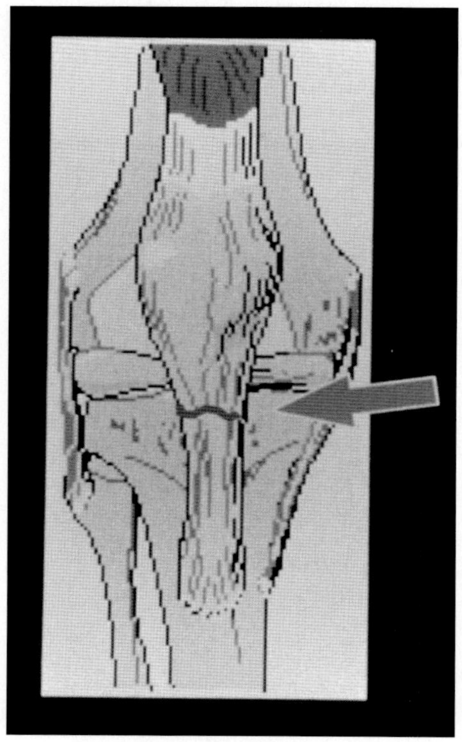

Figure 28.11. Patellar tendon rupture (arrow).

the fat pad for exposure. Also, excessive removal of the patellar bone or tibial bone may weaken the tendon attachment.[48]

Despite trying to prevent this complication, the incidence has been reported to be between 0.17% and 1.4%.[7,50] These figures include the intraoperative and early and late postoperative periods. Other causes of early rupture include knee manipulation, and it has increased frequency with previous knee operations. Later disruptions can occur if the patient falls, resulting in hyperflexion of the knee. Patients who receive systemic steroids or who have connective tissue disease, such as rheumatoid arthritis, lupus, or diabetes mellitis are at higher risk of rupture. Other factors include a higher incidence with distal patellar realignment procedures, constrained implants, and component malalignment, which puts extra stress on the patellar tendon, resulting in rupture.

Treatment may be unsatisfactory, and if this is the case, a knee arthrodesis may be the final outcome. However, attempts at treating this problem have included operative and nonoperative measures and have had various degrees of success. Nonoperative treatment is usually not successful. It includes immobilization or the use of a double upright drop-lock knee brace. Various surgical treatment options have been attempted for repair, including direct suture repair, internal fixation of an avulsed bone fragment, extensor mechanism allograft, bovine xenograft,[50] Dacron graft, fascia lata graft, hamstring autograft, and a gastrocnemius flap. The following is a review of some of these techniques.

If no defect is present in the tendon, then a direct suture repair may be attempted. Rand[50] reviewed 18 patients who had repair with various techniques. None of the patients who had suturing and only half who had a staple repair had a successful outcome. Rand also studied those patients treated with observation and immobilization, but again this did not lead to high rates of healing. Abril,[51] however, reported good results in two cases of direct repair of the tendon to bone with Bunnell suturing and placement of the sutures into a bone tunnel chiseled into the tibial tubercle, and then neutralizing the repair with a tension band wire.

Other techniques need to be considered if a gap exists in the patellar tendon. Finn[52] described the use of a medial gastrocnemius flap in seven patients. Improvement in range of motion and decreased extensor lag was reported. Another advantage of this technique is that it allows for improved soft tissue coverage. The procedure involves extending the previous midline incision distally and just medial to the tibia. A plane is developed between the medial gastrocnemius and soleus. The medial gastrocnemius is divided distally at the Achilles tendon and left attached proximally, preserving the medial sural artery. It is then transposed to cover the tibial tubercle and sutured to the anterior compartment fascia. The patellar tendon and the anterior aspect of the joint capsule are sutured to the medial border of the flap. The patient is then casted for 6 weeks.

Multiple graft methods have been utilized for reconstruction. Our center uses a similar technique to the one described by Ecker[53] with good results. This method involves transfer of the semitendinosus, with or without reinforcement with the gracilis and supplemented with a heavy gauge wire (Fig. 28.12). A midline incision is made, followed by exposure of the semitendinosus and gracilis tendons at the pes aserinus. The tendons are then harvested with a tendon stripper, but left attached to the pes anserinus. Two large drill holes are made to accommodate the tendon in the distal patella, and an oblique hole is made through the tibial tubercle. The semitendinosus is inserted through the tibial tubercle hole and then through the patella lateral to medial. The gracilis is passed medial to lateral through the patella. The tendons are tightened and sutured to each other. The repair is protected by the heavy gauge wire placed through the distal pole of the patella. The patient is casted for 6 weeks. At this stage, the wire is removed and the knee is manipulated under general anesthesia.

Other graft materials include bovine xenograft, fascia lata, and Dacron graft. Lanzetta[54] reviewed the use of fascia lata strips, but found it to lack the strength of

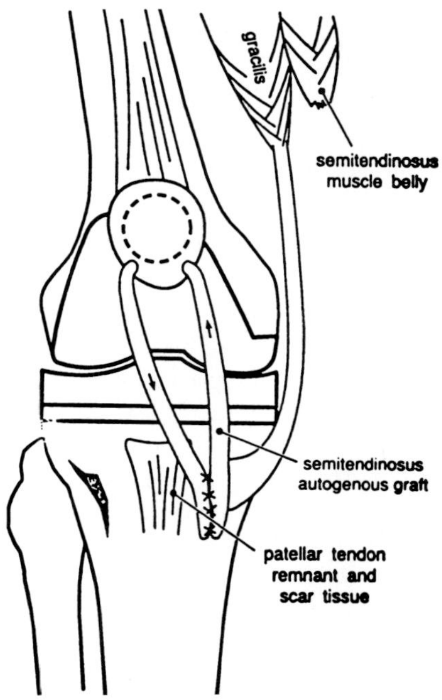

Figure 28.12. Semitendinosus reconstruction of a ruptured patellar tendon. The gracilis tendon can be used in addition for extra supplementation.

intact tendons. Levin[55] presented a case report of patellar tendon reconstruction using a Dacron graft, through longitudinal holes in the patella and tibial tubercle, with good results in this patient.

For more severe cases, Emerson[56,57] published good results in 15 patients with the use of an extensor mechanism allograft. The allograft consisted of the tibial tubercle, patellar tendon, resurfaced patella, and quadriceps tendon, which were freeze-dried or fresh frozen. Twelve had full passive extension, with six having no extensor lag and an average range of motion of 106 degrees postoperatively. Complications included one graft rupture, one patellar component loosening, and one fracture. Zanotti[58] described a less extensive technique with a good outcome in a case report of a less severely involved patient; an allograft bone-tendon-bone complex was used. The allograft bone is attached to the patient's patella and the other end is secured by a screw into the tibial tubercle.

CONCLUSION

Extensor mechanism problems are frequent and can result in early or late failure of a total knee arthroplasty. Serious technical consideration should be given to this area of knee joint replacement in order to achieve successful results.

References

1. Doolittle KH. Patellofemoral problems following total knee arthroplasty. *Orthop Rev* 1988;17:696–702.
2. Clayton ML. Patellar complications after total condylar arthroplasty. *Clin Orthop* 1982;170:152–155.
3. Mochizuki RM. Patellar complications following total knee arthroplasty. *J Bone Joint Surg* 1979;61A:879–883.
4. Moreland JR. ICLH replacement of the knee: 1977 and 1978. *Clin Orthop* 1979;145:47–59.
5. Leblanc JM. Patellar complications in total knee arthroplasty: a literature review. *Orthop Rev* 1989;18:296–304.
6. Ranawat CS. The patellar joint in condylar knee arthroplasty: pros and cons based on 5–10 year follow-up observations. *Clin Orthop* 1986;205:93–99.
7. Bourne RB. Extensor mechanism complications following total knee arthroplasty. *J Arthroplasty* 1987;2(2):135–140.
8. Reilly DJ, Marten M. Experimental analysis of the quadriceps muscle force and patellofemoral joint reaction force for various activities. *Acta Orthop Scand* 1972;43:126.
9. Dennis D. *Extensor mechanism problems in total knee arthroplasty.* Instr Course Lect 1997;46:171–180.
10. Hozack WJ. The patellar clunk syndrome: a complication of posterior stabilized total knee arthroplasties. *Clin Orthop* 1989;241:203–208.
11. Keblish PA, Varma AK, Greenwald AS. Patellar resurfacing or retention in total knee arthroplasty. A prospective study of patients with bilateral replacements. *J Bone Joint Surg* 1994;76(6):930–937.
12. Beight JL. Patellar clunk syndrome following posterior stabilized total knee arthroplasty: results of treatment. Paper presented at the Knee Society, San Francisco, 1993.
13. Cameron HU. The patella in total knee arthroplasty. *Clin Orthop* 1982;165:197–199.
14. Grace JN. Fracture of the patella after total knee arthroplasty. *Clin Orthop* 1988:230:168–175.
15. Windsor RE. Patellar fractures in total knee arthroplasty. *J Arthroplasty* 1989;4 Suppl:S63–67:563–567.
16. Kraay MJ. Patellar fracture and breakage. In: Fu F, Horner C, Vince K (eds). *Knee Surgery*. Baltimore: Williams & Wilkins, 1994:1473–1482.
17. Reuben JD. Effect of patellar thickness on patella strain following total knee arthroplasty. *J Arthoplasty* 1991;6:251–258.
18. Rand JA. Technique of patellar resurfacing in total knee arthroplasty. *Tech Orthop* 1988;3:57–66.
19. Goldstein SA. Patellar surface strain. *J Orthop Res* 1986;4:372–377.
20. Insall G. The total condylar knee prosthesis: a report of 220 cases. *J Bone Joint Surg* 1979;61A:173–180.
21. Scott RD. Stress fractures of the patella following duopatellar total knee arthroplasty with patellar resurfacing. *Clin Orthop* 1982;170:147–151.
22. Goldberg VM. Patella fracture type and prognosis in condylar total knee arthroplasty. *Clin Orthop* 1988;236:115–122.
23. Simmons E Jr. Patella alta and recurrent dislocation of the patella. *Clin Orthop* 1992;274:265–269.
24. Insall G. Rotational landmarks and sizing of the distal femur in total knee arthroplasty. *Clin Orthop Rel Res* 1996;331:35–45.
25. Whiteside L. Femoral rotational alignment based on the AT axis in total knee arthroplasty in a valgus knee. *J Bone Joint Surg* 1995;77A(9):1331–1334.
26. Campbell DG. Early patellofemoral revision following total knee arthroplasty. *J Arthroplasty* 1995;10(3):287–291.
27. Lotke P. Management of extensor mechanism complications. In: Current Concepts in Joint Replacement. Orlando, FL: 1997.
28. Williams RM. New treatment of recurrent patellar dislocation. *Orthop Rev* 1992;21(11):1329–1332.
29. Scott RD. Pros and cons of patellar resurfacing in total knee replacement. *Orthop Trans* 1980;4:328.
30. Sledge CB. Total knee arthroplasty experience at the

Robert Breck Brigham Hospital. *Clin Orthop* 1979; 147:78.

31. Steinberg J. Tissue culture model of cartilage breakdown in rheumatoid arthritis. *Biochem J* 1979;180:403.
32. Brick GW, Scott RD. The patellofemoral component of total knee arthroplasty. *Clin Orthop* 1988;231:163–178.
33. Levai JP. Why not resurface the patella? *J Bone Joint Surg* 1983;65B:447–451.
34. Picetti JD. The patellofemoral joint after total knee arthroplasty without patellar resurfacing. *J Bone Joint Surg* 1990;72A:1379–1382.
35. Abraham W. Should the patella be resurfaced in arthroplasty? *Clin Orthop* 1988;236:128–134.
36. Ewald FC. Duopatella total knee arthroplasty in rhematoid arthritis. *Orthop Trans* 1978;2:202.
37. Hofman GO. Pathomechanics of the patellofemoral joint following total knee arthroplasty. *Clin Orthop* 1987;224:251–259.
38. Sledge CB. Long joint complications after total knee arthroplasty with or without resurfacing of the patella. *J Bone Joint Surg* 1993;75A(5):674–681.
39. Bourne RB. Resurfacing vs. not resurfacing the patella during total knee replacement. *Clin Orthop Rel Res* 1995;321:156–161.
40. Scott RD. Prosthetic replacement of the patellofemoral joint. *Orthop Clin North Am* 1979;10:129.
41. Rae PJ. Patellar resurfacing in total condylar knee arthroplasty. *J Arthroplasty* 1990;5:259–265.
42. Berry DJ. Isolated patellar component revision of total knee arthroplasty. *Clin Orthop* 1986;286:110–115.
43. Buechel FF. Patellar tendon bone grafting for patellectomized patients having total knee arthroplasty. *Clin Orthop* 1991;271:72–78.
44. Bayley JC. Failure of the metal-backed patellar component after total knee replacement. *J Bone Joint Surg* 1988;70A:668–674.
45. Bayley JC. Further observation of metal-backed patella component failure. *Clin Orthop* 1988;236:82–87.
46. Rosenberg AG. Patellar component failure in cementless total knee arthroplasty. *Clin Orthop* 1988;236:106–114.
47. Stulberg SD. Failure mechanisms of metal-backed patella components. *Clin Orthop* 1988;236:88–105.
48. Gustillo RB. Quadriceps and patellar tendon ruptures following total knee arthroplasty. In: Rand JA, Doerr LD (eds). *Total Arthroplasty of the Knee*. Rockville, MD: Aspen, 1987:41–47.
49. Whiteside LA. Exposure in difficult total knee arthroplasty using tibial tubercle osteotomy. *Clin Orthop* 1995;321:32–35.
50. Rand JA. Patella tendon rupture after total knee arthroplasty. *Clin Orthop Rel Res* 1989;244:233–238.
51. Abril JC, Alvarez L, Vallejo JC. Patella tendon avulsion after total knee arthroplasty. *J Arthroplasty* 1995;10(3):275–279.
52. Finn HA. Medial gastrocnemius transposition flap for the treatment of disruption of the extensor mechanism after total knee arthroplasty. *J Bone Joint Surg* 1997;79A(6):866–873.
53. Ecker ML. Late reconstruction of the patella tendon. *J Bone Joint Surg* 1979;61A(6):884–886.
54. Lanzetta A. *Arch Orthop* 1962;75:606–613.
55. Levin P. Reconstruction of the patella tendon using a Dacron graft. *Clin Orthop Rel Res* 1976;118:70–72.
56. Emerson RH. Extensor mechanism reconstruction with an allograft after total knee arthroplasty. *Clin Orthop Rel Res* 1994;303:79–85.
57. Emerson RH. Reconstruction of patellar tendon rupture after total knee arthroplasty with an extensor mechanism allograft. *Clin Orthop Rel Res* 1990;260:154–161.
58. Zanotti RM. Use of patellar allograft to reconstruct a patella tendon deficient knee after total knee arthroplasty. *J Arthroplasty* 1995;10(3):271–274.

Chapter 29

FRACTURES AROUND TOTAL KNEE PROSTHESES

David A. Padden and Michael A. Mont

As an inevitable consequence of the ever-increasing number of knee arthroplasty procedures performed, complications have arisen that often require knowledge and understanding of combined disciplines such as trauma and reconstruction. Periprosthetic fractures around a total knee prosthesis, although occurring uncommonly (incidence from 0.3% to 2.0% in multiple large studies),[1–8] are potentially devastating injuries that may yield a poor implant result. Because of the relative paucity of these fractures and inherent difficulty in comparing most published studies, no established treatment regimen has been uniformly defined. This chapter enumerates a number of key points in preventing and managing these fractures.

TYPE AND NATURE OF POSTOPERATIVE PERIPROSTHETIC FEMUR AND TIBIA FRACTURES

Postoperative fractures around a total knee prosthesis typically occur as a result of low-energy trauma. They are most common in the elderly female patient with osteoporosis. An association with rheumatoid arthritis,[1–3,5,6] corticosteroid use, and neurologic disorders have also been observed. These fractures have been reported to occur anywhere from early in the postoperative period (within 4 weeks) to more than 10 years after surgery, with most occurring between 2 and 4 years.[1,2,4,5,7,9,10] Anatomically, most authors have defined femoral periprosthetic fractures as those occurring up to 15 cm from the joint line.[8,11] This definition has not been applied in the literature to tibial fractures. In this chapter we define both tibial and femoral periprosthetic fractures as occurring within 15 cm of the joint line (Fig. 29.1).

Appropriate evaluation requires a thorough history and physical examination, in addition to standard radiographs. Irrespective of the radiographic evaluation, the surgeon should determine if the patient can tolerate surgical intervention or whether nonoperative treatment is more appropriate. The functional performance of the knee arthroplasty prior to the fracture should be determined.

Physical examination should include a thorough check for concurrent injuries. Focus should be directed to an assessment of the injured limb, including a thorough neurovascular examination as well as an evaluation of the soft tissue envelope both proximal and distal to the knee. Previous skin incisions should be noted. Open wounds, areas of skin breakdown, and, in rare instances, fracture blisters may need to be addressed prior to or in conjunction with definitive fracture management.

Thorough radiographic assessment of periprosthetic fractures around the knee requires standard anteroposterior and lateral radiographs. Long-leg views including the hip, knee, and ankle should be obtained when possible. Often, patients may have additional ipsilateral arthroplasties or other implants that may limit treatment options, or require special-order implants, devices, or bone grafts for fixation or revision (Fig 29.2). This kind of information must be known prior to surgical intervention. Additionally, previous radiographs prior to the fracture should be reviewed with attention focused on alignment, bone quality and stock, implant fixation, and evidence of prosthetic wear. A patient with a loose prosthesis will not do well regardless of fracture healing, and

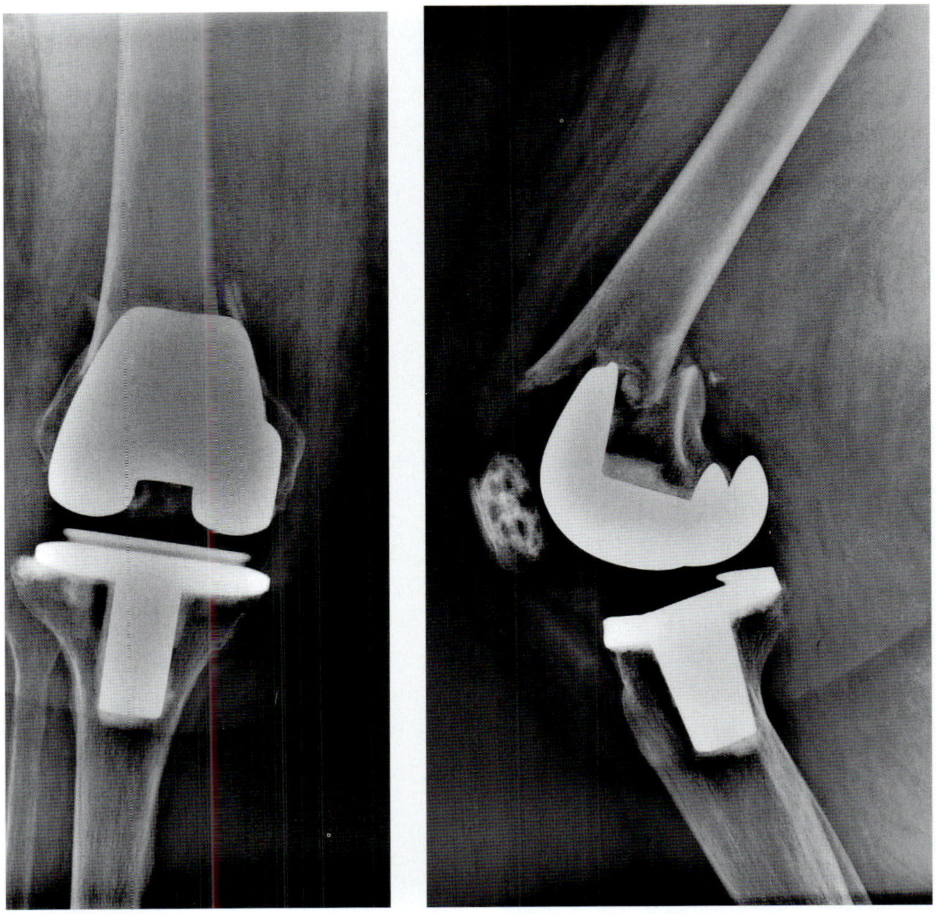

A B

Figure 29.1. A and B: Typical radiographic appearance of a supracondylar femoral fracture above a well-fixed total knee arthroplasty.

this should be understood by both patient and surgeon prior to embarking on any treatment plan.

Periprosthetic supracondylar femur fractures are far more commonly encountered than periprosthetic tibial fractures. The incidence of supracondylar femur fractures after total knee arthroplasty is approximately 1%, with rates ranging from 0.5% to 2.0% in various large series.[1–3,5,6,8] In one large series of periprosthetic tibial fractures consisting of 15 patients from the Mayo Clinic in the late 1970s, this complication represented 1.7% of a group of 705 knee replacement patients.[7] However, recent data from the same institution identified only 71 postoperative tibial fractures between 1970 and 1985, representing only 0.4% of the 17,727 total knee arthroplasties performed during that period.[4] This apparent decline in the incidence of these fractures remains unexplained but might be secondary to some of the preventative measures that are discussed later in this chapter.

Due to the relative paucity of data on reporting of these fractures, no absolute guidelines have been established concerning fracture classification or what constitutes appropriate management.[4,12–15] Several investigators have applied the Neer classification[14] for distal femur fractures to distinguish femoral fracture types in total knee arthroplasties. This classification divides supracondylar fractures into types 1, 2A, 2B, and 3 based on the degree of displacement, direction, and comminution. Type 1 fractures are nondisplaced (less than 5 mm displacement or 5 degrees of angulation). Type 2 fractures are displaced, and are subdivided depending on the direction of proximal femoral shaft displacement into medial (2A) or lateral (2B) types. Type 3 fractures include displacement combined with a significant degree of comminution. However, for the purpose of this discussion, based on our experience as well as our review of the literature, fractures will be classified as either type 1 (nondisplaced Neer 1) or type 2 (displaced and/or comminuted Neer 2 and 3). Both of these groups can then be further subdivided into knees with well-fixed components (A) or loose components (B). No attempt will be made to classify periprosthetic tibial

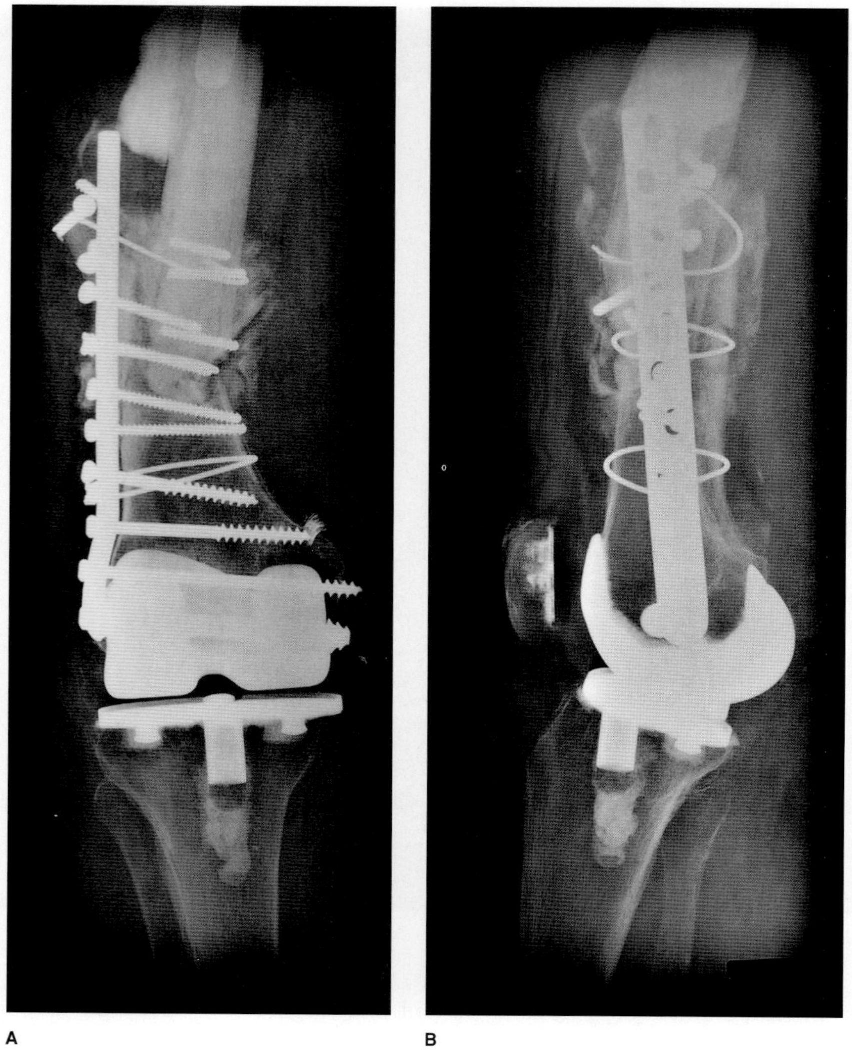

Figure 29.2. **A** and **B**: An ipsilateral cemented revision total hip arthroplasty may compromise fixation and contribute to a nonunion and loss of reduction.

fractures, as most of these are associated with loose components requiring revision. The other rare tibial fractures involving the shaft, spine, or tuberosity are usually treated nonoperatively or in a manner similar to fractures not associated with total knee prosthetic components.

PREVENTION OF PERIPROSTHETIC FACTORS AROUND TOTAL KNEE PROSTHESES

As the technique of total knee arthroplasty has been refined with later-generation instrumentation systems as well as newer prostheses, attempts to prevent complications associated with the procedure have focused on technical points other than those related to patient selection. The importance of accurate and meticulous surgical technique cannot be understated in the overall success of total knee arthroplasty. They are of major importance in the frail, osteopenic, medically fragile, or neurologically impaired individual to whom periprosthetic fractures primarily afflict and in whom minor errors in technique can lead to this complication.

Early in the history of total knee arthroplasty, several authors observed a relationship between a properly positioned prosthesis and a good result.[16,17] This point would appear to take on added significance in the prevention of periprosthetic tibial fractures, as a number of authors have demonstrated a significant association between varus angulation and tibial stress fractures.[7,16,18–20]

The role of breeching of the anterior femoral cortex (notching) and its association with supracondylar fractures of the femur was initially presented by Culp and co-workers,[3] who found a 29.2% decrease in polar moment of inertia with 3-mm notches of the anterior cortex. In addition, they found that 27 periprosthetic femoral fractures were associated with a notched anterior femoral cortex out of a series of 61 fractures (44%). However, Ritter and associates[10] reported a much larger series of 570 knees, of which 138 (24.2%) had notching in excess of 3 mm, in which only one periprosthetic fracture had occurred at 2- to 10-year follow-up. Because of the rarity of this complication, no firm conclusion can be derived from these series concerning the role of notching or the rate of fracture after notches. Based on our own experience and that reported in the literature, we cannot offer guidelines concerning the need for any prophylactic measures such as bracing or restricted weight bearing or activity to be used after notching. At the present time, we would not recommend any alteration in therapy or weight-bearing status in patients with notched femurs.

Gentle handling of tissues in the revision setting and in the treatment of the ankylosed joint is necessary as both of these scenarios are associated with increased rates of periprosthetic fractures. In the revision setting, overall bone stock and the quality of bone stock present are often compromised, and thus the use of excessive forces in implant removal, impaction, reaming, and trial reductions is likely to have a large impact on the remaining bone. The ankylosed joint, with its increased stresses on the distal femoral metaphysis, requires similar care in the prevention of fracture. Manipulation of these joints should be performed gently, and revision often requires wide exposure with additional techniques such as quadriceps muscle turndown or tibial tubercleplasty utilized as necessary.

TREATMENT, MANAGEMENT, AND SALVAGE OF FRACTURES AROUND TOTAL KNEE PROSTHESIS

FEMORAL FRACTURES

The treatment of supracondylar femur fractures ipsilateral to a total knee prosthesis must be managed on an individual basis. Advocates for either initial nonoperative management or early operative intervention may be found in the literature.[2,3,5,11,21–23] In studies by Delport and coworkers[11] and Hirsch and associates,[22] traction and casting were reported to provide for successful patient outcome in most cases. In contrast, Short and coworkers[23] discouraged closed treatment and recommended open reduction and internal fixation. Similarly, Bogach and associates[2] advised internal fixation of these fractures after attaining poor results in their patients treated nonoperatively. In 1987, Culp and coworkers[3] reported on the largest series to date. In this multicenter study, they compared the clinical outcome of 31 fractures treated with surgery versus 30 fractures treated without surgery and they concluded that initial secure internal fixation and early range-of-motion was the treatment of choice. However, subsequent reports have demonstrated success with nonoperative treatment,[5,12,24,25] once again indicating that controversy exists concerning the preferred treatment of these fractures.

Type I (nondisplaced) fractures should initially be treated nonoperatively with either a cast or a cast-brace (Fig. 29.3). The patient must be able to ambulate safely with appropriate precautions until union has occurred. Restriction to minimal toe-touch weight bearing (20% of body weight) for balance is advisable. It is imperative that follow-up radiographs be periodically obtained to ensure that displacement does not occur during this treatment method. Early range-of-motion exercises should be utilized and maintained throughout the course of treatment. Although the results of bracing and early knee motion have not been well documented in the literature, Chen and coworkers,[21] in a pooled metanalysis series (25 of 30 cases) tabulated that nonoperative treatment resulted in an 83% success rate. Unfortunately, the paucity of data regarding operative treatment of type I fractures makes exact recommendations for nonoperative treatment or comparisons to operative treatment impossible.

Nonoperative management of these fractures avoids the potential surgical risks such as deep infection, perioperative death, nonunion, and malunion. However, these risks must be weighed against the potential pitfalls of nonoperative management. Although there appears to be a similar incidence of malunion and/or nonunion in both surgical and nonsurgical groups, several authors have reported greater loss of motion following nonoperative treatment.[2,3,6] Immobilization in nonsurgically treated patients in these reports ranged from 3 to 12 weeks. It is likely that this period of immobilization not only affected the patients' return to prefracture range of motion, but also placed these patients at increased risk for deep vein thrombosis, pulmonary embolism, pressure sores, as well as psychological deterioration.

Despite these potential risks, nonoperative management of nondisplaced periprosthetic femur fractures should be sought as a primary treatment modality in this population. As cast-bracing devices and techniques continue to improve, the period of immobilization has decreased and will likely lead to even greater success than has been reported historically. Furthermore, if nonoperative treatment fails to achieve a satisfactory outcome, Chen and colleagues[21] reported that the patients can be salvaged with an operative procedure secondarily performed. They found an 89% success rate (17 of 19

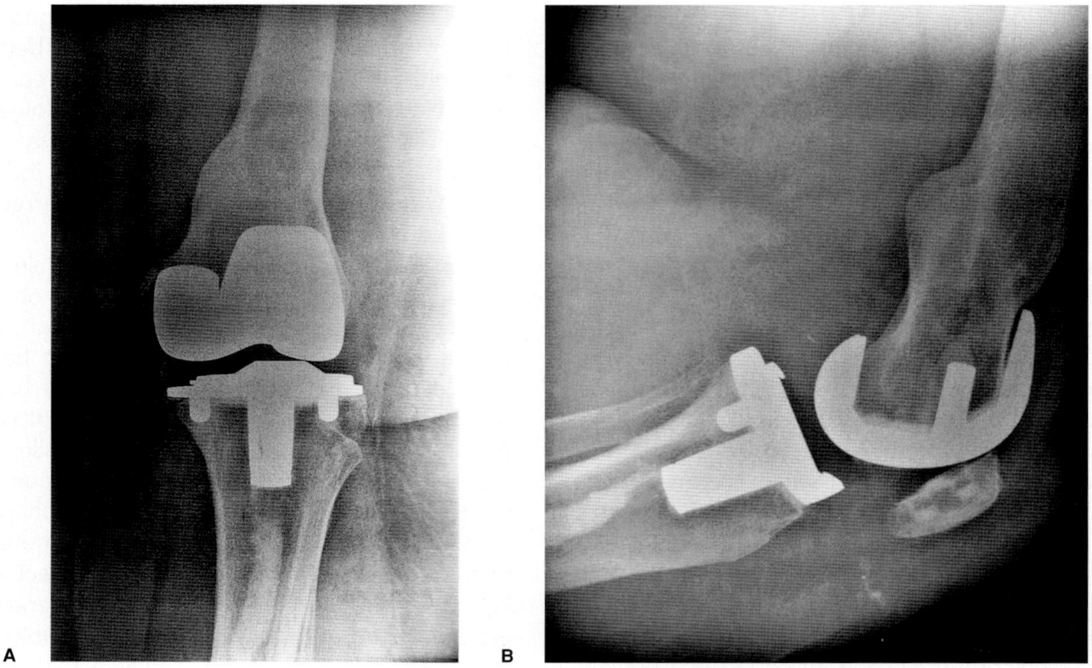

Figure 29.3. **A** and **B**: Healed periprosthetic supracondylar femoral fracture treated with casting followed by cast-brace.

cases) after salvage operations for patients initially treated with nonsurgical intervention. The treatment of type II fractures (displaced/comminuted) is less well defined. Prosthetic loosening in this scenario should be treated with revision arthroplasty. However, with a well-fixed femoral component, the results of open reduction and internal fixation versus traction or casting have not been shown to result in statistically different results.[21] Open reduction and internal fixation should be sought if the patient is unable to tolerate prolonged bed rest, if bone is of sufficient quality to maintain fixation, if the surgeon is technically able to perform the procedure, or if the patient has multiple or bilateral fractures. Traction followed by casting is a viable option if the patient can tolerate bed rest, acceptable alignment is both achievable and maintainable, bone is of poor quality precluding internal fixation, or if there is an unacceptably high risk of infection.

Many forms of operative treatment have been employed in the fixation of periprosthetic femur fractures. Open reduction and internal fixation with various plates and screws, external fixators, intramedullary rods, and revision prostheses, have all been utilized in various settings to achieve a successful result. Regardless of the technique chosen, acceptable fracture alignment and stability must be obtained to allow for early knee motion and partial weight bearing if possible. Prior to selection of an implant or fixation device, the surgeon must consider the degree of displacement and angulation, the overall extremity alignment, bone quality, bone damage in the distal condylar fragment, and both the knee implant in place as well as other implants in the ipsilateral limb.

PLATE AND SCREW FIXATION

Fracture plates, condylar buttress plates, blade plates, and condylar screws may all be utilized by the surgeon if sufficient bone is available in the distal fragment to obtain rigid fixation (Fig. 29.4). Although the condylar screw and blade plate provide the most rigid fixation, a condylar buttress plate provides greater flexibility if multiple fracture lines exist in the distal fragment. If fracture stability is not evident after the application of one of these plates, additional fixation with cortical bone, allograft, bone cement, double plating, or additional allograft strutting should be performed. If at least four bicortical screws cannot be obtained in the proximal fragment secondary to a previous hip implant, the plate should overlap the hip implant proximally by at least 2½ cortical diameters and fixation supplemented with cerclage wires as necessary.

Good clinical results with plate and screw fixation have been obtained by several authors.[18,26–28] Healy and associates[26] found a 90% of fractures healing rate

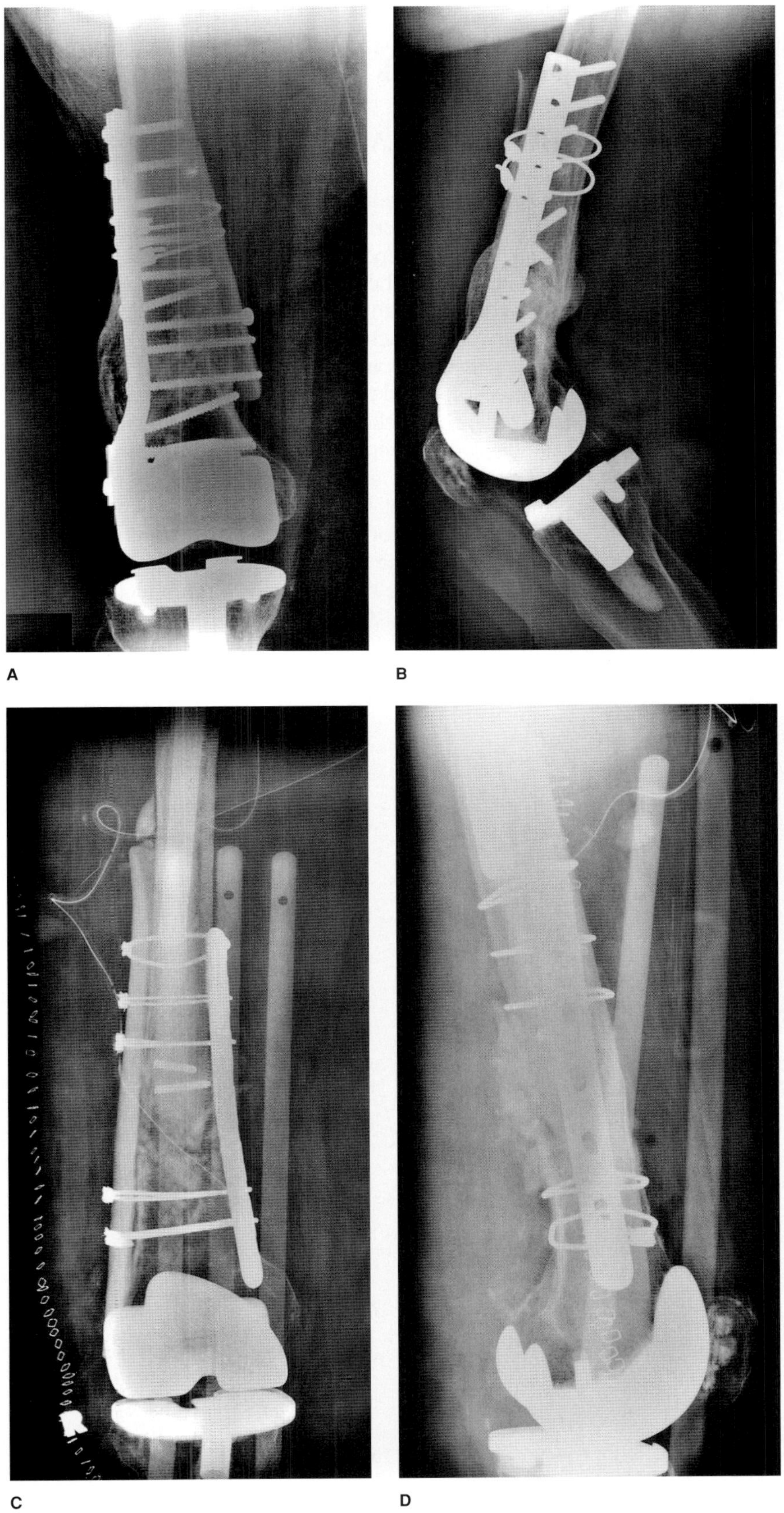

Figure 29.4. **A** and **B:** Healed periprosthetic fracture treated with condylar buttress plate and allograft strut. **C** and **D:** Example of Fig. 29.2 after takedown of nonunion. Fixation obtained with use of allograft strut, plate, liberal bone graft, and multiple cerclage wires.

(18 of 20) and demonstrated comparable Knee Society scores with the use of a blade plate, condylar screw, or buttress plate. Zehntner and Ganz[28] also reported successful results with the use of the condylar buttress plate in all six patients. They described the use of polymethylmethacrylate bone cement as an adjunct to fixation in highly osteopenic bone, and cautioned against the extensive medial periosteal stripping required for double plating. Regardless of the plate and/or screw system chosen, rigid fixation, limited periosteal dissection, and adjunctive measures including liberal use of bone grafting, supplemental cement, and secondary strutting with allograft or plates, should be utilized to maintain reduction.

EXTERNAL FIXATION

Although external fixation has been employed in a limited number of case reports to obtain alignment of periprosthetic supracondylar femur fractures, for the most part it is contraindicated.[6] Pin-site infections are an inevitable consequence of external fixators. The proximity of these pins to the prosthesis in order to allow for range of motion, with the subsequent risk of prosthetic infection, make this technique highly undesirable.

INTRAMEDULLARY ROD FIXATION

The use of intramedullary rod fixation, either flexible or rigid, has been described recently by several authors (Fig. 29.5).[29–33] The reported numbers involving these fixation devices is rather low, and thus neither technique can be considered the gold standard in fixation of supracondylar femur fractures proximal to total knee arthroplasties. Several points must be emphasized, based on the literature, to aid the surgeon in the use of these rods. Rush rods and Zickel nails are better suited for minimally displaced fractures with little or no comminution. They must provide enough stability to allow early range of motion, without loss of reduction if they are to be employed. Supracondylar rods placed in a retrograde fashion through the intercondylar space in the femoral component require knowledge of intercondylar distance and nail diameter. At least two locking screws should

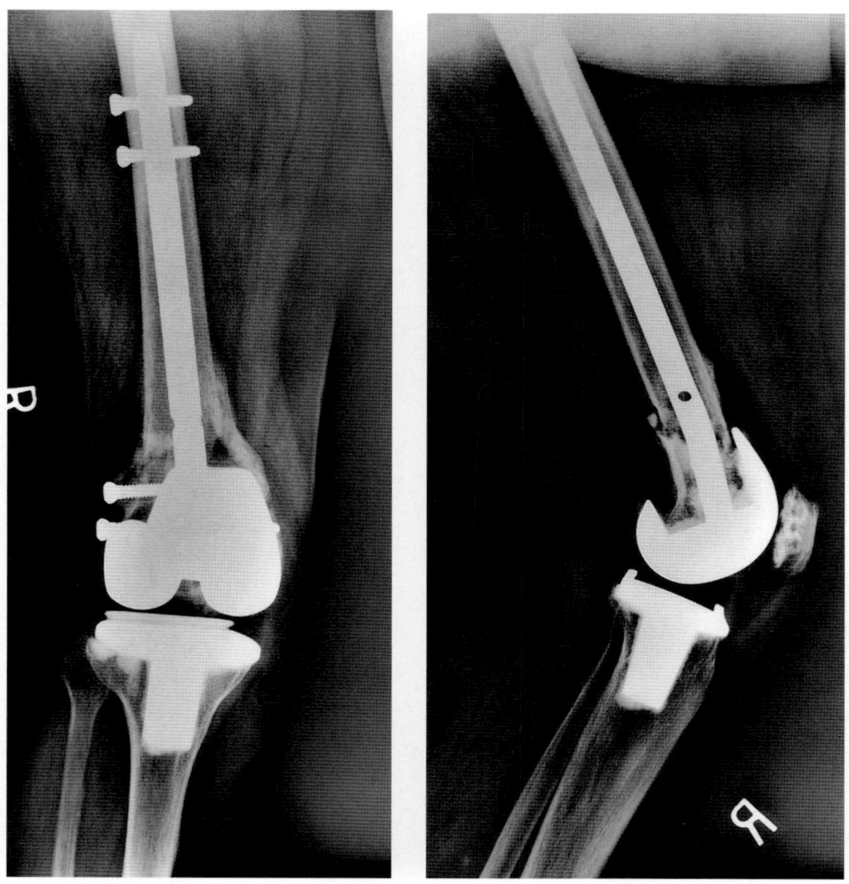

A B

Figure 29.5. **A** and **B**: Union of fracture in Fig. 29.1 after treatment with locked supracondylar intramedullary femoral nail.

be obtained in the distal fragment, and preferably the rod should pass the isthmus for additional stability. The advantages of intramedullary techniques include minimal disturbance of fracture hematoma, little or no periosteal stripping, rigid fixation, and decreased operative time. Complications include rod migration, femoral shortening, nonunion, loss of motion, and infection. It is likely that with the use of reamed nails, nonunion rates can be brought to a minimal level with this technique.

FEMORAL COMPONENT REVISION

Revision of the femoral component to a long-stemmed or custom component may be performed for treatment of these fractures.[18,30,34] The decision to revise immediately or obtain fracture healing initially followed by delayed revision depends on both the surgeon's skill level and patient characteristics. Preoperative planning should take into consideration the possible need for highly constrained prostheses, custom-made tumor prostheses, or custom-made revision prostheses. If custom-made tumor prostheses are utilized, careful attention to rotation and length should be ensured, and step-cutting of the allograft should be performed to obtain further rotational stability.

TIBIAL FRACTURES

Periprosthetic tibial fractures are hypothesized to commonly occur as a result of fatigue failure of the tibia secondary to axial malalignment and improper orientation of early components.[7,16,20,35,36] The present-day metal-backed components and improved alignment techniques have made this complication quite rare. Revision of the tibial component to a long-stemmed prosthesis with or without the use of wedges has been reported to provide a satisfactory result for this complication.[4,7,36] Fractures below the level of the prosthesis in the diaphysis of the tibia may be treated with conventional orthopedic techniques including casting or cast-bracing for nondisplaced fractures. For displaced on comminuted cases, external fixation, internal fixation, a variety of intramedullary techniques (Rush pins, Enders nails), or revision to a long-stemmed revision component can be utilized. The paucity of data concerning these complications does not lead to the conclusion of any clear-cut advantage of one technique over another. Hence, treatment options should be based on the medical condition of the patient, bone quality, stability of the prosthesis, and the surgeon's skill.

CONCLUSION

Periprosthetic femoral or tibial fractures around total knee prostheses are rare complications. Treatment is based on assessment of various patient factors including their medial condition, as well as a careful radiographic evalutation. In general, nondisplaced fractures can be treated nonoperatively. Displaced fractures may be treated by a variety of techniques, taking into account the prior prosthetic function, proximity of the fracture, stability of the components, and overall bone quality.

References

1. Aaron RK, Scott R. Supracondylar fracture of the femur after total knee arthroplasty. *Clin Orthop* 1987;219:136–139.
2. Bogoch E, Hastings D, Gross A, et al. Supracondylar fractures of the femur adjacent to resurfacing and Macintosh arthroplasties of the knee in patients with rheumatoid arthritis. *Clin Orthop* 1988;229:213–220.
3. Culp RW, Schmidt RG, Hanks G, et al. Supracondylar fracture of the femur following prosthetic knee arthroplasty. *Clin Orthop* 1987;222:212–222.
4. Felix NA, Stuart MJ, Hanssen AD. Periprosthetic fractures of the tibia associated with total knee arthroplasty. *Clin Orthop* 1997;345:113–124.
5. Figgie MP, Goldberg VM, Figgie HE, et al. The results of treatment of supracondylar fracture above total knee arthroplasty. *J Arthroplasty* 1990;5:267–276.
6. Merkel KD, Johnson EW. Supracondylar fracture of the femur after total knee arthroplasty. *J Bone Joint Surg* 1986;68A:29–43.
7. Rand JB, Coventry MB. Stress fractures after total knee arthroplasty. *J Bone Joint Surg* 1980;62A:226–232.
8. Sisto DJ, Lachiewicz PF, Insall JN. Treatment of supracondylar fractures following prosthetic arthroplasty of the knee. *Clin Orthop* 1985;196:265–272.
9. Cain PR, Rutash HE, Wissinger HA, et al. Periprosthetic femoral fractures following total knee arthroplasty. *Clin Orthop* 1986;208:205–214.
10. Ritter MA, Faris PM, Keating EM. Anterior femoral notching and ipsilateral supracondylar femur fracture in total knee arthroplasty. *J Arthroplasty* 1988;3:185–187.
11. Delport PH, Van Audekerck R, Martens M, et al. Conservative treatment of ipsilateral supracondylar fracture after total knee arthroplasty. *J Trauma* 1982;24:864.
12. Engh GA, Ammeen DJ. Periprosthetic fractures adjacent to total knee implants. *J Bone Joint Surg* 1997;79A:1100–1113.
13. Lewis PL, Rorabeck CH. Periprosthetic fractures. In: England GA, Rorabeck CH (eds). *Revision Total Knee Arthroplasty*. Baltimore: Williams & Wilkins, 1997:275–295.
14. Neer CS, Grantham SH, Shelton ML. Supracondylar fractures of the adult femur. *J Bone Joint Surg* 1967;49A:591.

15. Schatzker J. Supracondylar fractures of the femur. In: Schatzker J, Tile M (eds). *The Rationale of Operative Fracture Care*. Berlin: Springer-Verlag, 1987:255–273.
16. Bryan RS, Peterson LFA, Combs JJ. Polycentric knee arthroplasty: a preliminary report of postoperative complications in 450 knees. *Clin Orthop* 1973;94:148–152.
17. Lotke PA, Ecker ML. Influence of positioning of prosthesis in total knee replacement. *J Bone Joint Surg* 1977;59A:77–79.
18. Cordeiro EN, Cota RC, Carazzato JG, et al. Periprosthetic fractures in patients with total knee arthroplasties. *Clin Orthop* 1987;252:182–189.
19. Kettelkamp DB, Nasca R. Biomechanics and knee replacement arthroplasty. *Clin Orthop* 1973;94:8–14.
20. Nogi J, Caldwell JW, Kavzlarich JJ, et al. Load testing of geometric and polycentric total knee replacements. *Clin Orthop* 1976;114:235–242.
21. Chen F, Mont MA, Bachner RS. Management of ipsilateral supracondylar femur fractures following total knee arthroplasty. *J Arthroplasty* 1994;9:521–526.
22. Hirsch DM, Bhalla S, Roffman M. Supracondylar fracture of the femur following total knee replacement. *J Bone Joint Surg* 1981;63A:162.
23. Short WH, Hootnick DR, Murray DG. Ipsilateral supracondylar femur fractures following knee arthroplasty. *Clin Orthop* 1981;158:111.
24. Ayers DC. Supracondylar fracture of the distal femur proximal to a total knee replacement. *Inst Course Lect* 1997;46:197–203.
25. Chmell MJ, Moran MC, Scott RD. Periarticular fractures after total knee arthroplasty: principles of management. *J Amer Acad Orthop Surg* 1996;4:109–116.
26. Healy WL. Tibial fractures below total knee arthroplasty. In: Insall JN, Scott WN, Scuderi GR (eds). *Current Concepts in Primary and Revision Total Knee Arthroplasty*. Philadelphia: Lippincott-Raven, 1996:163–167.
27. Moran MC, Brick GW, Sledge CB, et al. Supracondylar femoral fracture following total knee arthroplasty. *Clin Orthop* 1996;324:196–209.
28. Zehntner MK, Ganz R. Internal fixation of supracondylar fractures after condylar total knee arthroplasty. *Clin Orthop* 1993;293:219–224.
29. Jabczanski FF, Crawford M. Retrograde intramedullary nailing of supracondylar femur fractures above total knee arthroplasty. A preliminary report of four cases. *J Arthroplasty* 1995;10:95–101.
30. McClaren AC, Dupont JA, Schroeber DC. Open reduction and internal fixation of supracondylar fractures above total knee arthroplasties using the intramedullary supracondylar rod. *Clin Orthop* 1994;302:194–198.
31. Murrell GAC, Nuhley JA. Interlocked supracondylar nails for supracondylar fractures after total knee arthroplasty: a new treatment method. *J Arthroplasty* 1995;10:37–42.
32. Ritter MA, Faris PM, Keating EM, et al. Rush rod fixation of supracondylar fractures above total knee arthroplasties. *J Arthroplasty* 1995;10:213–216.
33. Rolston LR, Christ DJ, Halpern A, et al. Treatment of supracondylar fractures of the femur proximal to a total knee arthroplasty. A report of four cases. *J Bone Joint Surg* 1995;77A:924–931.
34. Kraay MJ, Goldberg VM, Figgie MP, et al. Distal femoral replacement with allograft/prosthetic reconstruction for treatment of supracondylar fractures in patients with total knee arthroplasty. *J Arthroplasty* 1992;7:7–16.
35. Kettelkamp DBL, Chao EY. A method for quantitative analysis of medial and lateral compression forces at the knee during standing. *Clin Orthop* 1972;83:202–213.
36. Kjaersgaard-Anderson P, Johl M. Ipsilateral traumatic supracondylar femoral and proximal tibial fractures following total knee replacements. A case report. *J Trauma* 1989;29:398–400.
37. Hood RW, Vanni M, Insall JN. The correction of knee alignment in 225 consecutive total condylar knee replacements. *Clin Orthop* 1981;160:94.

Chapter 30

PATELLAR FRACTURES IN TOTAL KNEE ARTHROPLASTY

Charles L. Nelson and Russell E. Windsor

As surgical technique and implants have improved, the longevity of femoral and tibial components and the clinical results following total knee arthroplasty have improved as well. The primary source of complications following total knee arthroplasty in many series has been related to the extensor mechanism or patellofemoral joint.[1–3] These complications have included unexplained anterior knee pain, patellar clunk syndrome, patellar instability, patellar component disassociation, patellar component wear, patellar loosening, quadriceps or patellar tendon rupture, and patellar fracture. Patellar resurfacing may decrease the incidence of anterior knee pain, and has decreased the rate of reoperation following total knee arthroplasty.[4–6] However, this may occur at the potential expense of increased rates of patellar implant–related complications including patellar component loosening, patellar subluxation or dislocation, and patellar fracture.[1,4,7,8]

The incidence of patellar fractures following total knee arthroplasty has ranged from 0% to 21%.[5,7,9–14] The incidence is likely artificially low in some series secondary to undetected asymptomatic fractures, limited follow-up, or inadequate imaging. The incidence may be artificially high in other series secondary to prosthetic designs or issues relevant to surgical technique. Patellar fractures represent a spectrum of disease from minimally displaced longitudinal stress fractures to widely displaced transverse or comminuted fractures associated with a significant extensor lag. Minimally displaced longitudinal stress fractures are generally treated nonoperatively and conservatively with excellent results.[12,15] Significantly displaced transverse or comminuted fractures often do poorly despite surgical interventions including open reduction and internal fixation with tension band or cerclage wiring, revision of the patellar component, and patelloplasty or patellectomy with repair of the extensor mechanism.[7,10–12,15]

TYPES OF PATELLAR FRACTURES FOLLOWING TOTAL KNEE ARTHROPLASTY

There are several methods by which patellar fractures have been classified in the past.[7,10,12,15] None of these systems alone is sufficient to predict prognosis or outline a treatment algorithm. Patellar fractures have been classified based on mechanism as traumatic or atraumatic fractures.[12,16] Some authors have described the fractures according to the degree of displacement as being displaced or nondisplaced. The criteria for displacement have varied from >5 mm to >2 cm.[7,11] Patellar fractures have also been classified according to fracture pattern, such as transverse, longitudinal, or comminuted.[11] A scheme has been developed that classifies these injuries into four major types: type I, fractures that do not involve the implant/cement composite or the extensor mechanism; type II, fractures that involve the implant/cement composite or extensor mechanism; type IIIA, inferior pole fractures with associated patellar ligament rupture; and type IIIB, inferior pole fractures without patellar ligament rupture.[15] Pure patellar fractures are also distinguished from fracture dislocations in this classification scheme.[15]

For the surgeon to properly characterize these injuries and decide on appropriate treatment, a thorough history, review of records, physical examination, and radiographic evaluation must be performed. The history is important in determining whether a fracture is traumatic, and how much associated energy was used to create it. The duration between the surgical procedure and fracture may help identify predisposing factors in atraumatic situations, i.e., not associated with an actual injury. A history of patellar subluxation or dislocation, either at or prior to the time of fracture, may identify technical or patient factors leading to it. A history of multiple prior knee surgeries, lateral retinacular release, and fat pad excision may create devascularization of the patella, potentially predisposing it to fracture. This compromised blood supply may also potentially decrease the likelihood of achieving union following internal fixation.

The physical examination is critical to the evaluation of these patients. The presence of a palpable defect and the presence of a significant extensor lag are poor prognostic factors for a good functional result with nonoperative treatment. Pain and tenderness may be associated with more displaced fractures with or without component loosening. Radiographic studies provide valuable information regarding degree of displacement, component loosening, fracture pattern and location, component positioning, and tibiofemoral alignment. In one study, implant alignment was shown to be related to the severity of patellar fractures following total knee arthroplasty, as well as to the results following treatment.[17] Bone scans may determine whether the fractured patella is avascular.[18,19]

PREVENTION OF PATELLAR FRACTURES FOLLOWING TOTAL KNEE ARTHROPLASTY

Treatment of patellar fractures following total knee arthroplasty begins with prevention. Generally accepted factors predisposing to patellar fracture following total knee arthroplasty include the following: (1) The incidence of patellar fractures following knee replacement is higher in series where the patella is resurfaced than in series where the patella is not resurfaced.[11] (2) The incidence of patellar fractures is higher following resurfacing in revision total knee arthroplasty than following resurfacing in primary total knee arthroplasty.[11] (3) Technical factors such as overresection or underresection of the patella may predispose to patellar fracture following total knee arthroplasties involving patellar resurfacing.

It is recommended for onset patellar resurfacing that resection of the patella be parallel to the anterior surface of the patella, leaving a thickness of 1 to 1.5 cm following resection.[7] The goal is a composite resurfaced patella of a thickness equal to the native patella prior to resection. The composite resurfaced patella should not be thicker than the native patella prior to resurfacing to avoid overstuffing the patellofemoral joint. In the setting of severe patellar erosion, such as in cases of advanced rheumatoid arthritis, some authors advocate obtaining a composite thickness of approximately 26 mm in males and 23 mm in females. These thicknesses are believed to be the normal respective native patellar thickness.[20] Resection of bone overhanging the patella can lead to weakening of the remaining structure and should be avoided.[7,11]

For inset patellar resurfacing, it is recommended that reaming be performed perpendicular to the anterior patellar surface, and that the starting point be medialized to the region of the center ridge to facilitate patellar tracking.[20] The goal is to restore the native patellar thickness with the composite structure following reaming, except in the case of severe patellar erosion where the goal is to obtain a composite thickness of approximately 26 mm in average size males and 23 mm in average size females as discussed above.

Technical factors such as failure to perform a lateral release or malrotation or malalignment of the tibial or femoral components can lead to patellar subluxation or dislocation, which can predispose to patellar fractures.[2,13] Assessing the need for a lateral release is controversial, with some authors recommending the "no-thumbs" technique,[21] which involves assessing patellar tracking without a thumb manipulating the patella. Other authors feel it is reasonable to check patellar tracking following placement of a towel clip or suture between the vastus medialis insertion and apex of the patella to simulate tracking of the patellofemoral mechanism following closure. The latter is our preference to avoid unnecessary lateral releases. The lateral release should be performed 1.5 to 2 cm lateral to the lateral edge of the patella, as previous studies have demonstrated that releasing the retinaculum less than 1.5 cm from the patella compromises the lateral patellar circulation.[3,22] Other factors that contribute to abnormal lateral patellar tracking with excessive contact pressures are internal rotation of the femoral component and medial rotatory positioning of the tibial component. Internal rotation of the femoral component in excess of the epicondylar axis will result in abnormal patellar forces developing from the lateral flange of the prosthesis. Medial rotation of the tibial component in a fixed-bearing design will create secondarily an excessive quadriceps angle of the patellar tendon, predisposing to dislocation, subluxation, or fracture. The surgeon should carefully assess these three factors to ensure proper patellar tracking.

Theoretical factors that may predispose to patellar fractures following total knee arthroplasty include the following: bone necrosis due to either disruption of the patellar blood supply or thermal effects of polymerizing polymethylmethacrylate (PMMA) cement; and other biomechanical factors, such as the creation of stress risers during patella preparation, and increased patellofemoral joint reaction forces.[11,12]

The blood supply to the human patella has been well described by Scapinelli.[23] The patella has both an extraosseous and an intraosseous arterial supply. The extraosseous blood supply involves a vascular anastomotic ring surrounding the patella with contributions from the supreme genicular, medial superior genicular, lateral superior genicular, medial inferior genicular, lateral inferior genicular, and anterior tibial recurrent arteries. The lateral and medial superior geniculate arteries were noted to join just superior to the patella and anterior to the quadriceps tendon. The lateral and medial inferior geniculate arteries, on the other hand, were noted to anastomose posterior to the patellar tendon in the fat pad to form the transverse infrapatellar artery. The intraosseous blood supply can be divided into two major systems: midpatellar vessels enter vascular foramina on the anterior surface of the middle third of the patella, and polar vessels enter the deep surface of the patella between the attachment of the ligamentum patellae and the articular surface.

A medial parapatellar approach, the approach most often utilized during total knee arthroplasty, disrupts the medial extraosseous blood supply to the patella (Fig. 30.1).[18] A lateral release may disrupt a portion of the lateral extraosseus blood supply as well. Subvastus and midvastus approaches during total knee arthroplasty may not disrupt the entire medial extraosseus blood supply to the patella. Excision of the fat pad may further disrupt the extraosseous blood supply by disrupting the transverse infrapatellar artery.[12] Theoretically, reduced

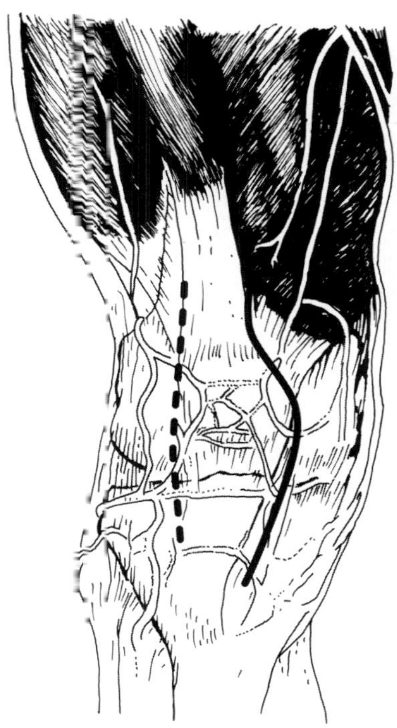

Figure 30.1. The blood supply to the human patella. The bold line depicts a standard medial parapatellar arthrotomy. The dashed line depicts a standard lateral retinacular release.

blood supply could result in inability to heal stress fractures and to an increased fracture rate following total knee arthroplasty. Postoperative bone scans have demonstrated decreased patellar perfusion following medial parapatellar arthrotomies with concurrent lateral releases.[18] However, clinical studies have failed to document whether lateral release and/or fat pad excision clinically predisposes to patellar fracture.[3,13,18]

Implants of greater constraint may create increased loads across the patellofemoral joint, predisposing to patellar fractures. Support for this hypothesis includes the higher rates of patellofemoral symptoms with early posterior stabilized designs compared with the total condylar prosthesis.[24] However, the higher fracture rates with posterior stabilized designs may be secondary to patients gaining greater flexion postoperatively and thereby generating increased forces across the patellofemoral joint.

Biomechanical studies have demonstrated that a large central fixation hole is associated with more strain than the peripheral three-peg designs, thereby potentially predisposing to patellar fracture.[7] In addition, some surgeons believe that an inset patella is at an increased risk of fracture over that of an onset patella secondary to the large central reaming that is performed during patellar preparation. Biomechanical studies comparing biconcave inset and three-peg onset patella both following preparation and following implantation have evaluated the theoretical risks of patellar fracture with these designs. Interestingly, these studies demonstrate that although the onset patella is stronger following preparation, the inset patella composite is stronger following implantation when tested using a three-point bending mode.[25] This suggests no increased predisposition to fracture with the inset patella, unless the component loosens. Clinical studies have had varying incidences of fractures using either design, and clinically there is no clear support of predisposition to patellar fracture associated with either design.

Most surgeons routinely resurface the patella by using an onset three-peg patella prosthesis, and should adhere to the principles outlined above. The patella may be resected freehand or with a patellar resection guide (Fig. 30.2), parallel to the anterior surface, leaving a minimum thickness of 1 to 1.5 cm. Patellar thickness should be measured before and after resection with the patellar trial component attached. If the trial patella composite is thicker than the native patellar dimension, and there is greater than 1 cm of patella remaining, the patella is resected again to avoid overstuffing the patellofemoral joint. The patellar component is positioned medially on the surface of the resected patella to facilitate proper patellar tracking. Every attempt should be made to preserve the lateral superior geniculate artery when doing a lateral release. A lateral retinacular release is

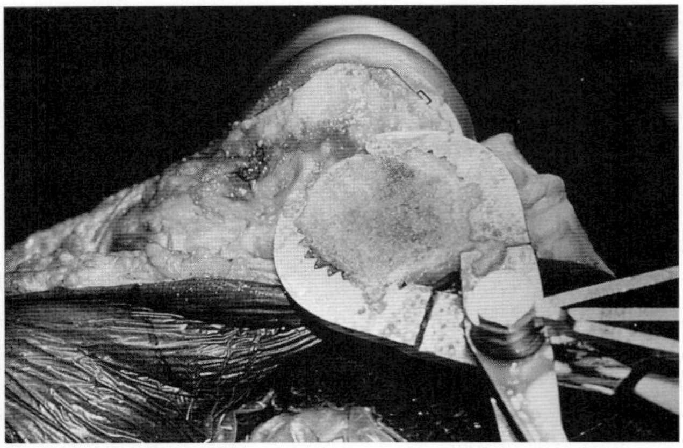

Figure 30.2. A patellar resection guide designed to facilitate ideal postresection patellar thickness parallel to the anterior surface of the patella. The goal is to avoid underresection leading to overstuffing the patellofemoral space, and overresection leading to a thin patella potentially predisposed to patellar fracture.

done 1.5 to 2 cm from the patella when the extensor mechanism does not track properly following a simulated closure as outlined above. Also, preservation of the fat pad during initial exposure of the lateral tibial plateau will help maximize the blood supply to the patella.

Femoral external rotation should be assessed with reference to the posterior femoral condyles, the epicondylar axis, and the midtrochlear line to avoid malrotation. In cases of severe posterior condylar erosion, the epicondylar axis is used as the reference point. The tibial component is independently positioned to face the medial third of the tibial tubercle to avoid inadvertent lateral rotation of the tibial tubercle following implantation. This maneuver is particularly important if a fixed-bearing total knee replacement design is utilized. In revision total knee arthroplasty, the patella is generally resurfaced only when there is adequate bone stock (at least 1 cm). However, with central erosion, it may be possible to implant an inset biconcave patella even if the central thickness is less than 1 cm.

TREATMENT, MANAGEMENT, AND SALVAGE OF PATELLAR FRACTURES FOLLOWING TOTAL KNEE ARTHROPLASTY

Management of patellar fractures following prior total knee arthroplasty procedures is dependent on the patient's presentation, symptoms, physical findings, and radiographs. Many postarthroplasty patellar fractures are noted incidentally on follow-up radiographs in asymptomatic patients. These fractures are best managed conservatively. In fact, nonoperative management is the standard of care for most patellar fractures occurring in patients with prior total knee arthroplasty procedures.[7,12] However, in some cases surgical intervention is necessary, with the goal of obtaining a satisfactory functional outcome.

Nonoperative management of postarthroplasty patella fractures is recommended for a spectrum of fractures including (1) asymptomatic or symptomatic stress fractures; (2) asymptomatic fractures noted incidentally on radiographs; (3) nondisplaced transverse, vertical, or comminuted fractures; and (4) some displaced comminuted and vertical fractures in which the extensor mechanism is intact functionally.[7,12] Nonoperative management of the above fractures assumes absence of associated patellar dislocation or component loosening (Fig. 30.3). Stress fractures, or asymptomatic fractures noted incidentally on radiographs require only observation.[7] Nondisplaced vertical, transverse, or comminuted fractures should be managed nonoperatively in a cylinder cast for 6 weeks.[7] The knee is placed in approximately 5 degrees of flexion in the cylinder cast to prevent excessive tension on the posterior capsule of the knee and to improve patient comfort. Full weight bearing is allowed in the cylinder cast. Isometric quadriceps and hamstring exercises can be instituted within the

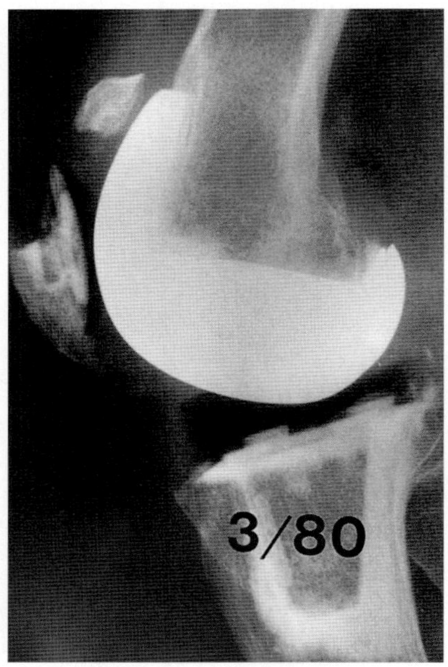

Figure 30.3. Superior pole patellar fracture. The patellar component appears to be well fixed. Because the patient has an intact extensor mechanism on physical examination, this fracture can be treated conservatively in a cylinder cast. The patellar fragment can be excised at a later time if it remains symptomatic.

cylinder cast when the acute pain has subsided. Physical therapy with gentle active and active assisted range of motion is begun following removal of the cylinder cast at 6 weeks. Isometric strengthening is continued, and isotonic strengthening is added once active flexion reaches 90 degrees. Displaced vertical and comminuted fractures can be managed nonoperatively in a cylinder cast for 6 weeks provided that the extensor mechanism is intact on clinical examination and their patellar component appears to be well fixed and aligned normally in the trochlear groove.

Surgical intervention is recommended for any patella fracture associated with a significant extensor lag. These include displaced transverse fractures, some displaced comminuted fractures, and inferior pole patellar fractures associated with disruption of the extensor mechanism.[7,11,15] Surgical intervention should be considered for patellar fractures with associated component loosening, malalignment, or patellar dislocation regardless of fracture pattern. Surgical options include open reduction and internal fixation of the patella with or without retention of the patellar component, partial patellectomy with or without placement of a new patellar component, and total patellectomy with reconstruction of the extensor mechanism. In cases having significant malalignment or malrotation of the femoral or tibial components, patellar subluxation or dislocation in association with a patellar fracture may only be corrected by revision total knee arthroplasty. The clinical results of postarthroplasty patellar fractures requiring operative intervention have for the most part not been good.[7,11,12,15]

Open reduction and internal fixation with repair of the patellar retinaculum is recommended for displaced transverse fractures demonstrating an extensor lag, provided that there is sufficient bone available for fixation.[7] Reduction and fixation are much more difficult compared with nonarthroplasty traumatic patellar fractures. The patellar bone may be sclerotic and nonviable secondary to prior surgical approaches and/or the toxic effects of PMMA cement. The patella will be thinner, and cement or the patellar component may interfere with internal fixation. Fixation can be acquired with longitudinal Kirschner wires and a tension band. However, in cases with severely compromised patellar bone stock, circlage wiring or patellectomy with reconstruction of the extensor mechanism may be required. If the patellar component is loose, in most cases, no new implant is replaced as the residual bone stock is usually insufficient. Because rigid internal fixation is usually not possible in these patients, we immobilize these patients in a cylinder cast for 6 weeks following internal fixation. This is followed by rehabilitation similar to nonoperatively treated postarthroplasty patellar fractures.

Displaced comminuted fractures associated with a significant extensor lag are in many cases not amenable to internal fixation.[7] For these injuries, circlage fixation with partial patellectomy and repair of the extensor mechanism is recommended, if possible. Salvage procedures include total patellectomy with repair of the extensor mechanism, or the use of a quadriceps tendon–patella–patellar tendon–tibial tubercle composite allograft to reconstruct the extensor mechanism in cases where repair of the extensor mechanism is impossible and the extensor lag is significant. The risks of utilization of these large bulk allografts include sepsis and late fatigue failure.

Inferior pole fractures associated with patellar tendon rupture can be managed with excision of the inferior pole fragment, and repair of the patellar tendon with a heavy nonabsorbable suture[15] (Fig. 30.4). The repair may be reinforced with either autograft tendon from the hamstrings, wire or merseline tape passed through drill holes in the patella, and tibial tubercle. Postoperative management and rehabilitation is dependent on the strength of the repair obtained. However, a more conservative approach is favored in this setting as decreased flexion is better tolerated and more salvageable than a significant extensor lag.

Following appropriate management of the patellar

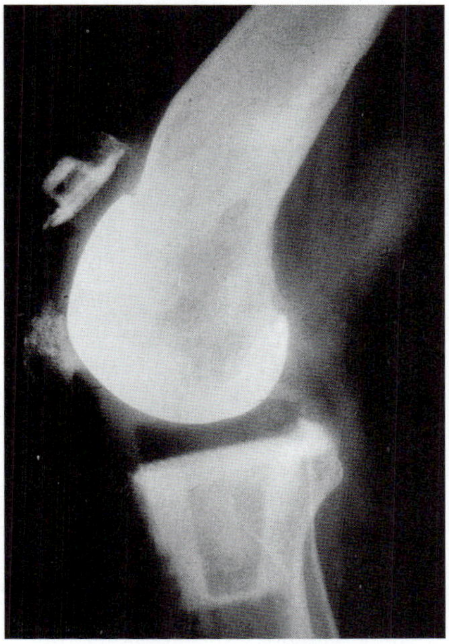

Figure 30.4. Traumatic inferior pole patellar fracture associated with disruption of the extensor mechanism. The patellar component appears well fixed. Union of the small inferior fragment in this setting is unlikely. Therefore, recommended treatment would involve partial patellectomy with repair or reconstruction on the patellar tendon.

fracture and repair of the extensor mechanism, careful examination of patellar tracking and component alignment and rotation are mandatory. If the patella, patellar remnant, or quadriceps tendon does not track centrally in the trochlea, there will be a tendency toward lateral subluxation or dislocation postoperatively, and refracture or unsatisfactory clinical outcomes may result (Fig. 30.5). Lateral retinacular release with or without medial imbrication may be sufficient.[26] However, in cases of significant tibial and/or femoral component malposition or malalignment, revision of the malaligned or malrotated component or components may be necessary. Figgie et al[17] noted that the poorest outcomes following postarthroplasty patellar fractures were noted in patients with tibiofemoral malalignment. Fracture dislocations of the patella are the fractures most likely to demonstrate significant component malalignment or malrotation.

CONCLUSION

No classification system is satisfactory for outlining treatment for postarthroplasty patellar fractures. Surgical intervention has been associated with less than optimal outcomes in the literature, and nonoperative management is recommended for most of these fractures. When surgical intervention is employed, the goals are to obtain stable fixation, preserve viable patellar bone stock, maintain patellar vascularity, repair the extensor mechanism, and rehabilitate the knee in a nonaggressive fashion. In cases where there is patellar dislocation with femoral and/or tibial component malalignment or malrotation, revision total knee arthroplasty may be necessary to obtain a satisfactory result.

The key to success of a total knee replacement is to preserve the full function of the extensor mechanism. A beautiful clinical result may be substantially compromised if insufficient attention is paid to patellar tracking and the factors that influence it. Proper selection of a total knee replacement design that clinically demonstrates good patellar tracking and mechanics is important. The surgeon must be mindful of the factors that contribute to proper patellofemoral mechanics. Patellar fracture will substantially impact the surgical outcome of an otherwise successful surgical exercise.

For the young, active patient or the morbidly obese individual, consideration might be given toward initially not resurfacing the patella, in an effort to prevent patellar fracture with a prosthesis in place. The patient must have an intact cartilage surface with osteoarthritis rather than rheumatoid arthritis. If the patient is informed that there may need to be a second procedure in the future to convert the patellar configuration to a resurfaced construct, sufficient time may be bought before severe patellar complications develop.

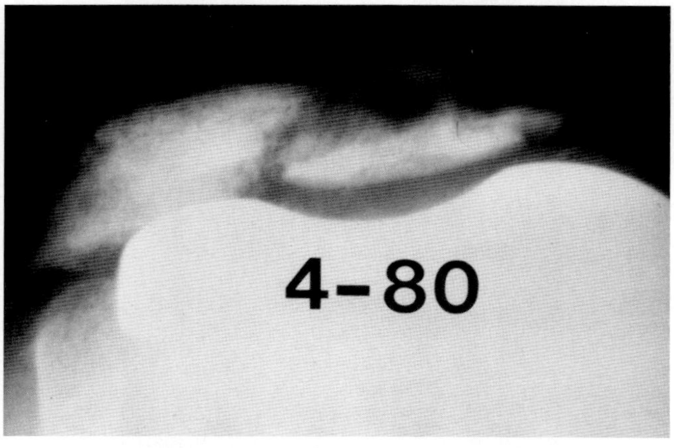

Figure 30.5. Example of a patella fracture with dislocation. Repair or reconstruction of the patella and/or extensor mechanism, or patellectomy would be unsuccessful without addressing the etiology of the instability. If the components are malrotated and soft tissue procedures are inadequate in restoring acceptable patellar or quadriceps tracking, revision total knee arthroplasty may be required in addition to treatment of the injury to the patella and extensor mechanism.

References

1. Keblish PA, Varma AK, Greenwald AS. Resurfacing of the patella in total knee arthroplasty. *J Bone Joint Surg* 1994;76B(6):930–937.
2. Goldberg VM, Figgie HE, Figgie MP. Technical considerations in total knee surgery, management of patella problems. *Orthop Clin North Am* 1989;20(2):189–199.
3. Kayler DE, Lyttle D. Surgical interruption of patellar blood supply by total knee arthroplasty. *Clin Orthop* 1988; 229:221–227.
4. Barrack RL, Wolfe MW, Waldman DA. Resurfacing of the patella in total knee arthroplasty. *J Bone Joint Surg* 1997;79A(8):1121–1131.
5. Ranawat CS. The patellofemoral joint in total condylar knee arthroplasty. *Clin Orthop* 1986;205:93–99.
6. Scott WN, Rubinstein M, Scuderi G. Results after knee replacement with a posterior cruciate-substituting prosthesis. *J Bone Joint Surg* 1988;70A:1163.
7. Windsor RE, Scuderi GR, Insall JN. Patella fractures in total knee arthroplasty. *J Arthoplasty* 1989;4(Suppl): S63–S67.
8. Picetti GD, McGann WA, Welch RB. The patellofemoral joint after total knee arthroplasty without patellar resurfacing. *J Bone Joint Surg* 1990;72A(10):1379–1382.
9. Cameron HU, Fedorkow DM. The patella in total knee arthroplasty. *Clin Orthop* 1982;165:197.

10. Clayton ML, Thirupathi R. Patellar complications after total condylar arthroplasty. *Clin Orthop* 1982;170:152–155.

11. Grace JN, Sim FH. Fracture of the patella after total knee arthroplasty. *Clin Orthop* 1988;230:168–175.

12. Hozack WJ, Goll SR, Lotke PA, et al. Treatment of patella fractures after total knee arthoplasty. *Clin Orthop* 1988; 236:123–127.

13. Ritter MA, Campbell ED. Postoperative patellar complications with or without lateral release during total knee arthroplasty. *Clin Orthop* 1987;219:163–168.

14. Insall JN, Scott WN, Ranawat CS. The total condylar knee prosthesis. *J Bone Joint Surg* 1979;61A:173.

15. Goldberg VM, et al. Patella fracture type and prognosis in condylar total knee arthroplasty. *Clin Orthop* 1988; 236:115–122.

16. Insall JN. Total knee replacement, in Insall JN (ed.) *Surgery of the Knee*. New York: Churchill Livingston, 1984:587.

17. Figgie HE 3d, Goldberg VM, Figgie MP, et al. The effect of alignment of the implant on fractures of the patella after condylar total knee arthroplasty. *J Bone Joint Surg* 1989;71A:1031–1039.

18. Scuderi GR, Scharf SC, Meltzer LP, et al. The relationship of lateral releases to patellar viability in total knee arthroplasty. *J Arthroplasty*. 1989;2(3):209–214.

19. Wetzner SM, Bezreh JS, Scott RD, et al. Bone scanning in the assessment of patellar viability following total knee replacement. *Clin Orthop* 1985;199:215–219.

20. Laskin RS. Patellar preparation: inlay technique. In: Scuderi G, Tria A (eds). *Surgical Techniques in Total Knee Arthroplasty*. New York: Springer-Verlag, 1999.

21. Scott RD. Prosthesis placement of the patellofemoral joint. *Orthop Clin North Am* 1979;10:129.

22. Merkow RL, Soudry M, Insall JN. Patellar dislocation following total knee arthroplasty. *J Bone Joint Surg* 1985;67A:1321–1327.

23. Scapinelli R. Blood supply of the human patella. *J Bone Joint Surg* 1967;49B(3):563–570.

24. Insall JN, Lachiewicz PF, Burstein AH. The posterior stabilized condylar prosthesis: a modification of the total condylar design. *J Bone Joint Surg* 1982;64A:1317.

25. Gomes LSM, et al. Bending strength of the patella with two methods of reaming and two designs of patellar prostheses. Paper presented at the 35th annual meeting of the Orthopaedic Research Society, Las Vegas, NV 1989: 14.

26. Mochizuki RM, Schurman DJ. Patellar complications following total knee arthroplasty. *J Bone Joint Surg* 1979; 61A(6):879–883.

Chapter 31

Soft Tissue Complications After Total Knee Arthroplasty

Fred D. Cushner, Susan Craig Scott, and W. Norman Scott

Of paramount importance to a successful total knee arthroplasty (TKA) is successful wound healing. Unfortunately, this is not always possible, and thus the goals of rapid rehabilitation and patient mobilization are not always achieved. Wound failure can lead to prosthesis infection, numerous surgical procedures, as well as an extended hospitalization. The patient's and surgeon's expectations are not met and frustration can occur for all parties involved.

This chapter focuses on wound healing problems, and discusses the anatomy, prevention, early recognition, and treatment options.

VASCULAR ANATOMY

Numerous studies have been undertaken to evaluate the blood supply to the tissue anterior to the knee.[1–5] The blood supply of this soft tissue is completely random, with perforating arteries from numerous vessels.[1–5] Because there are no underlying muscle layers or intermuscular septa, a pathway for direct arterial perforators is not present. Therefore, the blood flow to the anterior knee is from the parapatellar anastomotic arterial ring in the form of terminal branches of arteries, in which all but one originates from the superficial femoral system.[1–5]

Six main arteries make up the extraosseous parapatellar anastomotic ring (Fig. 31.1). The medial and lateral superior genicular vessels, medial and lateral inferior genicular vessels, supreme genicular and anterior tibial recurrent artery, as well as a branch of the profunda femoris are the major vessels in the anastomotic ring. Both the superior and inferior vessels arise from the popliteal artery and maintain the soft tissue in immediate proximity to the joint. It is through these terminal branches that any contribution to the local skin is provided. Interruption of these primary vessels and subsequent local ischemia may cause potential anastomotic communications and additional flow.[6]

In addition to these intrinsic vessels, three additional extrinsic vessels supplement the arterial soft tissue. The first are branches of the profunda femoris, which consists of branches that not only supply the rectis femoris, vastus intermedius, and vastus lateralis, but also send perforating branches to the overlying skin and through the dermal plexus, supplying the skin in the superior region of the interior knee.

The second extrinsic vessel is the supreme genicular vessel. This branch of the superficial femoral artery leaves this vessel in the adductor canal before branching into the musculoarticular branch and the saphenous artery. It is the musculoarticular branch that runs medially in the vastus medialis before meeting the superior medial genicular artery to supply the medial aspect of the joint and medial and superior aspect of the overlying skin.

The saphenous artery travels inferiorly, passes inferior to the sartorius tendon, and ends in a terminal vessel that supplies the skin just below the medial tibial plateau. The third extrinsic vessel is a recurrent branch of the anterior tibial artery. This branch of the popliteal artery eventually joins branches of the lateral inferior genicular artery to supply the skin overlying and lateral to the patella ligament.

Thus, it can be seen that a plentiful random blood supply exists, and in most situations a single incision in a healthy individual presents few problems in wound healing. Unfortunately, not all incisions for TKAs are primary and not all knees are free of previous incisions.

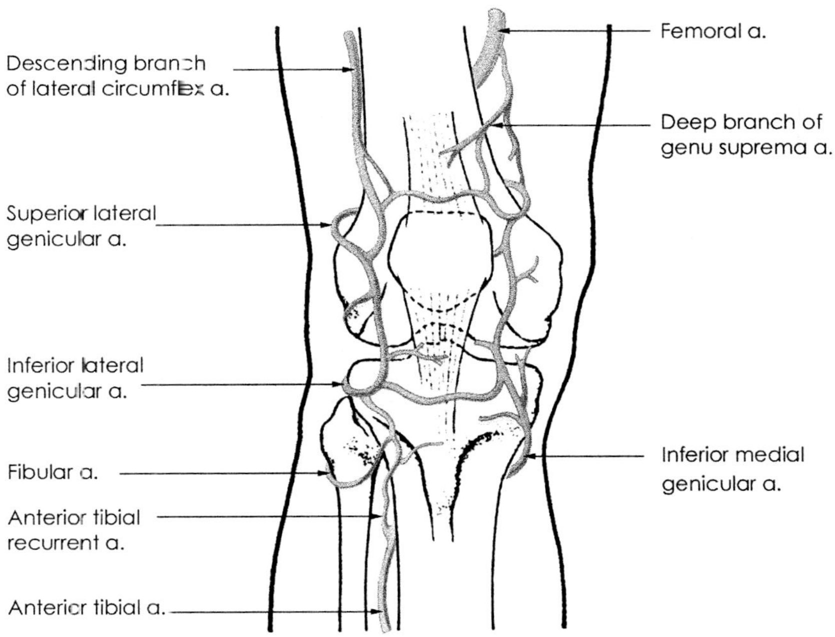

Figure 31.1. Knee arterial circulation.

It is incisions in a compromised skin tissue envelope that can lead to TKA wound problems.

PREVENTION OF WOUND PROBLEMS

Total knee arthroplasties are performed on a variety of patients. Unfortunately, the wound healing potential of all TKA candidates is not identical. This section focuses on those preoperative factors that could lead to skin compromise at the time of the indicated TKA.

Patient Factors

A thorough medical history as well as physical examination is required prior to a TKA. Although often the emphasis is on a patient's pulmonary and cardiac status, emphasis must also be placed on the patient's potential wound healing of the TKA incision. Calcified popliteal vessels and signs of arterial sclerosis or venous insufficiency should be identified at this visit. If needed, vascular reconstruction should be undertaken prior to the performance of the indicated TKA. Factors that adversely affect wound healing can also be identified prior to surgery and avoidance of these factors, or attempts to correct these patient factors can be done prior to this planned surgery.

For example, anemia has been identified in the past as a potential factor for defective wound healing.[7,8] It is commonly thought that wound healing could be jeopardized with a hematocrit less than 35%.[9] Theories on the mechanism of defective wound healing include a decreased wound oxygen tension secondary to the anemia as well as a nutritional component that leads to a deficiency anemia. Hypovolemia may also play a role. Heughan et al[9] concluded that mild or moderate uncomplicated anemia in an otherwise healthy individual does not impair oxygen delivery to the wound and, therefore, did not require transfusion in these patients in the hope of stimulation of wound healing. This does not mean anemia should be ignored. Anemia, secondary to a deficiency such as iron, should be corrected with supplementation. Aside from anemia, proper hydration is essential, with several studies showing a decrease in wound problems when proper hydration is obtained.[10,11] Because of the blood loss associated with the TKA procedure as well as the immunosuppression effect of allogeneic transfusions, erythropoietin supplementation may also be considered to help avoid infection that does lead to wound healing difficulties.

As mentioned above, nutrition plays an important role in wound healing. Decreased oxygen levels (less than 3.5 g/dL) as well as a total lymphocyte count (less than 1,500) may make a patient more prone to wound failure.[12,13] Patients with obesity may also be at risk for wound complications.[14,15] Obesity may place the patient at more risk not only from an exposure standpoint, in which more vigorous skin flap retraction is required, but also from soft tissue devascularization. Unfortunately, controlling obesity prior to TKA is often difficult and emphasis should be on obtaining improved skin handling at the time of the procedure. Large medial and lateral flaps must be avoided at all costs.

One factor that can be controlled preoperatively is cigarette smoking, which does have a direct inhibitory affect on the microcirculation of the dermis. Nicotinic acid as well as its breakdown product, cotinine, are potent vasoconstrictors, and it is this vasoconstrictor effect that impairs wound healing.[2] Cotinine is stored in body fat and is still released for weeks after cessation of smoking. Therefore, cigarette smoking should cease at least 3 weeks, not days, prior to surgery.[16–18]

Systemic conditions are very difficult to control and must also be considered. While it is often difficult to separate the effect of diabetes from other concurrent factors such as age and obesity, diabetes may also play a role in wound healing. While epithelialization is not impaired, collagen synthesis and gain in wound tensile strength are impaired in the diabetic patient.[12] Early capillary ingrowth into the healing wound may also be reduced.[19] Patients with rheumatoid arthritis are thought to be at more risk for wound problems, but this effect may be related to anemia and nutritional factors as well as a history of steroid use. It is the authors' experience that rheumatoid patients have thin atrophic skin, and caution must be utilized to protect the skin throughout the procedure, including the application and removal of adherent surgical drapes.

One last patient factor to consider is the use of corticosteroids. This drug class interferes at several points in the healing cycling.[2,19,20] For example, a decrease of fibroblast proliferation[20] as well as a reduction in collagen age clearance from the healing wound has been noted.[21,22] The relationship between steroid usage and wound healing has not been universally noted, with both Wilson et al[14] and Garner et al[23] finding no correlation between the dose of steroid or the duration of its use and the time for complete wound healing. Garner et al did note that with long-term steroid usage (over 3 years), there was a higher rate of wound infections as well as a longer time to heal.[23] Ideally, one would like to eliminate corticosteroids prior to total knee arthroplasty, but unfortunately the diseased state often does not allow steroid elimination. The surgeon should realize the increased risk of wound problems with long-term steroid use and take necessary precautions as outlined below.

Local Factors

One of the most difficult problems that faces the knee surgeon is the knee with multiple previously placed incisions. It is not unusual to encounter previously placed incisions from high tibial osteotomy, open medial or lateral meniscectomies, and fracture treatment. Numerous studies have shown that the multiple-incision knee has an increased risk of wound healing difficulties.[2,14,24] Even a brief review of the vascular anatomy shows how previously placed incisions injure the anastomotic network that supplies the anterior aspect of the knee.[2,25] Problems can arise not only from an avascular skin bridge between the new and old incisions, but also from decreased subcutaneous tissue and associated adherent skin.

TISSUE EXPANDERS

As can be seen, not all patient factors can be corrected prior to surgery and not even the best of surgeons can erase the effect of previously placed incisions. In these cases at our institution, we have relied on a soft tissue expansion prior to the indicated TKA. It is now standard at our institution to utilize tissue expanders when it is felt that the quality and viability of soft tissues could be compromised. This may occur to previous poorly placed skin incisions or may be secondary to trauma that caused an increased adherence of the skin to the tibial plateau below. Although criteria for using tissue expanders may be subjective, any patient with adherent immobile skin or numerous previously placed skin incisions is considered a candidate for skin expansion. Severe angular deformities with a rotation component are also considered candidates for this procedure. Patients with increased angular deformities must also be considered for expansion since correction of the angular deformity may lead to insufficient skin for coverage.

Gold et al[26] reported on the first 10 patients utilizing this technique. In this study, the expanders were gradually expanded over an average of 64.5 days and all wounds healed without incident. To date, over 40 knees have been prophylaxed with tissue expansion.

TECHNIQUE OF TISSUE EXPANSION

Expander insertion is performed under local anesthesia using a mixture of Xylocaine (0.05%) and 1 to 1,000,000 epinephrine. A total of approximately 300 mL is injected into the subcutaneous space until blanching of the subcutaneous skin is created. A small incision is then made in line with the planned arthrotomy incision. Typically, two 200-mL expanders are utilized and are oriented at 90 degrees to each other. Placement can be arranged to accommodate existing incisions. A subcutaneous pocket is then created for placement of the tissue-expanding balloon. Once it is placed, the patient is admitted for 24 hours and then knee immobilized for 1 week. After 1 week, gradual expansion is begun. On average, 10% of the expanded value is done weekly. Capillary refill (less than 5 seconds) and patient comfort are monitored so that more volume can be injected if tolerated by the patient. At the time of revision, we like to wait 2 weeks from the last expander injection. Expanders are easily removed at the time of surgery and the skin is plentiful. Trimming of excess skin can be done at the time of closure if excess skin is present. Subcutaneous drains can also be utilized to decrease hematoma in this previously expanded pocket.

Once the skin has been expanded, the surgeon must choose between using an old incision or creating a new one. When possible, the incision deemed most adequate is utilized. The tissue expanders enhance the vascularity of the flap, safely allowing the old incision to be utilized. When a prior incision is not adequate, a new longitudinal incision is chosen. If redundant excess skin is present, the skin bridge between the prior incision and the new incision can be excised and the remaining edges reapproximated.

This technique has been successful in primary TKAs, and there have been case reports of success in revision TKA[27] and infected TKA.[28] By allowing primary closure without tension, this technique allows for immediate postoperative range of motion and ability to perform standard rehabilitation protocols with the avoidance of difficult and delay-inducing reconstructive procedures.

Others have found this technique successful in wound difficulties. Riederman and Noyes[29] describe the use of tissue expanders in five patients with severe end-stage patellofemoral arthrosis. Tissue expanders were utilized prior to a Maquet osteotomy because of previously placed incisions, and no wound complications were noted.

While complications of skin expansion such as hematoma, infection, prosthesis exposure, and prosthesis failure do exist, by utilizing the above technique these complications have been avoided at our institution.[26]

By allowing primary closure without tension, the use of tissue expanders allows for nearly immediate range of motion (ROM), with the ability to perform the standard rehabilitation protocols and avoidance of the need for reconstructive procedures.

SURGICAL TECHNIQUE

Surgical technique may play a role in the prevention of wound problems. An adequate incision length should be chosen to avoid excessive skin tension. The skin edges should also be handled with care to avoid disruption of the perforating arteries emanating from the subcutaneous fascial layer. Large flaps should be avoided at all costs. If necessary, flaps must be created as deeply as possible to preserve the blood supply from the dermal plexus. When possible, a lateral release should be avoided since numerous studies have shown that a lateral retinacular release decreases skin oxygen tension and increases the risk of wound complications. If a lateral release is required, preserving the superior genicular vessel may be helpful in avoiding problems.

Wound closure should be atraumatic and the resulting closure should be under no tension. Although emphasis is on aggressive continuous passive motion (CPM) and early ROM, should there be any signs of skin compromise or decreased skin circulation, therapy should be delayed.

TECHNICAL FACTORS

One of the most important aspects of preventing wound problems is a correctly placed skin incision. Johnson et al[30,31] have evaluated transcutaneous oxygen tension measurements for a variety of incisions and found the presence of a medial-side predominance for cutaneous circulation. Thus, they concluded that the lateral wound edge showed lower oxygen tension for all incisions initially, but would return to preoperative levels by postoperative day 8. Therefore, a medial incision that creates a large lateral base flap should be avoided.

For a knee with no previous incisions, a midline incision should be chosen. This midline incision begins approximately one hand breadth below the patella slightly medial to the center of the quadriceps tendon. The incision must be long enough to allow complete joint exposure. Standard surgical techniques such as avoidance of excessive retraction or skin flaps, atraumatic handling of the skin edges, and good hemostasis to avoid hematomas should be standard for all procedures. Excessive retraction, with heavy instruments, crushing clamps, and heavy tooth forceps should also be avoided so as not to push marginal but viable skin to compromise. If there is any question about skin viability, retraction should be removed periodically during the procedure, even without deflating the tourniquet. The sustained crushing effect of retractors on skin accordioned on itself increases local edema and compromises local blood flow.

Problems arise when previously placed incisions must be incorporated into the planned surgical incision. Incisions near the midline can be incorporated into the new knee incision and previous far medial and far lateral incisions can often be avoided in their entirety. Transverse incisions can be crossed, in most instances, at 90-degree angles without a threat of compromise.[25,32,33] Caution should be utilized when encountering wide scars with minimal subcutaneous tissue, for this may be a sign of injury to the underlying dermal plexus.[25] Suture utilization in closure may also play a role. A subcuticular polydioxane showed 20% more suture reaction when compared to subcutaneous polygolic acid. Therefore, the use of polydioxane should be avoided.[34]

Unfortunately, not all previous incisions can be avoided. When the skin bridge is less than 2.5 cm, the knee may be more at risk for skin necrosis.[35] It is for these types of situations that tissue expander use must be considered.

Previously at our institution a sham (incision) was used to identify those patients with increased risk of a wound necrosis.[36] A planned incision is made and performed to the depth of the subcutaneous tissue, flaps are elevated, and then the wound is closed in a standard fashion. If this incision heals without incident, a TKA can be performed with greater confidence. If the wound fails to heal, local measures are utilized to obtain healing without the added pressure of an exposed prosthesis.

One last point to consider is the role of the patella lateral release and its effect on wound healing. It is felt that a lateral retinacular release with a standard medial parapatellar approach will transect the superior and inferior genicular vessels on the medial as well as the lateral side, thus compromising the prepatellar skin. Johnson et al[10] noticed a decrease in the skin oxygen tension as well as an increase in the superficial drainage and infection rates when a lateral release was performed and the lateral vessels were sacrificed. Thus, it is best to avoid a lateral release as discussed in other areas of this text. By obtaining proper component rotation as well as maintaining proper patella prosthesis height, the incidence of lateral release can be markedly reduced. If a lateral release is necessary, it is recommended that the lateral superior genicular vessel be preserved if possible. The lateral release should also be performed utilizing an all-inside technique so that a large lateral flap can be avoided.

POSTOPERATIVE FACTORS

Prevention of wound problems must include a discussion of the postoperative modalities utilized in the role, if any, in wound compromise. CPM has been advocated as a method to increase knee ROM following TKA and its usage is common at many institutions. Johnson[37] found a decrease in skin oxygen tension when the CPM past 40 degrees was utilized during the first 3 postoperative days. This is in contrast to Yashar,[38] who found clinically no increased wound problems when an acceleration of flexion from 70 to 100 degrees was utilized immediately in the recovery room. Although immediate CPM is utilized commonly without difficulty, patients with compromised skin circulation who are at increased risk of wound infection perhaps should go at a slower pace than those who are not at risk.

Avoidance of hemarthrosis formation is thought to be important in decreasing wound healing problems. It is felt that a large hematoma not only serves as a culture medium for infection, but also may compromise the skin viability. To accomplish hemostasis a tourniquet deflation is often performed prior to closure to visualize and cauterize perforating arteries that may lead to hemarthrosis formation. Not all authors find tourniquet deflation necessary, however, with some showing increased bleeding when intraoperative tourniquet deflation was performed.[39] Abdel-Salem and Eyres,[40] in a prospective randomized study, found that when no tourniquet was utilized, blood loss was still increased over that of the control group, but less postoperative pain and fewer superficial infections were encountered.

Another area of debate rests with the usage of postoperative drains. Holt et al[41] examined blood loss and wound problems in drained and nondrained groups. Forty percent of the undrained knees and none of the drained knees required dressing reinforcement; the undrained knees also had a higher incidence of ecchymosis. These authors concluded that drains are effective in preventing the accumulation of blood in the surrounding soft tissues. Not all authors agree with these conclusions. Crevoisier et al[42] examined 32 patients in drained and undrained groups. They concluded that there is no advantage to closed suction drainage usage. This was a small study, probably of insufficient size to draw a definitive conclusion on risk of wound infection since it occurs in less than 1% of cases. Ovadin et al[43] looked at 58 knees, and while there was little difference in the rate of infection, more serous drainage was noted in the undrained group. Therefore, at our institution we utilize postoperative drains not only for hemarthrosis avoidance, but also for the reinfusion benefits. With the use of reinfusion drains, the allogeneic transfusion rate has been reduced to approximately 2% for a unicompartmental knee. Drains are removed on postoperative day 1. Drinkwater and Neil[44] have shown a decrease in bacterial colonization when drains are removed during this 24-hour period.

There has been some concern over bleeding complications associated with postoperative deep vein thrombosis (DVT) prophylaxis.[46–48] It should be noted that bleeding complications have been noted with not only placebo, but also low molecular heparin and Coumadin usage. Stulberg et al[45] evaluated 638 TKAs and noticed a wound complication rate of 18.1%, with 10.6% having culture-negative drainage. Increased bleeding has also been noted with low molecular weight heparin, with bleeding complications of 2% to 5% noted in the literature. Bleeding problems are mutifactorial and perhaps some wound complications can be avoided with careful hemostasis, meticulous closure, as well as proper dosing of prescribed prophylaxis agents.

As can be seen, wound complications can be prevented or decreased by understanding of the vascular anatomy and how it relates to the patient's wound characteristics as well as techniques used as mentioned above.

TREATMENT

If prevention fails, the surgeon is left with treating the wound complication that occurred while attempting preservation of the prosthesis and acceptable range of motion. Treatment, therefore, is dependent on the type of wound complication that occurs, such as prolonged serous drainage, tense hematoma, superficial soft tissue necrosis, and full-thickness necrosis. These complications can occur both with and without the presence of an infection. As discussed in previous chapters, deep prosthetic infections must be ruled out, and if not present, prevented from developing through local wound care and judicious, but correct, antibiotic usage.

Prolonged Serous Drainage

Prolonged serous drainage often occurs following TKA. The question remains of when to explore the wound. If excessive erythema or purulence is not noted, these wounds can be initially observed. This drainage may be secondary to a large hematoma or subcutaneous hematoma. If drainage is not resolved by 5 to 7 days, surgical evaluation may become necessary.[25] The hematoma may adversely affect the wound, as will any increasing soft tissue tension as well as releasing the toxic breakdown products of hemoglobin. The surgeon should consider the continuation of CPM modalities as well as limit physical therapy while this wound is being observed. It should be noted that not all prolonged drainage is noninfected. The incidence of infection develops in the chronically serous drainage knee and it ranges from 17% to 50%.[49–51] Not all authors agree with initial observation of these serous drainage wounds. Weiss and Krackow[49] reported on early intervention of eight draining TKAs and concluded that early intervention may prevent a deep tissue prosthetic infection.

Tissue Hematoma

While a tense hematoma that is not draining can occur, initially observation is appropriate. With any signs of local skin compromise, increased pain, or limited range of motion, a surgical exploration can be performed. Once again, CPM and physical therapy may be limited during this observation period.

Superficial Soft Tissue Necrosis

Superficial infections are those wound problems that do not penetrate to the level of the prosthesis and bone. This category would include the benign stitch abscess that improves with only a suture debridement and dressing change as well as superficial soft tissue infections secondary to cellulitis. A superficial infection should be treated aggressively with cultures obtained prior to the initiation of antibiotics for the presumed organism. CPM and physical therapy should be discontinued and surgical exploration may be needed to rule out deep penetration.

Despite aggressive treatments, superficial infection may lead to skin necrosis. Initially necrosis less than 3 cm can be treated with local wound debridement under anesthesia and immobilization.[52] All dead tissue must be removed even if this results in the prosthesis exposure. If under surgical exploration the infection is noted to be superficial, then local coverage techniques may be adequate, but if the prosthesis becomes exposed, then the treatment is like that of a major skin necrosis (see below).

Treatment of the superficial necrosis begins with local wound care. This would include not only antibiotic prophylaxis, but also local debridement and observation. During this period where the skin viability is questionable, a wound can declare itself. In the absence of infection, tissue debridement can wait until the eschar separates. During this period, the wound may be contracting, which aids the surgeon by decreasing coverage needs. Small wounds can be allowed to heal by secondary intention. Benefits of healing by secondary intention is avoidance of a surgical procedure as well as the ability to continue with the range of motion, both active and passive, for the TKA.

Skin graft is indicated when the time for untreated healing would be longer than the postoperative 5 to 7 days of healing for a routine skin graft. Skin graft viability requires the penetration of vascular buds from the underlying wound bed, and proper immobilization is needed for this to occur. For the skin grafts to be viable, the infection must also be controlled with decreased bacterial counts noted.

A third option for treatment of superficial necrosis would be the use of a local fasciocutaneous flap. Hallock[53] described six patients with successful soft tissue coverage utilizing this technique. This author states that the fasciocutaneous flap should not be utilized when gross infection or the prosthesis is exposed.

Full-Thickness Soft Tissue Necrosis

The most serious of the wound problems encountered with TKA is full-thickness necrosis. This involves deep penetration of the soft tissue with exposure of the joint prosthesis. Coverage options are complex and would include either advancement of the local tissue or transfer of distant tissue in the form of a free flap.

Due to the complex nature of this problem, often prosthesis removal is required. An early plastic surgery consultation is also required to handle these difficult skin management issues. While options include local random or fasciocutaneous flaps, in practice it is a rotational gastrocnemius flap or free flap that are currently utilized to obtain closure. Simple closure over an exposed prosthesis is doomed to failure.[54]

Salvage with the gastrocnemius flap is well described in the literature.[55–58] Usually, it is the medial head of the gastrocnemius muscle because of its wide arc of motion once it is detached distally from its insertion into the Achilles tendon. The lateral gastrocnemius can be utilized for lateral coverage while the medial gastrocnemius is used for defects around the patella and tibial tubercle. These flaps can be utilized for necrosis in approximately two-thirds of the tibia while the distal one-third tibia lesions would require free flap coverage.

For those knees in which gastrocnemius flaps are not adequate, such as large defects with an exposed prosthesis, coverage can be accomplished with a free tissue transfer of the latissimus dorsi muscle, rectus abdominis muscle, or a scapular free flap. All these methods have been described and have been found reliable for this purpose.[2] Gerwin et al[59] treated 12 patients with an exposed prosthesis with a medial gastrocnemius flap and achieved 92% healing. Markovich et al[60] described their experience with muscle flap coverage. The results of five latissimus dorsi free flaps, six medial gastrocnemius flaps and two rectus abdominis free flaps was 100% wound revascularization and prosthesis retention of 83%. The worst results, as expected, were for flaps utilized to treat an infected prosthesis.

CONCLUSION

Wound problems are not always avoidable in TKA despite meticulous surgical technique and closure and postoperative care. Some wound difficulties and necrosis will occur. The key is to identify those patients at risk, identify preoperative factors if possible, and aggressively treat wound problems if they do occur. Despite occurrence of significant wound problems, prosthesis retention with acceptable functioning can still be maintained.

References

1. Scapinelli R. Studies on the vasculature of the human knee. *Acta Anat* 1968;70:305–331.
2. Craig SM. Soft tissue considerations in the failed total knee arthroplasty. In: Scott WN (ed). *The Knee*, vol 2. St. Louis: Mosby-Yearbook, 1994:1279–1295.
3. Abbott LC, Carpenter WF. Surgical approaches to the knee joint. *J Bone Joint Surg* 1945;27:277–310.
4. Bjorkstrom S, Goldie IF. A study of the arterial supply of the patellae in the normal state, in chondromalacia patellae and in osteonecrosis. *Acta Orthop Scand* 1980;51:63–70.
5. Waisbrod H, Treiman N. Intra-osseous venography in patellofemoral disorders: a preliminary report. *J Bone Joint Surg* 1980;62B:454–456.
6. Taylor GI, Palmer JH. The vascular territories (angiosomes) of the body: experimental study and clinical applications. *Br J Plast Surg* 1987;40:113.
7. Arey LB. Wound healing. *Physiol Rev* 1966;16:327.
8. Glenn F, Moore SW. The disruption of abdominal wounds. *Surg Gynecol Obstet* 1941;72:1041.
9. Heughan C, Chir B, Grislis G, Hunt JK. The effect of anemia on wound healing. *Ann Surg* 1974;179:163.
10. Johnson DD, Eastwood DM. Lateral patellar release in knee arthroplasty: effect on wound healing. *J Arthroplasty* 1992;7(suppl):407–431.
11. Archauer BM, Black KS, Litke DK. Transcutaneous pO_2 in flaps: a new method of survival prediction. *Plast Reconst Surg* 1980;65:738–745.
12. Ecker ML, Lotke PA. Postoperative care of the total knee patient. *Orthop Clin North Am* 1989;20:55–62.
13. Dickhaut SC, DeLee JL, Pase CP. Nutritional statistics. Importance in predicting wound healing after amputation. *J Bone Joint Surg* 1984;66A:71–75.
14. Wilson MG, Kelley K, Thornhill TS. Infection as a complication of total knee replacement arthroplasty: risk factors and treatment in sixty-seven cases. *J Bone Joint Surg* 1990;72A:878–883.
15. Cruse PJ, Foord R. A five-year prospective study of 23,649 surgical wounds. *Arch Surg* 1973;107:206–210.
16. Benowitz NL, Jacob P III. Daily intake of nicotine during cigarette smoking. *Clin Pharmacol Ther* 1984;35:494.
17. Benowitz NL, Koyt F, Jacob P. Influence of nicotine on cardiovascular and hormone effects of cigarette smoking. *Clin Pharmacol Ther* 1984;36:74.
18. Benowitz NL, Kuyt F, Jacob P 3d, et al. Cotinine disposition and effects. *Clin Pharmacol Ther* 1983;34:664.
19. Klein NE, Cox LU. Wound problems in total knee arthroplasty. In: Fu FH, Harner CD, Vince KG, et al (eds). *Knee Surgery*, vol 2. Baltimore: Williams & Wilkins, 1994:1539–1552.
20. Green JP. Steroid therapy and wound healing in surgical patients. *Br J Surg* 1965;52:523–525.
21. Wahl LM. Hormonal resolution of macrophage collagenase activity. *Biochem Biophys Res Commun* 1977;74:838–845.
22. Werb Z. Biochemical actions of glucocorticoids on macrophages in culture. *J Exp Med* 1978;147(6):1695–1712.

23. Garner RW, Mowot AG, Hazleman BL. Wound healing after operations on patients with rheumatoid arthritis. *J Bone Joint Surg* 1973;55B(1):134–144.

24. Grogan TJ, Dores F, Rolling J, Amstutz HC. Deep sepsis following total knee arthroplasty. *J Bone Joint Surg* 1986;68A(2):226–234.

25. Dennis PA. Wound complications in total knee arthroplasty. *Inst Course Lect* 1997;46:165–169.

26. Gold DA, Scott SC, Scott WN. Soft tissue expansion prior to arthroplasty in the multiply operated knee—a new method of preventing catastrophic skin problems. *J Arthroplasty* 1996;11(5):512–521.

27. Santore RF, Kaufman D, Robbins AJ, Dabezies EJ. Tissue expansion prior to revision total knee arthroplasty. *J Arthroplasty* 1997;12(4):475–478.

28. Namba RS, Diao E. Tissue expansion for staged reimplantation of infected total knee arthroplasty. *J Arthroplasty* 1997;12(4):471–474.

29. Riederman R, Noyes FR. Soft tissue skin expansion of contracted tissues prior to knee surgery. *Am J Knee Surg* 1991;4(4):195–199.

30. Johnson DD. Midline or parapatellar incision for knee arthroplasty. A comparative study of wound inability. *J Bone Joint Surg* 1988;70B(4):656–658.

31. Johnson DD, Houshton TA, Redford P. Anterior midline or medial parapatellar incision for arthroplasty of the knee. A comparative study. *J Bone Joint Surg* 1986; 68B(5):812–814.

32. Ecker ML, Lotke PA. Wound healing complications. In: Rand JA (ed) *Total Knee Arthroplasty*. New York: Raven Press, 1993:403–407.

33. Windsor RE, Insall JN, Vince KE. Technical consideration of total knee arthroplasty after proximal tibial osteotomy. *J Bone Joint Surg* 1988;70A:547–555.

34. Casha JN. Suture reaction following skin closure with subcuticular polydioxanone in total knee arthroplasty. *J Arthroplasty* 1996;11(7):859–861.

35. Rosenberg AG. Surgical technique of posterior cruciate sacrificing and preserving total knee arthroplasty. In: Rand JA (ed). *Total Knee Arthroplasty*. New York: Lippincott-Raven, 1993:115.

36. Rothause KO. Plastic and reconstructive surgery. In: Insall JN (ed). *Surgery of the Knee*, vol 2. New York: Churchill-Livingstone, 1993:1200–1201.

37. Johnson DD. The effect of continuous passive motion on wound healing and joint mobility after total knee arthroplasty. *J Bone Joint Surg* 1990;78(A):421–426.

38. Yashar AA. Continuous passive motion with accelerated flexion after total knee arthroplasty. *Clin Orthop* 1997; 345:38–43.

39. Faralli VJ, Lotke PA, Orenstein E. Blood loss after total knee replacement effects of early motion. Paper presented at the 55th annual meeting of AAOS, February 1988.

40. Abdel-Salam A, Eyres KS. Effects of tourniquet during total knee arthroplasty. A prospective randomized study. *J Bone Joint Surg* 1995;77B(2):250–253.

41. Holt BT, Parks NL, Ensh GA, Lawrence JM. Comparison of closed suction drainage and no drainage after primary total knee arthroplasty. *Orthopaedics* 1997;20(12): 1121–1124.

42. Crevoisier XM, Reber P, Noesberger B. Is suction drainage necessary after total joint arthroplasty? A prospective study. *Arch Orthop Trauma Surg* 1998; 117(3):121–124.

43. Ovadin D, Luger E, Bickels J, Menachem A, Dekel S. Efficacy of closed wound drainage after total joint arthroplasty. A prospective randomized study. *J Arthroplasty* 1997;12(3):317–321.

44. Drinkwater CJ, Neil MJ. Optimal timing of wound drain removal following total joint arthroplasty. *J Arthroplasty* 1995;10(2):185–189.

45. Stulberg BN, Insall JN, Williams GW, Ghelman B. Deep vein thrombosis following total knee replacement. *J Bone Joint Surg* 1984;66A(2):194–201.

46. Levine MN, Gent M, Hirsh J, et al. Ardeparin (low molecular weight heparin) vs. graduated compression stockings for the prevention of venous thromboembolism. A randomized trial in patients undergoing knee surgery. *Arch Intern Med* 1996;156:851–856.

47. Leclerc JR, Geerts WN, DesJardins L, et al. Prevention of venous thromboembolism (WTE) after knee arthroplasty—a randomized double-blind trial comparing a low molecular-weight heparin fragment (Enoxaparin) to warfarin. *Blood* 1992;84:246a.

48. Spiro TE, Fitzgerald RH, Trowbridge AA, et al. Enoxaparin—a low molecular weight heparin and warafin for the prevention of venous thromboembolic disease after elective knee replacement surgery. *Blood* 1994;84:246a.

49. Weiss AP, Krackow KA. Persistent wound drainage after primary total knee arthroplasty. *J Arthroplasty* 1993;8: 285–289.

50. Bergstrom S, Krutson K, Lidgren L. Treatment of infected knee arthroplasty. *Clin Orthop* 1989;245:173–178.

51. Insall J, Aglietti P. A five to seven-year follow-up of unicondylar arthroplasty. *J Bone Joint Surg* 1980;62A: 1329–1337.

52. Sculco TP. Local wound complications after total knee arthroplasty. In: Ranawat C (ed). *Total Condylar Knee Arthroplasty: Technique, Results and Complications*. New York: Springer-Verlag, 1985:194–196.

53. Hallock GG. Salvage of total knee arthroplasty with local fasciocutaneous flaps. *J Bone Joint Surg* 1990;72(B): 1236–1239.

54. Bergstrom S, Carlsson A, Relander M, Kuntson K, Lindgren L. Treatment of the exposed knee prosthesis. *Acta Orthop Scand* 1987;58:662–665.

55. Eckhardt JJ, Lesavoy MA, Dubrow TJ, Wackyum PA. Exposed endo-prosthesis. *Clin Orthop* 1990;251:220–229.

56. Hemphill CS, Ebert FR, Muench AG. The medial gastrocnemius muscle flap in the treatment of wound complications following total knee arthroplasty. *Orthopaedics* 1992;15(4):477–480.

57. Peled IJ, Franki U, Wexler MR. Salvage of exposed knee prosthesis by gastrocnemius myocutaneous flap coverage. *Orthopedics* 1983;6(10):1320–1322.

58. Salibian AH, Sanford HA. Salvage of an infected total knee prosthesis with medial and lateral gastrocnemius muscle flaps. *J Bone Joint Surg* 1983;65A(5):681–684.

59. Gerwin M, Rothaus KU, Windsor RE, et al. Gastrocnemius muscle flap coverage of exposed or infected knee prosthesis. *Clin Orthop* 1993;286:64–70.

60. Markovich G, Dorr LD, Klein NE, McPherson EJ, Vince KG. Muscle flaps in knee arthroplasty. *Clin Orthop* 1995;321:122–130.

Section VII

Miscellaneous Complications in Knee Surgery

Chapter 32

Osteochondral Lesions of the Knee

Jürgen Toft

Of all the complications that can occur in connection with joint surgery, damage to the articular cartilage surfaces ranks among the most debilitating and the most complicated to heal. As articular cartilage defects have a tendency to impair joint function, every attempt has to be made to restore the integrity of articular cartilage surfaces. Sometimes, following joint injury, there is a potential for self-healing, traces of which we often see in arthroscopic examinations. Most of the time, however, the healing potential is insufficient and a process of continuing degradation of the articular cartilage surface is instituted. The "rub-off" from the articular surfaces causes subclinical or clinical inflammation of the joint, which in turn impairs joint lubrication, thus preventing self-limitation of the process. At this point, the patient's main complaint is not pain but reduced function, especially in sports activities.

In the early stages of articular cartilage degradation the condition is often misdiagnosed as an early stage of osteoarthritis and treated with antiinflammatory medication and physiotherapy. Not infrequently, the joint damage is enhanced by such a regimen, because pain and swelling are suppressed by the use of drugs, and physiotherapy delivers loads to the joint surfaces that they can no longer tolerate. If there is any clinical suspicion of substantial articular cartilage damage, the next logical step would be to evaluate the quality of the joint's surfaces arthroscopically and, on the basis of these findings, formulate a treatment strategy. The "wait-and-see" attitude, often dictated by the fear of litigation, is not a good guideline in dealing with articular cartilage defects.

The armamentarium of surgical techniques utilized in dealing with chondral lesions comprises shaving chondroplasty, subchondral bone drilling or microfracturing, abrasion arthroplasty, osteochondral grafting, and cartilage cell transplantation. Some of these procedures are well accepted by the orthopedic community, whereas others have a reputation of being either unpredictable or experimental.[1] The same applies to postoperative protocols, where opinion also varies widely as to the duration of non–weight-bearing periods and the onset and type of physiotherapy.

In this chapter I report my experience in dealing with articular cartilage lesions, which is based on a total of 18,000 knee surgeries. Some of my presentation contradicts the mainstream of orthopedic thought, and what is worse for some believers in the orthopedic orthodoxy is that I fail to cite supporting scientific evidence. Sometimes, when the truth comes along in a different robe, it can hardly be recognized, and some have difficulty accepting it if it is not presented with pie-charts and chi-square tests. Nonetheless, I still hope that there will be some benefit from my contribution to both patients and colleagues alike.

IATROGENIC DAMAGE TO ARTICULAR CARTILAGE

Damage to the articular surfaces caused by the use of mechanical instruments does occur, but the frequency and severity of such damage depends on the surgeon's experience and dexterity. Superficial damage such as scuffing or little cuts in the articular cartilage surface have been shown to stay stationary and not result in matrix degradation or even osteoarthritis.[2] More severe damage to articular cartilage and even underlying bone has been reported from the use of surgical lasers.[3] To date there is no firm evidence of a beneficial effect of the laser on articular cartilage, but there is clear evidence of detrimental effects when energy output, angulation, and distance to the surface are not carefully controlled.[4]

POSTOPERATIVE DAMAGE TO ARTICULAR CARTILAGE

Some of the more severe complications involving articular cartilage stem from infection and arthrofibrosis. The damage from infection is mainly toxic and chondrolytic, whereas arthrofibrosis damages articular cartilage through nutrition barriers formed by fibrous tissue membranes that cover articular cartilage surfaces. As far as preventing infections is concerned, the one-shot perioperative administration of a wide-range antibiotic is considered a valid prophylactic measure.

Epidemiologic or cost considerations should not stand in the way of prioritizing the safety of an individual patient. If infection does occur, arguments of cost-effectiveness and epidemiology will be overthrown anyway. So why take the risk?

To prevent arthrofibrosis certainly is not always possible but its occurrence can be minimized by good timing and preparation for surgery. In anterior cruciate ligament (ACL) surgery, for instance, the incidence of arthrofibrosis has been shown to be increased in acute surgery.[5] Although there is evidence also to the contrary, the majority of surgeons feel that delayed surgery is preferable. Links have also been postulated with sympathetic reflex dystrophy, which makes prevention of arthrofibrosis even trickier. Especially in the light of concomitant cartilage lesions, it seems highly advisable to delay surgery and prepare the patient properly, because in those cases aggressive postoperative rehabilitation would be incompatible with the goal of articular cartilage repair.

LATE COMPLICATIONS INVOLVING ARTICULAR CARTILAGE

Articular cartilage damage due to biomechanical aberrations such as occur with unattended ACL tears, following total meniscectomy, and following unattended patellar dislocation, as well as fractures healed in malalignment, are well documented in the literature. These complications occur late in the process, often decades after the initial injury, and they often result in severe degrees of osteoarthritis.

The principles of prevention are obvious, and with due attention to all existing pathologies and with present-day techniques of correcting them, in the future we will see fewer and fewer of those disabling, severe osteoarthrites.

PITFALLS IN DIAGNOSING COMPLICATIONS INVOLVING ARTICULAR CARTILAGE

In our era of high-tech medicine the patient's history is sometimes grossly undervalued. Most of the time, a suspicion of articular cartilage damage can be formulated from what the patient reports. As mentioned earlier, pain is not the leading symptom in articular cartilage lesions. In the early stages it is a feeling of early joint fatigue, a feeling of congestion in the joint following exercise and slight feelings of stiffness after longer periods of rest. Visible and palpable swelling can also be present in the early stages of cartilage degradation, but depending on the absorption capacity of the synovium, the symptom can also be absent in spite of severe articular cartilage damage. Some patients may reduce their articular cartilage down to bone without ever experiencing any pain. Sometimes, when confronted with magnetic resonance imaging (MRI) evidence of complete articular cartilage loss in a knee compartment, the patient finds it hard to believe that his or her knee should be in such a poor state of health. With pain not being a major factor in cartilage lesions and clinical examination being very uncertain in this area, MRI and arthroscopy have become all the more valuable.

While the accuracy of the MRI for detecting partial-thickness cartilage lesions is limited, it has a place in detecting subchondral bony changes such as osteonecrosis and for the selection of candidates for abrasion arthroplasty. The pitfall here is to renounce the use of the MRI for reasons of cost-effectiveness and "pie-sharing" problems with the radiologists. In my view, MRI does have a place in the diagnosis and treatment planning of chondral and osteochondral lesions, and provides some of the pertinent answers not even arthroscopy can give. However, the arthroscope remains the most important tool in diagnosing articular cartilage damage. Here, the pitfall is not so much in underdiagnosing or not diagnosing articular cartilage lesions, but in the disbelief that something sensible can be done about it. The conclusions that will be drawn from an arthroscopic examination will largely depend on the surgeon's concepts of healing and repairing such defects. In this context, looking is not equivalent to seeing.

SALVAGE PROCEDURES FOR ARTICULAR CARTILAGE DEFECTS

Principles of Cartilage Healing

It is widely recognized that articular cartilage cannot substitute volume losses with its original tissue, i.e., hyaline cartilage.[6] This observation has led to the wrong conclusion that articular cartilage cannot heal at all. Although it is admitted that fibrocartilaginous healing can occur following perforation of subchondral bone, appositional mechanisms of cartilage healing are generally rejected.[7] In my experience, such appositional fibrocartilaginous healing of chondral defects does occur in much the same way as fibrocartilage is formed on the edges of meniscal tissue cuts. I came across this principle of healing quite accidentally when, years ago, a visiting surgeon was asking me about a filled defect on a medial femoral condyle in a case where a cruciate ligament replacement was performed 6 months following a joint debridement. I maintained that this was the result of previous abrasion arthroplasty and only after the surgeon insisted on seeing the original surgical videotape it became apparent that the reparative tissue had formed following a shaving chondroplasty, with no measures on the subchondral bone at all.

This observation came like a revelation to me, and over the years the surgical and rehabilitational principles of achieving such a result at all times have been developed. This tissue, once formed, stays in place over long periods of time and acts like a seal to prevent the damaged articular cartilage from further degrading. They also help normalize the joint's metabolism and lubrication. But even in the case of complete loss of articular cartilage in cases of advanced osteoarthritis, it is possible to re-create thick and mechanically resistant weight-bearing surfaces that also last over long periods of time and that, in analogy to total knee replacement, may be termed as "bioprostheses."[8]

ARTICULAR CARTILAGE REPAIR THROUGH SHAVING CHONDROPLASTY

As elaborated in the previous section, appositional reparative growth of fibrocartilage on articular cartilage defects can be stimulated by shaving chondroplasty (Fig. 32.1). The secret here is to shorten the cartilage stumps in such a way that they are left neither too long nor too short. One pitfall in dealing with shaving chondroplasty is doing the shaving too superficially. In such a case, even if everything else is done correctly, the blood clot from which the fibrocartilaginous plug is formed cannot attach itself firmly enough.

The same applies to the misconcept of articular cartilage smoothing where it might be felt that the smoother the cartilage following shaving, the better. Here, too, the blood clot doesn't have any chance of attaching itself to the treated surface, so that repair will not occur.

Other misconceptions preventing repair from occurring involve the postoperative management. Two major killers of cartilage repair are early rehabilitation and insufficient length of non–weight bearing. In my experience, physical therapy should not be instituted before the ninth postoperative week. In the meantime, only continuous passive motion should be allowed.[9] A period of 8 weeks of non–weight bearing and of another 4 weeks of partial weight bearing should be observed.

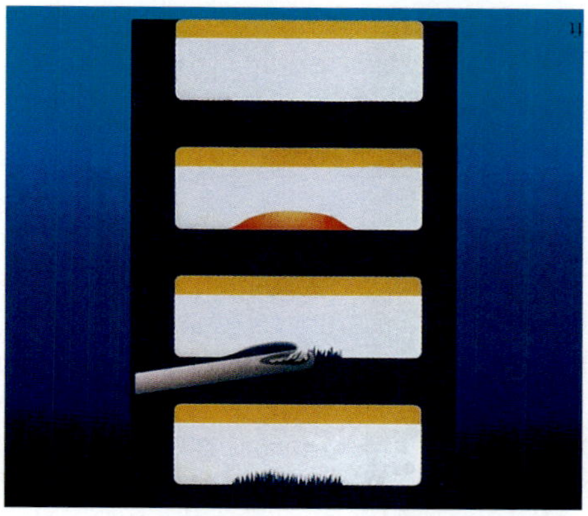

Figure 32.1. The concept of appositional articular cartilage repair. Cartilage trimming utilizing a shaver to prepare surface for blood clot attachment. Unimpeded conversion of blood clot into fibrocartilage is ensured by proper rehabilitational protocol.

In my experience it has been shown to be a fallacy that there is a difference in the postoperative protocol between shaving chondroplasty and abrasion arthroplasty. The times of non–weight bearing and other supportive measures do not differ at all between these two treatment entities. The pitfall here is to give in to what I might term as market pressures, meaning that such long non–weight-bearing periods may be a product difficult to sell to the patient. If healing is the prime goal for the patient, the surgeon should never avoid telling the patient the whole truth, even if the patient might be tempted to find another surgeon who will not require such hardships from him.

Another pitfall in connection with healing articular cartilage defects is the "don't-touch" ideology that one finds among a section of the orthopedic community. Not trusting the possibility of a sensible outcome from what they do with articular cartilage defects, these surgeons believe that by not touching the lesion they are at least not making it worse. In the short term, this may be true. Looked at from a long-term perspective, however, they are doing a disservice to the patient. Most of these lesions are not self-limiting, and over time the patient will go from bad to worse and the treatment options will become fewer and fewer, sometimes ending up in total knee replacement that would not have been necessary had the right measures been taken in due time. Another pitfall is thinking that such measures, even if you do believe in them, are of no use in older patients anymore. In my own experience, this is not true either. These principles apply irrespective of the patient's age, and I have arthroscopic evidence of such repair even on patients in their nineties.

CARTILAGE REPLACEMENT

Although the fibrocartilaginous layer that forms on bare bone following abrasion arthroplasty cannot be looked at as a true replacement, in many ways it serves as a replacement tissue (Fig. 32.2). I pay homage to the inventor of the technique, Dr. Lanny L. Johnson,[8] of East Lansing, Michigan. After learning the principles of abrasion arthroplasty from Dr. Johnson almost 20 years ago, I have become one of his staunchest disciples in continuing and further developing this remarkable technique of biologic resurfacing. Unfortunately, the technique has not met with the favorable response that it deserves, a fact that is due to a number of reasons. First, Dr. Johnson was very cautious and critical of his own work and set limitations on the technique that made it appear to be of limited clinical value. Second, he was heavily criticized for not providing sufficient scientific data to support his work. Other authors failed to repeat his excellent results and the conclusion was drawn that the technique is unpredictable and cannot be universally recommended. With so much criticism, it is small wonder that the majority of orthopedic surgeons felt on insecure ground when utilizing and confessing to abrasion arthroplasty.

My experience with abrasion arthroplasty is based on about 4,000 cases between 1980 and 1998. I share the fate of Dr. Johnson in not supplying unequivocal scientific data proving the validity of the concept and I am facing the same criticism in the orthopedic community as he did. The fact that I have not given up the technique in 18 years may suffice for those who are open to listen and want to try it themselves. I have successfully utilized abrasion arthroplasty in cases of severe osteoarthritis with complete loss of articular cartilage involving the totality of the medial and/or lateral femoral condyles and tibial plateaus (Figs. 32.3 and 32.4). I stopped respecting factors such as size of the lesion or age of the patient. I found that no matter how big the lesion is, fibrocartilaginous healing will always take place, provided proper surgical technique and postoperative management were ensured. In cases of axial de-

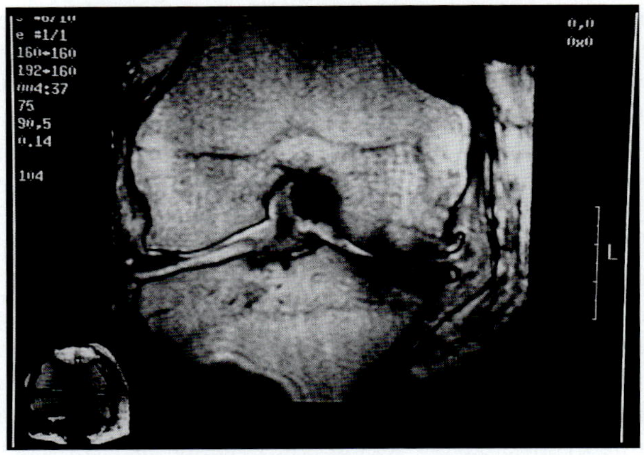

Figure 32.3. Preoperative magnetic resonance imaging (MRI) showing complete loss of articular cartilage in the medial compartment with substantial bony eburnation. As an alternative to partial or total knee joint replacement a decision is made in favor of abrasion arthroplasty.

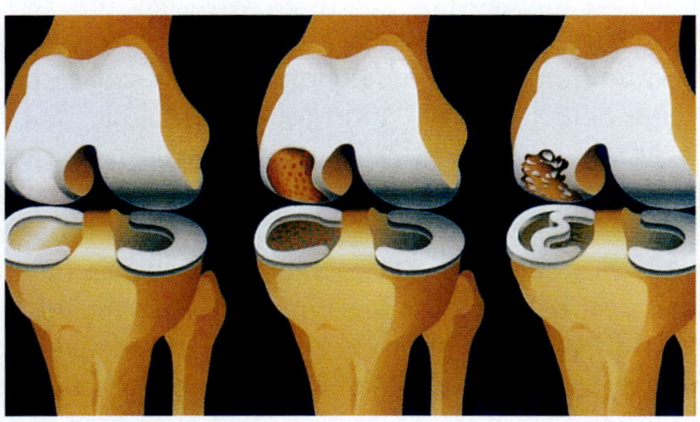

Figure 32.2. The concept of abrasion arthroplasty. Bare bone as well as adjacent irreparable third-grade cartilage lesions are included in the abrasion area to produce a uniform "salt-and-pepper" aspect of the surface. Additional microfractures or Pridie drillings may be required. If performed properly, including proper rehabilitation, the result will be a complete refill with reparative tissue.

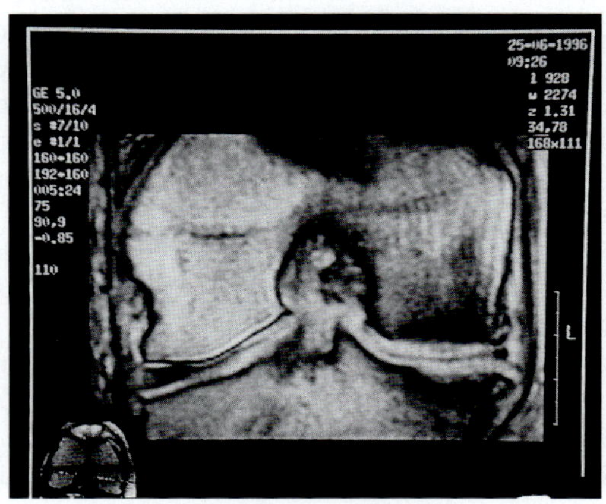

Figure 32.4. MRI of the same patient as in Fig. 32.3 8 months postoperatively, demonstrating thick and mature layers of reparative tissue sitting firmly on femoral and tibial bone. Radiographically this translates into the reappearance of a joint line.

formity, corrective osteotomy was performed, either at the time of abrasion arthroplasty or 6 weeks later if the time budgeted for simultaneous corrective osteotomy was considered insufficient.

In some patients with only slight angular deformities, the osteotomy was performed between 6 and 12 months postoperatively. In many patients, to whom osteotomy was suggested, it has never been performed and some of these patients are still doing well even 10 years after abrasion arthroplasty. Some of those patients have retained their fibrocartilage, and some have not. Even many of those who have not retained the reparative tissue are doing well, the reason for which is unclear.

What are the pitfalls with abrasion arthroplasty? The first pitfall is not believing in the concept and not using it. I daresay that a large number of patients could be saved from total or partial knee replacement and could be given at least 10 years of good joint function without any artificial device by utilizing the concept of abrasion arthroplasty. If combined with osteotomy, this period can be prolonged substantially. In addition, with a repaired osteoarthritic knee the patient can return to sports activities that he could never dream of with a total knee replacement. So we are not only talking about giving more years to that knee but also about giving more quality to the patient's life.

The next pitfall involves doing abrasion arthroplasty halfheartedly, thinking that by doing it very superficially one is doing less harm and one is better off if it does not work. The principle that applies here is, Nothing ventured, nothing gained. The key is to stay well inside cortical bone but still expose the bone's vascularity evenly and over the whole surface (Figs. 32.5 and 32.6).

In addition, one should not hesitate to remove thin layers of severely damaged and loose articular cartilage that does not have any potential for fibrocartilaginous healing, because the underlying layer is unstable on the bone. Hesitating to increase the size of the lesion and of bony exposure is another pitfall that might doom the surgery to failure. The severely damaged articular cartilage surfaces that one didn't have the courage to remove might be the cause of continuous inflammation that in turn creates a poor environment metabolically and thus inhibits fibrocartilaginous reparative growth on the bone. The goal should be not only to get rid of actual irritants in the joint, but also to make sure that there will be no future "troublemakers" staying or developing in the joint.

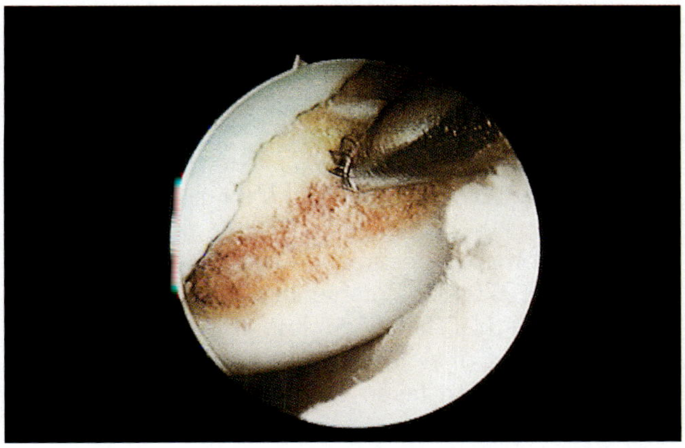

Figure 32.5. Arthroscopic view of a circumscribed lesion down to bone on the medial femoral condyle in a middle-aged male. Abrasion arthroplasty almost completed with exception of one little surface to the upper left.

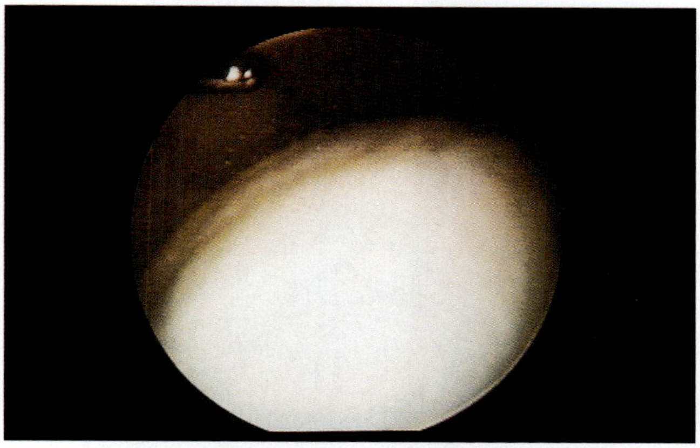

Figure 32.6. Same patient as in Fig. 32.5 1 year later with defect completely filled, the filling substance being recognizable only by slight color changes and a seam between the adjacent hyaline cartilage and the repair tissue. The patient is completely symptom free.

In connection with abrasion arthroplasty all intra- and extraarticular pathologies have to be addressed in order to respect this principle. In the histories that I take from my patients, but also in the international literature, I often experience a combination of overcautious surgery and overaggressive postoperative rehabilitation. For a successful cartilage repair and long-lasting results this has to be turned upside down; surgeons should be aggressive with the surgical measures and extremely cautious and soft with the rehabilitational program.

Summarizing the benefits of abrasion arthroplasty, I would emphasize that it does work if performed properly and if rehabilitation is in keeping with the principles of healing. Biomechanical factors such as maldistribution of compressive forces and/or instability have to be addressed simultaneously (Figs. 32.7 and 32.8). And last but not least, by performing abrasion arthroplasty with or without osteotomy and/or stabilization surgeons are not burning any bridges; in case of failure, they can always proceed to other salvage procedures such as total knee replacement.

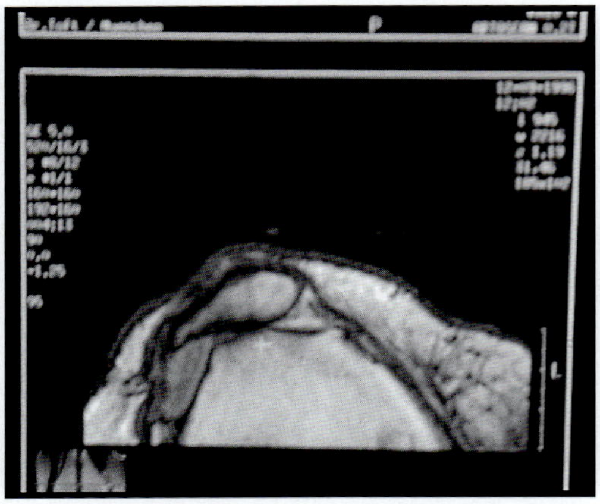

Figure 32.7. Female patient with chronic subluxation of patella and complete loss in the patellofemoral joint following previous recurrent dislocations of the patella. In spite of the severity of the condition, a decision was made in favor of abrasion arthroplasty, lateral release, and tibial tubercle transfer.

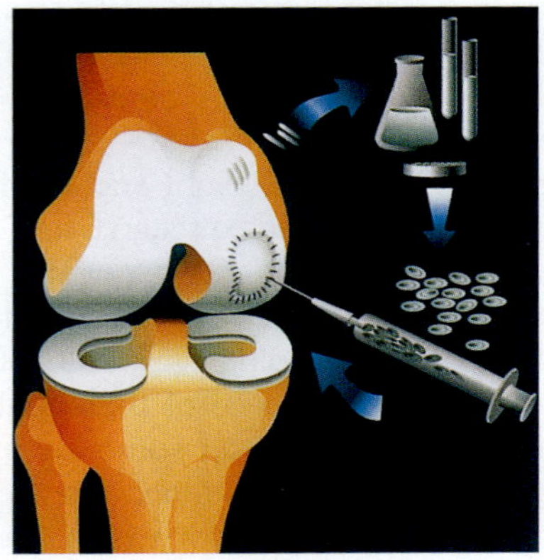

Figure 32.9. Schematic representation of cartilage cell transplantation. The patient's own multipled cartilage cells are used in an open surgery where the defect is cleaned and covered with a flap of periosteum that is sutured to the rim of adjacent hyaline cartilage, thus forming a kind of "incubator" for the transplanted cells.

CARTILAGE CELL TRANSPLANTATION

Thanks to the work of Peterson and Brittberg, which was published in the *New England Journal of Medicine* in 1994, a new concept has been added to the armamentarium of cartilage surgery.[10] In a procedure that involves harvesting of the patient's own cartilage material arthroscopically and then isolating the cartilage cells to multiply them to a point to be reintroduced into the patient's knee (Fig. 32.9), it was possible to produce a reparative tissue that, hystologically, comes very close to genuine hyaline cartilage. The disadvantage is the necessity for open knee joint surgery and its limitation to smaller size defects that are surrounded by a healthy rim of hyaline articular cartilage. The authors emphasize that the technique is not suitable for ostheoarthritis cases and for defects larger than 6 cm^2. The method may have a potential, though, for young patients with traumatic damage to circumscribed areas of articular cartilage in the weight-bearing surfaces, particularly on the femoral condyles.

The technique is less applicable in the patellofemoral joint, where, according to the authors, results are inferior, and also in the tibial plateau. For all its limitations, the know-how that is being accumulated in replicating cartilage cells and using them for reimplantation seems to be valid. The real quantum leap will probably come when this technique can be used arthroscopically. Whether the tissue generated by the technique will stand the test of time remains to be seen. Anecdotal reports of the physical state of such tissues probed arthroscopically 2 years postoperatively have demonstrated this tissue still to be very soft and immature.

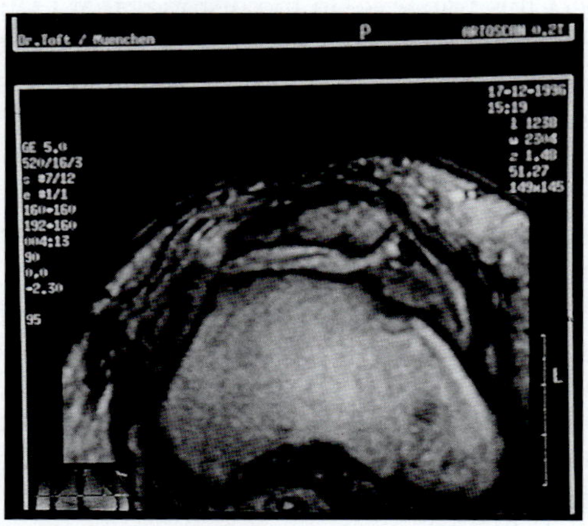

Figure 32.8. Same patient as in Fig. 32.5 6 months postoperatively demonstrating regrowth of reparative tissue both on the patellar back surface and on the trochlea, as well as the centrally sitting patella.

OSTEOCHONDRAL GRAFTING

Another promising technique was developed in the 1960s and 1970s by Wagner in Germany. It involves osteochondral transfer from less important areas to more important ones inside the same knee joint. This technique has been taken up recently by arthroscopic surgeons utilizing special instrumentation to harvest osteochondral cylinders and then perform a graft exchange from the good area to the bad area and vice versa (Fig. 32.10).

My experience with this technique is limited to about 20 cases, 15 of which did very well clinically, arthro-

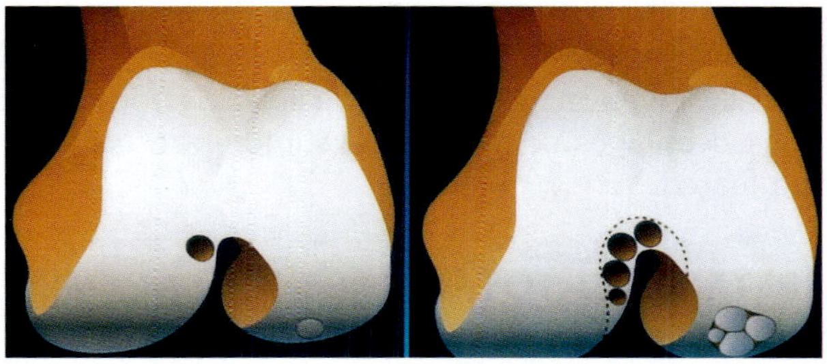

Figure 32.10. Graphic representation of osteochondral grafting. Grafting of osteochondral cylinders from mechanically less important areas to the main weight-bearing area of the knee. The technique is especially useful for osteochondritis dissecans and osteonecrosis of the femoral condyles.

scopically, and at MRI checkup. The remaining five were still symptomatic; two showed partial absorption of the transplanted cylinders, two showed fibrocartilaginous conversion of the transplanted cartilage, and one was symptomatic for no obvious reason. I have used this technique very successfully for osteochondrotic defects in younger patients and for osteonecroses in older patients where, surprisingly, the transplanted cylinders did survive the transfer.

For all the inherent positive potential that seems to be associated with this technique, the limitations for its use are similar to those for cartilage cell repair. The obvious advantage is the possibility of utilizing the technique arthroscopically and of transferring healthy subchondral bone together with the patient's own articular cartilage including its collagenous matrix. The pitfall here is with properly sizing the cylinders needed to fill any given defect and with harvesting the cylinders flush and perpendicularly to obtain an optimal fit with the surrounding surface. Another complication involves the tapping in of the cylinder, at which time the articular cartilage surface may be damaged mechanically.

In addition, it is sometimes difficult to control the depth of tapping in, because the sleeve has no firm support on the surrounding articular cartilage surface and has to be held freely by hand, which involves a certain risk of either tapping it too deeply or not deeply enough. Further improvement of the instrumentation will most probably eliminate these shortcomings.

ADDRESSING FAULTY BIOMECHANICS

When it comes to repairing articular cartilage defects or healing osteoarthritic cartilage loss, the key is not only to repair those defects in the short term, but also to ensure that the result will last over long periods of time. To maximize chances for a lasting result, biomechanical factors have to be taken into account as well. In

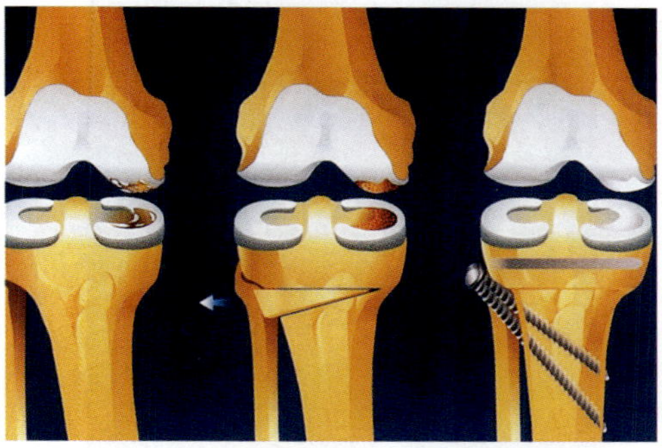

Figure 32.11. Graphic representation of high tibial osteotomy in combination with abrasion arthroplasty. The combination of abrasion arthroplasty and osteotomy improves surgical results and also saves time for the patient, because both repair processes can heal at the same time.

cases of varus or valgus deformities, corrective osteotomies (Fig. 32.11) should be considered, preferably at the time of the first surgery. Sometimes it is claimed that osteotomy alone will also do the trick. As far as pain is concerned, this may even be true. As far as joint function is concerned, this is certainly not true. The result can be significantly improved if not only the long axis of the leg is corrected, but also the "potholes" on the articular surfaces are refilled. The key here is not just to reduce intraarticular rub-off and degradation, but preferably to eliminate it completely.

In terms of patellofemoral biomechanics, additional lateral retinacular release (Fig. 32.12) and even tibial tubercle transfer (Fig. 32.13) might be necessary to protect the reparative tissue over the long term. In addition to the aforementioned maldistribution of compressive forces, instability from collateral and/or cruciate ligaments plays a role in the development of osteoarthritic changes in the knee. Whereas the previous practice was not to perform ACL replacement in older and osteoarthritic patients, the opinion is now swinging around to the belief that even for the osteoarthritic knee stability will be beneficial. I have never observed any age limits and I have always felt that to have an osteoarthritic knee is bad enough and that it does not have to be left unstable, too.

As opposed to the mainstream in the orthopedic community, I have never used the patellar tendon graft for osteoarthritic patients, feeling that a graft twice as stiff as the natural ACL cannot be a good choice in a joint where the femoral condyles underwent considerable deformation. Maybe some of the disillusionment with ACL replacement in osteoarthritic patients stems from utilizing patellar tendon as opposed to other more elastic materials such as semitendinosus tendon. Depending on the amount of additional instabilities and on

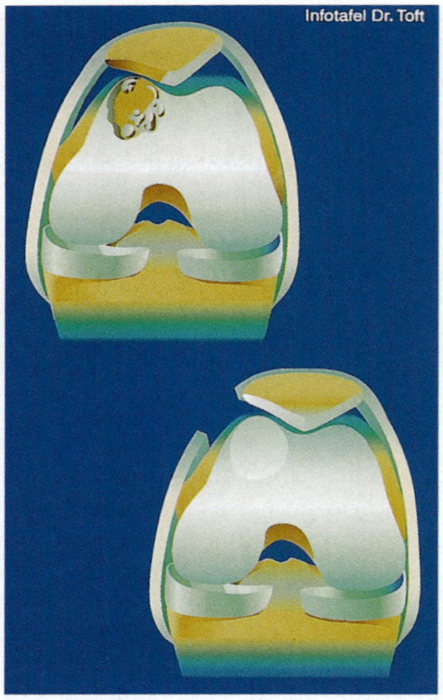

Figure 32.12. Graphic representation of the lateral release procedure. Decompressing and realigning the patella relative to the trochlea is a useful adjunct to corrective measures about the knee and helps protect the newly formed reparative tissue following both shaving chondroplasty and abrasion arthroplasty.

the patient's body weight, I would either use a double-looped or a quadrupled semitendinosus graft (Fig. 32.14), which, according to laboratory testing, shows an elasticity similar to that of the natural ACL. Here, too, the pitfall is in refusing to address the problem of instability early in the disease process. This is another example of the "wait-and-see" philosophy's being detrimental to the patient's health. Especially with today's minimally invasive techniques in replacing torn ACLs, the disadvantages of open ACL surgery are no longer to be feared.

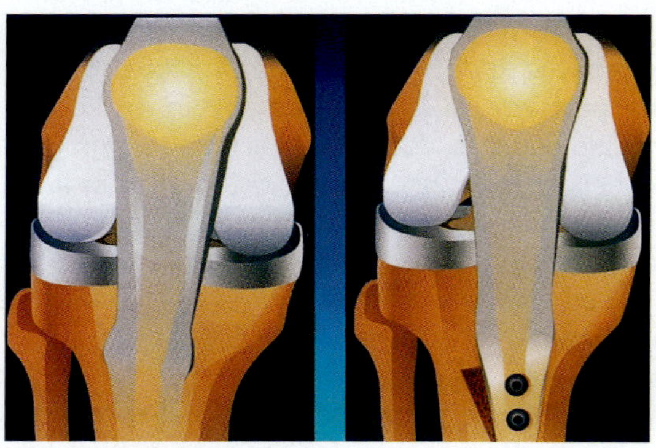

Figure 32.13. Graphic representation of tibial tubical transfer. In cases of significantly increased Q-angles, a lateral retinacular release would be insufficient to ensure long-lasting fibrocartilaginous healing in the patellofemoral joint. In such cases the additional medial transfer of the tibial tubercle is mandatory.

PARTIAL AND TOTAL KNEE REPLACEMENT

There are cases where the choice will be to use artificial components to replace lost articular cartilage to restore joint function. In this context, the rheumatoid patient comes to mind, but also the old, the weak, and the uncooperative patient as well. In such cases, and when there is substantial bone loss or severe axial deformity, possibly combined with severe and multidirectional instability, nobody would argue the necessity for total knee replacement.

There is, however, a large "gray zone" of indications where total or partial knee replacement could be circumvented or at least postponed significantly by utilizing techniques that aim at repair and restoration of articular cartilage tissue volume. That this is possible has been proven by experience. How it works and under which circumstances the results become more predictable has been elaborated on. To be more efficient with articular cartilage defects, the treating orthopedic surgeon should equip himself with a wide range of surgical procedures that he can use to achieve the best possible results for his patients.

PITFALLS IN REHABILITATION

No matter what mechanism of repair we're looking at, the key to success is the proper use of rehabilitational measures. Dictated by early functional treatment modal-

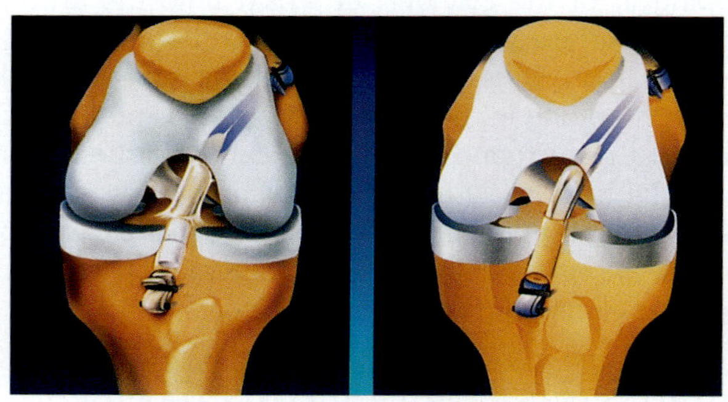

Figure 32.14. Graphic representation of the quadrupled semitendinosus plasty for anterior cruciate ligament (ACL) replacement. In the osteoarthritic knee the graft choice should be in favor of the semitendinosus tendon, which is less stiff than the patellar tendon and thus does not cause stress risers between the contacting articular surfaces.

ities that have been developed for ligament surgery to help collagenous structures reorient themselves in scar tissue, this concept, beneficial for ligament surgery, has been translated into other types of joint surgery. Unfortunately, the principle of early functional rehabilitation is detrimental to achieving the repair response that we want and need in dealing with articular cartilage defects. This applies to the same extent to both shaving chondroplasty and abrasion arthroplasty. The key here, in my experience, is to keep the patient away from the physiotherapist for about 2 months postoperatively. During that time, continuous passive motion is beneficial and absolutely sufficient.

Only after the repair response has matured to a point where the tissue will withstand compressive and sheer forces without risking damage can the focus shift back to muscular rehabilitation. In the first stage following shaving chondroplasty and/or abrasion arthroplasty the muscles have to be "sacrificed." Once the knee has healed and repaired itself, rebuilding the muscle will not cause a major problem.

If, on the other hand, the reparative response is incomplete or even absent, the muscles will never come back completely and the outcome will not be what it could have been had these principles been heeded. Advice such as "The patient should weight bear as tolerated" should be a thing of the past. Pain tolerance is not the question. Insufficient or absent repair of articular cartilage defects would not be felt by patients in the early postoperative stages. They would be felt when the patients think they are ready to return to more aggressive types of activities and then feel the limitations in the same way they felt them prior to surgery. Here again the surgeon has to be courageous to confront the patient's understandable desire for quick solutions, which, when they concern articular cartilage damage, are not at hand.

CONCLUSION

When confronted with articular cartilage lesions we should aim at restoring normal anatomy, normal physiology, and normal function as completely as possible. To achieve this, we have to utilize the necessary surgical and rehabilitational means that ensure a maximum probability of a good and long-lasting result. Together with the articular cartilage problem, additional pathologies such as axial deviations, patellar malalignment, and ligament instabilities have to be addressed with minimally invasive techniques.

Considerations of cost-effectiveness, fear of litigation or peer criticism, and maximal patient comfort should not be primary in the decision-making process. The key is to interrupt an otherwise vicious circle as completely as possible. This may involve a lot of surgery, a lot of time, and a lot of patience, on the part of both the patient and the doctor. In the long term, though, the prospect of having and keeping patients happy will outweigh the difficulties in achieving this goal. Surgeons should never be governed by the fear of losing the patient. Once they are prepared to lose the patient, because they believe in what they are doing and the patient does not, most of the time they will not lose the patient. And if they do lose the patient in the first place, they will get him back at a later stage when it turns out that the easy way did not do the trick.

References

1. Bert JM, Maschka K. The arthroscopic treatment of unicompartmental gonarthrosis: a five-year follow-up study of abrasion arthroplasty plus arthroscopic debridement and arthroscopic debridement alone. *Arthroscopy* 1989; 5:25–32.
2. Mankin HJ. The reaction of articular cartilage to mechanical injury. *J Bone Joint Surg* 1982;64A:460–466.
3. Small NC. Complications in arthroscopy: the knee and other joints. Commitee on Complications of the Arthroscopy Association of North America. *Arthroscopy* 1986;2:253–258.
4. Lane J, Amiel M, Monosov A, et al. Matrix assessment of the articular cartilage surface after chondroplasty with the holmium:YAG laser. *Am Orthop Soc Sports Med* 1997;25:560–569.
5. Shelbourne KD, Wilckens JH, Mollabashy A, et al. Arthrofibrosis in acute anterior cruciate ligament reconstruction: the effect of timing of reconstruction and rehabilitation. *Am J Sports Med* 1991;19:332–336.
6. Mankin HJ, Mow VC, Buckwater JA, et al. Form and function of articular cartilage. In: Simon SR (ed). Orthopaedic Basic Science. Rosemont, IL: *AAOS*, 1994:1–44.
7. Allen AA, Fealy S, Panariello R, et al. Chondral injuries. *Sports Med Arthrosc Rev* 1996;4:51–58.
8. Johnson LL. Arthroscopic abrasion arthroplasty historical and pathologic perspective: present status. *Arthroscopy* 1986;2:54–69.
9. Salter RB, Simmonds DF, Malcom BW, et al. The biological effect of continuous passive motion on the healing of full-thickness defects in articular cartilage. *J Bone Joint Surg* 1980;62A:1232–1251.
10. Brittberg M, Lindahl A, Nilsson A, Peterson L. Treatment of deep cartilage defects in the knee with autologous chondrocyte transplantation. *N Engl J Med* 1994;331: 889–895.

Chapter 33

CARTILAGE CELL TRANSPLANTATION

Lars Peterson

Articular cartilage injuries on weight-bearing areas of the knee do not heal and may progress into osteoarthritis by enzymatic digestion and mechanical wear.[1,2] The search for complete healing of articular cartilage injuries with hyaline regeneration is still ongoing. Chondral injuries could heal with either repair tissue or regeneration. "Repair tissue" means a filling of the defect with tissue not identical to hyaline cartilage; "regeneration" means a repair tissue identical to normal hyaline cartilage.

The repair tissue should be able to fill and seal off the damaged area and to withstand mechanical wear over time. The regenerating tissue should be included in the natural turnover of normal cartilage over time. At present, there is no optimal treatment of chondral injuries.

The use of the culture technique for chondrocyte transplantation was made possible by the work of Chesterman and Smith,[3] who were the first to isolate and culture chondrocytes free of matrix. In 1984, for the first time, results of autologous chondrocyte transplantation in a rabbit model were presented, showing hyaline cartilage repair.[4] This animal model was used in further studies in Gothenburg, Sweden, with confirmation and improvement of the results.[5]

Since 1985, work has been going on with human chondrocyte cell culture technique. In 1987 the ethical committee of the medical faculty of the University of Gothenburg approved a clinical pilot study using autologous cultured chondrocyte transplantation in chondral defects of the human knee (Fig. 33.1). The first results of this technique in treating chondral lesions in the human knee were presented in 23 patients in October 1994.[6] In 14 out of 16 patients treated for chondral injuries on the femoral condyles, the results were good to excellent. More than 500 patients have been treated in Sweden with autologous chondrocyte transplantation, and worldwide more than 1,500 patients have been treated with this technique.

INDICATION FOR AUTOLOGOUS CHONDROCYTE TRANSPLANTATION

Autologous chondrocyte transplantation is indicated in patients of ages 15 to 55 years with focal femoral articular cartilage injuries of 10 to 40 mm in diameter extending down to the subchondral bone. Contained lesions with normal cartilage surrounding the excised defect have a better prognosis than uncontained lesions extending to the synovial lining of the joint (Fig. 33.2).

Medial and lateral femoral condyle lesions with varus or valgus deformities need a correction with osteotomy to change the compressive forces acting on the compartments. Isolated femoral condyle defects with anterior cruciate ligament (ACL) deficiency are recommended for autologous chondrocyte transplantation along with ACL reconstruction.

The decision based on the indications for autologous chondrocyte transplantation is made during arthroscopic evaluation. Visualization, probing, and assessment of the depth and size of the defect are done as well as a complete arthroscopic examination. If the indications are found, cartilage is harvested for chondrocyte cell culturing.

CLINICAL EVALUATION

A history of any trauma or repetitive loading and a careful record of previous surgery are important. A thor-

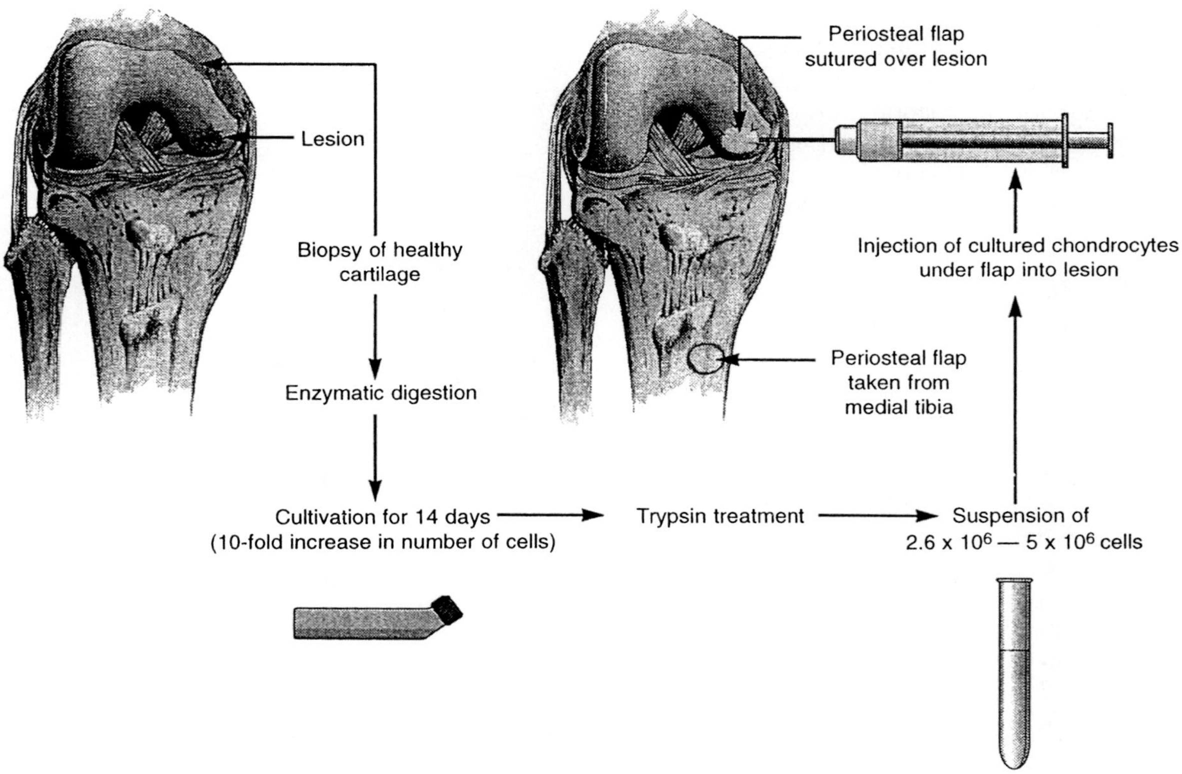

Figure 33.1. Autologous chondrocyte transplantation.

ough clinical examination is performed, including signs of local tenderness, swelling, range of motion, and crepitations. Varus or valgus deformities are examined as well as patella malalignment or instability. Clinical tests of ligament instability are performed. Standing x-rays are taken of the knee in extended position and in 45 degrees of flexion. X-rays with the hip-knee-ankle axes should also be taken. Any abnormal weight-bearing axes should be corrected, and slightly overcorrected by 2 to 3 degrees. Magnetic resonance imaging (MRI) could provide additional information of the joint status.

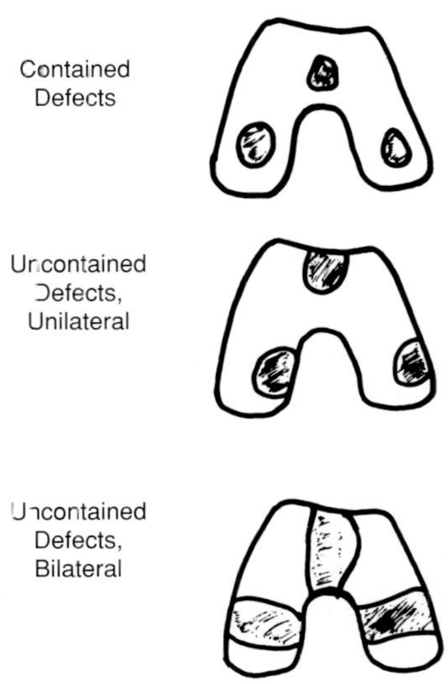

Figure 33.2. Examples of contained, unilateral, and bilateral uncontained defects.

ARTHROSCOPIC EVALUATION

Under general anesthesia, a complete stability test of the knee is done, comparing with the healthy side and the previous findings. A complete examination of the joint has to be done, including all articular cartilage surfaces, the synovial lining, the menisci, the cruciate ligaments, and any fragments, osteophytes, or loose bodies present. Undiagnosed intraarticular pathology is critical and could interfere with the indications and the results. Visualization, probing, and assessment of the depth, size, and location of the cartilage injury should be performed. The opposing articular surface should be normal, or at most only fibrillation or superficial fissuring are found.

During the arthroscopy, the planning of the transplantation is started and different surgical approaches are considered as well as the technical details of the intended debridement of the defect, and containment of the defect subchondral bone condition. Meniscus lesions should be treated arthroscopically, but after the harvesting of cartilage for cell culturing. Loose bodies and cartilage fragments should be removed before harvesting of cartilage. No debridement or only gentle debridement of the injury is performed at this point.

ARTHROSCOPIC HARVESTING OF CARTILAGE

Cartilage is harvested from the upper medial or upper lateral femoral condyle on minor weight-bearing areas. It could also be harvested from the intercondylar notch. In 98% of our cases, the cartilage is harvested from the upper medial femoral condyle. With the arthroscope in the lateral portal and the probe in the medial portal, access to the areas is evaluated. If there is any interference with a medial plica, this may have to be resected before harvesting the cartilage. With a curette or special instruments, three or four slices of cartilage sized 3 to 4 mm × 10 to 12 mm are taken from the upper medial femoral condyle and are large enough for defects up to 8 to 12 cm^2. The slices should extend into the subchondral bone plate, including some subchondral bone, and extend to the synovial lining. This will allow fibrous ingrowth as well as synovial ingrowth for covering of the harvest area.

The healing time for the harvest area is about 3 months. The area will be covered by fibrous tissue. In over 600 patients who have had cartilage removed for cell culturing, there have not been any complications or late symptoms. Optimal harvesting of cartilage is of greatest importance for the success of the cell culturing. Optimal cell quality is necessary for an optimal result of the procedure.[6]

SURGICAL PROCEDURE

The patient is under general anesthesia or spinal anesthesia. There is a tourniquet-controlled bloodless field. The arthrotomy starts with a minor parapatellar incision. The joint is opened and the defect area is identified. The defect area is carefully examined for size, depth, and grade of the lesion. The surgical approach to the lesion is assessed and if necessary the incision is increased to be able to perform an optimal surgical procedure.

Excision and Debridement of the Defect

The injured area should be excised with vertical edges and include all the damaged area with fissures running from the defect. A radical excision is the key to success (Fig. 33.3). Trochlear lesions may be angulated on

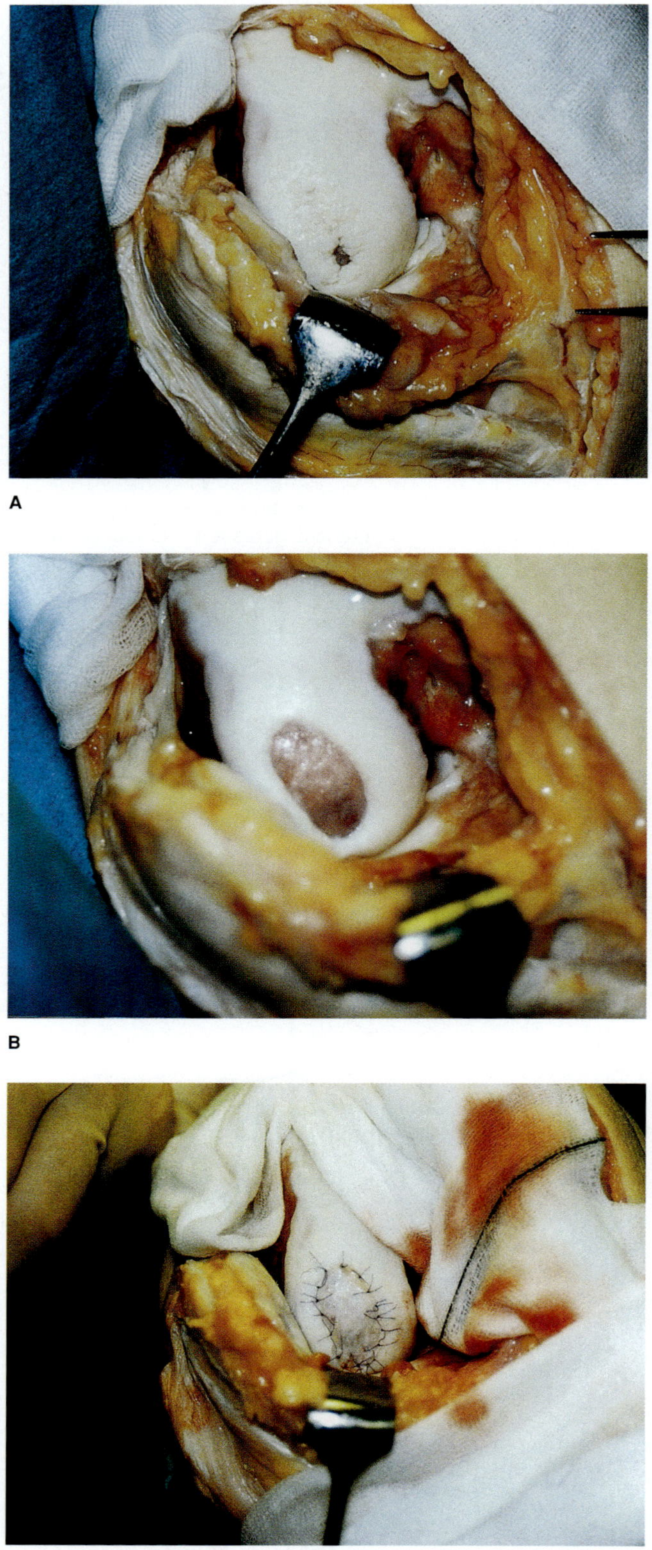

Figure 33.3. **A:** Lesion of the medial femoral condyle. **B:** Radical excision, including damaged tissue. **C:** Defect covered with periosteal flap.

the anterior and posterior edges to minimize catching in the early postoperative period. Gentle debridement of the excised area should be carefully carried out down to the subchondral bone with sharp curettes. Bleeding should be avoided as it will introduce fibroblasts and stem cells into the repair area, with fibrocartilage formation resulting.

Measurement of the Defect

Measurement of the defect should include the longest diameter of the excised defect and its longest perpendicular diameter. The use of a template for determining the exact size of the defect is recommended (Fig. 33.4).

Periosteal Harvesting

With increasing age and inactivity, the periosteum atrophies and sometimes becomes so thin that it is not possible to harvest or is of such poor quality that it cannot be used.

Periosteum is recommended to be harvested from the upper medial tibia, distal to the pes anserinus and the medial collateral ligament insertions. Another location for periosteal harvesting is proximal to the articular surfaces of the medial or lateral femoral condyles, where the periosteum is thicker. This harvesting area needs a synovial incision and a subsynovial dissection down to the periosteum. The periosteum in these locations is covered by numerous small vessels, which should be carefully cauterized after the incision and removal of the periosteal flap.

There is a risk for bleeding in the harvesting area, especially on the femur, and this could cause problems in the postoperative rehabilitation with swelling, adhesions, and arthrofibrosis.

In our experience the proximal medial tibia is the optimal and safest area for periosteal flap harvesting, and only three complications with hematomas in over 500 patients have occurred. Evacuation of the hematomas is required. No long-term negative effects have been seen.

Through a separate incision from the upper medial

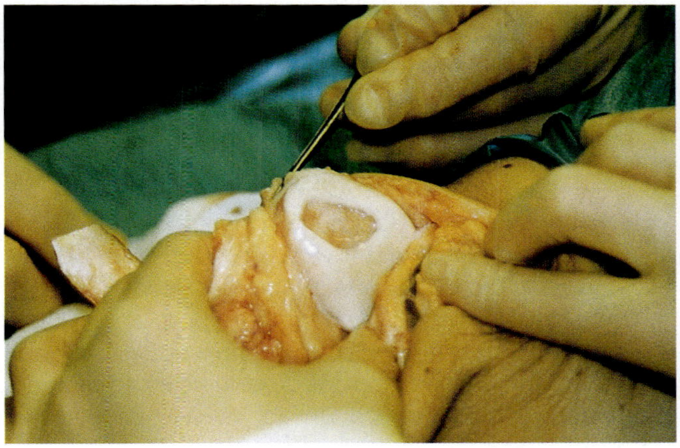

A

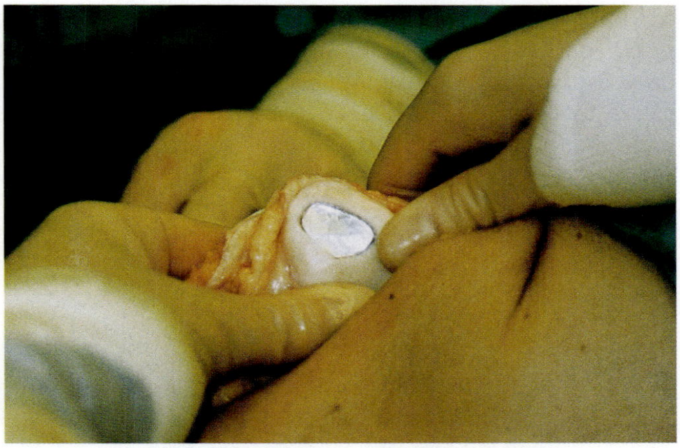

B

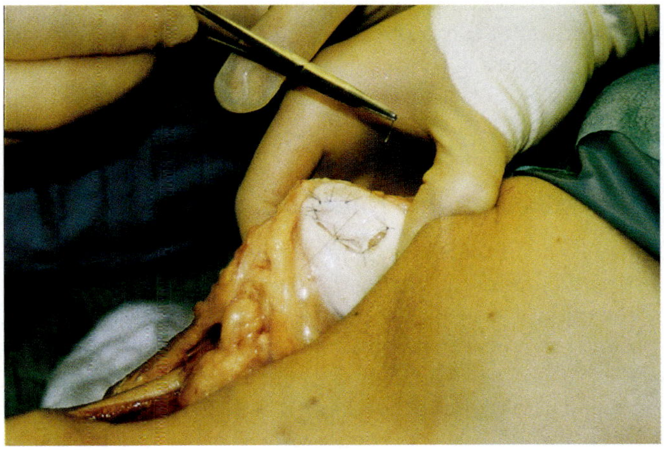

C

Figure 33.4. **A:** Radical excision of lesion. **B:** Use a template for sizing the periosteal flap. **C:** Periosteal flap after suturing to the defect.

tibia, clean the periosteum of fat and fibrous tissue. Avoid making any rifts in the periosteum. Then measure or use the template for sizing of the periosteum. Oversize the periosteal flap by adding 1 to 2 mm to the periphery of the intended flap. Incise the periosteum and use a sharp elevator to remove the periosteal flap, starting distally and going proximally with small movements to avoid rifts in the periosteum. Mark the side of the periosteum to be able to identify the cambium layer. Keep the periosteal flap moist with saline.

Suturing of the Periosteal Flap

The debridement is checked and any debrides remaining are removed. Place the periosteal flap with the cambium layer facing the subchondral bone of the defect. Use 5-0 or 6-0 resorbable sutures and start anchoring the flap with four sutures in each corner. Then place the sutures with 5- to 6-mm intervals and try to place the knot on the vertical edge, minimizing friction. Grasp with the suture at least 5 to 6 mm into normal cartilage. Use fibrin glue to seal the intervals between the sutures. Avoid fibrin glue in the defect adhering the periosteum to the subchondral bone. Wait for 60 seconds for sealing with fibrine glue. Leave an opening in the upper part of the defect for injection (Fig. 33.5). Introduce in this opening a soft catheter with a syringe with saline to check for any leakage by slow injection into the defect. If necessary, add another suture at any leaking spot and recheck. Then aspirate the saline and check with some air in the syringe that there is no fixation of the periosteum to the subchondral bone, closing off the defect.

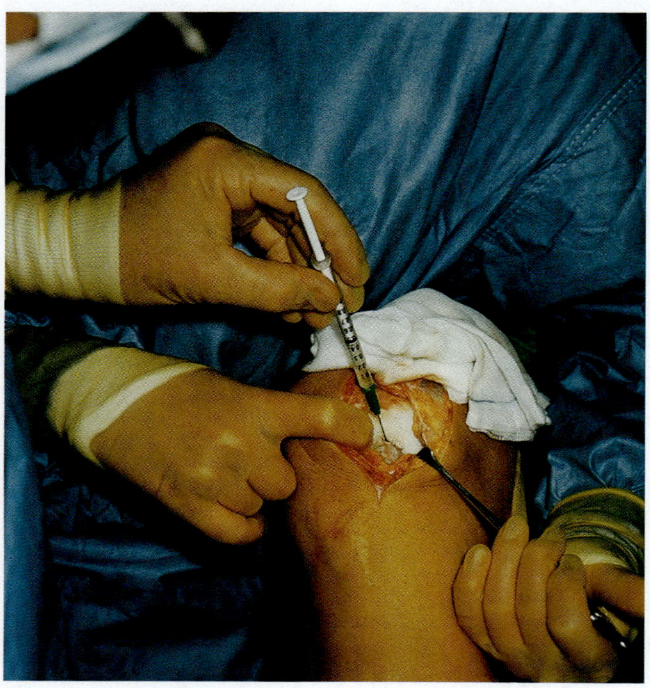

Figure 33.5. Opening for injection of chondrocytes.

Implantation of the Cells

Introduce in the opening at the upper edge of the defect a soft catheter. Place the catheter distal to the defect and gently inject the cells and slowly withdraw the syringe proximally. When the fluid appears in the opening at the injection site, close the injection site with a suture and with fibrin glue to seal off the defect (Fig. 33.5). Then close the joint in separate layers. When needed, use a drainage without suction in the joint.

POSTOPERATIVE TREATMENT

Place a bandage from the foot to over the knee. Six hours after surgery, use a continuous passive motion (CPM) machine with a range of motion of 0 to 40 degrees, and continue CPM as long as it is comfortable for the patient. Prophylactic antibiotics are given for 48 hours. Isometric quadriceps training and range of motion training is started the day after surgery. Mobilization with weight bearing of 30 to 40 pounds for the first 6 weeks is started the day after surgery. Gradually increase the weight bearing until full weight bearing is reached within the following 6 weeks.

Functional training in water could be started when the wound is healed. Bicycling on a stationary bike with low resistance could be started when 90 degrees of knee flexion is achieved. Gradually increase the resistance during bicycling and continue with outdoor bicycling. Skating, rollerblading, or cross-country skiing is a good intermediate rehabilitation before going back to running. Running could be started on an individual basis with short distances on flat surfaces at 6 to 9 months. Return to competitive sports is allowed after individual assessment including arthroscopic evaluation, usually at the earliest at 6 months, depending on the type of sport and the injury.[7]

OTHER SURGICAL CONSIDERATIONS

The ACL-Deficient Knee

If ACL instability is present, the ACL should be reconstructed either at the same time as the chondrocyte transplantation or at the same time as the harvesting is performed, using the arthroscopic technique for ACL reconstruction. The chondrocyte transplantation could probably take place between 3 and 6 months later or when the patient has recovered his knee function.

Varus or Valgus Deformity

Varus deformity with a medial femoral condyle lesion should be evaluated with hip-knee-ankle x-rays and weight-bearing x-rays with extended knees and in 45-degree flexion. High tibial osteotomy is used to correct the varus deformity. In a valgus deformity, if a minor correction of less than 8 degrees is needed, we use a high tibial varus osteotomy. If a major correction of a valgus deformity is needed, a distal femoral osteotomy is recommended. The osteotomy, when needed, could be performed either at the same time as the arthroscopic evaluation and the harvesting of cartilage or at the same time as the autologous transplantation is performed, which I prefer.

COMPLICATIONS

General

No serious general complications have been seen in the first 500 patients. There have been no deep infections, no deep thrombosis, no chronic swelling, and no chronic synovitis.

Local and Periosteal

Local complications with periosteal fibrillation of the fibers left on the periosteum have been seen in fewer than 10% of the patients who have had arthroscopic evaluation. Periosteal fibrillation, when symptomatic, causes crepitations and sometimes swelling. The complication is managed with gentle shaving of the fibrillation (Fig. 33.6).

Hypertrophic Periosteum

Hypertrophic periosteum occurs due to friction at motion. The hypertrophic tissue of the periosteum overlaps from the repair area to the normal cartilage in the direction of motion. On the femur it is always seen anterior or posterior to the defect. This overlapping hypertrophic periosteum gives symptoms such as crepitations or clicking, or in some rare cases catching or locking. Pain and swelling sometimes are present, and have been seen in about 20% of 46 patients who had a second arthroscopy. They are symptomatic in less than 50% of patients (Fig. 33.7). Sometimes there could be a local hypertrophy of the periosteum that has to be debrided down to the level of the surrounding cartilage.

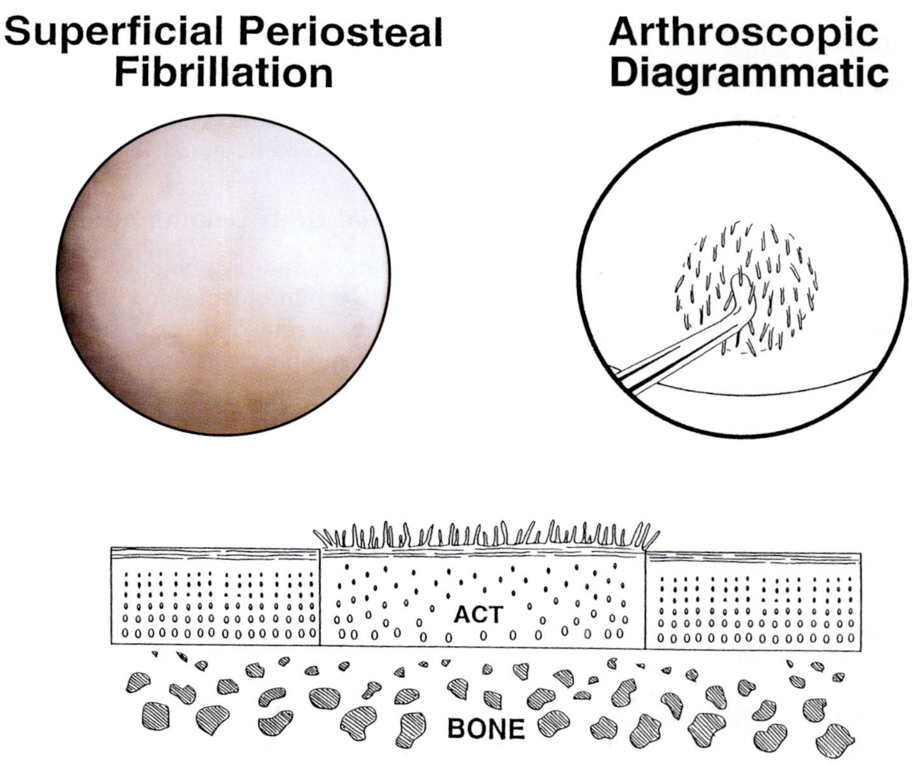

Figure 33.6. Periosteal fibrillation. Arthroscopic insert, showing periosteal fibrillation.

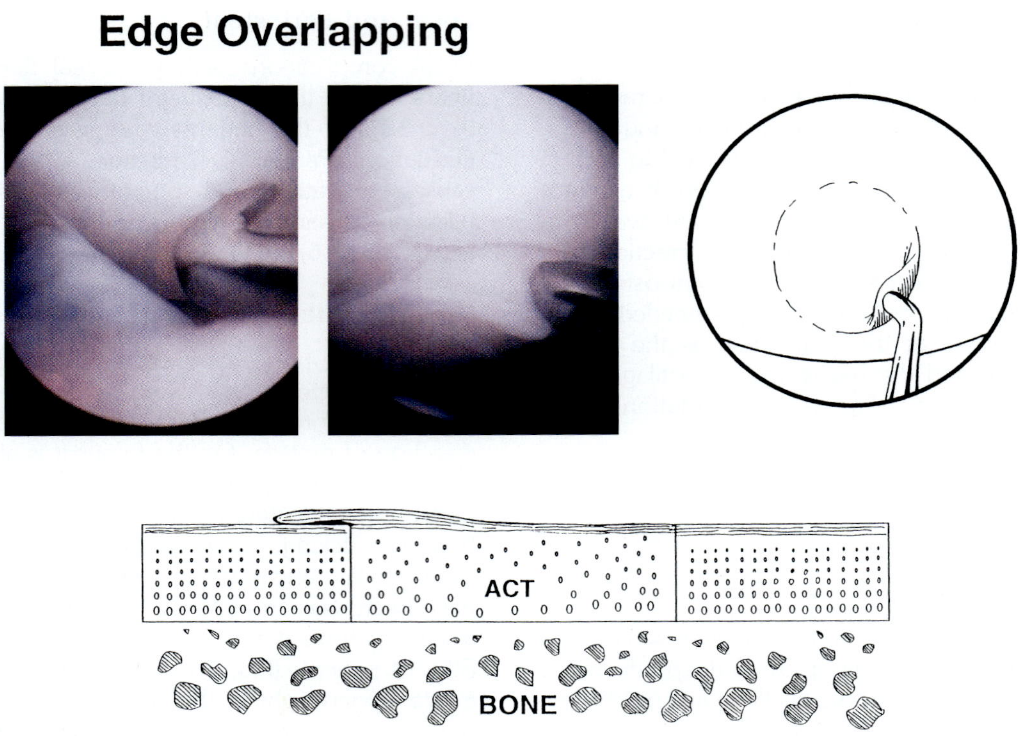

Figure 33.7. Periosteal edge overlapping. Arthroscopic insert to the right. Edge overlapping from repair area to normal surrounding cartilage.

Periosteal Delamination

The periosteum could delaminate from the underlying repair tissue due to friction or to vigorous activity in too early a stage of the repair period. It could either be partial or total (Fig. 33.8).

Partial Delamination

Partial delamination means that less than 50% of the periosteal flap has been delaminated. The patients experience clicking or catching and sometimes pain and swelling. The avulsed flap should be gently debrided, especially if it is a minor delamination.

Total Delamination

Total delamination includes more than 50% of the periosteum and could be attached or detached. If it is detached, it will appear as a loose body and should be extracted arthroscopically. If the periosteum is still attached, it should be removed completely. The underlying repair tissue should be left, as it still has the capacity of filling the defect, which is stimulated by motion to form a new surface. Filling of the defect will continue by repair activity. No long-term negative results have been seen from partial or total delamination.

Graft Delamination

Graft delamination means a loosening of the graft from the subchondral bone and from the surrounding cartilage. It could be either partial or total (Fig. 33.9).

Partial Graft Delamination

A partial graft delamination could be marginal with less than 10 mm of loosening of the graft in the attachment to the surrounding cartilage and the underlying bone. The marginal delamination should be excised and the defect left. If the partial delamination is larger than 10 mm, the graft should be debrided gently and cartilage for retransplantation should be taken. Four patients have had a second transplantation after partial graft delamination.

Total Graft Delamination

A total graft delamination is a serious complication. So far it has been diagnosed in only two cases due to reinjury. In both cases the patients experienced locking, pain, and swelling after an acute distortion of the knee. The delaminated graft should be removed and the patient should be retransplanted with autologous chondrocyte transplantation. The two patients with a total

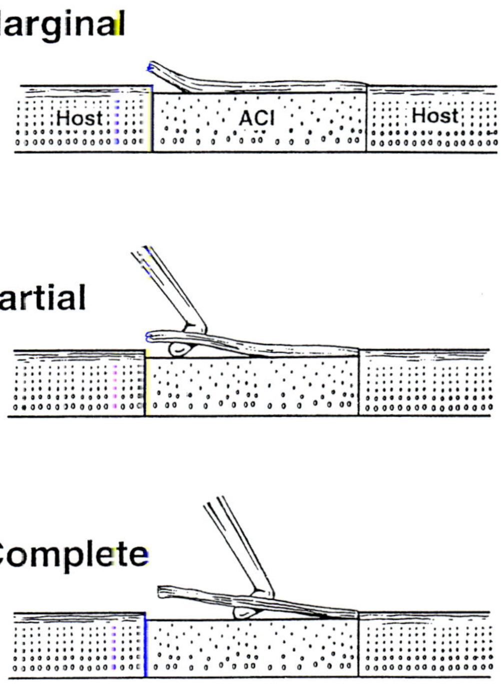

Figure 33.8. Periosteal delamination.

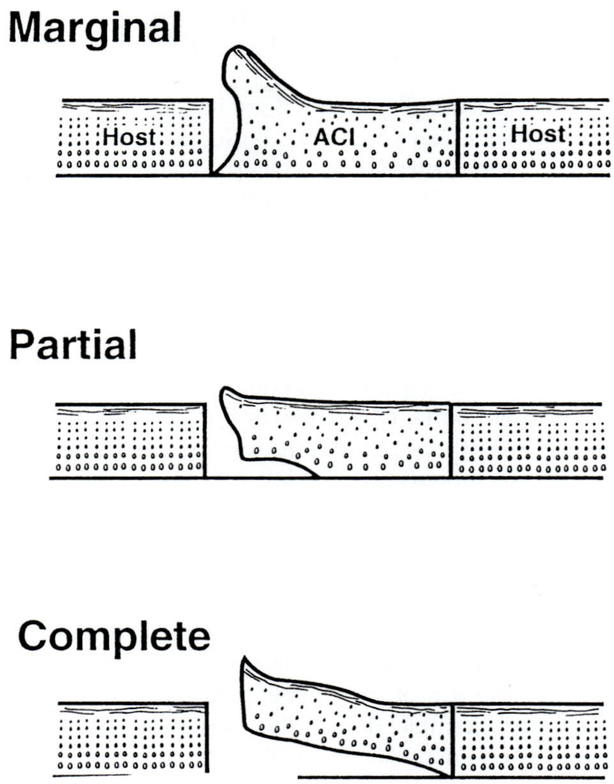

Figure 33.9. Graft delamination.

graft delamination who have been retransplanted have recovered after the second surgery with good results.

Adhesions and Arthrofibrosis

Restricted range of motion has occurred in six patients who have undergone arthroscopic debridement and mobilization. All of the patients have regained full range of motion. In the Cartilage Repair Registry there were adhesions and arthrofibrosis reported in the first 50 patients 2 years postsurgery in 3% and detachment or delamination in 5%.

Reoperations were performed in 7% due to shaving and trimming on the operated area, manipulation and lysis of adhesions in 2.5% and reimplantation in 1%. The total reoperation rate in the Cartilage Repair Registry was about 10%, of which 5% were directly related to the procedure as is in accordance with our reoperation rate.

PITFALLS

Selection of Patients

To avoid pitfalls, it is of utmost importance to keep to the original indications for autologous chondrocyte transplantation. Only grade I articular cartilage injuries on the opposing surface could be allowed for autologous chondrocyte transplantation. Do not transplant kissing lesions with deeper involvement. To start, the surgeon should select simple cases, and there is definitely a learning curve for this procedure.

From our personal experience, of the first five patients operated with this technique, three were failures. Before trying larger defects or more complicated cases with ACL reconstruction, osteotomy, etc., the surgeon should perform at least 10 simple cases. It is very important that the surgeon evaluate and decide the indications from his own arthroscopic examination and not from videotapes of other surgeons. It is very important in the beginning to start with defects located not too far back on the femoral condyle, because of the technical problems with posterior attachment of the periosteal flap on the femoral condyle. If varus or valgus deformity is present, affecting the injured side, osteotomy has to be considered either before or at the same time as transplantation. If ligament insufficiency is present, ligament reconstruction should be performed. Do not use this technique on kissing lesions on the tibia-femoral joint. The opposing articular surface should only have superficial fibrillation (grade I). Osteoarthritis is not an indication.

SURGICAL TECHNIQUE FOR INTRALESIONAL OSTEOPHYTES

Intralesional osteophytes or a bone formation in the subchondral bone can sometimes be found as an effect of repair or more often after drilling, microfracturing, or abrasion arthroplasty. The bony prominence remains after careful debridement of the damaged cartilage and may interfere with the attachment of the periosteal flap. The best management of a prominent osteophyte in the debrided area is to gently tap it down into the subchondral bone to the level of the surrounding subchondral bone. This will avoid bleeding and leave no rough or prominent bone, which may occur after debriding the osteophyte with curettes. Fibrous plugs left after drilling or microfracturing could be left debrided down to the subchondral bone level.

It must be emphasized that any damaged cartilage and fissures extending from the damaged area have to be included in the excised defect. The debridement down to subchondral bone has to be done very gently and carefully to avoid bleeding. Bleeding should be minimized by the use of epinephrine sponges put into the defect, for example during the harvesting of the periosteal flap. Punctual use of fibrin glue for hemostasis or electrocoagulation could be tried to stop the bleeding. The surgeon should try to avoid uncontained lesions initially. In unilateral uncontained lesions, careful suturing to the synovial lining should be performed, if possible, or attachment of the periosteal flap by suturing through small drill holes through the bone for anchoring the periosteum.

REHABILITATION

It is very important for the patient to strictly follow the rehabilitation program. But a fast and aggressive rehabilitation with too early and too heavy a dynamic strength training with resistance could jeopardize the transplanted area and could cause a delamination or hypertrophic overlapping of the periosteum. Too early a return to competitive sports, especially contact sports, impact sports, or cutting sports, should be avoided.

In professional athletes, return to training and competition should be allowed after a clinical evaluation, muscle strengths tests, functional tests, as well as arthroscopic evaluation of the hardness, filling, and attachment of the repair tissue.

SALVAGE PROCEDURES

The salvage procedure in a failure due to delamination of the graft or reinjury or any other graft failure should be reoperation with autologous chondrocyte transplantation as the first choice. If that for some reason is not possible, and the patient is young and the symptoms are serious with reduced function, microfracturing or multiple drilling along with abrasion, arthroplasty could be a salvage procedure. In our experience this should not be performed before a second chondrocyte transplantation has been tried. In older patients, artificial joint replacement may be considered on an individual basis.[10]

For patients requiring total menisectomy combined with varus or valgus deformity, it should include an osteotomy for correction of the weight-bearing center of the joint either before or at the same time as the chondrocyte transplantation.

At present we have no statistics on the importance of total or partial meniscectomy. Further follow-up studies should answer those questions. The use of allograft meniscal transplantation is not indicated, to our knowledge. At present we cannot recommend meniscal allograft in combination with chondrocyte transplantation; we recommend osteotomy in those cases.

CONCLUSION

Autologous chondrocyte transplantation has been performed for more than 10 years in Sweden, and over 500 patients have been operated in Sweden and over 1,500 worldwide. No serious adverse effects or complications have been reported. Adhesions, arthrofibroses, and periosteal complications have been the most common. Most adhesions, arthrofibroses, and periosteal complications can be treated with athroscopic debridement and mobilization technique without any long-term negative effects. There is a 5% reoperation rate. Graft delamination could be managed with reoperation with autologous chondrocyte transplantation. Previous surgery, such as total meniscectomy, abrasion arthroplasty, multiple drilling, and microfracturing, may affect the end result, but sufficient data are not available at present.

No severe general complications have been reported. No intraarticular infections have been diagnosed in over 1,500 patients treated with autologous chondrocyte transplantation. The local complications that have been reported have been low in frequency, and have been possible to treat with arthroscopic procedures, and in the few cases of delamination of the graft, retransplantation with autologous chondrocyte transplantation has been possible with good results so far.

It seems that autologous chondrocyte transplantation from the present experience of over 10 years as the longest follow-up, and with over 1,500 patients operated worldwide, is a safe procedure.

References

1. Mankin HJ. The response of articular cartilage to mechanical injury *J Bone Joint Surg* 1982;64A:460–466.
2. Buckwalter JA, Rosenberg LC, Hunziker EB. Articular cartilage: composition, structure, response to injury and methods of facilitating repair. In: Ewing JW (ed). *Articular Cartilage and Knee Joint Function:* Basic Science and Arthroscopy. New York: Raven Press, 1990:19–56.
3. Chesterman PJ, Smith AU. Homotransplantation of articular cartilage and isolated chondrocytes: an experimental study in rabbits. *J Bone Joint Surg* 1968;50B:184–197.
4. Peterson L, Menche D, Grande D, et al. Chondrocyte transplantation—an experimental model in the rabbit. In: Transactions from the 30th Annual Orthopaedic Research Society, Atlanta, February 1984. Palantine, IL: Orthopaedic Research Society, 1984:284(abst).
5. Brittberg M, Nilsson A, Lindahl A, Ohlsson C, Peterson L. Rabbit articular cartilage defects treated with chondrocytes. *Clin Orthop Rel Res* 1996;326:270–283.
6. Brittberg M, Lindahl A, Ohlsson C, Isaksson O, Peterson L. Treatment of deep cartilage defects in the knee with autologous chondrocyte transplantation. *N Engl J Med* 1994;331:889–895.
7. Minas T, Peterson L. Chondrocyte transplantation. *Oper Tech Orthop* 1997;7(4):323–333.
8. Blevins T, Steadman R, Rodrigo J, Silliman J. Treatment of articular cartilage defects in athletes: an analysis of functional outcome and lesion appearance. *Orthopaedics* 1998;21(7):761–768.

Chapter 34

ARTHROFIBROSIS FOLLOWING KNEE SURGERY (ARTHROSCOPIC/OPEN)

John C. Richmond

Restriction of motion or arthrofibrosis following knee surgery remains a potentially disastrous complication of any knee injury or surgical procedure. Loss of motion has been described as a potential complication of virtually any knee operation from as minor as diagnostic arthroscopy to major ligament or fracture reconstruction.[1–7] Generally, the frequency of arthrofibrosis is correlated to the magnitude of the surgical procedure and the duration, if any, of postoperative immobilization, and inversely correlated to the time between injury and surgery.

Arthrofibrosis can be subdivided into four categories based on the motions that are limited (Table 34.1): (1) Flexion deformity, or lack of extension, is poorly tolerated, with loss of as little as 10 degrees of extension leading to pain, limp, and patellofemoral arthrosis. (2) Extension deformity, or lack of flexion, has been most commonly encountered through the years. Small limitations of flexion (5 to 15 degrees) remain a common sequela of many major knee procedures, and are tolerated well, even in athletes. When flexion is limited to 125 degrees, often the only symptom will be inability to squat. As flexion becomes limited to 110 degrees or less, significant difficulties with activities of daily living result, particularly sitting in confined spaces, going down stairs, or athletic participation. (3) Combined flexion-extension deformity, with loss of both flexion and extension and limitation of patella mobility (patella entrapment), can progress to category 4, which is potentially the most problematic. (4) Patella infera and infrapatella contracture syndrome (IPCS), which was first described by Paulos et al,[2] is an abnormal fibrosclerotic healing response resulting in patella entrapment. It has come to be used for those patients who get a progressive shortening of the patellar tendon leading to a patella infera.[8] This can lead to development of patellofemoral arthrosis over a short period of time (2 to 6 months), if the patient continues to walk with a bent knee gait.[2,4,6]

It is also logical to subdivide arthrofibrosis into the presumed etiology. We can currently identify several potential common etiologies, including mechanical, inflammatory, and biologic. Mechanical causes include immobilization, malpositioned ligament grafts, or displaced tissues (e.g., locked meniscal fragment or misplaced fracture fragment).[9–12] Potential inflammatory causes include infection or inflammatory arthropathies.[13–15] Our preliminary work has identified the abnormal expression of multiple growth factors associated with arthrofibrosis as a possible biologic cause as well as the potential common pathway resulting from mechanical or inflammatory conditions.[16–18]

BIOLOGY OF SCAR

Understanding the biologic mechanism of normal scar formation in response to injury or surgery is important in approaching arthrofibrosis. Normal healing entails a series of successive and interrelated processes including cell migration and proliferation, neovascularization, extracellular matrix deposition, and the proliferation of cells to reconstitute the injured tissue.[19–22] A number of different growth factors regulate these processes. Those growth factors that currently have been identified as playing a role in wound healing are listed in Table 34.2. These growth factors are produced by cells that are adjacent to or migrate to an injury. Their expression is normally highest at the time of active tissue repair and declines upon healing. Mature scar tissue does not normally express these growth factors.[20,23,24]

Table 34.1. Types of arthrofibrosis based on motion limitation and patella mobility

Type	Extension loss (degrees)	Flexion loss (degrees)	Patella mobility
1	>5	None	Normal
2	None	>25	Limited inferior glide
3	>10	>25	Limited in all planes
4	>10	>30	Patella infera

Current research has shown abnormal expression of some of these growth factors in a number of fibroproliferative disorders including fibrous dysplasia, aggressive fibromatosis, palmar fibromatosis (Dupuytren's disease), and arthrofibrosis.[16–18,25–27] Immunohistochemistry also indicates a similarity of these conditions to adhesive capsulitis of the shoulder.[23] In vitro, manipulation with the blocking of platelet-derived growth factor-A (PDGF-A), transforming growth factor-β (TGF-β), and insulin-like growth factor-I (IGF-I) has been shown to inhibit the proliferation fibroblasts in cell cultures from primary arthrofibrosis of the knee.[16–18]

Also of note is the in vitro stimulation of fibroblasts from palmar fibromatosis by cyclic strain.[29] Alman and coworkers[29] have shown that fibroblasts from Dupuytren's disease respond differently to cyclic loading in tissue culture than do normal fibroblasts. There is a significant increase in the proliferation of these abnormal fibroblasts, possibly mediated by PDGF, when they are strained repetitively that is not seen in normal fibroblasts. As noted above, Dupuytren's fibroblasts and those from arthrofibrosis share some abnormal molecular biologic mechanisms. This should alert us to understand that aggressive stretching in some stiff joints, particularly during the inflammatory phase of patella entrapment syndrome, may actually aggravate the scarring.[6]

Healing without scar formation would eliminate arthrofibrosis. This occurs in the fetus, where dermal wound healing occurs more rapidly, with normal dermal architecture and without scar. In response to a wound,

Table 34.2. Growth factors involved in wound healing

Platelet-derived growth factors	PDGF-A
	PDGF-β
Transforming growth factors	TGF-α
	TGF-β
Insulin-like growth factors	IGF-I
	IGF-II
Acidic fibroblast growth factor	aFGF
Basic fibroblast growth factor	bFGF
Epidermal growth factor	EGF

adult fibroblasts produce a large amount of collagen aligned in parallel bundles, which are laid down perpendicular to the epidermis. This is the pattern that makes a scar. Fetal fibroblasts also respond to a wound by migration, proliferation, and collagen production. Fetal fibroblasts, however, produce collagen in a pattern that is indistinguishable from the reticular pattern of normal skin. This appears to be an intrinsic property of the fetal fibroblast that is associated with a differential expression of the collagen I gene.[30] The potential manipulation of growth factors or gene expression in the future may allow us to prevent or more easily treat the problems of arthrofibrosis.

PREVENTION OF ARTHROFIBROSIS

While prevention of arthrofibrosis at present is beyond our skills, we must strive to minimize the frequency and severity of this devastating complication. Although the details of reducing arthrofibrosis following each specific procedure are covered in those individual chapters, there are important generalities to discuss here, including reducing mechanical limitations to motion while optimizing the timing of surgery, and rehabilitation.

Mechanical Issues

Virtually every series on the treatment of arthrofibrosis identifies anterior cruciate ligament (ACL) reconstruction as the most frequent cause of arthrofibrosis.[1–7] While primary (or biologically induced) arthrofibrosis may result from ACL reconstruction, more commonly it results from a mechanical problem.[31–35] Often this is a suboptional graft position or excessive tensioning of a nonanatomic graft (Fig. 34.1). The more common positioning errors are (1) anterior placement of the tibial drill hole leading to notch impingement; and (2) femoral drill hole placement that is too anterior, resulting in a short overall intraarticular graft. There is an interplay between ACL graft placement and tensioning technique. Several authors feel that the optimal technique for tensioning patellar tendon grafts, to obtain reproducibly stable knees, with full range of motion (ROM), is to apply high initial tensions to the graft with the knee at full extension.[36,37] This will ensure that full extension is not limited by the graft. If any other technique for tensioning is used, then the surgeon must be able to obtain full passive extension of the knee intraoperatively.

Limiting extension early on following ACL reconstruction may lead to the proliferation of a fibrovascular nodule of scar anterior to the graft or "cyclops" nodule.[31] This scar may result from organization of the hematoma anterior to the graft and can be substantially reduced in incidence by promoting early full extension

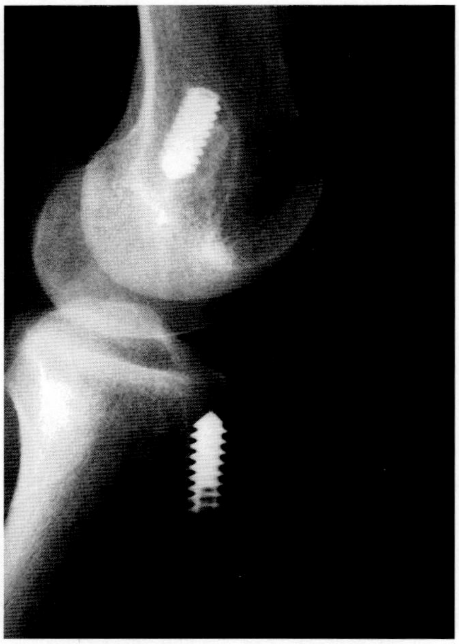

Figure 34.1. Lateral view of a misplaced ACL graft. This excessively anterior position will often result in limited motion of the knee both in extension and flexion.

of the knee (including normal hyperextension) in the immediate postoperative period.

Immobilization is no longer used following ACL reconstruction, but continues to be part of the postsurgical protocols for other procedures. As in ACL reconstruction, immobilization following other surgical procedures leads to an increased risk of arthrofibrosis when compared with early mobilization. This has been noted in many procedures including patellar realignment, posterior cruciate ligament reconstruction, repair of tibial spine fractures, meniscal repair, and complex multiligament reconstruction following knee dislocation.[9–12,38–43] While immobilization for short periods does offer protection to various structures from undue stress, longer periods of immobilization are associated with a myriad of deleterious effects, including stiffness, loss of strength of ligaments, and articular surface damage.[44–46] One must be cognizant of the potential of harm from immobilization when considering its use.

Continuous passive motion (CPM) has been suggested as a means to reduce the risk of arthrofibrosis following surgery. Its use has been studied for several different procedures, and although of significant benefit in some cases, it is not universally helpful. CPM has been of most benefit following total knee arthroplasty where the risk of arthrofibrosis requiring manipulation can be substantially reduced by its use (from 10% to 0% in one study).[47] CPM after patella realignment has also reduced the risk of arthrofibrosis.[38] Many studies on the use of CPM following arthroscopically assisted ACL reconstruction have shown no improvement in motion when CPM is used.[48–51]

Inadvertent limitation of motion may result from quadriceps weakness and an extensor lag. This is intertwined with the issues of timing of surgery, following injury. If a patient cannot actively fully extend his/her knee preoperatively, the risk of limitation of extension postsurgery is increased.

Future mechanical means to reduce adhesions may involve the use of hyaluronic acid products as either a film or a gel that could act as a barrier to block adhesion formation. Hyaluronic acid films have been proven to reduce intraabdominal adhesions following bowel surgery.[52,53] In unpublished work, we demonstrated in a rabbit knee model that hyaluronic acid films can reduce the number and density of adhesions that form following synovectomy. The use of hyaluronic acid products in high-risk surgical procedures on the knee may, in the future, reduce the chance of arthrofibrosis.

Inflammatory Issues

We are limited in our ability to change the inflammatory response that may lead to arthrofibrosis following most surgical procedures. Although there may be an inflammatory component to the issue of early surgery following injury, this subject is covered under timing issues (see below). The expansion of arthroscopic techniques over the past two decades has significantly reduced the need for knee arthrotomies. There has been a steady evolution of rehabilitation techniques during this same period. The performance of a given procedure arthroscopically should reduce the risk of limitation of motion compared to open techniques. This is highlighted when one looks at synovectomy for inflammatory synovitis where the rates of lost motion following open synovectomy range from 30% to 60% and only 1% to 5% following arthroscopic synovectomy.[13–15]

The pharmacologic methods for reducing inflammation postsurgery are somewhat limited and have not been shown to effect the risk of significant fibroarthrosis. The perioperative use of nonsteroidal antiinflammatory drugs (NSAIDs) has been associated with decreased postoperative narcotic analgesics usage as well as increased early motion (up to 3 weeks postsurgery).[54,55] Oral corticosteroids have also been demonstrated to reduce the demand for postoperative analgesics and speed the recovery from a number of arthroscopic procedures.[56,57] Since most surgical procedures have a relatively low risk of arthrofibrosis and there are significant potential risks related to oral corticosteroids (e.g., gastrointestinal ulceration and osteonecrosis), the routine perioperative use of oral corticosteroids is not encouraged. The carefully considered use of oral corticosteroids can be entertained in those situations where there is a high risk postoperative of arthrofibrosis (see Treatment, below).[6]

The intraarticular use of corticosteroids at the time of surgery has been associated with a significant increase in the risk of septic arthritis.[58] Although intraarticular corticosteroids offer a potential means of reducing postoperative arthrofibrosis, this risk of sepsis probably precludes the routine use of intraarticular corticosteroids at the time of surgery, except in very high risk procedures.

Cryotherapy has also been proposed as a means of reducing postoperative inflammation, pain, and swelling. Although results of several studies have been contradictory, cold therapy may reduce swelling and pain for several days postsurgery. There is no evidence to indicate that there is a long-term reduction in the risk of postsurgical arthrofibrosis.[59–62]

For unclear reasons, there is an increased risk of arthrofibrosis following ACL/medial collateral ligament (MCL) injury treated with early ACL reconstruction and repair of the MCL tear when the MCL tear is proximal.[63] This may be due to mechanical issues associated with repair of the MCL proximal to the joint knee, but may also relate to local inflammatory factors.

Timing Issues

Most reports on the issues of timing of surgery and arthrofibrosis have dealt with ACL injuries. A number of factors have contributed to this, including the feeling from the 1980s that there was a "golden period" of 2 weeks following ACL tear for optimal results with reconstruction. Shelbourne et al[64] and Mohtadi et al[65] in 1991 were the first to focus on the issues of timing of early ACL reconstruction and the risk of arthrofibrosis. They noted the association of earlier surgery and a high risk of motion problems. Delaying surgery until motion has recovered, until quadriceps control of the leg allows full active extension, and until the acute hemarthrosis has resolved significantly reduces the risk of postoperative arthrofibrosis requiring arthroscopy and/or manipulations.[66] While it is possible to achieve excellent results with surgery within the first 3 weeks following injury, if aggressive rehabilitation protocols are used, it is at a cost of 6% of patients requiring additional surgical procedures to regain motion.[67]

Timing of surgery, return of motion preoperatively, and the risk of motion limitations have been particularly problematic in the patient with an ACL tear and a locked bucket-handle meniscal tear. A three-stage approach with early meniscal repair, followed by rehabilitation to regain full motion, and then delayed ACL reconstruction has been very helpful in reducing the risk of arthrofibrosis.[11]

There are certain injuries such as knee dislocations and intraarticular fractures for which early surgical treatment is favored. In these cases, both the timing and the magnitude of the procedure can contribute to a high rate of stiffness requiring manipulation. The rate of manipulation following early treatment of knee dislocation, even with early protected mobilization, was greater than 50% in two recent series.[41,42] Unfortunately, to delay these procedures to improve motion will significantly compromise long-term stability and function. In Noyes and Barber-Westin's[42] series, only 25% of patients with late reconstructions could return to sports without symptoms, while more than 70% of acute reconstructions had no limitations at sport. The surgeon should anticipate this risk of stiffness and be prepared for early manipulation and/or arthroscopic arthrolysis.

TREATMENT

While prevention of arthrofibrosis is our goal, it is at present not fully attainable. Our current best treatment of arthrofibrosis is early recognition and aggressive treatment with the hope of preventing the joint surface arthrosis that can develop quickly in the patellofemoral joint with IPCS.[4,6,8] It is important that the orthopedic surgeons and physical therapists treating the knee recognize, early on, those patients not progressing appropriately with motion following injury or surgery.

Radiographs should be obtained when motion problems are recognized, to identify any mechanical impediment that needs correction to regain motion. These mechanical problems are most often the suboptimal placement of graft tunnels or hardware in ACL reconstructions (Fig. 34.1). Bony blocks to motion may also occur in malreduced fractures.[10] While it is difficult to confront the issue that an ACL tunnel location is the cause of limitation of motion, it is imperative that early treatment be undertaken to prevent patellofemoral arthrosis. It is better for the long-term health of the knee to perform an early removal of a misplaced ACL graft, allow the patient to regain full motion, and then perform an anatomically correct reconstruction, than it is to struggle with physical therapy and casting when this is doomed to fail.

Paulos et al[2,6] were among the first to recognize the early inflammatory stage that can be a sign of primary arthrofibrosis that will go on to IPCS. This may present as a knee that is hot and swollen in the region of the patellar tendon and fat pad. Early limitation of patella mobility, particularly superior glide, is often present. These patients have limitation of both flexion and extension, and although the scarring may be secondary to a mechanical factor, this may also be the beginning of primary arthrofibrosis, which can be particularly hard to treat. Although there has been no scientific study to confirm it, we have noted this to be more common in patients who are redheads and have fair complexion, particularly those who are keloid formers. We have been able to successfully treat this early inflammatory phase in some patients with a short course of high-dose oral corticosteriods or less commonly NSAIDs.[6] Overly aggressive stretching in this inflammatory stage seems to aggravate the inflammatory response in most patients (see Biology of Scar, above). Gentle nonforceful mobilization done actively by the patient is appropriate.[6,29]

Various authors have recognized many different patterns of arthrofibrosis.[1–3,6,8,31,33,68,69] While there are numerous classifications that have been proposed, a simple four-class schema based on motion limitation and patella mobility (Table 34.1) includes the information necessary to plan treatment, nonoperative or surgical. Our treatment algorithm is given in Fig. 34.2. It is applicable to arthrofibrosis types 1 to 3, but not to type 4, after the development of patella infera. The surgery performed depends on the type of arthrofibrosis, as outlined below.

If a patient does not come to full extension equal to the other knee (including physiologic hyperextension) early on after injury or surgery, then scar may form anterior in the notch or between the fat pad and the notch.[31,33] This is particularly so with ACL reconstructions but not limited to ACL surgery. This is type 1 arthrofibrosis. Once imaging studies have eliminated a mechanical cause, then treatment should be instituted. When recognized within the first few months after the index injury or procedure, mechanical stretching may alleviate the problem. Among the techniques that can be employed are dynamic extension splints, dropout casts, extension boards (Fig. 34.3), and serial extension casting. Serial extension casting must be employed cautiously due to the risk of articular surface damage from both immobilization and the pressure of forced extension, and casts should be changed at least every other day. By 4 months from the index procedure, these techniques are likely to be of limited value due to the maturity of the scar tissue, and surgical treatment is advised. Also, if there is a lack of progress at any time using these mechanical means, then early surgery is indicated.

The surgical treatment of arthrofibrosis is directed at removing any mechanical impediment to motion, removing significant areas of scarring, and restoring normal patella mobility and location. The extent of the surgery as well as the postoperative rehabilitation vary greatly from type 1 to type 4.

In type 1 arthrofibrosis, the arthroscopic treatment has proven quite successful. Flexion deformities of as little as 5 to 8 degrees can cause symptoms of limp or anterior knee pain. As limitations approach 10 degrees or more, the likelihood of symptoms increases. Surgery is indicated for any patient with anterior knee pain or flexion deformity $\geq$10 degrees. The arthroscopic findings are typically scarring anterior in the notch, or between the fat pad and the notch or anterior tibia. The "cyclops syndrome" described by Jackson and Schaefer[31] represents a variant of these findings following ACL reconstruction, where a nodule of scar is pedun-

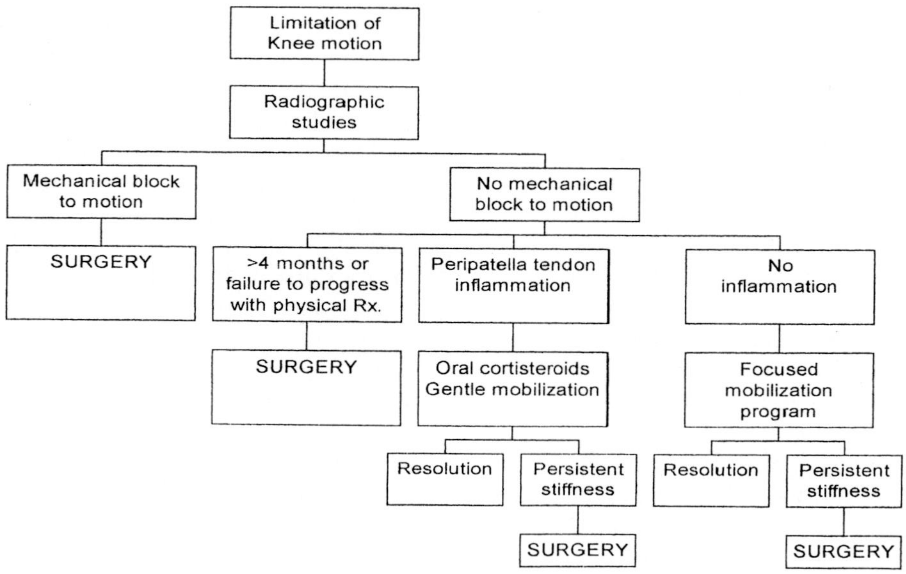

Figure 34.2. Algorithm for management of arthrofibrosis.

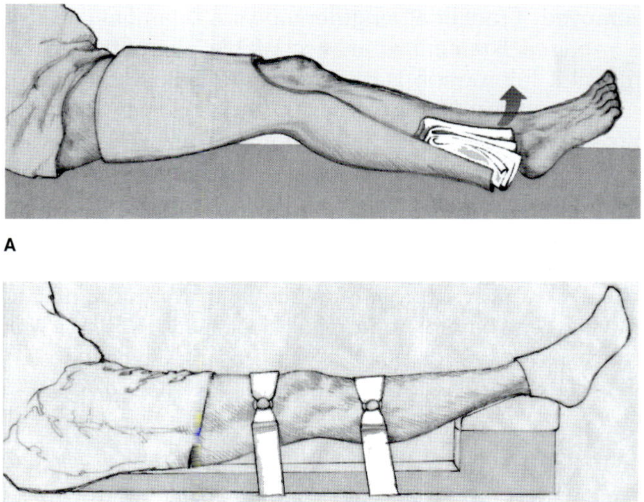

A

B

Figure 34.3. Dropout casts **(A)** or extension boards **(B)** may be used to gain extension early on, following injury or surgery.

culated and may cause mechanical type symptoms of clunking. At surgery, one must be careful to expand the notchplasty if an impinging ACL graft is identified. Multiple adhesions are rarely encountered in the suprapatella pouch in type 1 arthrofibrosis, but must be removed if seen.[6] These bands can limit the proximal excursion of the quadriceps muscle and inhibit the patient from regaining active extension postsurgery. If full extension is not reached intraoperatively by removing intraarticular scar, then any extrasynovial scar anterior to the tibia must be removed. This can be done arthroscopically or through a small open incision.[6,33]

Following surgery for type 1 arthrofibrosis, the patient can be managed as an outpatient or in a short-stay unit. Early full passive extension must be maintained for the first 7 to 10 days postoperatively. This can be accomplished by bracing and daily physical therapy. If CPM is used, one has to be very careful that full extension (including physiologic hyperextension) is attained in the machine in order to prevent notch scarring from recurring. In those patients for whom full extension is difficult at the end of surgery, casting in maximum extension for 24 to 48 hours, followed by physical therapy and the use of mechanical stretching devices (stretching board, dynamic splint, drop-out cast) is of benefit. Rarely will surgical release of posterior capsular structures be required.[4,6,8,33]

Type 2 arthrofibrosis, where only flexion is limited, usually results from immobilization in extension and is associated with suprapatella scarring. It can also occur when the quadriceps mechanism is scarred extraarticularly to the femur. The patella is not entrapped and only limited in inferior excursion. This is rare following ACL reconstruction with current early motion protocols. If not responsive to physical therapy, then surgical treatment is indicated. While some authors have recommended manipulation under anesthesia for this condition,[70] we favor arthroscopic lysis and resection of adhesions prior to manipulation, particularly in cases occurring 4 months or more after the index procedure. By this time any adhesion that has formed to an articular cartilage surface may be strong enough to avulse hyaline cartilage.[44,45]

Type 2 arthrofibrosis should be surgically treated via the arthroscope. The findings at surgery are a suprapatella pouch filled with multiple adhesions. Rarely is the pouch obliterated by scar. All visible scar should be resected.[1,3,4] While motorized shavers have been the traditional means for doing this, the newer radiofrequency electrocautery devices work well and are hemostatic. A blunt obturator or curved ¼-inch osteotome can be used to free the distal quadriceps from the femoral shaft at the completion of the arthroscopy. This helps to restore the normal volume of the suprapatella pouch.[4] Manipulation into full flexion completes the procedure. If a tourniquet has been utilized, it should be deflated prior to manipulation.

As opposed to type 1 arthrofibrosis, where CPM and postoperative drains are rarely necessary, they are important in the surgical treatment of extension contractures. Depending on the volume of drainage encountered, the drains can be removed early (after a few hours) or maintained for 24 to 48 hours. CPM machines should be set for maximum tolerated ranges (both flexion and extension).[4,6] Pain management can be an issue postoperatively with any type of arthrofibrosis and femoral nerve blocks help significantly in the perioperative period.

Types 3 and 4 arthrofibrosis are the spectrum of patella entrapment syndrome (PES) extending to IPCS.[2,4,6,8,33] Aggressive stretching through physical therapy or manipulation under anesthesia are contraindicated. This is particularly so when the peripatella region and fat pad are actively inflamed and hot. Forceful stretching only worsens the problem. Only when the inflammatory phase has resolved through time or with oral corticosteroids, and the patient has good quadriceps control, should surgery be performed.[6] Type 3 arthrofibrosis is differentiated from type 4 by the presence of patella infera in type 4. Noyes et al[8] have demonstrated that there is a wide normal variation between individuals in the ratio of patellar tendon to patella height (range 0.75 to 1.46), but virtually no variation from the left to right sides in the same person. Left to right flexed knee comparison radiographs of the patellar tendon length are indicated to identify patella infera.[8] For those patients with more than 8 mm of shortening of the patellar tendon, a DeLee-type tibial tubercle osteotomy (Fig. 34.4) will be necessary to restore the patella toward its normal location.[2,6]

Open or arthroscopic surgical techniques can be employed in the release of types 3 and 4 arthrofibrosis, depending on the comfort and skill of the surgeon.[1–8,33] In either case, all intraarticular adhesions must be resected, lateral and medial releases performed, and all scar between the patella and the anterior tibial plateaus removed. The retropatellar tendon bursa should be freed and the patellar tendon released to the level of its insertion on the tibial tubercle. Any mechanical block to motion, particularly a malpositioned ACL graft, must be removed. Fractional lengthening of a ligament graft or a repaired ligament is an acceptable alternative to removal if full motion is obtained on the operating table.

The arthroscopic treatment of types 3 and 4 arthrofibrosis requires a systematic approach whereby a working area is established bluntly, intercondylar notch and fat pad scarring removed, and the gutters and suprapatella pouch cleared. The patella and quadriceps mechanisms are then freed by lateral and medial releases, blunt elevation of the quadriceps from the anterior, medial, and lateral femoral surfaces, and lysis of the retropatellar tendon bursa. The notch should be assessed if the location or impingement of an ACL graft is in

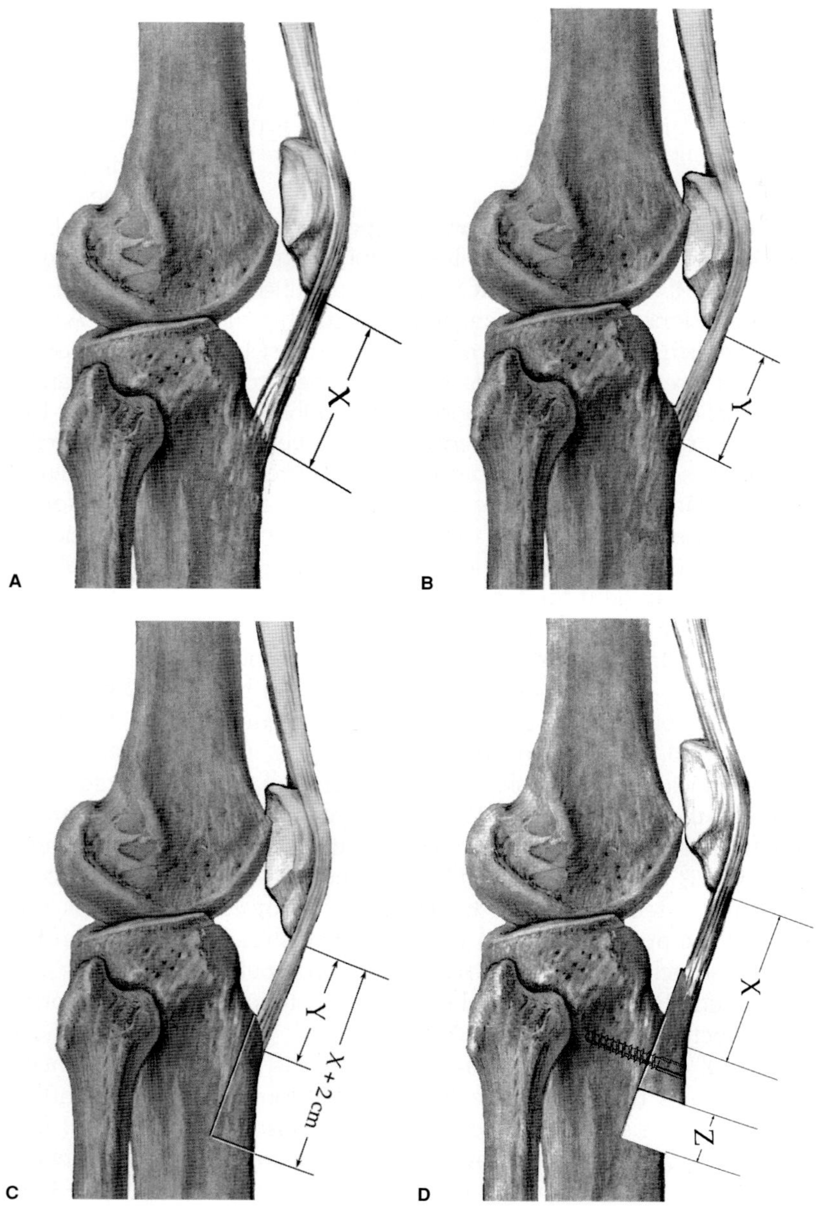

Figure 34.4. Technique for DeLee osteotomy. **A:** The normal patellar tendon length (X) measured from the noninjured knee. **B:** The length of the shortened patellar tendon (Y) is measured. **C:** The overall length of the short patellar tendon plus osteotomy should be 2 cm longer than the normal tendon. This will allow 2 cm of bone contact after the slide. The angle of the osteotomy should be 30 to 40 degrees from the long axis of the tibia. **D:** Osteotomy completed and proximally moved tibial tubercle is internally fixed with a screw.

question. Notchplasty followed by partial release or resection of the ACL graft is performed if full extension cannot be obtained.[4]

While extracapsular bands from the patella to the femur have been described, the blind release of the quadriceps from the femur in conjunction with the lateral release has been adequate to treat these if present, without specifically exposing them (Fig. 34.5).[1,4]

The DeLee-type tibial tubercle slide osteotomy will restore a patella infera to its normal location, but will not restore normal function to the patellofemoral articulation, which often remains painful for the long term.[4,6] This is probably due to both the articular surface damage and the markedly shortened patellar tendon, which has little or no flexibility. Even with bone grafting of the defect, patients who resume high activity levels after this osteotomy are prone to stress fractures at the point the tubercle was advanced from (Fig. 34.6).

Postoperative care includes draining the knee and early motion, including CPM. Cryotherapy should be utilized. Femoral nerve blocks can be a valuable adjunct for pain control in the first 48 hours postsurgery. Patella mobilization as well as electrical stimulation to regain quadriceps control are helpful adjuncts to maintain motion. If serial casting is utilized to gain extension, the casts should be changed at least daily and mobilization of the patella and flexion performed with a physical therapist.[33] If warmth develops in the anterior knee, a 3- to 4-week tapered course of high-dose oral corticosteroids is indicated.[6]

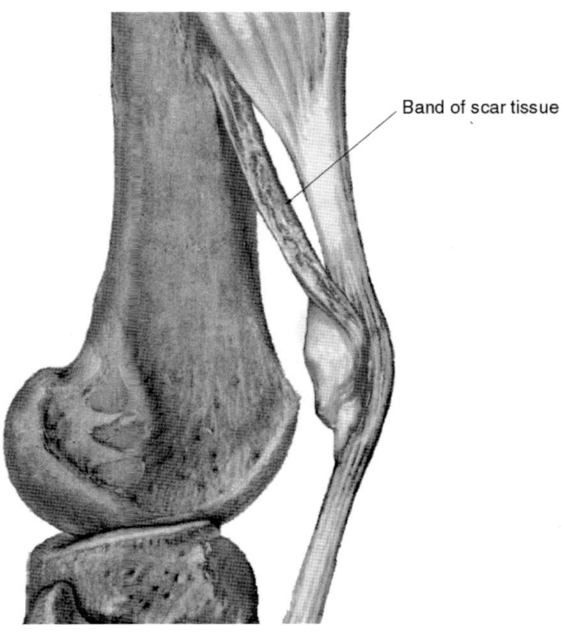

Figure 34.5. Extracapsular band from lateral patella to anterolateral femur.

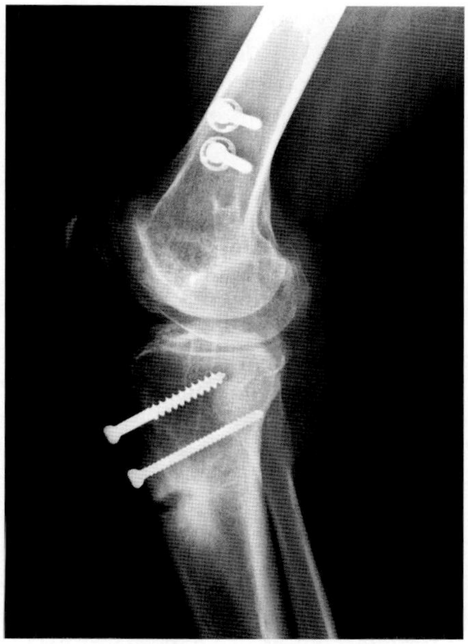

Figure 34.6. Marked stress reaction around site of tubercle slide in an aggressive athlete who went back to running sports 6 months after a DeLee osteotomy.

Results

Most series report return of normal or near-normal range of motion and long-term function following the treatment of types 1 or 2 arthrofibrosis. The results of treatment of the syndrome of patella entrapment to infrapatellar contraction are far less satisfactory.[1–8,31,33] Patients with patella entrapment without patella infera can be expected to gain substantial motion both in flexion (average ~ 30 degrees) and extension (average ~14 degrees). The recovery of function is less predictable, often necessitating reduction in athletic activity. Patellofemoral pain and crepitance are frequent. Those patients who have patella infera rarely resume normal function, in spite of gains in motion similar to those in patients with less severe patella entrapment.

CONCLUSION

Significant reduction in the frequency of arthrofibrosis following knee injury and surgery has occurred by recognition of the contribution of the timing of surgery following injury and the use of postsurgical rehabilitation protocols that promote knee motion and patella mobility.[1–8,31–35] Early recognition of developing mobility problems is key to reducing the risk of chronic limitation of mobility, articular surface damage, and decreased function. All physicians and physical therapists involved in the treatment of the knee must be aware of arthrofibrosis and recognize motion problems. The type of arthrofibrosis should be identified and treatment instituted. If an inflammatory stage of patella entrapment is recognized, mechanical treatment should not be aggressive, and oral corticosteroid use may be an important adjunct to reduce inflammation prior to surgical treatment.[6]

While nonoperative treatment is indicated early on (before 4 months) after the index injury or surgery, the surgical treatment should not be delayed if progress is not being made or a mechanical block is identified. The surgical treatment, open or arthroscopic, is based on removing intraarticular adhesions, releasing extraarticular scar, eliminating mechanical blocks to motion, and restoring both patella mobility and position. Failure to accomplish any of these will lead to persistent motion limitation and the risk of articular surface damage. Postsurgical rehabilitation protocols need to maintain early motion and patella mobility while encouraging return of quadriceps function. CPM use can be important in maintaining flexion gained at arthrolysis.

Future directions in the prevention and treatment of arthrofibrosis may include identification of the molecular biologic mechanisms at the origin of excessive scar.[16–18,29,30] Blocking these pathways in high-risk patients has the promise of further reduction in the rates of arthrofibrosis following knee injury and surgery. Mechanical means using hyaluronic acid gels or films to limit adhesions may also have promise in the prevention and treatment of arthrofibrosis.[52,53]

References

1. Sprague NJ, III, O'Connor RL, Fox JM. Arthroscopic treatment of postoperative knee fibroarthrosis. *Clin Orthop Rel Res* 1982;166:165–172.
2. Paulos LE, Rosenberg TD, Drawbert J, et al. Infrapatellar contracture syndrome. An unrecognized cause of knee stiffness with patella entrapment and patella infera. *Am J Sports Med* 1987;15(4):331–341.
3. Parisien JS. The role of arthroscopy in the treatment of postoperative fibroarthrosis of the knee joint. *Clin Orthop Rel Res* 1988;229:185–192.
4. Richmond JC, Assal MA. Arthroscopic management of arthrofibrosis of the knee, including infrapatellar contraction syndrome. *Arthroscopy* 1991;7(2):144–147.
5. Cosgarea AJ, DeHaven KE, Lovelock JE. The surgical treatment of arthrofibrosis of the knee. *Am J Sports Med* 1994;22(2):184–191.
6. Paulos LE, Wnorowski DC, Greenwald AE. Infrapatellar contracture syndrome diagnosis, treatment, and long-term follow-up. *Am J Sports Med* 1994;22(4):440–449.
7. Klein W, Shah N, Gasse A. Arthroscopic management of postoperative arthrofibrosis of the knee joint: indication, technique, and results. *Arthroscopy* 1994;10(6):591–597.
8. Noyes FR, Wojtys EM, Marshall MT. The early diagnosis and treatment of developmental patella infera syndrome. *Clin Orthop Rel Res* 1991;265:241–252.
9. Harner CD, Irrgang JJ, Paul J, et al. Loss of motion after anterior cruciate ligament reconstruction. *Am J Sports Med* 1992;20(5):499–506.
10. Berg EE. Comminuted tibial eminence anterior cruciate ligament avulsion fractures. Failure of arthroscopic treatment. *Arthroscopy* 1993;9(4):446–450.
11. Shelbourne KD, Johnson GE. Locked bucket-handle meniscal tears in knees with chronic anterior cruciate ligament deficiency. *Am J Sports Med* 1993;21(6):779–782.
12. Graf BK, Ott JW, Lange RH, et al. Risk factors for restricted motion after anterior cruciate reconstruction. *Orthopedics* 1994;17(10):909–912.
13. Smiley P, Wasilewski SA. Arthroscopic synovectomy. *Arthroscopy* 1990;6(1):18–23.
14. Ogilvie-Harris DJ, Basinski A. Arthroscopic synovectomy of the knee for rheumatoid arthritis. *Arthroscopy* 1991;7(1):91–97.
15. Klein W, Jensen K. Arthroscopic synovectomy of the knee joint: indication, technique, and follow-up results. *Arthroscopy* 1988;4(2):63–71.
16. Richmond JC, Alman BA, Pojerski M. Growth factor expression in arthrofibrosis. *Arthroscopy* 1996;12(3):352–353.
17. von Deck MD, Richmond JC, Alman BA. Arthrofibrosis: a potential treatment based on growth factor manipulation. *Arthroscopy* 1997;13(3):393–394.
18. Richmond JC, Alman BA, von Deck MD. Growth factor expression in arthrofibrosis: a review and preliminary study. Unpublished paper.
19. Grotendorst GR, Grotendorst CA, Gilman T. Production of growth factors (PDGF and TGF-β) at the site of tissue repair. *Prog Clin Biol Res* 1988;266:47–54.
20. Steefnos H, Lossing C, Hansson HA. Immunohistochemical demonstration of endogenous growth factors in wound healing. *Wounds* 1990;2:218–226.
21. Antoniades HN, Galanopoulos T, Neville-Golden J, et al. Injury induces in vivo expression of PDGF and PDGF-receptor mRNAs in skin epithelial cells and PDGF mRNA in connective tissue fibroblasts. *Proc Natl Acad Sci USA* 1991;88:565–569.
22. Antoniades HN, Galanopoulos T, Neville-Golden J, et al. Expression of growth factor and receptor mRNAs in skin epithelial cells following acute cutaneous injury. *Am J Pathol* 1993;142:1099–1110.
23. Ross R, Raines EW, Bowen-Pope DF. The biology of platelet derived growth factor. *Cell* 1986;46:155–169.

24. Whitby DJ, Ferguson MWJ. Immunohistochemical localization of growth factors in fetal wound healing. *Dev Biol* 1991;147:207–215.

25. Alman BA, Goldberg MJ, Nabor SP, et al. Aggressive fibromatosis. *J Pediatr Orthop* 1992;12:1–10.

26. Alman BA, Nabor SP, Terek RM, et al. Platelet derived growth factor in fibrous musculoskeletal disorders: a study of pathologic tissue sections and primary cell cultures. *J Orthop Res* 1995;13:66–77.

27. Terek RM, Jiranek WA, Goldberg MJ, et al. The expression of platelet-derived growth-factor gene in Dupuytren contracture. *J Bone Joint Surg* 1995;77A(1):1–9.

28. Bunker TD, Anthony PP. The pathology of frozen shoulder. A Dupuytren-like disease. *J Bone Joint Surg* 1995; 77B(5):577–583.

29. Alman BA, Greel DA, Ruby LK, et al. Regulation of proliferation and platelet-derived growth factor expression in palmar fibromatosis (Dupuytren contracture) by mechanical strain. *J Orthop Res* 1996;14(5):722–728.

30. Gallivan K, Alman BA, Moriarty KP, et al. Differential collagen I gene expression in fetal fibroblasts. *J Pediatr Surg* 1997;32(7):1033–1036.

31. Jackson DW, Schaefer RK. Cyclops syndrome: loss of extension following intraarticular cruciate ligament reconstruction. *Arthroscopy* 1990;6(3):171–178.

32. Fisher SE, Shelbourne KD. Arthroscopic treatment of symptomatic extension block complicating anterior cruciate ligament reconstruction. *Am J Sports Med* 1993; 21(4):558–564.

33. Shelbourne KD, Johnson GE. Outpatient surgical management of arthrofibrosis after anterior cruciate ligament surgery. *Am J Sports Med* 1994;22(2):192–197.

34. Lane JG, Daniel DM, Stone ML. Graft impingement after anterior cruciate ligament reconstruction. Presentation as an active extension "thunk." *Am J Sports Med* 1994; 22(3) 415–417.

35. Reider B, Belniak RM, Preiskorn DO. Arthroscopic arthrolysis for flexion contracture following intra-articular reconstruction of the anterior cruciate ligament. *Arthroscopy* 1996;12(2):165–173.

36. Bach BR, Jones GT, Sweet FA, et al. Arthroscopy-assisted anterior cruciate ligament reconstruction using patellar tendon substitution. Two- to four-year follow-up results. *Am J Sports Med* 1994;22(6):758–767.

37. Nabors ED, Richmond JC, Vannah WM, et al. Anterior cruciate ligament graft tensioning in full extension. *Am J Sports Med* 1995;23(4):488–492.

38. Fulkerson JP, Becker GJ, Meaney JA, et al. Anteromedial tibial tubercle transfer without bone graft. *Am J Sports Med* 1990;18(5):490–497.

39. Austin KS, Sherman OH. Complications of arthroscopic meniscal repair. *Am J Sports Med* 1993;21(6):864–869.

40. Fanelli GC, Giannotti BF, Edson CJ. Current concepts review. The posterior cruciate ligament arthroscopic evaluation and treatment. *Arthroscopy* 1994;10(6):673–688.

41. Shapiro MS, Freedman EL. Allograft reconstruction of the anterior and posterior cruciate ligaments after traumatic knee dislocation. *Am J Sports Med* 1995;23(5): 580–587.

42. Noyes FR, Barber-Westin SD. Reconstruction of the anterior and posterior cruciate ligaments after knee dislocation. *Am J Sports Med* 1997;25(6):769–778.

43. Sallay PI, Poggi J, Speer KP, et al. Acute dislocation of the patella. A correlative pathoanatomic study. *Am J Sports Med* 1996;24(1):52–60.

44. Evans EB, Eggers GWN, Butler JK, et al. Experimental immobilization and remobilization of rat knee joints. *J Bone Joint Surg* 1960;42A(5):737–758.

45. Enneking WF, Horowitz M. The intra-articular effects of immobilization on the human knee. *J Bone Joint Surg* 1972;54A(5):973–985.

46. Frank CB. Ligament healing: current knowledge and clinical applications. *J Am Acad Orthop Surg* 1996;44(2): 74–83.

47. Ververeli PA, Sutton DC, Hearn SL, et al. Continuous passive motion after total knee arthroplasty. Analysis of cost and benefits. *Clin Orthop Rel Res* 1995;321: 208–215.

48. Richmond JC, Gladstone J, MacGillvray J. Continuous passive motion after arthroscopically assisted anterior cruciate ligament reconstruction: comparison of short-versus long-term use. *Arthroscopy* 1991;7(1):39–44.

49. Rosen MA, Jackson DW, Atwell EA. The efficacy of continuous passive motion in the rehabilitation of anterior cruciate ligament reconstruction. *Am J Sports Med* 1992;20(2):122–127.

50. Witherow GE, Bollen SR, Pinczewski LA. The use of continuous passive motion after arthroscopically assisted anterior cruciate ligament reconstruction: Help or hindrance? *Knee Surg Sports Traumatol Arthrosc* 1993; 1(2):68–70.

51. McCarthy MR, Yates CK, Anderson MA, et al. The effects of immediate continuous passive motion on pain during the inflammatory phase of soft tissue healing following anterior cruciate ligament reconstruction. *J Orthop Sports Phys Ther* 1993;17(2):96–101.

52. Becker JM, Dayton MT, Fazio VW, et al. Prevention of postoperative abdominal adhesions by a sodium hyaluronate-based bioresorbable membrane: a prospective, randomized, double-blind multicenter study. *J Am Coll Surg* 1996;183:297–306.

53. Burns JW, Colt MJ, Burgess LS, et al. Preclinical evaluation of Sperafilm bioresorbable membrane. *Eur J Surg* 1997;suppl 577:40–48.

54. Nelson WE, Henderson RC, Almekinders LC, et al. An evaluation of pre- and postoperative nonsteroidal anti-inflammatory drugs in patients undergoing knee arthroscopy. A prospective, randomized, double-blinded study. *Am J Sports Med* 1993;21(4):510–516.

55. Rasmussen S, Thomsen S, Madsen SN, et al. The clinical effect of naproxen sodium after arthroscopy of the

knee. A randomized, double-blind, prospective study. *Arthroscopy* 1993;9(4):375–380.

56. Vargas JH, Ross DG. Corticosteroids and anterior cruciate ligament repair. *Am J Sports Med* 1989;17(4):532–534.
57. Highgenboten CL, Jackson AW, Meske NB. Arthroscopy of the knee. Ten-day pain profiles and corticosteroids. *Am J Sports Med* 1993;21(4):503–506.
58. Armstrong RW, Bolding F, Joseph R. Septic arthritis following arthroscopy. Clinical syndromes and analysis of risk factors. *Arthroscopy* 1992;8(2):213–223.
59. Cohn BT, Draeger RI, Jackson DW. The effects of cold therapy in the postoperative management of pain in patients undergoing anterior cruciate ligament reconstruction. *Am J Sports Med* 1989;17(3):344–349.
60. Daniel DM, Stone ML, Arendt DL. The effect of cold therapy on pain, swelling, and range of motion after anterior cruciate ligament reconstructive surgery. *Arthroscopy* 1994;10(5):530–533.
61. Edwards DJ, Rimmer M, Keene GCR. The use of cold therapy in the postoperative management of patients undergoing arthroscopic anterior cruciate ligament reconstruction. *Am J Sports Med* 1996;24(2):193–195.
62. Konrath GA, Lock T, Goitz HT, et al. The use of cold therapy after anterior cruciate ligament reconstruction. A prospective, randomized study and literature review. *Am J Sports Med* 1996;24(5):629–633.
63. Robins AJ, Newman AP, Burks RT. Postoperative return of motion in anterior cruciate ligament and medial collateral ligament injuries. Effect of medial collateral ligament rupture location. *Am J Sports Med* 1993;21(1):20–25.
64. Shelbourne KD, Wilckens JH, Mollabashy A, et al. Arthrofibrosis in acute anterior cruciate ligament reconstruction. The effect of timing of reconstruction and rehabilitation. *Am J Sports Med* 1991;19(4):332–336.
65. Mohtadi NGH, Webster-Bogaert S, Fowler PJ. Limitation of motion following anterior cruciate ligament reconstruction. A case-control study. *Am J Sports Med* 1991;19(6):620–625.
66. Shelbourne KD, Foulk DA. Timing of surgery in acute anterior cruciate ligament tears on the return of quadriceps muscle strength after reconstruction using an autogenous patellar tendon graft. *Am J Sports Med* 1995;23(6):686–689.
67. Hunter RE, Mastrangelo J, Freeman JR, et al. The impact of surgical timing on postoperative motion and stability following anterior cruciate ligament reconstruction. *Arthroscopy* 1996;12(6):667–674.
68. Murakami S, Muneta T, Ezura Y, et al. Quantitative analysis of synovial fibrosis in the infrapatellar fat pad before and after anterior cruciate ligament reconstruction. *Am J Sports Med* 1997;25(1):29–34.
69. Mariani PM, Santori N, Rovere P, et al. Histological and structural study of the adhesive tissue in knee fibroarthrosis: a clinical-pathological correlation. *Arthroscopy* 1997;13(3):313–318.
70. Dodds JA, Keene JS, Graf BK, et al. Results of knee manipulations after anterior cruciate ligament reconstructions. *Am J Sports Med* 1991;19(3):283–287.

Section VIII

Unusual Complications in Knee Surgery from Around the World: Case Reports

Chapter 35.1

Patellar Fracture After Anterior Cruciate Ligament Reconstruction with Bone–Patellar Tendon–Bone Graft

Antonio Miguel

The bone–patellar tendon–bone graft is considered the gold standard in anterior cruciate ligament (ACL) reconstruction.[1] The advantages of taking the central third of the patellar tendon are its grip force and the bone-to-bone fixation that favors a faster healing.[2] Patellar tendon grafts can result in the following complications: patellofemoral pain, patellar tendinitis and patellar fracture, as well as extensor mechanism weakness.[3] The morbidity rate of the patellar graft is currently a very controversial topic, but the English-language literature still considers the use of the central third of the patellar tendon the gold standard.

CASE REPORT

An 18-year-old man whose recreational physical activity consisted of baseball, soccer, football, and mountain cycling presented with major symptoms of knee swelling and a sensation of instability. He reported that on October 15, 1992, during a baseball game, he was trying to steal second base. When he reached out to touch the base, his right foot remained fixed on the ground due to the spike shoes, which resulted in a valgus knee flexion. He heard a "pop" and experienced severe pain and functional disability. His knee swelled mildly at that moment and he was taken off the playing field. Cryotherapy was applied but the following day his right knee was much more swollen. He presented at the emergency room, where arthrocentesis was performed and a red intraarticular fluid was drawn out. He wore a splint for 1 week.

When he presented at our clinic 3 weeks after the injury, we found anterior instability of the right knee, with a 2+ Lachman, a 3+ pivot shift, and a 3+ anterior drawer in neutral position. The varus/valgus exploration at 0 and 30 degrees was negative, without posterior displacement of the tibia. We performed an arthrometry and found a 7-mm difference in the maximum manual shift, as compared with the healthy knee. X-rays in four projections were taken and showed an alligned and correctly positioned patella. Arthroscopically assisted ACL reconstruction surgery was suggested with an autologous bone–patellar tendon–bone free graft. Laboratory tests were all within normal ranges.

Surgery was performed on November 25, 1992. General anesthesia was given to the patient, tourniquet pressure was 250 mm Hg, and the 10-mm-wide graft was harvested from the central third of the patellar tendon. Graft length was 25 mm at the level of the tibia and 25 mm at the patellar level. The graft was harvested using an oscillating saw, and no complications occurred. The Johnson & Johnson template was used to attach the ligament to both the tibial and the femoral aspects. The graft was fixed with three no. 5 Ethibon sutures on the tibial and femoral aspects; an 11-mm staple with spikes was used on the tibial and femoral portions. The patient started an accelerated rehabilitation program right away with the continuous passive mobilizer.

Hospital stay was 2 days; total weight bearing on the right pelvic limb with crutches was allowed upon discharge. A home rehabilitation program was indicated, allowing initially only quadriceps contraction exercises as well as flexion and extension, so as to achieve the latter in a 6- to 8-week period. Total flexion was achieved at 6 weeks and total extension at 8 weeks. Then closed-chain exercises with resistance were started, and the patient was allowed to jog at 10 weeks. He had a satisfactory course.

However, 5 months after surgery he was jogging on

the beach and stepped into a hole, which caused forced flexion of the right knee. He felt a pop inside the knee, experienced severe pain, and had functional disability. We saw him at the emergency room, where we clinically diagnosed transverse patellar fracture (Fig. 35.1.1). This diagnosis was proven with anteroposterior (AP) and lateral x-rays. Internal fixation was performed on the same day with two parallel Kirschner wires and a figure-8–shaped AO (Association Osteosynthèse) wire cerclagé (Fig. 35.1.2). We had the patient use the continuous passive mobilizer immediately and allowed full weight-bearing with crutches. At 6 weeks he had achieved total knee flexion and extension, and he started closed-chain exercises with resistance. He did well and the strength of his right quadriceps was quite good. Five months after this, however, he complained of anterolateral knee pain. During the exploration we found protrusion of the fixation wire used to treat the fracture. Since complete healing of the patella had been achieved, we decided to surgically remove the osteosynthesis material as well as the staple used to fix the reconstruction graft on the anteromedial aspect of the tibia.

The patient has done well so far. He resumed his recreational physical activities, especially soccer during the weekends and 10 km of mountain cycling daily. X-rays showed total patellar healing; the axial projection with Merchant's technique did not show patellar displacement and no decrease was observed in joint spaces. Strength of the affected leg is 100% relative to the healthy leg as seen during a jump test.

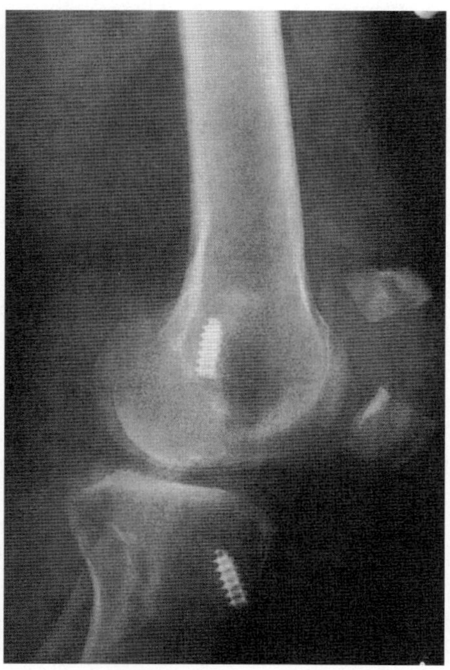

Figure 35.1.1. Lateral view of the transverse patellar fracture of the right knee.

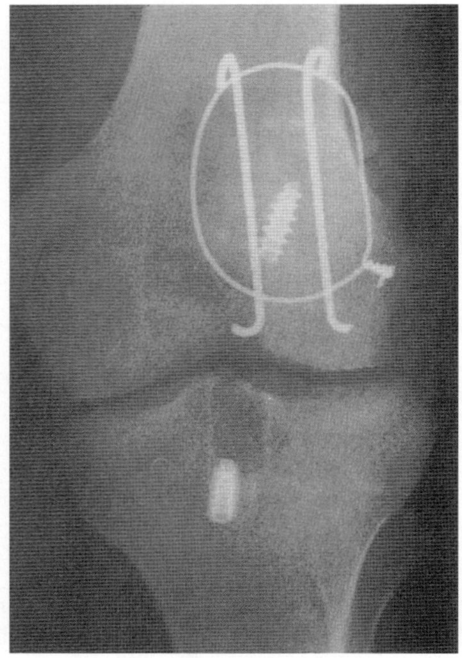

Figure 35.1.2. Lateral view after the internal fixation with parallel kirschner wires and a figure-8-shaped Association Osteosynthèse (AO) wire cerclage of the right knee.

DISCUSSION

The bone–patellar tendon–bone autologous graft is very popular and is still recognized as the gold standard for ACL reconstruction. Some methods and instrumentation have been suggested to avoid the complication of late patellar fracture.[4,5] Patellar fracture usually has one of the following two configurations: a longitudinal fracture resulting from the use of an osteotome to remove the patellar bone fragment from its bed,[6] or a fracture that occurs a few months after surgery and is caused by a low-energy movement. The preexisting relation between a crack and a late fracture has never been reported.[4] Only 25 cases of fracture have been reported as late complications of ACL reconstruction.[7] Christen and Jakob[8] reported six cases with cracks after ACL reconstruction, five of them arthroscopically and one with an open approach. The patellar rupture occurred at the moment of harvesting the bone graft at the donor site. All cases underwent internal fixation with transverse screws and one was treated using nonabsorbable suture cerclage, and the remaining three did not require additional treatment. Some of the causes of fractures associated with patellar graft harvesting during ACL reconstruction are the inaccurate cuts made with the oscillating saw, the misuse of osteotomes, and a patellar graft that is too long. Whenever an abnormal cut is detected, it should be immediately treated with internal fixation and a cancellous graft to avoid delayed healing, and a less aggressive rehabilitation program should be followed.[8] I once did too deep and too long a cross-sectional cut. Internal fixation was used with two Kirschner pins and an AO wire cerclage. The patient was put in the continuous passive mobilizer to prevent a delayed ACL reconstruction surgery. The outcome at 5 years is good, and no complications of the fracture have occurred.

References

1. Fu HF, Schulte RK. Anterior cruciate ligament surgery. State of the art. *Clin Orthop* 1996;325:19–24.
2. Newton PO, Horibe S, Woo SL-Y. Experimental studies on anterior cruciate ligament. Autografts and allografts. Mechanical studies. In: Daniel DM, Akeson WH, O'Conner JJ (eds). *Knee Ligaments: Structure, Function, Injury, and Repair*. New York: Raven Press, 1990:389–399.
3. Aglie Hip P, Buzzi R, Zaccherotti G. Patellar tendon versus semitendinosus and gracilis in anterior cruciate ligament reconstruction. Paper presented at the 18th annual American Orthopaedic Society for Sports Medicine meeting, abstracts and outlines, San Diego, CA, 1992:29–30.
4. Carson WG. A new technique of harvesting patellar tendon autografts for anterior cruciate ligament reconstruction. *Arthroscopy* 1991;4:368–374.
5. Johnson D. Practical arthroscopy. *News Letter* 1998; 1(3):241.
6. Graf B, Uhr F. Complications of intra-articular anterior cruciate reconstruction. Clin Sports Med 1988;7:835–848.
7. Carpenter JE, Kasman R, Matthews LS. Fractures of the patella. *J Bone Joint Surg* 1993;75:1550–1561.
8. Christen B, Jakob RP. Fractures associated with patellar ligament grafts in cruciate ligament surgery. *J Bone Joint Surg* 1992;74B:617–619.

Chapter 35.2

UNUSUAL COMPLICATIONS OF PERSISTENT KNEE JOINT INFECTION FOLLOWING ARTHROSCOPIC ANTERIOR CRUCIATE LIGAMENT RECONSTRUCTION

M. Noda, M. Kurosaka, S. Yoshiya, and K. Mizuno

A postoperative infection following an arthroscopic procedure is a rare complication. Even if it occurs, an acceptable outcome can usually be obtained by an appropriate treatment during the acute phase. Nevertheless, once an infection persists for a certain period, it may cause a chronic impairment of the knee. This chapter presents a case of persistent infection after anterior cruciate ligament (ACL) reconstruction using a prosthetic ligament. This stubborn infection resisted repeated debridement and administration of various antibiotics. We performed daily intraarticular irrigation with a 10% povidone-iodine solution, resulting in a subsidence of the infection.

CASE REPORT

A 26-year-old man injured his right knee while participating in an American Football game on September 17, 1989. Arthroscopic ACL reconstruction using the iliotibial band augmented with a polypropylene braid [Kennedy ligament augmentation device (LAD): 3M, Minneapolis, MN], and repair of the medial collateral ligament and medial meniscus were performed in another hospital on September 29 (Fig. 35.2.1). Four days after the surgery, the patient complained of severe knee pain with significant swelling and local heat. Body temperature rose to 39.0°C, and *Staphylococcus epidermidis* was identified by the culture of the superficial wound drainage. Antibiotics were administered intravenously to treat the suspected acute postoperative infection. Despite this treatment, symptoms continued, and therefore arthroscopic debridement and continuous suction and drainage were initiated at 5 weeks after the surgery. Since secretion persisted from the tibial drill hole, additional extraarticular debridement in and around the exit of the tibial drill hole was performed twice. Despite all these procedures, the infection continued. Open debridement of the knee joint and removal of the Kennedy LAD was conducted at more than 2 months after the onset of infection. Additionally, extraarticular debridement around the medial parapatellar skin incision and removal of all the hardwares were performed a week later. The culture of the specimens taken at debridement revealed methicillin-resistant *Staphylococcus aureus* (MRSA). Since continuous discharge was noted with positive culture from the wound at 3½ months after the initial operation, the patient was referred to our institution.

On our first examination of the patient, the knee was found swollen with local heat, and five fistulas were identified, one at the superior-lateral, two at the superior-medial, and two at the inferior-medial aspects of the knee (Fig. 35.2.2). Among them one tibial fistula, located in the center of the tibial exposed bone, appeared to directly communicate with the intraarticular space through the drill holes made at the time of the reconstructive surgery. A plain radiograph showed diffuse periarticular bony atrophy, and moderate joint space narrowing (Fig. 35.2.3). Pneumofistelography revealed the fistulas connected to the joint cavity (Fig. 35.2.4).

Since administration of more than 10 kinds of antibiotics, such as vancomycin HCL, amikacin sulfate was attempted for 3 months without any remarkable sign of healing, we decided to perform intraarticular irrigation through the fistula with a 10% povidone-iodine solution in conjunction with copious saline irrigation. This was done twice daily for 10 weeks, and no antibiotics were administered during this period. The level of C-reactive protein (CRP) and erythrocyte sedimentation rate (ESR)

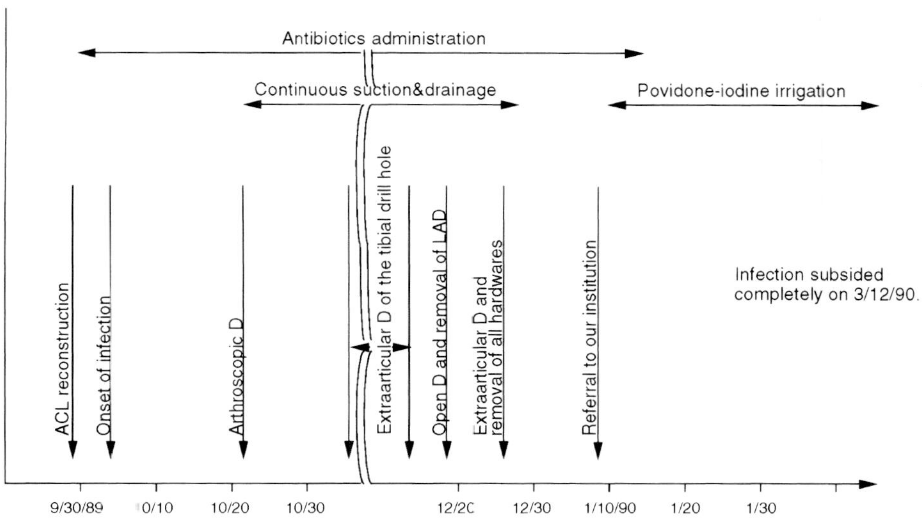

Figure 35.2.1. Outline of treatment given to the patient. D, debridement; LAD, ligament augmentation device.

decreased from 4.2 to 0.3 mg/dL, and from 149 to 15 mm/h, respectively. Consequently, the intraarticular infection subsided and granulation tissue gradually formed around the fistulas. All fistulas finally closed completely and were covered with the epithelium.

At 5-year follow-up, there was no sign of recurrent infection. Range of knee motion was restricted from −10 to 90 degrees, and minimum anterior instability was noted with moderate arthrosis. The patient did not complain of pain on level walking, but could not participate in athletic activities.

DISCUSSION

Postoperative complications of arthroscopic surgery such as effusion, contracture, losing broken instruments, and infection were reported in the literature,[1–5] of which infection is the most devastating complication. The re-

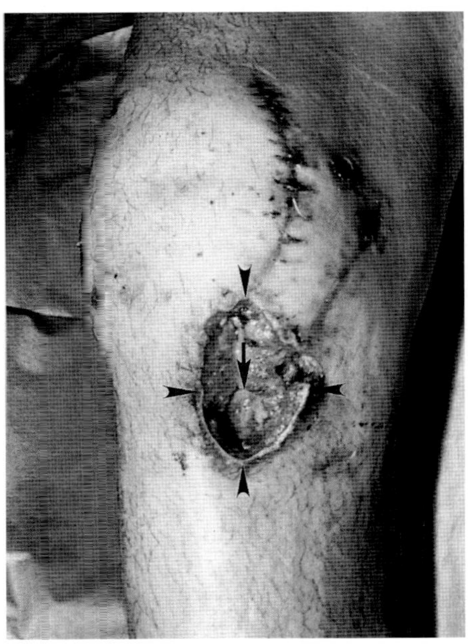

Figure 35.2.2. Clinical image of the infected knee. Note the open wound (arrowheads). One tibial fistula (arrow), located in the center of the tibial exposed bone, appeared to directly communicate with the intraarticular space through the drill holes made at the time of reconstructive surgery.

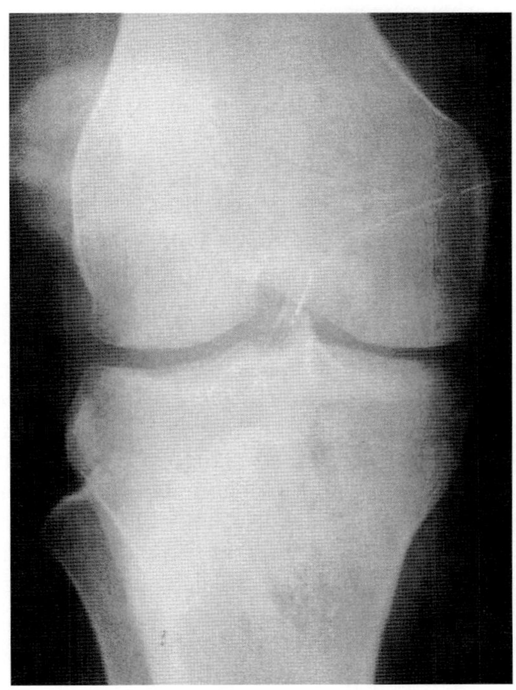

Figure 35.2.3. A plain radiograph revealed diffuse periarticular bony atrophy and moderate joint space narrowing.

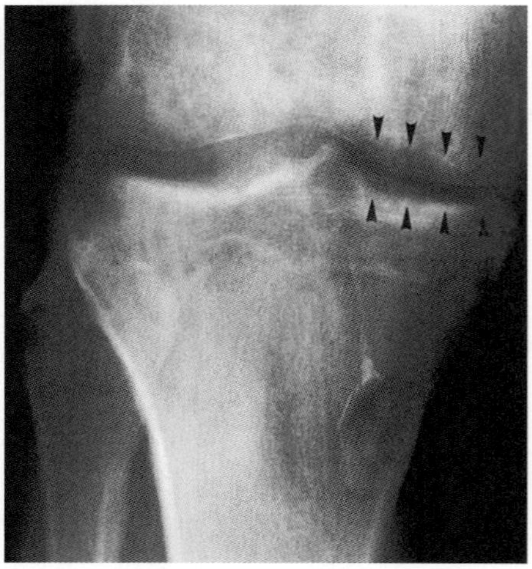

Figure 35.2.4. Pneumofistulography through an inferomedial tibial drill hole demonstrated air (arrowheads) at the medial joint space.

ported infection rate is as low as 0.1% among all the series of arthroscopic procedures including diagnostic arthroscopy.[6] Several factors are recognized as engendering infections, such as intraarticular steroid injections, long operation time, the usage of prosthetic materials, and combined procedures.[6,7] The infection rate significantly increases to 0.5% to 2.7% among ACL reconstructive procedures with prosthetic ligaments.[1,5,8–10]

There have been nine cases of postoperative infection of ACL reconstruction detailed in the English-language literature to the best of our knowledge.[7,11,12] These patients showed slightly limited range of motion, and six patients were reported to have minimal to negligible pain in daily activities.

TREATMENT OF PRIMARY INFECTION

If infection cannot be controlled in the acute phase, it is generally recommended to remove the prosthetic ligament together with intraarticular debridement. In previous reports, more than 70% of the cases required removal of prosthetic ligaments.[5,10,11] As long as an artificial ligament is retained in the infected joint, it may work as a focus for the infection. Moreover, thorough removal of infected and necrotic tissue from the bony tunnel is technically demanding. The longer the articular cartilage is exposed to the leukocytic fibrinoid tissue, the more a destructive change results. Therefore, surgeons should be decisive in removing prosthetic materials when an infection cannot be controlled. Also, extraarticular debridement including removal of all the hardwares should be done earlier when extraarticular infection is suspected. Postoperative infection with ACL reconstruction can develop extraarticularly, since Barrett and Field[10] suggested that presence of the LAD could act in a "wick effect," indicating that superficial infection could spread intraarticularly through the bony tunnel. To detect extraarticular puruloid accumulation in the early phase, a careful physical examination is mandatory. Williams et al[7] also reported that magnetic resonance imaging is useful to visualize extraarticular fluid collection. We conclude that, in this case, extraarticular infection could have influenced subsequent healing, as thorough debridement of this spot was not done for 3 months.

Intraarticular irrigation with a 10% povidone-iodine solution was selected to treat the persistent infection in our case. Povidone-iodine was reported to be an extremely potent microbicidal agent, even against MRSA, although it is not generally recommended for use with intraarticular infections.[13,14] This solution can be harmful to synovial tissue and the articular cartilage as well[15]; thus, the degeneration and destruction of intraarticular tissue are inevitable. Since previous debridement had been conducted five times and high-dose administration of different antibiotics did not result in an infection-free joint, we selected this treatment at the risk of joint degeneration.

At the 5-year follow-up, there was a moderate arthrosis noted, with limited range of motion. However, the infection had subsided completely. Since the patient was only 31 years old at follow-up, some future deterioration of joint function will be unavoidable. However, we believe that his knee function is as good as could possibly be obtained considering the previous tenacious infection.

CONCLUSION

This chapter described an unusual case in which a persistent knee infection occurred after an arthroscopic anterior cruciate ligament reconstruction. After removal of the prosthetic ligament, the infection was brought under control by intraarticular irrigation with 10% povidone-iodine solution.

References

1. Andersen HN, Bruun C, Sondergard-Petersen PE. Reconstruction of chronic insufficient anterior cruciate ligament in the knee using a synthetic Dacron prosthesis—a prospective study of 57 cases. *Am J Sports Med* 1992; 20:20–23.

2. Fujikawa K, Iseki F. Anterior cruciate ligament reconstruction with the Leeds-Keio artificial ligament. *Bull Hosp Jt Dis Orthop Inst* 1991;51:140–154.

3. Klein W, Jensen KU. Synovitis and artificial ligaments. *Arthroscopy* 1992;8:116–124.
4. Olson EJ, Kang JD, Fu FH, Georgescu HI, Mason GC, Evans CH. The biochemical and histological effects of artificial ligament wear particles: in vitro and in vivo studies. *Am J Sports Med* 1988;16:558–570.
5. Paulos LE, Rosenberg TD, Grewe SR, Tearse DS, Beck CL. The Gore-Tex anterior cruciate ligament prosthesis—a long term follow-up. *Am J Sports Med* 1992;20:246–252.
6. Armstrong RW, Bolding F, Joseph R. Septic arthritis following arthroscopy: clinical syndrome and analysis of risk factors. *Arthroscopy* 1992;8:213–223.
7. Williams RJ III, Laurencin CT, Warren RF, Speciale AC, Brause BD, O'Brien S. Septic arthritis after arthroscopic anterior cruciate ligament reconstruction. *Am J Sports Med* 1997;25:261–267.
8. Bolton CW, Bruchman WC. The Gore-Tex expanded polytetrafluoroethylene prosthetic ligament—an in vitro and in vivo evaluation. *Clin Orthop* 1985;196:202–213.
9. Park JP, Grana WA, Chitwood JS. A high-strength Dacron augmentation for cruciate ligament reconstruction—a two-year canine study. *Clin Orthop* 1985;196:175–185.
10. Barrett GR, Field LD. Comparison of patella tendon versus patella tendon/Kennedy ligament augmentation device for anterior cruciate ligament reconstruction: study of results, morbidity, and complications. *Arthroscopy* 1993;9:624–632.
11. Indelicato PA, Pascale MS, Huegel MO. Early experience with the Gore-Tex polytetrafluoroethylene anterior cruciate ligament prosthesis. *Am J Sport Med* 1989;17:55–62.
12. Kohn D. Case report: unsuccessful arthroscopic treatment of pyarthrosis following anterior cruciate ligament reconstruction. *Arthroscopy* 1988;4:287–289.
13. Goebel ME, Drez D Jr, Heck SB, Stoma MK. Contaminated rabbit patellar tendon grafts—in vivo analysis of disinfecting methods. *Am J Sports Med* 1994;22:387–391.
14. Michel D, Zach GA. Antiseptic efficacy of disinfecting solutions in suspension test in vitro against methicillin-resistant *Staphylococcus aureus*, *Pseudomonas aeruginosa*, and *Escherichia coli* in pressure sore wounds after spinal cord injury. *Dermatology* 1997;195:36–41.
15. Bertone AL, McIlwraith CW, Jones RL, Norrdin RW, Radin MJ. Povidone-iodine lavage treatment of experimentally induced equine infectious arthritis. *Am J Vet Res* 1987;48:712–715.

Chapter 35.3

Malunion of Tibial Spine Avulsion of the Anterior Cruciate Ligament Causing a Block to Extension

Ponky Firer

Avulsion fractures of the anterior cruciate ligament's attachment to the tibial plateau including the spines is a recognized injury in the immature skeleton. Recommended forms of treatment include closed reduction and immobilization in full extension[1,2]—the fracture being held in place by the femoral condylar contact in this position—or open reduction and internal fixation.[3–6] As most fractures are immobilized in full extension after reduction, a fixed flexion deformity is a rare but described complication of malunion.

CASE REPORT

An $11\frac{1}{2}$-year-old girl fell off a skateboard, injuring the left knee (November 1996). Despite suitable x-rays (Fig. 35.3.1) and a hemarthrosis being drained, diagnosis of a type III avulsion fracture[7] was missed. She was sent for physiotherapy, but because of lack of extension, which persisted $2\frac{1}{2}$ months after her injury, the physiotherapist referred her back to her doctor and she was ultimately referred to an orthopedic surgeon. The correct diagnosis was made, and she had an open surgical procedure through an anteromedial arthrotomy (February 1997). Operative notes obtained from the surgeon state that the "cavity from which the avulsion had come was curetted and the fragment replaced into position, and fixed with a screw inserted from anteriorly, just proximal to the growth plate." She was immobilized in a cast for 6 weeks, but no mention was made in the notes about the status of her extension, or the position of the knee in the cast. Further physiotherapy followed removal of the cast. Postoperative x-rays showed that the fracture was still not adequately reduced (Fig. 35.3.2).

The patient was referred to the author 11 months following the initial injury (October 1997), as her parents were concerned about her gait, lack of extension, and especially the future of the knee if it was left as it was. The patient hardly experienced any pain, there being only slight discomfort anteromedially when attempting full extension. She had noticed this at physiotherapy after the operation.

Her examination confirmed a fixed flexion deformity. On the uninjured right knee she hyperextended to 8 degrees, and on the injured left knee she had a 10-degree fixed flexion deformity, i.e., there was a side-to-side deficit of 18 degrees. Her prone heel height difference was 110 mm. There was a 5-degree loss of flexion on the injured left side. Her patella mobility was only slightly decreased compared to the right knee when tested with both knees equally flexed. The Lachman test revealed a 4- to 5-mm difference, with the left knee being greater than the right. A KT-1000 test was not done.

The rest of the knee examination was entirely normal, there being no other ligamentous laxity and no sign of meniscal injury. The only tender area was along the anteromedial joint space and a solid-feeling block to extension was obtained when attempting to extend the knee. Computed tomography (CT) scan showed the united avulsed fragment still to be impinging on the femoral condyle (Fig. 35.3.3). The previously inserted screw was also noted.

Corrective surgery was carried out at the beginning of November 1997. Arthroscopy was carried out to confirm the impingement (Fig. 35.3.4A) and to ensure there were no further intraarticular problems, which there weren't. A "kiss lesion" causing damage (Fig. 35.3.4B) was seen on the lateral femoral condyle.

Through the old anteromedial incision the screw was removed. The area of the avulsion was osteotomized in

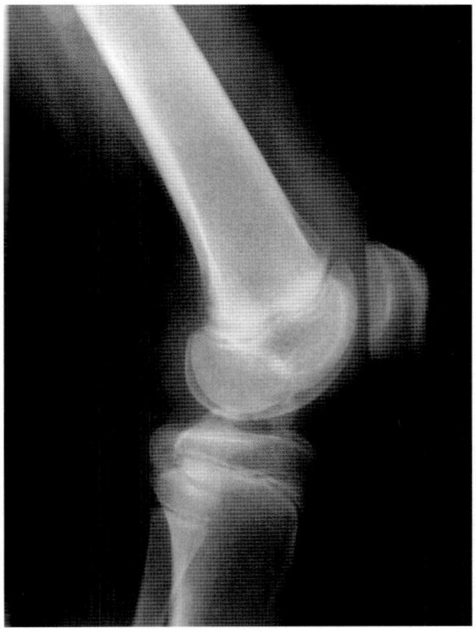

Figure 35.3.1. X-ray taken after initial injury. Avulsed type III fragment readily seen (November 1996).

a cube-shaped block, keeping a 7- to 8-mm thickness of underlying cancellous bone attached to the articular fragment and its attached anterior cruciate ligament. The bed from which the block had been removed was then deepened with a small burr and curettes until the block countersunk into its normal anatomic position,

A

B

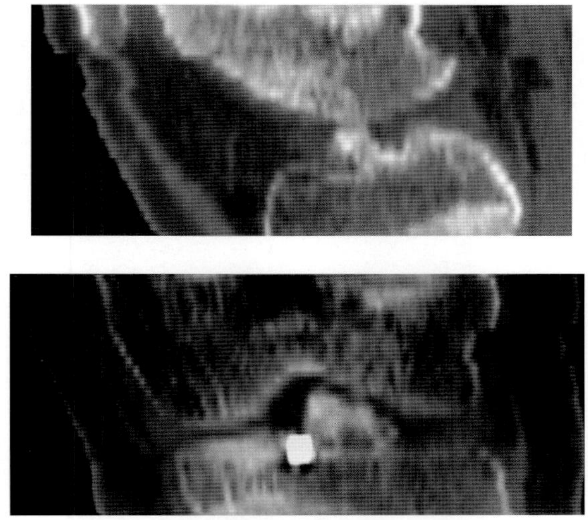

Figure 35.3.3. **A:** On computed tomography (CT) scan, anteroposterior (AP) reconstruction showed impingement of fragment. **B:** Lateral reconstruction showed impingement of fragment.

with the edges of the articular cartilage surfaces flush with the rest of the plateau. With this in place the knee could be extended an extra 10 to 15 degrees (from an 18-degree deficit). Gentle manipulation allowed the knee to regain full extension.

The block was held in its bed by a no. 2 nonabsorbable suture passed through 1.5-mm drill holes from

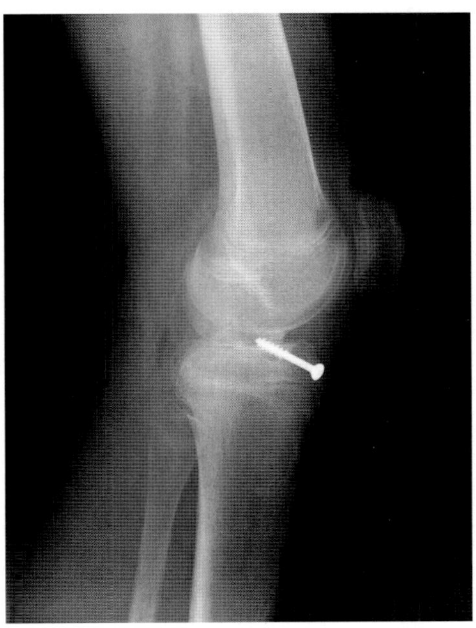

Figure 35.3.2. Postoperative x-ray after initial reduction and fixation. Fragment nail positioned (February 1997)

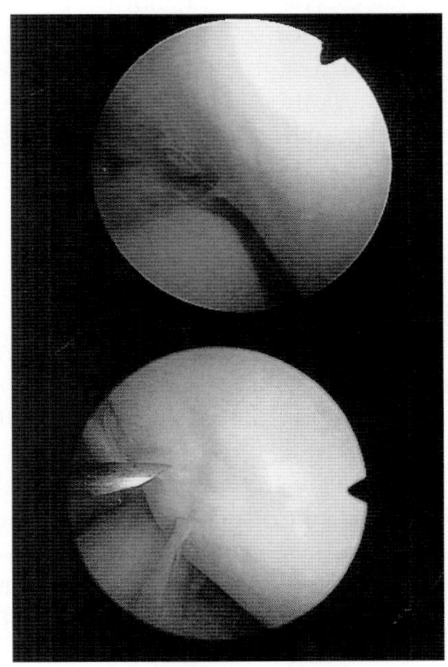

Figure 35.3.4. **A:** Arthroscopic view of impinging fragment. **B:** Kiss lesion on lateral femoral condyle.

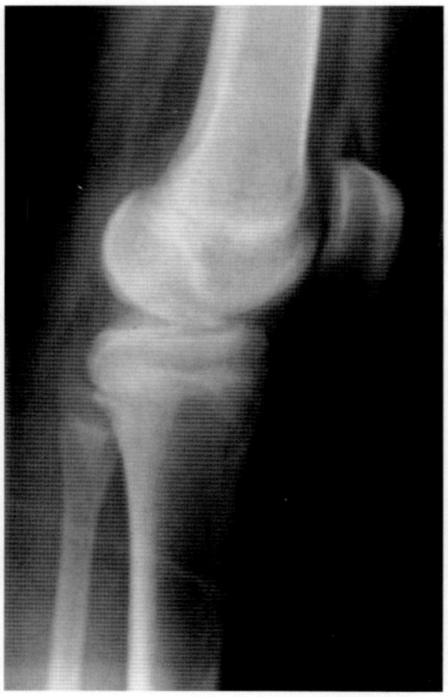

Figure 35.3.5. Postoperative x-ray showing reduced fragment and full extension in cast (November 1997).

below (adjacent to the tibial tubercle); sutures were tied over a button on the anterior cortex of the tibia. After closure the knee was immobilized in maximum extension in a plaster cast. X-rays showed reduction of the fragment (Fig. 35.3.5). The cast was removed at 6 weeks, and the knee was at full hyperextension equal to the other knee. The patient, however, missed physiotherapy follow-up for 2 of the subsequent 4 weeks and regressed to a 5-degree lack of full hyperextension. After further physiotherapy she has progressed to a 15-mm heel height difference, i.e., 2-degree lack of full hyperextension.

DISCUSSION

Avulsion fractures of the tibial spines in the immature skeleton are more frequent than intraligamentous ruptures of the anterior cruciate ligament. They must be suspected in an injured knee with a hemarthrosis for which no other cause can be found. A degree of malunion in conservatively treated patients is probably not uncommon, with slight displacement occurring but having no ill effects, as full extension is achieved easily. Most of these injuries (9 out of 11 in the author's experience) have had a residual increase to the Lachman sign at late follow-up. These have been between 3- and 5-mm side-to-side differences on Lachman and KT-1000 testing. However, all have had a solid end point; six of nine had negative pivot shifts and three had a glide. None had functional instability. It would seem that the anterior cruciate ligament undergoes some plastic deformation under load before the failure occurs at the bony insertion, pulling up the block off the tibial plateau. Laxity has occurred even with perfect anatomic reduction.

The surgery in this case was not difficult but required meticulous dissection of the fragment and a large-enough block needed to be taken to ensure fixation in a good base of bone for healing.

It is essential, whether treating this condition conservatively or by open reduction, that full extension is achieved.

CONCLUSIONS

The lessons learned from this case are the following:

1. X-rays must be carefully studied if a hemarthrosis is found.
2. Fat should be specifically looked for after drainage of a hemarthrosis—and will always be found in avulsion fractures.
3. A positive Lachman test would have been found, if conducted, leading to suspicion of an anterior cruciate ligament or anterior cruciate ligament avulsion injury in this age group.
4. Any knee that is not improving its loss of extension within 2 weeks of treatment must be reassessed by a specialist.

This rare complication of loss of extension due to a malunited avulsion fracture has been successfully treated by osteotomy and refixation in a normal position.

References

1. Clark HO. Discussion on fracture of the tibia involving the knee-joint. *Proc R Soc Med* 1935;28:1035–1050.
2. Garcia A, Neer CS II. Isolated fractures of the intercondylar eminence of the tibia. *Am J Surg* 1958;95:593–598.
3. Lee HG. Avulsion fracture of the tibial attachments of the cruciate ligaments. Treatment by operative reduction. *J Bone Joint Surg* 1937;19:460–468.
4. Meyers MH, McKeever FM. Follow-up notes. Fracture of the intercondylar eminence of the tibia. *J Bone Joint Surg* 1970;52A:1677–1684.
5. Roth PB. Fracture of the spine of the tibia. *J Bone Joint Surg* 1928;10:509–518.
6. Zaricznyj B. Avulsion fracture of the tibial eminence. Treatment by open reduction and pinning. *J Bone Joint Surg* 1977;59A:1111–1114.
7. Meyers MH, McKeever FM. Fracture of the intercondylar eminence of the tibia. *J Bone Joint Surg* 1959;41A: 209–222.

Chapter 35.4

Arthroscopic Anterior Cruciate Ligament Reconstruction Using a Bone-Tendon-Bone Patellar Ligament Graft: Complications of Femoral Press-Fit Anchoring

Harald Boszotta

Though commonly used for fixation of the bone-tendon-bone (BTB) graft in anterior cruciate ligament (ACL) reconstruction, interference screw fixation may be associated with considerable complications, so that press-fit anchoring has been suggested as a suitable alternative.[1–8] The press-fit technique employed in our department is based on the use of an oscillating hollow saw, allowing for the standardized removal of a BTB graft with cylindrical bone blocks. On account of their cylindrical shape and the specific transtibial endoscopic technique used, these bone blocks provide for optimal press-fit anchoring with excellent primary stability. This chapter describes the particular complications encountered with arthroscopic femoral press-fit anchoring and discusses methods for standardizing procedures and avoiding such complications.

CASE REPORTS

Case 1

Six months after sustaining a trauma, a 20-year old patient undergoes surgery for an ACL-deficient knee. The procedure is performed under general anesthesia and application of a pneumatic tourniquet. Following arthroscopic debridement, the tibial tunnel is placed as usual using a 9.5-mm oscillating hollow drill. With the knee flexed approximately 90 degrees, the femoral tunnel is drilled in the transtibial technique using an 8-mm hand reamer over a 2-mm guidewire. Next, the graft is harvested with an 8.4-mm oscillating hollow saw. The graft is removed together with two cylindrical bone blocks (diameter 8.4 mm), introduced into the joint using a stay suture, and the patellar bone block is plugged into the femoral tunnel under arthroscopic vision. Excessive intraoperative resistance to plugging results in fracture of the bone block, which is discovered in the intraoperative radiograph (Fig. 35.4.1). Insufficient anchorage necessitates the additional use of an interference screw after reversal of the graft. The screw is introduced from the anteromedial direction after removal of one-half of the bone block.

Case 2

Two years after sustaining a trauma, a 32-year-old woman undergoes ACL reconstruction for instability problems. Following extensive debridement and visualization of the cruciate ligament insertions, the tibial tunnel is drilled using an oscillating hollow saw. The femoral tunnel, placed as far dorsal as possible, is drilled in transtibial technique. Following harvest of the graft together with two cylindrical bone blocks by means of the hollow saw, the BTB graft is introduced and the patellar bone block is plugged into the femoral tunnel under arthroscopic vision. Intraoperatively, no problems are encountered. With the knee flexed approximately 15 degrees, the graft is finally fixed under adequate tension over a medial screw head on the femur head. Intraoperative arthroscopic evaluation revealed no problems, with the patellar ligament graft showing the usual posi-

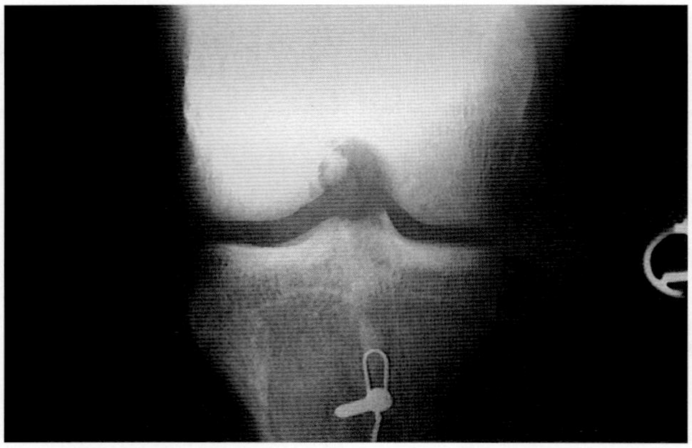

Figure 35.4.1. Block fracture due to difficulties in plugging.

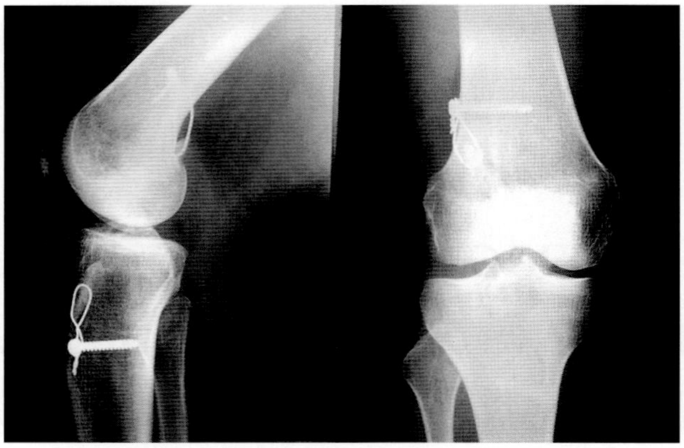

Figure 35.4.3. Postoperative radiographs after over-the-top fixation.

tion and adequate tension. However, the intraoperative radiograph revealed dorsal canting of the femoral bone block into the popliteal space, requiring a revision of the femoral anchorage from the lateral over-the-top position to ensure sufficiently load-stable anchoring (Figs. 35.4.2 and 35.4.3).

DISCUSSION

Stable and secure graft fixation is of special importance, in particular with regard to early postoperative functional rehabilitation. High primary stability and safe healing of the graft must be ensured. However, the commonly used method of interference screw fixation has been associated with a large number of possible complications including graft damage upon screw insertion, secondary damage due to misplacement or graft protrusion, bone block fragmentation, breaking of the femoral cortical bone, delayed healing and screw divergence with reduced pullout strength.[1–8]

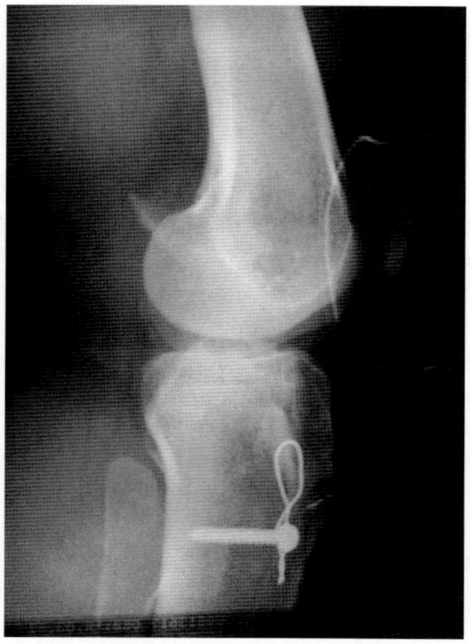

Figure 35.4.2. Dorsal canting of bone block.

In their articles, McGuire et al[9] and Bush et al[3] discuss the importance of tibial tunnel positioning for the placement of the femoral tunnel in endoscopic transtibial technique. The same also applies for the arthroscopic femoral press-fit technique. Adequate flexion of approximately 90 degrees is an essential prerequisite for the placement of both the tibial and femoral tunnel. This will not only ensure a virtually rectangular bone block/ligament angulation in terminal extension, but also avoid damage to the dorsal cortical femur. While such flexion appears to be ideal for femoral press-fit anchoring, increasing knee flexion may be associated with problems upon insertion of interference screws.[7–9]

Three possible primary complications may be identified in the use of arthroscopic femoral press-fit technique:

1. problems upon insertion of the femoral bone block,
2. insufficient anchorage due to inadequate bone block/ligament angulation,
3. insufficient anchorage as a result of a trough-shaped tunnel at the condylar roof of the femur.

Problem 1 can be avoided by using a template allowing for adequate preparation of the patellar bone block prior

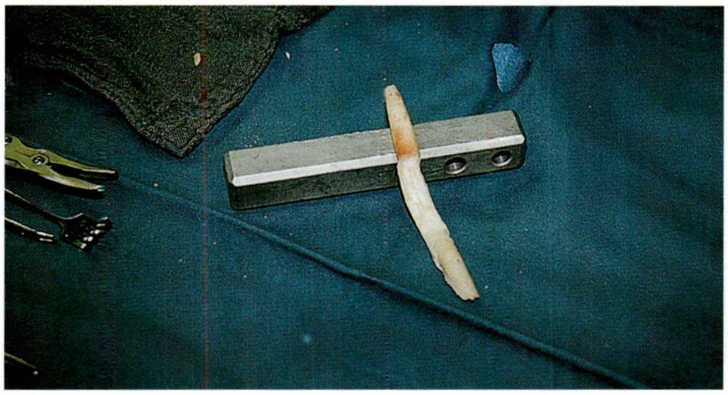

A

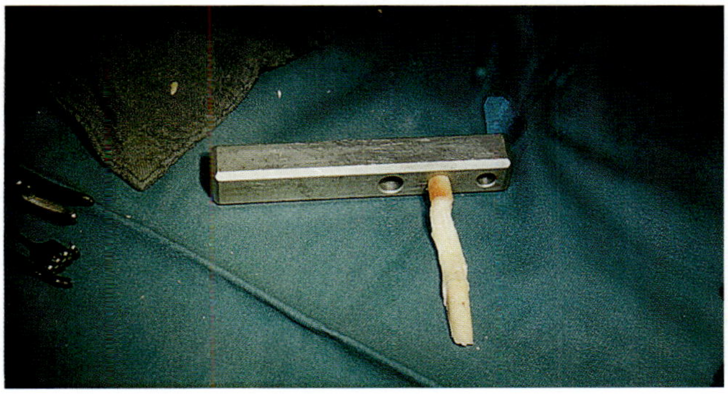

B

Figure 35.4.4. Template for standardized preparation of the patellar bone block.

to introduction into the knee joint, so that half of the trimmed bone block slides into the femoral tunnel by the pull of the stay sutures (Fig. 35.4.4). Thus, the end of the bone block may be plugged in under arthroscopic vision without any associated risk of canting or fracture. Use of an excessively long bone block must be avoided and bone quality should be adequately considered when preparing the bone block.

Distal-end fissures of the inserted bone block associated with reduced pullout strength may be experienced if plugging proves difficult.[10] In addition, bone block/ligament angulation is critical for femoral press-fit anchoring and should be 60 to 90 degrees in terminal extension, which can be achieved by adequate knee flexion when placing the femoral tunnel. Ideally, the procedure should be performed at 90-degree knee flexion, ensuring a 90-degree polylactic acid (PLA) in terminal extension.

The problem of an excessively dorsal placement of the femoral tunnel may be encountered with any endoscopic technique and may be avoided by sufficient flexion and use of transtibial target drill units serving as guidance for the central guidewire of the cannulated reamer.[3,9] Prior to final placement, an impression on the dorsolateral condyle roof may be placed to verify adequate positioning. Considering the methods for standardizing surgical procedures discussed above, arthroscopic femoral press-fit technique provides an adequate, low-risk alternative to interference screw fixation.

CONCLUSION

During a period of 6 years (1992–1997) 528 arthroscopic anterior cruciate ligament (ACL) reconstructions using patellar ligament grafts in press-fit technique were performed. Block fracture consequent to difficulties in plugging, canting of the bone block in intercondylar space, dorsal canting into the popliteal space due to excessively dorsal placement of the femoral tunnel, as well as insufficient anchorage due to excessively flat plug/ligament angulation were encountered in seven of these cases (1.3%) and constitute the specific complications of femoral press-fit anchoring. Methods for standardizing techniques and avoiding such complications were described.

References

1. Bach BR. Potential pitfalls of Kurosaka screw interference fixation for ACL surgery. *Am J Knee Surg* 1989;2: 76–82.
2. Arciero RA. Endoscopic anterior cruciate ligament reconstruction: complication of graft rupture and a method of salvage. *Am J Knee Surg* 1996;9:27–31.
3. Bush-Joseph CA, Bach BR, Bryan J. Posterior cortical violation of the femoral tunnel during endoscopic anterior cruciate ligament reconstruction. *Am J Knee Surg* 1995; 8:130–133.
4. O'Donnell JB, Scerpella TA. Endoscopic anterior cruciate ligament reconstruction: modified technique and radiographic review. *Arthroscopy* 1995;11:577–584.
5. Berg EE. Autograft bone–patella tendon–bone plug comminution with loss of ligament fixation and stability. *Arthroscopy* 1996;12:232–235.
6. Franco GM, Bach BR, Bush-Joseph CA. Intraarticular placement of Kurosaka interference screws. *Arthroscopy* 1994;10:412–417.

7. Brodie JT, Torpey BM, Donald GD, Bade HA. Femoral interference screw placement through the tibial tunnel: a radiographic evaluation of interference screw divergence angles after endoscopic anterior cruciate ligament reconstruction. *Arthroscopy* 1996;12:435–440.

8. McGuire DA, Wolchok JC. Consistent and accurate graft passage and interference screw guide wire placement during single incision anterior cruciate ligament reconstruction. *Arthroscopy* 1997;13:526–529.

9. McGuire DA, Hendricks SD, Grinstead GL. Use of an endoscopic aimer for femoral tunnel placement in anterior cruciate ligament reconstruction. *Arthroscopy* 1996;12:26–31.

10. Boszotta H. Arthroskopische femorale Press-fit Fixation des Lig patellae–Transplantates beim Ersatz des vorderen Kreuzbandes: Experimentelle Grundlagen und Operationstechnik *Arthroskopie* 1997;10:583–587. Boszotta H. Arthroscopic anterior cruciate ligament reconstruction using a patellar tendon graft in press-fit-technique: surgical technique and follow-up. *Arthroscopy* 1997;13:332–339.

Chapter 35.5

Complications in Anterior Cruciate Ligament Reconstructive Surgery

Giancarlo Puddu and Vittorio Franco

This chapter presents two case reports that we observed in the past few years. They are both patients operated on for anterior cruciate ligament (ACL) reconstruction. The first case is a patient who had a difficult postoperative recovery because of a painful articular "click" localized at the superomedial pole of the patella, which often occurred during recurrent swellings. After a long series of arthrocentesis and delayed therapeutic decisions, only a second-look arthroscopic identified the cause and solved the problem.

The second case is an unlucky chain of events from a routine ACL reconstruction to a functional disaster of the knee joint. The wrong timing of surgery probably was the main reason why a malign infrapatellar contracture syndrome developed and engendered its worst consequences. Of these two patients, only the first underwent the index surgical procedure in our hospital. The second came to us after she had been operated on for ACL reconstruction, and reoperated with a salvage procedure by the same surgeon, in another hospital.

In the past 30 years the reconstruction of ACL-deficient knees, at the beginning an open procedure and then arthroscopically assisted, has become the most popular operation in knee surgery and probably in operative sports medicine. It's not surprising that many articles in the orthopedic literature focus on this subject, including the basic science and biomechanics, proposals for new surgical techniques, and accelerated protocols of rehabilitation. However, several possible surgical complications have been reported, including arthrofibrosis,[1] reflex sympathetic dystrophy, deep vein thrombosis,[2] loss of motion,[2] septic arthritis, osteomyelitis, graft failure,[2,3] patellar tendon rupture,[4] patellar subluxation,[1] intraoperative and postoperative patellar fracture,[5] popliteal artery laceration, saphenous nerve injury, patellar tendinitis, intraarticular placement of bone plug, bone plug nonunion, interference screw damage of graft, and supracondylar femoral fracture.[6,7]

CASE REPORT 1: INTRAARTICULAR FEMOROPATELLAR PAINFUL CLICK AFTER ACL RECONSTRUCTION

A 38-year-old man had a ski accident and ruptured the ACL of his right knee in March 1996. The patient, after diagnosis of the complete ligament tear, was submitted to a preoperative protocol of rehabilitation. During the following 3 weeks he performed the physical therapy assisted by a therapist, including isometric exercises, range of motion (ROM) exercises, closed kinetic chain exercises, massages, and antiinflammatory applications.[8] The day of surgery (April 2, 1996) he arrived at the operation in good physical condition, with normotrophic and normotonic quadriceps and full ROM without intraarticular swelling.

The operation, arthroscopically aided, was performed by the senior author. It consisted of the reconstruction of the torn ligament by means of one-third bone–patellar tendon–bone autograft. The femoral tunnel was drilled with outside-inside technique and the graft fixation was accomplished by interference screwing. No additional surgery needed.

The early postoperative period was normal. We have been following the same rehabilitation program since the beginning of the 1990s.[8] The patient starts with continuous passive motion (CPM) from the first postoperative day and normally reaches 90 degrees of flexion at the 5th day and 120 degrees at the end of the 2nd week.[9]

Isometric quadriceps sets varying the degrees of hip and knee flexion (since 1994 assisted by a muscular biofeedback device[10]) combined with partial weight-bearing walking exercises represent the core of the muscle rehabilitation program during the first 15 post-operative days. Compared with the average ROM, the patient showed, from the beginning, a slowdown trend; at the end of the first month he was able to bend the knee up to 110 degrees only. Since the first days, when CPM started to flex the knee, he felt an internal painful "click," probably referable to the patellofemoral joint in correspondence to the superomedial pole of the patella. Moreover he had a swollen knee for a long time after the operation despite the three arthrocenteses that we did to evacuate the synovial fluid in the first 2 months.

In July, 3 months after the operation, the patient had a stable but swollen and painful knee, and the ROM was fully regained. He especially complained of the pain in climbing or descending stairs and because his knee started to swell as soon as he tried to perform physical work or exercise. The pain seemed to be positively influenced by the presence of the intraarticular swelling. When he rested from physical efforts, some days continuously, the joint was able to resume its normal proportions, producing a sharp increase of the anterior knee pain.

At the physical examination it was possible to palpate a sort of "click" at the superomedial pole of the patella while the patient started to flex the knee; the fingering of the proximal edge of the patella while the click was produced resulted in the patient feeling pain. Magnetic resonance imaging (MRI) examination showed the neoligament with a normal signal, well recognizable for the whole intraarticular length. The femoral and tibial attachments appeared isometrically compatible, and there were no signs of intercondylar impingement and no hypertrophic tissue with the characteristics of the cyclops syndrome was present. The menisci and the articular surfaces were normal. The radiologist pointed out the presence of a cartilaginous flap rising from the medial side of the trochlea (Fig. 35.5.1). That flap could be related to the painful click we palpated during the physical examination.

The patient was prepared for a second-look arthroscopic, which we performed at the end of July. We assessed the reconstructed ligament, which looked fine; the menisci were intact and the articular surfaces, too, but the lateral facet of the patella presented a superficial lesion of the cartilage. That lesion corresponded to a synovial adhesion (type A of the Perugia-Mariani classification[11]) that looked like a plica that originated from the lateral capsule and inserted medially to the trochlea (Fig. 35.5.2).

This never-before-seen structure was the only abnormal finding. We couldn't demonstrate a conflict between the patella and the plica during the knee flexion. Probably the liquid irrigation of the joint, which distended the capsule, prevented the contact and the articular click. We excised the plica with the shaver and ended the arthroscopic examination. An articular suction drainage was left in place for 24 hours.

In the postoperative period the patient had a swollen knee for about 2 weeks. The swelling slowly subsided and he recovered quickly the normal ROM. At the last follow-up, just before Christmas, he had regained his normal muscular ability, the operated knee was dry, and he had a full active ROM. The painful click disappeared.

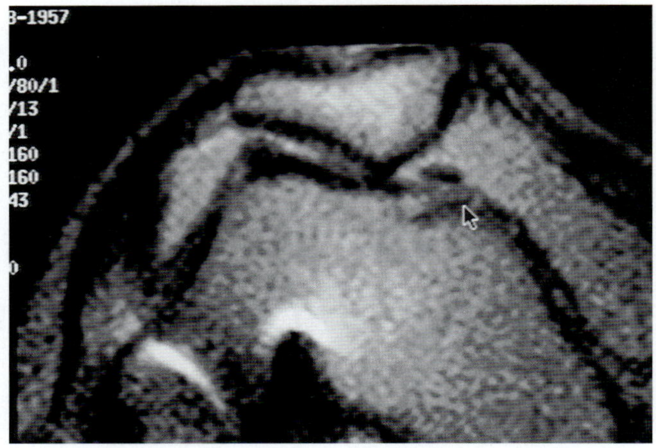

Figure 35.5.1. Magnetic resonance imaging (MRI) scan of the patellofemoral joint. The black arrow points to the cartilaginous flap rising from the medial side of the trochlea.

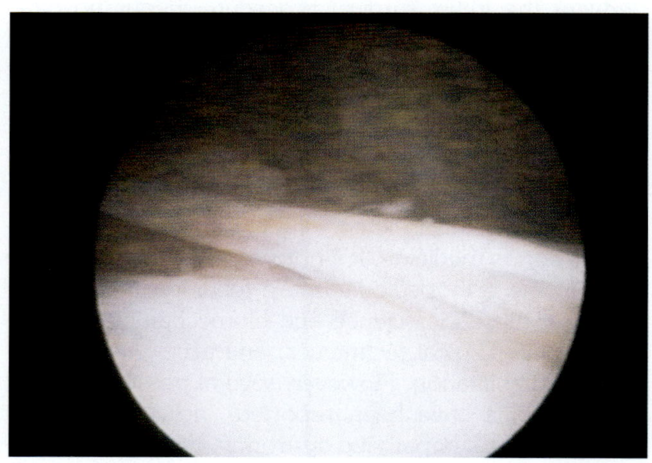

Figure 35.5.2. Arthroscopic look of the synovial adhesion as it originates from the medial capsula and inserts medially on the trochlea.

Discussion

Compared with other cases complicated by a difficult postoperative recovery, this reconstructed knee had a peculiar behavior different from all the rest in our experience. The problem seemed to be the articular swelling combined with the consequent inability to improve the ROM according to our rehabilitation protocol, but what mainly disturbed the patient was the painful click he felt each time he started to flex the knee. His discomfort was paradoxally reduced by the intraarticular distention; the more swollen the knee, the less evidence of a painful click. This is now easily explained by an obvious consideration: the pain originated in a conflict between the patella and the strange synovial plica at the first degrees of flexion; the synovial fluid present in the swollen knee increased the distance between the floating patella and the trochlea, preventing any contact, any mechanical click, and, consequently, any pain. The secondary arthroscopy with the excision of the abnormal plica solved the problem.

Conclusion

It is difficult to say whether the plica was already present at the first operation or was a consequence of it. We don't know if a more accurate examination of the patellofemoral joint would have made it possible to avoid the postoperative troubles, but this experience taught us to take seriously any complaint of the patient, especially when there is a correspondence between what is subjective and what is objective. In this case we could probably have performed the second arthroscopy two months earlier with real benefit to the patient.

CASE REPORT 2: HOW INCORRECT TIMING OF SURGERY CAN TRANSFORM A ROUTINE ACL RECONSTRUCTION INTO A FUNCTIONAL DISASTER

The second patient, a 17-year-old girl, had a knee sprain because of a fall while skiing on February 26, 1991. Many specialists examined her in the first 2 weeks after the trauma without finding a ligamentous lesion. The last specialist diagnosed a complete ACL tear and recommended surgical reconstruction. Although 6 weeks went by after the trauma before she was admitted to the hospital for surgery, no rehabilitation program was prescribed for her.[12] The result was that the girl arrived in the operating room with a stiff joint (ROM between 30 and 90 degrees of flexion). On April 12, she was operated on for ACL reconstruction with a bone–patellar tendon–bone autograft performed arthroscopically. The femoral tunnel was drilled from outside-inside. The ACL tear was isolated and no additional surgery required. After the operation the knee was protected by a femorotibial brace locked at 30 degrees of flexion. No motion was allowed until the 15th postoperative day.

When CPM was started, the joint looked swollen and painful. At the same time, the patient underwent a very aggressive physical rehabilitation. The next 4 months her knee was passively forced to extend and flex not less than 5 hours every day. There was a clear delay compared with the average ROM values. The patient was not able to go over 30 to 90 degrees of flexion. The CPM device was abandoned after 6 weeks, and only passive, aggressive, ROM exercises manually assisted by the therapist were prescribed. She was allowed to do partial weight-bearing walking 20 days after the operation and to walk without crutches after another 20 days. She could only limp and was in pain in the stance phase of the gait.

Because of the unacceptable result, her physician, who had performed the reconstruction, decided to improve the ROM with a closed manipulation under general anesthesia. On August 30 the surgeon attempted to improve the range of motion by forcing both the extension and the flexion, but, because extension was judged to be the main problem, the knee was immobilized in an extension cast for 15 days. Immediately after the operation, the limit of the maximum extension had been moved up to 10 degrees from the full extension. One week later they attempted to fully extend the knee by cutting and extending the plaster, and were able to force the knee to once more reach the target of 0 degrees (full extension). But this further increased the suffering of the patient, weakening her capacity to contribute to the recovery. When she returned for cast removal to the outpatient clinic, the cast was precut and when she was again in physical therapy it was removed. The knee was still flexed about 30 degrees, exactly the same as before manipulation, and swollen as it had always been, starting from the operation, but what now worried the therapist was the new abnormal swelling in the posterolateral aspect of the distal two-thirds of the thigh. This swelling had the look and all the characteristics of a huge hematoma, and it hurt the patient with a sharp unbearable pain.

Three days later she was admitted to the hospital. The intention of the physician was to evacuate the hematoma by means of a small incision, but the damage was found to be much more serious than what had been believed. An uncontrollable hemorrhage obliged him to do an emergency operation. From an extended posterolateral approach the surgeon explored the anterolateral and posterolateral compartments of the thigh, where he found significant muscular damage involving both the gastrocnemius at the femoral origin and the biceps femoris with a subtotal lesion. The posterior articular capsule was torn, too. The hematoma was evacuated and the hemorrhage halted; the muscular and the capsular damage was left unrepaired because of the risk of scarring retraction. After the operation the knee was again immobilized with a femorotibial cast in extension.

The patient remained in the hospital because of her poor general condition. She needed blood transfusions and medical therapy. For the first 15 postoperative days no physical therapy was administered, and only after this time was she able to start with very mild general exercises. She left the hospital after 30 days without a cast. Unluckily, the ROM was worsened by the cast up to joint mobility of only few degrees (between 15 and 30 degrees of flexion). The partial progress of the extension deficit from 30 to 15 degrees had provided hope that an acceptable result with the physical therapy was still possible. She started again with CPM, and again she dedicated many hours a day to the assisted rehabilitation. Her situation didn't change during the following year, and the patient arrived at our clinic at the end of October 1992. At the physical examination the knee showed a 15-degree extension deficit. The active ROM was between 15 and 25 degrees. A severe quadriceps atrophy was associated with a significant antalgic gait. The patellar mobility was reduced. We observed a significant loss of superoinferior (passive and active) patellar glide, associated with the complete absence of passive patellar tilt. On the x-rays there was evidence of severe femorotibial and patellofemoral chondral damage (Fig. 35.5.3). The lateral view showed a shortened patellar tendon with obvious patella infera (Fig. 35.5.4).

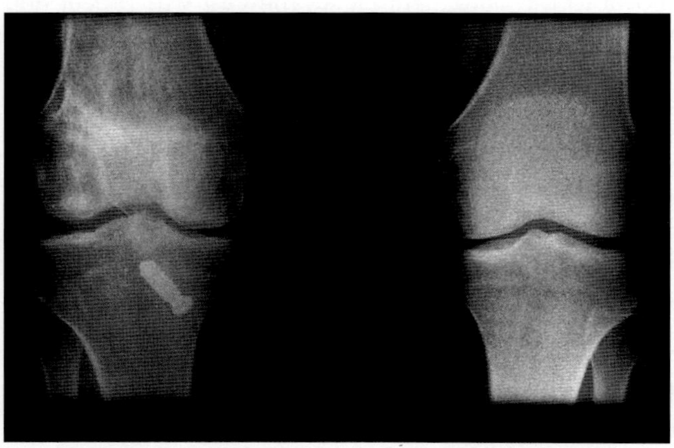

Figure 35.5.3. On this anteroposterior (AP) view severe chondral damages of the femorotibial surfaces are evident. The comparison with the healthy knee makes the picture still more dramatic.

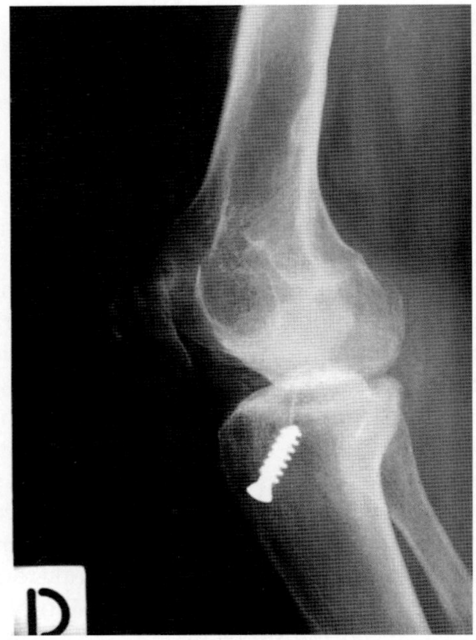

Figure 35.5.4. The lateral view shows a shortened patellar tendon with obvious patella infera.

The patient underwent her third operation on November 3, 1992. The operation, performed by the senior author, consisted of the following steps:

1. extended longitudinal skin incision and large medial parapatellar access to the joint;
2. lateral release of the patellofemoral retinacular;
3. arthrolysis with debridement of all adhesions that were between the articular surfaces of the patellofemoral joint or that obliterated the entire suprapatellar pouch and the medial and lateral recess (Fig. 35.5.5);
4. subtotal excision of the sclerotic fat pad;
5. debridement of all intercartilaginous adhesions in the femorotibial compartment;
6. extraarticular release of all femoral metaphysis from the surrounding soft tissues with particular attention to the lateral and posterolateral side of the bone, where we recognized the effects of the previous salvage procedure; at this point of the operation the knee had gained 90 degrees of flexion, and the extension deficit was reduced to 10 degrees;
7. osteotomy of the tibial tuberosity with the tendon attachment;
8. removal of the remnant of the reconstructed-ACL and consequent notchplasty;

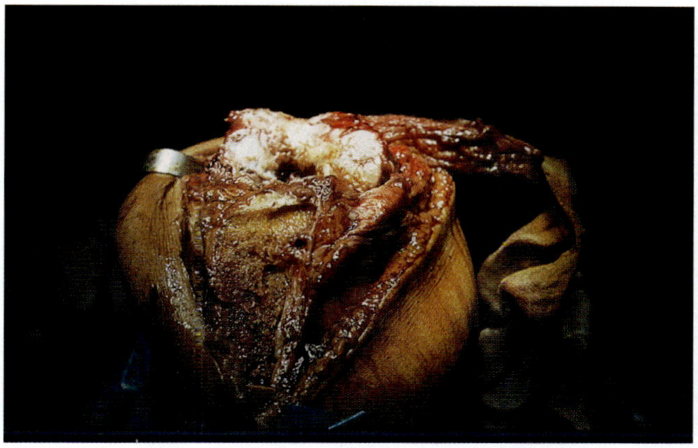

Figure 35.5.5. The fibrotic tissue filled with tenacious adhesions of all the joint recesses. No articular surface has been spared by widespread lesions of the cartilage.

9. proximal reposition of the tuberosity, about 1.5 cm higher (Fig. 35.5.6).

At the end of the operation the ROM increased from less than 5 degrees to 130 degrees. The result was very satisfactory, but the chondral damage remained. The patient started, immediately after the operation, with a CPM device (Toronto Mobilimb) from −10 to 120 degrees ROM for 16 to 18 hours per day. She had continuous analgesic infusion from a peridural catheter left in situ for 7 days. During the 6 to 8 hours a day free from the passive motion, we tried to preserve the extension, forcing the knee by means of a dropout cast slightly modified from that presented by Paulos et al.[13] Nonaggressive physical therapy completed the therapeutic postoperative program beginning on the second day. The therapist came twice a day, focusing on improving the active ROM and the muscular control of the limb.

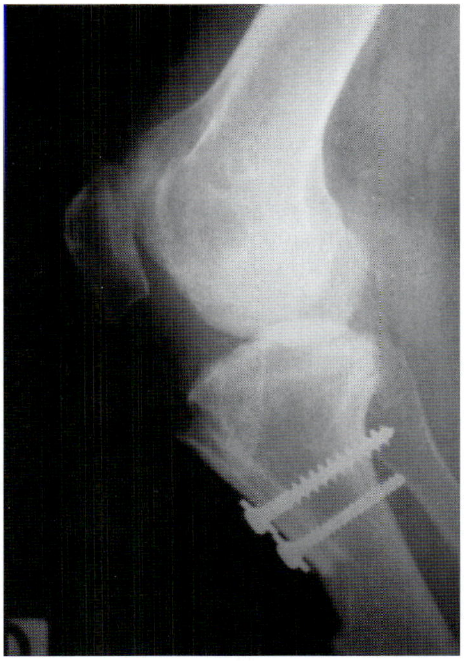

Figure 35.5.6. The restored patellar height on the postoperative x-rays.

The patient started partial weight bearing while walking almost immediately, and she reached full weight bearing after the first postoperative month. We closely followed the patient during the first year after the operation, and then at least once a year thereafter. When the stitches were removed after 2 weeks, the ROM had already increased to 90 degrees. In the following 3 months we recorded a slight worsening of the extension. After the 6th postoperative month a very slow increase in flexion started, reaching a maximum of 100 degrees. One year after the operation, the patient was able to walk without limping, to climb or descend stairs, and to sit down normally. The ROM was stabilized at 10 to 100 degrees.

We evaluated the long-term results 2 years later. We used the knee ligament standard evaluation form from the IKDC (International Knee Documentation Committee).[14] The patient's subjective assessment was the best grade (A = normal); all the objective results were in the two lowest grades (C and D = abnormal and severely abnormal). We classified a very good subjective result in the poor category. Three years later we reevaluated the patient. This time the subjective assessment was "abnormal," and the others remained the same. The x-ray examination showed an evident increase in chondral damages, and further narrowing of both the patellofemoral and femorotibial joints, giving the impression of a condemned knee (Fig. 35.5.7).

Discussion

It's hard to say where the first error was in this case and how it influenced the outcome. But we identify the unrecognized infrapatellar contracture syndrome (IPCS) as the first error, which made operating on a knee with a ROM of only 30 to 90 degrees of flexion even less appropriate, because the surgeon had waited for about 6 weeks from the time of the trauma. The postoperative program of rehabilitation, compared with present programs,[8,15] waited too long after the operation before beginning. Nowadays no surgeon would wait for 2 weeks before starting with CPM, and no surgeon would leave a reconstructed knee immobilized at 30 degrees of flexion.

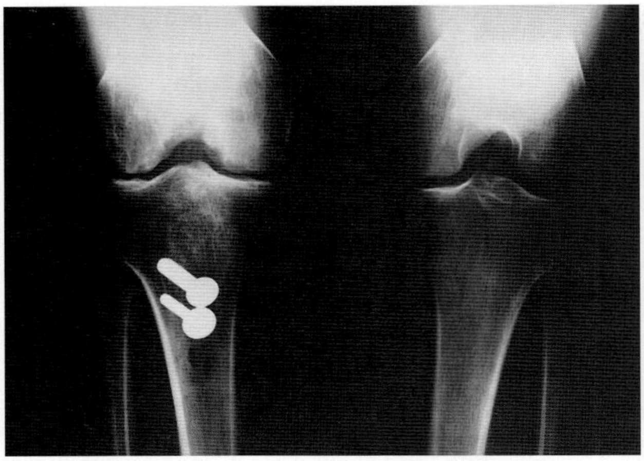

A

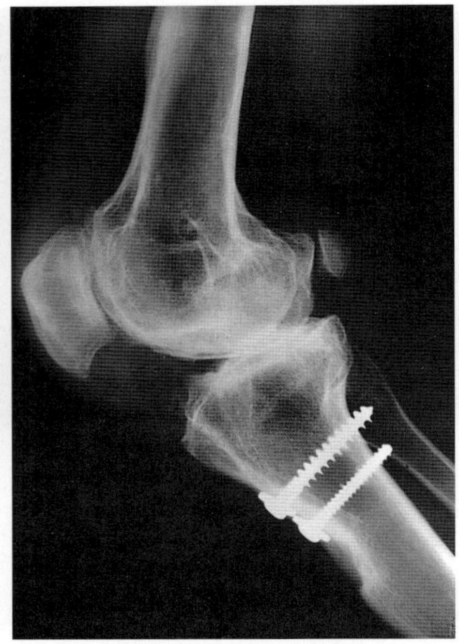

B

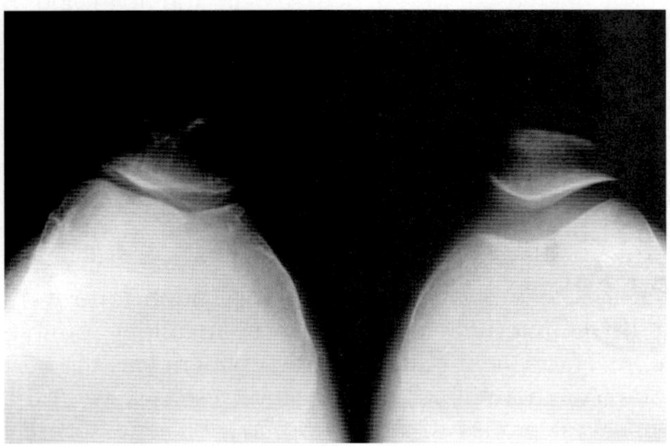

C

Figure 35.5.7. The joint condition in the x-rays 5 years after the last procedure: **(A)** 45-degree posteroanterior flexion weight-bearing view. (Used, with permission, from Rosenberg TD, Paulos LE, Parker RD, et al. The forty-five degree posteroanterior flexion weight-bearing radiograph of the knee. *Journal of Bone and Joint Surgery* 1988; 70A:1479–1483.) **(B)** lateral view, **(C)** axial view.

During the operation, after the ACL reconstruction, could the knee be passively fully extended? The extension deficit had always been the major problem and we cannot know whether this problem would have remained even if the knee had been moved immediately.

According to Paulos et al,[13,16] treatment recommendations include aggressive rehabilitation, antiinflammatory medications, and transcutaneous electrical nerve stimulation (TENS) or other antalgic physical applications. Then the patient goes on to the second active stage of IPCS, and it is mandatory to discontinue continuous manual manipulation, forced passive motion, or traction, because all these maneuvers cause recurrent inflammation and pain, thus worsening the disease process at this stage. They did not understand in time that a malign IPCS was occurring in the operated knee. The rest of the history was a consequence of that fact. The patient continued daily with 5 hours or more of aggressive physical therapy, passing through an inopportune forced closed manipulation with disastrous consequences and the relative salvage procedure 3 weeks later.

Not even after this second operation was the program changed, as the intensive sessions of physical therapy started again and went on for another year. When we visited the patient for the first time she was out of the active stage of the IPCS. But the intensive therapy she underwent for the past year put her knee in a subacute condition, to the point that the physical examination corresponded in many respects to an acute inflamed joint. The knee was swollen and very painful, and no residual patellar mobility remained in either the superior-inferior or medial-lateral directions. The presence of an abrupt step-off at the distal attachment of the patellar tendon to the tibial tubercle resembled the "shelf sign" descripted by Paulos et al.[13]

At the operation we couldn't perform only a salvage procedure, such as the proximal transposition of the tibial tubercle attachment, which was absolutely essential; we also tried to restore as much as possible the joint function and the articular congruence of the knee. We were unable to obtain a satisfactory result. This was evident from the beginning, during the operation and immediately after. The IKDC form confirms those early impressions. The last x-ray examination has the same adverse prognostic value (Fig. 35.5.7). Nevertheless the patient leads a normal life, except for no sports activities.

Conclusion

The correct timing of ACL reconstruction is crucial. IPCS can always occur with a patellar tendon graft. To be unprepared to recognize its signs makes this syndrome disastrous for knee function. In the presented case we'll never know if a timely performed intraarticular and extraarticular debridement and release would have been able to avoid the problem, but we can be sure that a correct diagnosis at the correct time would have prevented the unwise manipulation to force the knee and most of the articular disaster.

References

1. Hughston JC Complications of anterior cruciate ligament surgery. *Orthop Clin North Am* 1985;16:237–240.
2. Small NC. Complications in arthroscopy: the knee and other joints. *Arthroscopy* 1986;2:253–258.
3. Bach BR Jr. Potential pitfalls of Kurosaka screw interference fixation for ACL surgery. *Am J Knee Surg* 1989; 2:76–82.
4. Bonamo JJ, Krinick RM, Sporn AA. Rupture of the patellar ligament after use of its central third for anterior cruciate reconstruction. *J Bone Joint Surg* 1984;66A: 1294–1297.
5. McCarroll JR. Fracture of the patella during a golf swing following reconstruction of the anterior cruciate ligament. *Am J Sports Med* 1983;11:26–27.
6. Noah J, Shermann OH, Roberts C. Fracture of the supracondylar femur after anterior cruciate ligament reconstruction using patellar tendon and iliotibial band tenodesis: a case report. *Am J Sports Med* 1992;20:615–618.
7. Ternes JP, Blasier RB, Alexander AH. Fracture of the femur after anterior cruciate ligament reconstruction with a GORE-TEX prosthetic graft: a case report. *Am J Sports Med* 1993;21:147–149.
8. Franco V, Selvanetti A, Gianni E, et al. Post-operatorio e riabilitazione. In: Puddu G, Cerullo G (eds). La Patologia del Legamento Crociato Anteriore: Diagnosi e Trattamento. Rome: Il Pensiero Scientifico Editore, 1994; 195–205.
9. Franco V, Cipolla M, et al. La mobilizzazione passiva continua nella chirurgia del ginocchio. *Il Ginocchio* 1994; 14:33–40.
10. Franco V, Pompili S, Flamini M, Puddu G. The effectiveness of the muscular biofeedback in the early postoperative time after anterior cruciate ligament reconstruction. Paper presented at the 7th ESSKA Congress, Budapest, 1986.
11. Perugia L, Mariani PP, De Carli A. Inquadramento clinico, valutazione diagnostica ed indicazioni terapeutiche delle rigidità post-traumatiche del ginocchio. *G Ital Ortop Traumatol* 1995;21(3 suppl):281–290.
12. Shelbourne KD, Wilckens JH, Mollabashy A, et al. Arthrofibrosis in acute anterior cruciate ligament reconstruction. The effect of timing of reconstruction and rehabilitation. *Am J Sports Med* 1991;19:332–336.
13. Paulos LE, Rosenberg TD, Drawbert J, et al. Infrapatellar contracture syndrome: an unrecognized cause of knee stiffness with patella entrapment and patella infera. *Am J Sports Med* 1987;15:331–341.
14. Hefti F, Muller W, Jakob RP, et al. Evaluation of knee ligament injuries with the IKDC form. *Knee Surg Sports Traumatol Arthrosc* 1993;1:226–234.
15. Shelbourne KD, Nitz PA. Accelerated rehabilitation following anterior cruciate ligament reconstruction. *Am J Sports Med* 1990;18:292–299.
16. Paulos LE, Daniel CW, Greenwald AE. Infrapatellar contracture syndrome. Diagnosis, treatment and long-term follow-up. *Am J Sports Med* 1994;22:440–449.
17. Rosenberg TD, Paulos LE, Parker RD, et al. The forty-five degree posteroanterior flexion weight-bearing radiograph of the knee. *J Bone Joint Surg* 1988;70A: 1479–1483.

Chapter 35.6

TENDINITIS/GRANULOMA POSTCENTRAL PATELLAR TENDON ARTHROSCOPY APPROACH

C.N. Van Dijk and R.K. Marti

CASE REPORT

A professional soccer player presented with chronic pain located over the patellar ligament of his left knee. There was no swelling and no joint effusion. Pain on palpation was located over the full length of the patellar ligament with the maximum point of tenderness located at its tibial insertion. Standard x-rays did not reveal pathology.

Treatment consisted of physiotherapy. After initial recovery, recurrence of sharp pain made return to competitive play impossible. Magnetic resonance imaging (MRI) was performed, which demonstrated a longitudinal segment of the patellar tendon that contained more water than the surrounding normal patella tissue (Fig. 35.6.1). An injection at the side of maximum tenderness was performed. After a prolonged period of rest, the player returned to competitive play, but sharp pain returned. A new MRI in the transverse direction again demonstrated a central segment in the patellar tendon over its full length (Fig. 35.6.2). The diagnosis again was a local tendinitis of the patellar tendon. A prolonged period of physiotherapy and rest was unsuccessful. A third MRI (Fig. 35.6.3) revealed the same pathology.

The patient was sent for a second opinion. On examination there was pain over the patellar tendon with its maximum point of tenderness located over the tuberosities. X-ray did not show abnormalities. A computed tomography (CT) scan was performed (Fig. 35.6.4), which revealed a small bony fragment that corresponded with the point of local tenderness. After removal, the patient was symptom free within a few weeks and returned to competitive play without any restriction and without recurrence of his symptoms.

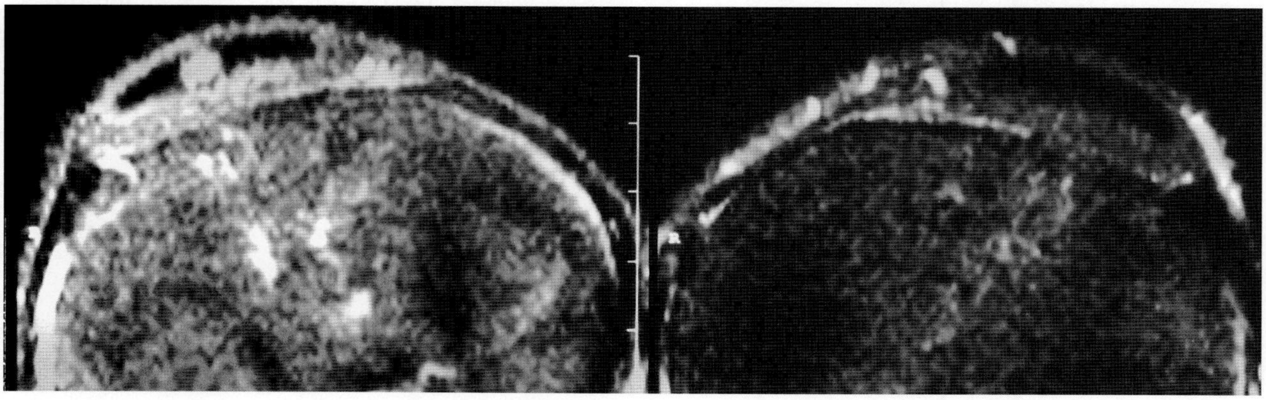

Figure 35.6.1. Axial MRI view of both knees at the level of the patellar ligament demonstrating a central segment in the patellar ligament containing more water than the surrounding normal patellar tissue. All axial sections of the whole length of the patellar ligament demonstrated this pathologic central section.

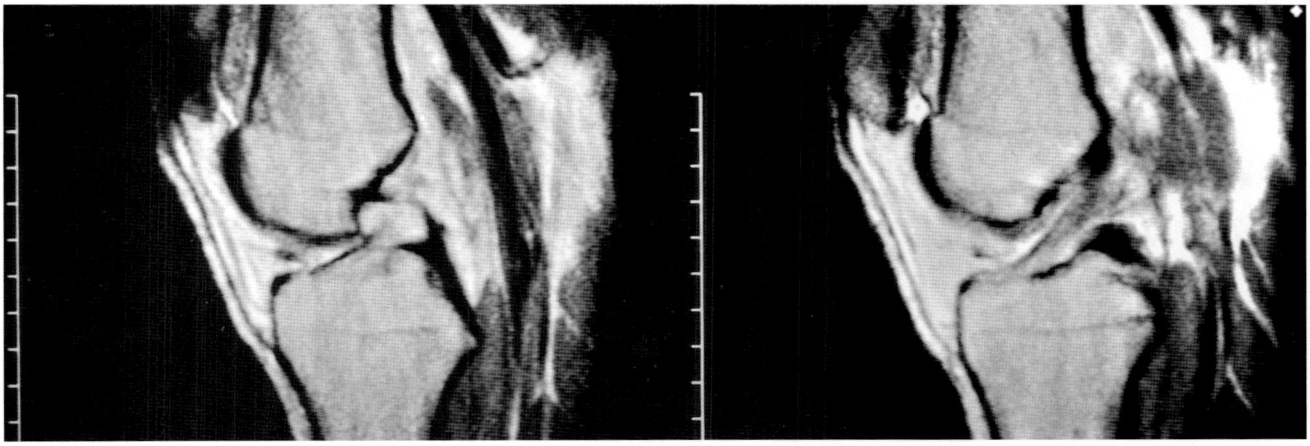

Figure 35.6.2. MRI in the transverse direction 4 months later, again demonstrating a longitudinal segment in the center of the patellar ligament containing more water.

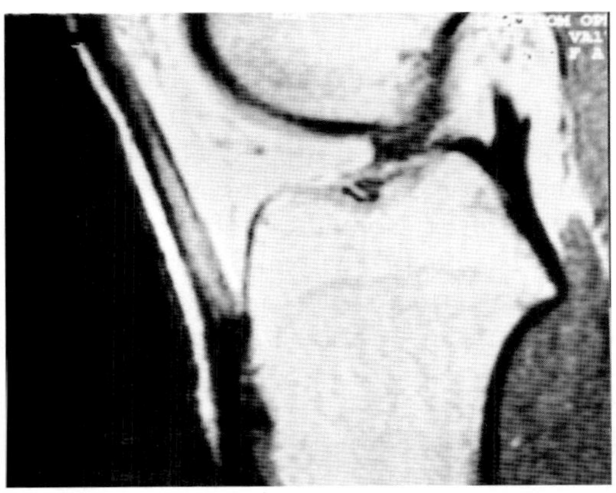

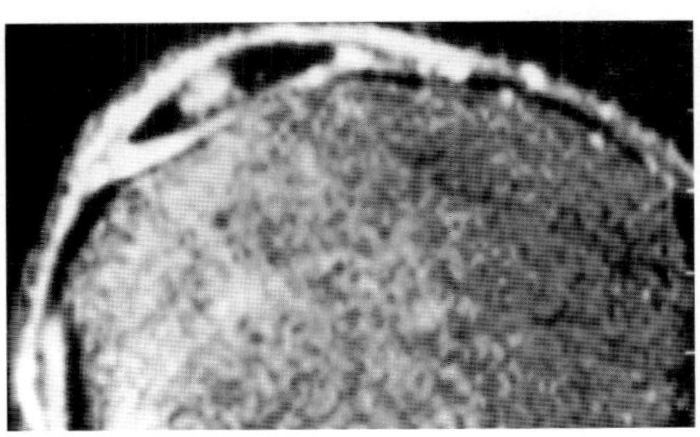

Figure 35.6.3. A new MRI 2 months later showing the same pathology.

DISCUSSION

MRI sometimes is believed to present a solution to all diagnostic problems. In this case of bony pathology, MRI gave information on secondary soft tissue involvement, thus contributing to the diagnosis and treatment.

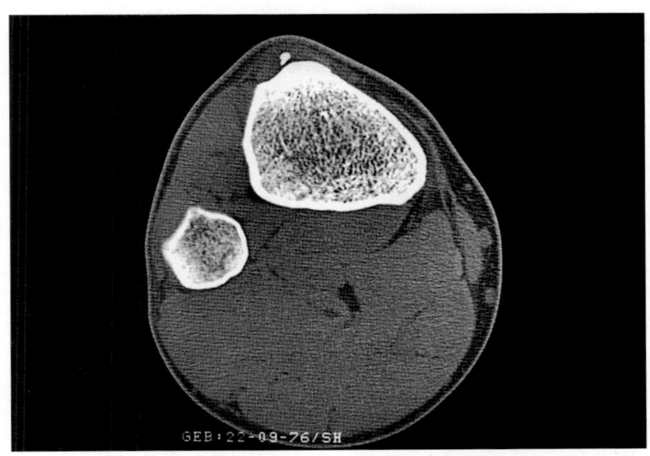

Figure 35.6.4. CT scan at the level of the tuberosities tibiae demonstrating a small bony fragment.

Chapter 35.7

Nonunited Avulsion Fracture of the Tibial Tubercle

C.V. Van Dijk and R.K. Marti

CASE REPORT

A professional soccer player underwent arthroscopic removal of a torn medial meniscus by means of a central patellar approach. He developed pain at the side of the patellar portal at the apex of the patella. Two injections of corticosteroid were administered. Over a 3-year period the complaints increased, which finally prevented him from performing at the highest level. On investigation there was pain over the medial/midinsertion of the patellar tendon to the patellar bone. Apart from some local swelling and localized pain on palpation, there were no other deformities. The x-ray did not reveal pathology. Magnetic resonance imaging (MRI) (Figs. 35.7.1 and 35.7.2) showed a large area of pathologic patellar ligament tissue consisting of the complete midmedial insertion (some 40% of the circumference of the patellar ligament). The pathologic part of the patellar tendon was excised after 6 weeks of plaster immobilization and protected mobilization, and the patient re-

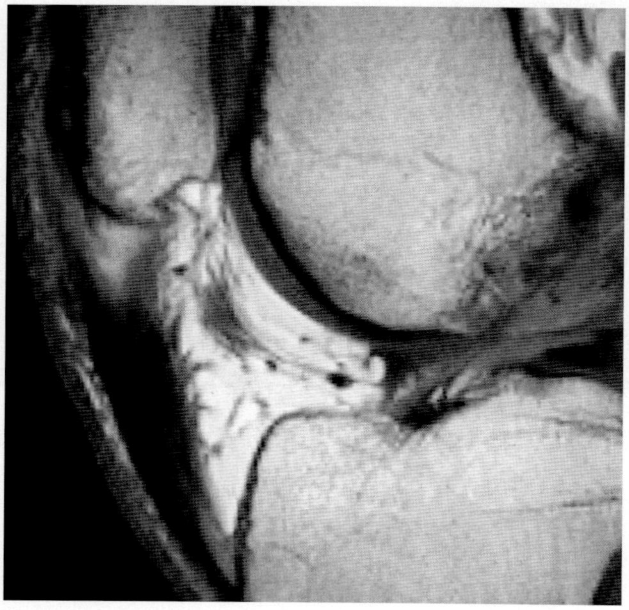

Figure 35.7.1. MRI showing a large area of pathologic tissue located at the apex of the patella (midmedial segment).

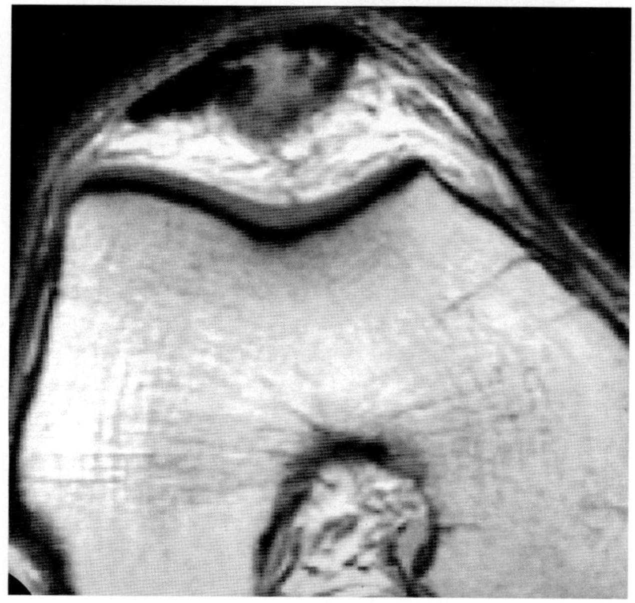

Figure 35.7.2. Axial MRI view through the patellar ligament just distal to the level of the apex of the patella showing a large area of pathologic tissue.

turned to the field 4 months after operation. Six months after the operation he was performing at the highest level.

DISCUSSION

The central patellar arthroscopic approach to the knee has been advocated by some authors.[1] Patellar tendinitis after this approach has been associated with the use of Cydex as the sterilization fluid of the arthroscopic instrument (Eriksson, personal communication). This professional soccer player, however, developed mechanical irritation and tendinitis, which did not resolve until excision of the pathologic tissue was performed.

Reference

1. Gillquist. Operative arthroscopy of the knee. In: McGinty JB (ed.) *Operative Arthroscopy*, 2nd ed. Philadelphia: Lippincott-Raven, 1995.

Chapter 35.8

KNEE MIGRATION OF TIBIAL ENDER NAILS: THE ARTHROSCOPIC SOLUTION

Ramon Cugat and Montserrat Garcia

The use of osteosynthesis instruments to fix fractures is common. However, in some cases a joint can be disturbed by one of these instruments,[1–3] as is described in this case. Under these circumstances, arthroscopy is a useful technique,[4] as it is shown in the present case.

CASE REPORT

A 49-year-old man presented in June 1985 to the first author with a history of pain in the left knee that made him lame on that foot. He explained that in 1984 he had suffered from an open fracture in the medial third–distal third of the left tibia and fibula. He had been treated surgically with intramedullary Ender nails. The postoperative period was fine until he started walking with weight bearing. It was then that pain occurred in the left knee.

The physical examination showed a correct axis of both lower limbs. The left patella shock test was positive. The temperature of the left knee was slightly higher than that of the right knee. The decubitus supinus position with full extension of the knee was uncomfortable for the patient. Discomfort disappeared with the knee flexed. The McMurray test was positive.

The radiological examination of the left leg showed:

perfect consolidation of the fracture,

slight Südeck bone dystrophy of the left knee,

both Ender nails' heads seemed to be inside the left knee joint.

Arthroscopy of the left knee was performed. Under epidural anesthesia the patient was placed in the decubitus supine position. Three portals were opened: anterolateral (AL), anteromedial (AM), and superomedial (SM). All the intraarticular structures were correct. But in the anterior area of the knee two metallic foreign bodies were found (Fig. 35.8.1). These were the Ender nails' heads and they were removed (Fig. 35.8.2). One of them was removed through the AM (Fig. 35.8.3) and the other through the AL portal.

After the arthroscopic surgery, pain, knee flexion contracture and swelling disappeared. The patient attended rehabilitation for 2 months, and after this period he returned to his usual work completely recovered.

DISCUSSION

Intramedullary fixation is commonly used for the treatment of different types of femur and tibial fractures.[5–9]

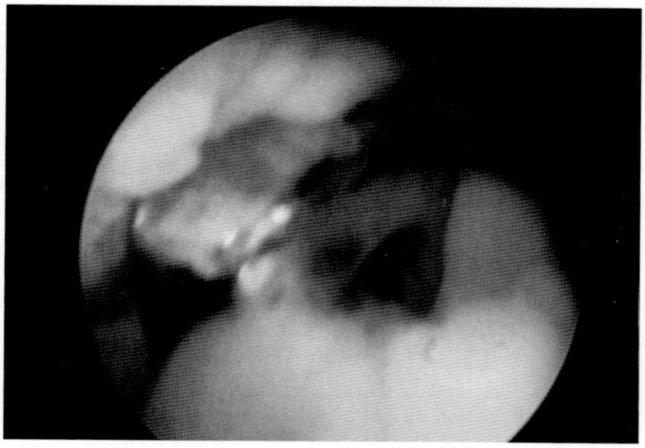

Figure 35.8.1. Arthroscopic view of the Ender nail's head in the anteromedial area of the left knee.

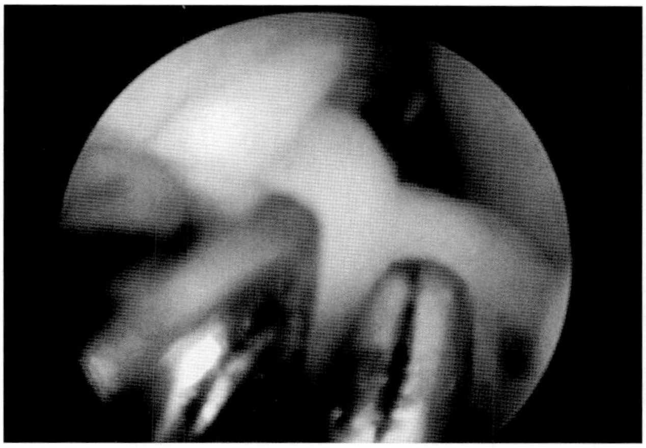

Figure 35.8.2. Arthroscopic view of the hook of the extractor in the head hole.

However, different authors have pointed out the possible migration of the nails inside the joint adjacent to the bone metaphysis.[10–12] The diagnosis and the removal of these foreign bodies can be performed with the arthroscopy technique.[13] Once the surgery is carried out, symptoms disappear, the postoperative period is comfortable and short, and the patient can return to work completely recovered.

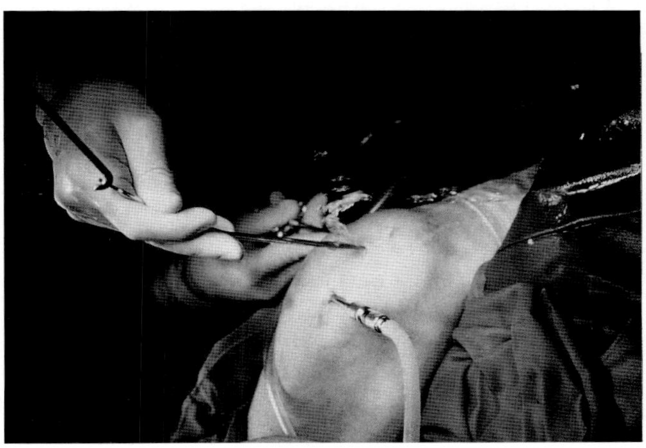

Figure 35.8.3. Extraction of the Ender nail through the anteromedial portal.

References

1. Chen YJ, Wu CC, Hsu RW, Shih CH. The intra-articular migration of the broken wire: a rare complication of circumferencial wiring in patellar fractures. *Keng I Hsuch* 1994;17:276–279.
2. Ritter MA, Meding JB. Intraarticular trochanteric wire migration following bilateral total hip arthroplasty. A case report. *Orthopaedics* 1988;11:1295–1297.
3. Pankovich AM, Tarabishy IE. Ender nailing of intertrochanteric and subtrochanteric fractures of the femur. *J Bone Joint Surg* 1980;62A:635–645.
4. Chapple CR, Porter KM. An unusual use for the arthroscope. *Injury* 1984;15:351–352.
5. Melis GC, Sotgiu F, Lepori M, Guido P. Intramedullary nailing in segmental tibial fractures. *J Bone Joint Surg* 1981;63A:1310–1318.
6. Charnley J. *The Closed Treatment of Common Fractures*, 3rd ed. London: Churchill-Livingstone, 1972.
7. Langard O, Bo O. Segmental tibial shaft fractures. *Acta Orthop Scand* 1976;47:351–357.
8. Masse Y, Aubriot JH, Lamotte N. Fractures diaphysaires de jambes traitées par enclouage à foyer fermé sans alésage. Étude d'une série de 521 cas. *Rev Chir Orthop* 1977;63:575–591.
9. Merle d'Aubigné R, Maurer P, Zucman J, Masse Y. Blind intramedullary nailing for tibial fractures. *Clin Orthop* 1974;105:267–275.
10. Holbrook JL, Swiontkowski MF, Sanders R. Treatment of open fractures of the tibial shaft: Ender nailing versus external fixation. *J Bone Joint Surg* 1989;71A:1231–1238.
11. Mayer L, Werbie T, Schwab JP, Johnson RP. The use of Ender nails in fractures of the tibial shaft. *J Bone Joint Surg* 1985;67A:446–455.
12. Pankovich AM, Goldflies ML, Pearson RL. Closed Ender nailing of femoral-shaft fractures. *J Bone Joint Surg* 1979;61A:222–232.
13. Cobbs KF, Berg EE. Arthroscopic advancement of a tibial nail. *Arthroscopy* 1997;13:763–766.

Chapter 35.9

Nonunion of a New High Tibial Osteotomy with Screw and Wire Fixation

Masaaki Ito and Hiroshi Narita

High tibial osteotomy is a commonly performed procedure for osteoarthritis. The external fixation is mainly used for this operation; however, it is impossible to avoid complications.[1–4] Pin-tract infection is the most common. A new internal fixation for high tibial osteotomy is used to prevent complications.

CASE REPORT

A 58-year-old woman had bilateral gonalgia for about 10 years, and could not walk more than 500 meters. Varus deformity was present. The right knee range of motion was 0 to 140 degrees, and the left knee was −10 to 110 degrees. The femoral tibial angle (FTA) in the supine position was 180 degrees on the right side and 186 degrees on the left side (Fig. 35.9.1). Medication and injection of hyaluronic acid was not effective. Arthroscopy was first performed on the left side, which was worse. The arthroscopic findings showed eburnation of the femoral condyle and tibia plateau. The lateral femoral condyle, tibia plateau, and lateral meniscus were intact.

We performed high tibial osteotomy using the Charnley transfixation-compression method. The FTA was improved from 186 to 167 degrees. The corrected valgus angle was 19 degrees (Fig. 35.9.2). Setting and straight leg raising (SLR) quadriceps examination was performed, and continuous passive motion was started on the day after the operation. One-fourth weight bearing was permitted at 2 weeks after the operation, and was increased by one-fourth every 2 weeks. At 5 weeks after the operation, discharge was found around the pins area. This patient had no immunodeficiency, diabetes mellitus, or rheumatoid arthritis. Antibiotics were given for superficial infection, which was not suppressed. At 6 weeks after the operation, the pins were removed and casting was performed.

The discharge soon stopped and union was performed. The FTA remained at 167 degrees. The symptoms on the left side improved, but the gonalgia on the right side became worse. At 4 months after the first operation on the left side, arthroscopy was performed, and we checked the lateral joint space. High tibial osteotomy was suitable. Reflecting on the superficial infection, we tried a new internal fixation, which was compressed with the screws and wire. The first dome osteotomy was performed, and two 3.2-mm Kirschner wires (K-wires) were placed through the proximal and distal fragments. The FTA was corrected by 11 degrees from 180 to 169 degrees.

Two 6.5-mm cannulated screws were inserted through the 3.2-mm K-wire, and fragments were fixed with a 2.0-mm cable passed through the cannulated screw (Fig. 35.9.3). Unfortunately, we made a crack at the lateral side of the proximal fragment. Casting was done for 4 weeks after the operation. Following the radiographic findings, another varus deformity, FTA of 173 degrees, and pseudoarthritis-like signs appeared. To recorrect FTA, curettage, and bone graft, two staple fixations were performed at 5 weeks after the first operation on the right side (Fig. 35.9.4). There was no infectious sign and the fragment was unstable and fixed firmly using screws and wire.

A cylinder cast was set for 10 weeks after the revision. At 3 months after the revision, varus and valgus instability persisted. A union was not achieved. Finally we performed total knee arthroplasty (TKA) with cement (Fig. 35.9.5). At 3 months after TKA, the patient had no severe pain and could walk.

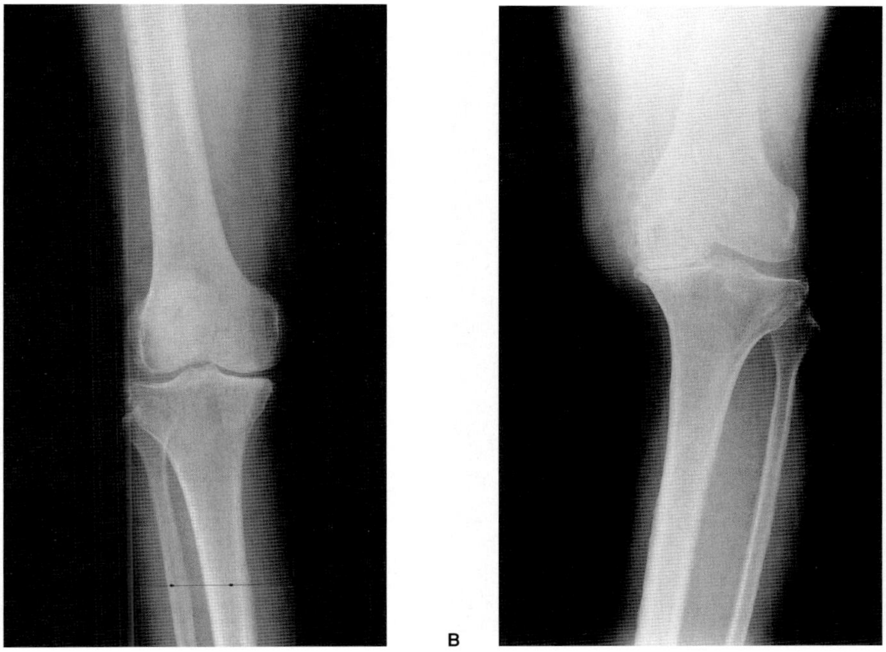

A B

Figure 35.9.1. Radiograph before operation. The femoral tibial angle (FTA) in the supine position was 180 degrees on the right side and 186 degrees on the left side.

DISCUSSION

The purpose of high tibial osteotomy is to avoid complications, to obtain a definite union, to correct the angle, and to achieve good results. In Japan, the medial side osteoarthritis of the knee is the main approach in patients who have varus deformity of the knee. High tibial osteotomy is a good method to correct varus deformity and to reduce mechanical stress on the medial joint space. We have mainly performed high tibial osteotomy using the Charnley transfixation-compression method in patients who had early-stage osteoarthritis of the knee. Complications of this operation are nonunion and infection. The rates of nonunion and infection are several percent.[1–4]

Rigid fixation of high tibial osteotomy is necessary to

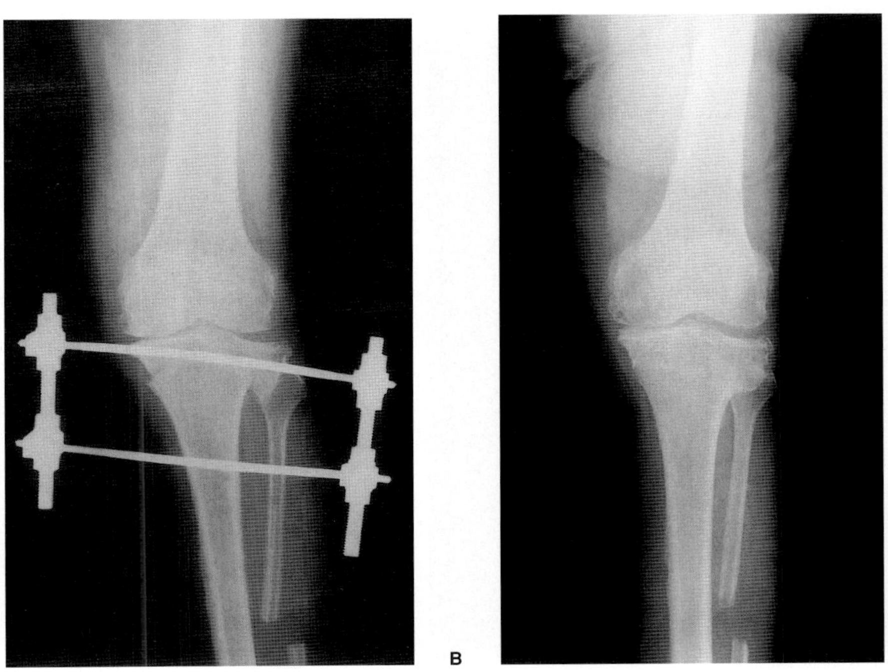

A B

Figure 35.9.2. Radiograph after the first operation on the left side. Charnley transfixation-compression method was performed. The FTA was improved from 186 to 167 degrees.

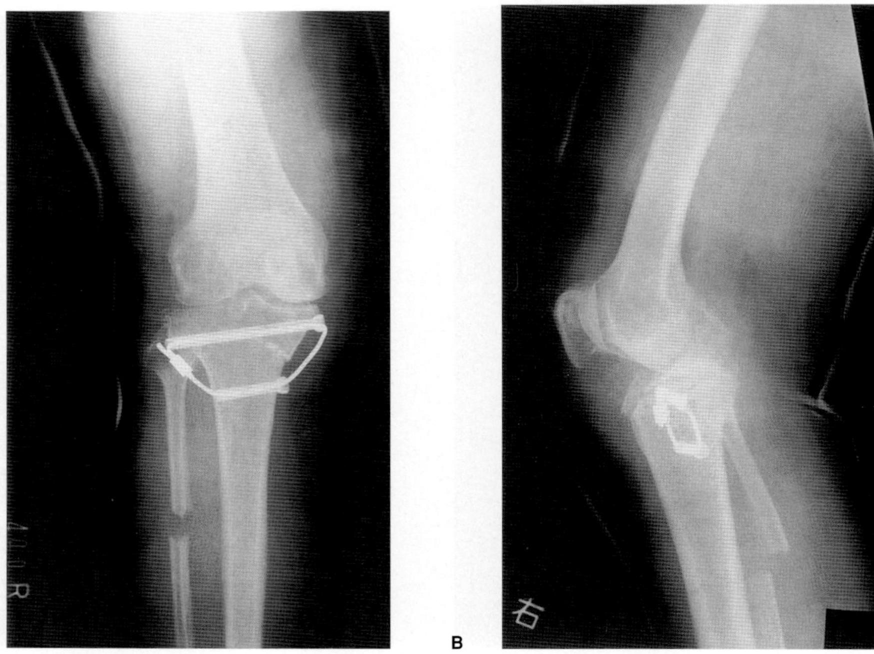

A B

Figure 35.9.3. New internal fixation using screw and wire.

obtain a union. The rate of so-called pin-tract infection is higher with external fixation than with internal fixation. In the present case, superficial infection occurred after the first high tibial osteotomy on the left side. We are concerned about infection. A new compression screw and wiring internal fixation method was used. This method, however, has a big disadvantage: we cannot measure the proper tension of the wire. It is not clear how many pounds the wire should be pulled to achieve union. High tension led to a crack in this case. The crack resulted in instability of the high tibial osteotomy. Our experience confirms that TKA after high tibial osteotomy is not easy and bone defect cannot be avoided.

The Charnley transfixation-compression method is satisfactory, but pin-tract infection may occur and patients cannot take a bath for 2 or 3 months. This screw

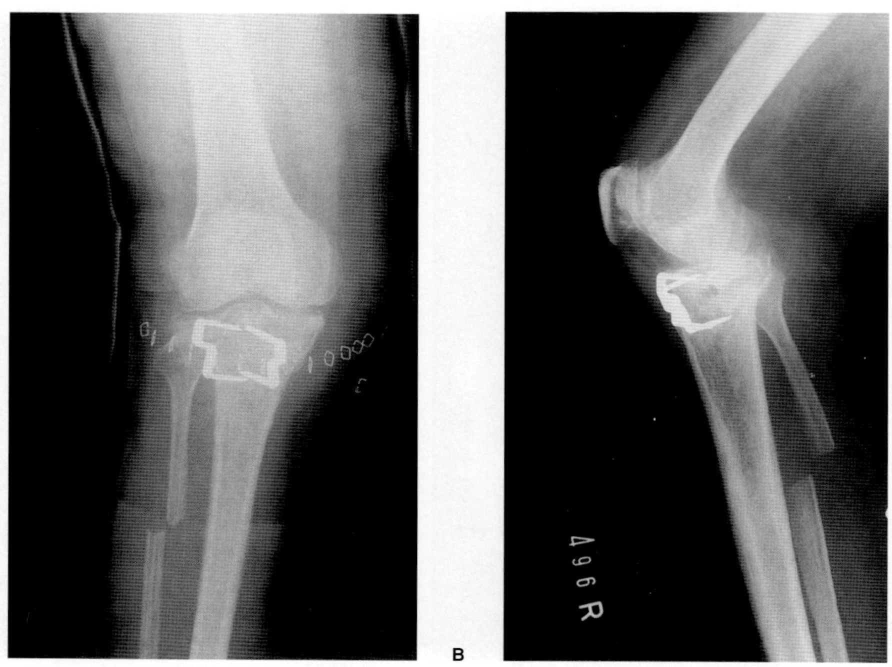

A B

Figure 35.9.4. Pseudoarthritis-like signs appeared. Curettage, bone graft, and two staple fixations were performed.

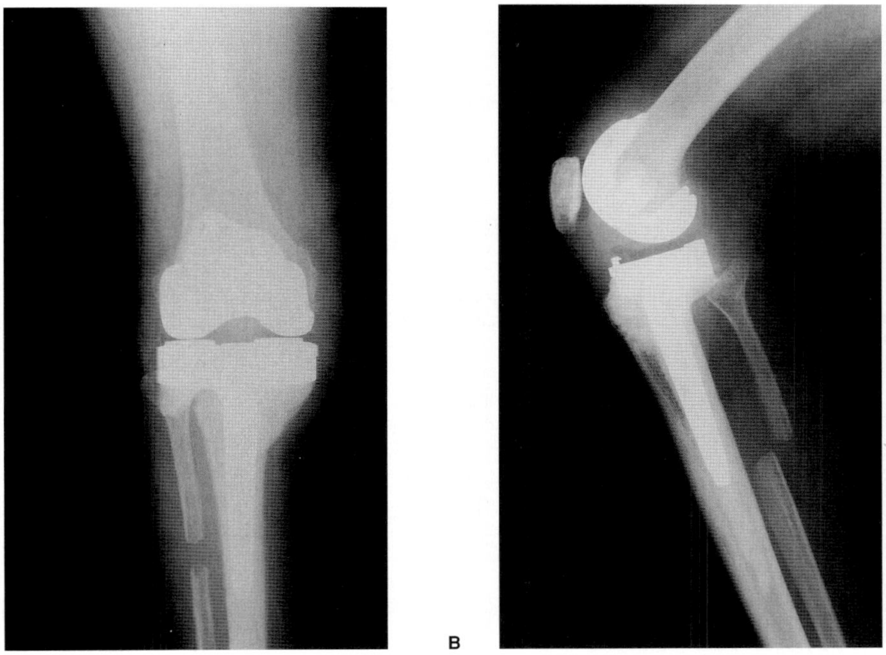
A B

Figure 35.9.5. It was impossible to achieve a union. Finally total knee arthroplasty was performed.

and wire-type fixation is improved, and proper tension of the wire is determined with a tension meter. This method is well established and gives good results.

CONCLUSION

The osteoarthritis of the medial joint space was usually done in Japan as a high tibial osteotomy using the Charnley transfixation-compression method. A new high tibial osteotomy with screw and wire fixation was performed; however, the fragment made a crack in the lateral tibial side. This case became a nonunion and total knee arthroplasty was performed.

References

1. Jackson JP, et al. The technique and complications of upper tibial osteotomy. *J Bone Joint Surg* 1974;56B: 236–245.
2. Robert WW, et al. The study of Maquet dome high tibial osteotomy. Arthroscopic-assisted analysis. *Clin Orthop* 1989;243:280–285.
3. Witonski D, et al. Outcome of treating osteoarthritic degenerative changes in the knee with high tibial osteotomy. Chir Narzadow Ruchu *Ortop Pol* 1994;59:39–43.
4. Tjornstrand B, et al. Results of surgical treatment for nonunion after high tibial osteotomy in osteoarthritis of the knee. *J Bone Joint Surg* 1978;60A:973–977.

Chapter 35.10

Osteolysis Associated with Polyethylene and Metallic Wear After Total Knee Arthroplasty

Dae Kyung Bae and Chang Moo Yim

Osteolysis has been an unrecognized complication after total knee replacement arthroplasty, despite the recognized problem of wear. The majority of patients did not undergo the revision procedure specifically to treat osteolysis. We report the case of a patient who was treated by the removal of the failed patellar component, an exchange of the worn tibial insert for thicker one, and cement filling for the defect area due to osteolysis on the margin of the tibial and femoral component after complete elimination of wear debris.

CASE REPORT

A 76-year-old woman had a primary right cemented total knee arthroplasty (Miller-Galante, Zimmer, Warsaw, IN) in 1989 for osteoarthritis. She had no problems with the right total knee arthroplasty and no symptoms appeared. Eight years after the original total arthroplasty of the right knee, crepitus developed after minor trauma. The swelling, pain, and crepitus in the knee joint increased gradually.

A preoperative physical examination revealed an effusion that had not been noted before and a sensation of grating of metal on metal when the knee was moved. A range of motion from 0 to 120 degrees of flexion was associated with a moderate grating sensation.

Radiographs of the knee were made shortly before the revision (Fig. 35.10.1). The oval-shaped soft tissue shadow due to metallosis is seen on the anterolateral part of the knee joint.

The right knee was reexplored on December 1, 1997. A dark serosanguineous fluid was evacuated from the joint and was sent for culture. An extensive reactive synovitis of gray-black hypertrophic and friable synovial tissue encased the joint cavity. The polyethylene portion of metal-backed patellar component was worn and broken (Fig. 35.10.2A). The corresponding area on the femoral component was worn due to metal-on-metal friction, causing burnishing of the distal weight-bearing articulating surface of the femoral component medially and laterally (Fig. 35.10.2B,C). Extensive pitting, discoloration, and surface erosion were present in the retrieved insert (Fig. 35.10.3).

The failed patellar component and polyethylene insert of tibial component were removed, and a radical debridement was carried out. The synovial tissue that contained considerable metal or polyethylene wear debris was excised as much as possible. The osteolytic portion of cancellous bone on the margin of the tibial and femoral component was removed by rongeur forceps and a curette (Fig. 35.10.4). The femoral and tibial component appeared to be solidly fixed after debridement. The defective area in the margin of the tibial and femoral component due to osteolysis was filled with cement (Fig. 35.10.5). An 11-mm tibial insert was replaced by a 13.5-mm tibial insert because of some laxity. After removal of the base plate of the patellar component, the remaining irregular bony area was shaved smooth (Fig. 35.10.6).

Bacteriologic cultures that were taken during the revision operation did not show any growth. At 3-month follow-up, the patient had a range of motion from 0 to 110 degrees of flexion and no pain.

DISCUSSION

Complications of total knee arthroplasty include patellar instability, polyethylene wear, prosthetic breakage or dissociation from metal backing, loosening, and osteo-

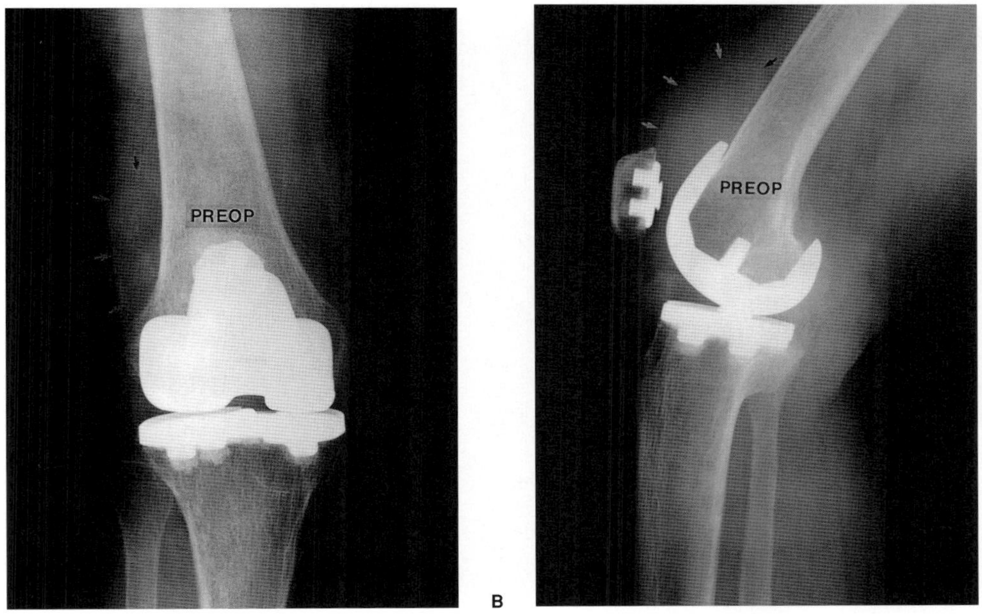

A B

Figure 35.10.1. Radiographs of the knee were made shortly before the revision. The soft tissue shadow due to metallosis (white and black arrows) can be seen in the anterolateral part of the knee joint on the anteroposterior **(A)** and lateral **(B)** radiograph.

lysis due to metallosis and wear debris. With the gradual resolution of other problems of total knee arthroplasty, osteolysis due to wear of polyethylene has become a major factor.

There have been many recent reports of failure of the patellar component in patients who had a total knee arthroplasty.[1,2] Berry and Rand[3] reported significant complication (31.8%) after an isolated patellar component revision of total knee arthroplasty. Because of the risk of subsequent patellar instability or wear, scrupulous attention to optimize patellar tracking is also required.

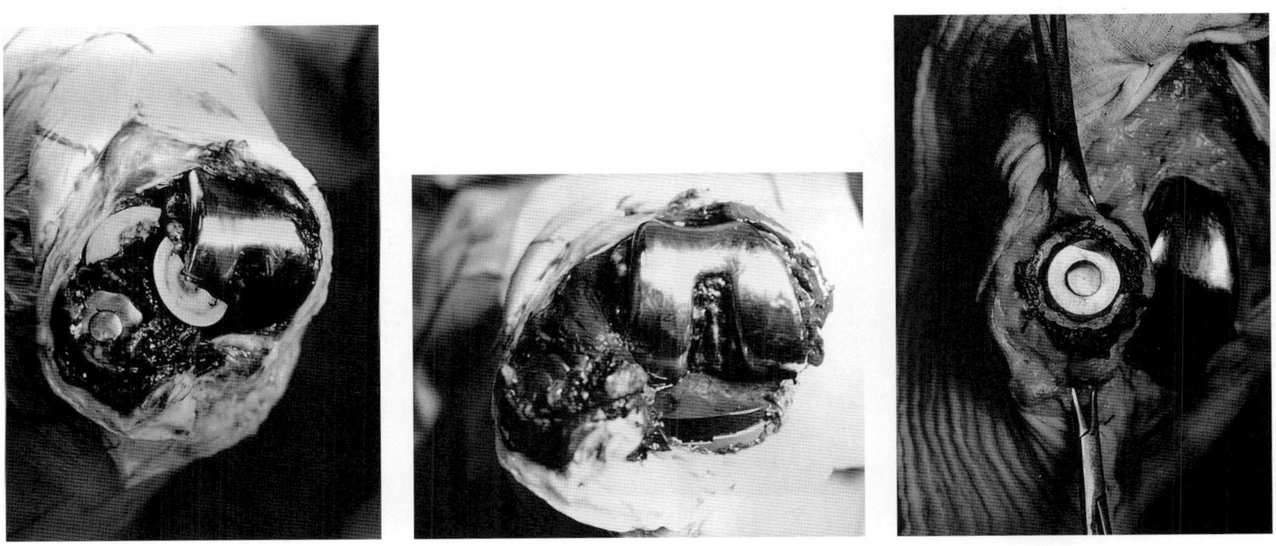

A B C

Figure 35.10.2. Intraoperative photographs revealing the extensive reactive synovitis of gray-black hypertrophic and friable synovial tissue, the patterns of a failure of polyethylene **(A)**, and the abrasion of the surface of the femoral component secondary to articulation with the metallic portion of the patellar implant **(B,C)**.

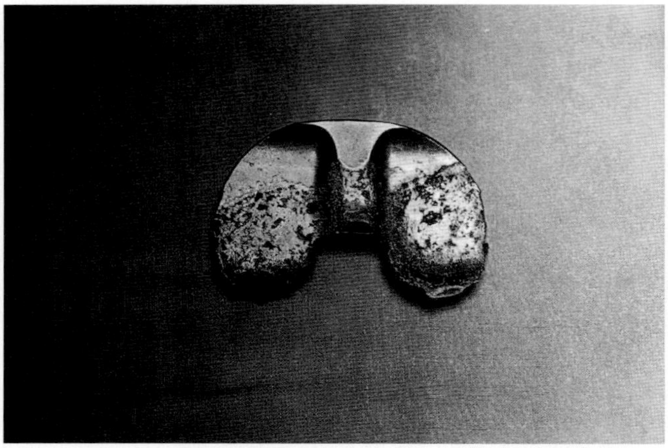

Figure 35.10.3. The polyethylene insert that was retrieved from the right knee, demonstrating extensive pitting, wear, and surface erosion of the polyethylene.

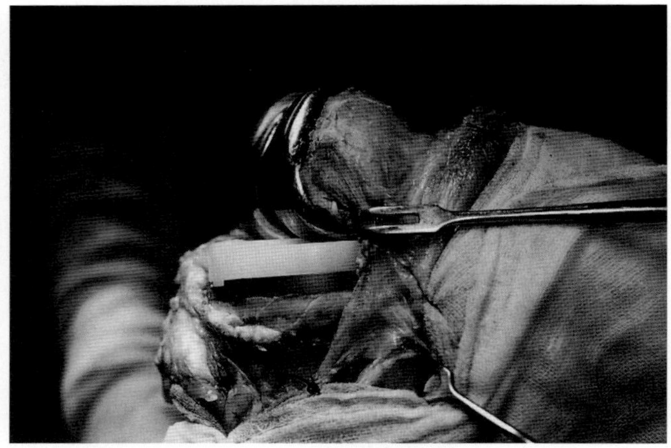

Figure 35.10.5. Intraoperative photograph revealing the defective area that was filled with cement in the margin of the tibial and femoral component.

Because of the paucity of previous reports on osteolysis associated with total knee arthroplasty, numerous studies have addressed these problems in an effort to identify contributing factors and to formulate guidelines for treatment. Peters and Engh[4] demonstrated a high prevalence (16%) of osteolysis after total knee replacements with a modular polyethylene tibial insert. According to Engh and Park,[5] osteolysis was frequently present on the tibial and femoral side of the total knee implant as well as beneath the patellar component. They emphasized the importance of revision that was based on the state of the component.

In our patient, a mechanical cause was also not likely, and we can only hypothesize that an inflammatory process, stimulated by the metallosis or polyethylene wear debris, or both, produced the osteolytic area.

Complications after revision knee arthroplasty, especially extensor mechanism and deep infection, are significantly more frequent than after primary total knee arthroplasty.[6] The clinical results of revision total knee arthroplasty also are not as good as the results of primary arthroplasty.[7]

Generally, revision total knee arthroplasty includes changing all three components: femoral, tibial, and patellar. In revision surgery, the major problem has been a large bone defect. There have been numerous suggestions for the treatment of bone defect: (1) filling the defect with acrylic cement, (2) using a long stem or aug-

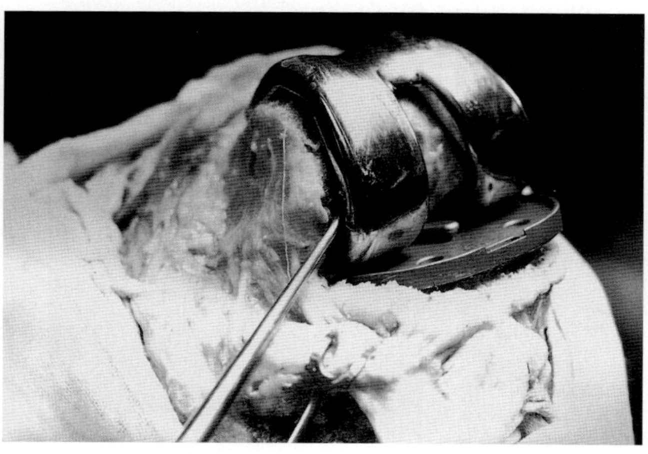

Figure 35.10.4. Intraoperative photograph revealing the osteolytic area on the margin of the tibial and femoral component that was removed by rongeur forceps and curette.

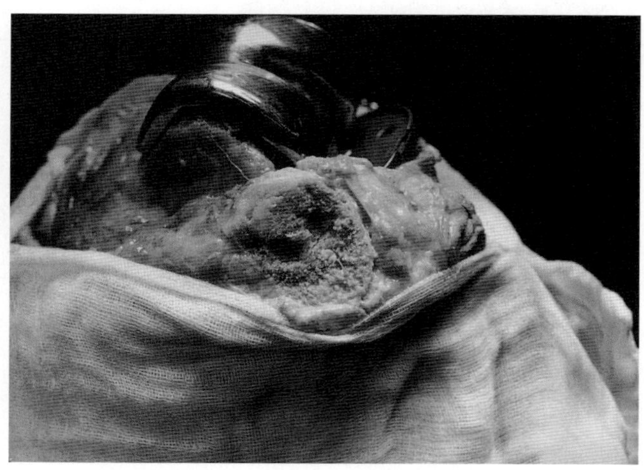

Figure 35.10.6. Intraoperative photograph revealing the smoothly shaved patellar area.

mentation device, and (3) using an allograft or custom prosthesis.[8–10] Engh and Park[5] reported a good outcome of different surgical options when confronted with osteolysis during a revision operation.

The advantage of changing all three components was complete removal of metal particles and wear debris. But the disadvantages include the substantial expense of revision components, the increased operative time and surgical risk, and the uncertainty of the long-term stability provided by bulk allografts.

Accordingly, surgeons have eliminated all sources of potential excessive wear debris as much as possible, and retained a stable tibial and femoral component. To prevent further osteolysis and to enhance the component stability, we performed cement filling on the osteolytic portion of cancellous bone curetted on the margin of the tibial and femoral component. Because of the possible complications, such as wear, that can occur between the damaged femoral component and revised patellar component, the patellar bone was shaved smooth only after removal of the patellar component without resurfacing.

Our methods of treatment have the advantages of minimal blood loss, lesser morbidity, and rapid recovery, especially in elderly patients. This is also a cost-effective approach that appeals to the patient because of its simplicity and short hospital stay. But the ultimate longevity of our method requires further follow-up.

CONCLUSION

A case was described of failure of a metal-backed patellar component and osteolysis associated with polyethylene and metallic wear after total knee arthroplasty. It was treated with our special technique, as described.

References

1. Brick GW, Scott RD. The patellofemoral component of total knee arthroplasty. *Clin Orthop* 1988;231:163–178.
2. Rosenberg AG, Andriacchi TP. Patellar component failure in cementless total knee arthroplasty. *Clin Orthop* 1988;236:106–114.
3. Berry DJ, Rand JA. Isolated patellar component revision of total knee arthroplasty. *Clin Orthop* 1993;286: 110–115.
4. Peters PC, Engh GA. Osteolysis after total knee arthroplasty without cement. *J Bone Joint Surg* 1992;74A: 864–876.
5. Engh GA, Park NL. Tibial osteolysis in cementless total knee arthroplasty: a review of 25 cases treated with and without tibial component revision. *Clin Orthop* 1994; 309:33–43.
6. Goldberg VM, Figgie MP. The results of revision total knee arthroplasty. *Clin Orthop* 1988;226:86–92.
7. Rand JA, Bryan RS. Results of revision total knee arthroplasty using condylar prostheses: a review of fifty knees. *J Bone Joint Surg* 1988;70A:738–745.
8. Brooks PJ, Walker PS. Tibial component fixation in deficient tibial bone stock. *Clin Orthop* 1984;184: 302–308.
9. Dorr LD, Ranawat CS. Bone graft for tibial defects in total knee arthroplasty. *Clin Orthop* 1986;205:153–165.
10. Windser RE, Insall JN. Bone grafting of tibial defects in primary and revision total knee arthroplasty. *Clin Orthop* 1986;205:132–137.

INDEX

ISBN 0-387-98294-9

EAN

9 780387 982946